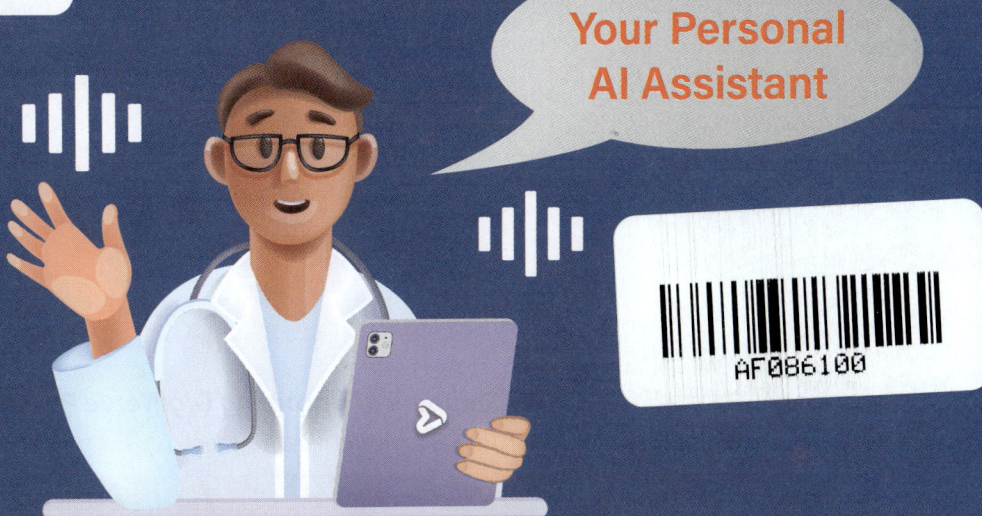

### List of QR Codes for Snippets of Upcoming DigiNerve Physiology Video Lectures
*(Register at EJaypee, scan the QR code and play the video)*

| S. No. | Topic | Chapter and page number |
|---|---|---|
| 1 | Active transport | Chapter 5, Page 29 |
| 2 | Stages of differentiation of red cells/erythropoiesis | Chapter 13, Page 80 |
| 3 | Transmission of impulse across neuromuscular junction | Chapter 26, Page 174 |
| 4 | Action potential of cardiac muscle | Chapter 27, Page 189 |
| 5 | Gastric secretion | Chapter 30, Page 235 |
| 6 | Events in cardiac cycle | Chapter 36, Page 294 |
| 7 | Components of normal ECG | Chapter 37, Page 303 |
| 8 | Oxygen hemoglobin dissociation curve | Chapter 53, Page 443 |
| 9 | Structure of juxtaglomerular apparatus | Chapter 58, Page 499 |
| 10 | Reabsorption in proximal convoluted tubule | Chapter 59, Page 510 |
| 11 | Mechanism of action of insulin | Chapter 69, Page 618 |
| 12 | Menstrual cycle | Chapter 76, Page 671 |
| 13 | Descending tract of spinal cord | Chapter 87, Page 775 |
| 14 | Types of EEG waves | Chapter 89, Page 795 |
| 15 | Differences between sympathetic and parasympathetic nervous system | Chapter 91, Page 815 |

# TEXTBOOK OF PHYSIOLOGY

### Concepts With Clinical Insights

**MANJINDER KAUR**
MBBS MD (Physiology) MAMS CMCL-FAIMER ACME
Additional Principal, Professor and Head
Department of Physiology
Geetanjali Medical College and Hospital
Udaipur, Rajasthan, India

*Co-author*
**SANGEETA NAGPAL**
MBBS MD (Physiology)
Professor
Department of Physiology
Maharishi Markandeshwar College of Medical Sciences and Research
Sadopur, Ambala, Haryana, India

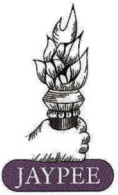

## JAYPEE BROTHERS MEDICAL PUBLISHERS

*The Health Sciences Publisher*
New Delhi | London

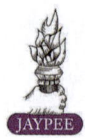

**Jaypee Brothers Medical Publishers (P) Ltd**

**Headquarters**
Jaypee Brothers Medical Publishers (P) Ltd
EMCA House, 23/23-B
Ansari Road, Daryaganj
New Delhi 110 002, India
Landline: +91-11-23272143, +91-11-23272703
+91-11-23282021, +91-11-23245672
Email: jaypee@jaypeebrothers.com

**Corporate Office**
Jaypee Brothers Medical Publishers (P) Ltd
4838/24, Ansari Road, Daryaganj
New Delhi 110 002, India
Phone: +91-11-43574357
Fax: +91-11-43574314
Email: jaypee@jaypeebrothers.com

**Overseas Office**
J.P. Medical Ltd
83 Victoria Street, London
SW1H 0HW (UK)
Phone: +44 20 3170 8910
Fax: +44 (0)20 3008 6180
Email: info@jpmedpub.com

Website: www.jaypeebrothers.com
Website: www.jaypeedigital.com

© 2025, Jaypee Brothers Medical Publishers

The views and opinions expressed in this book are solely those of the original contributor(s)/author(s) and do not necessarily represent those of editor(s) and Publisher of the book.

All rights reserved. No part of this publication may be reproduced, stored or transmitted in any form or by any means, electronic, mechanical, photocopying, recording or otherwise, without the prior permission in writing of the publishers.

All brand names and product names used in this book are trade names, service marks, trademarks or registered trademarks of their respective owners. The publisher is not associated with any product or vendor mentioned in this book.

Medical knowledge and practice change constantly. This book is designed to provide accurate, authoritative information about the subject matter in question. However, readers are advised to check the most current information available on procedures included and check information from the manufacturer of each product to be administered, to verify the recommended dose, formula, method and duration of administration, adverse effects and contraindications. It is the responsibility of the practitioner to take all appropriate safety precautions. Neither the publisher nor the author(s)/editor(s) assume any liability for any injury and/or damage to persons or property arising from or related to use of material in this book.

This book is sold on the understanding that the publisher is not engaged in providing professional medical services. If such advice or services are required, the services of a competent medical professional should be sought.

Every effort has been made where necessary to contact holders of copyright to obtain permission to reproduce copyright material. If any have been inadvertently overlooked, the publisher will be pleased to make the necessary arrangements at the first opportunity.

**Inquiries for bulk sales may be solicited at:** jaypee@jaypeebrothers.com

*Textbook of Physiology*

First Edition: **2025**

ISBN: 978-93-5696-364-1

*Printed at: Samrat Offset Pvt. Ltd.*

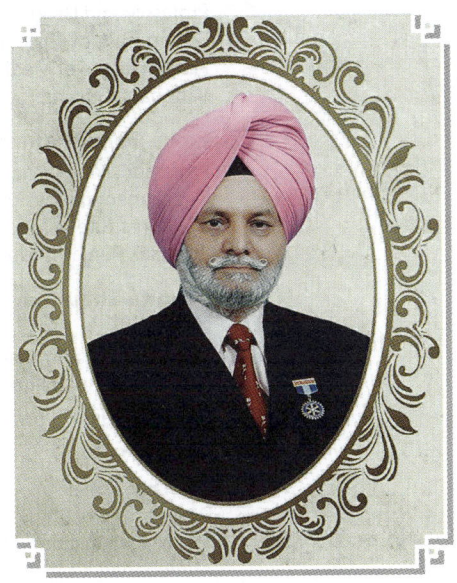

### *'My Dream Book'*
## DEDICATED TO

The permanent source of inspiration, my late father, *Dr OPS Kande*. He was a visionary leader, thorough professional, and an excellent human. He was an anesthesiologist by profession who had not only treated critically sick patients in his ICU but also given them new life, hope, and purpose in life. He stood up for our medical fraternity, whenever needed, as our leader par excellence. He raised his voice to fight against violence against doctors and female foeticide. His moto in life had been to serve the humanity with compassion, empathy, and love.

# CONTRIBUTORS

**Anish S Singhal**
Assistant Professor
Department of Physiology
All India Institute of Medical Sciences
Bibinagar, Telangana, India

**Anupinder Thind**
Assistant Professor
Department of Physiology
All India Institute of Medical Sciences
Bhatinda, Punjab, India

**Naren Kurmi**
Professor
Department of Physiology
Geetanjali Medical College and Hospital
Udaipur, Rajasthan, India

**Neeraj Mahajan**
Associate Professor
Department of Physiology
Smt NHL Municipal Medical College
Ahmedabad, Gujarat, India

**Omlata Bhagat**
Professor
Department of Physiology
All India Institute of Medical Sciences
Jodhpur, Rajasthan, India

**Pratibha Mehta**
Professor
Department of Physiology
American Institute of Medical Sciences
Udaipur, Rajasthan, India

**Puja Dullo**
Professor and Head
Department of Physiology
Parul Institute of Medical Science and Research
Vadodara, Gujarat, India

**Richa Ghay Thaman**
Professor
Department of Physiology
SGRD Institute of Medical Sciences and Research
Amritsar, Punjab, India

**Sangita Chauhan**
Professor
Department of Physiology
Pacific Medical College and Hospital
Udaipur, Rajasthan, India

**Shaista Saiyad**
Associate Professor
Department of Physiology
Smt NHL Municipal Medical College
Ahmedabad, Gujarat, India

**Suman Sharma**
Professor
Department of Physiology
Geetanjali Medical College and Hospital
Udaipur, Rajasthan, India

# NATIONAL ADVISORY BOARD

## Andhra Pradesh

**Ameerunnisa Begum**
Professor and Head, Department of Physiology
Kurnool Medical College
Kurnool, Andhra Pradesh, India

**Geetanjali**
Professor and Head, Department of Physiology
Andhra Medical College
Visakhapatnam, Andhra Pradesh, India

**Lakshmi Divya**
Assistant Professor, Department of Physiology
Guntur Medical College
Guntur, Andhra Pradesh, India

**Madhavi Latha**
Professor and Head, Department of Physiology
NRI Academy of Medical Sciences
Vijayawada, Andhra Pradesh, India

**Satish Pundik**
Additional Professor, Department of Physiology
AIIMS
Mangalagiri, Andhra Pradesh, India

**Sreekanth**
Professor and Head, Department of Physiology
PSIMS, Gannavaram
Andhra Pradesh, India

**Sujatha**
Professor and Head, Department of Physiology
ACSR Medical College
Nellore, Andhra Pradesh, India

**Suresh Babu**
Professor and Vice Principal, Department of Physiology
Gayatri Medical College
Visakhapatnam, Andhra Pradesh, India

**Syamala Devi**
Professor and Head, Department of Physiology
KIMS Medical College
Amalapuram, Andhra Pradesh, India

## Chandigarh

**Anumeha Bhagat**
Associate Professor, Department of Physiology
Government Medical College
Chandigarh, India

## Chhattisgarh

**Alakh Ram Verma**
Professor and Head, Department of Physiology
Government Medical College
Mahasamund, Chhattisgarh, India

**Manish Goyal**
Associate Professor, Department of Physiology
Rajmata Shrimati Devendra Kumari Singhdeo
Government Medical College
Ambikapur, Chhattisgarh, India

**SK Diwedi**
Associate Professor and Head, Department of Physiology
Government Medical College, Jagdalpur
Chhattisgarh, India

**Sheshnarayan Chandrakar**
Assistant Professor, Department of Physiology
Government Medical College
Mahasamund, Chhattisgarh, India

## Delhi

**Mohd Iqbal Alam**
Professor and Head, Department of Physiology
Hamdard Institute of Medical Science and Research
Jamia Hamdard
New Delhi, India

## Goa

**Sandip Sardessai**
Professor and Head, Department of Physiology
Goa Medical College
Bambolim, Goa, India

## Gujarat

**Dharitri Parmar**
Senior Professor, Department of Physiology
Government Medical College
Surat, Gujarat, India

**Geetanjali Purohit**
Professor and Head, Department of Physiology
Swaminarayan Institute of Medical Science and Research
Kalol, Gandhinagar, Gujarat, India

**Jasmin Parmar**
Associate Professor, Department of Physiology
Shri MP Shah Government Medical College
Jamnagar, Gujarat, India

**Jitendra Patel**
Associate Professor, Department of Physiology
GMERS Medical College
Vadnagar, Gujarat, India

**Neeta Mehta**
Senior Professor, Department of Physiology
BJ Medical College and Civil Hospital
Ahmedabad, Gujarat, India

## Haryana

**Anil Kumar Pandey**
Professor and Dean, Department of Physiology
ESIC Medical College and Hospital Faridabad
Haryana, India

**Deepti Dwivedi**
Associate Professor, Department of Physiology
Faculty of Medicine and Health Sciences, SGT University
Gurugram, Haryana, India

**Nimarpreet Kaur**
Professor, Department of Physiology
Faculty of Medicine and Health Sciences, SGT University
Gurugram, Haryana, India

**Shivani Agarwal**
Professor and Head, Department of Physiology
ESIC Medical College and Hospital
Faridabad, Haryana, India

## Karnataka

**Ashwini**
Professor and Head, Department of Physiology
MR Medical College
Gulbarga, Karnataka, India

**Gurcharan**
1st year PG, Department of Physiology
Kasturba Medical College
Mangalore, Karnataka, India

**Jnaneshwar Shenoy**
Head, Department of Physiology
Father Muller Medical College
Mangalore, Karnataka, India

**Lavanya S**
Assistant Professor, Department of Physiology
Rajarajeshwari Medical College and Hospital
Bengaluru, Karnataka, India

**Pallavi LC**
Associate Professor, Department of Physiology
Kasturba Medical College, MAHE
Manipal, Karnataka, India

**Preethi Hegde**
Assistant Professor, Department of Physiology
KS Hegde Medical Academy
Mangalore, Karnataka, India

**Suman Veerappa Budihal**
Associate Professor, Department of Physiology
Kasturba Medical College
Mangalore, Karnataka, India

**Vinodini NA**
Associate Professor, Department of Physiology
Kasturba Medical College
Mangalore, Karnataka, India

**Vishrutha KV**
Professor and Head, Department of Physiology
Srinivas Institute of Medical Sciences and Research Centre
Mangalore, Karnataka, India
Madhya Pradesh

**Ajay Bhatt**
Professor and Head, Department of Physiology
MGM Medical College
Indore, Madhya Pradesh, India

**Anita Choudhary**
Professor and Head, Department of Physiology
Rd Gardi Medical College
Ujjain, Madhya Pradesh, India

**Sahebrao K Sadawarte**
Professor and Head (Ex. Dean), Department of Physiology
People's Medical College
Bhopal, Madhya Pradesh, India

## Maharashtra

**Abhay Naik**
Associate Professor, Department of Physiology
Topiwala Nair Medical College
Mumbai Central, Maharashtra, India

**Amit Faida**
Head, Department of Physiology
LTMC
Mumbai, Maharashtra, India

**Anand Govind Joshi**
Professor and Head, Department of Physiology
Krishna Vishwa Vidyapeeth
Karad, Maharashtra, India

**Anita Mandare**
Assistant Professor, Department of Physiology
Rajarshi Chhatrapati Shahu ji Maharaj GMC
Kolhapur, Maharashtra, India

**Anupriya Deshpande**
Professor and Head, Department of Physiology
Prakash Institute Health Sciences
Islampur, Maharashtra, India

**Arun Kowale**
Dean, Department of Physiology
SSPM Medical College
Kasal-Sindhudurg, Maharashtra, India

## NATIONAL ADVISORY BOARD

**Anuradha Joshi**
Professor and Head, Department of Physiology
Bharati Vidyapeeth Medical College
Pune, Maharashtra, India

**Ashwini Patil**
Professor and Head, Department of Physiology
Symbiosis Medical College for Women
Pune, Maharashtra, India

**Atish Pagar**
Professor, Department of Physiology
Bharati Medical College
Sangli, Maharashtra, India

**AR Joshi**
Professor and Head, Department of Physiology
Vedantaa Institute of Medical Sciences
Palghar, Maharashtra, India

**DN Shenvi**
Professor and Head, Department of Physiology
Seth GS Medical College Parel
Mumbai, Maharashtra, India

**Deepa S Nair**
Professor and Head, Department of Physiology
MIMER Medical College
Talegaon, Maharashtra, India

**Girish Thakare**
Head, Department of Physiology
Government Medical College
Jalgaon, Maharashtra, India

**Hemlata Bipin Munjappa**
Associate Professor, Department of Physiology
Bharati Vidyapeeth Medical College and Hospital
Sangli, Maharashtra, India

**Indira Anil Kurane**
Professor and Head, Department of Physiology
BKL Walawalkar Rural Medical College
Ratnagiri, Maharashtra, India

**Kiran Buge**
Professor, Department of Physiology
Vikhe Patil Medical College
Ahmednagar, Maharashtra, India

**Krishnakant Patil**
Dean, Department of Physiology
Smt Kashibai Navale Medical College
Pune, Maharashtra, India

**Lalita Chandan**
Head, Department of Physiology
HBTC Medical College
Mumbai, Maharashtra, India

**MS Karandikar**
Professor, Department of Physiology
Dr DY Patil Medical College
Pune, Maharashtra, India

**Madhu Karandikar**
Associate Professor, Department of Physiology
Bharati Vidyapeeth Medical College
Pune, Maharashtra, India

**Meena Parekh**
Professor and Head, Department of Physiology
Bharati Vidyapeeth Medical College and Hospital
Sangli, Maharashtra, India

**Mukund Bhaskarrao**
Associate Professor, Department of Physiology
Dr Shankarrao Chavan Government. Medical College
Nanded, Maharashtra, India

**Nikhil Gode**
Associate Professor , Department of Physiology
Government Medical College
Alibag, Maharashtra, India

**Nitin Babanrao Dhokane**
Associate Professor, Department of Physiology
Government Medical College
Oros-Sindhudurg, Maharashtra, India

**Padmaja R Desai**
Professor and Head, Department of Physiology
DY Patil Medical College
Kolhapur, Maharashtra, India

**Prafulla Ratanlal Chandak**
Professor, Department of Physiology
SMBT Medical College
Nashik, Maharashtra, India

**Pranjali Parikshit Muley**
Professor, Department of Physiology
Datta Meghe Medical College
Nagpur, Maharashtra, India

**Pranjali Shinde**
Head, Department of Physiology
ACPM Medical College
Dhule, Maharashtra, India

**Pravin Shekokar**
Associate Professor (Medical Superintendent), Department of Physiology
Government Medical College
Akola, Maharashtra, India

**Priya Mardikar**
Professor and Head, Department of Physiology
Smt Kashibai Navale Medical College
Pune, Maharashtra, India

**Rakhee Tirpude**
Professor, Department of Physiology
NKPSIMS and Research Centre
Nagpur, Maharashtra, India

**Rajkumar S Sood**
Professor and Head, Department of Physiology
Dr DY Patil Medical College
Pune, Maharashtra, India

**Ranjana Shimoga**
Head, Department of Physiology
DUPMC
Jalgaon, Maharashtra, India

**Rita Khadkikar**
Head, Department of Physiology
MGM Medical College
Navi Mumbai, Maharashtra, India

**Sandeep Gundre**
Head, Department of Physiology
Government Medical College
Nandurbar, Maharashtra, India

**Sangita R Phatale**
Professor and Head, Department of Physiology
MGM'S Medical College
Sambhaji Nagar, Maharashtra, India

**Satish Waghmare**
Professor, Department of Physiology
Dr Vasantrao Pawar Medical College Hospital and Research Centre
Nashik, Maharashtra, India

**Shashank Jadhav**
Professor and Head, Department of Physiology
Chhatrapati Sambhaji Maharaj Government Medical College and Hospital
Satara, Maharashtra, India

**Smita Ajay Kumar Shinde**
Associate Professor, Department of Physiology
Bharati Vidyapeeth Medical College and Hospital
Sangl, Maharashtra, India

**Smita Wagh**
Professor, Department of Physiology
ACPM Medical College
Dhule, Maharashtra, India

**Sonali Pande**
Professor, Department of Physiology
TNMC and BYL Nair Hospital
Mumbai Central, Maharashtra, India

**Sunil Kolekar**
Professor and Head, Department of Physiology
Bharat Ratna Atal Bihari Vajpayee Medical College
Pune, Maharashtra, India

**Sunita Handergulle (Birajdar)**
Professor and Head, Department of Physiology
SRTR Government Medical College
Ambajogai, Maharashtra, India

**Sunita Nighute**
Professor and Head, Department of Physiology
Vikhe Patil Medical College
Ahmednagar, Maharashtra, India

**Sunita Subhash Dhule**
Associate Professor, Department of Physiology
SRTR Government Medical College
Ambajogai, Maharashtra, India

**Surendra Shivalkar**
Associate Professor, Department of Physiology
Grant Government Medical College
Mumbai, Maharashtra, India

**Sushma Pande**
Professor and Head, Department of Physiology
Dr PDM Medical College
Amravati, Maharashtra, India

**Syeda Afroz**
Professor and Head, Department of Physiology
Government Medical College
Chh. Sambhaji Nagar, Maharashtra, India

**VS Mantur**
Associate Professor, Department of Physiology
SSPM Medical College and Lifetime Hospital
Padve, Maharashtra, India

**Vaishali M Paunikar**
Professor, Department of Physiology
Jawaharlal Nehru Medical College
Sawangi -Wardha, Maharashtra, India

**Vijay Kumar Gupta**
Assistant Professor, Department of Physiology
Dr DY Patil Medical College
Navi Mumbai, Maharashtra, India

**Vinod Kathore**
Professor and Head, Department of Physiology
DBVP Rural Medical College
Ahmednagar, Maharashtra, India

## *Punjab*

**Avjot K Miglani**
Head, Department of Physiology
Punjab Institute of Medical Science
Jalandhar, Punjab, India

**Babita Bansal**
Associate Professor, Department of Physiology
Gian Sagar Medical Hospital and College
Rajpura, Punjab, India

**Deepinder Kaur**
Head, Department of Physiology
SGRD Medical College and Hospital
Amritsar, Punjab, India

**Harkirat Kaur**
Professor and Head, Department of Physiology
SGRD Medical College and Hospital
Amritsar, Punjab, India

**Jaspreet Takkar**
Head, Department of Physiology
Gian Sagar Medical Hospital and College
Rajpura, Punjab, India

**Meena Arora**
Associate Professor, Department of Physiology
Punjab Institute of Medical Science
Jalandhar, Punjab, India

**Rajiv Sharma**
Professor, Department of Physiology
GGS Medical College and Hospital
Faridkot, Punjab, India

**Ruchika Garg**
Professor, Department of Physiology
Adesh Institute of Medical Science and Research
Bathinda, Punjab, India

**Sangeeta Gupta**
Assistant Professor, Department of Physiology
Government Medical College
Amritsar, Punjab, India

**Suchet**
Head, Department of Physiology
BR Ambedkar State Institute of Medical Science
Mohali, Punjab, India

**Sukhjinder Kaur Dhillon**
Professor, Department of Physiology
SGRD Medical College and Hospital
Amritsar, Punjab, India

### *Rajasthan*

**BK Binawara**
Senior Professor and Head, Department of Physiology
SPMC
Bikaner, Rajasthan, India

**Garima Bafna**
Senior Professor, Department of Physiology
JLN Medical College
Ajmer, Rajasthan, India

**Islam Khan**
Assistant Professor, Department of Physiology
Government Medical College
Alwar, Rajasthan, India

**Jyotsna Shukla**
Senior Professor, Department of Physiology
SMS Medical College
Jaipur, Rajasthan, India

**Kamla Choudhary**
Associate Professor, Department of Physiology
Dr Sampurnanand Medical College (SNMC)
Jodhpur, Rajasthan, India

**Meghshyam Sharma**
Professor and Head, Department of Physiology
RNT Medical College
Udaipur, Rajasthan, India

**Sheshav Somani**
Professor and Head, Department of Physiology
RVRS Government Medical College
Bhilwara, Rajasthan, India

**Suresh Kumar Goyal**
Senior Professor and Head, Department of Physiology
Government Medical College
Dausa, Rajasthan, India

**Varsha Gupta**
Professor, Department of Physiology
SMS Medical College
Jaipur, Rajasthan, India

### *Telangana*

**Abdul Raoof Omer Siddiqui**
Associate Professor, Department of Physiology
Osmania Medical College
Hyderabad, Telangana, India

**D Joya Rani**
Professor and Head, Department of Physiology
PMRIMS College
Hyderabad, Telangana, India

**GS Prema**
Professor, Department of Physiology
Gandhi Medical College
Hyderabad, Telangana, India

**Mohd Abdul Hannan Hazari**
Professor and Head, Department of Physiology
DCMS
Hyderabad, Telangana, India

**Mujahid Mohammad**
Professor, Department of Physiology
Mamata Academy of Medical Sciences
Hyderabad, Telangana, India

**P Shiva Shankar**
Assistant Professor, Department of Physiology
Medicity Medical College
Hyderabad, Telangana, India

**Raghavendra Sherikar**
Professor, Department of Physiology
Malla Reddy Medical College for Women
Hyderabad, Telangana, India

**SP Srinivas**
Associate Professor, Department of Physiology
Gandhi Medical College
Hyderabad, Telangana, India

### *Uttar Pradesh*

**Bharti Bhandari Rathore**
Professor and Head, Department of Physiology
Government Institute of Medical Science
Grater Noida, Uttar Pradesh, India

**Bindu Garg**
Professor and Head, Department of Physiology
SRMS
Bareilly, Uttar Pradesh, India

**JK Bajpai**
Professor and Head, Department of Physiology
Varun Arjun Medical College
Shahjahanpur, Uttar Pradesh, India

### Namita
Assistant Professor, Department of Physiology
Rajarshi Dashrath Autonomous Medical College
Ayodhya, Uttar Pradesh, India

### Narendra Gupta
Professor and Head, Department of Physiology
Rajshree Medical College and Research Centre
Bareilly, Uttar Pradesh, India

### Naveen Gaur
Professor and Head, Department of Physiology
GS Medical College
Hapur, Uttar Pradesh, India

### Niraj Srivastava
Professor and Head, Department of Physiology
Rama Medical College
Hapur, Uttar Pradesh, India

### Ranjan Kumar Dixit
Associate Professor, Department of Physiology
Madhav Prasad Tripathi Medical College
Siddharth Nagar, Uttar Pradesh, India

### Sameer Srivastava
Professor, Department of Physiology
Maharshi Vashishtha Autonomous Medical College
Basti, Uttar Pradesh, India

### Shashank Shekhar Sinha
Professor, Department of Physiology
Rajarshi Dashrath Autonomous Medical College
Ayodhya, Uttar Pradesh, India

### Shreyasi Vaksh
Professor and Head, Department of Physiology
Government Medical College
Pilibhit, Uttar Pradesh, India

### Shomi Anand
Associate Professor, Department of Physiology
ASMC
Gonda, Uttar Pradesh, India

### Sumit Garg
Professor and Head, Department of Physiology
Saraswati Institute of Medical Sciences
Hapur, Uttar Pradesh, India

## *Uttarakhand*

### Neeru Garg
Head, Department of Physiology
Graphic Era Medical College
Dehradun, Uttarakhand, India

# PREFACE

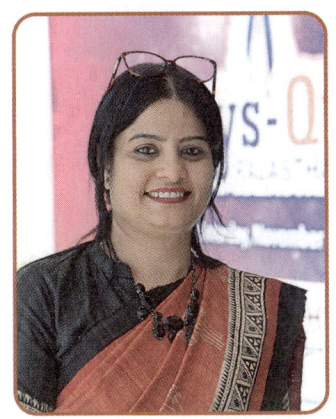

In the vast expanse of medical education, one foundational subject stands out as the bedrock upon which the understanding of the human body is built: Physiology. It is the science that delves into the intricate workings of our biological systems, revealing the marvels of how our bodies function, adapt, and respond to the myriad stimuli of life. As stewards of knowledge and educators, it is our solemn duty to transmit this understanding to the next generation of healthcare professionals, equipping them with the tools and insights necessary to navigate the complexities of human physiology with confidence and competence.

This textbook is our humble attempt to fulfill that duty, to provide students with a beacon of clarity amidst the often-daunting landscape of medical education. It is crafted with an unwavering commitment to providing an enriching, accessible, and holistic learning experience in the field of Medical Physiology. Rooted in the structure of the competency-based curriculum provided by the National Medical Commission, this book meticulously covers basic concepts and their application in clinical conditions. It is our belief that by grounding our teachings in the framework established by esteemed medical authorities, we ensure that our students are equipped with the knowledge and skills necessary to excel in their academic pursuits and future careers.

Central to the design of this textbook is a commitment to inclusivity and accessibility. We recognize that students come from diverse backgrounds and possess varying levels of prior knowledge. Therefore, every effort has been made to present complex concepts in a clear, concise, and engaging manner. Each chapter is structured to enable students to engage in experiential learning through clinical scenarios and case-based learning modules. These practical applications not only reinforce theoretical concepts but also enhance understanding by providing real-world context.

Moreover, this textbook goes beyond mere dissemination of information; it empowers students to assess their own learning through a variety of assessment tools. At the end of each chapter, students will find review questions, critical thinking prompts, and multiple-choice questions designed to reinforce learning and stimulate deeper understanding. Additionally, different types of puzzles are included to maintain student interest and engagement throughout the learning process.

In the spirit of fostering a well-rounded educational experience, we also emphasize the importance of early clinical exposure for clinical physiology. We believe that practical experiences complement theoretical learning and enhance the overall learning experience. Therefore, we encourage students to seek out opportunities for hands-on learning in clinical settings, where they can apply the knowledge gained from this textbook in real-world scenarios.

Furthermore, we recognize the value of supplementary resources in enriching the educational experience. To that end, we recommend viewing the video lectures available on DigiNerve for an in-depth explanation of Physiology. These lectures provide additional insights and explanations that complement the content presented in this textbook, offering students a more comprehensive understanding of the subject matter.

As we embark on this journey together, it is important to acknowledge the countless individuals who have contributed to the creation of this textbook. From esteemed colleagues whose expertise has enriched its content to dedicated students whose curiosity and enthusiasm have served as a constant source of inspiration, this textbook is a testament to the collaborative spirit that defines the academic community.

To our students, both past and present, we extend our deepest gratitude. It is to you, dear students, that we dedicate this textbook, with the hope that it may serve as a guiding light on your educational journey. May it empower you to explore the wonders of Medical Physiology and make a meaningful difference in the world.

In the words of Maya Angelou, *"When you learn, teach. When you get, give."* It is our sincere hope that the knowledge contained within these pages will not only enrich your understanding of Medical Physiology but also inspire you to share your insights with others, thus perpetuating a cycle of learning and growth that transcends boundaries and enriches lives.

With deepest gratitude and warmest wishes,

**Manjinder Kaur**

# ACKNOWLEDGMENTS

In the creation of this Medical Physiology textbook, I am deeply grateful to **The Almighty God**, whose divine guidance and inspiration have illuminated every step of this journey.

To my father, **Dr OPS Kande**, whose legacy of passion and relentless pursuit of excellence continues to fuel my ambitions. His presence remains a constant source of inspiration even from the heavens above.

To my mother, **Mrs Surinder Kaur**, your teachings of patience and perseverance have been my guiding light. Her unwavering belief in hard work and dedication has shaped my approach to achieving each goal, one step at a time.

To my esteemed teacher and guide, **Dr Gurbachan Kaur Ahuja**, your love for Physiology and relentless quest for knowledge have ignited a similar passion within me. Her mentorship has been instrumental in laying the foundation of my understanding in the field of Medical Physiology.

To our Chairman, **Shri JP Agarwal Sir** and entire the management of **Geetanjali University** and **Geetanjali Medical College and Hospital, Udaipur**, Rajasthan for encouragement, support and belief in me. He had been a guiding light, motivating and inspiring for excellence in this field. He has shown us that by hard work, constant efforts and following our dreams, we can actually transform them into reality.

To my husband, **Dr Harpreet Singh**, who have been my pillar of strength, supporting me through my tough times, throughout this journey. His encouragement and belief in my abilities had been like the lamp which brightened up my gloomy days. He had always been the wind beneath my wings, which lifted me to the newer heights, not only during this project but through all walks of life, personal and professional.

To my daughter, **Ms Muskan Singh**, her resilience and support during this arduous journey have been invaluable. Her insights from a student's perspective have greatly enriched the content of this book. Her positive encouragement at times, when I was low, made me wonder at her wisdom and maturity. Thank you dear, for always being there for me.

To my son, **Mr Guntesh Singh**, for his unwavering support amidst his own challenges, I am deeply grateful. His strength and assistance have been a source of immense comfort.

To my coauthor, **Dr Sangeeta Nagpal** (Professor, Maharishi Markandeshwar College of Medical Sciences and Research, Ambala, Haryana), your shared vision and dedication to creating a comprehensive yet accessible textbook have been instrumental in realizing this project.

I extend my heartfelt appreciation to **Dr Suman Sharma** (Professor, Geetanjali Medical College, Udaipur, Rajasthan), **Dr Naren Kurmi** (Professor, Geetanjali Medical College, Udaipur, Rajasthan), **Dr Sangita Chauhan** (Professor, Pacific Medical College, Udaipur, Rajasthan), **Dr Pratibha Mehta** (Professor, American Institute of Medical Sciences, Udaipur, Rajasthan) **Dr Richa Ghay Thaman** (Professor, SGRDIMSAR, Amritsar, Punjab), **Dr Puja Dullo** (Professor and Head, PIMSR, Vadodara, Gujarat), **Dr Omlata Bhagat** (Professor, AIIMS, Jodhpur, Rajasthan), **Dr Shaista Saiyad** (Associate Professor, NHL Medical College, Ahmedabad, Gujarat), **Dr Neeraj Mahajan** (Associate Professor, Smt NHL Municipal Medical College, Ahmedabad, Gujarat), **Dr Anish S Singhal** (Assistant Professor, AIIMS, Bibinagar, Hyderabad), and **Dr Anupinder Thind** (Assistant Professor, AIIMS, Bhatinda, Punjab), and all others whose invaluable contributions have enriched this work.

To my diligent content editor, **Dr Aditya Tayal** (Editorial Manager—Content Strategy), for his persistent encouragement and unwavering support, which have been indispensable. He is truly an invaluable angel, who helped me transforming **"My Dream Book"** to reality.

I convey my sincere thanks to **Shri Jitendar P Vij** (Group Chairman), **Dr Madhu Choudhary** (Director—Educational Publishing) and **Mr Rishi Sharma** (Director Marketing) of M/s Jaypee Brothers Medical Publishers (P) Ltd, New Delhi, India for giving this opportunity and believing in me.

Last but not the least, **Mr Deepak Saxena** (Typesetter), **Mr Gopal Singh Kirola** (Graphic Designer), and **Mr Anil Singh** (Proofreader) of M/s Jaypee Brothers Medical Publishers (P) Ltd, New Delhi, India for their help in the formatting and their experienced technical assistance in developing this project.

With sincere gratitude,

**Manjinder Kaur**

# CONTENTS

## Section 1: General Physiology

1. **Mammalian Cell**    3
   - Cell   3
   - Nucleus   3
   - Mitochondria   3
   - Cell Membrane/Plasma Membrane/Unit Membrane   6
   - Cell Adhesion Molecules (CAMs)   7

2. **Homeostasis**    10
   - Regulation of Homeostatic Mechanisms   10
   - Feedback Mechanisms   10
   - Feed Forward Mechanism   12
   - Importance of Homeostatic Control Mechanisms   13
   - Gain in Homeostatic Control   13

3. **How Do Cells Communicate?**    16
   - Intercellular Connections   16
   - Mechanism of Action of Chemical Messengers   17

4. **Apoptosis: Physiology and Mechanisms**    23
   - Mechanism of Apoptosis   23
   - Situations in which Apoptosis Occur   24
   - Differences between Apoptosis and Necrosis   24
   - Effects of Dysregulated Apoptosis (Too Little/Too Much)   25

5. **Transport Across Cell Membranes**    26
   - Proteins Involved in Transport Across Cell Membrane   26
   - Classification of Mechanism of Transport Across Cell Membrane   26
   - Passive Transport   26
   - Active Transport   29

6. **Body Fluids and Compartments**    33
   - Body Fluids   33
   - Composition of ECF and ICF   34
   - Measurement of Body Fluid Volumes   34
   - Regulation of Body Fluid Volume and Tonicity   37
   - Fluid Replacement Therapy   37

7. **Acid-base Balance**    40
   - Physiological Significance of pH of Body Fluids   40
   - Regulation of pH of the Body Fluids   41
   - Role of Lungs and Kidneys in pH Regulation   41
   - Clinical Assessment of Acid-Base Balance   44

8. **Membrane Potentials of Excitable Tissues**    48
   - Resting Membrane Potential   48
   - Action Potential in Excitable Tissues   50

9. **Applications of Cellular Physiology in Health and Research**    55
   - Methods used to Demonstrate the Functions of the Cells and its Products   55
   - Methods used to Demonstrate the Cellular Communications   57

## Section 2: Hematology

10. **Introduction to Blood**    65
    - Functions of Blood   65
    - Composition of the Blood   65
    - Physiological Significance of Each Component of the Blood   66
    - Physical Characteristics of Blood   67

11. **Plasma Proteins**    69
    - Origin of the Plasma Proteins   69
    - The Normal Levels of Plasma Proteins   69
    - Types of Plasma Proteins   69
    - Functions of Plasma Proteins   69
    - Variations in the Levels of Plasma Proteins   70
    - Plasmapheresis   71

12. **Hemoglobin**    73
    - Synthesis of Hemoglobin   73
    - Structure of Hemoglobin   73
    - Types of Hemoglobin   74
    - Forms of Hemoglobin   75
    - Normal Values, Variation and Functions of Hemoglobin   75
    - Functions   75
    - Fate/Breakdown of Hemoglobin   76
    - Applied Aspects/Clinical Correlates   76

13. **Erythrocytes: Formation and Function**    79
    - Erythrocytes   79
    - Functions of Erythrocytes   80
    - Erythropoiesis   80

14. **Physiology of Anemia**    85
    - Anemia   85
    - Iron Deficiency Anemia   86
    - Macrocytic Anemia   88
    - Hemolytic Anemia   91

15. **Physiology of Jaundice**    96
    - Classification of Jaundice   97
    - Diagnosis of Jaundice   98
    - Physiological Jaundice   98

16. **Leukocytes and their Formation**   101
    - General Structure of a Leukocyte   101
    - Leukopoiesis (Formation of Leukocytes)   101
    - Counts   103
    - Monocyte Macrophage System/Reticuloendothelial System (RES)   106

17. **Basics of Immunity**   109
    - Functions of Immunity   109
    - Classification of Immunity   109
    - Cell Mediated Immunity   110
    - Humoral Immunity   112
    - Immunoglobulin (Ig)   113
    - Types of Humoral/Immune Responses   114
    - Complement System   115
    - Some Other Applications of Immunity   116

18. **Platelets: Structure, Formation and Functions**   120
    - Formation of Platelets/Thrombopoiesis   120
    - Functional Structure of Platelets   120
    - Functions of Platelets   121
    - Clinical Significance   122
    - Antiplatelet Drugs   124

19. **Hemostasis**   127
    - Definition of Hemostasis   127
    - Mechanism of Hemostasis   127
    - Temporary Hemostasis (Platelet Plug Formation)   128
    - Clot Retraction   131
    - Disorders of Hemostasis   133
    - Hemophilia   134
    - Von Willebrand Disease   135
    - Approach to Bleeding Disorders Diagnosis   135

20. **Blood Groups**   138
    - ABO System of Blood Grouping   138
    - Rh Blood Grouping System   139
    - Blood Groups Testing   141

21. **Blood Banking and Blood Transfusion**   145
    - Blood Collection   145
    - Blood Typing and Crossmatching   145
    - Screening for Diseases   146
    - Proper Storage Procedures   146
    - Importance of Blood Transfusions   147
    - Risks and Complications of Blood Transfusions   147
    - Ethical and Legal Considerations   148

## Section 3: Nerve and Muscle Physiology

22. **Neurons and Neuroglia**   155
    - Structure of a Neuron   155
    - Classification of Neurons   156
    - Neuroglia   156

23. **Nerve Growth Factor and Cytokines**   159
    - Nerve Growth Factor   159
    - Brain-derived Neurotrophic Factor   159
    - Neurotropin-3, Neurotropin-4/5   160
    - Other Factors Affecting Neuronal Growth   160

24. **Nerve Fibers and their Properties**   161
    - Structure of an Axon   161
    - Classification of Nerve Fibers   162
    - Axonal Transport   162
    - Properties of Nerve Fibers   163

25. **Degeneration and Regeneration of Peripheral Nerves**   167
    - Grading of Nerve Injury   167
    - Changes in the Nerve After the Injury   167
    - Changes in the Cell Body of Neuron   167
    - Changes in Proximal and Distal Stumps   167
    - Factors Influencing Regeneration of Nerve   169
    - Diagnosis of Nerve Injury   170

26. **Neuromuscular Junction**   172
    - Physiological Anatomy of the Neuromuscular Junction   172
    - Transmission of Impulse Across Neuromuscular Junction   174
    - Drugs Acting on Neuromuscular Junction   176
    - Disorders of Neuromuscular Junction   176

27. **Muscle: Structure, Properties and Physiology of Muscle Contraction**   182
    
    **Structure of the Muscle**   182
    - Skeletal Muscle   182
    - Muscle Proteins   182
    - Myofilaments in Smooth Muscles   186
    
    **Sarcotubular System of the Muscle**   187
    - Skeletal Muscle   187
    - Cardiac Muscle   187
    - Smooth Muscle   188
    
    **Excitability (Electrical Properties of the Muscles)**   188
    - Action Potential of Skeletal Muscle   189
    - Action Potential of the Cardiac Muscle   189
    - Electrical Properties of Smooth Muscle   190
    
    **Contractility**   190
    - Physiology of Muscle Contraction in Skeletal Muscle   190
    - Contraction in Cardiac Muscle   193
    - Contraction in Smooth Muscle   194
    
    **Relationship of Electrical and Contractile/Mechanical Response of Muscles**   195
    - Skeletal Muscle   195
    - Cardiac Muscle   195
    - Smooth Muscle   196
    
    **Contractile Properties of Different Types of Muscles**   196
    - Properties of Skeletal and Cardiac Muscles   196
    
    **Types of Muscle Contractions**   200
    - Recording of Isotonic and Isometric Contractions   201
    - Series Elastic Component   201
    
    **Energy Sources of Muscle Contraction**   202
    - Adenosine Triphosphate   202
    - Creatine Phosphate   202
    - Oxidative Phosphorylation   202
    
    **Disorders of Muscles/Muscular Dystrophy**   203

## Section 4: Gastrointestinal System

**28. Organization of Gastrointestinal System**    **211**
- Physiological Anatomy of GI System   211
- Smooth Muscles of GIT   212
- Migrating Motor Complexes (MMC)   213
- General Principles of Gastrointestinal Secretions   213
- General Principles of Gastrointestinal Motility   215
- Regulation of GI Functions (Secretions and Motility)   215
- Gastrointestinal Reflexes   217
- Physiology of Splanchnic Circulation   218
- Functions of Splanchnic Circulation   218
- Immune Apparatus of Gut   220
- Intestinal Flora/Gut Microbiota   221
- Gut-Brain Axis   221

**29. Digestion in Oral Cavity and Esophagus**    **224**
- Oral Cavity/Mouth   224
- Salivary Secretion   225
- Physiology of Mastication (Chewing)   228
- Physiology of Swallowing/Deglutition   228
- Digestion of Food in Oral Cavity   230

**30. Physiology of Digestion in Stomach**    **233**
- Functional Anatomy of Stomach   233
- Functions of Stomach   234
- Gastric Secretion   235
- Regulation of Gastric Secretion   237
- Gastric Motility   237
- Regulation of Gastric Emptying   239
- Digestion and Absorption in Stomach   239
- Disorders of Stomach   240
- Gastric Function Tests   241

**31. Physiology of Digestion in Small Intestine (Including Pancreas)**    **245**
- Anatomy of Small Intestine and Pancreas   245
- Secretions of Pancreas and Small Intestine   246
- Pancreatic Secretion   246
- Secretions of Small Intestine   249
- Motility of Small Intestine   251
- Digestion and Absorption in Small Intestine   251
- Disorders of Pancreas and Small Intestine   252
- Pancreatic Function Tests   252

**32. Physiology of Hepatobiliary System**    **255**
- Functional Anatomy of Liver   255
- Functions of Liver   256
- Biliary Secretion   257
- Mechanism of Biliary Secretion   258
- Regulation of Bile Secretion   258
- Bile Salts   259
- Enterohepatic Circulation   260
- Choleretics and Cholagogues   260
- Role of Bile in Digestion of Fats   260
- Disorders of Liver and Gallbladder   260
- Liver Function Tests   262

**33. Physiology of Digestion in the Large Intestine**    **264**
- Functional Anatomy of Large Intestine   264
- Functions of Large Intestine   265
- Secretion of Large Intestine   265
- Colonic Motility   266
- Defecation   267
- Digestion and Absorption in Large Intestine   269
- Composition of Feces   269
- Physiological Importance of Dietary Fibers   269
- Clinical Correlation: Large Intestinal Disorders   269

**34. Physiology of Digestion and Absorption of Nutrients**    **274**
- Digestion and Absorption   274
- Digestion and Absorption of Carbohydrates   275
- Digestion and Absorption of Proteins   276
- Digestion and Absorption of Fats   277
- Absorption of Water, Minerals and Trace Elements (Sodium, Chloride, Calcium, Bicarbonate)   278
- Disorders of Digestion and Absorption   279

## Section 5: Cardiovascular System

**35. Functional Anatomy of Heart**    **287**
- External Anatomy   287
- Internal Anatomy   287
- Functions of Cardiovascular System   290

**36. Cardiac Cycle**    **293**
- Cardiac Cycle Time   293
- Methods to Study Cardiac Cycle   293
- Mechanical Events in the Cardiac Cycle   294
- Description of Events in Cardiac Cycle   294
- Pressure and Volume Changes in Left and Right Heart   296
- Overview of Cardiac Cycle   297
- Applied Physiology   299

**37. Basics of Electrocardiography**    **302**
- Components of Normal ECG   303
- Intervals   306
- Segments   307
- Recording of ECG   307

**38. Physiological Basis of Abnormalities of Electrocardiogram**    **314**
- Heart Rate   314
- Rhythm   314
- Disorders of Rhythm   316
- Disorders of Conduction   317
- First Degree Heart Block   317
- Second Degree Heart Block   317
- Complete Heart Block   317
- Sick Sinus Syndrome   318
- Axis Deviation   319
- Chamber Enlargement   319
- Myocardial Infarction   319
- Electrolyte Disturbances in ECG   319

## 39. Circulation and Hemodynamics — 324
- Circulatory System   324
- Hemodynamics   326

## 40. Cardiovascular Regulatory Mechanisms — 333
- Higher Centers in Brain and Brainstem for Cardiovascular Regulation   333
- Classification of Cardiovascular Regulatory Mechanisms   333
- Short-term Regulatory Mechanisms   333
- The Lie Detector Polygraph Test   337
- Intermediate Term Regulation   338
- Long-term Regulation   338

## 41. Heart Rate and Regulation — 342
- Heart Rate   344

## 42. Cardiac Output — 347
- Measurement of Cardiac Output   347
- Factors Affecting Cardiac Output   349
- Variations in Cardiac Output   349
- Regulation of Cardiac Output   350
- Cardiac Function Curves   351

## 43. Venous Return and its Regulation — 354
- Factors Affecting the Venous Return   355

## 44. Blood Pressure and its Regulation — 358
- Determinants of Blood Pressure   358
- Measurement of Blood Pressure   359
- Factors Affecting Blood Pressure   360
- Regulation of Blood Pressure   360
- Applied Aspects   362

## 45. Coronary Circulation — 365
- Coronary Blood Flow   365
- Blood Flow in the Coronaries   366
- Pecularities of Coronary Blood Flow   366
- Factors Affecting Coronary Circulation   367
- Regulation of Coronary Blood Flow   367
- Coronary Artery Disease (CAD) or Ischaemic Heart Disease (IHD)   368

## 46. Blood Flow in Systemic Circulation: Arterial, Capillary, Venous and Lymphatic Circulation — 374
- Components of Systemic Circulation   374
- Arterial Circulation (From Heart to Capillaries)   375
- Microcirculation and Capillary Circulation   375
- Venous Circulation (From Capillaries to Heart)   378
- Lymphatic Circulation   379

## 47. Physiological Basis of Cardiovascular Diseases — 383
- Shock   383
- Cardiac Failure   386

## Section 6: Respiratory Physiology

## 48. Functional Anatomy of Respiratory System — 395
- Functional Anatomy of the Respiratory Tract   395
- Nonrespiratory Functions of the Respiratory System   401

## 49. Mechanics of Pulmonary Ventilation (Chest Movements, Pressure Changes, Alveolar Surface Tension, Compliance, Airway Resistance) — 404
- Mechanics of Respiration   404
- Muscles of Respiration   405
- Mechanism of Inspiration   405
- Mechanism of Expiration   407
- Pressure Gradients   407
- Lung Compliance   408
- Surface Tension   411
- Surfactant   411
- Infant Respiratory Distress Syndrome   413
- Adult Respiratory Distress Syndrome   414
- Airway Resistance   414
- Work of Breathiing   415

## 50. Pulmonary Ventilation (Diffusion of Gases Across Respiratory Membrane) — 418
- Diffusion of Gases ($O_2$ and $CO_2$)   418
- Diffusion Capacity   420
- Inspired, Alveolar and Expired Air   421
- Ventilation-Perfusion Ratio ($V_A/Q$)   422
- Physiological Shunt   423
- Dead Space Air   423

## 51. Pulmonary Function Tests — 426
- Spirometry   426
- Static Lung Volumes and Capacities vs Dynamic Lung Volumes and Capacities   427
- Pulmonary Ventilation   430
- Other Methods for Assessment of PFT   431

## 52. Pulmonary Circulation — 434
- Physiological Anatomy of Pulmonary Circulation   434
- Blood Volume and Flow in Pulmonary Circulation   436
- Functions of Pulmonary Circulation   438
- Pulmonary Edema   438
- Pleural Effusion   439

## 53. Transport of Respiratory Gases (Oxygen and Carbon Dioxide) — 442
- Transport of Oxygen   442
- Oxygenation of Hemoglobin   443
- Oxygen Hemoglobin Dissociation Curve   443
- Oxygen Release in Tissues at Rest   446
- Oxygen Consumption   447
- Co-Efficient of Utilization of $O_2$   447
- Vehicles for the Transport of Oxygen: A Comparison of Plasma, Hemoglobin and Whole Blood   447
- Transport of Carbon Dioxide   447
- Carbon Dioxide Dissociation Curves   448

## 54. Regulation of Respiration — 453
- Nervous Regulation   454
- Chemical Regulation   457
- Nonchemical Regulation   459
- Breath Holding   460

## 55. Respiration in Special Conditions (In Different Barometric Pressures) — 463
- High Altitude Physiology   464
- Space Physiology   468
- Deep-Sea Diving   470

### 56. Physiological Basis of Respiratory Disorders — 475
- Hypoxia  475
- Dyspnea  477
- Asphyxia  478
- Cyanosis  479
- Periodic Breathing  480
- Bronchial Asthma  482
- Chronic Obstructive Pulmonary Disease  483
- Respiratory Failure  484

## Section 7: Renal Physiology

### 57. Functional Anatomy of Kidney — 491
- Kidney  491
- Nephron  492
- Functions of Kidneys  494
- Renal Blood Flow  494

### 58. Juxtaglomerular Apparatus and Renin-angiotensin Aldosterone System — 499
- Juxtaglomerular Apparatus  499
- Renin-angiotensin Aldosterone System (RAAS)  501

### 59. Formation of Urine (Glomerular Filtration, Tubular Reabsorption and Secretion, Concentration of Urine) — 505
- Glomerular Filtration  505
- Concentration of Urine  514
- Role of Antidiuretic Hormone  516

### 60. Renal Function Tests (Including Plasma Clearance) — 524
- Blood Tests  524
- Tests to Assess Glomerular Filtration Rate (GFR)  526
- Estimation of Renal Blood Flow  528
- Renal Tubular Function Tests  528
- Radiographic Technique/IVP  529
- Urine Analysis  530

### 61. Physiological Basis of Diuretics and Renal Disorders — 533
- Diuretics  533
- Acute Renal Failure (ARF)/Acute Kidney Injury (AKI)  534
- Chronic Renal Failure (CRF)/Chronic Kidney Disease (CKD)  537
- Dialysis/Artificial Kidney  539
- Renal Transplantation  540

### 62. Urinary Bladder and its Applied Physiology — 543
- Functional Anatomy of Urinary Bladder  543
- Urodynamic Studies (Cystometery and Radiographic Technique)  545
- Neurogenic Bladder  546

## Section 8: Endocrine Physiology

### 63. Endocrine System and Hormones — 555
- Hormones  555
- Classification of Hormones  555
- Mechanism of Hormone Action  555
- Principles of Endocrinal Disorders  561

### 64. Physiology of Bone and Calcium Regulation — 564
- Physiology of Calcium Regulation  564
- Calcium Dysregulation  566
- Hormonal Control of Calcium Level  569

### 65. Physiology of Hypothalamus — 577
- Functional Anatomy  577
- Functions of Hypothalamus  578

### 66. Physiology of Pituitary Gland — 585
- Functional Anatomy  585
- Hormones of Pituitary Gland  585
- Growth Hormone  586
- Disorders of Anterior Pituitary Gland  588
- Hormones of Posterior Pituitary Gland  590
- Diabetes Insipidus (DI)  591
- Oxytocin  593

### 67. Thyroid Gland — 597
- Functional Anatomy of Thyroid Gland  597
- Hormones of Thyroid Gland  597
- Functions  598
- Biosynthesis of Thyroid Hormone  598
- Transport in Blood  599
- Mechanism of Action of Thyroid Hormones  599
- Actions of Thyroid Hormone  599
- Metabolism of Thyroid Hormones  600
- Regulation of Thyroid Hormone Secretion  600
- Disorders of Thyroid Gland  600
- Thyroid Function Tests  604

### 68. Physiology of Adrenal Gland — 607
- Physiological Anatomy of Adrenal Gland  607
- Mineralocorticoids (Aldosterone)  608
- Glucocorticoid (Cortisol, Corticosterone)  609
- Disorders of Adrenocortical Hormones  612
- Adrenal Function Tests  614

### 69. Glucose Homeostasis: Role of Endocrine Pancreas — 617
- Insulin  617
- Diabetes Mellitus  619
- Diabetic Ketoacidosis  622
- Hyperosmolar Nonketotic Coma  622
- Glucagon  623
- Somatostatin  623

### 70. Physiology of Thymus and Pineal Gland — 627
**Thymus  627**
- Physiological Anatomy  627
- Factors Affecting Thymus  628
- Clinical Significance  628

**Pineal Gland  629**
- Physiologic Anatomy of Pineal Gland  629
- Physiology of Pineal Gland  629
- Function of Pineal Gland  629
- Mechanism of Secretion of Melatonin  629
- Functions of Melatonin  629
- Clinical Significance  630

71. **Metabolic Syndrome (A Self-Directed Learning Module)** 632
    - Introduction to Metabolic Syndrome 632
    - Diagnostic Criteria 632
    - Pathophysiology 633
    - Lifestyle Modifications and Management 633
    - Associated Complications 634
    - Psychiatry Component 635

## Section 9: Reproductive Physiology

72. **Reproductive Physiology and Endocrinology** 641
    - Hypothalamo-Pituitary-Gonadal Axis 641
    - Reproductive Hormones 641
    - Mechanism of Action 645
    - Transport and Metabolism 646
    - Regulation of Secretion of Hormones 646

73. **Sex Determination and Sex Differentiation of Embryo** 648
    - Sex Determination 648
    - Sex Differentiation 649
    - Disorders of Sexual Development 649
    - Chromosomal Anomaly 651

74. **Life Cycle of Reproductive Physiology** 655
    - Puberty (Adolescence) 655
    - Tanner's Classification/Sexual Maturity Rating 655
    - Disorders of Adolescence 657
    - Castration/Gonadectomy (Removal of Gonads) 657
    - The End of Reproductive Period (Menopause and Andropause) 658

75. **Reproductive Physiology in Males** 661
    - Functional Anatomy of Male Reproductive System 661
    - Microscopic Anatomy of Testis 661
    - Functions of Testes 663
    - Structure of Sperm 664
    - Seminal Vesicle 665
    - Prostate Gland 665
    - Semen 665
    - Disorders Related to Spermatogenesis, Resulting in Male Infertility 666

76. **Reproductive Physiology in Females** 670
    - Functional Anatomy of Female Reproductive System 670
    - Oogenesis (Formation of Ovum) 670
    - The Female Sexual Cycle (Menstrual Cycle) 671
    - Uterine Changes 675

77. **Physiology of Pregnancy and Lactation** 679
    - Physiology of Conception 679
    - Pregnancy 681
    - Placental Hormones 683
    - Parturition 685
    - Lactation 688

78. **Contraception** 692
    - Rhythm Method 692
    - Lactational Amenorrhea Method 693
    - Barrier Methods 693
    - Intrauterine Device 693
    - Oral Contraceptives Pills 694
    - Other Methods 694

## Section 10: Neurophysiology and Special Senses

79. **Organization of Nervous System** 701
    - Central Nervous System 701
    - Brain 701
    - Functional Anatomy of Brain and Spinal Cord 701

80. **Synapse** 711
    - Types of Synapse 711
    - Structure and Functioning of the Synapse 712
    - Properties of Synapse 713

81. **Neurotransmitters** 718
    - Small Molecule Neurotransmitters 718
    - Large Molecule Neurotransmitters 720

82. **Physiology of Sensory Receptors** 723
    - How are Sensations Carried and Recognized? 723
    - Receptors 723
    - Properties of Receptors 725

83. **Postural Reflexes and their Regulation** 730
    - What is a Postural Reflex? 730
    - The Postural Muscles 730
    - Postural Reflexes Integrated at Different Levels of CNS 731

84. **Cerebral Cortex** 742
    - Functional Anatomy of Cerebral Cortex 742
    - Lobes of Cerebrum 742
    - Communication between Both the Cerebral Hemispheres 749
    - Cerebral Dominance 749

85. **Thalamus** 752
    - Structure and Nuclei of Thalamus 752

86. **Role of Cerebellum and Basal Ganglia (Motor Planning, Programming and Execution)** 755
    - Cerebellum 756
    - Basal Ganglia 761
    - Summary of Motor Programming and Planning in Motor Execution 766

87. **Spinal Cord and the Pathways between Cerebrum and Peripheral Parts of Body** 769
    - Functional Anatomy 769
    - Organization of Spinal Cord 769
    - Sensory Tracts: Ascending Tracts of Spinal Cord 771
    - Spinocerebellar Tracts 775
    - Motor Tracts: The Descending Tracts of Spinal Cord 775
    - Some Common Lesions of Spinal Cord 778
    - **Pain and Analgesia System** 781
    - Pain 781
    - Analgesia System 783

## 88. Reticular Activating System (RAS)   787
- Anatomy and Structure of RAS   787
- Functions of RAS   787

## 89. Physiology of Limbic System, Speech, Memory, EEG and Sleep   789
- Physiology of Emotions—the Limbic System   789
- Physiology of Speech   791
- Physiology of Learning and Memory   792
- Physiology of Electroencephalography   795
- Physiology of Sleep   799

## 90. Vestibular System   805
- Vestibular Apparatus   805
- Functions of Vestibular Apparatus   807
- Vestibular Pathways and Connections   809
- Vestibular Nuclei   809
- Vestibular Reflexes   810
- Disorders Associated with Vestibular Apparatus   811

## 91. Autonomic Nervous System   814
- Organization of Autonomic Nervous System   814
- Parasympathetic Nervous System   815
- Sympathetic Nervous System   815
- Fight or Flight Response   818
- Levels of Control of the Autonomic Nervous System   818
- Working of Autonomic Nervous System   818
- Feedback Mechanism in the Autonomic Nervous System   819

## 92. Cerebral Blood Flow   823
- Functional Anatomy of Cerebral Blood Flow   823
- Physiology of Cerebral Circulation   824
- Cerebrovascular Accidents (CVA)/Stroke   825
- Metabolism in Brain   825

## 93. Physiology of Olfaction   827
- Smell or Olfaction   827
- Mechanism of Olfaction   828
- Sniffing   832
- Adaptation of Olfactory Receptors   832
- Disorders Related to Olfaction   832
- Method of Quantitative Estimation of the Sense of Smell Using an Olfactometer   833

## 94. Physiology of Taste Sensation (Gustatory Sensation)   836
- Functional Anatomy of Tongue   836
- Transduction of Gustatory Stimuli   838
- Factors Affecting Taste Sensation   838
- Mechanism of Gustatory Transduction   839
- Taste Pathways   840
- Applied Aspect   841

## 95. Physiology of Vision   844
- Anatomy of Eye   844
- Genesis of Electrical Activity in Retina   850
- Photoreceptor Potentials   851
- Responses to Bipolar, Amacrine and Horizontal Cells   854
- Response Pattern of Ganglion Cells   855
- Responses of Neurons in Lateral Geniculate Bodies and Visual Cortex   857
- Visual Pathway   857
- Principles of Optics   860
- Eye Movements   865

## 96. Physiology of Hearing   870
- Sound Waves   870
- Functional Anatomy of Ear   872
- Electrical Responses in the Hair Cells   877
- Central Auditory Pathway   881
- Physiology of Hearing Defects/Deafness   883

# Section 11: Integrated Physiology

## 97. Temperature Regulation and Adaptation   891
- Normal Human Body Temperature   891
- Heat Producing and Heat Dissipating Mechanisms of the Body   892
- Regulation of Temperature (or Adaptation to Heat and Cold)   893

## 98. Physiology of Physical Activity (Sedentary Lifestyle and Exercise)   898
- Recognizing Sedentary Behavior   898
- Classification of Exercise   900
- Physiological Effects of Exercise   901
- Response to Exercise   903
- Long-term Adaptation of Exercise   904
- Exercise in Extreme Climate (Heat and Cold)   904

## 99. Physiology of Infancy   910
- Developmental Milestones   910
- Importance of Understanding Infant Physiology   910
- Physiological Changes in Infants   913

## 100. Physiology of Aging, Free Radicals and Antioxidants   920
- Theories of Aging   920
- Physiological Changes Associated with Ageing   921
- Role of Free Radicals   921
- Antioxidants: Mechanisms and Importance   922
- Strategies to Mitigate Aging and Oxidative Stress   923

## 101. Physiology of Yoga and Meditation   925
**Yoga and Meditation   925**
- Physiology of Stress   925
- Yoga   926
- Process of Meditation   928
- Integrating Yoga and Meditation for Health and Wellness   929

## 102. Brain Death   931
- Concept and Criteria   931
- Implications   931

*Appendix (AETCOM 1 and 2)*   935

*Answers to Crossword Puzzles*   939

*Index*   941

# COMPETENCY TABLE

| Number | Competency: The student should be able to | Core (Y/N) | Chapter number | Page number |
|---|---|---|---|---|
| PY1.1 | Describe the structure and functions of a mammalian cell | Y | 1 | 3 |
| PY1.2 | Describe and discuss the principles of homeostasis | Y | 2 | 10 |
| PY1.3 | Describe intercellular communication | Y | 3 | 16 |
| PY1.4 | Describe apoptosis—programmed cell death | Y | 4 | 23 |
| PY1.5 | Describe and discuss transport mechanisms across cell membranes | Y | 5 | 26 |
| PY1.6 | Describe the fluid compartments of the body, its ionic composition and measurements | Y | 6 | 33 |
| PY1.7 | Describe the concept of pH and buffer systems in the body | Y | 7 | 40 |
| PY1.8 | Describe and discuss the molecular basis of resting membrane potential and action potential in excitable tissue | Y | 8 | 48 |
| PY1.9 | Describe and discuss the methods used to demonstrate the functions of the cells and its products, its communications and their applications in Clinical care and research | Y | 9 | 55 |
| PY2.1 | Describe the composition and functions of blood components | Y | 10 | 65 |
| PY2.2 | Discuss the origin, forms, variations, and functions of plasma proteins | Y | 11 | 69 |
| PY2.3 | Describe and discuss the synthesis and functions of Haemoglobin and explain its breakdown. Describe variants of haemoglobin | Y | 12 | 73 |
| PY2.4 | Describe RBC formation (erythropoiesis and its regulation) and its functions | Y | 13 | 79 |
| PY2.5 | Describe different types of anaemias and Jaundice | Y | 14<br>15 | 85<br>96 |
| PY2.6 | Describe WBC formation (granulopoiesis) and its regulation | Y | 16 | 101 |
| PY2.7 | Describe the formation of platelets, functions, and variations | Y | 18 | 120 |
| PY2.8 | Describe the physiological basis of haemostasis and, anticoagulants. Describe bleeding and clotting disorders (Haemophilia, purpura) | Y | 19 | 127 |
| PY2.9 | Describe different blood groups and discuss the clinical importance of blood grouping, blood banking and transfusion | Y | 20<br>21 | 138<br>145 |
| PY2.10 | Define and classify different types of immunity. Describe the development of immunity and its regulation | Y | 17 | 109 |
| PY3.1 | Describe the structure and functions of a neuron and neuroglia; Discuss Nerve Growth Factor and other growth factors/cytokines | Y | 22<br>23 | 155<br>159 |
| PY3.2 | Describe the types, functions and properties of nerve fibers | Y | 24 | 161 |
| PY3.3 | Describe the degeneration and regeneration in peripheral nerves | Y | 25 | 167 |
| PY3.4 | Describe the structure of neuro-muscular junction and transmission of impulses | Y | 26 | 172 |
| PY3.5 | Discuss the action of neuro-muscular blocking agents | Y | 26 | 172 |
| PY3.6 | Describe the pathophysiology of Myasthenia gravis | Y | 26 | 172 |
| PY3.7 | Describe the different types of muscle fibres and their structure | Y | 27 | 182 |
| PY3.8 | Describe action potential and its properties in different muscle types (skeletal and smooth) | Y | 27 | 182 |
| PY3.9 | Describe the molecular basis of muscle contraction in skeletal and in smooth muscles | Y | 27 | 182 |
| PY3.10 | Describe the mode of muscle contraction (isometric and isotonic) | Y | 27 | 182 |
| PY3.11 | Explain energy source and muscle metabolism | Y | 27 | 182 |
| PY3.12 | Explain the gradation of muscular activity | Y | 27 | 182 |
| PY3.13 | Describe muscular dystrophy: myopathies | Y | 27 | 182 |

| Number | Competency: The student should be able to | Core (Y/N) | Chapter number | Page number |
|---|---|---|---|---|
| PY3.17 | Describe Strength-duration curve | Y | 27 | 182 |
| PY4.1 | Describe the structure and functions of digestive system | Y | 28 | 211 |
| PY4.2 | Describe the composition, mechanism of secretion, functions, and regulation of saliva, gastric, pancreatic, intestinal juices and bile secretion | Y | 29<br>30<br>31<br>32<br>33 | 224<br>233<br>245<br>255<br>264 |
| PY4.3 | Describe GIT movements, regulation and functions. Describe defecation reflex. Explain role of dietary fibre | Y | 29<br>30<br>31<br>33 | 224<br>233<br>245<br>264 |
| PY4.4 | Describe the physiology of digestion and absorption of nutrients | Y | 29<br>34 | 224<br>274 |
| PY4.5 | Describe the source of GIT hormones, their regulation and functions | Y | 28 | 211 |
| PY4.6 | Describe the Gut-Brain Axis | Y | 28 | 211 |
| PY4.7 | Describe and discuss the structure and functions of liver and gall bladder | Y | 32 | 255 |
| PY4.8 | Describe and discuss gastric function tests, pancreatic exocrine function tests and liver function tests | Y | 30<br>32 | 233<br>255 |
| PY4.9 | Discuss the physiology aspects of: peptic ulcer, gastro-oesophageal reflux disease, vomiting, diarrhoea, constipation, Adynamic ileus, Hirschsprung's disease | Y | 30<br>31<br>33 | 233<br>245<br>264 |
| PY5.1 | Describe the functional anatomy of heart including chambers, sounds; and Pacemaker tissue and conducting system. | Y | 35 | 287 |
| PY5.2 | Describe the properties of cardiac muscle including its morphology, electrical, mechanical and metabolic functions | Y | 27 | 182 |
| PY5.3 | Discuss the events occurring during the cardiac cycle | Y | 36 | 293 |
| PY5.4 | Describe generation, conduction of cardiac impulse | Y | | |
| PY5.5 | Describe the physiology of electrocardiogram (E.C.G), its applications and the cardiac axis | Y | 37 | 302 |
| PY5.6 | Describe abnormal ECG, arrythmias, heart block and myocardial Infarction | Y | 38 | 314 |
| PY5.7 | Describe and discuss hemodynamics of circulatory system | Y | 39 | 324 |
| PY5.8 | Describe and discuss local and systemic cardiovascular regulatory mechanisms | Y | 40 | 333 |
| PY5.9 | Describe the factors affecting heart rate, regulation of cardiac output and blood pressure | Y | 41<br>42<br>43<br>44 | 342<br>347<br>354<br>358 |
| PY5.10 | Describe and discuss regional circulation including microcirculation, lymphatic circulation, coronary, cerebral, capillary, skin, foetal, pulmonary and splanchnic circulation | Y | 45<br>46<br>52<br>92 | 365<br>374<br>434<br>823 |
| PY5.11 | Describe the patho-physiology of shock, syncope and heart failure | Y | 47 | 384 |
| PY6.1 | Describe the functional anatomy of respiratory tract | Y | 48 | 395 |
| PY6.2 | Describe the mechanics of normal respiration, pressure changes during ventilation, lung volume and capacities, alveolar surface tension, compliance, airway resistance, ventilation, V/P ratio, diffusion capacity of lungs | Y | 49<br>50<br>51 | 404<br>418<br>426 |
| PY6.3 | Describe and discuss the transport of respiratory gases: Oxygen and Carbon dioxide | Y | 53 | 442 |
| PY6.4 | Describe and discuss the physiology of high altitude and deep sea diving | Y | 55 | 463 |
| PY6.5 | Describe and discuss the principles of artificial respiration, oxygen therapy, acclimatization and decompression sickness. | Y | 55 | 463 |
| PY6.6 | Describe and discuss the pathophysiology of dyspnoea, hypoxia, cyanosis asphyxia; drowning, periodic breathing | Y | 56 | 475 |

| Number | Competency: The student should be able to | Core (Y/N) | Chapter number | Page number |
|---|---|---|---|---|
| PY6.7 | Describe and discuss lung function tests and their clinical significance | Y | 51 | 426 |
| PY7.1 | Describe structure and function of kidney | Y | 57 | 491 |
| PY7.2 | Describe the structure and functions of juxta glomerular apparatus and role of renin-angiotensin system | Y | 58 | 499 |
| PY7.3 | Describe the mechanism of urine formation involving processes of filtration, tubular reabsorption and secretion; concentration and diluting mechanism | Y | 59 | 505 |
| PY7.4 | Describe and discuss the significance and implication of renal clearance | Y | 60 | 524 |
| PY7.5 | Describe the renal regulation of fluid and electrolytes and acid-base balance | Y | 7 | 40 |
| PY7.6 | Describe the innervations of urinary bladder, physiology of micturition and its abnormalities | Y | 62 | 543 |
| PY7.7 | Describe artificial kidney, dialysis and renal transplantation | Y | 61 | 532 |
| PY7.8 | Describe and discuss renal function tests | Y | 60 | 524 |
| PY7.9 | Describe cytometry and discuss the normal cystometrogram | Y | 62 | 543 |
| PY8.1 | Describe the physiology of bone and calcium metabolism | Y | 64 | 524 |
| PY8.2 | Describe the synthesis, secretion, transport, physiological actions, regulation and effect of altered (hypo and hyper) secretion of pituitary gland, thyroid gland, parathyroid gland, adrenal gland, pancreas and hypothalamus | Y | 64<br>65<br>66<br>67<br>68<br>69 | 524<br>578<br>586<br>597<br>607<br>618 |
| PY8.3 | Describe the physiology of Thymus and Pineal Gland | Y | 70 | 628 |
| PY8.4 | Describe function tests: Thyroid gland; Adrenal cortex, Adrenal medulla and pancreas | Y | 67<br>68<br>69 | 597<br>607<br>618 |
| PY8.5 | Describe the metabolic and endocrine consequences of obesity and metabolic syndrome, Stress response. Outline the psychiatry component pertaining to metabolic syndrome. | Y | 71 | 632 |
| PY8.6 | Describe and differentiate the mechanism of action of steroid, protein and amine hormones | Y | 63 | 555 |
| PY9.1 | Describe and discuss sex determination; sex differentiation and their abnormities and outline psychiatry and practical implication of sex determination | Y | 73 | 648 |
| PY9.2 | Describe and discuss puberty: onset, progression, stages; early and delayed puberty and outline adolescent clinical and psychological association | Y | 74 | 655 |
| PY9.3 | Describe male reproductive system: functions of testis and control of spermatogenesis and factors modifying it and outline its association with psychiatric illness | Y | 75 | 661 |
| PY9.4 | Describe female reproductive system: (a) functions of ovary and its control; (b) menstrual cycle—hormonal, uterine and ovarian changes | Y | 76 | 670 |
| PY9.5 | Describe and discuss the physiological effects of sex hormones | Y | 72<br>75 | 641<br>661 |
| PY9.6 | Enumerate the contraceptive methods for male and female. Discuss their advantages and disadvantages | Y | 78 | 692 |
| PY9.7 | Describe and discuss the effects of removal of gonads on physiological functions | Y | 74 | 655 |
| PY9.8 | Describe and discuss the physiology of pregnancy, parturition and lactation and outline the psychology and psychiatry-disorders associated with it | Y | 77 | 679 |
| PY9.9 | Interpret a normal semen analysis report including (a) sperm count, (b) sperm morphology and (c) sperm motility, as per WHO guidelines and discuss the results | Y | 75 | 661 |
| PY9.10 | Discuss the physiological basis of various pregnancy tests | Y | 77 | 679 |
| PY9.11 | Discuss the hormonal changes and their effects during perimenopause and menopause | Y | 74 | 655 |

| Number | Competency: The student should be able to | Core (Y/N) | Chapter number | Page number |
|---|---|---|---|---|
| PY10.1 | Describe and discuss the organization of nervous system | Y | 79 | 701 |
| PY10.2 | Describe and discuss the functions and properties of synapse, reflex, receptors | Y | 80<br>82<br>83 | 711<br>723<br>730 |
| PY10.3 | Describe and discuss somatic sensations and sensory tracts | Y | 87 | 769 |
| PY10.4 | Describe and discuss motor tracts, mechanism of maintenance of tone, control of body movements, posture and equilibrium and vestibular apparatus | Y | 83<br>86<br>87<br>90 | 730<br>755<br>769<br>805 |
| PY10.5 | Describe and discuss structure and functions of reticular activating system, autonomic nervous system (ANS) | Y | 88<br>91 | 787<br>814 |
| PY10.6 | Describe and discuss Spinal cord, its functions, lesion and sensory disturbances | Y | 87 | 769 |
| PY10.7 | Describe and discuss functions of cerebral cortex, basal ganglia, thalamus, hypothalamus, cerebellum and limbic system and their abnormalities | Y | 84<br>85<br>86<br>89 | 742<br>752<br>755<br>789 |
| PY10.8 | Describe and discuss behavioural and EEG characteristics during sleep and mechanism responsible for its production | Y | 89 | 789 |
| PY10.9 | Describe and discuss the physiological basis of memory, learning and speech | Y | 89 | 789 |
| PY10.10 | Describe and discuss chemical transmission in the nervous system. (Outline the psychiatry element) | Y | 81 | 718 |
| PY10.12 | Identify normal EEG forms | Y | 89 | 789 |
| PY10.13 | Describe and discuss perception of smell and taste sensation | Y | 93<br>94 | 827<br>836 |
| PY10.14 | Describe and discuss patho-physiology of altered smell and taste sensation | Y | 93<br>94 | 827<br>836 |
| PY10.15 | Describe and discuss functional anatomy of ear and auditory pathways and physiology of hearing | Y | 96 | 870 |
| PY10.16 | Describe and discuss pathophysiology of deafness. Describe hearing tests | Y | 96 | 870 |
| PY10.17 | Describe and discuss functional anatomy of eye, physiology of image formation, physiology of vision including colour vision, refractive errors, colour blindness, physiology of pupil and light reflex | Y | 95 | 844 |
| PY10.18 | Describe and discuss the physiological basis of lesion in visual pathway | Y | 95 | 844 |
| PY10.19 | Describe and discuss auditory and visual evoke potentials | Y | 95<br>96 | 844<br>870 |
| PY11.1 | Describe and discuss mechanism of temperature regulation | Y | 97 | 891 |
| PY11.2 | Describe and discuss adaptation to altered temperature (heat and cold) | Y | 97 | 891 |
| PY11.3 | Describe and discuss mechanism of fever, cold injuries and heat stroke | Y | 97 | 891 |
| PY11.4 | Describe and discuss cardio-respiratory and metabolic adjustments during exercise; physical training effects | Y | 98 | 898 |
| PY11.5 | Describe and discuss physiological consequences of sedentary lifestyle | Y | 98 | 898 |
| PY11.6 | Describe physiology of Infancy | N | 99 | 910 |
| PY11.7 | Describe and discuss physiology of aging; free radicals and antioxidants | N | 100 | 920 |
| PY11.8 | Discuss and compare cardio-respiratory changes in exercise (isometric and isotonic) with that in the resting state and under different environmental conditions (heat and cold) | Y | 98 | 898 |
| PY11.10 | Interpret anthropometric assessment of infants | N | 99 | 910 |
| PY11.11 | Discuss the concept, criteria for diagnosis of Brain death and its implications | Y | 102 | 931 |
| PY11.12 | Discuss the physiological effects of meditation | N | 101 | 925 |

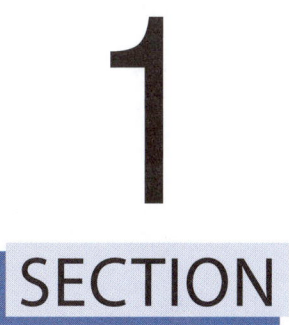

# GENERAL PHYSIOLOGY

## Section Outline

**Chapter 1:** Mammalian Cell
**Chapter 2:** Homeostasis
**Chapter 3:** How Do Cells Communicate?
**Chapter 4:** Apoptosis: Physiology and Mechanisms
**Chapter 5:** Transport Across Cell Membranes
**Chapter 6:** Body Fluids and Compartments
**Chapter 7:** Acid-base Balance
**Chapter 8:** Membrane Potentials of Excitable Tissues
**Chapter 9:** Applications of Cellular Physiology in Health and Research

# Mammalian Cell

**CHAPTER 1**

### COMPETENCY ADDRESSED
**PY1.1:** Describe the structure and functions of a mammalian cell.

###  LEARNING OBJECTIVES
**At the end of this chapter, the learner should be able to:**
- Define a cell.
- Enumerate the cell organelles.
- Describe the structure and functions of all cell organelles.
- Describe the structure and functions of cell membrane.
- Describe the functions of cell membrane proteins.
- Describe physiological significance of cell adhesion molecules (CAM).
- Describe the molecular motors.
- Describe the physiological basis of disorders of cell organelles.

## CELL

The structural and functional unit of living organism is known as cell **(Fig. 1.1)**.

The three principle constituents of a cell are **(Tables 1.1A and 1.1B)**:
1. Cytoplasm and its organelles
2. Cell membrane
3. Nucleus

## NUCLEUS (FIG.1.3)

- It is a spherical structure which controls all the cellular activities and reproduction of cells
- It has double layer nuclear membrane, has large pores by which macromolecules like ribonucleic acid (RNA) can pass through.
- The chromosomes are present inside the nucleus, which are made-up by deoxyribonucleic acid (DNA), on which genes are present.
- **A gene** is a portion of deoxyribonucleic acid (DNA) molecule responsible for transmission of hereditary characteristics across the generations.
- It contains **nucleolus** responsible for the synthesis of RNA (transcription) for the ribosome. This RNA moves to cytoplasm and regulates the synthesis of protein (translation) by the cell.

## MITOCHONDRIA (FIG. 1.4)

- It is the major site of aerobic respiration
- Contains the enzymes responsible for biological oxidation, enzymes for citric acid cycle and respiratory chain oxidation

**Table 1.1A:** Principle constituents of the cell.

| CYTOPLASM | | |
|---|---|---|
| **Organelles** | **Inclusion bodies** | **Cytoskeleton** |
| Permanent components of cell | Temporary component of cell | Network of fibers |
| • Contain enzymes which participate in the cellular metabolic activity<br>• Cell organelles are mitochondria, endoplasmic reticulum, Golgi apparatus, ribosome, lysosomes, peroxisomes, etc. | They include lipid droplets, secretary granules, melanin pigment, lipofuscin | It include microtubules, microfilaments and intermediate filaments |

**Table 1.1B:** Cytoskeleton.

| CYTOSKELETON (Fig. 1.2): Is formed by a network of fibrillar proteins organized as filaments and tubules | | |
|---|---|---|
| **Microtubules** | **Intermediate filaments** | **Microfilaments** |
| • They are made-up of two globular protein α and β tubulin<br>• They provide structural strength to the cell<br>• Kinesin and dyneins are known as molecular motors; which help in movement of molecules through the microtubules<br>• They form tracts on which chromosomes, mitochondria and secretory granules move from one part of the cell to another (intracellular transport)<br>• Cilia and flagella, present on cell surface are also the type of microtubules which are responsible for the locomotion of cells<br>• Centrioles and mitotic spindles of cells undergoing mitosis are also examples of stiff microtubules | • Intermediate filaments are strong ropelike structure<br>• Along with the microtubules they provide strength and support to the fragile tubulin structures<br>• All the cells have intermediate filament and they predominantly serve the function of mechanical support<br>• Some cells have special intermediate filaments, e.g., neurofilaments in neurons, desmin in the muscle cells<br>• Proteins of intermediate filaments are specific so they are use as cellular markers | • These microfilaments, when present in the outer zone of cytoplasm (ectoplasm), it provides elastic support to the cell<br>• The actin and myosin microfilaments when present inside the muscle cells, forms the contractile apparatus<br>• They are responsible for cell movement<br>• Actin, along with integrin receptors form focal adhesion complexes, responsible for cell adhesion<br>• These microfilaments form microvilli, which increase the surface area for absorption |

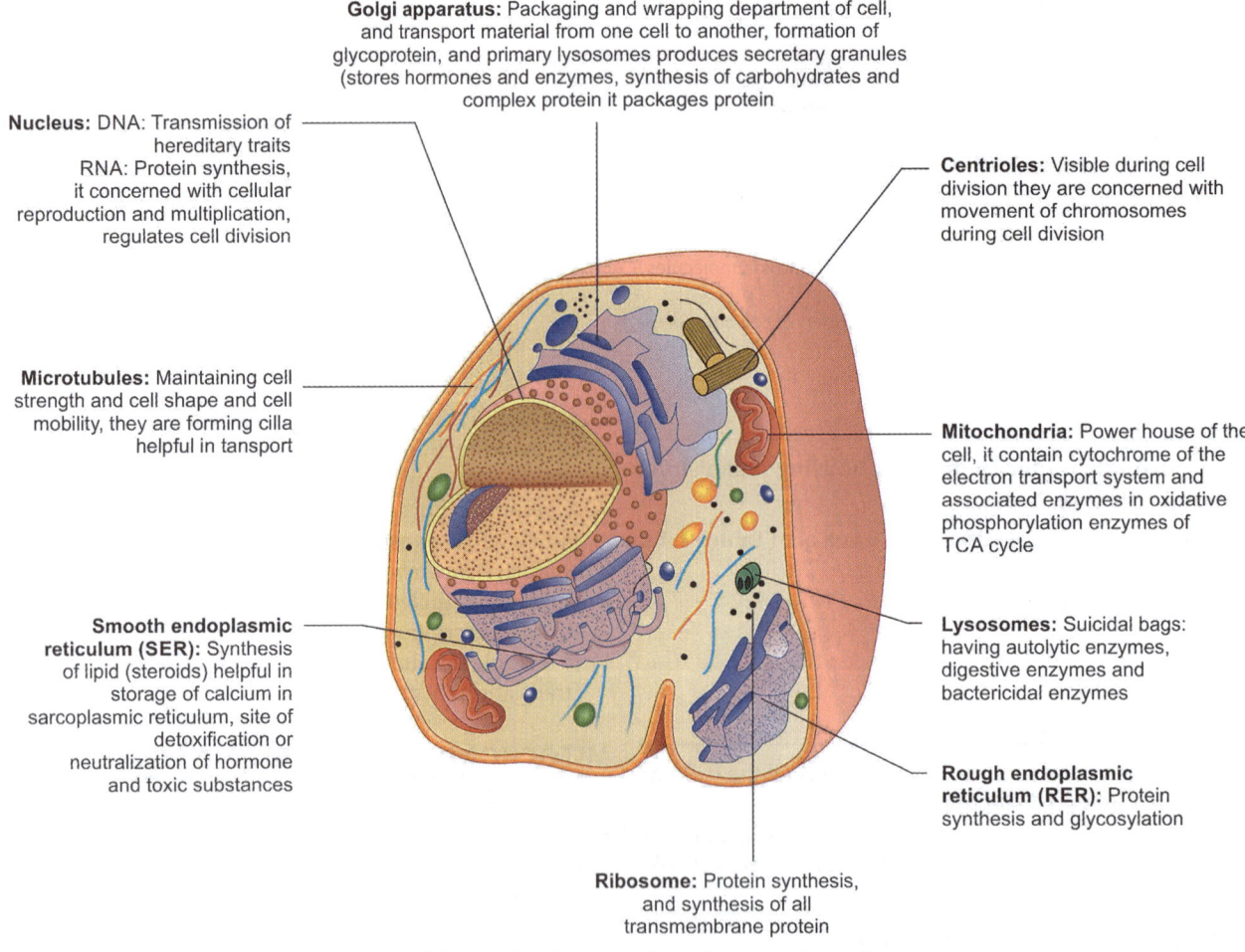

**Golgi apparatus:** Packaging and wrapping department of cell, and transport material from one cell to another, formation of glycoprotein, and primary lysosomes produces secretary granules (stores hormones and enzymes, synthesis of carbohydrates and complex protein it packages protein

**Nucleus:** DNA: Transmission of hereditary traits RNA: Protein synthesis, it concerned with cellular reproduction and multiplication, regulates cell division

**Centrioles:** Visible during cell division they are concerned with movement of chromosomes during cell division

**Microtubules:** Maintaining cell strength and cell shape and cell mobility, they are forming cilla helpful in tansport

**Mitochondria:** Power house of the cell, it contain cytochrome of the electron transport system and associated enzymes in oxidative phosphorylation enzymes of TCA cycle

**Smooth endoplasmic reticulum (SER):** Synthesis of lipid (steroids) helpful in storage of calcium in sarcoplasmic reticulum, site of detoxification or neutralization of hormone and toxic substances

**Lysosomes:** Suicidal bags: having autolytic enzymes, digestive enzymes and bactericidal enzymes

**Rough endoplasmic reticulum (RER):** Protein synthesis and glycosylation

**Ribosome:** Protein synthesis, and synthesis of all transmembrane protein

**Fig. 1.1:** Functional organization of a mammalian cell.

- It also synthesizes the membrane bound proteins.
- The inner membrane of mitochondria has cristae, rich in many enzymes like cytochrome b, c, a, NADH dehydrogenase, succinate dehydrogenase etc.
- The inner cavity of the mitochondrion is filled with a matrix that contains large quantities of dissolved enzymes necessary for extracting energy from nutrients. It has short life span and has a self-replicative capacity.

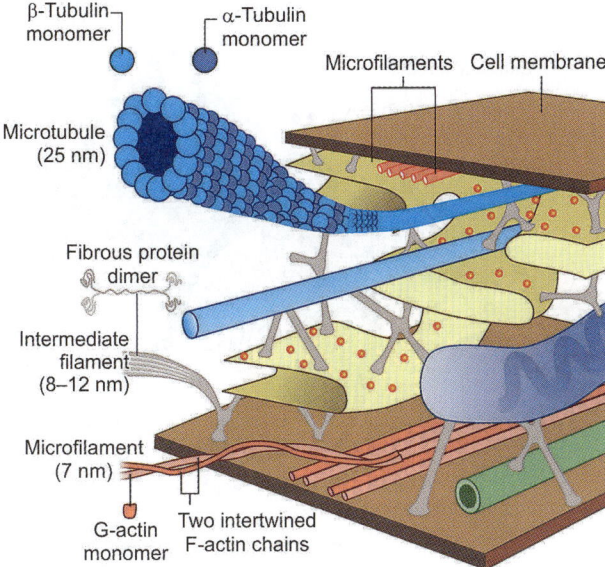

**Fig. 1.2:** Cell cytoskeleton.

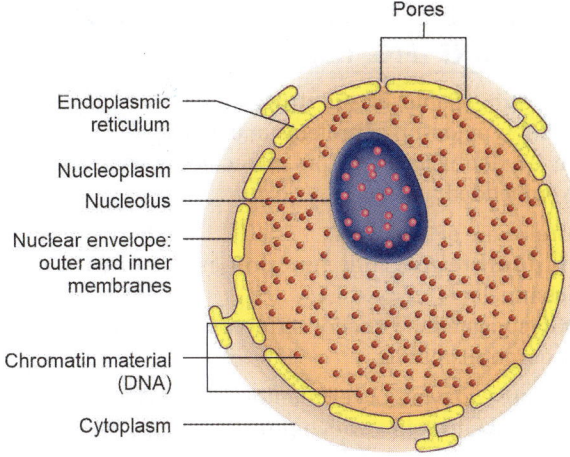

**Fig. 1.3:** Cell nucleus.

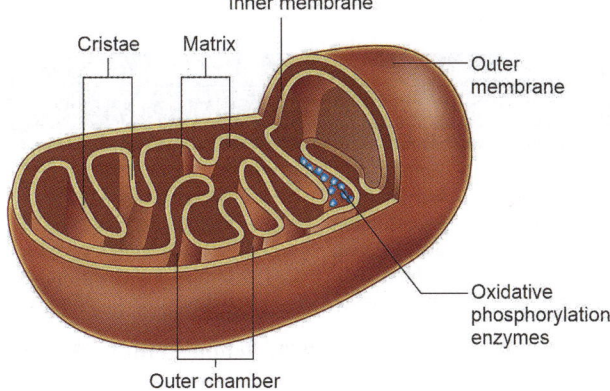

**Fig. 1.4:** Mitochondrion.

The mitochondrial DNA (mtDNA) has the *maternal inheritance*. Hence, the mitochondrial disorders are also inherited from the mother to off springs. The patients with mitochondrial disorders present with the following clinical symptoms:

- **Fatigue and weakness:** Patients often experience persistent fatigue and muscle weakness due to insufficient energy supply to muscle cells, impairing their ability to sustain physical activity.
- **Exercise intolerance:** Individuals with mitochondrial diseases may exhibit intolerance to exercise, as their muscles are unable to meet the increased energy demands during physical exertion.
- **Neurological symptoms:** Neurological manifestations are prevalent due to the high energy requirements of the brain. Patients may present with seizures, developmental delays, cognitive impairment, movement disorders, and neuropathies.
- **Cardiomyopathy:** Dysfunction of cardiac muscle cells due to energy depletion can lead to cardiomyopathy, resulting in symptoms such as heart failure, arrhythmias, and sudden cardiac death.
- **Ophthalmologic abnormalities:** Mitochondrial diseases often affect the optic nerve and retinal cells, leading to vision impairment, optic atrophy, and ophthalmoplegia.
- **Gastrointestinal dysfunction:** The gastrointestinal tract, reliant on energy for proper function, may be affected, resulting in symptoms such as dysmotility, recurrent vomiting, diarrhea, and failure to thrive.
- **Endocrine dysfunction:** Hormone-producing organs like the pancreas and thyroid may be impacted, leading to diabetes mellitus, thyroid dysfunction, and other endocrine disorders.
- **Multi-organ involvement:** Mitochondrial diseases can affect multiple organ systems simultaneously, resulting in a wide array of symptoms that vary in severity and presentation among affected individuals.

**Peroxisomes/microbodies/subcellular respiratory organelles:** It contains oxidases, it destroys certain product formed from $O_2$, e.g., $H_2O_2$ (toxic to the cell). The catalase enzyme reduces the $H_2O_2$ to nontoxic end products.

> *How peroxisomes protects us from free radical injuries (oxidative stress)?*
> Peroxisomes protects from oxidative stress due to the presence of the enzyme catalases which destroy $H_2O_2$, a potent oxidant and one of the most important agent of oxidative stress.

**Lysosomes:** Lysosomes are membrane-bound vesicular organelles which are formed by the breaking off from the Golgi apparatus. The lysosomes contains various *digestive enzymes* helpful in digesting damaged cellular structures, food particles that have been ingested by the cell and unwanted matter such as bacteria.

> **Lysosomal storage diseases:** Congenital absence of lysosomal enzymes leads to the accumulation of partially digested cellular materials known as inclusion bodies which interfere with the normal functioning of the cell and produces diseases.
> **Examples:** Gaucher disease, Tay-Sachs disease.
> **Zellweger syndrome:** Peroxisomes may be absent or abnormal.

# CELL MEMBRANE/PLASMA MEMBRANE/UNIT MEMBRANE (FIG. 1.5)

It is a thin, pliable, elastic structure 7.5 to 10 nanometers thick. It is made-up of proteins and lipids.

It is a double layer of lipid molecules in which proteins are embedded.

**Proteins** are of two types:
1. **Lipoproteins:** They function as enzymes and ion channels
2. **Glycoproteins:** Function as receptors for hormones and neurotransmitters

There are two types of cell membrane proteins:
1. *Integral proteins*, which protrude all the way through the membrane
2. *Peripheral proteins*, which are attached only to one surface of the membrane and do not penetrate all the way through.

| Arrangement of the proteins in the cell membrane (55%) | | |
|---|---|---|
| Intrinsic protein | Extrinsic/peripheral protein | Transmembrane protein |
| Serve as enzyme anchored to the cytoskeleton of the cell | • Helpful in formation of cytoskeleton<br>• Serve as cell adhesion molecules (CAM) | • Present in the entire thickness of cell membrane<br>• Act as channels, carriers, pumps and receptors<br>• It has antigenic property |

**Lipids** are phospholipids (25%), cholesterol (13%) and glycolipids.
- **Head end:** Polar/hydrophilic end, soluble in water and face the exterior of the cell as shown in **Figure 1.6**.
- **Tail end:** Nonpolar/hydrophobic end, insoluble in water, facing interior of cells as shown in **Figure 1.6**.

**Carbohydrates:** They are present with combination of protein or lipid. The entire outside surface of the cell often has a loose carbohydrate coat called the *glycocalyx*.
- They have a negative electrical charge, which is helpful in repels other negatively charged objects.
- It is helpful to attaching cells to one another.
- Many of the carbohydrates act as *receptors* for binding hormones, such as insulin.
- Some carbohydrate helps in immune reactions.

**Functions of cell membrane:**
- Protective sheath for cell organelles
- Digestive function
- It has quality of selective permeability due to lipids it forming major barrier for the water soluble molecules like electrolytes, urea and glucose and fat soluble substances $O_2$, fatty acids alcohol can easily pass
- Cell membrane has high insulating capacity
- It forms the basis of intercellular junctions
- It maintains constant and distinct intracellular environment
- It maintains cell volume

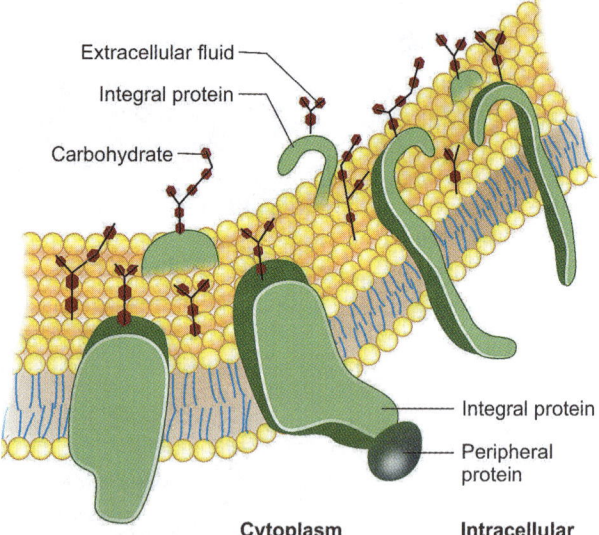

**Fig. 1.5:** Structure of cell membrane showing phospholipid bilayer with proteins (peripheral and integral).

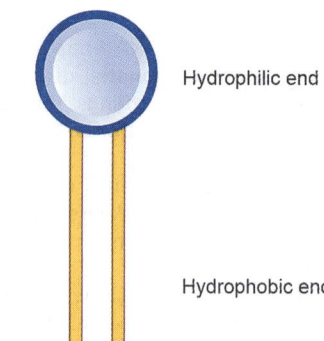

**Fig. 1.6:** Polar and nonpolar ends of lipid molecule.

- It helps in recognition of foreign cells and antigen so they can be phagocytized

> **What is the importance of selective permeability of cell membrane?**
> It is helpful in maintaining the difference of composition between extracellular fluid and intracellular fluid.

**Some important points to remember:**
- Acid phosphatase is used as a marker for lysosomal activity.
- Acrosomes, located on the head of spermatozoa is a specialized lysosomes it plays important role in penetration of ovum by sperm.
- $O_2$, $CO_2$, $N_2$, Lipid, steroid hormone, alcohol can dissolve in tail end and move rapidly across the membrane.
- Ions, glucose are slowly move across the cell membrane.
- Fluidity of membrane is due to presence of cholesterol so that cell changes its shape without disruption of their cell integrity.

## CELL ADHESION MOLECULES (CAMs)

**Definition:** These are the adhesion molecules by which cells attach to other cells and to basal lamina. They are responsible for transfer of signals into and out of cells.

**Types:**
- **Integrin:** Bind to various receptors
- **IgG:** Bind to various antigen
- **Cadherin:** $Ca^{2+}$ dependent molecule helpful in cell-to-cell adhesion
- **Selectin:** Bind to carbohydrates
- **Laminin:** It is present in extracellular matrix and it is essential for maintaining tissue structure and regulating cellular behavior.

**Functions:**
- They have important role in embryonic development
- Formation of nervous system
- They hold tissue together in adults
- They play important role in inflammation and wound healing
- They are responsible for metastasis of tumor
- They transmit signals into and out of the cells

| MOLECULAR MOTORS (Fig. 1.7): Helpful in movement of different protein, organelles and other cell part to all parts of the cell | |
|---|---|
| Microtubules based molecular motor | Actin based molecular motors |
| Produce motion along microtubules | Produce motion along the actin filaments |
| Conventional kinesin and dynein | Myosin |
| Kinesin involved in cell division and dynein is responsible for beating action of cilia and flagella | It forms cross bridges to the actin molecule with myosin head and responsible for contraction, contraction of intestinal villi and cell migration |

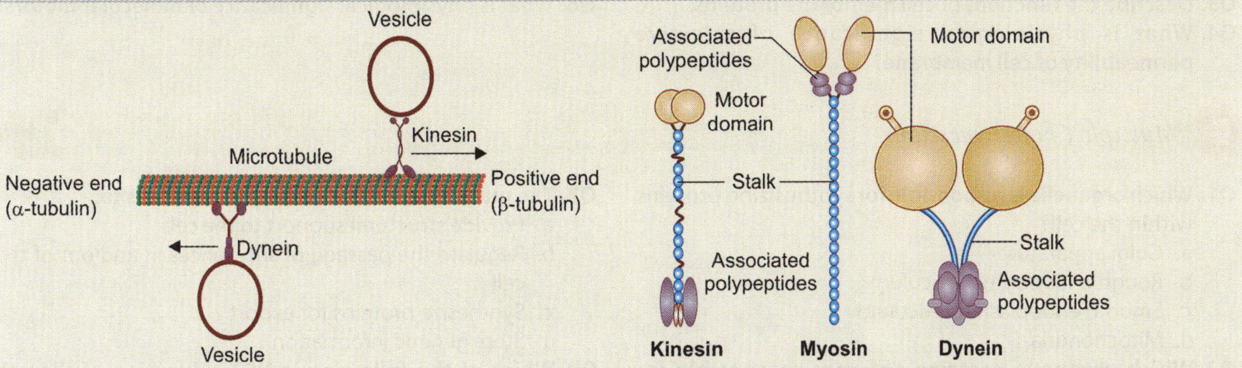

**Fig. 1.7:** Molecular motors: kinesin, myosin and dynein.

| Cell organelles | Active in |
|---|---|
| Mitochondria | Metabolically active cells, e.g., liver and cardiac muscle |
| RER | Cells active in protein synthesis, e.g., Russell's bodies of plasma cell, Nissl granules of nerve cells, acinar cells of pancreas |
| SER | Leydig cells, cells of adrenal cortex |
| Golgi apparatus | Exocrine glandular cells |
| Lysosomes | Cells involved in phagocytic activity, e.g., neutrophil, macrophages |
| Peroxisomes | Hepatocytes and tubular epithelium cells |
| Ribosomes | In growing cells/in cells actively synthesizing proteins |

## SUMMARY

**Introduction to cells:** The chapter begins with an overview of cells as the fundamental units of life, outlining their basic characteristics and importance in biological systems.
- **Cell organelles:** A detailed enumeration of cell organelles is provided, highlighting their diversity and specialized functions within the cell.
- **Structure and functions of cell organelles:** Each organelle is examined in depth, elucidating its structure and role in cellular processes. From the powerhouse mitochondria to the protein synthesis hub of the ribosomes, readers gain a comprehensive understanding of how these structures contribute to cellular function.
- **Cell membrane:** The structure and functions of the cell membrane, including its composition and selective permeability, are explored. Emphasis is placed on its crucial role as a barrier between the internal cellular environment and the external milieu.
- **Cell membrane proteins:** The functions of various proteins embedded within the cell membrane are discussed, ranging from transporters and receptors to enzymes and structural proteins. Their diverse roles in cellular communication, signaling, and homeostasis are highlighted.
- **Cell adhesion molecules (CAM):** The physiological significance of CAMs in cell-cell and cell-extracellular matrix

interactions is examined. Their role in tissue development, immune response, and pathological conditions is explored, shedding light on their importance in maintaining tissue integrity and function.
- **Molecular motors:** An overview of molecular motors, including motor proteins such as kinesin and dynein, is provided. Their role in intracellular transport, cell division, and muscle contraction is discussed, emphasizing their indispensable function in cellular dynamics.
- **Physiological basis of organelle disorders:** The chapter concludes with a discussion on the physiological basis of disorders associated with cell organelles. From lysosomal storage diseases to mitochondrial dysfunction, readers gain insight into how abnormalities in organelle structure and function can lead to pathological conditions, providing a link between cellular biology and human health.

## LET US SEE, HOW MUCH YOU HAVE LEARNT?

 *Review Questions*

Q1. Describe the functions of each of the cell organelles.
Q2. Draw a well labeled diagram of cell membrane.
Q3. Describe the functions of cell membrane proteins.
Q4. What is physiological significance of selective permeability of cell membrane?
Q5. What is physiological significance of cell adhesion molecules?
Q6. What is physiological significance of molecular motors?

 *Multiple Choice Questions*

Q1. Which organelle is responsible for synthesizing proteins within the cell?
 a. Golgi apparatus
 b. Rough endoplasmic reticulum
 c. Smooth endoplasmic reticulum
 d. Mitochondria

Q2. Which organelle contains enzymes responsible for breaking down cellular waste and debris?
 a. Golgi apparatus
 b. Endoplasmic reticulum
 c. Lysosome
 d. Nucleus

Q3. Which organelle is involved in energy production through aerobic respiration?
 a. Golgi apparatus
 b. Endoplasmic reticulum
 c. Lysosome
 d. Mitochondria

Q4. Which organelle is responsible for storing calcium ions and lipid synthesis?
 a. Golgi apparatus
 b. Endoplasmic reticulum
 c. Lysosome
 d. Nucleus

Q5. Which organelle is responsible for maintaining cell shape and providing structural support?
 a. Golgi apparatus
 b. Endoplasmic reticulum
 c. Cytoskeleton
 d. Mitochondria

Q6. The cell membrane is composed primarily of:
 a. Phospholipids and proteins
 b. Nucleic acids and proteins
 c. Carbohydrates and lipids
 d. Proteins and cholesterol

Q7. The main function of the cell membrane is to:
 a. Provide structural support to the cell
 b. Regulate the passage of substances in and out of the cell
 c. Synthesize proteins for export
 d. Store genetic information

Q8. Which of the following is NOT a function of the cell membrane?
 a. Cell signaling
 b. Cell adhesion
 c. Energy production
 d. Selective permeability

Q9. Integral membrane proteins are primarily involved in:
 a. Cell adhesion
 b. Transport of molecules across the membrane
 c. Signal transduction
 d. Lipid synthesis

Q10. Receptor proteins on the cell membrane are important for:
 a. Cell adhesion      b. Cell signaling
 c. Maintaining cell shape   d. Energy production

Q11. Channel proteins facilitate the movement of which type of molecules across the cell membrane?
 a. Large proteins     b. Ions
 c. Lipids            d. Nucleic acids

Q12. Cell adhesion molecules (CAMs) are important for:
 a. Transporting molecules across the cell membrane
 b. Maintaining cell shape
 c. Binding cells together
 d. Energy production

Q13. Which of the following is a physiological role of CAMs?
 a. Enhancing cell signaling
 b. Breaking down cellular waste
 c. Facilitating muscle contraction
 d. Promoting tissue integrity and wound healing

Q14. Molecular motors are responsible for:
   a. Synthesizing proteins
   b. Facilitating cell movement and transport of organelles
   c. Breaking down cellular waste
   d. Regulating gene expression

Q15. Kinesin and dynein are examples of molecular motors involved in:
   a. Muscle contraction
   b. Mitosis and cell division
   c. Synaptic transmission
   d. Lipid synthesis

Q16. Disorders of cell organelles can result from:
   a. Mutations in nuclear DNA only
   b. Mutations in mitochondrial DNA only
   c. Mutations in both nuclear and mitochondrial DNA
   d. Environmental factors only

Q17. Which of the following statements regarding mitochondrial disorders is true?
   a. Mitochondrial disorders are solely caused by mutations in nuclear DNA
   b. Mitochondrial disorders affect only a single organ system in the body
   c. Symptoms of mitochondrial disorders are always consistent among affected individuals
   d. Mitochondrial disorders can result from mutations in either mitochondrial DNA or nuclear DNA

Q18. Which of the following is a common symptom of mitochondrial disorders?
   a. High blood pressure
   b. Joint pain
   c. Muscle weakness
   d. Visual disturbances

## ANSWERS

1. b    2. c    3. d    4. b    5. c    6. a    7. b    8. c    9. b    10. b    11. b    12. c    13. d    14. b
15. b    16. c    17. d    18. c

# Homeostasis

**CHAPTER 2**

**COMPETENCY ADDRESSED**
PY1.2: Describe and discuss the principles of homeostasis.

**LEARNING OBJECTIVES**
At the end of this chapter, the learner should be able to:
- Define homeostasis.
- Describe the various homeostatic control mechanisms.
- Describe gain in homeostatic control.

## DEFINITION

Homeostasis is defined as a self-regulating process by which an organism can maintain internal stability while adjusting to changing external conditions.

When these homeostatic mechanisms fail, the normal physiology is disrupted, and a disease process sets in.

The concept of a stable internal environment or *'milieu interior'* was first introduced by the French physiologist *Claude Bernard* in the nineteenth century.

This ability of an organism to maintain a stable internal environment for the proper functioning of the body. It was later termed as *Homeostasis by WB Cannon* in the twentieth century, where Homeo means *'same'* and stasis means *'standstill'*.

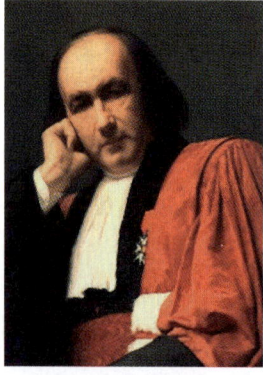
**Claude Beranard**
Coined the term 'milieu interior'

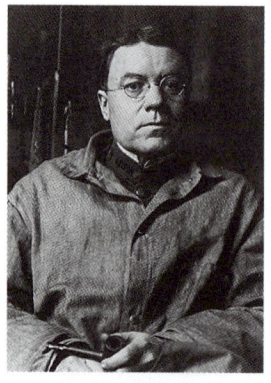
**WB Cannon**
Coined the term 'homeostasis'

## REGULATION OF HOMEOSTATIC MECHANISMS

The regulatory mechanisms act in a manner to maintain the constancy of the internal environment.

They follow a basic structure of the control system, described below. It consists of three units, the sensor (receptor), center (reference set point) and effector (target) **(Fig. 2.1)**.

Depending on the output/response, the regulatory mechanisms are divided into the feedback and feed forward mechanisms **(Fig. 2.2)**:

## FEEDBACK MECHANISMS

The feedback mechanisms are further classified as negative and positive feedback mechanisms.

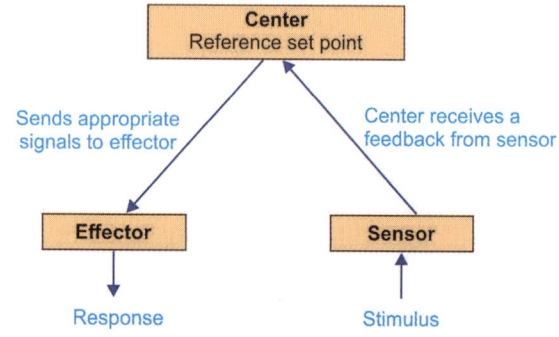
**Fig. 2.1:** Hemostatic regulatory mechanism.

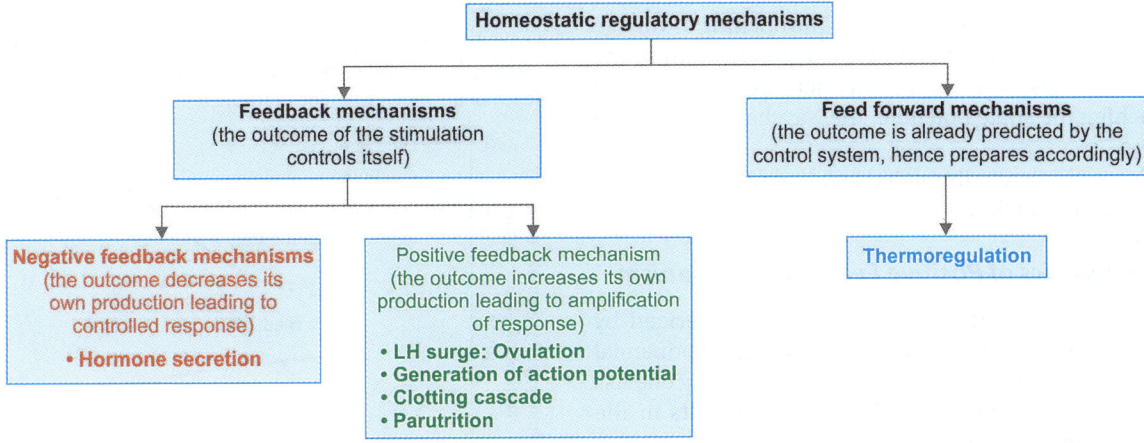

**Fig. 2.2:** Feedback mechanism and feed forward mechanism.
(LH: luteinizing hormone)

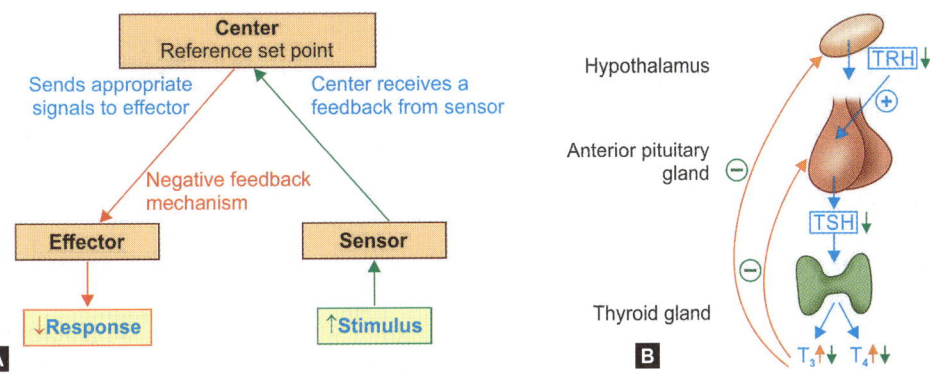

**Figs. 2.3A and B:** (A) Negative feedback mechanism; (B) Regulation of secretion of the thyroid hormones by the negative feedback mechanism.
(TRH: thyrotropin-releasing hormone; TSH: thyroid stimulating hormone)

## Negative Feedback Mechanism

When a variable *decreases its own production* by sending negative signals to control center. It is known as negative feedback mechanism **(Fig. 2.3A)**.

Most of the regulatory mechanism operates through the negative feedback mechanism.

Examples:
- Regulation of secretion of a hormone **(Fig. 2.3B)**
- Water homeostasis

Disadvantages of negative feedback mechanism
- It is often incomplete/and not precise
- Error in the response may occur
- Too much feedback results in instability

## Positive Feedback Mechanism (Fig. 2.4)

When a variable *stimulates the homeostatic mechanism to increase its own production* by sending positive signals to the control center, it sets up a positive feedback loop. This is a self-limiting process which terminates after the intended result is obtained.

Example:
- **LH surge:** The estrogen levels peak 2 days before ovulation setting up the positive feedback loop, which increases the levels of Luteinizing hormone (LH). This

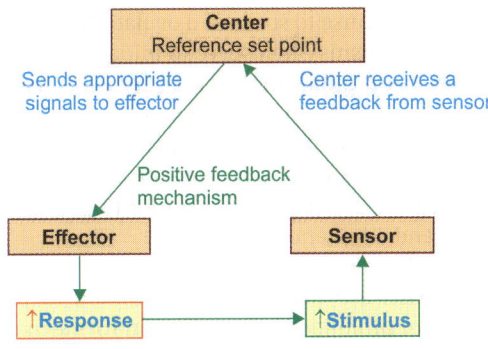

**Fig. 2.4:** Positive feedback mechanism.

  results in ovulation on the day 14 (the intended action), after which the levels of LH and estrogen decreases.
- **Parturition reflex:** Similarly, the oxytocin stimulates the full-term gravid uterus to contract for the birth of baby. The descent of baby into cervical canal of uterus further intensifies the uterine contractions till the baby is delivered (the intended action). After which the positive feedback is blocked, and the uterus relaxes.
- **Lactation:** Here also, suckling at the breast by the baby sets up a positive feedback loop resulting in milk let down.
- **Clotting mechanism:** This mechanism also involves a positive feedback based cascade reaction till the clot is formed and the hemostasis is achieved.

- **Generation of action potential:** The opening of voltage gated $Na^+$ channels result in the depolarization of the nerve or muscle till all the channels are opened. After reaching the spike potential, the $Na^+$ channels begin to close.
- Release of calcium through ryanodine receptors during muscle contraction.

### Characteristics of Positive Feedback Mechanism

The positive feedback mechanism is characterized by *amplification* of the initial stimulus resulting in exponential increase in the response. It results in the following effects:
- The exponential increase in response results in the formation of nonlinear response curve, which is characterized by increasing steepness or acceleration over time, rather than reaching a stable equilibrium.
- Positive feedback mechanisms often lead to deviation from a steady state. Instead of restoring the system to its original state, positive feedback drives the system away from equilibrium, potentially leading to rapid changes or transitions to new states or event.
- Positive feedback mechanisms creates a self-perpetuating cycle where the output of the process reinforces the initial stimulus, leading to further amplification of the response. This cycle continues until external factors intervene or the process reaches a physiological limit.
- They are prevalent in biological systems and play critical roles in various physiological processes.
  Examples: blood clotting cascade, uterine contractions during childbirth, action potential generation, hormone release in response to stress and ovulation.
- These mechanisms often serve to initiate or accelerate specific biological processes, facilitating rapid responses to environmental changes or internal stimuli. While they can lead to abrupt changes or transitions, positive feedback loops are essential for driving critical physiological processes and promoting organismal survival and adaptation.
- Despite their destabilizing nature, positive feedback mechanisms are often tightly regulated to prevent excessive or prolonged responses. Control mechanisms, such as threshold levels or feedback inhibition, help modulate the intensity and duration of positive feedback loops, ensuring appropriate physiological outcomes.
- If the positive feedback cycles are not tightly regulated, it may result in the unfavorable results, hence most of the regulatory mechanisms are controlled by negative feedback mechanisms.

> **Why do most of the feedback control mechanisms operate via negative feedback instead of positive feedback?**
> The positive feedback control sets in a vicious circle of self-propagation and instability. It is useful only under a few situations which are brief and self-limiting like blood clotting, action potential, LH surge during ovulation and parturition.

Apart from these, positive feedback mechanisms, for the conditions which are not self-limiting, can even lead to the death of an individual. For example:

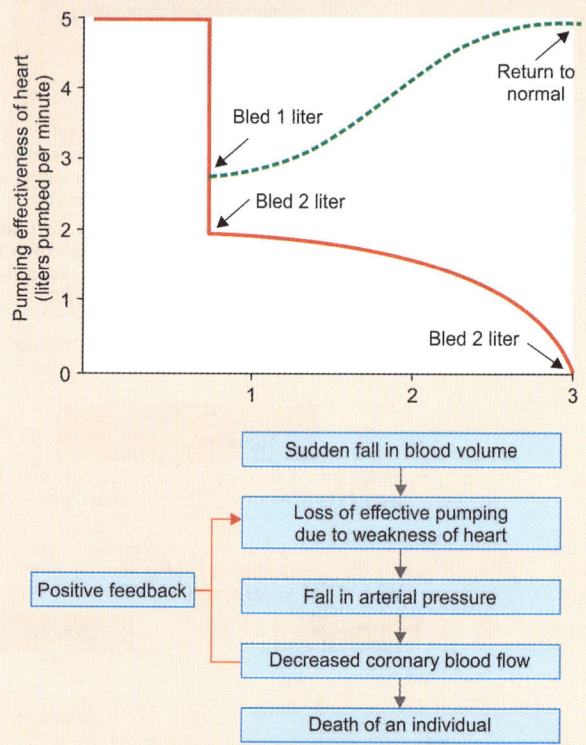

If a patient suddenly loses 2 L of blood, the blood volume suddenly falls. This leads to fall in arterial pressure decreasing coronary blood blow. This can lead to the death of an individual. Whereas, the negative feedback mechanism brings about stability and maintains the balance in various body systems.

## FEED FORWARD MECHANISM (FIG. 2.5)

A feed forward response is not a true homeostatic control mechanism as it is the anticipatory response of the body to any external stimulus thus preparing the body for it. It works in association with feedback control systems.

This results in the preparatory adjustments of the body in anticipation of predicted changes.

The feed forward mechanism is seen in regulation of temperature, where the body begins to adapt

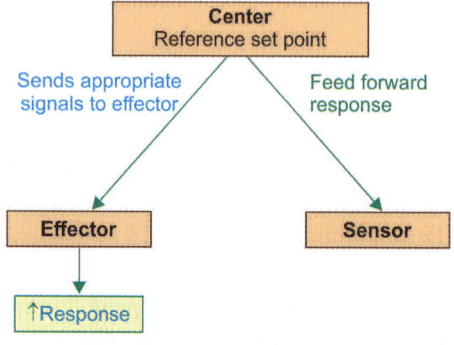

**Fig. 2.5:** Feed forward mechanism.

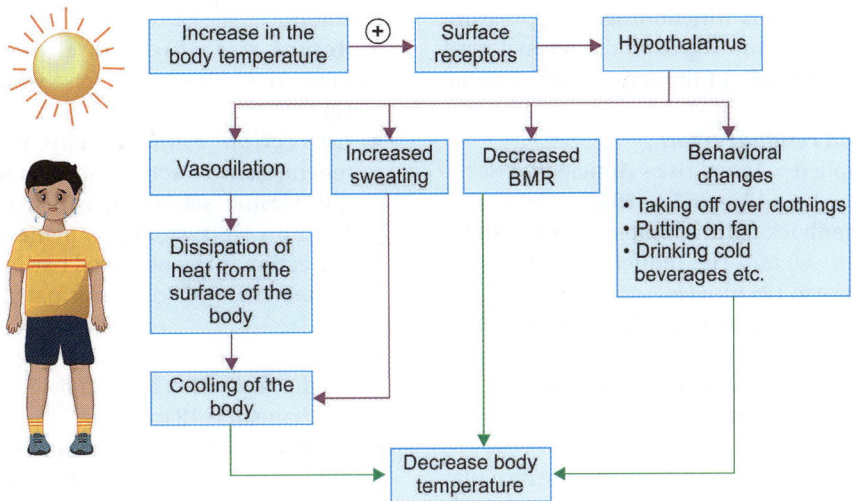

**Fig. 2.6:** Feed forward mechanism in regulation of body temperature.
(BMR: basal metabolic rate)

according to the predicted changes in the environmental temperature along with the feedback from the cutaneous receptors **(Fig. 2.6)**.

Feed forward mechanism is capable of overcoming the disadvantages of feedback control mechanism.

## IMPORTANCE OF HOMEOSTATIC CONTROL MECHANISMS

The internal environment of the body is made up of the ECF compartment which comprises about 20% of the body weight and includes the plasma, fluid present around the cells, i.e., the interstitial fluid and the transcellular fluid (Refer to Chapter 6 for the detailed study of the fluid distribution in the body compartments).

It is very essential to keep certain variables constant in our body like the BP, temperature, pH, osmolarity, availability of the hormones, ionic distribution across the cell membrane, etc. for the optimum functioning of the bodily processes and this is achieved through the homeostatic mechanism **(Fig. 2.7)**.

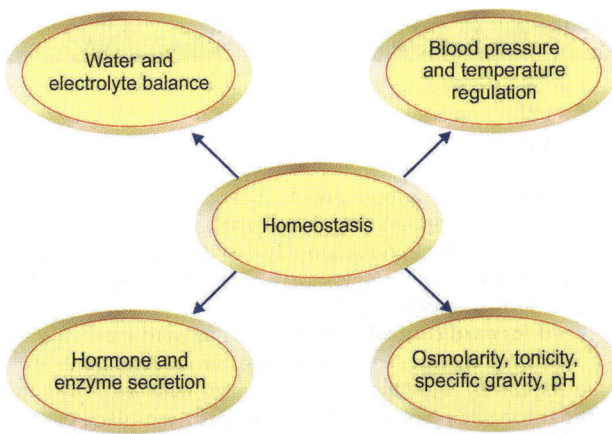

**Fig. 2.7:** Importance of homeostatic control mechanism.

*What are the factors that maintain homeostasis?*
- Regulation of temperature
- Delivery of nutrients, oxygen, and hormones
- Removal of metabolic and other waste products
- Maintenance of pH, water and electrolyte balance
- Maintenance of blood pressure

There are many self-disciplined regulatory mechanism in the body that operate on the principle of feedback mechanism.

## GAIN IN HOMEOSTATIC CONTROL

It aims that every system works to maintain a stable internal environment. It is important to strictly maintain the pH, temperature, osmolarity in the body so that all the bodily processes can function smoothly. Any disruption or change in the milieu interior should be eliminated and each parameter should be brought back to normal set point. In a nutshell, it determines the efficiency of homeostatic control mechanism.

This efficiency of each system is quantified in terms of the gain of the homeostatic mechanism

$$\text{Gain} = \frac{\text{Correction applied}}{\text{Residual error}}$$

A higher the gain indicates more efficient homeostatic mechanism, i.e., correction applied is more and residual error is less.

Example:
1. **Scenario description:** A large volume of blood is transfused into a person.
   - In the first scenario, the person's baroreceptor pressure control system is not functioning. As a result, the arterial pressure rises from the normal level of 100 mm Hg up to 175 mm Hg. This defines the expected rise in arterial pressure.
   - In the second scenario, the same volume of blood is injected into the same person, but this time the

baroreceptor system is functioning. The pressure increases only by 25 mm Hg, from the normal level of 100 mm Hg. This defines the actual rise in arterial pressure.

- **Correction and residual error:**
  Correction applied = Actual rise – Anticipated rise
  = 125 – 175 = –50 mm Hg
  Hence, the feedback control system has caused a "correction" of –50 mm Hg, reducing the pressure from 175 mm Hg to 125 mm Hg.
  Residual error = Anticipated rise – Correction applied
  = 175 – 50 = 25 mm Hg
  There remains an increase in pressure of +25 mm Hg, which is termed the "error."

- **Calculation of gain:**
  The gain of the system is calculated using the formula:
  Gain = Correction applied/Residual error
  = 50/25 = –2 mm Hg
  In this case, the correction is –50 mm Hg and the error is +25 mm Hg. Therefore, the gain of the person's baroreceptor system for controlling arterial pressure is –50 divided by +25, which equals –2.

- **Interpretation of gain:**
  ♦ A gain of –2 indicates that a disturbance that increases or decreases arterial pressure does so only one-third as much as it would if the control system were not present.
  ♦ In other words, the baroreceptor system reduces the effect of disturbances on arterial pressure by a factor of 1/3.
  ♦ This example illustrates the effectiveness of the baroreceptor pressure control system in regulating arterial blood pressure and reducing the impact of external disturbances. It highlights how the gain of the system quantifies its ability to minimize deviations from the desired set point.

2. Another example, routinely seen, is rise in blood pressure of an individual after exercise. What should be the gain if the anticipated rise in blood pressure after exercise is 150 mmHg and the actual rise is only 138 mmHg?
Anticipated rise in BP: After exercise, it was expected that the blood pressure (BP) would increase to 150 mm Hg.

Solution:
- **Actual rise observed:** However, the observed increase in BP after exercise was only up to 138 mm Hg.
- **Correction applied:** The baroreceptor reflex mechanism is activated to maintain BP close to the normal set point, which is typically around 120 mm Hg systolic. To achieve this, it applies a correction to the observed rise in BP.
  Correction applied = Anticipated rise – Actual rise
  = 150 mm Hg – 138 mm Hg
  = 12 mm Hg
  So, the correction applied by the baroreceptor reflex mechanism is 12 mm Hg.
- **Residual error:** The residual error represents the difference between the anticipated rise in BP and the corrected BP after the reflex mechanism has acted.
  Residual error = Anticipated rise – Correction applied
  = 150 mm Hg – 12 mm Hg
  = 138 mm Hg
  Therefore, the residual error is 138 mm Hg.
- **Calculation of gain:** The gain represents how effectively the reflex mechanism corrects the deviation in BP. It's calculated as the ratio of the correction applied to the residual error.
  Gain = Correction applied/residual error
  = 12 mm Hg/138 mm Hg
  ≈ 0.087
  So, the gain in this case is approximately 0.087. This indicates that for every 1 mmHg increase in the residual error (deviation from the set point), the reflex mechanism corrected by approximately 0.087 mm Hg.

Depending on the efficiency, the homeostatic mechanisms are classified as high and low gain systems, which are enumerated below:
♦ *High gain systems:*
  ♦ Kidney body fluid mechanism in regulating the BP is a very efficient system with a gain of
  ♦ Temperature regulating mechanism
♦ *Low gain systems:*
  ♦ Baroreceptor reflex mechanism

## SUMMARY

- Homeostasis refers to the ability of biological systems to maintain internal stability and balance despite external changes. It involves the regulation of various physiological variables such as body temperature, blood pressure, pH levels, and glucose concentrations within a narrow range conducive to optimal cellular function. Homeostasis is crucial for the survival and proper functioning of organisms, ensuring that internal conditions remain relatively constant despite fluctuations in the external environment.
- Homeostatic control mechanisms maintain internal stability by detecting deviations from set points and initiating appropriate responses to restore balance. These mechanisms can be broadly categorized into feedback and feed forward control systems.
- **Feedback control systems:** Feedback mechanisms monitor the output of a system and adjust it to maintain stability. Negative feedback loops are the most common type, where the response opposes the initial deviation from the set point. Positive feedback loops amplify deviations, but they are typically limited in biological systems to specific processes like childbirth or blood clotting.
- **Feed forward control systems:** Feed forward mechanisms anticipate changes in internal or external conditions and preemptively adjust the system's output to minimize deviations from the set point before they occur. These mechanisms

operate based on predictive cues rather than feedback from the current state of the system.
- **Gain in homeostatic control systems** represents the sensitivity and effectiveness of the system in maintaining internal stability. It quantifies the relationship between the correction applied by the control mechanism and the remaining error or deviation from the set point.
- **Calculation of gain:** Gain is calculated as the ratio of the correction applied to the remaining error. A higher gain indicates greater sensitivity and effectiveness in correcting deviations from the set point. Conversely, a lower gain suggests a less responsive control system.
- **Interpretation of gain:** A positive gain indicates amplification of deviations from the set point, which is rare in biological systems. Negative gain signifies corrective action, where the control system opposes deviations from the set point, restoring stability. The magnitude of the gain reflects the degree to which the control system counteracts deviations and maintains internal balance.

## LET US SEE, HOW MUCH YOU HAVE LEARNT?

### Review Questions

**Q1.** Define homeostasis and describe the various feedback mechanisms.

**Q2.** What is gain in homeostatic control? Illustrate one example.

### Critical Thinking Case-Based Questions

**Q1.** A 30-year-old woman started her regular morning run. As she laced up her running shoes and stepped outside, her body began to make adjustments in anticipation of the physical activity. Despite not having started running yet, her heart rate increased slightly, and she feels more alert and ready for exercise.

Based upon this scenario, answer the following questions:
a. Which homeostatic control mechanism got activated in this condition?
b. Explain the physiological responses initiated by the body.

### Multiple Choice Questions

**Q1.** What is homeostasis?
 a. The process of cell division
 b. The ability of biological systems to maintain internal stability
 c. The breakdown of complex molecules into simpler ones
 d. The movement of substances across a semipermeable membrane

**Q2.** Which type of homeostatic control system operates by anticipating changes in internal or external conditions and preemptively adjusting the system's output?
 a. Negative feedback control system
 b. Positive feedback control system
 c. Feed forward control system
 d. Reactive control system

**Q3.** In a negative feedback control system, the response to a deviation from the set point:
 a. Amplifies the deviation further
 b. Opposes the deviation, restoring stability
 c. Ignored the deviation
 d. Mimics the deviation

**Q4.** What does gain in homeostatic control systems represent?
 a. The ability to detect changes in the external environment
 b. The sensitivity and effectiveness in maintaining internal stability
 c. The magnitude of the response to a stimulus
 d. The rate of metabolic reactions

**Q5.** How is gain calculated in homeostatic control systems?
 a. Ratio of the correction applied to the remaining error
 b. Difference between the set point and the deviation
 c. Rate of change in the system output
 d. Ratio of the stimulus to the response

**ANSWERS**
 **1.** b   **2.** c   **3.** b   **4.** b   **5.** a

# How Do Cells Communicate?

**CHAPTER 3**

### COMPETENCY ADDRESSED
**PY1.3:** Describe intercellular communication.

### LEARNING OBJECTIVES
**At the end of this chapter, the learner should be able to:**
 Describe various intercellular and intracellular modes of communication.
 Describe the mechanism of intracellular signaling pathways.

We have studied about the cells, tissues and organ systems but you must be wondering that how these cells communicate with each other. Before we understand the various cellular signaling pathways or other complex things, we must understand that how these cells are connected to each other.

## INTERCELLULAR CONNECTIONS (FIG. 3.1 AND TABLE 3.1)

### Physical Connections

The cells can be physically connected to other cells through intercellular junctions:
- Tight junctions/zona occludens
- Adherent junctions/zona adherens

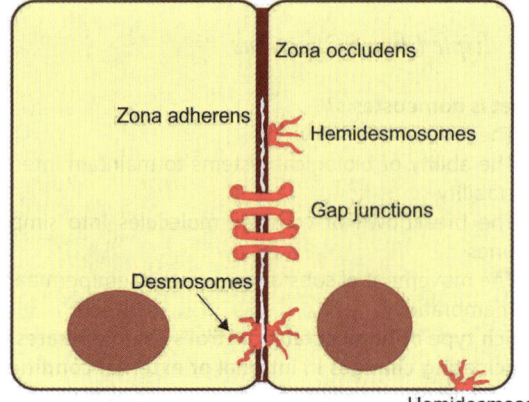

**Fig. 3.1:** Different intercellular connections.

**Table 3.1:** Types of physical cell connections.

|  | **Zona occludens** | **Zona adherens** | **Gap junctions** | **Desmosomes** | **Hemidesmosomes** |
|---|---|---|---|---|---|
| **Type of junction** | Tight junction | Adherent junction | Tunnel between adjacent cells | Filamentous connections between adjacent cells | Filamentous connections between adjacent cells |
| **Structural peculiarity** | • It is created by the close apposition of cell membranes of the adjacent cells<br>• There is no intercellular space between the cells | • It is a continuous structure on the basal side of tight junctions<br>• Some intercellular space is present between the cells | • These are characterized by the pore/tunnel like connections between the adjacent cells<br>• Intercellular space is very thin (around 4 nm) | • Thickening of apposed portions of cell membranes of adjacent cells<br>• Intermediary filamentous fibers are attached to the thickenings, radiating from them | Look like half desmosomes |

*Contd...*

Contd...

|  | Zona occludens | Zona adherens | Gap junctions | Desmosomes | Hemidesmosomes |
|---|---|---|---|---|---|
| Protein channels/ proteins | Transmembrane proteins: occludin, junctional adhesion molecules, and claudins | Cadherins | Connexon (consists of six protein subunits called as connexins) | Cadherins | Integrins |
| Location | • Apical margins of epithelia in intestinal and renal tubular mucosa<br>• Choroid plexus forming blood brain barrier<br>• In testis forming blood testicular barrier | Lateral and basal sides of the cells | Smooth muscles, cardiac muscles | Present in areas of shearing stress | Present in areas of shearing stress |
| Function | Acts like a barrier for transport of many molecules (esp. proteins) but permits passage of ions, solutes through paracellular transport | Provides attachment to intracellular microfilaments | Rapid propagation of electrical impulses from one cell to another. Permits the passage of ions, sugars, amino acids, etc. | Maintenance of tissue architecture | Maintenance of tissue architecture |

- Gap junctions
- Desmosomes/hemidesmosomes

**Clinical correlation: Connexons**
Experimental studies on animal models have shown that connexin deletions have resulted in electrophysiological defects in heart and predisposes to host of abnormalities like sudden cardiac death, cataract, hearing loss, abnormal bone development.

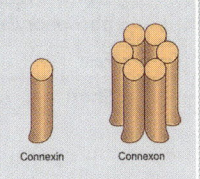

## Chemical Connections

These cells are chemically connected through chemical messengers, resulting in the communication between them.
- Hormones (autocrine, paracrine, endocrine glands) (**Fig. 3.2**, **Table 3.2**)
- Neurotransmitters (**Table 3.3**)

These chemical messengers bring about their action by binding to the receptors, which may be present of the surface of the cells (in case of lipid insoluble chemicals like protein-based substances) or inside the cells (for lipid soluble substances). Let's study the classification of these chemical messengers (both the neurotransmitters as well as the hormones.

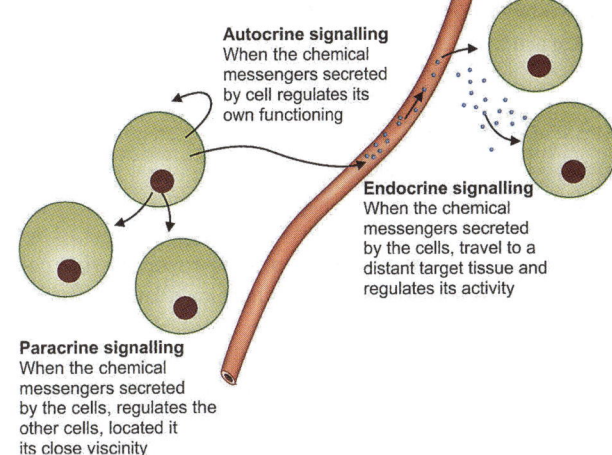

**Fig. 3.2:** Hormones and cell communications.

## MECHANISM OF ACTION OF CHEMICAL MESSENGERS

The chemical messengers (hormones and neurotransmitters) act on the target tissues by binding to the specific receptors. The location of these receptors depends

**Table 3.2:** Classification of hormones.

|  | Amine hormones | Peptide hormones | Steroid hormones |
|---|---|---|---|
| Examples | • **Iodinated** → Thyroxine<br>• **Non-iodinated**<br>  ▪ Epinephrine<br>  ▪ Norepinephrine<br>  ▪ Dopamine<br>  ▪ Serotonin | • **Insulin family:** *Insulin, IGF-I*<br>• **GH family:** *GH, Prolactin, HPL*<br>• **Glycoprotein:** *LH, FSH, TSH, hCG*<br>• **Secretin family:** *Secretin, Glucagon, VIP, GIP*<br>• **Others:** *ANP, Calcitonin, CCK, ADH, ACTH, PTH* | • **Adrenal cortex:** *Mineralocorticoids, Glucocorticoids*<br>• **Gonadal hormones:** *Estrogen, Progesterone, Testosterone*<br>• **1,25-Dihydrocholecalceferol (DHCC)** |
| Precursor | Tyrosine | Amino acids | Cholesterol |
| Mechanism of hormone action | • Thyroxine → act via intracellular, intranuclear receptors<br>• Catecholamines → Act via receptors on plasma membrane | Act via receptors on plasma membrane | Act via intracellular, intracytoplasmic receptors |

**Table 3.3:** Classification of neurotransmitters.

|  | Class I | Class II | Class III | Class IV |
|---|---|---|---|---|
| Neurotransmitter | Acetyl Choline | Amines (NE, Epinephrine, Dopamine, Serotonin, Histamine) | Amino acids (GABA, Glycine, Glutamate, Aspartate) | Nitric Oxide (NO) |
| Receptors | Nicotinic and muscarinic receptors, present on the plasma membrane | α and β receptors, present on the plasma membrane | Specific receptors, present on the plasma membrane | Specific receptors, present on the plasma membrane |

**Table 3.4:** Classification of chemical messengers.

|  | Chemical messengers that can cross the plasma membrane | Chemical messengers that cannot cross the plasma membrane |
|---|---|---|
| Type of biomolecule | Lipid derivative | Protein/peptide molecules |
| Lipid solubility | Lipid soluble/lipophilic | Lipid insoluble |
| Example of chemical messenger | • All steroid hormones like cortisol, progesterone, estrogen, testosterone, etc.<br>• Thyroid hormones | • All protein or peptide hormones like growth hormone, insulin, pituitary hormones, etc.<br>• Neurotransmitters |
| Receptors | Located inside the cell (intracellular receptors) | Located on the cell/plasma membrane |
| Second messenger | Not required | Required (various second messengers are $Ca^{+2}$, cAMP, etc.) |
| Site of action | Act on DNA which results in formation of new proteins | Acts on receptor resulting in activation of ion channels, G protein coupled receptor activation resulting in phosphorylation of proteins |
| Onset of action | Slow | Fast |
| Duration of action | Prolonged | Short |

upon the ability of these chemicals to cross the cell membrane, hence dividing these chemicals into two broad groups **(Table 3.4)**.

Based on above classification, the illustrated mechanism of receptor activation is shown in **Figures 3.3 and 3.4**.

## Mechanism of Action of Hormones Acting on Receptors Located Inside the Cell

Hormones that act on intracellular receptors typically include steroid hormones (e.g., cortisol,

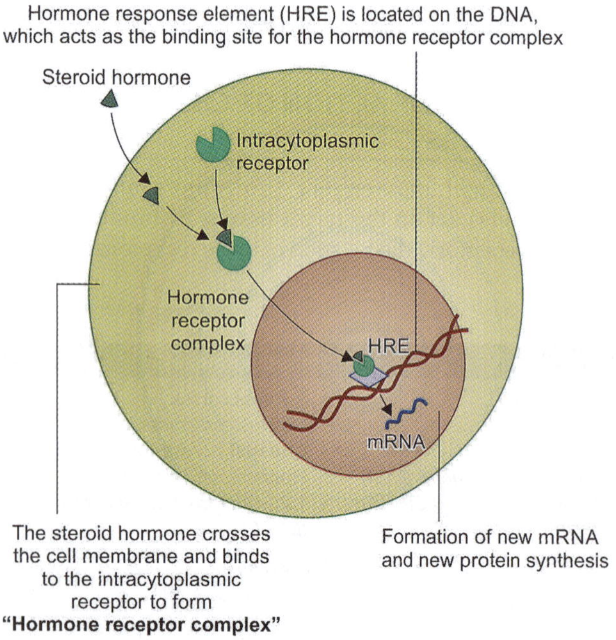

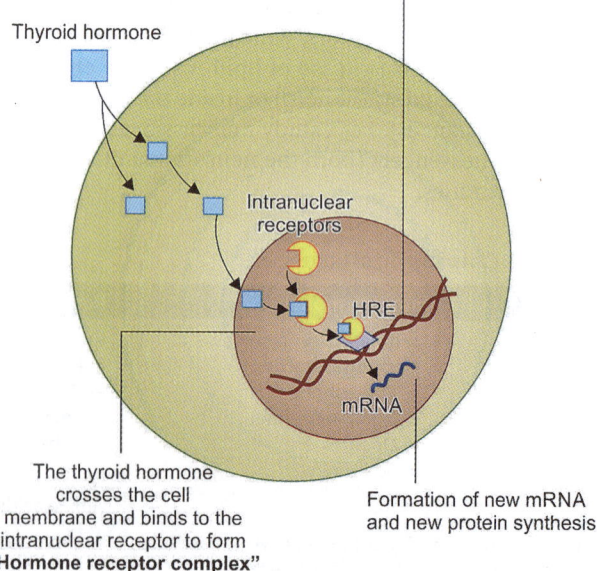

**Fig. 3.3:** Mechanism of action of steroid hormones.

**Fig. 3.4:** Mechanism of action of thyroid hormones.

estrogen, testosterone) and thyroid hormones (e.g., triiodothyronine, thyroxine). These hormones are lipid-soluble and can diffuse across the cell membrane to bind with specific intracellular receptors located in the cytoplasm or nucleus. Lipid-soluble hormones diffuse through the cell membrane and enter the target cell. Once inside the cell, the hormone binds to its specific intracellular receptor, forming a hormone-receptor complex. These receptors are often located in the cytoplasm (for steroids) or nucleus (for thyroxine). Upon binding, the hormone-receptor complex undergoes conformational changes, leading to activation of the receptor. In the case of receptors located in the cytoplasm, the hormone-receptor complex may translocate into the nucleus. Within the nucleus, the hormone-receptor complex binds to specific DNA sequences known as *hormone response elements (HREs)* or hormone regulatory elements (HREs), which are typically located in the promoter regions of target genes. Binding of the hormone-receptor complex to HREs regulates the transcription of target genes. This can either enhance (transcriptional activation) or inhibit (transcriptional repression) gene expression, depending on the specific hormone and target gene. Transcriptional activation results in the synthesis of mRNA from the target genes. The newly synthesized mRNA is then translated into proteins, leading to changes in cellular function or metabolism. The proteins synthesized as a result of hormone-induced gene transcription mediate the cellular response to the hormone. This response may involve changes in cell growth, differentiation, metabolism, or other physiological processes.

## Mechanism of Action of Hormones Acting on Receptors Located on Cell Membranes

(*Catecholamines and peptide hormones* act on receptors of plasma membrane because they are hydrophilic and cannot cross the cell membrane).

Classification of receptors located on plasma membrane:
- **Receptors acting as ion channels (Fig. 3.5):** In this type the receptors act as ligand-gated ion channels. These ion channels get activated when the ligand/

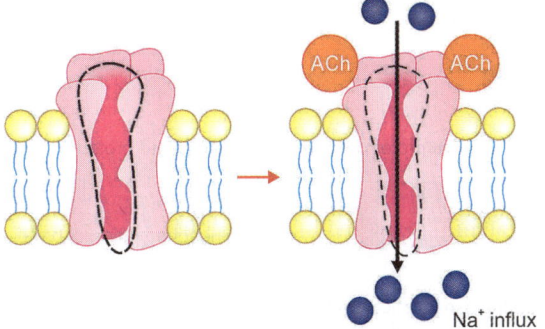

**Fig. 3.5:** Receptor acting as ligand gated ion channels.

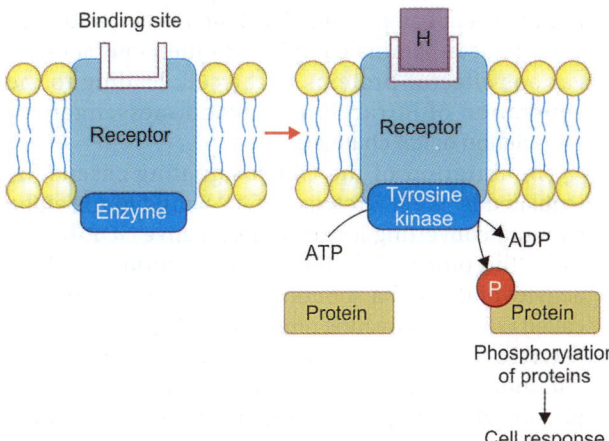

**Fig. 3.6:** Receptor acting as enzyme.

chemical binds to the receptor and brings about the conformational change in the receptors resulting in the movement of the ions across the cell membrane. **Example:** ACh gated sodium channels present in neuromuscular junction ($N_M$ receptors) and in autonomic ganglia ($N_N$ receptors)
- **Receptors acting as enzymes (Fig. 3.6):** These receptors are linked to the enzymes on the intracellular surface. Upon binding with their specific ligands, enzyme-linked receptors undergo conformational changes that activate their enzymatic activity, leading to the phosphorylation or dephosphorylation of intracellular proteins. This enzymatic activity allows for the amplification and regulation of cellular signaling pathways, playing crucial roles in various physiological processes such as cell growth, differentiation, and metabolism. Examples of enzyme-linked receptors include receptor tyrosine kinases for insulin, IGF-1.
- **G protein coupled receptors** are a large family of cell surface receptors involved in transmitting signals from the extracellular environment to the inside of the cell. They play a crucial role in regulating various physiological processes such as sensory perception, neurotransmission, hormone response, and immune response.

Structurally, GPCRs consist of a single polypeptide chain that spans the cell membrane seven times, forming seven transmembrane alpha helices. This arrangement creates an extracellular N-terminus and an intracellular C-terminus, along with three extracellular loops and three intracellular loops. The ligand-binding site is typically located on the extracellular loops.

When a ligand (such as a hormone, neurotransmitter, or light-sensitive molecule) binds to the extracellular domain of the GPCR, it induces a conformational change in the receptor. This change triggers the activation of an associated heterotrimeric G protein, which consists of three subunits: alpha, beta, and gamma.

The activated G protein undergoes a dissociation process, where the GTP-bound alpha subunit separates from the beta-gamma complex. Both the alpha subunit and the beta-gamma complex can then interact with various effector proteins in the cell, leading to the generation of intracellular second messengers or modulation of ion channels.

The duration of the GPCR signaling cascade is regulated by the hydrolysis of GTP bound to the alpha subunit, converting it back to its inactive GDP-bound form. This process is facilitated by the intrinsic GTPase activity of the alpha subunit or by regulatory proteins called GTPase-activating proteins (GAPs).

Overall, GPCRs play a fundamental role in cellular communication and are involved in a wide range of physiological and pathological processes, making them important targets for drug development in various therapeutic areas. It acts via four different pathways, described below:

- *Via adenylyl cyclase/cAMP pathway (Fig. 3.7)*
  - ACTH
  - ADH
  - FSH, LH
  - TSH
  - Parathormone
  - Glucagon
  - Calcitonin
  - β-adrenergic catecholamines
- *Via ion channel (Fig. 3.8)*
- *Via PLC; $IP_3$/DAG pathway (Fig. 3.9)*
  - GnRH
  - TRH
  - Oxytocin
  - Somatostatin
  - α-adrenergic catecholamines
- *JAK/STAT pathway (Growth Hormone) (Fig. 3.10)*

**Second messenger:** It is the chemical messenger, present/generated inside the cell, resulting in activation of

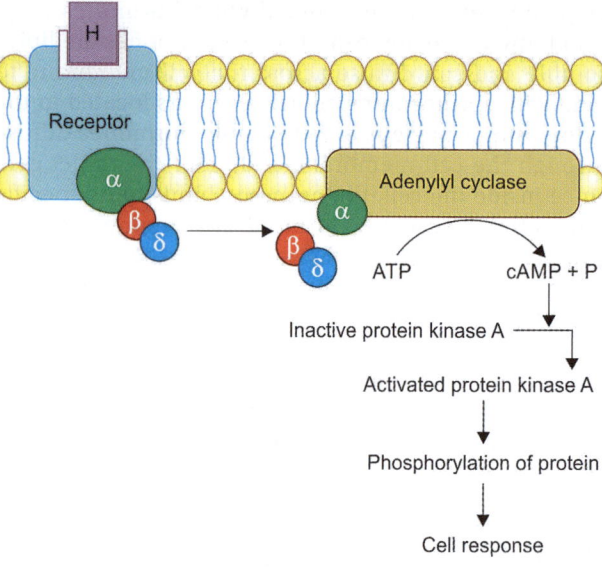

**Fig. 3.7:** cAMP pathway.

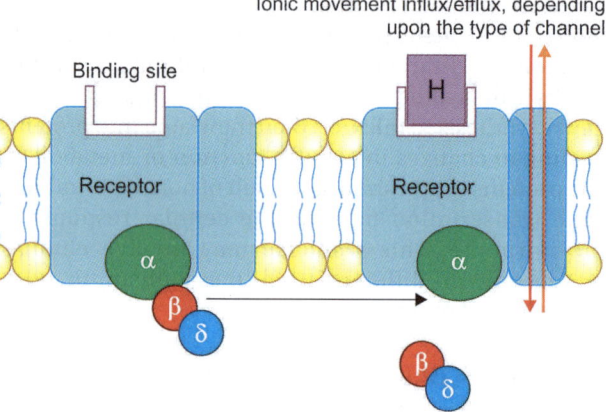

**Fig. 3.8:** G-protein coupled ion channel.

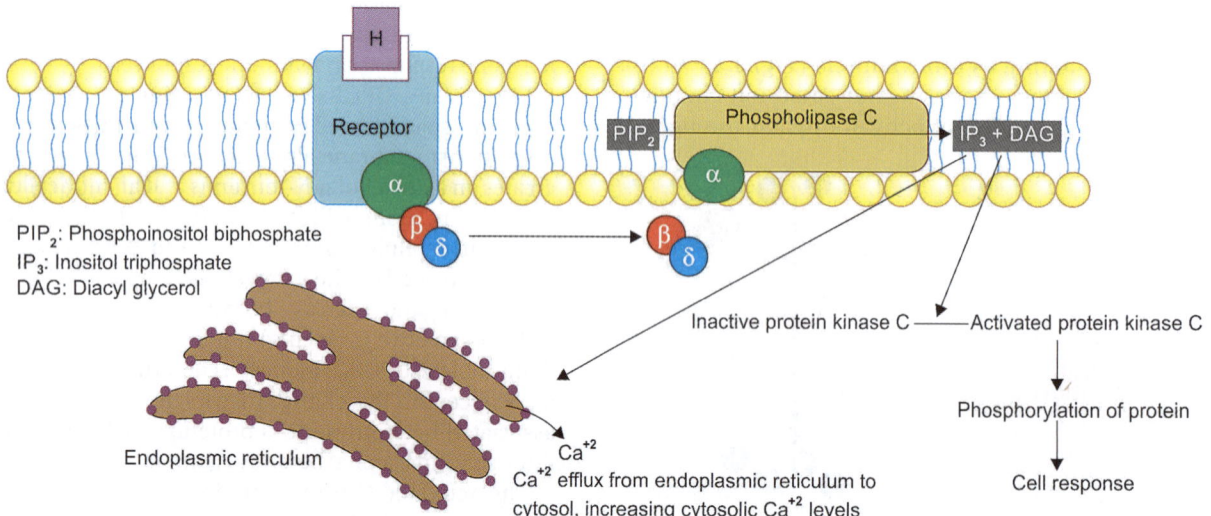

$PIP_2$: Phosphoinositol biphosphate
$IP_3$: Inositol triphosphate
DAG: Diacyl glycerol

$Ca^{+2}$ efflux from endoplasmic reticulum to cytosol, increasing cytosolic $Ca^{+2}$ levels

**Fig. 3.9:** G-protein coupled PLC- $IP_3$/DAG pathway.

cytosolic proteins. It is required to bring about the action of those chemical messengers which cannot cross the plasma membrane, hence referred to as 'first messengers'. Various second messengers are calcium, cAMP, $IP_3$ and DAG.

**G-protein**: These are small proteins formed by three subunits: α, β and δ. When the first messenger binds to the receptor, these G-proteins get activated. During activation, the α-subunit separates from the rest of two subunits (β and δ). The α-subunit either binds to the enzyme (adenylyl cyclase or phospholipase C) or activates the ion channels. Hence, it brings about the desired effects of the first messenger. Further, this α-subunit can be of two types: $α_s$ or $α_i$.

- $α_s$: It has the stimulatory effect
- $α_i$: It has the inhibitory effect

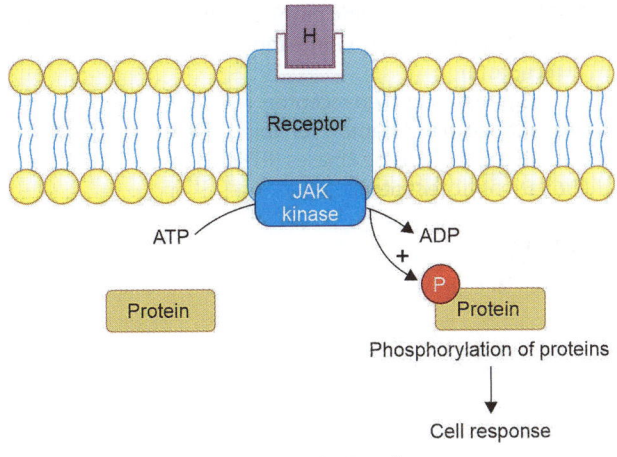

**Fig. 3.10**: JAK/STAT pathway.
(JAK/STAT: Janus kinase/signal transducer)

## SUMMARY

In this chapter, we have learnt various ways in which the cells communicate with each other. It begins by exploring direct intercellular communication mechanisms, such as gap junctions, which facilitate the direct exchange of ions, small molecules, and signaling molecules between adjacent cells. The discussion then expands to cover paracrine signaling, where cells release signaling molecules into the extracellular fluid to influence nearby cells, and endocrine signaling, which involves the secretion of hormones into the bloodstream to reach distant target cells. Additionally, the chapter explores cellular signaling, prevalent in nervous systems, where neurotransmitters are released across synaptic gaps to transmit signals between neurons. Through detailed examples and illustrations, readers gain a comprehensive understanding of the diverse intercellular communication strategies employed by organisms.

Beginning with an overview of the cellular components involved in signaling pathways, including receptors, second messengers, and effector proteins. The extracellular signals are received by cell surface receptors, leading to the activation of intracellular signaling molecules and the propagation of the signal to the nucleus or other cellular targets. Various types of intracellular signaling pathways are explored, including G protein-coupled receptors (GPCRs), receptor tyrosine kinases (RTKs), and intracellular receptors for lipid-soluble hormones.

## LET US SEE, HOW MUCH YOU HAVE LEARNT?

### Review Questions

**Q1.** Enumerate various intercellular junctions. Describe the sites and examples of intercellular junctions.

**Q2.** What are the various modes of intercellular communication?

**Q3.** Describe the mechanism of action of the lipid soluble hormones (steroids and thyroid hormones).

**Q4.** Describe the mechanism of action of hormones acting via G protein coupled receptors.

**Q5.** What is a second messenger? What are the functions of second messenger?

### Multiple Choice Questions

**Q1.** Which of the following directly facilitates the exchange of ions and signaling molecules between adjacent cells?
  a. Paracrine signaling    b. Endocrine signaling
  c. Gap junctions    d. Synaptic signaling

**Q2.** What type of signaling involves the release of signaling molecules into the extracellular fluid to influence nearby cells?
  a. Endocrine signaling    b. Autocrine signaling
  c. Paracrine signaling    d. Juxtacrine signaling

**Q3.** In nervous systems, what type of signaling is characterized by the release of neurotransmitters across synaptic gaps?
  a. Endocrine signaling    b. Paracrine signaling
  c. Autocrine signaling    d. Synaptic signaling

**Q4.** Which cellular component is responsible for receiving extracellular signals in signal transduction pathways?
  a. Second messengers    b. Effector proteins
  c. Receptors    d. Nucleus

**Q5.** Which type of signaling pathway involves the activation of intracellular signaling molecules by cell surface receptors?
   a. G protein-coupled receptors (GPCRs)
   b. Intracellular receptors for lipid-soluble hormones
   c. Receptor tyrosine kinases (RTKs)
   d. Synaptic receptors

**Q6.** What is the primary function of second messengers in intracellular signaling?
   a. Transcription of genes
   b. Direct activation of effector proteins
   c. Amplification and propagation of signals
   d. Transport of signaling molecules across the cell membrane

**ANSWERS**
   **1.** c   **2.** c   **3.** d   **4.** c   **5.** a   **6.** c

# Apoptosis: Physiology and Mechanisms

**CHAPTER 4**

**COMPETENCY ADDRESSED**

PY1.4: Describe apoptosis—programmed cell death.

**LEARNING OBJECTIVES**

**At the end of this chapter, the learner should be able to:**
- Define apoptosis.
- Discuss the physiological significance of apoptosis.
- Discuss the mechanism of apoptosis.
- Describe physiological significance of apoptosis.
- Distinguish between necrosis and apoptosis.
- Explain the effect of disordered apoptosis process.

## INTRODUCTION

The several trillions of cells that make up the body function as a highly organized community where the number of cells is maintained by regulating both the rate of cell division and the rate of cell death. They go through a **suicide/programmed cell death** when they are no longer required or pose a harm to the organism.

### Definition

Apoptosis (Greek word **apo** "away" + **ptosis** "fall") is an orderly cell death that results in disassembly and phagocytosis of the cell before any leakage of its contents occurs, and neighboring cells usually remain healthy.

### Functional Significance

Due to apoptosis, billions of cells die every hour and are replaced by new cells, even in adults. In healthy people, however, the creation of new cells often balances out programmed cell death. Otherwise, the tissues of the body would excessively shrink or grow. This biological mechanism **successfully eliminates unwanted cells** while preserving the balance of cells in the human body.

## MECHANISM OF APOPTOSIS

Senescent cells, near death activate intrinsic enzymes and degrade their own nuclear DNA and cytoplasmic proteins

↓

Activation of **caspases**, a group of cysteine proteases

↓

Cells shrinks and become smaller in size

↓

Cytoplasm and organelles becomes tightly packed

↓

Nuclear chromatin shrinks and become condensed at center or at periphery (**Pyknosis**)

↓

Chromatic material disintegrate and becomes fragmented (**Karyorrhexis**)

↓

Cells starts to form **blebs** on its surface and starts to break into small fragments called **apoptotic bodies**. These bodies have portions of cytoplasm, organelles and nuclear fragments

↓

These apoptotic bodies are eaten up by **phagocytes**

**Initiator caspases:** Caspase 2, 8, 9, 10
**Executioner caspases:** Caspase 3, 6, 7

> **Apoptosis does not elicit inflammation**
> This is because apoptotic bodies have intact membrane and prevent any content to be leaking out into interstitium. Also, apoptotic bodies are quickly recognized and removed by phagocytes and neighboring cells usually remain healthy.

> *Which of the following is not a characteristic of apoptosis?*
> 1. Causes tissue inflammation.
> 2. Nuclear degradation in apoptosis is ordered.
> 3. Apoptosis involves cell shrinkage.
> 4. Apoptosis ends with phagocytosis.
> 5. Apoptotic cells fragment into apoptotic bodies.

## SITUATIONS IN WHICH APOPTOSIS OCCUR

### Physiological Apoptosis

Occurs as a part of normal physiological development or adult tissue homeostasis.

**Examples of physiological apoptosis:**
- Apoptosis is a key **regulator** of **development:**
  - It is a process that occurs frequently during development and in adulthood. Many neurons are created in the central nervous system (CNS), and then they are destroyed during **remodeling** that takes place **throughout development** and **synapse creation**.
  - It is utilized to **get rid** of **undesirable cells** in the early **stages of development.** For instance, during development, the webs between the fingers and toes go through apoptosis to separate the digits from one another.
  - Through the course of the **fetus's sexual development**, it results in the regression of duct systems *(Mullerian or Wolfian duct)*.

> *What will happen if there is absence of apoptosis during embryonic development ?*
> Absence of apoptosis results in malformation of digits.

- **Involution of hormone dependent tissues:**
  - Cyclical sloughing of lining of uterus (endometrium) that causes **menstruation**.
  - **Atresia of follicles** of ovary in menopause.
  - **Regression of breast parenchyma after lactation** during weaning.
- Apoptosis occurs in epithelia in cells that are no longer connected to the basal lamina and to nearby cells. This is what causes the **enterocytes** that are **shed** from the tips of intestinal villi to die.
- It causes **death of inflammatory cells** after their functions are over.
- In the immune system, apoptosis removes **self-reactive lymphocytes**.

### Pathological Apoptosis

- Occurs as a part of disease process. Cells can undergo apoptosis when damaged or involved in a disease process.
- It is needed to **destroy** those cells which represent **threat** to the **integrity** of an organism.
- **Injured cells** that can't be repaired
- **Misfolded protein**
- Cell **infected** with virus
- Killing of **tumor** cells

## DIFFERENCES BETWEEN APOPTOSIS AND NECROSIS

See **Table 4.1**.

> *Why does necrosis cause inflammation?*
> 1. Plasma membrane ruptures and the cellular contents escape to the extracellular space.
> 2. Loss of water results in significant cell shrinkage.
> 3. Hypoproteinemia causing capillary leakage causes inflammation.
> 4. Chemical leaking to the extracellular space.

**Table 4.1:** Differences between apoptosis and necrosis.

| Apoptosis | Necrosis |
|---|---|
| Apoptosis, or programmed cell death, is a form of cell death that is generally triggered by normal, healthy processes in the body | Necrosis is the premature death of cells triggered by acute injury |
| Programmed | Unprogrammed |
| Natural cell death | Unnatural cell death |
| Cell membrane intact | Cell membrane destroyed |
| No leakage of cytoplasm | Leakage of cytoplasm |
| Adjacent cells are not affected | Affect adjacent group of cells |
| Does not evoke inflammatory response | Evokes inflammatory response |
| Leads to cell death with cell shrinkage, pyknosis, and karyorrhexis | Leads to cell death with karyolysis, pyknosis, karyorrhexis |
| May be pathological or Physiological | Always pathological |

# EFFECTS OF DYSREGULATED APOPTOSIS (TOO LITTLE/TOO MUCH)

- **Deficient apoptosis:**
  - Cancer
  - Autoimmune disorders
  - Failure of normal deletion of unwanted cell population during development can produce a range of abnormalities. **Example:** Failure of the normal deletion of interdigital tissue leads to syndactyly.
- **Excessive apoptosis:**
  - Neurodegenerative disease like Alzheimer's and Parkinson's disease
  - Ischemic heart disease (MI)

## SUMMARY

- This chapter commences with a clear and concise definition of apoptosis, the programmed cell death mechanism crucial for maintaining tissue homeostasis and eliminating unwanted or damaged cells. It elucidates the controlled and orderly nature of apoptosis, which distinguishes it from necrosis, highlighting key features such as cell shrinkage, chromatin condensation, and formation of apoptotic bodies.
- Apoptosis plays an important role in tissue remodeling, immune system regulation, and the maintenance of cellular homeostasis, underscoring its indispensable role in health and disease.
- It provides a comprehensive overview of the two main pathways: intrinsic (mitochondrial) pathway and extrinsic (death receptor) pathway.
- The activation of caspases, the central executioners of apoptosis, and the interplay of pro-apoptotic and anti-apoptotic factors regulating cell fate.
- Hence, apoptosis contributes to the removal of unwanted or damaged cells, preventing the accumulation of aberrant cells that could lead to disease states such as cancer.
- Necrosis is characterized by cellular swelling, membrane rupture, and inflammation, often associated with pathological conditions and tissue damage, whereas apoptosis is a controlled process vital for development and tissue remodeling.
- Dysregulated apoptosis processes. It discusses how abnormalities in apoptosis can lead to various pathological conditions, including cancer, autoimmune diseases, and neurodegenerative disorders. By exploring the consequences of disrupted apoptotic pathways, readers gain a deeper understanding of the importance of maintaining the delicate balance of cell death and survival in physiological contexts.

## LET US SEE, HOW MUCH YOU HAVE LEARNT?

 *Review Questions*

**Q1.** Define apoptosis. Describe the mechanism involved in apoptosis.

**Q2.** What is the physiological significance of apoptosis?

 *Multiple Choice Questions*

**Q1.** Which of the following best describes apoptosis?
  a. Uncontrolled cell proliferation
  b. Programmed cell death
  c. Cellular swelling and rupture
  d. Inflammatory response in tissues

**Q2.** What is the primary physiological significance of apoptosis during embryonic development?
  a. Promotion of cell proliferation
  b. Removal of excess or unwanted cells
  c. Induction of inflammation
  d. Maintenance of tissue integrity

**Q3.** In which of the following processes does apoptosis play a crucial role?
  a. Tissue regeneration
  b. Inducing cellular hypertrophy
  c. Immune cell activation
  d. Cancer progression

**Q4.** Which pathway of apoptosis involves the activation of caspases by signals from within the cell, such as DNA damage or cellular stress?
  a. Intrinsic pathway
  b. Extrinsic pathway
  c. Necrotic pathway
  d. Autophagic pathway

**Q5.** Dysregulated apoptosis is associated with the development of:
  a. Neurodegenerative disorders
  b. Increased tissue regeneration
  c. Enhanced immune response
  d. Promotion of cell differentiation

### ANSWERS
**1.** b  **2.** b  **3.** a  **4.** a  **5.** a

# Transport Across Cell Membranes

**CHAPTER 5**

### COMPETENCY ADDRESSED
**PY1.5:** Describe and discuss transport mechanisms across cell membranes.

###  LEARNING OBJECTIVES
**At the end of this chapter, the learner should be able to:**
- Enumerate and describe the membrane transport proteins.
- Classify mechanism of transport across cell membrane.
- Define and describe simple and facilitated diffusion.
- Define and describe Gibbs Donnan effect.
- Define and describe diffusion.
- Define and describe primary and secondary active transport.
- Classify vesicular transport.
- Describe exocytosis, endocytosis and transcytosis.

There is a significant difference in the composition of extracellular fluid (ECF) and intracellular fluid (ICF). Cell membrane plays a vital role in maintaining this difference. There is frequent movement of substances across cell membrane. In this chapter we will discuss about various mechanism involved in transport of molecule/atom/ion across cell membrane.

## PROTEINS INVOLVED IN TRANSPORT ACROSS CELL MEMBRANE (FIGS. 5.1 AND 5.2)

The various proteins present in the cells membrane help in the transport of substances, either by functioning as channels or carrier proteins.
- **Channels:** The channels are specific for the transport of specific substances/ions like water channels, ion channels, etc.
- **Carrier proteins:** Depending on the use of ATP, they further divided into:
    - ATP dependent: $Na^+ K^+$ ATPase pump
    - ATP independent pump: This transport can be in the same direction (Symport).
    - Example: Sodium glucose linked transport (SGLT).

In the opposite direction. Example: $Na^+ H^+$ exchanger/antiport.

## CLASSIFICATION OF MECHANISM OF TRANSPORT ACROSS CELL MEMBRANE

See **Table 5.1**.

## PASSIVE TRANSPORT

### Diffusion
- Diffusion is the random movement of molecules where molecules move in all directions, but the net movement is from a zone of high concentration to zone of low concentration.
- Generally, semipermeable membrane is not required for diffusion. But, in living being, plasma membrane significantly influences the process of diffusion.
- "Electrochemical gradient of the substance" is the driving force for the movement of molecules of the substance.
- Molecules move from the zone of high concentration to zone of low concentration. In case of ionic molecule,

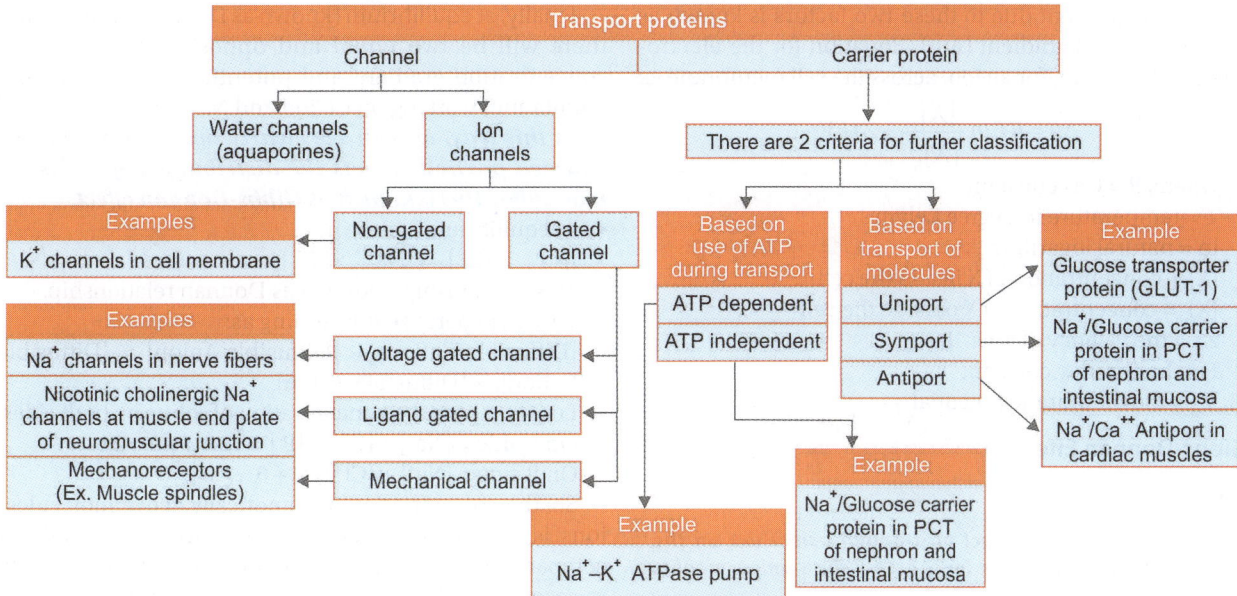

**Fig. 5.1:** Protein involved in transport across cell membrane.
(PCT: proximal convulated tubule)

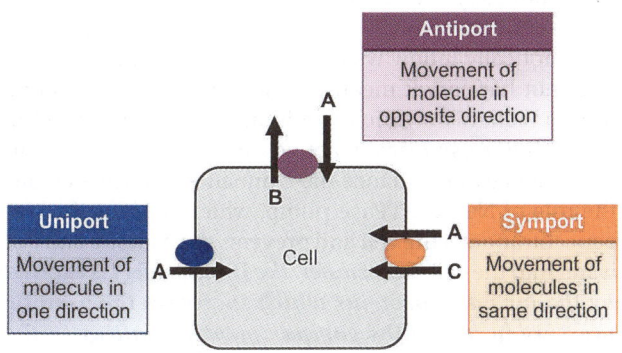

**Fig. 5.2:** Diagrammatic representation of uniport, symport and antiport.

**Table 5.1:** Mode of transport across cell membrane.

| Types | Passive transport | Active transport |
|---|---|---|
| Energy use | No energy is required | Energy is required |
| Direction of transport of substance | Along electrochemical gradient of substance | Against electrochemical gradient of substance |
| Classification | 1. Diffusion-<br>  a. Simple diffusion<br>  b. Facilitated diffusion<br>2. Osmosis | 1. Primary active transport<br>2. Secondary active transport<br>3. Vesicular transport:<br>  a. Endocytosis<br>  b. Exocytosis<br>  c. Transcytosis |

diffusion is also influenced by potential difference across the zones of diffusion.

## Simple Diffusion

**Diffusion of Neutral Molecules**

- Lipid soluble molecules can easily diffuse through the cell membrane.
- Water soluble molecules diffuse through various protein channels present in the membrane. Opening of these channels may be controlled by membrane potential, neurotransmitter, hormone, or any other chemical substance.
- Rate of diffusion across membrane is explained by Fick's law of diffusion:

$$\text{Rate of diffusion} = \frac{-DA\Delta C}{T}$$

Here, A = Surface area of membrane

T = Thickness of membrane
$\Delta C$ = Concentration gradient
D = Diffusion coefficient

- –ve sign indicates that the direction of diffusion is from high concentration area to low concentration area.
- Rate of diffusion is proportional to the concentration gradient of the substance. So, as the concentration difference across the membrane increases, the rate of diffusion also increases. It does not follow the saturation kinetics.
- As simple diffusion is not mediated by any carrier protein, there is no chance of competitive inhibition.

**Diffusion of Ions**

Because of charge on the diffusing particle, diffusion depends on two factors:
1. Concentration gradient
2. Electrical/potential gradient

The net gradient due to these two factors is known as electrochemical gradient ($\Delta\mu_x$). Equation for the electrochemical gradient, for an ion, across the cell membrane is:

$$\Delta\mu = RT \ln \frac{[X]_i}{[X]_o} + ZxFV_m$$

where, R = Gas constant
T = temperature in degree Kelvin
ln = natural logarithm
$[X]_i$ = concentration of X inside the cell
$[X]_o$ = concentration of X outside the cell
Zx = the valency of ions
F = the Faraday constant
$V_m$ = the membrane potential

### Gibbs-Donnan Effect

*What would be the effect of a nondiffusible ion on the distribution of diffusible ions, across the semipermeable membrane?*

Here is an example, there are two compartments A and B containing solution A and B, in the respective compartments. Have a look at the composition of solution at beginning. This membrane is permeable for Na$^+$, K$^+$ and Cl$^-$ but impermeable for P$^-$ anion. After diffusion and on reaching the equilibrium, *what would be the final composition of solution A and B* (Figs. 5.3A and B)?

For Na$^+$, there is no electrochemical gradient across membrane. So, Na$^+$ would not diffuse in the starting. For P$^-$, there is concentration gradient, but membrane is impermeable. So P$^-$ cannot diffuse. For Cl$^-$, there is a concentration gradient across cell membrane. So, *which ion will diffuse at start?* It would be Cl$^-$ ion. It will diffuse from solution B to solution A. This diffusion will start creating a potential difference across cell membrane. Side A and side B would be at –ve and +ve potential, respectively. This potential difference will oppose the diffusion on Cl$^-$ ions. On the other hand, this increasing potential difference would lead to diffusion of Na$^+$ from side A to side B.

Finally, at equilibrium (known as Donnan equilibrium), there will be two equal and opposite forces (due to concentration gradient and potential difference across membrane) working on Cl$^-$ ion and Na$^+$ ion.

*In this way, we can see clearly that a nondiffusible charged particle affects the distribution of diffusible molecules. This is known as Gibbs-Donnan effect.*

- At equilibrium state-
  $[Na^+]_A \times [Cl^-]_A = [Na^+]_B \times [Cl^-]_B$
  This relationship is known as Donnan relationship.
  We can generalize this finding as:
  $[\text{Diffusible Cation}]_A \times [\text{Diffusible Anion}]_A = [\text{Diffusible Cation}]_B \times [\text{Diffusible Anion}]_B$
- Let's compare the concentration of solute on both sides.
  On A side = $[Na^+] + [Cl^-] + [P^-] = 12 + 3 + 9 = 24$
  On B side = $[Na^+] + [Cl^-] = 6 + 6$

So, the concentration of osmotically active molecules/ions is present in greater concentration on A side as compared to B side. Nearly same kind so situation is present in case of a cell. Where cell is equivalent to side A. Cell contains nondiffusible intracellular –ve charged proteins and nucleic acids. Side B is equivalent to side B. Same kind of "osmotically active molecule concentration disparity" is present between ICF and ECF. Logically, it should lead to osmotically inflow water inside the cell. But actually it does not happen. It means, these there, should be some other mechanism which would attempt to decrease the intracellular osmotically active molecule concentration and which would balance the Donnan effect. Here comes the role of Na$^+$ K$^+$ ATPase pump, which reduces the Na$^+$ concentration of the cell and prevents the osmotic entry of water into the cell. *Remember, the Donan effect is exerted by the ions and proteins which increases the osmotic pressure in any of the compartments, resulting in the osmotic movement of water towards that side.*

### Facilitated Diffusion (Fig. 5.4)

- Carrier molecules of cell membrane are required for diffusion of molecules.

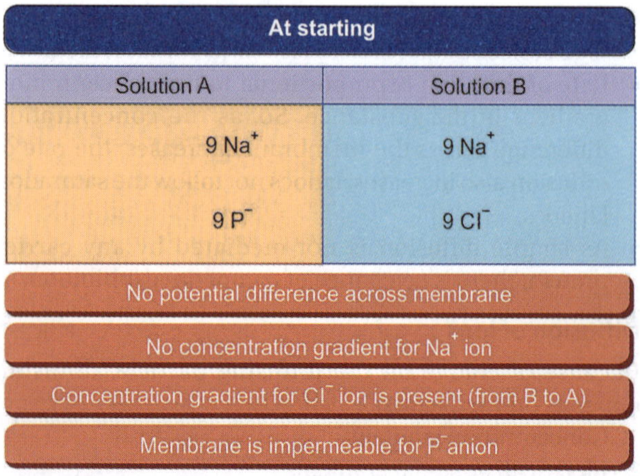

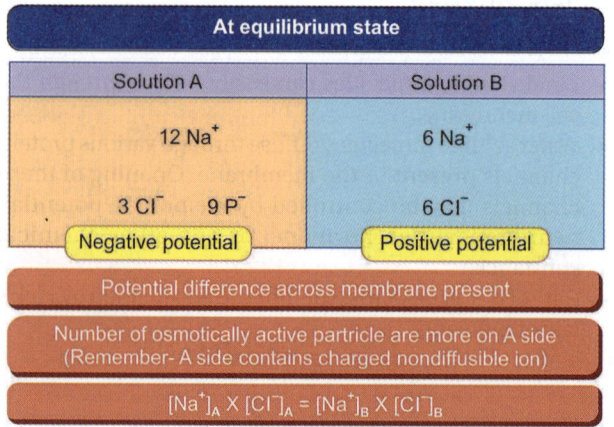

**Fig. 5.3A:** Understanding Gibbs-Donnan effect at starting.

**Fig. 5.3B:** Understanding Gibbs-Donnan effect at equilibrium state.

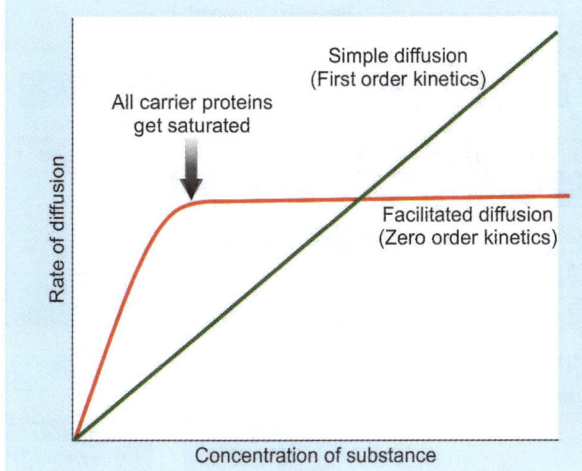

**Fig. 5.4:** Saturation kinetics—primary vs. secondary diffusion.

- Number of carrier molecules is the limiting factor for increase in rate of diffusion along with the increase in the concentration gradient. So, it follows the saturation kinetics.
- As this diffusion involves carrier molecule, it could be competitively inhibited.

## Osmosis

- It is movement of water across the semipermeable membrane from low concentrate solution to high concentrated solution.
- Rate of osmosis depends on concentration gradient of solute across the membrane.
- *What is the cause of osmosis?*
    - There is continuous and random movement of water molecules. This movement is responsible for the kinetic energy of water molecules. This energy is expressed as water potential. As a convention, its value in pure water form is zero (at standard temperature and zero external pressure).
    - In a solution, concentration of water molecules is less as compared to pure water. Along with this, there is interaction between solute molecules and water molecules. These factors lead to decrease in water potential.
    - We can say that water potential is inversely proportional to concentration of solution.
    - During the process of osmosis, due to difference in water potentials of solutions, water moves from the zone of higher water potential (low concentrated solution) to the zone of low water potential (high concentration solution).

## ACTIVE TRANSPORT

- Protein carriers, present in plasma membrane, are involved.

- Energy is utilized during movement of substance (atom/ion/molecule).
- Substance is transported against the electrochemical gradient.
- Follow saturation kinetics.
- Carrier proteins are substrate specific.
- Competitive and noncompetitive inhibition of active transport is possible.

### Primary Active Transport

- During transport, energy is directly obtained from the ATP breakdown.
- Example of primary active transport—*$Na^+/K^+$ ATPase pump*.
    - $Na^+/K^+$ ATPase is a transmembrane enzyme. It is consist of alpha (α) and beta (β) subunits. It translocates 3 $Na^+$ from cytoplasm to intercellular space and 2 $K^+$ from intercellular space to the cytoplasm. This translocation process takes place at an expense of 1 ATP. So, one $Na^+/K^+$ ATPase cycle leads to net loss of one positive charged ion from the cell. In this way, this pump is electrogenic in nature and it also decreases the concentration of osmotically active substance in the cell. Now if we apply the principle of osmosis, cell should get shrunken because of exosmosis (due to Na/K ATPase pump induced less concentration of osmotically active particle in the cell). But, in real, cell does not shrink. It means, there must be some other mechanism which is showing opposite effect on the cell (i.e., increasing the concentration of osmotically active molecules in the cell). This occurs due to Gibbs Donnan effect.

### Secondary Active Transport

- The energy required for the transport of a substance from its low concentration zone to its high concentration zone is obtained from the energy released during movement of some other substance from its high concentration zone to its low concentration zone.
- **Example:** $Na^+$/glucose symport—this is involved in glucose absorption in intestine and PCT of nephron **(Fig. 5.5)**.

As its name suggests, $Na^+$/glucose symport transport (SGLT) $Na^+$ and glucose from ECF to cytoplasm. Glucose concentration is more in cytoplasm as compared to ECF. Glucose is transported against the concentration gradient. So, it requires energy. On the other hand, $Na^+$ concentration is more in ECF as compared to cytoplasm.

In this way, $Na^+$ moves along its concentration gradient and releases potential energy stored in its concentration gradient. If we think logically, there must be some mechanism which would be responsible for the formation of $Na^+$ gradient. As this $Na^+$ gradient stores potential energy, there must be expenditure of some energy during formation of this $Na^+$ gradient. In this case, it is $Na^+/K^+$ ATPase, which

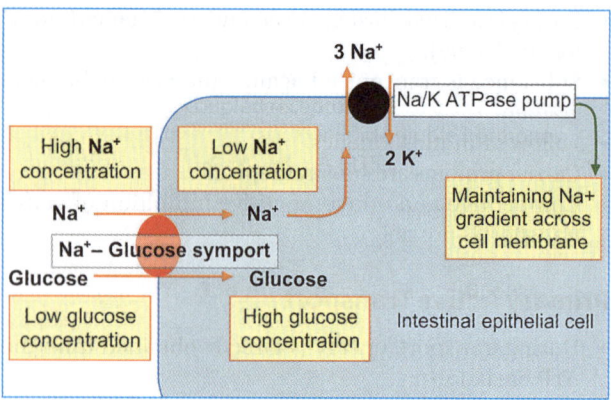

**Fig. 5.5:** Na$^+$-glucose symport (example of secondary active transport).

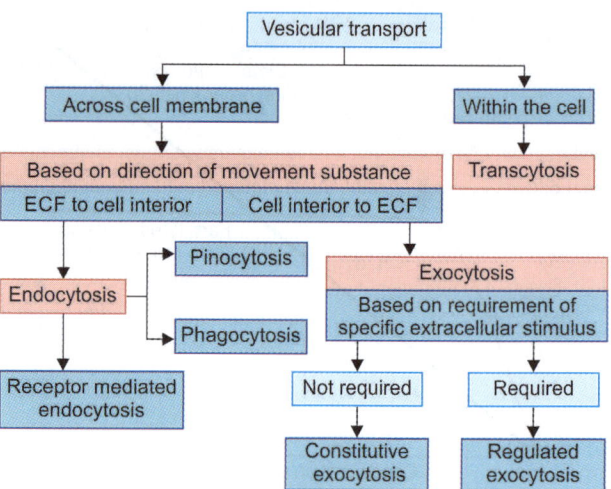

**Fig. 5.6:** Types of vesicular transport.

is responsible for creation for this Na$^+$ gradient. In this way, ATP, utilized at Na$^+$/K$^+$ ATPase, indirectly supply energy required for the transport of glucose.

## Vesicular Transport

It involves vesicle mediated transport of substance either from ECF to cell interior or vice versa.

### Types of Vesicular Transport (Fig. 5.6)

- **Endocytosis** is a process in which a part of plasma membrane gets internalized and forms a vesicle. Later, this vesicle pinches off from the cell membrane and migrates in the cell.
  - *Pinocytosis/cell drinking:* In this type on endocytosis, vesicle transports solution/fluid from ECF to cell interior.
  - *Phagocytosis/cell eating:* Phagocytosis is involved in transport on macromolecules or micro-organisms from ECF to cell interior by specific cell.
  - *Receptor-mediated endocytosis (Fig. 5.7):* As its name suggests, cell membrane have substance specific receptors containing region known as coated pits. Once the receptor specific substance attaches to the receptor, that zone of cell membrane gets engulfed by endocytosis and form vesicle. During this process *clathrin* helps in vesicle formation and adaptin protein acts as interlink between receptor and clathrin protein. *Dynamin*, a guanosine triphosphate (GTPase), facilitates the separation of vesicle from the plasma membrane. After endocytosis, adaptin and clathrin proteins get recycled for further use. The remaining vesicle gets fused with appropriate cell organelle like lysozyme.
- **Exocytosis** is a process in which cytoplasmic vesicle migrates to the cell membrane and later, fusion of vesicle membrane cell membrane takes place. This leads to expulsion of vesicle content in ECF.
  - *Constitutive exocytosis:* It involves continuous exocytosis from the cell without any dependency on any extra cellular controlling factor. Example- release of mucous from intestinal mucous cells.

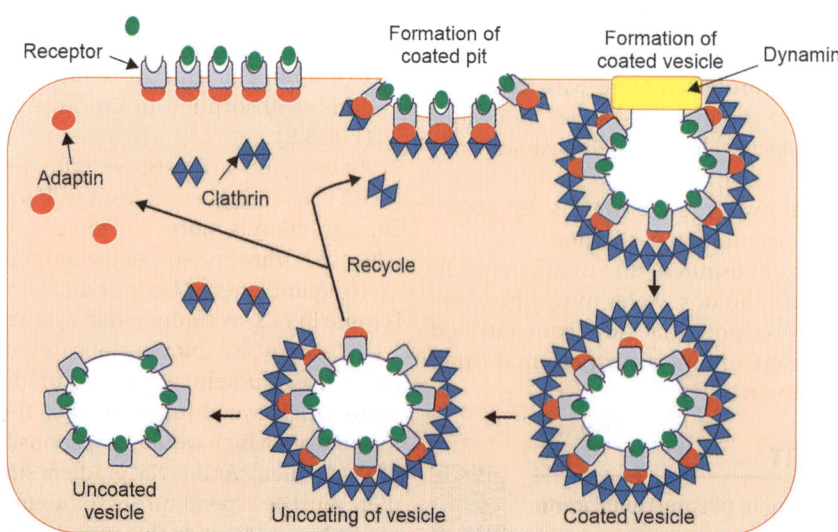

**Fig. 5.7:** Mechanism of receptor-mediated endocytosis.

- **Regulated exocytosis:** This type of exocytosis is controlled by extracellular factors like hormones, chemicals, neurotransmitter. This kind of transport takes place in secretion of glands (endocrine as well as exocrine), release of neurotransmitter from neurons. On appropriate stimulus vesicle (containing presynthesized molecules) moves toward the cell membrane and releases chemicals by exocytosis.
- **Transcytosis:** It involves intracellular transport of substance by vesicle.

### Clinical correlation
Inactivation of $Na^+/K^+$ ATPase causes increase in osmolarity inside the cell which leads to endosmosis and increase in cell size. This scenario is evident in the RBCs of stored blood. During storage period, blood glucose gets utilized in cell respiration in RBC. So, gradually there is depletion in ATP (outcome of cell respiration). It will lead to inactivation of $Na^+/K^+$ ATPase in RBC. It results in endosmosis and increase in size of RBC.

## SUMMARY

In this chapter, we have learnt that:
- Different types of transport proteins, including channels, carriers, and pumps, are described here, elucidating their structures, functions, and mechanisms of action.
- The diverse mechanisms by which molecules traverse cell membranes: passive and active transport, outlining their respective characteristics and providing examples to illustrate each process.
- The concept of diffusion, a fundamental process governing the movement of molecules in biological systems, is explored in depth. Simple diffusion and facilitated diffusion are defined and dissected, highlighting their similarities, differences, and the role of transport proteins in facilitated diffusion.
- The Gibbs Donnan effect, a phenomenon influencing the distribution of ions across semipermeable membranes.
- Key principles of diffusion, such as Fick's law and factors influencing diffusion rates, are elucidated to provide a comprehensive understanding of this fundamental process.
- Primary and secondary active transport mechanisms are elucidated in this chapter, providing insights into how cells utilize energy to transport molecules against concentration gradients. The chapter also explores the roles of ATP and ion gradients in primary active transport and the coupling of transport processes in secondary active transport.
- Vesicular transport processes, crucial for the uptake and secretion of large molecules and particles by cells, are classified and discussed. Readers gain an understanding of the different types of vesicular transport, including endocytosis, exocytosis, and transcytosis, along with their physiological significance.
- The intricate mechanisms of exocytosis, endocytosis, and transcytosis with detailed descriptions of each process, including the formation of vesicles, membrane fusion events, and regulatory mechanisms, provide readers with a comprehensive understanding of vesicular transport in cellular physiology.

## LET US SEE, HOW MUCH YOU HAVE LEARNT?

### Review Questions

Q1. Enumerate and describe the mechanism of transport across cell membrane.
Q2. Define Osmosis. What are the factors affecting osmosis?
Q3. Define diffusion. What are the differences between simple and facilitated diffusion?
Q4. Describe Gibbs-Donnan effect.
Q5. Describe primary and secondary active transport with appropriate examples.
Q6. How does balance between activities of Gibbs Donnan effect and $Na^+/K^+$ ATPase pump maintain cell size?
Q7. Describe the mechanisms of vesicular transport.

### Multiple Choice Questions

Q1. Which type of membrane transport protein requires the expenditure of energy to move molecules against their concentration gradient?
    a. Channel protein      b. Carrier protein
    c. Pump protein      d. Receptor protein

Q2. Simple diffusion is primarily driven by:
    a. ATP hydrolysis
    b. Membrane proteins
    c. Concentration gradient
    d. Electrical potential

Q3. Which of the following best describes the Gibbs Donnan effect?
    a. Movement of molecules from an area of high concentration to an area of low concentration
    b. Unequal distribution of ions across a semipermeable membrane due to ion impermeability
    c. Active transport of ions against their concentration gradient
    d. Facilitated diffusion of ions through membrane channels

**Q4. Fick's law of diffusion describes the relationship between diffusion rate and:**
a. Membrane potential
b. Concentration gradient
c. ATP concentration
d. Vesicular transport

**Q5. Which of the following is an example of facilitated diffusion?**
a. Movement of water through aquaporin channels
b. Movement of oxygen across the lipid bilayer
c. Movement of ions through voltage-gated channels
d. Movement of glucose through carrier proteins

**Q6. Primary active transport involves the direct use of:**
a. ATP
b. Electrochemical gradient
c. Secondary messengers
d. Co-transport proteins

**Q7. Which vesicular transport process involves the secretion of molecules from a cell?**
a. Exocytosis
b. Endocytosis
c. Transcytosis
d. Pinocytosis

**Q8. Endocytosis involves the:**
a. Uptake of extracellular fluid and solutes by the cell
b. Secretion of molecules from the cell
c. Fusion of vesicles with the plasma membrane
d. Transport of molecules from the Golgi apparatus to the cell surface

**Q9. Transcytosis combines elements of:**
a. Exocytosis and endocytosis
b. Simple and facilitated diffusion
c. Primary and secondary active transport
d. Channel and carrier proteins

**Q10. Which membrane transport process requires the presence of specific receptor proteins on the cell membrane?**
a. Simple diffusion
b. Exocytosis
c. Endocytosis
d. Osmosis

## ANSWERS

1. c    2. c    3. b    4. b    5. d    6. a    7. a    8. a    9. a    10. c

# Body Fluids and Compartments

## CHAPTER 6

### COMPETENCY ADDRESSED
**PY1.6:** Describe the fluid compartments of the body, its ionic composition and measurements.

### LEARNING OBJECTIVES
At the end of this chapter, the learner should be able to:
- Describe the importance of normal body fluid compartments and regulation of fluid volume, tonicity and pH.
- Describe the role of serum electrolytes in maintaining normal body functioning.
- Analyze the various disturbances in the fluid homeostasis through different case scenarios.
- Briefly describe the regulation of fluid volume and tonicity.

## BODY FLUIDS

The primary constituent of the living body is the water, which comprises 65–70% of the body weight. The body water is distributed in our body in such a way that every cell contains water inside its membrane and it is bathed in a watery medium, which consists of ions and nutrients for maintenance of the internal environment of the body (Figs. 6.1 and 6.2).

- The total amount of water present inside and outside the cells is called ***total body water (TBW)***. An average adult man weighing 70 kg has 40 to 45 L of water. The water content of the body decreases with age hence an infants has higher water content than an adult. The water content in an obese individual is less as compared to a lean person because the adipose tissue contains less fluid. The males have higher body water as compared to the females.

**Why elderly are more prone to dehydration as compared to adults?**
The elderly are more prone to dehydration because of decreased total body water with the advancing age.

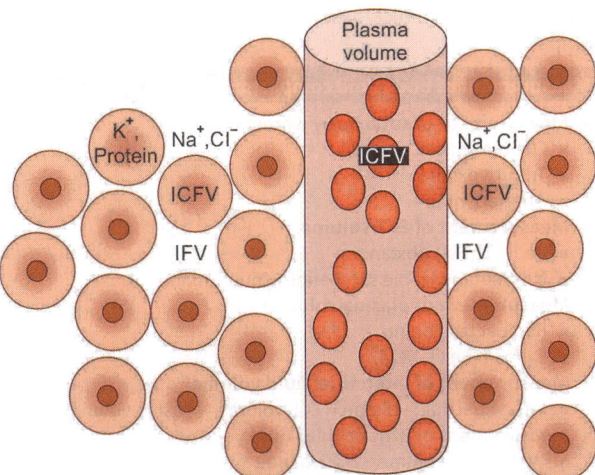

**Fig. 6.1:** Distribution of fluid volumes in various body fluid compartments.
(ICFV: intracellular fluid volume)

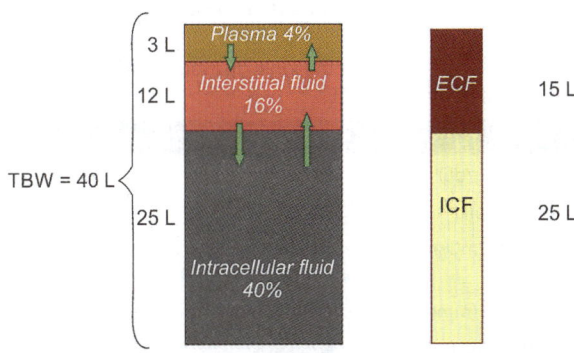

**Fig. 6.2:** Distribution of water in various body fluid compartments.
(ECF: extracellular fluid; ICF: intracellular fluid)

**Why the infants are more prone to dehydration as compared to adults?**

Though the infants have more body water as compared to adults but still they are more prone to dehydration because of the less body surface area.

- The amount of water present inside the cells is called *intracellular fluid (ICF)*. It comprises of 2/3rd of total body water or 40% of the body weight.
- The amount of water present outside the cells is called *extracellular fluid (ECF)*. It comprises of 1/3rd of total body water or 20% of the body weight. The various body fluid compartments comprising of ECF are:
  - *Interstitial fluid/tissue fluid (ISF):* The water present around the cells.
  - *Plasma:* The water present inside the blood vessels is called intravascular fluid. Since the main fluid component of intravascular fluid is plasma. The term **plasma (PV)** is used instead of intravascular fluid.
  - *Transcellular fluid (TCF):* The fluid present in the visceral cavities light pleural fluid, pericardial fluid, synovial fluid, etc.

Hence, ECF = PV + ISF + TCF

## COMPOSITION OF ECF AND ICF

The ECF and ICF are separated by the cell membrane showing the difference in the ionic composition in both the compartments, as shown in **Figure 6.3** and **Table 6.1**.

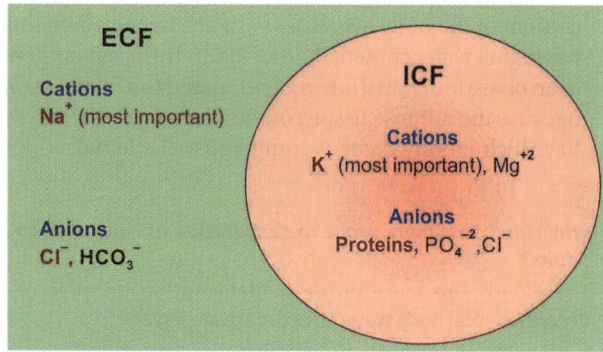

**Fig. 6.3:** Ionic distribution in ECF and ICF.

**Table 6.1:** Normal values of the ionic distribution and physical attributes of body fluids (ECF).

|  | Normal value | Normal range |
|---|---|---|
| Glucose (mg/dL) | 85 | 75–95 |
| Acid-base (pH) | 7.4 | 7.3–7.5 |
| Osmolality (mOsm/L) | Specific gravity normal value: 300 |  |
| Sodium ion (mmol/L) | 142 | 132–146 |
| Potassium ion (mmol/L) | 4.2 | 3.8–5.0 |
| Chloride ion (mmol/L) | 108 | 103–112 |
| Bicarbonate ion (mmol/L) | 28 | 24–32 |

## MEASUREMENT OF BODY FLUID VOLUMES

The measurement of the body fluid volumes is based on *Dilution principle*

$$V = \frac{m}{c}\ ml$$

where, 'm' is amount of substance injected in the fluid, and 'c' is the concentration of that substance after being dissolved in the fluid.

Since the mass of the injected substance tend to distribute/metabolize/excreted, we use the difference of initial and final amount of the indicator substance measured in the compartment, whose volume has to be determined. So the formula becomes,

$$V = \frac{A1 - A2}{C}$$

where, V = volume of fluid compartment
A1 = amt of indicator injected in fluid
A2 = amt of indicator removed by metabolism or excretion
C = conc of indicator in fluid

Based on this principle, the indicator is injected into the specific body fluid compartment. It is allowed to distribute evenly in the entire compartment and then the samples are taken to get the values of *A1, A2* and *C*. The choice of indicator substances used, depend upon the compartment under study and its biosafety **(Table 6.2)**. Various indicators, specifically used for each compartment are shown in **Table 6.3**:

**Table 6.2:** Characteristics of indicator substance.

| Characteristics of material/indicator injected |
|---|
| • Nontoxic |
| • Mix evenly |
| • Easy to measure |
| • No effect of its own on distribution of water/other substances |
| • Should stay in the compartment in which it is injected |
| • Unchanged by the body |

**Table 6.3:** Various indicator substances used for various body compartments.

| Measurement of body fluid compartments |
|---|
| • **Measurement of total body water**: |
| ▪ Deuterium oxide ($D_2O$) |
| ▪ Tritium oxide |
| ▪ Aminopyrine |
| • **Measurement of ECF volume**: |
| ▪ Radioactive substances |
| ▪ Nonmetabolizable saccharides: inulin, mannitol |
| • **Measurement of plasma volume**: |
| ▪ Radioactive iodine |
| ▪ Evan's blue (T-1824) |
| • **Measurement of interstitial fluid volume**: |
| ▪ Interstitial fluid volume = ECF volume − Plasma volume |
| • **Measurement of intracellular fluid volume**: |
| ICF Vol = TBW volume − ECF volume |
| • **Blood volume:** If plasma volume is measured then: |
| Total blood volume = $\dfrac{Plasma\ volume \times 100}{100 - Hematocrit}$ |

- **Measurement of total body water:** The indicator substance should evenly distribute through all the body fluid compartments.
- **Measurement of ECF volume:** The indicator substance should evenly distribute through extracellular fluid compartment only. It should not be able to cross the cell membrane, and not have any distribution in the cells.
- **Measurement of plasma volume:** The indicator substance should evenly distribute through the intravascular compartment but should not diffuse out of it. Hence, the indicator used is the one, which binds to the plasma proteins (as they cannot cross the capillary membrane), is used.
- **Measurement of interstitial fluid volume:** It is not possible to measure the ISFV directly. Hence it is indirectly measured by subtracting PV from ECF volume.
- **Measurement of intracellular fluid volume:** It is also not possible to measure the ICFV directly. Hence it is indirectly measured by subtracting ECF volume from TBW.
- **Blood volume:** Once the plasma volume is known, blood volume can be calculated as plasma makes 55% of whole blood.
  Blood volume = Plasma volume × 1/1−hematocrit

*What happens to body fluid osmolality and tonicity in clinically relevant situations like diarrhea, dehydration, water intoxication, etc.?*

To answer the above question, you must understand the *fluid movement across compartments*.

The ICF is separated from the ECF by the **cell membrane**, which is selectively permeable for the ionic and fluid movement. Hence, the transport of substances between these two compartments is governed by the principles of transport across cell membrane, viz., active and passive transport.

However, the intravascular compartment plasma volume (PV) is separated from the interstitial fluid (ISF) by **the capillary basement membrane** which is governed by the principles of capillary fluid dynamics/Starling's forces.

> **Remember**
> - Intracellular fluid and extracellular fluid is separated by cell membrane, which is semipermeable. Transport is through active and passive transport.
> - Intravascular compartment and Interstitial fluid of ECF; are separated by capillary membrane, which is freely permeable to fluid and electrolytes.

Hence, the movement of water across these compartments depends on many factors. It will be better understood if study these compartments on the *Darrow-Yannet diagram (D-Y diagram)* showing the tonicity and volume of the fluid compartments **(Fig. 6.4)**.

In this diagram, we observe that the tonicity of all the compartments remains same, which governs the fluid movement across the compartments. The loss of water from the body due to dehydration or excessive water ingestion immediately affects the ECF volume. The changes in ICF take some time to reflect.

After this basic understanding, we can sum it up as follows:
- The intracellular and extracellular fluid compartments are separated by cell membrane which has the following characteristics:
  - It is freely permeable to movement of water across the membrane
  - It is impermeable to Na$^+$ and Cl$^-$ (not penetrating solutes)

Since, Na$^+$ and Cl$^-$ are the most abundant impermeable and osmotically active ions of the extracellular fluid, they influence the osmolality of the ECF compartment.

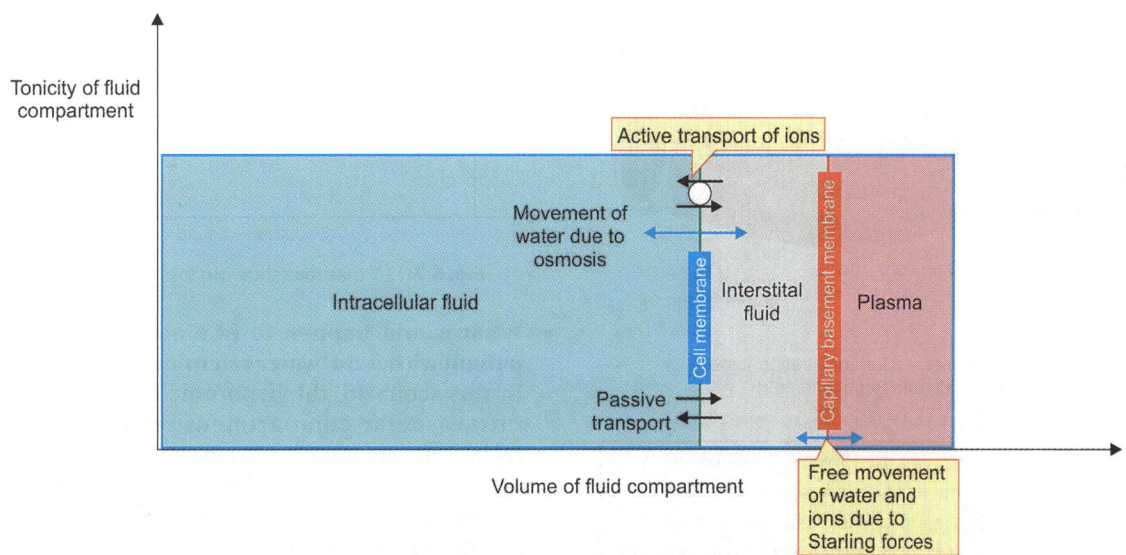

**Fig. 6.4:** D-Y diagram showing the distribution of body fluid compartments and the representation of tonicity and volume on graphical axis.

> **What will happen to intracellular volume in a patient of hypernatremia?**
> Hypernatremia means, increased sodium levels in ECF. It will increase the osmolality of ECF, the water which is freely permeable moves from ICF to ECF, hence shrinking the cell size/reducing the intracellular volume
> **Why the cell size increases in a patient of hyponatremia? (Answer yourself)**

The intracellular fluid volume is affected by the presence of various types of solutes present in ECF. Let us consider a rapidly penetrating osmotically active solute (e.g., Urea); added to ECF. **How do you think, it will affect the ICFV?**

> **Rapidly penetrating solutes:** Urea
> They rapidly enter the cells, equilibrating the osmotic concentration across the cell membrane. Hence, does not affect the cell volume.
> **Slowly penetrating solutes:** Glycerol
> They slowly enter the cells, equilibrating the osmotic concentration across the cell membrane slowly. They produce the initial osmotic effect, resulting in movement of water from the cell into ISF and then slowly normalizing the cell volume.
> **Not penetrating solutes:** Sodium, Chloride
> They do not enter the cells, creating the osmotic gradient across the cell membrane. Hence, it results in movement of water outside the cell resulting in cell shrinkage.

- The interstitial fluid volume and plasma are separated by capillary membrane, which is freely permeable to almost the soluble substances except plasma proteins. Hence, the concentration of plasma proteins affects the osmolality between plasma and interstitial fluid, by affecting the colloid osmotic pressure. The movement of water between these two compartments is regulated by Starling forces **(Fig. 6.5)**.

Looking back into some clinically relevant scenarios, let us discuss the concept of fluid volume changes in them:

- **What would happen to ECF and ICF volume in a patient of severe water loss or dehydration due to sweating?**

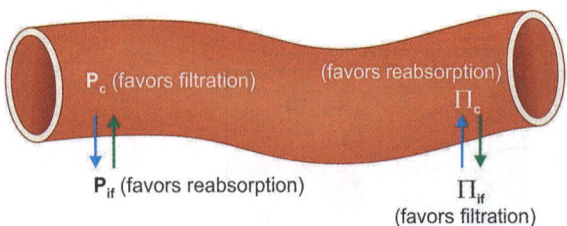

Net filtration pressure = (Sum of filtration forces) − (Sum of all reabsorptive forces)
= $(P_c + \Pi_{if}) - (P_{if} + \Pi_c)$

> $P_c$: Capillary hydrostatic pressure
> $P_{if}$: Interstitial fluid hydrostatic pressure
> $\Pi_c$: Capillary colloid osmotic pressure
> $\Pi_{if}$: Interstitial fluid colloid osmotic pressure

**Fig. 6.5:** Starling forces for regulation of fluid movement.

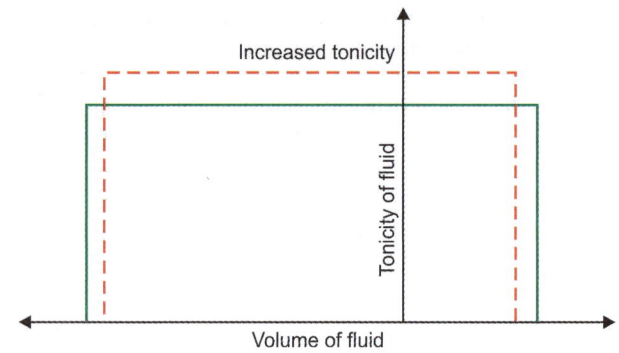

**Fig. 6.6:** D-Y diagram showing loss of hypotonic fluid from the body. (The solid lines indicate the normal distribution of water in body fluid compartments, dashed lines indicate the clinical condition being discussed)

In severe dehydration, the person loses water from the extracellular fluid (hypotonic fluid loss) **(Fig. 6.6)** resulting in the increased tonicity of the ECF. Sustained higher tonicity of ECF can further result in the movement of water from the cells into the ECF, shrinking ICF volume also. Hence the D-Y diagram will show shrinkage of ECF and ICF along with increased tonicity of body fluids. Similar condition is seen in alcoholism, Formation of dilute urine (diabetes insipidus, etc.).

- **What would happen to ECF and ICF volume in a patient with acute blood loss/hemorrhage?**
In hemorrhage, there is loss of isotonic whole blood resulting in loss of only extracellular fluid volume **(Fig. 6.7)**. Since the tonicity of the ECF remains same, the intracellular fluid volume is not affected; only ECF volume is affected. Similar condition is seen in severe diarrhea, vomiting, etc.

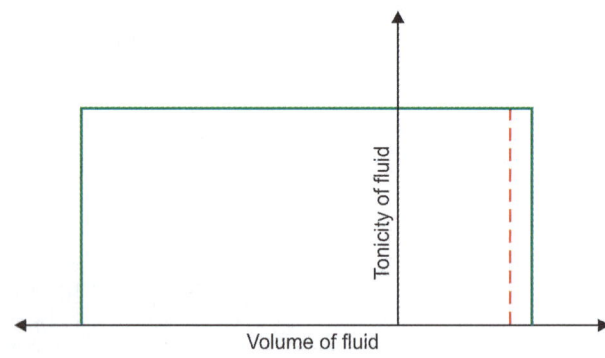

**Fig. 6.7:** D-Y diagram showing loss of isotonic fluid.

- **What would happen to ECF and ICF volume in a patient with fluid/water retention?**
In this scenario, the hypotonic fluid present in the intravascular compartment raises the capillary hydrostatic pressure, raising the net filtration pressure at the capillary membrane (Starling Forces) **(Fig. 6.8)**. The increased hypotonic ECF volume, as compared to ICF, results in movement of water into the cells; increasing the ICF volume also. However, the net tonicity of the body fluids is reduced. This pattern of water distribution

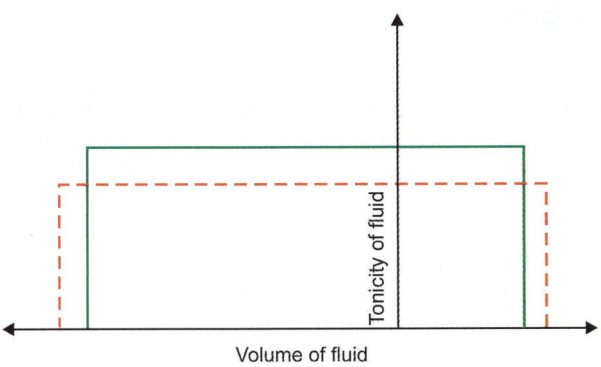

**Fig. 6.8:** D-Y diagram showing water retention.
(Similar findings will be seen in infusion of hypotonic fluids or primary adrenal insufficiency)

will also be seen in hypotonic fluid infusion and primary adrenal insufficiency.
- **What would happen to ECF and ICF volume in a patient with excessive salt ingestion or hypertonic saline infusion?**
Excessive salt ingestion/hypertonic saline infusion would result in the movement of water from the cells into the interstitial and the intravascular spaces **(Fig. 6.9)**, hence resulting in contraction of ICF volume and expansion of ECF volume. The salt/hypertonic solution raises the tonicity of the body fluids.

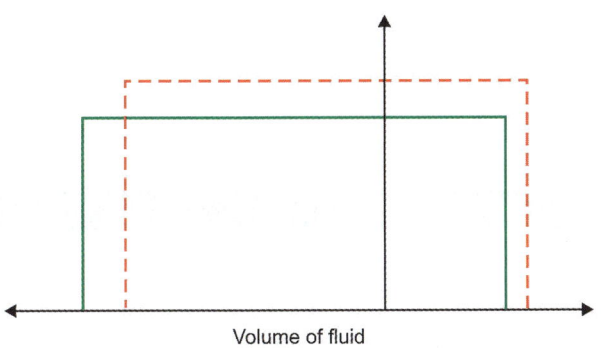

**Fig. 6.9:** D-Y diagram showing hypertonic solution.

## REGULATION OF BODY FLUID VOLUME AND TONICITY

The body fluids play a vital role in the maintenance of proper cellular function and homeostatic control. Any deviation in the pH, volume and tonicity of the body fluids could result significant deterioration of the cellular activity affecting the physiological functions of body. Hence, a tight regulation of fluid homeostasis is very important, which is brought about by the following mechanisms:
- Fluid transport across the compartments (ICF and ECF).
- Osmotic transport of water equalizing the concentration of solutes on both sides of membrane.
- **Role of kidneys:** Through filtration, reabsorption and secretion of various electrolytes, water and metabolites, the kidney play an important role in water and electrolyte homeostasis.
- **Role of hormones:** Various hormones play an important role in the regulation of water and electrolytes in our body like:
    - Antidiuretic hormone (ADH) secreted from posterior pituitary gland results is conservation of water in the body
    - Aldosterone secreted from adrenal cortex results in retention of sodium and water in the body
    - Atrial natriuretic peptide (ANP) released by heart promotes sodium and water excretion in urine resulting in decrease in fluid volume, helping to lower the arterial pressure.
- **Thirst mechanism:** Whenever the body fluid volume decreases or there is increase in tonicity, the osmoreceptors sense the change in tonicity and activate the hypothalamic thirst center. The individual hence drinks the water to restore the fluid volume of the body.

If a person experiences an imbalance in pH, fluid volume and tonicity, the body prioritizes the correction of pH over volume and tonicity; because many cellular functions operate in a very narrow range of pH. Regulation of pH is discussed in Chapter 7. The correction in pH is closely followed by correction in fluid volume and then tonicity. Once the pH is regulated, the fluid volume is maintained to ensure proper arterial pressure and tissue perfusion. The tonicity is corrected, usually along with the volume. However, in situations where tonicity becomes a primary concern (e.g., hypertonic or hypotonic conditions), the body adjusts fluid intake and output, as well as electrolyte levels, to restore tonicity to normal levels. Hormones such as ADH and aldosterone also contribute to tonicity regulation by influencing water and electrolyte reabsorption in the kidneys. To sum up, while pH regulation takes precedence due to its critical role in cellular function, volume and tonicity regulation closely follow to maintain overall homeostasis. These processes are intricately linked and often occur simultaneously to ensure optimal functioning of the body's internal environment.

## FLUID REPLACEMENT THERAPY

Fluid replacement therapy refers to the administration of fluids to maintain or restore hydration and electrolyte balance in individuals who are dehydrated, have lost fluids due to illness or injury, or require supplemental fluids for medical reasons.

### Types of Fluids

#### *Crystalloids*

**Definition**

Crystalloid solutions contain small molecules that can pass freely through cell membranes. They are composed of water and electrolytes in varying concentrations.

### Indications

- **Isotonic crystalloids (e.g., normal saline, lactated ringer's solution):** Used for volume expansion, intravascular fluid replacement, and maintenance hydration in patients with dehydration, hypovolemia, and ongoing fluid losses.
- **Hypertonic crystalloids (e.g., hypertonic saline):** Used in specific clinical situations such as severe hyponatremia, cerebral edema, and traumatic brain injury to rapidly increase serum sodium levels and reduce cerebral edema.
- **Hypotonic crystalloids (e.g., 0.45% saline):** Used cautiously in patients with mild dehydration or hypernatremia to provide free water and correct electrolyte imbalances.

## *Colloids*

### Definition

Colloid solutions contain larger molecules, such as starches or proteins, which remain within the intravascular space and exert oncotic pressure to help retain fluid.

### Indications

- **Synthetic colloids (e.g., hydroxyethyl starch, dextran):** Used for volume replacement in patients with hypovolemia due to hemorrhage, burns, or surgery when crystalloids alone are insufficient.
- **Natural colloids (e.g., albumin):** Used in patients with hypoalbuminemia or hypo-oncotic states to maintain intravascular volume and improve tissue perfusion.

## SUMMARY

- The human body comprises various fluid compartments, including intracellular and extracellular spaces, which must be maintained within narrow ranges for optimal health.
- Regulation of fluid volume, tonicity, and pH is crucial for preserving cellular integrity, facilitating enzymatic reactions, and supporting overall homeostasis.
- Mechanisms such as renal regulation, hormonal signaling, and thirst sensation play pivotal roles in ensuring the balance of fluid compartments and pH levels.
- Serum electrolytes, including sodium, potassium, chloride, calcium, and magnesium, are vital for numerous physiological processes such as nerve conduction, muscle contraction, and acid-base balance.
- Maintaining appropriate electrolyte levels is imperative for preserving cellular membrane potential, osmotic balance, and overall organ function.
- Disturbances in electrolyte concentrations can lead to various health issues, emphasizing the importance of their regulation and monitoring.
- Fluid volume and tonicity are regulated through intricate physiological mechanisms involving the kidneys, hormonal signaling, and thirst sensation.
- The kidneys play a central role in adjusting fluid volume and electrolyte concentrations through processes such as filtration, reabsorption, and excretion.
- Hormones like antidiuretic hormone (ADH), aldosterone, and atrial natriuretic peptide (ANP) modulate renal function to maintain fluid balance and tonicity.

## LET US SEE, HOW MUCH YOU HAVE LEARNT?

### *Review Questions*

Q1. Describe normal body fluid compartments crucial for health.
Q2. Regulation of volume and tonicity vital for cellular integrity and homeostasis.
Q3. Renal, hormonal, and sensory mechanisms involved in maintaining balance.
Q4. What will happen to the body fluid volume of a patients with acute gastroenteritis?
Q5. Why infants are more prone to dehydration?
Q6. What will happen to the body fluid volume in a person from acute gastroenteritis?
Q7. Why do you prescribe re-hydration solution (containing salt and glucose together) for correcting the fluid depletion in a person?
Q8. What will happen, to the body fluid volume, if you inject the 1 liter of 5% dextrose intravenous infusion in a person?

### *Multiple Choice Questions*

Q1. A 65-year-old patient with congestive heart failure presents to the emergency department with complaints of increasing shortness of breath and swelling in the lower extremities. On examination, the patient appears edematous, with crackles heard on auscultation of the lungs. Laboratory tests reveal decreased serum sodium levels. Which of the following mechanisms is most likely contributing to the fluid imbalance in this patient?
 a. Increased secretion of antidiuretic hormone (ADH)
 b. Decreased secretion of atrial natriuretic peptide (ANP)
 c. Impaired renal filtration
 d. Excessive intake of hypertonic fluids

**Q2.** A 30-year-old athlete participates in an intense marathon race during a hot summer day. Following the race, the athlete experiences muscle cramps, dizziness, and fatigue. Upon evaluation, laboratory tests show elevated serum sodium levels. What is the most likely cause of the fluid imbalance in this individual?
a. Excessive loss of electrolytes through sweating
b. Overhydration with hypotonic fluids
c. Decreased secretion of aldosterone
d. Hypersecretion of antidiuretic hormone (ADH)

**Q3.** A 45-year-old patient with chronic kidney disease presents with complaints of excessive thirst and frequent urination. Laboratory investigations reveal increased serum potassium levels and metabolic acidosis. Which of the following mechanisms is likely responsible for the observed fluid imbalance in this patient?
a. Deficient secretion of antidiuretic hormone (ADH)
b. Impaired renal reabsorption of water
c. Elevated secretion of aldosterone
d. Inadequate excretion of potassium and acid by the kidneys

**Q4.** Which of the following hormones is primarily responsible for promoting water reabsorption in the kidneys, thereby influencing fluid volume regulation?
a. Aldosterone
b. Antidiuretic hormone (ADH)
c. Atrial natriuretic peptide (ANP)
d. Parathyroid hormone (PTH)

**Q5.** During dehydration, which of the following physiological responses is most likely to occur to maintain fluid balance?
a. Decreased secretion of aldosterone
b. Increased production of atrial natriuretic peptide (ANP)
c. Enhanced release of antidiuretic hormone (ADH)
d. Decreased renal reabsorption of water

**Q6.** Which of the following electrolytes is predominantly found in the extracellular fluid compartment and plays a critical role in regulating osmotic pressure and fluid balance?
a. Potassium
b. Chloride
c. Magnesium
d. Phosphate

**Q7.** In response to increased blood volume and pressure, which hormone is secreted by the heart to promote sodium and water excretion by the kidneys, thus aiding in fluid volume regulation?
a. Aldosterone
b. Antidiuretic hormone (ADH)
c. Atrial natriuretic peptide (ANP)
d. Parathyroid hormone (PTH)

**Q8.** Which of the following mechanisms is primarily responsible for maintaining the osmotic balance between intracellular and extracellular fluids?
a. Sodium-potassium pump
b. Active transport of glucose
c. Passive diffusion of water
d. Facilitated diffusion of ions

**Q9.** Which of the following intravenous fluid therapies would be most appropriate for a patient who has undergone surgery and requires maintenance hydration?
a. 0.9% sodium chloride (normal saline)
b. 5% dextrose in water (D5W)
c. Lactated Ringer's solution
d. Hypertonic saline (3% NaCl)

**Q10.** In the management of severe dehydration, which intravenous fluid therapy is most appropriate to restore intravascular volume and correct electrolyte imbalances?
a. 0.9% sodium chloride (normal saline)
b. 5% dextrose in water (D5W)
c. Hypotonic saline (0.45% NaCl)
d. Balanced crystalloids (e.g., Plasma-Lyte)

**ANSWERS**

1. a   2. a   3. d   4. b   5. c   6. b   7. c   8. a   9. c   10. a

# Acid-base Balance

**CHAPTER 7**

### COMPETENCY ADDRESSED
**PY1.7:** Concepts of pH and buffer systems in the body.

### LEARNING OBJECTIVES
**At the end of this chapter, the learner should be able to:**
- Define pH and buffer.
- Discuss the different types of buffers to maintain pH.
- Discuss the role of kidney in maintaining the acid-base balance.
- Describe the derangements of pH in terms of respiratory and metabolic acidosis and alkalosis.
- Describe the effect of pH disturbance on various physiological processes.

Though this chapter is extensively covered by the text books of biochemistry, I feel that the basic knowledge about the pH and buffer systems of body is essential to understand the basic physiological processes of the body. In simple words, we will be talking about the acidity ($H^+$ concentration) of blood and its importance in carrying out physiological processes.

Acid-base balance is one of the most important homeostatic mechanism in the body as most of our enzymatic reactions are pH specific and become deranged with minor alterations in pH. *The normal pH range of our body system is between 7.35 and 7.45.*

To understand the concept of pH, we have to revisit our basics from the Chemistry.

pH stands for "potential of hydrogen." It is a measure of the acidity or alkalinity of a solution, indicating the concentration of hydrogen ions ($H^+$) present in the solution. The pH scale ranges from 0 to 14, where:
- pH values less than 7 indicate acidity (higher concentration of $H^+$ ions).
- pH values equal to 7 indicate neutrality (equal concentration of $H^+$ and $OH^-$ ions).
- pH values greater than 7 indicate alkalinity (higher concentration of $OH^-$ ions).

The pH scale is logarithmic, meaning that a change of one unit on the pH scale represents a tenfold change in the concentration of hydrogen ions. It represents negative logarithm of $H^+$ concentration.

$$pH = -\log [H^+]$$

Hence, pH $\alpha$ $1/H^+$

## PHYSIOLOGICAL SIGNIFICANCE OF pH OF BODY FLUIDS

The normal physiological range of pH is 7.35 to 7.45. Hence, it becomes very clear that the average pH of our body fluids is alkaline (above 7). If pH falls below 7.35, it is referred as acidosis and an increase in pH above 7.45 is referred as alkalosis. This narrow range of pH is essential for many physiological processes mentioned below **(Table 7.1)**:
- It regulates the optimum enzymatic activity required for most of the physiological processes.
- It is essential for maintaining integrity and functions of cells, such as protein synthesis, ion transport and cell signaling.

**Table 7.1:** pH of different body fluids.

| | $H^+$ concentration (mEq/L) | pH |
|---|---|---|
| Extracellular fluid<br>• Arterial blood<br>• Venous blood<br>• Interstitial fluid | <br>$4.0 \times 10^{-5}$<br>$4.5 \times 10^{-5}$<br>$4.5 \times 10^{-5}$ | <br>7.40<br>7.35<br>7.35 |
| Intracellular fluid | $1 \times 10^{-3}$ to $4 \times 10^{-5}$ | 6.0–7.4 |
| Urine | $3 \times 10^{-2}$ to $1 \times 10^{-5}$ | 4.5–8.0 |
| Gastric HCl | 160 | 0.8 |

- Proper pH is required for delivery of oxygen to the tissues.
- pH can influence the immune functions of the body by modulating the antimicrobial peptides, immune cell migration, etc.
- pH of the gastrointestinal fluids varying from 2 to 8 in different parts of the GIT, helps in proper digestion of the food.

## REGULATION OF pH OF THE BODY FLUIDS

Body is constantly under a threat of an imbalance between the acid-base balance as a large amount of acid is produced daily due to the ongoing metabolic activities in the body as well as due to the dietary intake of proteins. The pH regulation is primarily done by a balance of activity of kidneys and lungs. The $HCO_3^-$ concentration is regulated mainly by the kidneys, whereas the $PCO_2$ in extracellular fluid is controlled by the rate of respiration.

Acids produced can be divided in two types:
1. Volatile acids
2. Nonvolatile acids

### Volatile Acids

Carbon dioxide ($CO_2$) is constantly produced in the body during the aerobic metabolic activities and during oxidation of carbohydrates, fats and proteins.

$$CO_2 + H_2O \xrightarrow{\text{Carbonic anhydrase}} H_2CO_3 \longrightarrow HCO_3^- + H^+$$
$$\xleftarrow{\text{Acidosis}}$$

In acidosis, i.e., when there is increased production of H⁺ (due to metabolic causes) the reaction shifts to the left (as shown by the red arrow) with the production of $CO_2$, which is a volatile gas and can be easily exhaled out through the lungs.

### Nonvolatile Acids

- **Lactic acid** is produced as a by-product of anerobic metabolism in the body
- **Uric acid** is produced as a by-product of metabolism of nucleic acid
- **Sulphuric acid** and **Phosphoric acid** are produced by excess protein diet

These acids are also known as fixed acids and add approximately 50–100 mEq/L of H⁺ to our body which can lower the pH and disrupt all the enzymatic activities.

But this does not happen due to the presence of the various buffer mechanisms. A buffer is defined as a system that resists changes in pH when an acidic or basic substance is added to it. Buffers are composed of a weak acid and its conjugate base (or a weak base and its conjugate acid) that can react with hydrogen ions (H⁺) or hydroxide ions (OH⁻) to maintain a relatively constant pH. Buffers are essential in biological systems to maintain the pH within a narrow range, which is crucial for proper enzyme function, cellular processes, and overall homeostasis.

There are three main buffer systems present in our body that regulate the acid-base balance and maintain a strict blood pH around 7.4.

These are as follows **(Table 7.2)**:
- Blood buffer system
- Respiratory buffer system
- Renal buffer system

## ROLE OF LUNGS AND KIDNEYS IN pH REGULATION

### Role of Lungs

- When the $CO_2$ levels are altered due to metabolic causes **(Fig. 7.1)**.
- When the $CO_2$ levels are not affected by metabolism. The patient is having the respiratory stimulation or depression **(Fig. 7.2)**.

Hence, it becomes clear that the primary lung disorders can result in acid-base disorders. In these conditions the kidneys remain the sole mechanism to combat the pH derangements.

### Role of Kidneys

Kidneys play an important and strong buffer system which balances the bicarbonate and H⁺ through three important buffer systems (discussed above). Our body produces 80 mEq/d of nonvolatile acids, which cannot be excreted

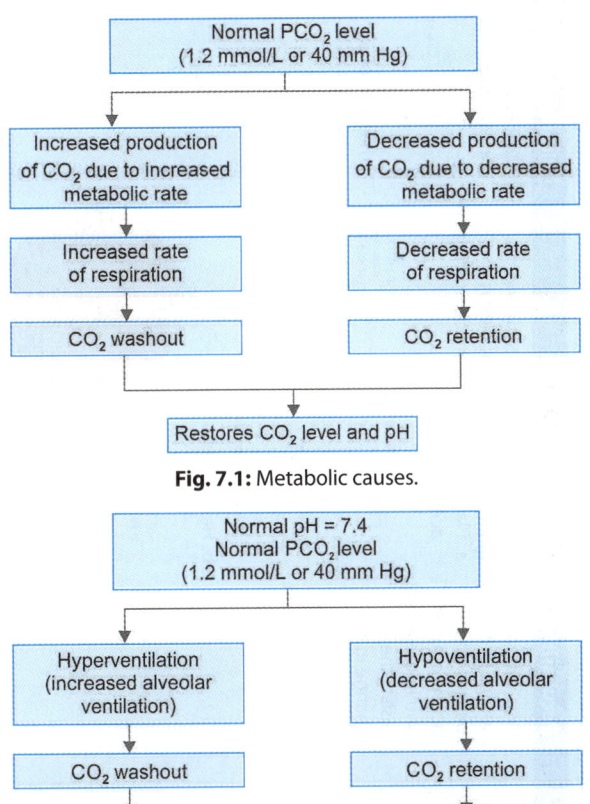

**Fig. 7.1:** Metabolic causes.

**Fig 7.2:** Respiratory causes.

**Table 7.2:** Details of buffer systems.

| Blood buffer system | Peculiarities | Protein buffer | Bicarbonate buffer | Phosphate buffer | Ammonia buffer |
|---|---|---|---|---|---|
| | Acts within seconds and binds with the acid produced and immediately resists the change in the pH | Include the plasma proteins and the buffering effect of hemoglobin<br>a. Plasma proteins are made up of amino acids<br><br>1) pH <7.35 (Acidosis) ↓pH ↑H⁺ — H⁺ + NH₂ → NH₃ (Correction of acidosis)<br>R—C—COOH<br>2) pH >7.45 (Alkalosis) ↑pH and ↓H⁺ — COO⁻ + H⁺ → ↑H⁺ (Correct alkalosis)<br><br>b. Hemoglobin<br>RBC: $CO_2 + H_2O$ → $H_2CO_3$ → $H^+ + HCO_3^-$<br>(The H⁺ binds of NH₂ group of globin protein) Attachment of H⁺ results in Bohr's effect<br>In lungs: $H \cdot Hb + O_2 → HbO_2 + H^+$<br>$H^+ + HCO_3^-$<br>$H_2CO_3$<br>$CO_2 + H_2O$<br>Excreted out | Most important buffer in the **Extracellular fluid** compartment<br><br>$CO_2 + H_2O \xrightarrow{\text{Carbonic anhydrase}} H_2CO_3 \rightarrow HCO_3^- + H^+$<br><br>It has a pK of 6.1 | Most important buffer in the **renal tubular fluid** and **intracellular** compartment<br>Excretes the H⁺ as $H_2PO_4^-$ which is a titratable acid<br>It has a pK of 6.8 | x |
| | Acts within few minutes Regulation is done by the respiratory centers resulting in hypoventilation or hyperventilation | x | pH <7.35 → Acidosis → Respiratory centers ⊕ → Hyperventilation → Washout of $CO_2$ → ↓$PCO_2$ → ↓$H_2CO_3$ → Correct acidosis | x | x |
| Renal buffer system | It is the most potent buffer as it leads to:<br>• Excretion of the H⁺<br>• Reabsorption of bicarbonate ($HCO_3^-$)<br>• Excretion of titratable acid | x | The bicarbonate buffer operates in PCT, thick ascending limb of loop of Henle and early DCT<br><br>Renal interstitial fluid — Tubular cells — Tubular lumen<br>K⁺/ATP/Na⁺ … $HCO_3^-$ + H⁺ ← $H_2CO_3$ ← Carbonic anhydrase ← $H_2O$ + $CO_2$ → $CO_2 + H_2O$<br>Na⁺ + $HCO_3^-$ | Renal interstitial fluid — Tubular cells — Tubular lumen<br>K⁺/ATP/Na⁺ … $HCO_3^-$ + H⁺ ← $H_2CO_3$ ← Carbonic anhydrase ← $H_2O$ + $CO_2$<br>Na⁺ + $NaHPO_4$ → H⁺ + $NaHPO_4$ → $NaH_2PO_4$ Excreted out<br>• When the H⁺ load becomes high enough to be handled alone by the bicarbonate buffer, the phosphate | Renal interstitial fluid — Proximal tubular cells — Tubular lumen<br>Glutamine → Glutamine → 2$HCO_3^-$ + 2$NH_4$ → $NH_4^+$ + Na⁺ → $NH_4^+$ + Cl⁻<br>• Glutamine enters the PCT, which gets metabolized to form two new |

*Contd...*

# CHAPTER 7: Acid-base Balance

Contd...

| Peculiarities | Protein buffer | Bicarbonate buffer | Phosphate buffer | Ammonia buffer |
|---|---|---|---|---|
| • Excretion of ammonium ion ($NH_4^+$) | × | In PCT, it handles the $H^+$ excretion from kidneys by:<br>• Sodium ion reabsorption in exchange for $H^+$ secreted<br>• Tubular reabsorption of $HCO_3^-$<br><br>*[Diagram: Type A intercalated cell showing $CO_2 + H_2O \to H_2CO_3 \to HCO_3^- + H^+$, with $H^+$ secreted into tubular lumen via ATP pump, $Cl^-$ exchange, and $K^+$ transport between renal interstitial fluid and tubular lumen]*<br><br>• In thick ascending limb of LOH and early DCT, active secretion of $H^+$ into the renal tubule | buffer takes up that extra load. The $H^+$ is removed by the $NaHPO^-$ in addition to bicarbonate buffer | bicarbonate ions and $NH_4^+$. The two bicarbonate ions are reabsorbed back into the blood while the $NH_4^+$ is secreted into lumen by $Na^+$-$NH_4^+$ exchanger. The $NH_4Cl$ is then excreted in the urine, removing the excess $H^+$<br><br>*[Diagram: Collecting tubular cells showing $CO_2 + H_2O \to H_2CO_3 \to HCO_3^- + H^+$ via Carbonic anhydrase; $NH_3$ diffuses into tubular lumen combining with $H^+$ to form $NH_4^+ + Cl^-$ excreted out; $Na^+/K^+$ ATP pump shown]*<br><br>• In collecting ducts, ammonia diffuses into the tubular lumen, where it reacts with secreted $H^+$ to form $NH_4^+$, which is then excreted in the urine<br>• For each $NH_4^+$ excreted, a new $HCO_3^-$ is formed in the tubular cells and returned to the blood<br>• The ammonia buffer is hence, the most potent buffer, which handles the pH of urine below 4.5<br>• The ammonia buffer aids the excretion of $H^+$ and formation of new $HCO_3^-$ – hence compliments the bicarbonate and phosphate buffer and increases the efficiency of renal buffer mechanism |

from lungs, hence the kidneys remain the mainstay for removing these acids. Kidneys use three basic mechanisms for pH regulation:
1. Secretion of $H^+$
2. Reabsorption of $HCO_3^-$
3. Formation of new $HCO_3^-$

The three buffer systems, discussed in **Table 7.1**, are:
1. **Bicarbonate buffer:** It is the most potent and basic buffer system, where the $CO_2$ combines with water to form $H_2CO_3$ in the presence of carbonic anhydrase, which further breaks down to form $H^+$ and $HCO_3^-$. The $HCO_3^-$ is reabsorbed back while $H^+$ is secreted into lumen by either of two ways:
   1. *$Na^+$-$H^+$ exchanger* in PCT. It can reduce the pH of tubular fluid to 6.7.
   2. *$H^+$ ATPase pump* in thick ascending limb of loop of Henle and Early DCT by the I cells (type A intercalated cells). Though it accounts for 5% of $H^+$ secretion, it is responsible for producing maximal acidic urine further reducing the tubular pH to 4.5.

> **FACTS**
> - 1 Liter of urine can excrete only 0.03 mEq of $H^+$.
> - To excrete 80 mEq of nonvolatile acids, 2,667 L of urine has to be passed.
> - Hence, to handle this excessive $H^+$ load, the other powerful buffer mechanisms come into play, such as phosphate and ammonia buffers.

2. **Phosphate buffer:** This buffer operates quite similar to bicarbonate buffer, but the $H^+$ instead of binding to filtered $HCO_3^-$, binds to phosphate ions ($NaHPO_4^-$). This leads to absorption of a new $HCO_3^-$ to the blood. *Under physiological limits, only 30–40 mEq/day of phosphates are available for $H^+$ buffering.*

3. **Ammonia buffer:** It is the most potent buffer systems out of all the renal buffer mechanisms. It results in the generation and reabsorption of new $HCO_3^-$. It operates in two different ways:
   1. ***In PCT, thick ascending limb of loop of Henle and early DCT:*** The glutamine enters the cells and gets metabolized through series of reactions to form two molecules of $HCO_3^-$ and $NH_4^+$. The $HCO_3^-$ is reabsorbed back into the blood, whereas the $NH_4^+$ is secreted into the tubules, which is excreted into the urine.
   2. ***In collecting ducts:*** The $H^+$ is secreted by the type A intercalated (I cells) into the tubular lumen. The $NH_3$ directly enters the lumen and combines with $H^+$ to form $NH_4^+$, which is excreted in urine.

## Changes in Urine during Acidosis

- The excessive $H^+$ results in complete absorption of $HCO_3^-$ and excessive excretion of $H^+$ in urine. This excessive $H^+$ can also be excreted as phosphate or ammonium salts.
- The chronic acidosis increases the $NH_4^+$ excretion.
- There is decrease in $HCO_3^-/H^+$ ratio of the tubular fluid.

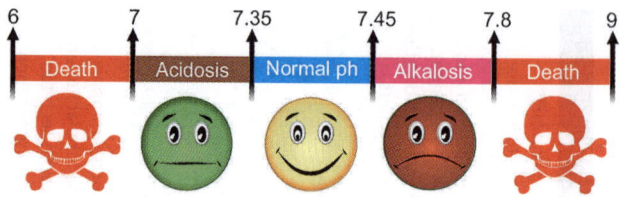

**Fig. 7.3:** Blood pH levels.

## Changes in ECF/Urine during Alkalosis

- Increase in ratio of $HCO_3^-/CO_2$ in extracellular fluid
- Increase in $HCO_3^-/H^+$ ratio of the tubular fluid

> **Renal tubular acidosis (RTA)**
> *Cause:* Defect in renal secretion of $H^+$ of reabsorption of $HCO_3^-$ or both occurring due to chronic renal failure, Addison's disease (aldosterone insufficiency), Fanconi's syndrome, etc.
> *Types:*
> - Impaired $HCO_3^-$ reabsorption
> - Impaired $H^+$ secretion into tubules
> 
> *Clinical findings:*
> - Decreased amount of net titratable acids in urine.
> - Increased acids in body fluids resulting in acidosis.

As discussed above, the pH of the blood is maintained between 7.35 and 7.45 by the above described regulatory buffer mechanisms. However, in certain metabolic or respiratory derangements the pH gets deranged resulting in the clinical conditions called as acidosis (pH <7.35) and alkalosis (pH >7.45) **(Fig. 7.3)**.

Depending on the cause of pH imbalance, the acidosis and alkalosis are further classified as respiratory and metabolic **(Table 7.3)**.

Various effects of acidosis and alkalosis are tabulated in **Table 7.4**.

## CLINICAL ASSESSMENT OF ACID-BASE BALANCE

- **Bicarbonate excretion:** It is calculated to find out the rate of removal of $HCO_3^-$ from blood. It is calculated as: *Urine flow rate × Urinary bicarbonate concentration*
- **Amount of new $HCO_3^-$ contributed to the blood:** It can be calculated by estimating the amount of secreted $H^+$ bound to nonbicarbonate urinary buffers.
- **pH of the blood:** The pH of the blood is measured to determine normal pH, acidosis or alkalosis.
- **Plasma $PCO_2$ and $HCO_3^-$ concentration:** Normal value of pH is 7.35–7.40, $H^+$ concentration is 40 mE/L, $PCO_2$ is 40 mm Hg and $HCO_3^-$ is 24 mEq/L. The levels of $PCO_2$ and $HCO_3^-$ in respiratory and metabolic pH disturbances is shown in table below:

|  | pH | $H^+$ | $PCO_2$ | $HCO_3^-$ |
|---|---|---|---|---|
| Normal | 7.4 | 40 mEq/L | 40 mm Hg | 24 mEq/L |
| Respiratory acidosis | ↓ | ↑ | ↑↑ | ↑ |
| Respiratory alkalosis | ↑ | ↓ | ↓↓ | ↓ |
| Metabolic acidosis | ↓ | ↑ | ↓ | ↓↓ |
| Metabolic alkalosis | ↑ | ↓ | ↑ | ↑↑ |

**Table 7.3:** Summary of respiratory/metabolic acidosis and alkalosis.

| | | Acidosis | Alkalosis |
|---|---|---|---|
| Respiratory | Causes | There is accumulation of $H^+$ due to **respiratory depression**, as the patient is not able to eliminated $CO_2$ from the body | There is excessive $HCO_3^-$ in the blood due to $CO_2$ wash out which occurs, when the patient is **hyperventilating** |
| | Compensatory mechanism | The kidneys excrete the excessive $H^+$ in urine | The kidneys decreases the $H^+$ excretion in urine, hence conserves it |
| Metabolic | Causes | • There is **excessive production** of nonvolatile acids due to metabolic disturbances. This leads to increased production of $H^+$ in the body<br>• **Ingestion** of acidic substances<br>• **Vomiting from deeper GIT** | • There is excessive $H^+$ loss resulting in $HCO_3^-$ excess in blood<br>• **Excessive vomiting** resulting in loss of $H^+$<br>• **Ingestion of alkali** |
| | Compensatory mechanism | Induces **hyperventilation** to remove the excessive $CO_2$ and hence tries to restore the pH | Causes respiratory depression, which can cause symptoms such as dizziness, lightheadedness, tingling sensations, and muscle cramps due to decreased levels of $CO_2$ in the blood |

**Table 7.4:** Effect of acidosis and alkalosis of different organs and physiological functions.

| | Acidosis | Alkalosis |
|---|---|---|
| **Cardiovascular system** | Decreased cardiac contractility, vasodilation, impaired response to catecholamines (which can result in decreased blood pressure and reduced tissue perfusion.) | • Decreased $Ca^{2+}$ levels in the blood, which may cause cardiac arrhythmias, muscle spasms, and tetany<br>• Vasoconstriction may result in increased blood pressure and reduced tissue perfusion |
| **Central nervous system** | Altered mental status, confusion, lethargy, and coma in severe cases | Altered neuronal excitability and neurotransmitter function, causing irritability, restlessness, confusion, and seizures. May also lead to decreased cerebral blood flow, exacerbating neurological symptoms |
| **Renal system** | Increase the excretion of hydrogen ions and reabsorb more bicarbonate ions to help regulate pH levels | • Reduces bicarbonate reabsorption and increase hydrogen ion excretion to help normalize pH levels<br>• Chronic alkalosis may lead to renal potassium wasting and hypokalemia, which can affect muscle function and lead to cardiac arrhythmias |
| **Musculo skeletal system** | • Muscle weakness and fatigue may occur due to impaired muscle contraction<br>• Chronic acidosis may also contribute to conditions such as osteoporosis by promoting the loss of calcium from bones to buffer the excess acid in the body | • Hypocalcemia resulting from alkalosis can lead to muscle cramps, tetany, and spasms<br>• Alkalosis also affects bone health by promoting calcium excretion, potentially leading to osteoporosis over time |
| **Gastro intestinal system** | • Nausea, vomiting, and abdominal pain<br>• Affects the absorption of nutrients and electrolytes in the intestines, leading to nutritional deficiencies and electrolyte imbalances | • Nausea, vomiting, and abdominal pain<br>• It interferes with digestion and nutrient absorption in the intestines |
| **Metabolism** | • Decreased glycolysis (due to increased insulin resistance), which in turn leads to increased gluconeogenesis (due to increased secretion of glucagon)<br>• Increased ketogenesis, increased protein catabolism<br>• Increased lipolysis as alternate substrates for energy | • Increased glycolysis (due to increased insulin sensitivity)<br>• Decreased secretion of glucagon causes decreased gluconeogenesis and glycogenolysis<br>• Decreased ketogenesis, decreased protein catabolism<br>• Inhibits lipolysis |
| **Management** | • Large amount of sodium bicarbonate or ammonium chloride is ingested by mouth<br>• Intravenous infusion of sodium lactate and sodium gluconate | |

- **Anion gap:** The anion gap represents *the difference between the measured cations (positively charged ions) and anions (negatively charged ions) in the blood plasma*. It is used to evaluate acid-base disorders, particularly metabolic acidosis.
  *The anion gap = $(Na^+ + K^+) - (Cl^- + HCO_3^-)$*
  In a normal state, the concentrations of cations and anions are balanced, resulting in a relatively low anion gap. *The normal anion gap ranges from 8–16 mEq/L.* However, when there's an excess of unmeasured anions, such as organic acids (e.g., lactate, ketones), the anion gap increases, indicating the presence of metabolic acidosis.

Conversely, some conditions can lead to a decreased anion gap, such as hypoalbuminemia or increased concentrations of unmeasured cations (e.g., hypercalcemia, hypermagnesemia).

If plasma $Cl^-$ increases in proportion to the fall in plasma $HCO_3^-$, the anion gap will remain normal. This is often referred to as *hyperchloremic metabolic acidosis. However, the normal anion gap, without the increase in $Cl^-$* levels can occur due to rise in other unmeasured anions.

Clinically, the anion gap is a valuable tool in diagnosing the underlying cause of metabolic acidosis (Ketoacidosis or lactic acidosis) and guiding appropriate treatment.

| Increased anion gap (normochloremia) | Normal anion gap (hyperchloremia) |
|---|---|
| Diabetes mellitus (ketoacidosis) | Diarrhea |
| Lactic acidosis | Renal tubular acidosis |
| Chronic renal failure | Carbonic anhydrase inhibitors |
| Aspirin (acetylsalicylic acid) poisoning | Addison's disease |
| Methanol poisoning | |
| Ethylene glycol poisoning | |
| Starvation | |

- **Acid-base nomogram (Fig. 7.4):** It is used for mixed acid-base disorder occurring due to two or more underlying causes. It can be used to predict type of pH disturbance as well as its severity. In this nomogram, we plot the following parameters pH, $HCO_3^-$ and $PCO_2$ after the full compensatory response to the disturbance has been established.

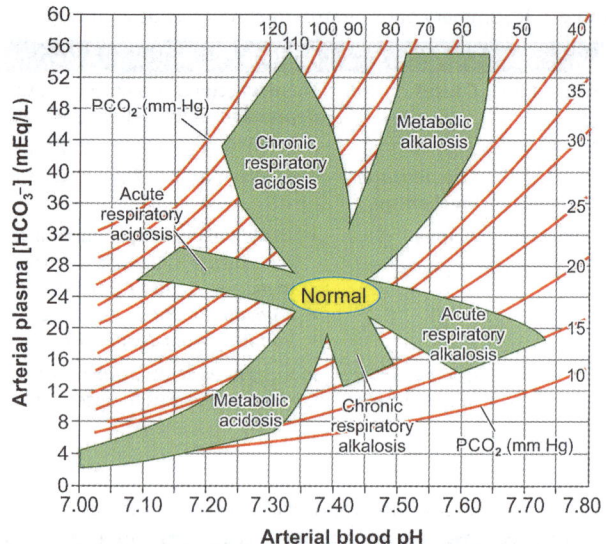

Fig. 7.4: Acid-base nomogram.

*Find out the type of respiratory disorder in the following conditions, using the acid-base nomogram:*

- pH = 7.30. Plasma $HCO_3^-$ concentration: 12 mEq/L, $PCO_2$ = 25 mm Hg
- pH = 7.15. Plasma $HCO_3^-$ concentration: 7 mEq/L, $PCO_2$ = 50 mm Hg
- pH = 7.60. Plasma $HCO_3^-$ concentration: 44 mEq/L, $PCO_2$ = 50 mm Hg

## SUMMARY

- pH is a measure of the acidity or alkalinity of a solution, representing the concentration of hydrogen ions ($H^+$) present. A lower pH indicates higher acidity, while a higher pH indicates higher alkalinity. Buffers are substances that resist changes in pH by accepting or donating hydrogen ions, helping to stabilize the pH of a solution.
- Buffers play a critical role in maintaining pH balance in biological systems. They can be categorized into two main types:
  1. Chemical buffers, such as bicarbonate, phosphate, and protein buffers, operate rapidly to minimize changes in pH by binding or releasing hydrogen ions.
  2. Physiological buffers, including the respiratory and renal systems, work more slowly but provide long-term regulation of pH by adjusting levels of carbon dioxide ($CO_2$) and bicarbonate ($HCO_3^-$) in the blood.
- The kidneys play a vital role in regulating acid-base balance by excreting hydrogen ions and reabsorbing bicarbonate ions. They also synthesize new bicarbonate ions and can generate ammonia to buffer excess acids. Renal regulation of acid-base balance is crucial for long-term pH homeostasis and complements the buffering capacity of other systems.
- Disruptions in pH balance can occur due to respiratory or metabolic factors:
  - Respiratory acidosis and alkalosis result from changes in carbon dioxide levels, leading to alterations in blood pH.
  - Metabolic acidosis and alkalosis stem from disturbances in bicarbonate levels or other metabolic processes, affecting blood pH.
- Understanding these derangements is essential for diagnosing and treating underlying conditions that cause acid-base imbalances.
- pH disturbances can impact numerous physiological processes:
  - **Enzyme activity:** Changes in pH can affect enzyme function, altering metabolic reactions.
  - **Respiratory and cardiovascular function:** pH imbalances can affect oxygen delivery, blood flow, and respiratory drive.
  - **Electrolyte balance:** pH disturbances can influence the distribution and regulation of electrolytes in the body.
  - **Nervous system function:** pH alterations can affect neuronal excitability and neurotransmitter release, impacting cognitive and motor function.
- Understanding the effects of pH disturbances on physiological processes is crucial for recognizing their clinical manifestations and guiding appropriate interventions.
- In conclusion, maintaining proper pH balance is essential for optimal physiological function, and disruptions can have far-reaching consequences on health. Understanding the mechanisms of pH regulation and the effects of pH disturbances is crucial for healthcare professionals in diagnosing, treating, and managing acid-base disorders.

# LET US SEE, HOW MUCH YOU HAVE LEARNT?

## Review Questions

Q1. Describe the significance of pH balance in biological systems and its importance for maintaining cellular function.

Q2. Explain how pH is regulated in the human body, considering the roles of buffers in respiratory system and kidneys.

Q3. Describe the mechanisms of action for two types of chemical buffers commonly found in the human body. Provide examples of how these buffers help maintain pH stability in different physiological environments.

Q4. Explain the concept of respiratory acidosis and respiratory alkalosis, including their causes, physiological effects, and potential treatments.

Q5. Compare and contrast metabolic acidosis and metabolic alkalosis in terms of their etiology, clinical manifestations, and diagnostic criteria. Describe the role of the kidneys in compensating for these acid-base disturbances.

Q6. What is the impact of pH disturbances on various physiological processes, including enzyme activity, respiratory function, electrolyte balance, and nervous system function?

Q7. Define a buffer and explain its role in maintaining pH stability.

Q8. Name two types of chemical buffers and describe how they function?

Q9. Briefly explain the role of the respiratory system in regulating pH balance.

Q10. What is the primary function of the kidneys in maintaining acid-base balance?

## Multiple Choice Questions

Q1. What does pH measure in a solution?
  a. Concentration of oxygen
  b. Concentration of hydrogen ions
  c. Concentration of carbon dioxide
  d. Concentration of bicarbonate ions

Q2. Which of the following is NOT a type of chemical buffer in the body?
  a. Bicarbonate buffer      b. Phosphate buffer
  c. Protein buffer          d. Respiratory buffer

Q3. What is the primary function of a buffer in biological systems?
  a. To regulate blood pressure
  b. To maintain electrolyte balance
  c. To stabilize pH levels
  d. To promote enzyme activity

Q4. Which system in the body helps regulate pH by adjusting carbon dioxide levels in the blood?
  a. Respiratory system      b. Renal system
  c. Endocrine system        d. Digestive system

Q5. A patient is hyperventilating due to anxiety. What acid-base disturbance is likely to occur?
  a. Respiratory acidosis    b. Respiratory alkalosis
  c. Metabolic acidosis      d. Metabolic alkalosis

Q6. Which of the following is a characteristic of metabolic acidosis?
  a. Decreased blood pH and increased bicarbonate levels
  b. Increased blood pH and decreased bicarbonate levels
  c. Decreased blood pH and decreased bicarbonate levels
  d. Increased blood pH and increased bicarbonate levels

Q7. A patient presents with vomiting and dehydration. What acid-base disturbance is likely to occur?
  a. Respiratory acidosis    b. Respiratory alkalosis
  c. Metabolic acidosis      d. Metabolic alkalosis

Q8. Which of the following physiological processes is NOT affected by pH disturbances?
  a. Enzyme activity         b. Respiratory function
  c. Electrolyte balance     d. Hormonal regulation

Q9. A patient with chronic kidney disease exhibits increased retention of hydrogen ions. What acid-base disturbance is likely to occur?
  a. Respiratory acidosis    b. Respiratory alkalosis
  c. Metabolic acidosis      d. Metabolic alkalosis

Q10. What is the main mechanism by which the kidneys regulate acid-base balance?
  a. Excreting bicarbonate ions
  b. Retaining hydrogen ions
  c. Adjusting carbon dioxide levels
  d. Excreting ammonia

Q11. A patient is admitted to the emergency department with symptoms of acute respiratory distress. Arterial blood gas analysis reveals a pH of 7.30, a partial pressure of oxygen ($PaO_2$) of 60 mm Hg, a partial pressure of carbon dioxide ($PaCO_2$) of 50 mm Hg, and a bicarbonate ($HCO_3^-$) level of 24 mEq/L. Using the acid-base nomogram, what is the most likely acid-base disturbance in this patient?
  a. Metabolic acidosis      b. Respiratory acidosis
  c. Respiratory alkalosis   d. Metabolic alkalosis

## ANSWERS

1. b   2. d   3. c   4. a   5. b   6. c   7. d   8. d   9. c   10. b   11. c

# Membrane Potentials of Excitable Tissues

**CHAPTER 8**

**COMPETENCY ADDRESSED**

**PY1.8:** Describe and discuss the molecular basis of resting membrane potential and action potential in excitable tissue.

**LEARNING OBJECTIVES**

At the end of this chapter, the learner should be able to:
- Define and describe diffusion potential.
- Define and describe Nernst potential.
- Explain molecular basis of resting membrane potential.
- Explain molecular basis of action potential in nerve fiber.

Excitable tissues are the one which can be stimulated by electrical, mechanical or chemical stimulus to produce a response. These excitable tissues can be classified as:
- Nervous tissue
- Muscular tissue: Skeletal muscle, cardiac muscle and smooth muscle
- Secretory cells

The excitability of these tissues depends on the voltage/potential difference across the cell membrane. Look at the unequal distribution of ions across the cell membrane:

This unequal distribution of ions across the cell membrane is due to *Gibbs-Donnan effect* (**Fig. 8.1**), which states that, '*in the presence of a nondiffusible ion, the concentration of diffusible ions is redistributed in a predictable way*' (**Figs. 8.2A and B**).

## RESTING MEMBRANE POTENTIAL

Resting membrane potential (RMP) is defined as the *potential difference across the cell membrane when the cell is **not stimulated**.*

### Reason for RMP

Cell membrane is selectively permeable for different ions, creating nonuniform distribution of ions across the

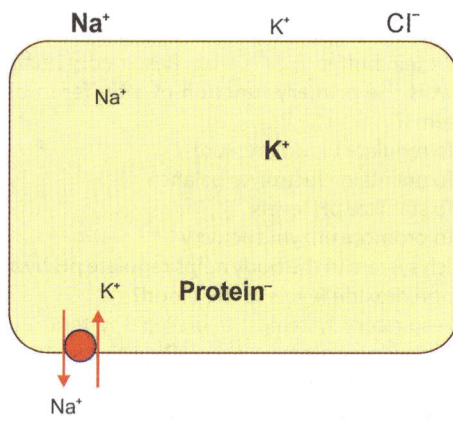

**Fig. 8.1:** Distribution of ions in ECF and ICF at rest. (**Note:** The size of font represents the concentration of the ion in that compartment).

cell membrane generates potential difference across the membrane. It is known as membrane potential.

Let's perform an experiment for understanding the concept of membrane potential (**Fig. 8.3**). In this experiment we have solution A and solution B. These solutions are separated by a selectively permeable membrane for K$^+$. We took 4 mmol KCl in solution A and 155 mmol KCl in solution B. In this way, solution A and solution B, are equivalent of K$^+$ composition in ECF and ICF, respectively. We have also added mannitol in solution

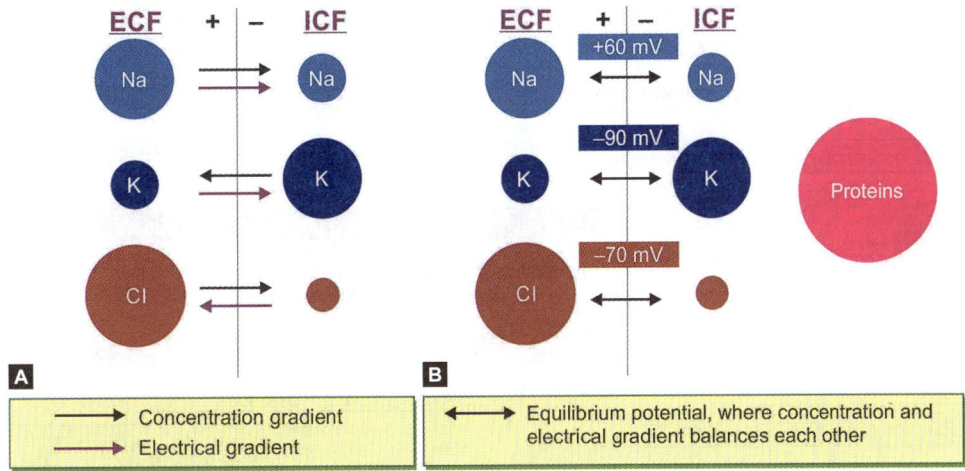

**Figs. 8.2A and B:** (A) Movement of diffusible ions according to concentration and electrical gradient; (B) Resultant equilibrium potential of each ion.

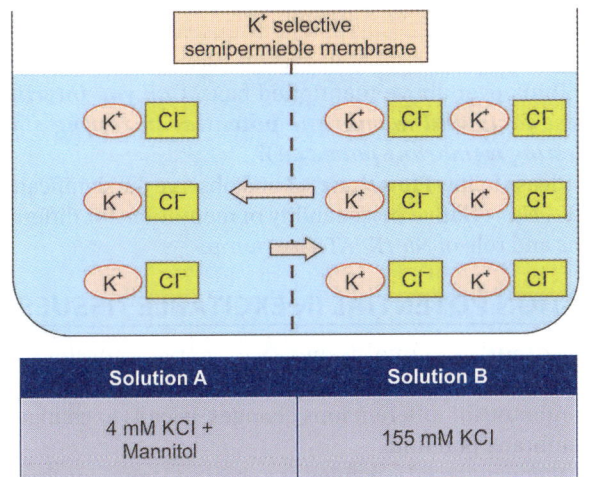

**Fig. 8.3:** An experiment showing the concept of resting membrane potential across the semipermeable membrane separating solution A and B.

A. This is to avoid osmotic movement of water across the membrane. Now let's think about the movement of $K^+$ ion across the membrane. *What are the forces which will regulate the movement of $K^+$?*

In previous chapters, we have studied that movement ion is controlled by electrochemical gradient. Now, just apply this concept on $K^+$. In starting, $K^+$ diffuses along it's concentration gradient, from solution B to solution A. *What would be the effect of this initial $K^+$ ions movement on the net charge in solution A and solution B?*

In solution B, because there is no diffusion of $Cl^-$ ions across the membrane, the concentration of $Cl^-$ ions would be more as compared to $K^+$. On the other hand, in solution concentration of $K^+$ would become more as compared to $Cl^-$ ion concentration. This ionic distribution would create electronegativity in solution A and electropositivity in solution B. As this potential difference is created due to diffusion of ion, it is known as *diffusion potential*. This potential difference would apply electrical force on $K^+$ from solution A to solution B, i.e., opposite to concentration gradient. Finally, at certain potential difference, when magnitude of both these opposite forces would become equal diffusion will stop, *equilibrium potential*. This potential is known as *Nernst potential* for the ion.

Experimentally, we can apply the same principle on mammalian cell for various ions. But the requirement will remain the same, i.e., the membrane should be permeable for particular ion. For example, if we take an example of nerve fiber and observe the Nernst potential for $K^+$, the Nernst potential is described by the following equation, known as Nernst equation:

$$\text{Nernst potential for } K^+ \text{ (mV)} = \pm 61 \times \text{Log} \frac{\text{Concentration of } K^+ \text{ in intracellular fluid}}{\text{Concentration of } K^+ \text{ in extracellular fluid}}$$

**Effect of multiple ions on membrane potential- Goldman-Hodgkin Katz Equation:**

In the previous we discussed about the diffusion potential which generates due to diffusion of one particular ion. We also followed a condition that the membrane should be permeable for that particular ion. But, most of the times, reality does not follow this limitation. Mostly, cell membrane is permeable for multiple types of ions. Of course, permeability of membrane might be different for various ions. *What will be scenario in this condition? Let's think....*As per the electromotive forces, diffusion of ions will take place. And finally, at certain membrane potential net current across the membrane will become zero. *This zero current represents an equilibrium state, when there would be no further diffusion of ions across the membrane.*

**Flowchart 8.1:** Significance of K⁺, Na⁺, relative permeability of membrane for different ions.

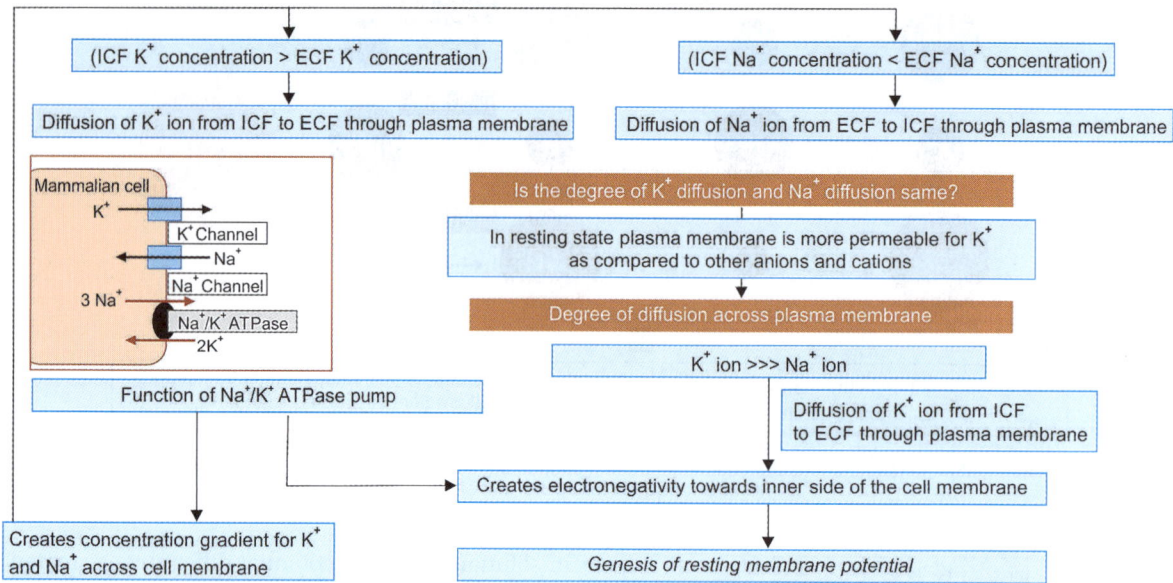

What do you that, in this equilibrium state, when multiple ions are involved, what are the factors on which membrane potential depend?

As this equilibrium potential/membrane potential is the outcome of diffusion of ions it depends on these factors:
- Charge on the ion
- Concentration of ions across the membrane
- Permeability of membrane for the ion. Goldman-Hodgkin Katz Equation takes account of all these factors and gives the membrane potential.

Let's take the example of any mammalian cell. Here, Ions under consideration are Na⁺, K⁺ and Cl⁻. ***Goldman-Hodgkin Katz Equation*** for the membrane potential for nerve fiber is:

Membrane potential (Millivolts) = $-61 \times \text{Log} \dfrac{C_{Na^+ in} P_{Na^+} + C_{K^+ in} P_{K^+} + C_{Cl^- o} P_{Cl^-}}{C_{Na^+ o} P_{Na^+} + C_{K^+ o} P_{K^+} + C_{Cl^- in} P_{Cl^-}}$

where
- $C_{Na^+ in}$ – Na⁺ in intracellular fluid
- $C_{Na^+ o}$ – Na⁺ in extracellular fluid
- $C_{K^+ in}$ – K⁺ in intracellular fluid
- $C_{K^+ o}$ – K⁺ in extracellular fluid
- $P_{Na^+}$ – Permeability of plasma membrane for Na⁺ ion
- $P_{K^+}$ – Permeability of plasma membrane for Na⁺ ion

This membrane potential is actually intracellular potential as reference to extracellular potential.

**Origin of resting membrane potential in excitable cell:**
Let's take example of nerve fiber.
- Due to leaky channels plasma membrane is relatively more permeable for K⁺ (as compared to other ions).
- **Ionic concentration:**
  - Na⁺ (ICF)—14 mEq/L; Na⁺ (ECF)—142 mEq/L
  - K⁺ (ICF)—140 mEq/L; K⁺ (ECF)—4 mEq/L
- Na⁺/K⁺ ATPase pump pumps three Na⁺ outside and two K⁺ ion inside the cell. So it is electrogenic in nature.

Think over above mentioned facts. *Can you interlink these facts and membrane potential in resting state (Resting membrane potential)?*

Please follow **Flowchart 8.1** and observe the significance of K⁺, Na⁺, relative permeability of membrane for different ions and role of Na⁺/K⁺ ATPase pump.

## ACTION POTENTIAL IN EXCITABLE TISSUES

In various excitable tissues (e.g., nerve, muscles), on appropriate stimulation, the permeability of plasma membrane for different ions changes. It leads to change in membrane potential.

Action potential is defined as a short and transient change in membrane potential after stimulation, which follows all or none principle and gets transmitted along the membrane.

### Physiological Basis of Nerve Action Potential

See **Figure 8.4, Table 8.1**.

### Phases of Action Potential

See **Figure 8.5, Table 8.1**.

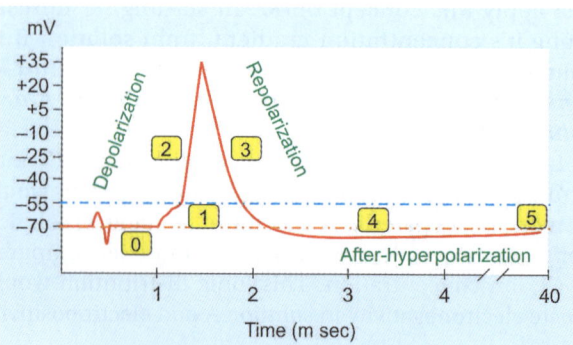

**Fig. 8.4:** Nerve action potential.

**Table 8.1:** Phases of action potential.

| Phase | Name | Physiological basis | Explanation |
|---|---|---|---|
| 0 | Resting potential | Mechanism already explained | The difference in the concentration of the ions across the cell membrane creates the electrical gradient (polarity) across the cell membrane. The intracellular and extracellular compartments behave as two poles. Hence, in this state cell membrane is termed as *polarized* |
| 1 | Local response | Stimulation opens limited number of $Na^+$ channel which, due to inflow of $Na^+$ ions, raises membrane potential up to threshold potential | Increase in the intracellular voltage below threshold |
| 2 | Rapid depolarization | Raising membrane potential up to threshold lead to further opening of many more number of $Na^+$ channel which are governed by positive feedback mechanism known as Hodgkin's cycle (Refer **Figure 8.6**) | Rapid increase in intracellular voltage above threshold voltage resulting in the action potential. It occurs either due to increase in positive ions inside the cells, due to $Na^+/Ca^{2+}$ influx or blockage of $K^+$ efflux |
| 3 | Repolarization | After attaining peak of depolarization, $Na^+$ channels starts to get close and $K^+$ channel starts to open which leads to out flow of $K^+$ ion. In this way membrane potential reaches up to resting membrane potential. During later part of depolarization voltage-gated $K^+$ channel starts to get close slowly | Decrease in intracellular voltage from the spike potential to RMP, is termed as *repolarization*. It occurs due to loss of intracellular positive ion/decrease in voltage. Increased $K^+$ efflux, results in repolarization |
| 4 | After hyperpolarization | Due to slow closure of $K^+$ channels, some extra $K^+$ ions leave the cell and further depolarize the cell | Decrease in the intracellular voltage below the RMP, i.e., increased electronegativity of cell is called as *hyperpolarization*. It occurs due to continued $K^+$ efflux |
| 5 | Attaining resting membrane potential | $Na^+/K^+$ ATPase pump activity bring back ion distribution to normal and membrane potential again attains resting membrane potential | The restoration of intracellular voltage to RMP due to continuous pumping of $Na^+/K^+$ ATPase pump and decreased permeability of the membrane to $K^+$ efflux |

**Note:** This entire concept of membrane potential is based on voltage change across the cell membrane. To understand, the difference in voltage/potential difference, across the cell membrane, at rest is called **as resting membrane potential.** This is due to unequal ionic distribution.

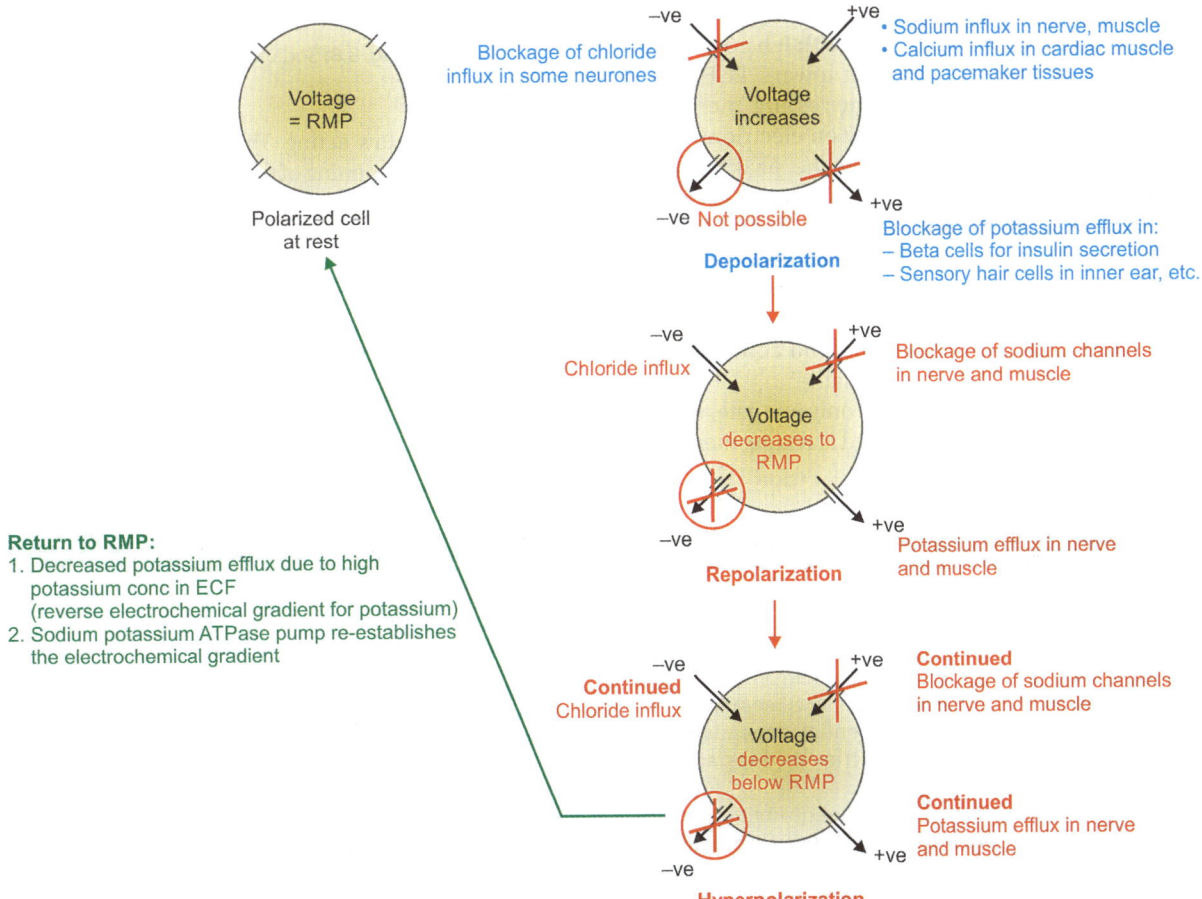

**Fig. 8.5:** Physiological basis of electrical changes in excitable tissues resulting in different phases of action potential.

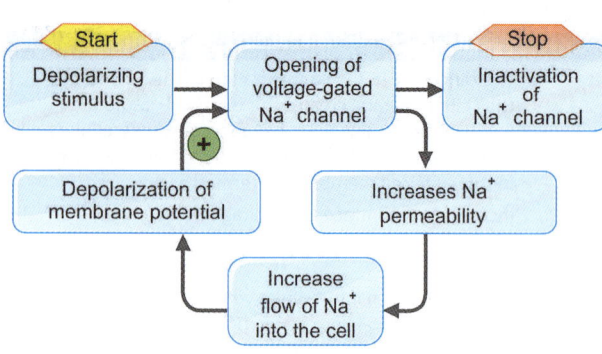

Fig. 8.6: Hodgkin's cycle.      Fig. 8.7: Voltage-gated K⁺ channel.

## Feedback Regulation of Voltage-gated Na⁺ Channel (Hodgkin's Cycle)

See **Figure 8.6**.

## Feedback Regulation of Voltage-gated K⁺ Channel

See **Figure 8.7**.

## Mechanism of Activation and Inactivation of Voltage-gated Na⁺ and K⁺ Channels

- **Voltage-gated Na⁺ channel (Fig. 8.8):** It has two gates:
  1. *Activation gate:* It is present toward ECF side of channel. It remains close at resting membrane potential. It gets open *rapidly* on electric stimulus. It remains open till attaining the peak of action potential. During depolarization phase, it closes and attains its starting position.
  2. *Inactivation gate:* It is present towards the ICF side of the channel. It remains open at the resting membrane potential. It is slow acting. It slowly starts to close during depolarization and completely get closed at peak of action potential.
- **Voltage-gated K⁺ channel:** It has only one gate, which is towards ICF side. It remains closed at resting membrane

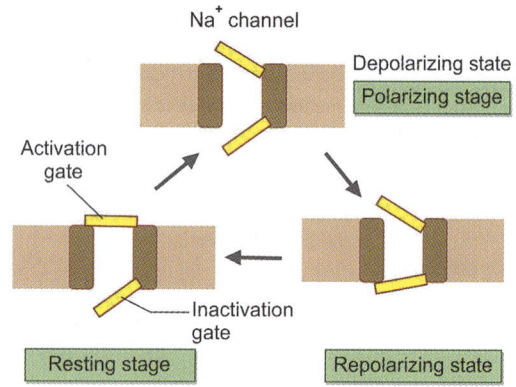

Fig. 8.8: Sodium channel.

potential. It is slow acting. The depolarization to cell is the stimulus for opening of this gate. It opens completely at peak of action potential and during late phase of depolarization, it starts to close *slowly*. It is slow closing allow extra K⁺ ion out of the cell and lead to after hyperpolarization.

## Cyclic Activity of Voltage-gated Na⁺ and K⁺ Channel during Action Potential

See **Figure 8.9**.

---

### SUMMARY

- Diffusion potential refers to the electrical potential difference across a membrane that arises from the unequal distribution of ions. This potential develops when ions move down their concentration gradient through ion channels, generating a net movement of charge across the membrane. The magnitude of the diffusion potential depends on the concentration gradient of the permeant ions and their respective permeabilities.
- The Nernst potential, also known as the equilibrium potential, is the membrane potential at which the electrochemical gradient for a specific ion is balanced, resulting in no net movement of that ion across the membrane. The Nernst equation calculates the equilibrium potential for a given ion based on its intra- and extracellular concentrations, as well as the charge on the ion.
- The resting membrane potential (RMP) is the steady electrical potential difference across the plasma membrane of excitable cells, such as neurons and muscle cells, in the absence of stimulation. The RMP is primarily maintained by the unequal distribution of ions across the membrane, with higher

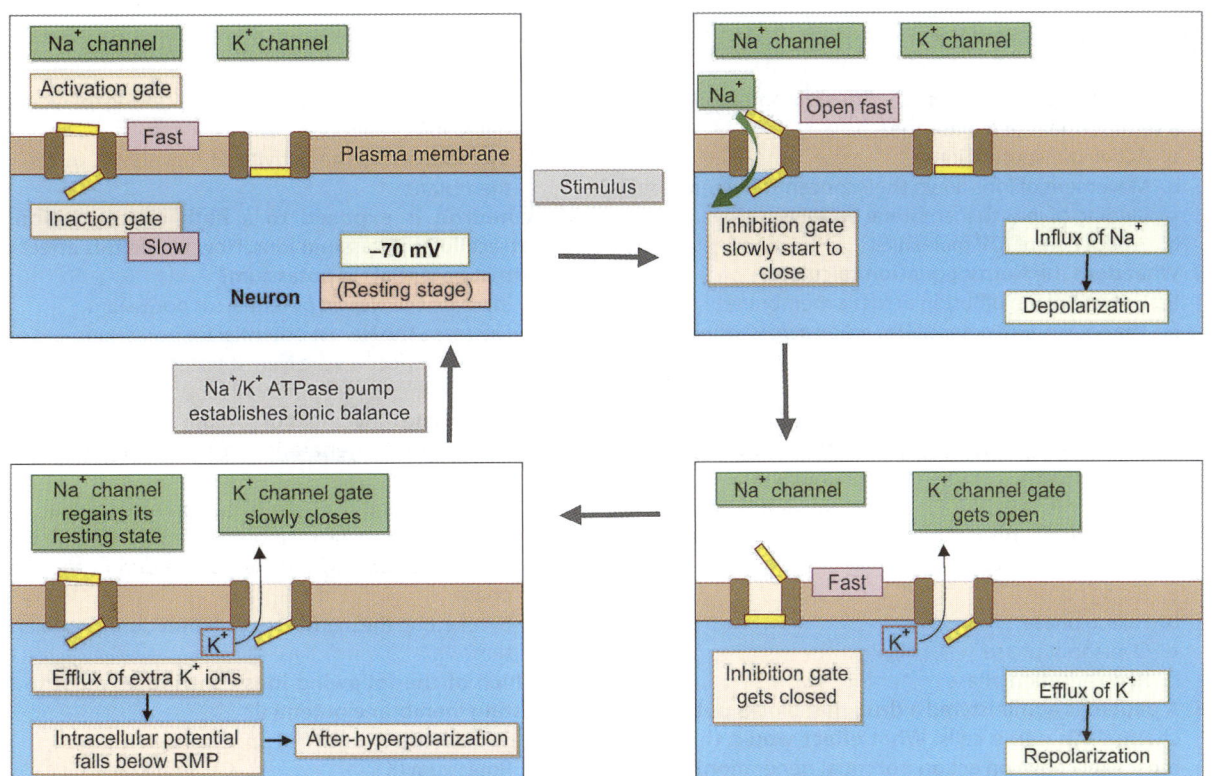

**Fig. 8.9:** Cyclic activity of voltage-gated Na+ and K+ channel.

concentrations of sodium (Na⁺) and chloride (Cl⁻) outside the cell and higher concentrations of potassium (K⁺) inside the cell. This uneven distribution of ions is established and maintained by ion pumps, such as the sodium-potassium ATPase pump, and ion channels, which selectively permit the movement of ions based on their electrochemical gradients.

- Action potential is a transient reversal of the membrane potential that propagates along the length of excitable cells, such as neurons. The molecular basis of action potential involves a sequence of events, including depolarization, repolarization, and hyperpolarization. Depolarization occurs when voltage-gated sodium channels open, allowing an influx of sodium ions, leading to a rapid increase in membrane potential. Repolarization is driven by the opening of voltage-gated potassium channels, leading to potassium efflux and the restoration of the membrane potential towards its resting state. Hyperpolarization occurs briefly due to prolonged potassium efflux before the sodium-potassium ATPase pump restores the ionic balance.

- In summary, understanding membrane potentials, including diffusion potential, Nernst potential, resting membrane potential, and action potential, is essential for comprehending the electrical excitability and signal propagation in neurons and other excitable cells. These concepts provide the foundation for elucidating the complex mechanisms underlying neuronal communication and neural function.

## LET US SEE, HOW MUCH YOU HAVE LEARNT?

*Review Questions*

**Q1.** Explain diffusion potential and how it forms across a semipermeable membrane. Give examples and their significance in cells.

**Q2.** Describe the Nernst equation and how it calculates an ion's equilibrium potential. What factors affect it, and how is it used in neurons and muscles?

**Q3.** Explain how the resting membrane potential is established and maintained in excitable cells. Discuss ion pumps, ion channels, ion gradients, and the effects of their alterations.

**Q4.** Describe the events in generating and propagating an action potential along a nerve fiber. Include the roles of voltage-gated sodium and potassium channels in depolarization, repolarization, and hyperpolarization.

## Multiple Choice Questions

**Q1.** What is the primary cause of diffusion potential across a semipermeable membrane?
  a. Active transport of ions
  b. Movement of ions down their concentration gradient
  c. Binding of ions to membrane proteins
  d. Production of ATP molecules

**Q2.** What does the Nernst equation calculate?
  a. The rate of ion diffusion across a membrane
  b. The equilibrium potential for an ion across a membrane
  c. The resting membrane potential of a neuron
  d. The action potential threshold in a nerve fiber

**Q3.** Which of the following ions primarily contributes to the establishment of the resting membrane potential?
  a. Sodium ($Na^+$)  b. Potassium ($K^+$)
  c. Chloride ($Cl^-$)  d. Calcium ($Ca^{2+}$)

**Q4.** During which phase of the action potential does depolarization occur?
  a. Rising phase
  b. Falling phase
  c. Overshoot phase
  d. Repolarization phase

**Q5.** A patient is administered a drug that blocks potassium channels in nerve cells. What effect would this drug most likely have on action potential generation?
  a. Decreased action potential frequency
  b. Increased action potential duration
  c. Reduced action potential threshold
  d. Enhanced action potential propagation

**Q6.** How does the Nernst potential contribute to the resting membrane potential of a neuron?
  a. By establishing an electrical gradient for ion movement
  b. By balancing the influx and efflux of ions across the membrane
  c. By regulating the opening and closing of voltage-gated ion channels
  d. By modulating the activity of ion pumps in the cell membrane

**Q7.** A neuron is exposed to a high concentration of extracellular potassium ions. How would this affect the Nernst potential for potassium?
  a. Increase the Nernst potential for potassium
  b. Decrease the Nernst potential for potassium
  c. Have no effect on the Nernst potential for potassium
  d. Reverse the Nernst potential for potassium

**Q8.** How does the movement of sodium and potassium ions contribute to the generation of an action potential in a nerve fiber?
  a. By maintaining the resting membrane potential
  b. By depolarizing the membrane during the rising phase
  c. By hyperpolarizing the membrane during the falling phase
  d. By resetting the membrane potential during repolarization

**Q9.** Which of the following ions contributes most to the resting membrane potential?
  a. Sodium ($Na^+$)  b. Chloride ($Cl^-$)
  c. Potassium ($K^+$)  d. Calcium ($Ca^{2+}$)

**Q10.** What is the equilibrium potential for an ion?
  a. The potential at which the ion concentration is equal inside and outside the cell
  b. The potential at which there is no net movement of the ion across the membrane
  c. The potential at which the ion concentration is maximal inside the cell
  d. The potential at which the ion concentration is minimal inside the cell

### ANSWERS

**1.** b  **2.** b  **3.** b  **4.** a  **5.** b  **6.** b  **7.** a  **8.** b  **9.** c  **10.** b

# Applications of Cellular Physiology in Health and Research

**CHAPTER 9**

### COMPETENCY ADDRESSED
**PY1.9:** Methods used to demonstrate the functions of the cells and its products, its communication and their applications in clinical care and research.

### LEARNING OBJECTIVES
**At the end of this chapter, the learner should be able to:**
- Describe the methods used to demonstrate the functions of the cells and its products.
- Describe the methods used to demonstrate the cellular communications.

## METHODS USED TO DEMONSTRATE THE FUNCTIONS OF THE CELLS AND ITS PRODUCTS

### Microscopy Techniques

**Principle:** Microscopic techniques enable visualization of cellular structures and processes at various resolutions.

**Aim:** The Aim of microscopy techniques is to observe and analyze cellular morphology, organelle distribution, and protein localization within cells.

**Procedure:**
- Light microscopy (Fig. 9.1):
  - *Bright-field microscopy:* Cells are observed under a bright field, allowing visualization of cell morphology.
  - *Phase-contrast microscopy:* Utilizes phase shifts to enhance contrast in transparent specimens, facilitating visualization of organelle distribution.
  - *Fluorescence microscopy:* Fluorescent dyes label specific proteins within cells, enabling observation of protein localization.
- Electron microscopy (Fig. 9.2):
  - Utilizes electrons instead of light, providing higher resolution images.
  - Allows visualization of subcellular structures such as mitochondria, endoplasmic reticulum, and cell membranes.

**Results:** Microscopy techniques yield detailed images of cellular structures and processes, aiding in understanding cellular organization and function.

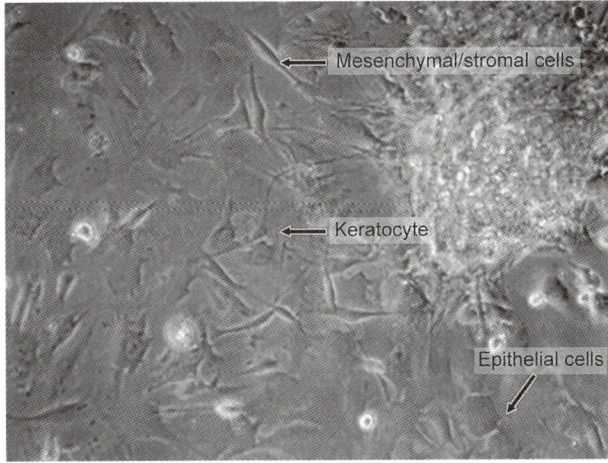

**Fig. 9.1:** Mouse eye cells observed under the light microscope showing mixed cell population of mesenchymal cells, keratocyte and epithelial cells.

**Utility in clinical practice:** Microscopy techniques are indispensable in clinical practice for:
- Diagnosis of cellular abnormalities such as irregular shape, size, and the arrangement of nuclei in malignancy.
- Monitoring disease progression at cellular and subcellular level.
- Studying cellular responses to treatments by localizing proteins.
- Advancing understanding of disease mechanisms as in Parkinsons disease, by using specific dyes, size, shape, and distribution of mitochondria is studied. Similarly

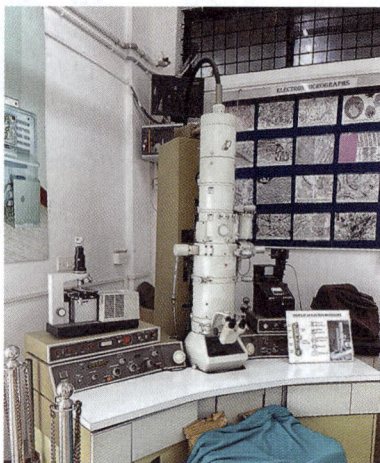

**Fig. 9.2:** A transmission electron microscope (TEM).

amyloid plaques and tau tangles are analyzed in Alzheimer's disease.

## Cell Fractionation and Biochemical Assays

**Principle:** Cell fractionation involves isolating various cellular components based on their size, density, or biochemical properties. Biochemical assays are then performed on these fractions to analyze cellular functions.

**Aim:** The Aim of cell fractionation and biochemical assays is to isolate cellular components and perform biochemical analyses to understand cellular functions such as enzymatic activities, metabolic pathways, and protein-protein interactions.

**Procedure:**
- **Cell component isolation:** Cellular components such as organelles or membranes are isolated through fractionation techniques.
- **Biochemical assays:**
  - *Enzyme activity assays:* Assess the activity levels of enzymes within isolated cellular fractions.
  - *Protein quantification:* Measure the concentration of proteins within the fractions.
  - *Metabolic profiling:* Analyze the metabolic pathways within the isolated fractions.

**Results:** Cell fractionation and biochemical assays yield insights into cellular functions by providing information on enzymatic activities, protein concentrations, and metabolic profiles within specific cellular components.

**Utility in clinical practice:** Cell fractionation and biochemical assays are valuable tools in clinical practice for:
- Understanding disease mechanisms at the cellular level, e.g., biochemical assays on lysosomal fractions can help understand diseases characterized by lysosomal storage, such as Tay-Sachs or Gaucher's disease.
- Identifying biomarkers for disease diagnosis and prognosis.
- Monitoring treatment responses by assessing changes in cellular function.

- Developing targeted therapies based on cellular pathways and interactions, e.g., targeting membrane proteins receptors or ion channels to alter cell signaling.

## Cell Culture and Cell-based Assays

**Principle:** Cell culture techniques enable the growth of cells *in vitro* under controlled conditions, providing a platform to study cellular processes in a controlled environment. Cell-based assays utilize cultured cells to assess cellular responses to various stimuli, drugs, or genetic manipulations.

**Aim:** The Aim of cell culture and cell-based assays is to manipulate and study cellular processes, assess cellular responses to different conditions, and gain insights into cell functions and signaling pathways.

**Procedure:**
- ***In vitro* growth conditions:** Cells are cultured *in vitro* under controlled conditions of temperature, humidity, and nutrient availability.
- **Cell-based assay types:**
  - *Proliferation assays:* The MTT (3-[4,5-dimethyl-thiazol-2-yl]-2,5 diphenyl tetrazolium bromide) assay is a colorimetric assay for measuring cell metabolic activity. It is based on the ability of nicotinamide adenine dinucleotide phosphate (NADPH)-dependent cellular oxidoreductase enzymes to reduce the tetrazolium dye MTT to its insoluble formazan, which has a purple color. It measures the rate of cell proliferation or growth under different conditions.
  - *Apoptosis assays:* 7-AAD, annexin V FITC and propidium iodide markers are used to assess the induction of programmed cell death in response to stimuli or treatments **(Fig. 9.3)**.
  - *Reporter gene assays:* Utilize reporter genes to monitor gene expression or cellular responses to specific stimuli.

**Results:** Cell culture and cell-based assays provide valuable information on cellular responses, proliferation rates,

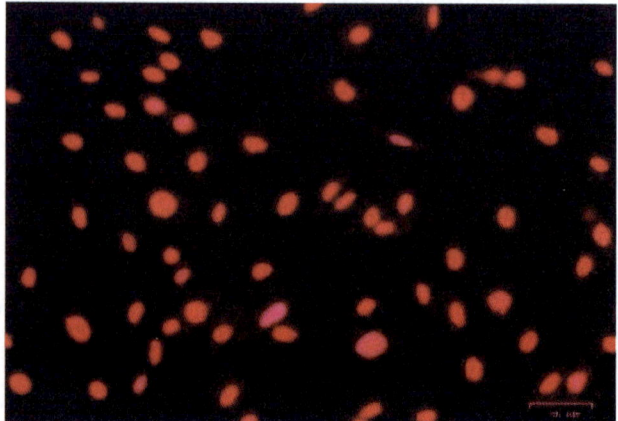

**Fig. 9.3:** Cells taking up red colored propidium iodide stain signifies dead cells.

apoptosis induction, and gene expression profiles under different conditions, contributing to our understanding of cellular functions and signaling pathways.

**Utility in clinical practice:** Cell culture and cell-based assays are crucial in clinical practice for:
- Screening potential drugs or therapeutics for efficacy and toxicity. For instance, the effectiveness of chemotherapeutic agents such as doxorubicin was extensively studied in various cancer cell lines before progressing to clinical trials. Similarly for products of cosmetic industry.
- Studying disease mechanisms and identifying therapeutic targets. For example, for instance, Vero cells (a type of kidney cell from African green monkeys) were used extensively to study SARS-CoV-2 replication and to test potential antiviral compounds.
- Advancing regenerative medicine and tissue engineering techniques. For example, techniques like CRISPR/Cas9. Scientists can introduce specific genetic changes into cultured cells and use cell-based assays to observe the outcomes on cellular behavior, protein expression, or disease phenotypes.

### Live Cell Imaging and Time-lapse Microscopy

**Principle:** Live cell imaging techniques enable the real-time visualization of dynamic cellular processes, including cell migration, cell division, and intracellular trafficking. Time-lapse microscopy facilitates the tracking of individual cells over time, offering insights into cell behavior and responses to stimuli.

**Aim:** The Aim of live cell imaging and time-lapse microscopy is to observe and analyze dynamic cellular processes, providing insights into cell behavior, interactions, and responses to environmental cues.

**Procedure:**
- **Real-time visualization techniques:** Utilize various imaging modalities such as fluorescence microscopy to observe dynamic cellular processes in real-time.
- **Long-term observation of cellular dynamics:** Employ time-lapse microscopy to capture images of cells at intervals over an extended period, allowing the tracking of individual cells and analysis of cellular dynamics.

**Results:** Live cell imaging and time-lapse microscopy yield valuable data on dynamic cellular processes, facilitating the understanding of cell behavior, interactions, and responses to stimuli.

**Utility in clinical practice:** Live cell imaging and time-lapse microscopy have significant utility in clinical practice for:
- Studying disease progression and treatment responses at the cellular level. For example, to monitor the movement of cancer cells in real time as they invade surrounding tissues or migrate through the body and response to chemotactic signals. Thus, is also useful in drug development and testing.

- Investigating cellular mechanisms underlying disease pathology. As in observing the formation of the mitotic spindle, alignment and separation of chromosomes, and cytokinesis. This is particularly valuable in genetic studies where mutations affecting these processes can be linked to diseases like cancer.
- Identifying potential targets for therapeutic intervention.

## METHODS USED TO DEMONSTRATE THE CELLULAR COMMUNICATIONS

### Molecular Biology Techniques

**Principle:** Molecular biology techniques involve the analysis of gene expression, protein levels, and post-translational modifications within cells. These techniques provide insights into transcriptional regulation, protein synthesis, and cellular signaling pathways.

**Aim:** The Aim of molecular biology techniques is to analyze gene expression and protein profiles to understand cellular functions and signaling pathways involved in various biological processes.

**Procedure:**
- **Gene expression analysis:**
  - Techniques are employed to quantify and analyze the expression levels of genes within cells.
  - ***RNA sequencing:*** Sequences RNA molecules to analyze gene expression patterns.
- **Protein analysis:**
  - Western blotting
  - Detects and quantifies specific proteins within cell lysates
  - Proteomics

**Results:** Molecular biology techniques yield valuable information on gene expression patterns, protein levels, and post-translational modifications within cells, providing insights into cellular functions and signaling pathways.

**Utility in clinical practice:** Molecular biology techniques play a critical role in clinical practice for:
- Identifying biomarkers for disease diagnosis and prognosis.
- Techniques like Western blotting, enzyme-linked immunosorbent assay (ELISA), and mass spectrometry are employed to measure protein levels in biological samples. These methods are fundamental in biomarker discovery, where specific proteins are associated with particular diseases. For example, increased levels of prostate-specific antigen (PSA) can be indicative of prostate cancer.
- Techniques such as quantitative PCR (qPCR) and RNA sequencing (RNA-seq) are used to analyze gene expression profiles in different types of cancer. By comparing the gene expression profiles of cancerous cells to those of normal cells, oncogenes can be identified. For instance, the identification of overexpressed HER2 in certain breast cancers.

- Monitoring disease progression and treatment responses at the molecular level.
- Developing targeted therapies based on molecular signatures. Techniques like flow cytometry and fluorescence microscopy are used to analyze signaling pathways by measuring the activation states of proteins involved in these pathways. For example, the use of fluorescent tags to visualize and measure the activity of kinases such as MAPK and PI3K helps in understanding the signaling mechanisms that control cell growth, division, and survival. Insights gained from these studies are crucial for developing drugs that target specific components of signaling pathways, such as kinase inhibitors in cancer therapy.

## Immunocytochemistry (ICC) and Immunohistochemistry (IHC) (Figs. 9.4 and 9.5)

**Principle:** Immunocytochemistry (ICC) and immunohistochemistry (IHC) involve targeting specific proteins within cells to visualize their localization and quantify their expression levels. ICC involves the staining of cells that have been fixed to a solid surface, such as a microscope slide or a culture dish. These cells are typically derived from cell cultures or cell suspensions.

IHC involves the staining of thin tissue sections obtained from formalin-fixed, paraffin-embedded (FFPE) tissue blocks or fresh-frozen tissue samples. This provides insights into protein function and cellular organization.

**Aim:** The Aim of ICC and IHC is to accurately label and detect specific proteins within cells/tissue, enabling their visualization and quantification.

**Procedure:**
- **Labeling techniques:** Antibodies conjugated to fluorescent probes or are used to target specific proteins within cells.
- **Applications in cellular analysis:**
    - The labeled proteins are visualized under a microscope to determine their localization within cells.
    - Quantification of protein expression levels is performed to analyze cellular processes and organization.

**Results:** Immunocytochemistry and immunofluorescence techniques provide detailed information on protein localization and expression levels within cells, contributing to our understanding of cellular function and organization.

**Utility in clinical practice:** Immunocytochemistry and immunofluorescence techniques have significant utility in clinical practice for:
- Identifying disease markers and cell signaling process within cells. For example, using these techniques to stain for proteins such as tau or beta-amyloid allows researchers to study their accumulation and the formation of pathological features like neurofibrillary tangles or plaques in Alzheimer's disease.
- Diagnosing diseases based on cellular abnormalities. ICC can be used to detect proteins involved in apoptosis,

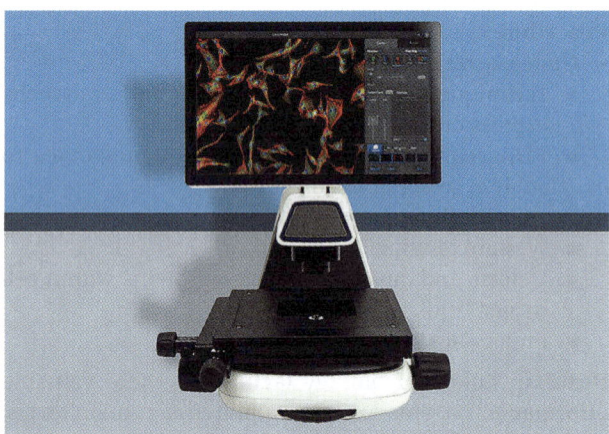

**Fig. 9.4:** A fluorescent microscope used to visualize live cells, fixed cells, tissue sections stained with fluorescent labeled antibodies.

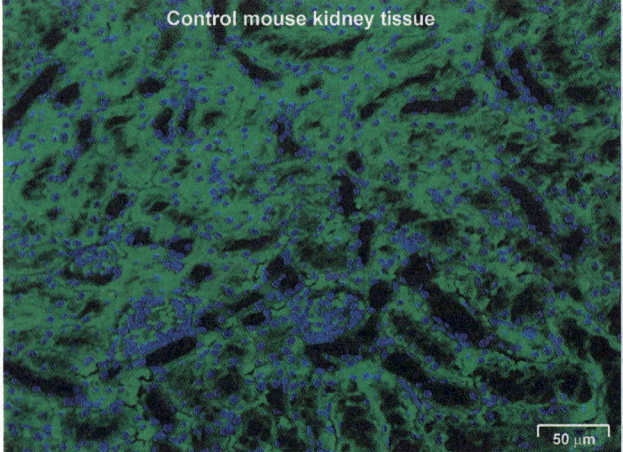 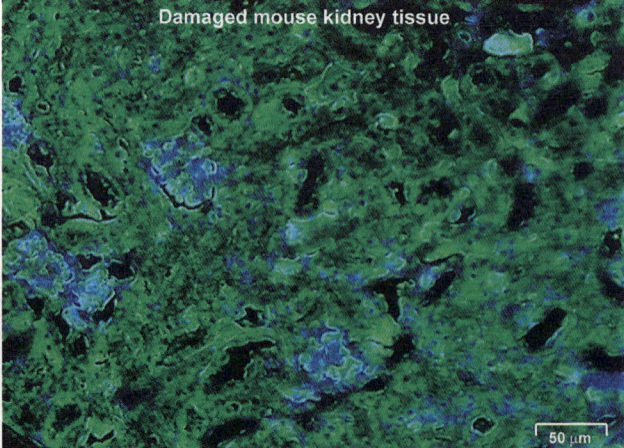

**Fig. 9.5:** Kidney tissue stained with laminin (Green Fluorescence) and Hoechst 3333 staining the nucleus (Blue). Laminin stains are less in normal kidney tissues showing low intensity, whereas in damaged kidney tissue shows increased fluorescent intensity representing increased laminin deposition leading to renal fibrosis.

such as caspases or Bcl-2 family proteins, within cultured cells. These techniques are also useful to identify and localize immune cells in inflammatory diseases like rheumatoid arthritis or multiple sclerosis.
- Monitoring treatment responses and developing targeted therapies. ICC and IHC are critical in the drug development, particularly in validating the potential of drug targets. For example, IHC is used to confirm the overexpression of a novel protein in cancer tissues compared to normal tissues.

## Electrophysiology

**Principle:** Electrophysiological techniques are employed to study the electrical properties of cells, focusing on membrane potential, ion channel activity, and synaptic transmission.

**Aim:** The Aim of electrophysiology is to understand the fundamental electrical characteristics of cells, particularly excitable cells like neurons and muscle cells, and to elucidate the mechanisms of cell-to-cell communication.

**Procedure:**
- **Techniques for electrical property study:** Utilize various methods such as patch-clamp recording and voltage-sensitive dye imaging to measure and manipulate the electrical activity of cells.
- **Applications in excitable cells:** Focus on studying the electrical properties of neurons and muscle cells to unravel mechanisms underlying cell-to-cell communication.

**Results:** Electrophysiological studies provide detailed insights into the electrical behavior of cells, aiding in the understanding of neuronal signaling, muscle contraction, and other physiological processes.

**Utility in clinical practice:** Electrophysiological techniques have significant utility in clinical practice for:
- Diagnosing and monitoring neurological disorders by assessing neuronal activity. Techniques such as patch-clamp recordings enable detailed studies of ion channels and measure the flow of ions through these channels under various conditions in neurons. Abnormalities in ion channel function can lead to neurological disorders. For instance, calcium channel dysfunction has been linked to epilepsy and bipolar disorder.
- Understanding muscle function. For example, techniques like electrocardiography (ECG) and intracardiac electrophysiology studies (EPS) are used to assess the electrical activity of the heart and to diagnose arrhythmias. Techniques such as electromyography (EMG) are used to study the electrical activity of muscle fibers.
- Guiding the development of treatments targeting electrical abnormalities in excitable cells.
- Advancing therapies such as deep brain stimulation for conditions like Parkinson's disease.
- Techniques like somatosensory evoked potential (SSEP), motor evoked potential (MEP), direct nerve stimulation (DNS), brain stem evoked potential (BERA), visual evoked potential (VEP) are commonly used intraoperatively for neurophysiological monitoring.

### SUMMARY

This chapter deals with various methods used to demonstrate, analyze and understand cellular functions and communications. Microscopy techniques are essential for visualizing cellular structures and processes, crucial for diagnosing diseases and monitoring treatment responses. Cell fractionation and assays allow for the isolation of cellular components and biochemical analysis, aiding in understanding disease mechanisms and developing targeted therapies. Cell culture and cell-based assays facilitate the growth of cells in vitro to study cellular responses to stimuli, crucial for drug screening. Live cell imaging and time-lapse microscopy provide real-time insights into dynamic cellular processes, important for understanding disease progression and cellular mechanisms. Molecular biology techniques analyze gene expression and protein levels, identifying biomarkers and developing targeted therapies. Lastly, Immunocytochemistry and Immunohistochemistry focus on protein localization within cells and tissues, helping diagnose diseases and monitor treatments, while electrophysiology examines the electrical properties of cells, critical for diagnosing neurological and muscle disorders, guiding treatment development and intraoperative neurophysiological monitoring. Each method offers unique insights, contributing significantly to medical science and clinical applications.

### LET US SEE, HOW MUCH YOU HAVE LEARNT?

 *Review Questions*

Q1. Explain how microscopy techniques can aid in the diagnosis of malignancies?

Q2. Describe the role of biochemical assays in understanding lysosomal storage diseases like Tay-Sachs or Gaucher's disease.

Q3. How can cell culture techniques assist in the development of chemotherapeutic agents? Provide an example.

Q4. What is the significance of live cell imaging in monitoring the movement of cancer cells?

Q5. List two utilities of immunocytochemistry (ICC) and immunohistochemistry (IHC) in clinical practice.

## Multiple Choice Questions

**Q1.** Which microscopy technique is particularly useful for studying the size, shape, and distribution of mitochondria in Parkinson's disease?
   a. Electron microscopy
   b. Phase contrast microscopy
   c. Fluorescence microscopy
   d. Light microscopy

**Q2.** Cell fractionation and biochemical assays help in developing targeted therapies by:
   a. Identifying immune cells
   b. Targeting membrane protein receptors or ion channels
   c. Measuring electrical activity of the heart
   d. Monitoring neuronal activity

**Q3.** Which of the following is NOT a utility of cell culture and cell-based assays in clinical practice?
   a. Screening potential drugs for efficacy and toxicity
   b. Studying electrical properties of neurons
   c. Advancing regenerative medicine techniques
   d. Identifying therapeutic targets

**Q4.** Live cell imaging and time-lapse microscopy are significant in clinical practice for:
   a. Identifying biomarkers for diseases
   b. Studying disease progression and treatment responses
   c. Diagnosing diseases based on cellular abnormalities
   d. Developing vaccines

**Q5.** Which electrophysiological technique is used intra-operatively for neurophysiological monitoring?
   a. Electrocardiography (ECG)
   b. Direct nerve stimulation (DNS)
   c. Patch-clamp recordings
   d. Western blotting

### ANSWERS
**1.** c   **2.** b   **3.** b   **4.** b   **5.** b

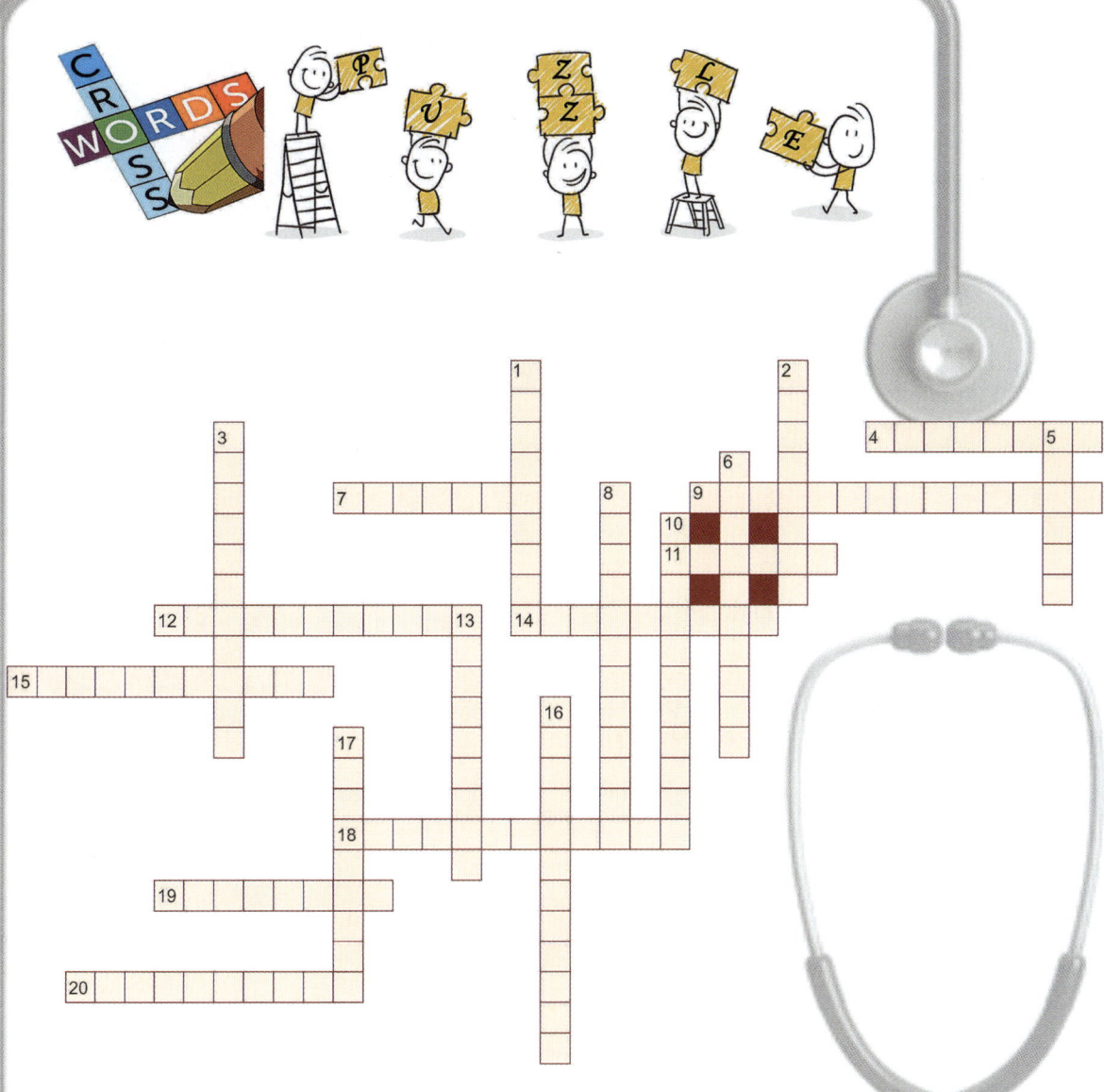

### Across

4. Contains enzymes that break down waste materials and cellular debris
7. Transport of water through a semipermeable membrane
9. Decrease in intracellular voltage from the spike potential to RMP
11. .......... oxide — Class IV neurotransmitter
12. Precursor for steroid hormones
14. Example of noniodinated amine hormone
15. The ability of biological systems to maintain internal stability
18. The process by which a cell engulfs particles to form an internal vesicle
19. Slowly penetrating solutes
20. Filamentous connections between adjacent cells

### Down

1. Specialized lysosomes, plays important role in penetration of ovum by sperm
2. Premature death of cells triggered by acute injury
3. Most potent and basic buffer system
5. Actin based molecular motor
6. Visible during cell division, concerned with movement of chromosomes
8. Made-up of two globular protein α and β tubulin
10. Membrane transport process requires the presence of specific receptor proteins on the cell membrane
13. A positive feedback loop resulting in milk let down
16. Solutions containing small molecules that can pass freely through cell membranes
17. Programmed cell death, a mechanism to remove damaged cells

# SECTION 2

# HEMATOLOGY

## Section Outline

**Chapter 10:** Introduction to Blood
**Chapter 11:** Plasma Proteins
**Chapter 12:** Hemoglobin
**Chapter 13:** Erythrocytes: Formation and Function
**Chapter 14:** Physiology of Anemia
**Chapter 15:** Physiology of Jaundice
**Chapter 16:** Leukocytes and their Formation
**Chapter 17:** Basics of Immunity
**Chapter 18:** Platelets: Structure, Formation and Functions
**Chapter 19:** Hemostasis
**Chapter 20:** Blood Groups
**Chapter 21:** Blood Banking and Blood Transfusion

# Introduction to Blood

**CHAPTER 10**

### COMPETENCY ADDRESSED
PY2.1: Describe the composition and functions of blood components.

### LEARNING OBJECTIVES
**At the end of this chapter, the learner should be able to:**
- Define blood.
- Enumerate the important functions of the blood.
- Describe the composition of the blood.
- Describe the physiological role of the various components of blood.
- Differentiate between blood, plasma and serum.

## FUNCTIONS OF BLOOD

Blood is the **fluid connective tissue**, present inside the blood vessels. The average blood volume is **5–6 liters**, amounting to **8%** of the total body weight. The blood serves the following functions:

- **Medium of transport**
  - For **respiratory gases** (oxygen and carbon dioxide) to and from the tissues
  - *Nutrients* (glucose, amino acids, vitamins, etc.) to the tissues.
  - *Waste products* from the tissues to the excretory organs (lactic acid, nitrogenous waste products, etc.)
  - *Hormones* from the endocrine glands to the target tissue
  - Various **inorganic ions** and electrolytes like $Na^+$, $K^+$, $Fe^{3+}$, $Cu^{2+}$, $HCO_3^-$, $H^+$, etc.
- **Storage:** It acts as a storehouse of many hormones, vitamins, electrolytes, etc.
  - Proteins in the form of plasma proteins
  - Free fatty acids
  - Bound form of hormones like cortisol bound to globulin
  - Ions and electrolytes
- Provides us **immunity** due to γ-globulins and complement system
- *Perfusion of the organs*: The blood flow to the organs maintains adequate perfusion of the organs for their proper functioning
- The hydrostatic pressure maintained by the blood volume is responsible for the **capillary fluid dynamics**. Maintains colloid osmotic pressure of blood due to Donnan effect.
- The plasma proteins and hemoglobin present in blood act as **buffer** for the pH regulation of blood.
- Blood forms and important component of the extracellular fluid.
- It helps in the maintenance of **body temperature**.
- The red iron pigment imparts the **red color** to the blood giving a healthy look to the person.

## COMPOSITION OF THE BLOOD

The blood is composed of the cellular elements and the fluid plasma.

On centrifugation of the whole blood, the cellular elements settle down at the bottom of the tube whereas the fluid portion comes on the top of the tube **(Fig. 10.1)** and is clearly differentiated into three layers:

- **Red blood cells**/erythrocytes form the bottom most layer which gets packed tightly hence called as the *packed cell volume* (PCV or hematocrit). The packed cell volume of a healthy individual ranges from **42%** to **45%.**
- Just above the packed erythrocytes, is present the *buffy layer*, which is mainly composed of *platelets and white blood cells/leukocytes*.
- On the **top** the layer of straw colored liquid is present which is called as *plasma*. Plasma is composed of water,

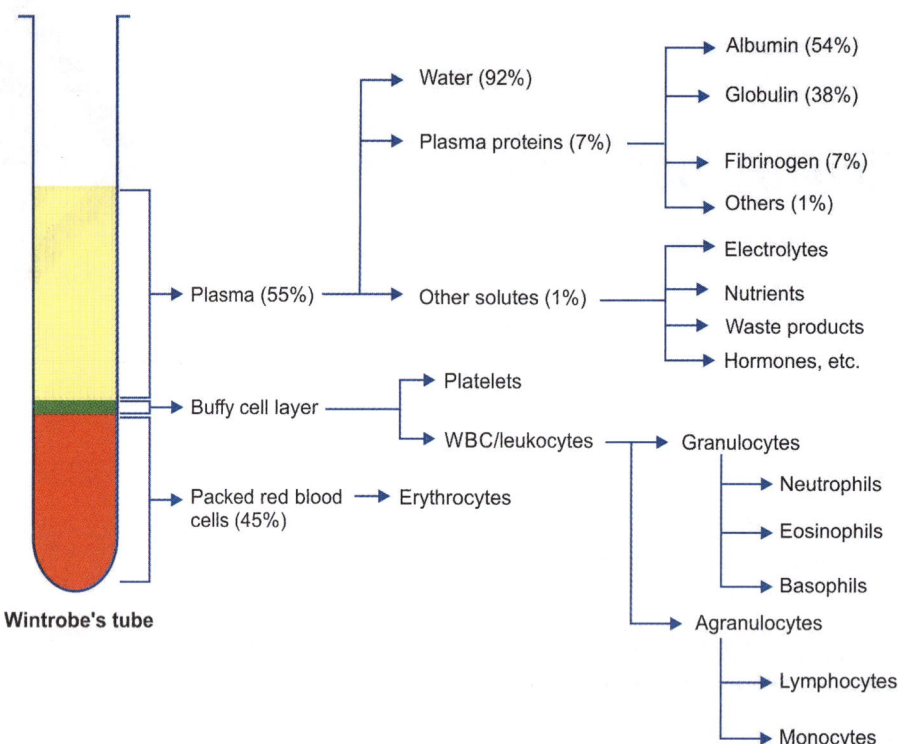

**Fig. 10.1:** Composition of whole blood.

organic compounds and inorganic ions. The plasma consists of the clotting factors, hence is capable of clotting. Plasma makes **55%** of the total blood volume.

## PHYSIOLOGICAL SIGNIFICANCE OF EACH COMPONENT OF THE BLOOD

- **Packed red cell volume:** This layer clearly indicates the volume of red blood cells present in the blood. **Decreased thickness** of packed erythrocytes indicates the **anemia**.
- **Buffy layer**
  - This layer is rich in the **platelets**/thrombocytes and the various growth factors secreted by them.
  - This buffy layer also contains the **leukocytes**. The thickness of this layer may increase in the presence of infection.
  - *Clinical significance:*
    - Due to the abundance of the platelet derived growth factor and other factors, it is used clinically for many therapeutic purposes in the form of **platelet rich plasma (PRP)**.
    - Certain **atypical cells** present in the buffy layer could be identified by making a blood smear from it, e.g., LE cells in systemic lupus erythematosus, **blast cells** in certain malignancies and premalignant and for identification of bacteria and fungi growing within the neutrophils.
- **Plasma:** It is the fluid portion of the blood. It is primarily composed of **water (92%)** and the major solid content is made by the **plasma proteins (7%)** and other **solutes (1%)**.

**Why do we use serum for various biochemical investigations of blood?**

The serum is a clear transparent liquid formed after the clotting of the whole blood. So, it is devoid of all kind of cellular elements of blood and clotting factors but it is rich in water and inorganic substances. Hence, serum can be used for the estimation of various substances like Creatinine, Uric acid, Cholesterol, etc.

Referring to **Figure 10.2**, the difference of whole blood, plasma and serum can be understood, that:
- If we allow the whole blood to clot, it will form *serum*.
- If we remove the cells from the whole blood by centrifugation we get *plasma*.
- If the plasma is allowed to clot, it will form *serum*.

Hence, we can say that the clear transparent liquid obtained after clotting (removal of cells and clotting factors) forms the serum.

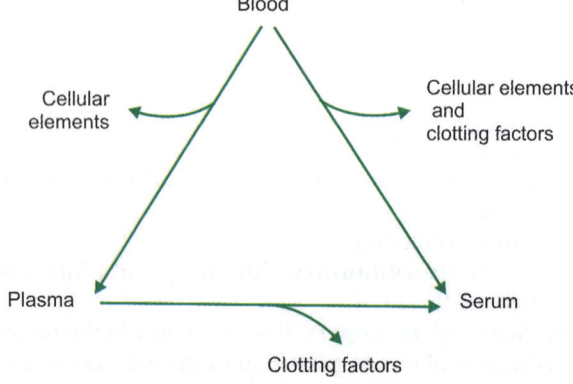

**Fig. 10.2:** Interrelation between blood, plasma and serum.

## PHYSICAL CHARACTERISTICS OF BLOOD

- Blood is a **colloidal suspension,** comprising of various cellular and non-cellular components.
- **Red** in color due to presence of red color iron containing pigment in the red blood cells.
- **Specific gravity/density (1.050):** It is determined by the number of cells and composition of plasma.
- **Osmolality of blood:** Normal osmolality of blood is around 300 mosm/L.
- **Osmotic fragility:** The red blood cell volume remains constant if the solute load of the intracellular and extracellular fluid is same, i.e., at 300 mosm/L. Depending on the solute load/osmolality of the fluids, they are classified as:
    - *Iso-osmotic/isotonic fluid:* The osmolality of fluid is 300 mosm/L.
    - *Hypotonic fluid:* The osmolality of fluid is less than 300 mosm/L.
    - *Hypertonic fluid:* The osmolality of the fluid is more than 300 mosm/L.
    - The erythrocytes tend to hemolyze if placed in hypotonic solutions. The osmolality at which the hemolysis begin is termed as the osmotic fragility.
- **Viscosity:** It is defined as the resistance to blood flow. The viscosity is primarily due to the plasma proteins especially *fibrinogen*. The viscosity of whole blood is four times that of water. The viscosity of plasma is less than whole blood and more than water. It is represented by '$\eta$'.
- **pH of blood:** The whole blood is slightly alkaline with the pH ranging from **7.35 to 7.45**. The pH of *venous blood is slightly less than the arterial blood due to the presence of $CO_2$ in it.*
- **Hematocrit:** The bottom layer of centrifuged blood is termed as hematocrit (discussed earlier).
- **Cell counts:**
    - *Erythrocytes:* Females: 4–4.5 million/cc, Males: 5–5.5 millions/cc
    - *Leukocytes:* 4,000–11,000/cc
    - *Platelets:* 1.5–3 lakh/cc

Various blood tests are used to find out the physical characteristics of blood. These characteristics have to be maintained within a strict range for a proper homeostatic control of various physiological functions of the body.

- Erythrocyte sedimentation rate (ESR)
- Packed cell volume (hematocrit)

## SUMMARY

- **Functions of the blood** are storage of various molecules, medium of transport, providing immunity, regulation of temperature and pH.
- **Components of blood** are:
    - *Plasma:* Liquid portion of blood, composed of water, electrolytes, proteins, hormones, and waste products. Plasma without clotting factors is called **serum**.
    - *Red blood cells (RBCs):* Carry oxygen and carbon dioxide, contain hemoglobin for gas exchange.
    - *White blood cells (WBCs):* Part of the immune system, defend against infections and foreign substances.
    - *Platelets:* Cell fragments involved in blood clotting, prevent excessive bleeding.

## LET US SEE, HOW MUCH YOU HAVE LEARNT?

### Review Questions

**Q1.** Describe the components of blood and their respective roles in maintaining physiological balance within the body.
**Q2.** Explain in detail the various functions of blood.
**Q3.** Write a note on the physical characteristics of blood.
**Q4.** Draw a well-labeled diagram showing various components of blood.
**Q5.** Define and classify osmotic fragility.

### Critical Thinking Case-Based Questions

**Q1.** An anemic patient presented to the laboratory for a comprehensive blood count and kidney function tests. Unfortunately, a technician mistakenly collected the blood sample in the wrong vial, leading to blood coagulation and leaving only serum for analysis.

a. What is the difference between plasma and serum?
b. Identify the specific test or tests that cannot be performed on coagulated blood in this context.
c. What are the properties of plasma? Write a note on its function as well.

### Multiple Choice Questions

**Q1.** What does the osmotic fragility of blood assess?
　a. Hemoglobin concentration
　b. Red blood cell membrane integrity
　c. White blood cell count
　d. Plasma viscosity

Q2. Which component of blood plays a key role in maintaining acid-base balance and transporting gases, nutrients, and hormones throughout the body?
   a. Red blood cells (RBCs)
   b. White blood cells (WBCs)
   c. Plasma
   d. Platelets

Q3. What factor primarily influences the viscosity of blood?
   a. Red blood cell count
   b. Plasma volume
   c. Platelet concentration
   d. White blood cell count

**ANSWERS**

1. b    2. c    3. a

# Plasma Proteins

**11 CHAPTER**

**COMPETENCY ADDRESSED**

**PY2.2:** Discuss the origin, forms, variations and functions of plasma proteins.

**LEARNING OBJECTIVES**

At the end of this chapter, the learner should be able to:
- Define the plasma proteins.
- Enumerate the various plasma proteins.
- Describe the physiological role of plasma proteins.
- Describe the effect of deficiency of plasma proteins on the body.
- Describe the importance of plasmapheresis as a treatment modality.

**Definition:** The dissolved proteins present in the plasma are called as the plasma proteins.

## ORIGIN OF THE PLASMA PROTEINS

The plasma proteins are formed in the liver, from the exchangeable amino acid pool.

The total amino acid pool is created by the protein intake its digestion and absorption, and is present in two major forms **(Fig. 11.1)**:
1. The exchangeable pool
2. The fixed pool

## THE NORMAL LEVELS OF PLASMA PROTEINS

The normal concentration of plasma proteins in blood ranges *between 6 and 8 g%, within average of 7 g%*.

The level of plasma protein *below 6 g%* is referred as hypoproteinemia.

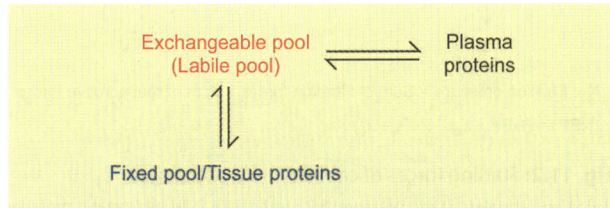

**Fig. 11.1:** Pools of plasma protein.

## TYPES OF PLASMA PROTEINS

Based on the structure and molecular weight, the plasma proteins are classified into **(Table 11.1)**:
- Albumin
- Globulin
- Fibrinogen

## FUNCTIONS OF PLASMA PROTEINS

### Albumin

- **Colloid osmotic pressure:** Albumin accounts for 70% of the colloid osmotic pressure of the plasma. The osmotic pressure exerted by albumin is primarily because of the Donnan effect exerted by the albumin molecules which are explained below:
  The albumin molecules are negatively charged, hence it has a capability to attract and retain sodium ions inside the vascular compartment. It also binds to some chloride ions which further increases the negative charge on the albumin molecules, further increasing the retention of sodium in the intra vascular compartment. This enhances the osmotic pressure exerted by the albumin molecules by 50%.
- **Transport of molecules:** It transport of many substances like bilirubin hormones metals vitamins and drugs.
- **Fat metabolism:** It helps in fat metabolism by binding to the fatty acids and keep them in a soluble form in

**Table 11.1:** Types of plasma proteins.

| | Albumin | Globulin | Fibrinogen |
|---|---|---|---|
| Molecular weight (Dalton) | 66,000 | 90,000–156,000 | 340,000 |
| Concentration in plasma (g%) | 4–5.5 | 1.5–3 | 0.3 |
| Half-life | 20 days | Few days to weeks | 3–5 days |
| Subtypes/categories | | $\alpha(\alpha_1, \alpha_2)$: $\alpha_1$-antitrypsin, $\alpha_2$-macroglobulin, haptoglobin<br>$\beta(\beta_1, \beta_2)$: Transferrin, complement system<br>$\gamma$: Immunoglobulins | |
| Synthesis | Liver at the rate of 150–250 mg/kg/day | Most of globulins are synthesized in liver<br>$\gamma$-globulins: Plasma cells | |
| Functions | • **Colloid osmotic pressure**<br>• **Storage** of organic compounds in blind form<br>• Acts as **carrier for transport** of organic and inorganic compounds<br>• Helps in **fat metabolism** | • Gamma globulin acts as antibody and confers humoral **immunity**<br>• Acts as a **carrier** for transport of many hormones and other organic and inorganic molecules<br>• Acts as a **storage** form for many hormones like cortisol, thyroxine etc. | • It is the **largest** plasma protein, hence it is primarily responsible for **viscosity** of blood<br>• It plays a very important role in the **clotting**, as it is the clotting factor I<br>• It is used for the determination of erythrocytes sedimentation rate (**ESR**) |

plasma. Hence, a patient of hypoalbuminemia may present with hyperlipidemia.
- **Storage:** It keeps the organic substances in the bound form in plasma. These substances are released as per the requirement of the tissues in a controlled fashion.

## VARIATIONS IN THE LEVELS OF PLASMA PROTEINS

Variations in normal plasma levels are tabulated in **Table 11.2**.

**Table 11.2:** Variations in normal plasma protein levels.

| | Increase | Decrease |
|---|---|---|
| Albumin | Acute dehydration | • Decreased intake of proteins<br>• Intestinal malabsorption<br>• Severe burns<br>• Liver failure<br>• Nephrotic syndrome<br>• Glomerulonephritis |
| Globulin | • $\alpha_1$-antitrypsin excess seen in inflammatory bowel disease<br>• Excessive $\alpha_2$-macroglobulin is seen in nephrotic syndrome due to loss of low molecular weight proteins in urine<br>• Haptoglobin rises in response to stress, infection, acute inflammation<br>• Transferrin levels rise in severe iron deficiency | • Malnutrition<br>• Immunodeficiency<br>• Nephrotic syndrome<br>• Haptoglobin levels decrease after hemolysis because it complexes with free hemoglobin and is cleared from circulation<br>• Corticosteroid treatment |

### A:G Ratio

Normal albumin:globulin ratio ranges from **1.5** to **2.5:1**. This ratio is altered in certain diseases resulting either from the decreased levels of albumin or increased levels of globulin. In acts as the diagnostic as well as the prognostic marker for many diseases.

### Deficiency of Plasma Proteins/Hypoproteinemia

- A higher risk of **chronic obstructive pulmonary disease** is observed in people with *congenital deficiency of $\alpha_1$-antitrypsin* on prolonged exposure to smoking, pollution or dust.
- Decreased levels of albumin in blood reduces the colloid osmotic pressure affecting the capillary fluid dynamics and resulting in edema, which is explained below:
  - According to the Starling forces of fluid exchange, the plasma proteins/albumin is mainly responsible for maintaining colloid osmotic pressure of blood. This COP ($\pi_c$) results in inward movement of the water in the capillaries (**Fig. 11.2**), hence balancing the

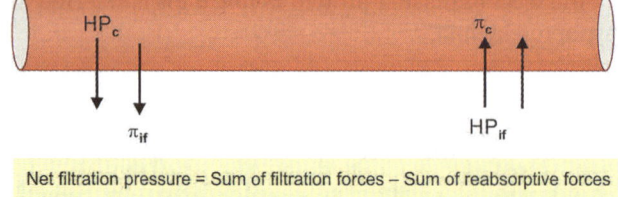

Net filtration pressure = Sum of filtration forces – Sum of reabsorptive forces
(NFP) = (HPc + $\pi_{if}$) – (HP$_{if}$ + $\pi_c$)

**Fig. 11.2:** Starling forces of capillary fluid exchange.
(HP$_c$: Capillary hydrostatic pressure; HP$_{if}$: Interstitial fluid hydrostatic pressure; $\pi_c$: Colloid osmotic pressure of capillary; $\pi_{if}$: Colloid osmotic pressure of interstitial fluid)

filtration due to hydrostatic pressure of capillaries (HP$_c$) and the COP ($\pi_{if}$) of interstitial fluid.
- If the NFP is positive, it indicates the net filtration occurring in the capillaries whereas the a negative value indicates the net reabsorption.
- In patients with hypoproteinemia, the COP ($\pi_c$) decreases and the net filtration pressure increases resulting in the movement of fluid from the intravascular compartment towards the interstitial fluid resulting in edema (**Fig. 11.3**).

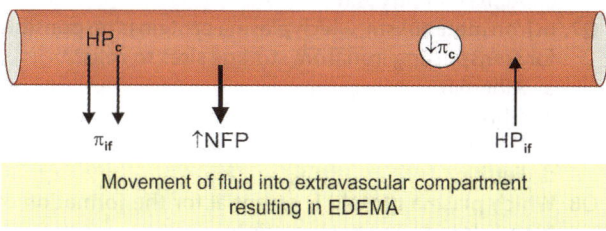

**Fig. 11.3:** Capillary fluid dynamics in hypoproteinemia.

- In case of severe hypoproteinemia, the edema will be severe; more prominent around the eyes (puffy eyes), as seen in the renal disease.

**Why the plasma protein level below 2 g%, is incompatible with life?**
At this concentration, the exchangeable pool gets completely exhausted and the fixed pool begins to mobilize. This results in cellular degradation and essential proteins are also not formed. However, protein supplementation is very helpful in this situation.

## PLASMAPHERESIS

It is a therapeutic intervention in which the blood is removed from the body and the plasma is separated from it. The separated cells are infused again in the body but the plasma is either removed, replaced or returned back after filtration. It is used as a therapy in many diseases but commonly used for removal of antibodies in the autoimmune diseases.

## SUMMARY

In this chapter, we have studied that:
- The dissolved proteins in the plasma are called the plasma proteins.
- These are broadly classified as albumin, globulin and fibrinogen.
- They are synthesized in the liver, hence their plasma concentration drops in the liver failure.
- These proteins are required for the maintenance of osmotic pressure of blood, transport of hormones, minerals and vitamins, immunity and many other functions.

## LET US SEE, HOW MUCH YOU HAVE LEARNT?

 *Review Questions*

### Long/Short Answer Questions

Q1. Define plasma proteins. Classify them. Describe the functions of the plasma proteins.
Q2. How does albumin maintain the colloid osmotic pressure?
Q3. What are Starling Forces? How does albumin affect the Starling Forces?

### Explain Why? (Reasoning Questions)

Q1. A patient of hypo-proteinemia develop edema?
Q2. What will happen, if a plasma protein falls below 2 g%?
Q3. Liver diseases affect the plasma proteins levels?
Q4. Kidney disorders affect the plasma protein levels?

 *Critical Thinking Case-Based Questions*

Q1. A 45-year-old male presented to the clinic with complaints of generalized edema, fatigue, and weight loss. His medical history revealed chronic liver disease with poor appetite and malnutrition for several months. A physical examination showed pitting edema in his lower extremities. Blood tests reveal significantly low serum protein and albumin levels. Urinalysis shows no significant proteinuria. Based on patient's symptoms and lab results, answer the following questions:
   a. Explain the physiological mechanisms leading to his hypoproteinemia.
   b. What are the potential causes of hypoproteinemia in this patient?

## Multiple Choice Questions

**Q1.** A patient presents with edema and low serum protein levels. Which of the following plasma proteins is primarily responsible for maintaining colloidal osmotic pressure in the blood?
   a. Albumin
   b. Fibrinogen
   c. Immunoglobulins
   d. Transferrin

**Q2.** A newborn is diagnosed with congenital hypogammaglobulinemia. Which of the following plasma proteins would most likely be deficient in this condition?
   a. Albumin
   b. Fibrinogen
   c. Immunoglobulins
   d. Ceruloplasmin

**Q3.** A patient with liver disease has prolonged clotting times and decreased blood clot formation. Which plasma protein deficiency is most likely contributing to this condition?
   a. Albumin
   b. Fibrinogen
   c. Transferrin
   d. Antithrombin III

**Q4.** A pregnant woman undergoes routine blood tests, revealing elevated levels of alpha-fetoprotein (AFP). What is the primary source of AFP production during pregnancy?
   a. Liver
   b. Placenta
   c. Fetal kidney
   d. Maternal blood cells

**Q5.** A patient presents with symptoms of autoimmune disease, including joint pain and skin rashes. Which plasma protein may be elevated in autoimmune conditions?
   a. Albumin
   b. C-reactive protein
   c. Ceruloplasmin
   d. Rheumatoid factor

**Q6.** Which of the following plasma proteins is commonly used as a biomarker for inflammation and infection?
   a. Albumin
   b. Fibrinogen
   c. C-reactive protein (CRP)
   d. Alpha-1 antitrypsin

**Q7.** In iron metabolism, which plasma protein is responsible for transporting iron from storage sites to cells?
   a. Albumin
   b. Fibrinogen
   c. Transferrin
   d. Ferritin

**Q8.** Which plasma protein is essential for the formation of blood clots during hemostasis?
   a. Albumin
   b. Fibrinogen
   c. Immunoglobulins
   d. Complement proteins

**Q9.** Inherited deficiencies of which plasma protein can lead to conditions such as hemophilia?
   a. Albumin
   b. Fibrinogen
   c. Factor VIII
   d. Plasminogen

**Q10.** Which plasma protein is primarily responsible for binding and transporting bilirubin in the bloodstream?
   a. Albumin
   b. Fibrinogen
   c. Ceruloplasmin
   d. Haptoglobin

**ANSWERS**

**1.** a  **2.** d  **3.** b  **4.** b  **5.** d  **6.** c  **7.** c  **8.** b  **9.** c  **10.** a

# Hemoglobin

**CHAPTER 12**

> **COMPETENCY ADDRESSED**
>
> **PY2.3:** Describe and discuss the synthesis and functions of hemoglobin and explain its breakdown. Describe variants of hemoglobin.

> **LEARNING OBJECTIVES**
>
> **At the end of this chapter, the learner should be able to:**
> - Describe the structure and synthesis of hemoglobin.
> - Describe the functions of hemoglobin.
> - Describe the variations of normal and abnormal hemoglobin.
> - Describe the normal values of hemoglobin and variations in the hemoglobin content.
> - Describe the breakdown and fate of hemoglobin.

## INTRODUCTION

Hemoglobin (Hb) is a complex conjugated, iron containing, protein present inside the red blood cells. In some lower animals, it is present dissolved in the plasma but in the higher animals, the erythrocytes act as the carrier of Hb.

> **What would happen, if hemoglobin was dissolved in the plasma?**
>
> Around 3% of hemoglobin present in the blood vessels, can cross the capillary membranes and extravasate into the interstitial fluid. Similarly, this much Hb would cross the glomerular capillaries and get filtered there resulting in hemoglobinuria (passage of hemoglobin in the urine). Hence, dissolved Hb and hemoglobinuria would result in following physiological effects in an individual:
> - Due to **dissolved Hb**:
>   - Increase in the blood **viscosity**
>   - Increase in the **peripheral resistance**
>   - Increase in systemic **arterial pressure**
>   - Increase in **afterload** for the left ventricle, resulting in **left ventricular hypertrophy** and eventually **failure**
>   - Affect the **colloid osmotic pressure** of intravascular compartment affecting the capillary fluid dynamics.
> - Due to **hemoglobinuria**:
>   - Presence of Hb in the tubular filtrate would **increase** the **colloid osmotic pressure** of the **bowman's** capsule.
>   - Hb would affect the tubular reabsorption at the PCT.
>   - Hb crystals would precipitate in the renal tubules, blocking of them and resulting in the **renal tubular necrosis** and eventually renal shut down.
>
> Not to worry, the Hb is enclosed in the erythrocytes which safely carry it to all the parts of the body without exerting all these effects and saving us from them.

> **FACT**
>
> Do you know, RBC can concentrate 34 g/100 mL of cells, but not beyond that because that is the maximum metabolic limit of Hb forming mechanism in the RBCs. Hence the RBC can never be hyperchromic!

## SYNTHESIS OF HEMOGLOBIN

The Hb molecule is primarily made-up of two moieties, Heme and Globin **(Fig. 12.1)**
- Heme moiety is made from Succinyl-CoA and Glycine to form the pyrrole ring
- Four pyrrole rings join to form the Protoporphyrin IX
- Protoporphyrin IX then combines with ferrous form of iron ($Fe^{2+}$) to form heme moiety
- Heme then combines with the two globin chains each ($\alpha$ or $\beta$) to form adult Hb (HbA)

## STRUCTURE OF HEMOGLOBIN

Now we know that Hb is formed of two basic moieties, hence the structure of Hb is also explained accordingly.

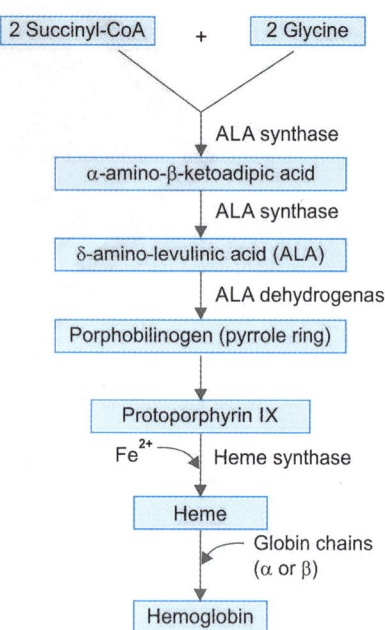

**Fig. 12.1:** Formation of hemoglobin.

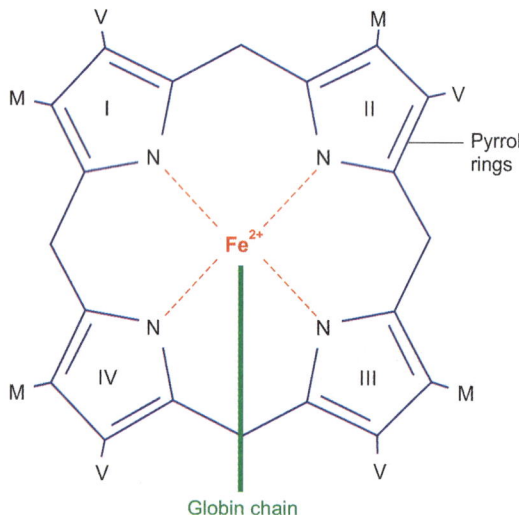

**Fig. 12.2:** Structure of Hb molecule.

Hence, the heme moiety is made-up four pyrrole rings with 4 ferrous ion in the center, connected to the four globin chains **(Fig. 12.2)**.

The different types of the globin chains, found in various types of Hb are:

- **Alpha ($\alpha$) chain:** It is the part of the adult ($\alpha_2\beta_2$) as well as the fetal ($\alpha_2\gamma_2$) Hb
- **Beta ($\beta$) chain:** 2$\beta$ chains are present in the adult Hb ($\alpha_2\beta_2$) only
- **Gamma ($\gamma$) chain:** Are found in the fetal Hb ($\alpha_2\gamma_2$) or Hb bart ($\gamma_4$)
- **Delta ($\delta$) chain:** These chains are found in a variant of adult Hb—HbA2($\alpha_2\delta_2$)

- **Epsilon ($\epsilon$) chain:** They are found in embryonic Hb, Gower type 1 and 2
- **Zeta ($\zeta$) chain:** They are found in embryonic Hb, Gower type 1

## TYPES OF HEMOGLOBIN (TABLE 12.1)

### Normal Types of Hemoglobins

- **HbA1 and HbA2 (Adult Hb):** The globin chains present in HbA1 are $\alpha_2\beta_2$ whereas in HbA2 are $\alpha_2\delta_2$. The HbA1 is most abundant Hb present in adults making up to 97% of Hb, while HbA2 makes the rest of it.
- **HbF (Fetal Hb):** It present in the fetal life and replaced by the adult Hb after the birth. The affinity of HbF for oxygen is much more than the adult Hb, hence it extracts the oxygen from the maternal blood and delivers to the fetus. Hence, the Oxygen Hb dissociation curve of HbF lies to the left of HbA1. *Presence of fetal Hb after birth is abnormal and indicates the failure to synthesize the $\beta$ chains ($\beta$-thalassemia).*
- **Embryonic Hb:** Gower Hb type 1 consists of two zeta and two epsilon chains ($\zeta_2\epsilon_2$) whereas Gower type 2 consisted of $\alpha_2\epsilon_2$ chains.
- **Hb Bart:** In this all the four globin chains are of $\gamma$ type ($\gamma_4$).

### Abnormal Hemoglobin (Hemoglobinopathies)

- **HbS:** Valine replaces the glutamic acid at the 6th position in $\beta$-globin chain. It is seen in sickle cell anemia.
- **HbC:** Lysine replaces the glutamate at 6th position of beta chain
- **HbD:** Glutamine replaces glutamic acid at 121 position of beta chain. It is referred to as HbD Punjab and HbD Los Angeles.
- **HbE:** It is also a beta chain variant hemoglobinopathy where the lysine replaces the glutamic acid at 26th

**Table 12.1:** Characteristics of different types of hemoglobin.

| Hemoglobin type | Characteristic |
|---|---|
| HbA1 | $\alpha_2\beta_2$ |
| HbA2 | $\alpha_2\delta_2$ |
| HbF | $\alpha_2\gamma_2$ |
| Gower type 1 | $\zeta_2\epsilon_2$ |
| Gower type 2 | $\alpha_2\epsilon_2$ |
| HbS | Valine replaces glutamic acid at the 6th position in $\beta$-globin chain |
| HbC | Lysine replaces glutamate at 6th position of beta chain |
| HbD | Glutamine replaces glutamic acid at 121 position of beta chain |
| HbE | Lysine replaces the glutamic acid at 26th position of beta chain |

position of beta chain. There is slight decrease in the production of beta chain resulting in mild thalassemia.

## FORMS OF HEMOGLOBIN

- **OxyHb:** This form of Hb exists when it is combined with oxygen molecules. It is important to understand that the Hb is oxygenated and not oxidized. *(Oxidation refers to loss of electrons and would change the valance of $Fe^{2+}$ to $Fe^{3+}$, as occurs in meth Hb)*.
- **CarbaminoHb:** The **carbon dioxide** reversibly **combines with globin chains** of Hb to form carbamino Hb. It forms an important means to transport the $CO_2$ from tissues to lungs.
- **CarboxyHb:** It is formed by an reversible combination of **carbon monoxide** (CO) with Hb by displacing the oxygen from it. This compound gives **cherry red color** to the blood. CO exposure occurs due to inhalation of CO from the automobile exhaust, cigarette smoke and other similar sources. It decreases the oxygen delivery to the tissues. Long-term exposure to CO can result in chronic hypoxia, demyelination and other effects on body. The half life of carboxyHb is 2 hours but it can be reduced by inhalation of 100% oxygen or hyperbaric oxygen.
- **MethHb:** When the ferrous ion is **oxidized** to ferric form, it reduces the affinity of Hb to bind with oxygen, reducing its capacity to bind with the oxygen resulting is hypoxia. Normally, the concentration of meth Hb is very low but it may increase with the consumption of some drugs or chemicals. If the concentration of methHb becomes more than 5 g%, it leads to bluish discoloration of mucosal membranes, the extremities called as cyanosis.
- **SulfHb:** The sulfur binds **irreversibly to the porphyrin ring** resulting in the formation of sulfHb. The oxygen carrying capacity of Hb reduces markedly and results in hypoxia.
- **CyanmethHb:** The *cyanide ions oxidize the $Fe^{2+}$ to $Fe^{3+}$* to form the cyanmethHb.
  - **Glycated hemoglobin (HbA1c):** The **valine** in residue at **β-chain** of hemoglobin binds **nonenzymatically** with **glucose** forming the glycated hemoglobin. HbA1c is clinically used to monitor the **long-term diabetic control** in patients with diabetes mellitus. It is calculated as the percentage of glycated Hb and the normal HbA1 and usually the levels of HbA1c remain **less than 4%** in **nondiabetic** individuals. An increased percentage of HbA1c indicates predisposition to development of diabetes mellitus or poor diabetic control/over last 3 months (*because life span of RBC is 120 days*). HbA1c levels of **5.7–6.4%** indicates that the person is **pre-diabetic** or he has **fairly good control**, if already a diagnosed case of diabetes mellitus.
  - HbA1c levels **more than 6.5%** indicate the presence of **overt diabetes mellitus** or **borderline controlled diabetes.**

## NORMAL VALUES, VARIATION AND FUNCTIONS OF HEMOGLOBIN

Normal values in different individuals is shown in **Table 12.2** and variations in Hb is shown in **Table 12.3**.

## FUNCTIONS

- **Transport of oxygen:** The main function of Hb is to transport oxygen to the tissues from the lungs. About 97% of oxygen is transported in the bound form. It **binds loosely to coordination bonds of the iron atom,** hence this combination is highly reversible. There are four iron atoms in a molecule of Hb, hence it binds to the **four molecules of oxygen**. It is worth noting that the oxygen binds as a molecule ($O_2$) and doesn't become the ionic oxygen. Hence, the combination of oxygen with Heme is called as **oxygenation**. The hemoglobin, after binding with oxygen is called as **oxyhemoglobin**.

  The whole blood contains around **15 g of Hb/100 mL** of blood in **men** and **14 g of Hb/100 mL of blood in women**. Hence, 100 mL of blood can carry around **20 mL of $O_2$ in men** and **19 mL of $O_2$ in women**.
- **Transport of carbon dioxide:** The carbon dioxide binds to the Hb and forms the carbaminoHb, though it's not an important way of carbon dioxide transport.

**Table 12.2 :** Normal values of hemoglobin.

| Males | 14–18 g/dL |
|---|---|
| Females | 12–16 g/dL |
| Newborns | 16–23 g/dL |
| Children (10 years) | 12–14 g/dL |

**Table 12.3:** Variations in Hb content.

(ADH: antidiuretic hormone)

| | Increase Hb content | Decreased Hb content |
|---|---|---|
| | **Physiological causes** | |
| 1 | High altitude | Infants and children |
| 2 | Newborns | Pregnancy |
| 3 | Excessive sweating | Old age |
| 4 | Hemoconcentration state | Hemodilutional states |
| | **Pathological causes** | |
| 1 | Severe diarrhea, vomiting resulting in hemoconcentration | Anemia |
| 2 | Hypoxia due to chronic lung or heart diseases | Chronic renal failure |
| 3 | Polycythemia vera | Excessive ADH secretion resulting in hemodilution |

- **Buffer:** It acts as an important buffer present in blood and maintains the minor fluctuations in the pH of the blood.
- It binds to the nitric oxide (a locally acting vasodilator substance released by the vascular endothelium, also called as endothelium derived relaxing factor) and destroys it.
- It imparts red color to the blood.

## FATE/BREAKDOWN OF HEMOGLOBIN

The RBC breakdown occurs in the spleen and Hb is released. The Hb is then broken down into heme and globin **(Fig. 12.3)**. The globin chains breakdown and are returned back to amino acid pool. However, the heme moiety undergoes following steps of degradation:
- Heme breaks down to **biliverdin** (a green pigment), by the action of enzyme **heme oxygenase**. The inorganic iron is returned to the body iron stores for resynthesis of Hb.
- Biliverdin is reduced to **bilirubin** (yellow pigment) by **biliverdin reductase**.
- Bilirubin then combines with albumin to form **Albumin-Bilirubin complex,** for transportation of bilirubin to the liver. This bilirubin is also called as **unconjugated** bilirubin, as it has not yet been conjugated in the liver.
- On reaching the **liver**, the bilirubin gets **detached from albumin**, some of it enters the circulation and reaches the kidneys but most of it gets conjugated with **UDP Glucuronic** acid to form **Bilirubin glucuronide**. This is called the **conjugated bilirubin.**
- The conjugated bilirubin is **secreted** into the **duodenum** through the bile. In the intestines, the conjugated bilirubin gets converted into **stercobilinogen**, a brown colored pigment. The **stercobilin is excreted in the feces** and is responsible for the brown color of the feces. *In the absence of this pigment, the person is going to pass clay colored stools (as seen in obstructive jaundice).*
- The other byproduct of conjugated bilirubin, **urobilinogen** (yellowish brown pigment) gets absorbed from intestines and are filtered in the **urine as Urobilin**. It is responsible for the yellowish color of the urine.

## APPLIED ASPECTS/CLINICAL CORRELATES

- **Thalassemia:** It is characterized by decreased or no synthesis of either of the globin chain. Depending on the type of globin chain affected, it classified as α-thalassemia and β-thalassemia.
    - *α-thalassemia:* There is defective synthesis of α-chains
    - *β-thalassemia:* There is defective synthesis of β-chains.
        - β-thalassemia minor: There is defective or decreased synthesis of β chains. There is increase in the HbF instead of HbA.
        - β-thalassemia major: There is complete absence of β-chains hence there is a very high amount of HbF instead of HbA.
        **Clinical features:**
            - Anemia
            - Hepatosplenomegaly
            - CBC shows mild anemia, reduced hematocrit and increased reticulocyte count

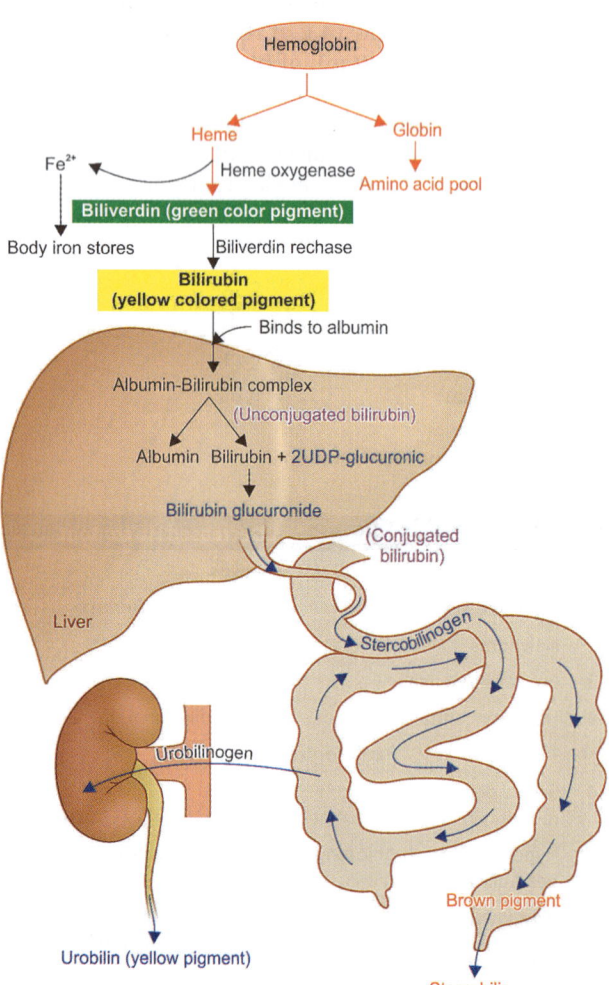

**Fig. 12.3:** Fate and excretion of hemoglobin.

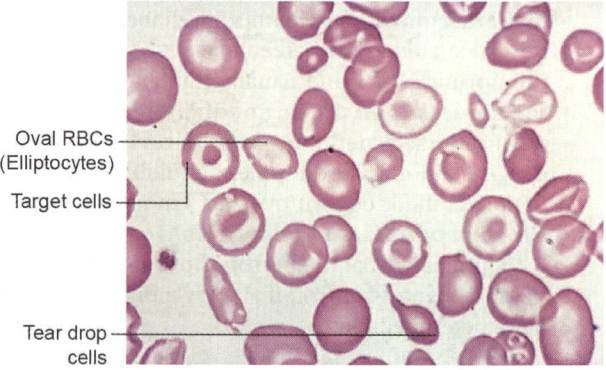

**Fig. 12.4:** Microcytic hypochromic cells.

- Signs of marrow expansion in severe cases like coarse facies, osteoporosis and osteopenia
- Peripheral blood film shows microcytic hypochromic anemia with anisopoikilocytosis and target cells (**Fig. 12.4**). Bone marrow shows erythroid hyperplasia
- **Anemia:** *See* **Chapter 14**
- **Jaundice (prehepatic/hemolytic):** *See* **Chapter 15.**

### SUMMARY

In this chapter we have learnt that the:
- Hemoglobin is an oxygen carrying molecule present in the red blood cells. It is made up of tetrapyrrole rings and 4 globin chains (2 alpha and 2 beta chains).
- The normal Hb concentration in males is 14–18 g/dL and in females it is 12–16 g/dL. It is higher in newborns.
- The Hb is of various types depending on the globin chains.
- The abnormal Hb (HbS, HbC) occurs due to the mutations in the globin chains. Thalassemia occurs, if one of the globin chains are not defective or absent.
- The Hb levels below normal are referred to as anemia.
- The Hb molecule when breaks down form the bile pigment and is excreted through bile into the duodenum, which is excreted out in feces and urine.

## LET US SEE, HOW MUCH YOU HAVE LEARNT?

### *Review Questions*

#### *Long/Short Answer Questions*

Q1. Describe the functions of hemoglobin.
Q2. What will happen if, the hemoglobin was dissolved in plasma instead of being packed in the RBCs?
Q3. Differentiate between HbA and HbF.
Q4. Describe the fate/breakdown of hemoglobin.

#### *Explain Why? (Reasoning Questions)*

Q1. In which condition, an adult person can have higher content of HbF? Describe why?
Q2. The newborn babies have high Hb content?
Q3. What will happen to the bilirubin content, if a person experiences massive hemolysis?
Q4. What will happen to the color of stool, if there obstruction to the flow of bile into the intestine and why?
Q5. What is the clinical significance of HbA1c?
Q6. What a patient of severe anemia does not show the signs of cyanosis?
Q7. What is the difference in oxidation and oxygenation of Hb?

### *Critical Thinking Case-Based Questions*

Q1. Suraj, a 58-year-old male, presented to the OPD with complaints of dark-colored urine and pale stools. He had a history of chronic hemolytic anemia. His lab tests reveal elevated levels of unconjugated bilirubin and low levels of urobilinogen in the urine. There is no significant elevation in liver enzymes.
a. Describe the physiological pathway of hemoglobin breakdown products once they reach the intestines.
b. Explain how abnormalities in this pathway could lead to Suraj's symptoms.
c. Why might Suraj have dark-colored urine if the levels of urobilinogen in his urine are low?

### *Multiple Choice Questions*

Q1. What is the primary function of hemoglobin?
  a. Maintaining blood sugar levels
  b. Facilitating blood clotting
  c. Transporting oxygen
  d. Regulating blood pressure
Q2. Which of the following components is essential for the synthesis of hemoglobin?
  a. Glucose        b. Iron
  c. Calcium        d. Vitamin C
Q3. Which part of the hemoglobin molecule binds to oxygen?
  a. Globin
  b. Heme group
  c. Iron ion
  d. Carbon dioxide
Q4. Hemoglobin is primarily synthesized in which of the following organs?
  a. Liver          b. Kidneys
  c. Bone marrow    d. Spleen
Q5. Which term refers to abnormal variations in hemoglobin structure due to genetic mutations?
  a. Hemostasis
  b. Hemophilia
  c. Hemoglobinopathies
  d. Hematopoiesis

**Q6.** In which of the following scenarios would an individual most likely experience a decrease in hemoglobin levels?
   a. Living at high altitudes
   b. Engaging in regular aerobic exercise
   c. Chronic blood loss
   d. Consuming iron-rich foods

**Q7.** A patient with a genetic mutation resulting in abnormal hemoglobin structure experiences difficulty breathing during physical exertion. Which condition is most likely present?
   a. Sickle cell anemia
   b. Thalassemia
   c. Polycythemia
   d. Hemochromatosis

**Q8.** An individual with low hemoglobin levels may exhibit which of the following symptoms?
   a. Pale skin
   b. Yellowing of the eyes
   c. Increased heart rate
   d. All of the above

**Q9.** During anemia, the body compensates by increasing the production of which hormone to stimulate red blood cell production?
   a. Insulin
   b. Erythropoietin
   c. Thyroxine
   d. Cortisol

**Q10.** Which dietary factor is most crucial for maintaining adequate hemoglobin levels?
   a. Vitamin D
   b. Vitamin B12
   c. Vitamin K
   d. Vitamin A

**Q11.** A patient presents with fatigue, shortness of breath, and pale skin. Laboratory tests reveal low hemoglobin levels. What is the most likely diagnosis?
   a. Iron deficiency anemia
   b. Sickle cell disease
   c. Thalassemia
   d. Hemochromatosis

**Q12.** A pregnant woman undergoes routine screening and is found to have elevated hemoglobin levels. What is the most likely reason for this finding?
   a. Increased oxygen demand during pregnancy
   b. Dehydration
   c. Excessive iron supplementation
   d. Genetic mutation

**Q13.** A patient presents with joint pain, fever, and jaundice. Blood tests reveal low hemoglobin levels and the presence of abnormal-shaped red blood cells. What condition is most likely present?
   a. Thalassemia
   b. Sickle cell anemia
   c. Hemochromatosis
   d. Polycythemia

**Q14.** A marathon runner participating in a high-altitude race experiences shortness of breath and dizziness. What physiological adaptation is occurring in response to the high altitude?
   a. Increased hemoglobin synthesis
   b. Decreased hemoglobin synthesis
   c. Increased red blood cell destruction
   d. Decreased oxygen affinity of hemoglobin

**Q15.** A patient with chronic kidney disease exhibits low hemoglobin levels. What is the most likely mechanism underlying this finding?
   a. Decreased erythropoietin production
   b. Increased erythropoietin production
   c. Impaired hemoglobin synthesis
   d. Excessive iron absorption

**ANSWERS**

1. c   2. b   3. b   4. c   5. c   6. c   7. a   8. d   9. b   10. b   11. a   12. a   13. b   14. a   15. a

# Erythrocytes: Formation and Function

## 13
CHAPTER

**COMPETENCY ADDRESSED**

**PY2.4:** Describe RBC formation (erythropoiesis and its regulation) and its functions.

**LEARNING OBJECTIVES**

**At the end of this chapter, the learner should be able to:**
- Describe the structure and functions of erythrocytes.
- Define erythropoiesis.
- Describe the sites and stages of erythropoiesis.
- Describe the regulation of erythropoiesis.

## ERYTHROCYTES

These anucleated biconcave disc-shaped cells, devoid of all cellular organelles and having the size of 7–7.8 µm, are also called as the red blood cells (RBCs). The main function of erythrocyte is to carry the Hb for an efficient gaseous exchange.

- Why do the RBCs lose their nucleus during the process of erythropoiesis?
- When is an erythrocyte called, fully saturated with Hemoglobin?
- If the RBCs do not have any cell organelles, then how do they metabolize substrates for their needs?
- If the size of mature RBC is around 7 µm, then how do they pass through the capillaries of 5 µm?

You will see further in the chapter, that the red cells lose their nucleus during the process of maturation. This occurs to accommodate more hemoglobin in the red cells. They not only lose the nucleus but also all the cellular organelles for the same reason. Hence, the erythrocytes depends primarily on the **glycolytic pathway** for the energy production; while the other source of energy production is **HMP shunt** pathway.

The red cell membrane has specific structural proteins (*ankyrin and spectrin*) which are responsible for their **biconcave** shape. In the **absence/defects** in these structural proteins, the red cells fail to retain the biconcave shape called as **spherocytosis** or **ovalocytosis** respectively.

These **biconcave discoid** red cells have a diameter of 7–7.8 µm and thickness of 2.5 µm at the periphery and 1 µm in the center **(Fig. 13.1)**.

This shape of the red cells enable them to **fold, squeeze and pass through the capillaries** (diameter of around 5 µm) with narrow lumen. If the red cells become spherical, they are no longer able to pass through these capillaries and result in hemolysis. Hence, **spherocytosis** is associated with **hemolytic anemia**.

The *red cell volume is around 90–95 µm$^3$* and is able to concentrate hemoglobin in cell cytoplasm up to 34 g/100 mL of cells.

Life span of RBC is *120 days* in circulation. After that the senescent red cells enter the splenic sinusoids and

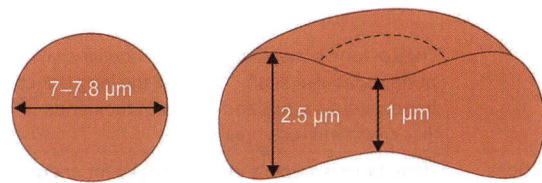

**Fig. 13.1:** Structure of red blood cell.

undergo hemolysis. The hemoglobin is broken down, out of which globin and heme iron is recycled, however the porphyrin ring is converted into biliverdin and bilirubin, which is then taken to liver bound to albumin. Bilirubin is conjugated with glucuronic acid and is secreted in bile (Chapter 12).

## FUNCTIONS OF ERYTHROCYTES

- The main function of the erythrocytes is to carry **hemoglobin**. Each cell is fully saturated with *28–32 pg of Hb, which amounts to about 33% of cell volume.* It is the maximum saturation as the cell reaches its metabolic limit here. Hence, the red cells can be normochromic or hypochromic, but never hyperchromic.
- It transports the **respiratory gases** in the combined form with Hb. If Hb is 100% saturated with oxygen, it can combine with **1.34 mL of oxygen/gram**. Hence, an average **man** carries around **20 mL** and average **woman** carries **19 mL of oxygen per 100 mL of blood.**
- Red cells contain large quantities of **carbonic anhydrase enzyme** which catalyzes the reaction between $CO_2$ and $H_2O$ to form $H_2CO_3$.
- It carries the **blood group antigens** on its cell membrane and provides the basis of blood group matching and transfusion.
- Radioisotope of **chromium labelled** red cells are used for measuring **volume** of **intravascular compartment**.

## ERYTHROPOIESIS

**Definition:** Formation of the red blood cells in bone marrow is called erythropoiesis.

The erythropoiesis takes place in the **red bone marrow** in adults.

**Bone marrow:** It is the hemopoietic raw material present in the medullary cavity of the bones. At birth, much of the bone marrow is vascular and is rich in the hemopoietic stem cells, but gradually, as the age advances the red bone marrow is replaced by the fat called as, the yellow bone marrow. In adults, red bone marrow is present at the ends of the long bones and the flat bones like skull bones, vertebrae, ribs, iliac crest and sternum. The differences in the red and the yellow bone marrow are given in **Table 13.1**.

The red bone marrow has three times more precursors of white blood cells than the red blood cells (**myeloid: erythroid = 3:1**), however in peripheral blood the ratio is reversed to **1:700** because the red cells have a much longer life span as compared to white blood cells.

**Table 13.1:** Differences in red and yellow bone marrow.

|  | **Red bone marrow** | **Yellow bone marrow** |
|---|---|---|
| Composition | Hematopoietic stem cells which forms the red and white blood cells and the platelets | Mostly composed of fats and contains stem cells that can become cartilage, fat or bone cells |
| Sites | Ends of long bones, flat bones (scapulae, skull bones, sternum, ribs and iliac crest) and vertebrae | The medullary cavities of all the long bones except their ends |
| Functions | Hemopoiesis: formation of blood cells | Stores fat for energy |

### Sites of Erythropoiesis

| Mesoblastic stage | In embryonic life | Mesoderm of yolk sac | All the other sites of erythropoiesis, except bone marrow, are called extramedullary sites. In adults the extramedullary erythropoiesis indicates bone marrow failure |
|---|---|---|---|
| Hepatic stage | After 5th week of intrauterine life | Liver and spleen | |
| After birth | Second trimester onwards | Bone marrow | |

### Stages of Differentiation of Red Cells/Erythropoiesis

See **Table 13.2**.

### Regulation of Erythropoiesis

Erythropoiesis is primarily regulated by *hypoxia*. Whenever there is tissue hypoxia, due to any cause, the rate of erythropoiesis increases through multiple factors. The most important hormone stimulated by hypoxia is *Erythropoietin* which influences the formation of red cells.

The various factors affecting erythropoiesis can be classified as:

### *Growth and Differentiation Inducers*

These are multiple proteins responsible for controlling the growth and reproduction of different stem cells. There are at least four types of growth inducers, but the most important is **Interleukin 3 (IL-3)**. The formation of these inducers is controlled by environmental factors like hypoxia (for RBCs), infections (for WBCs), etc.

### *Environmental Factors*

As discussed earlier, the **prime regulator** of erythropoiesis is **hypoxia**. In situations like high altitude or other conditions which decrease the dissolved oxygen in the blood (lung diseases resulting in the decreased diffusion), tissue hypoxia results in the release of erythropoietin and increased formation of red cells. Hence, people living at high altitudes and even newborn babies (due to intrauterine hypoxia) have a high RBC count.

**Table 13.2:** Stages of differentiation of red cells.

| Name of erythroblast stage | Cell morphology | Cell diameter | Cytoplasmic characteristics | Nuclear characteristics | Hemoglobin | Summary |
|---|---|---|---|---|---|---|
| Hemocytoblast | | 18–23 µm | Blue basophilic cytoplasm | Prominent nucleus with mitotic activity. Nucleoli present | Absent | • 7 days to form mature RBC<br>• **Size:** Decreases, from 18–23 µm to 7 µm<br>• **Nucleus:** Condenses, pyknotic, disappears<br>• **Hb:** Appears in intermediate normoblast<br>• **Cytoplasm:** Increase in amount, staining changes from basophilic to acidophilic<br>• **Mitosis:** Stops after intermediate normoblast |
| Proerythroblast pronormoblast | | 14–19 µm | Blue basophilic cytoplasm | Prominent nucleus with mitotic activity. Nucleoli present | Absent | |
| Early normoblast | | 11–17 µm | Blue basophilic cytoplasm | Active mitosis present. Nucleus condenses and shows *'wheel spokes appearance'* | Starts forming but the concentration is very low to be stained | |
| Intermediate normoblast | | 10–14 µm | Due to the appearance of hemoglobin in this stage, the staining character of cytoplasm begins to change from basophilic to acidophilic. Hence at this stage it picks up both the stains hence shows polychromatic staining pattern | Nucleus further condenses and decreases in size and begins to appear as a *'checker board'* | Amount of Hb increases and becomes identifiable. Hence, Hb appears during this stage | |
| Late normoblast | | 7–10 µm | Cytoplasm stains pink/eosinophilic | Nucleus further condenses and takes *'cart wheel appearance'* | Hb concentration rises further | |
| Reticulocyte | | 7–7.5 µm | Cytoplasm stains pink/eosinophilic. There is a fine reticular meshwork present in cytoplasm | **Nucleus gets extruded** out at this stage | Increases | |
| Erythrocyte | | 7–7.5 µm | Cytoplasm stains pink/eosinophilic | Nucleus is *absent* | Fully saturated with hemoglobin | |

*Why does the RBC count increase at high altitudes?*

*Why do the newborns have a high RBC count/high hemoglobin content?*

*Why the patients with long standing cardiac failure/lung disease have high RBC count?*

*Why does a patient with chronic renal disease is anemic?*

## Hormonal Factors

- **Erythropoietin:** It is a **glycoprotein** hormone (molecular weight 34,000), secreted primarily by **kidney (90%)** (probably from fibroblast like interstitial cells surrounding the tubules in the cortex and medulla) and rest by **liver**. Decreased oxygenation of renal tissue due to hypoxia, low blood volume, lung diseases, other hormones like norepinephrine, epinephrine and some prostaglandins, increases the levels of *hypoxia inducible factor 1 (HIF-1)*, a transcription factor for hypoxia inducible genes. HIF binds to *hypoxia response element* in the *erythropoietin gene* and produces **mRNA**, which leads to *synthesis of erythropoietin* (Fig. 13.2).

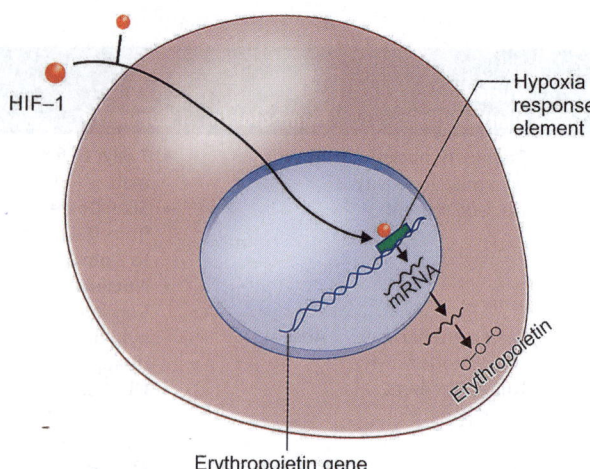

**Fig. 13.2:** Formation of erythropoietin.
(HIF-1: hypoxia inducible factor 1)

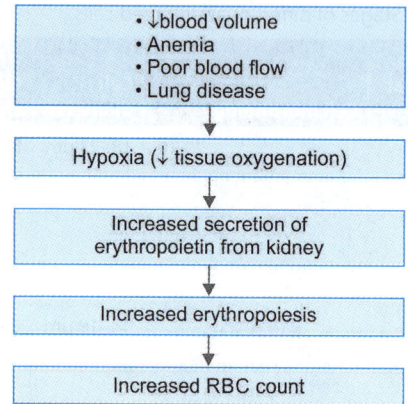

**Fig. 13.3:** Factors contributing to increase in RBC count.

The erythropoietin production begins **within minutes** to hours but it's **peak** production within **24 hours**. The red cells, however begin to appear in the circulation **after about 5 days**. This shows that the erythropoietin **stimulates** the production of **proerythroblasts** from the hemopoietic stem cell. It increases the speed of erythropoiesis. It acts through cytokine receptors present on the cell membrane of the target cells.

*Mechanism of action of erythropoietin (Fig. 13.3):*
- It stimulates progenitor cells and early precursors of erythrocytes
- It increases hemoglobin synthesis
- It acts on stem cells to promote their transformation towards erythroid series
- It stimulates the early release of reticulocytes into blood (increases reticulocyte count in the peripheral blood)

- **Thyroxine:** It is an important hormone synthesized by the thyroid gland is responsible for the maintenance of the basal metabolic rate of our body. This hormone also **stimulates** the production of RBCs by increasing the overall rate of growth.
- **Testosterone:** It is the male reproductive hormone which **stimulates** the erythropoiesis and is responsible for the higher RBC count in the males as compared to females.

*Why males have higher RBC count as compared to females?*

### Dietary Factors

- **Proteins:** The availability of proteins determine the rate of erythropoiesis, as they are required for the **synthesis of the globin chains of Hb.** Hence, the patients of hypoproteinemia, suffer from chronic anemia.

*Why patients with long standing hypoproteinemia suffer from chronic anemia?*

- **Minerals:** Various minerals like **iron, cobalt and manganese** are required for erythropoiesis.
- **Vitamins:** Vitamin B12 and **folic acid** are required for nuclear maturation during the erythropoiesis. Both these vitamins act as the methyl carriers and results in condensation of nucleus. In the absence of any of these vitamins, the nuclear maturation lags behind the cytoplasmic maturation. The cell size remains larger than the mature RBCs; resulting in the formation of macrocytes. Some of the RBCs remain nucleated, which are called as megaloblasts, hence the name Megaloblastic anemia.

## SUMMARY

In this chapter, we have learnt that:
- The erythrocytes, also called as the red blood cells are anucleated cells formed in the bone marrow which carries the oxygen bound to the hemoglobin present inside them.
- The process of formation of erythrocytes is called the erythrocytosis. In the embryonic stage, it takes place in yolk sac while in fetus it takes place in liver and spleen. Both these are extramedullary sites of erythropoiesis. However, second trimester onwards till the rest of life after birth, the hemopoiesis takes place in bone marrow (medullary site).
- The red cell formation takes place through various stages beginning from a large hemocytoblast cell to proerythroblast, early, intermediate and late normoblast, reticulocyte and erythrocyte. It is completed in 7 days in bone marrow. The cell size decreases, nucleus shrinks, becomes pyknotic and gets extruded from the cell after late normoblast stage.
- The Hb appears in intermediate normoblast stage.
- The erythropoiesis is regulated by the secretion of erythropoietin hormone.
- Other factors affecting erythropoiesis are hypoxia, mineral and proteins.

## LET US SEE, HOW MUCH YOU HAVE LEARNT?

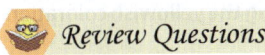
### Review Questions

#### Long/Short Answer Questions

Q1. Define erythropoiesis. Describe the stages of erythropoiesis with emphasis on cell size, cytoplasmic changes and nuclear changes.
Q2. Describe the factors affecting the erythropoiesis.
Q3. Describe the regulation of erythropoiesis.
Q4. Describe the release, mechanism of action and functions of erythropoietin.

#### Explain Why? (Reasoning Questions)

Q1. RBCs lose their nucleus during the process of erythropoiesis?
Q2. When is an erythrocyte called, fully saturated with hemoglobin?
Q3. If the RBCs do not have any cell organelles, then how do they metabolize substrates for their needs?
Q4. If the size of mature RBC is around 7 μ̈, then how do they pass through the capillaries of 5 μ?
Q5. Why does the RBC count increases at high altitudes?
Q6. Why do the newborns have a high RBC count/high hemoglobin content?
Q7. Why the patients with long standing cardiac failure/lung disease have high RBC count?
Q8. Why does a patient with chronic renal disease is anemic?
Q9. Why males have higher RBC count as compared to females?
Q10. Why patients with long standing hypoproteinemia suffer from chronic anemia?

### Critical Thinking Case-Based Questions

Q1. A 50-year-old male reported with complaints of fatigue, shortness of breath, and dizziness. His medical history revealed chronic kidney disease (CKD), which had been progressively worsening over the past few years. Blood tests indicated a significantly low hemoglobin level and reduced red blood cell (RBC) count, consistent with anemia. Further tests show decreased serum erythropoietin levels. Depending upon the given case scenario, answer the following:
   a. Explain how chronic kidney disease can lead to anemia through the disruption of erythropoietin regulation?
   b. What role does erythropoietin play in the regulation of erythropoiesis?
   c. What are the mechanism of actions of erythropoietin?

### Multiple Choice Questions

Q1. What is the primary function of erythrocytes?
   a. Transporting oxygen
   b. Fighting infections
   c. Producing hormones
   d. Regulating body temperature
Q2. What is the lifespan of a typical human erythrocyte?
   a. 60 days            b. 90 days
   c. 120 days           d. 150 days
Q3. Which component of erythrocytes is responsible for oxygen transport?
   a. Hemoglobin         b. Nucleus
   c. Mitochondria       d. Endoplasmic reticulum
Q4. Which organ is primarily responsible for the production of erythrocytes?
   a. Liver              b. Kidneys
   c. Bone marrow        d. Spleen
Q5. What is the shape of a mature human erythrocyte?
   a. Round              b. Cuboidal
   c. Discoid            d. Spherical
Q6. Which condition is characterized by a decreased number of erythrocytes?
   a. Anemia             b. Leukemia
   c. Thrombocytopenia   d. Hemophilia
Q7. How does carbon monoxide poisoning affect erythrocytes?
   a. It increases their lifespan
   b. It decreases their ability to carry oxygen
   c. It enhances their oxygen-carrying capacity
   d. It has no effect on erythrocytes
Q8. Which hormone stimulates the production of erythrocytes?
   a. Insulin            b. Thyroxine
   c. Erythropoietin     d. Adrenaline
Q9. What is the average volume of an erythrocyte?
   a. 80–90 fl           b. 120–140 fl
   c. 150–160 fl         d. 180–190 fl
Q10. Which nutrient is essential for the synthesis of hemoglobin in erythrocytes?
   a. Vitamin C          b. Iron
   c. Vitamin D          d. Vitamin B12
Q11. A patient presents with pale skin, fatigue, and shortness of breath. Lab results show low levels of hemoglobin. Which condition is most likely?
   a. Iron deficiency anemia
   b. Sickle cell anemia
   c. Polycythemia
   d. Aplastic anemia

Q12. A marathon runner experiences dehydration and electrolyte imbalances during a race. How might this affect their erythrocyte function?
   a. Decreased oxygen transport
   b. Increased oxygen transport
   c. No effect on oxygen transport
   d. Increased lifespan of erythrocytes

Q13. A patient with kidney disease is prescribed erythropoietin injections. What is the intended effect of this treatment?
   a. Stimulate erythrocyte production
   b. Decrease erythrocyte count
   c. Increase platelet count
   d. Improve white blood cell function

Q14. A newborn infant is diagnosed with jaundice due to excessive breakdown of erythrocytes. Which pigment accumulates in the skin causing the yellowish coloration?
   a. Bilirubin
   b. Melanin
   c. Carotene
   d. Hemoglobin

Q15. A person living at high altitudes may have increased erythrocyte levels compared to a person at sea level. What is the physiological reason for this adaptation?
   a. Increased oxygen affinity of hemoglobin
   b. Decreased oxygen affinity of hemoglobin
   c. Increased production of erythropoietin
   d. Decreased production of erythropoietin

**ANSWERS**

1. a   2. c   3. a   4. c   5. c   6. a   7. b   8. c   9. b   10. b   11. a   12. a   13. a   14. d
15. c

# Physiology of Anemia

**CHAPTER 14**

**COMPETENCY ADDRESSED**

PY2.5: Describe different types of anemias and jaundice.

**LEARNING OBJECTIVES**

At the end of this chapter, the learner should be able to:
- Define anemia.
- Classify anemia according to morphological, clinical and etiological classification.
- Describe physiological basis of clinical features of anemia.
- Describe pathophysiology of Iron deficiency anemia.
- Describe the sources, absorption, transport of iron.
- Describe pathophysiology of megaloblastic anemia.
- Describe pathophysiology of different types of hemolytic anemia with special emphasis on G-6-PD deficiency.
- Describe the clinic-laboratory profile of different types of anemias.

## ANEMIA

### Definition of Anemia

Anemia is defined as *the decrease in the oxygen carrying capacity of the blood* which may or may not be accompanied with decreased hemoglobin or RBC count.

### Classification of Anemia

There are different ways to classify anemia, depending upon the clinical presentation, etiology or morphology of the red blood cells. Lets quickly go through all the three types of classifications:

- **Clinical classification:** It is the widely used classification for categorization of anemia on the basis of hemoglobin.
  - *Mild anemia:* Hemoglobin level is between 10–12 g%
  - *Moderate anemia:* Hemoglobin level is 7–10 g%
  - *Severe anemia:* Hemoglobin level is 5–7 g%
  - *Life threatening:* Hemoglobin level is <5 g%
- **Morphological classification (Fig. 14.1):** It is based on the morphology of the red blood cells seen on the peripheral blood fil and also calculated as per the red cell indices (mean corpuscular volume (MCV) and mean corpuscular hemoglobin concentration (MCHC)). Based on these two indices, the morphological classification is done as shown in **Table 14.1**.

**Table 14.1:** Morphological classification of anemia.

| | Hypochromic (Hb conc. <33%) | Normochromic (Hb conc. ≥33%) |
|---|---|---|
| Microcytic (cell size <7 μ) | Iron deficiency anemia | Thalassemia, chronic disease |
| Normocytic (cell size = 7 μ) | Anemia of chronic diseases like chronic kidney disease, chronic gastrointestinal diseases | Acute blood loss Hemolytic anemia Aplastic anemia |
| Macrocytic (cell size >7 μ) | Malnutrition | Liver disease, vitamin B12 deficiency |

*Why don't we see the hyperchromia in the RBC?*

- **Etiological classification:** This classification is based on the cause of anemia **Table 14.2**.

### Clinical Features

Clinical presentation of these patients is primarily due to acute of chronic hypoxia occurring due to decreased oxygen carrying capacity of blood.

### *General Presentation (Fig. 14.2)*

- Easy fatigue and loss of energy (Most common)
- Weakness

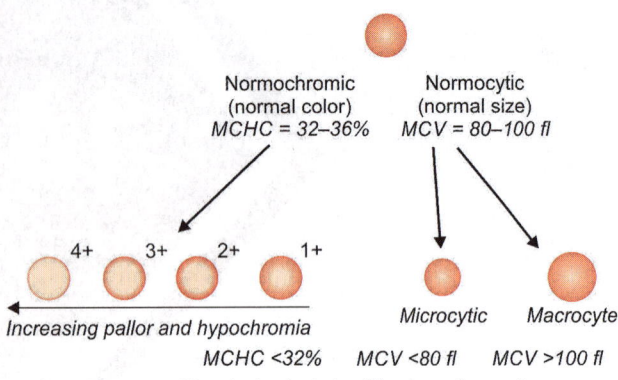

Fig. 14.1: Morphological classification of anemia.

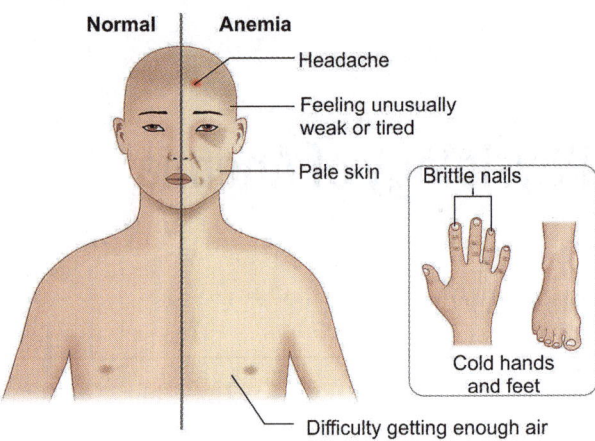

Fig. 14.2: Clinical features of anemia.

- Pale skin
- Cold hands and feet
- Light-headedness
- Shortness of breath especially on exertion
- Anxiety, depression, irritability
- Dizziness
- Poor performance
- Leg cramps
- Reduced exercise tolerance
- Hair loss which are easy to break

### Signs due to Effect on Cardiovascular System

- **Tachycardia:** It occurs as a response to tissue hypoxia occurring in anemia. The sympathetic overactivity increases the heart rate in an attempt to increase the cardiac output and hence improve the tissue oxygenation.
- **Hyperdynamic state with increased cardiac output (Increased blood flow):** According to the physiological explanation, a decrease in red blood cells (RBCs) lowers the viscosity, which decreases peripheral resistance and enhances tissue blood flow.
- **Systolic murmur:** The reason of the systolic flow murmur is hyperdynamic circulation. When a large volume of blood passes through a normal cardiac valve, the laminar blood flow is disrupted, creating noise and turbulence. It is heard in severe anemia.

- **Increased cardiac workload during activity:** It is due to increase workload on heart. Heart is working more to pump adequate oxygen to the body resulting in increased workload on heart.
- **Decreased oxygen reserve for exercise:** Anemic patient has difficulty during exercise because of limited ability to increase $O_2$ delivery to the active tissues.

## IRON DEFICIENCY ANEMIA

The anemia occurring due to deficiency of iron in the diet or due to increased loss of heme iron (increased blood loss due to bleeding disorder of parasitic infestation) results in iron deficiency anemia (IDA). It is *most common cause of anemia* in India, especially in infants, growing children, women and elderly.

### Etiopathogenesis

- **Dietary deficiency:**
  - Infants on exclusive breast feeding beyond 6 months
  - Deficient iron in diet
- **Decreased absorption from GIT:**
  - Decreased HCl secretion
  - Inflammation of GIT

Table 14.2: Etiological classification of anemia.

| Increased blood loss | | Increased breakdown of red cells (Hemolysis) | | Decreased synthesis of red cells | |
|---|---|---|---|---|---|
| Acute | Chronic | Intracorpuscular defect | Extracorpuscular defect | Increased demand | Decreased production |
| **Acute blood loss:**<br>• Trauma<br>• Surgery | **Bleeding:**<br>• Piles<br>• Esophageal varices<br>• Abnormal uterine bleeding<br>**Parasites:**<br>Hookworm infestation | **Defects in red cell membrane:**<br>• Hereditary spherocytosis<br>• Hereditary ovalocytosis<br>**Defects in red cell enzymes:**<br>• G-6-PD deficiency<br>• Pyruvate kinase deficiency<br>**Defects in hemoglobin:**<br>• Thalassemia<br>• Sickle cell anemia | **Nonimmune mediated:**<br>• Splenomegaly<br>• Chronic malaria<br>• Burns<br>• Drug induced<br>**Immune mediated:**<br>• Incompatible blood transfusion<br>• Hemolytic disease of newborn | • Children<br>• Adolescents<br>• Pregnancy<br>• Lactation | **Deficiency of nutrients:**<br>• Iron deficiency anemia<br>• Folic acid deficiency anemia<br>• Vitamin B12 deficiency anemia<br>• Deficiency of proteins, cobalt and other nutrients<br>**Autoimmune anemia:**<br>Pernicious anemia<br>**Defects in bone marrow:**<br>• Aplastic anemia<br>• Pure red cell aplasia |

- Decreased absorption due to chelation with calcium/phytates
- **Increased demand:**
  - Growing children
  - Pregnancy
  - Lactation
- **Increased loss:**
  - Chronic bleeding: Hemorrhoids (Piles), abnormal uterine bleeding
  - Parasitic infestation: Hookworm infestation

## Clinical Features

All the features of tissue hypoxia are seen in iron deficiency anemia also. Apart from these, some specific signs worth remembering are
- **Pica:** Craving to eat non-food items like chalk, clay etc.
- **Koilonychia (Fig. 14.3):** Spooning of the nails/concavity in the nails

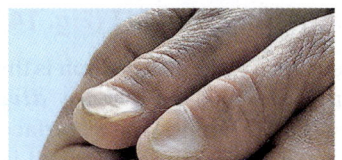

**Fig. 14.3:** Koilonychia.

> **CLINICAL CASE SCENARIO**
> A 42-year-old woman presents with history of progressive fatigue and breathlessness on exertion, is unable to climb a flight of stairs with stopping. She is vegetarian. Her menstrual cycles are regular with heavy bleeding. Her CBC reports reveal Hb: 7.2 g/dL, Hematocrit (%): 21.6, RBC: 3.5 million/cm$^3$, MCV: 89 fL, MCHC%: 39. Iron profile shows decreased serum iron, ferritin and transferrin saturation. Total iron binding capacity (TIBC) is increased.
> Justify your diagnosis with clinico-laboratory findings.
> *Note:* To study the case based scenario, refer to author's Early Clinical Exposure in Clinical Physiology.

### Laboratory Findings of IDA

See **Table 14.3**.

### Dietary Sources of Iron

- Non Heme iron: Green leafy vegetables, legumes, nuts, seeds, etc.
- Heme Iron: Meat, liver, sea food, etc.

The daily requirement of iron in adults is recommended as:
- In men and non-menstruating women: 8 mg
- In menstruating women: 18 mg
- In pregnant women: 27 mg

**Table 14.3:** Laboratory findings of iron deficiency anemia (IDA).

| Laboratory parameter | In IDA | Normal values |
|---|---|---|
| Red blood cell count | ≤4 million/cc | 4–4.5 million/cc in females<br>5–5.5 million/cc in males |
| Hemoglobin content | ≤12 g% | 12–14 g% in females<br>13–15 g% in males |
| Packed cell volume | ≤40% | 42–45% |
| Erythrocyte sedimentation rate | >20 mm at the end of 1st hour | <15 mm at the end of 1st hour in males<br>< 20 mm at the end of 1st hour in females |
| **Red cell indices** | | |
| MCV | ≤78 fL | 78–96 fL |
| MCH | ≤27 pg | 27–33 pg |
| MCHC | ≤33% | 33–37% |
| Peripheral blood film | Microcytic hypochromic red cells | Normocytic normochromic red cells |
| Serum ferritin levels | ≤10 µg/L | 20–200 µg/L in females<br>30–300 µg/L in males |
| Total iron binding capacity | Increased | 250–450 µg/L |
| Serum transferrin levels | Raised | 215–380 mg/dL |
| Percentage saturation of transferrin | <16% | 33% |

## Absorption of Iron from GIT (Fig. 14.4)

The main site for the absorption of iron is the duodenum. The duodenal mucosal cell has a *divalent metal transporter (DMT-1)* on its apical surface. The *Ferric reductase* converts $Fe^{3+}$ into $Fe^{2+}$, which is transported inside the mucosal cell by the DMT-1. The heme iron is transported by another transporter protein *heme carrier protein (HCP-1)*. The heme is converted to $Fe^{2+}$ by *heme oxygenase ($HO_2$)*. Some of the $Fe^{2+}$ combines with ferritin and stays in the enterocyte. This gets lost in the stool, whenever the enterocytes are sloughed off or renewed. Majority of $Fe^{2+}$ is transported into interstitial fluid by *ferroportin (FPN-1)*. The transferrin binds to the $Fe^{3+}$ instead of $Fe^{2+}$, hence another membrane proteins *Hephaestin (Heph)* converts $Fe^{2+}$ to $Fe^{3+}$. Hence the $Fe^{3+}$ binds to *transferrin*, which gets saturated up to 33% and enters the blood stream.

The iron is stored in our body as hemoglobin (70%), myoglobin (3%) and rest as ferritin in various tissues bound to apoferritin. *Apoferritin* is also present in enterocytes. Ferritin may also be present in the lysosomal membrane called *hemosiderin*. Serum iron levels in males is **130 µg/L** and in females is **110 µg/L**.

### CLINICAL CASE SCENARIO

A 46-year-old male presented to the medicine OPD with reddish discoloration of skin and hair along with the complaint of pain in right hypochondrium and joint pains. On further exploration it was revealed that he had been receiving repeated blood transfusions for thalassemia. His laboratory investigations show increased serum iron levels and low total iron binding capacity. His liver enzymes are deranged, suggesting the liver involvement. His fasting blood sugar and HBA1c are also raised indicating the diabetes in the patient. What is your probable diagnosis? Justify your answer.

This patient is suffering from **hemochromatosis** due to repeated blood transfusions resulting in iron overload and hence resulting in these symptoms of liver and pancreatic involvement. The reddish discoloration of skin and hair due to deposition of hemosiderin in these tissues. The diabetes in these patients has a specific name **"Bronze diabetes"** owing to the reddish discoloration of body.

## MACROCYTIC ANEMIA

It is defined as the decreased oxygen carrying capacity of blood due to decreased hemoglobin with macrocytosis (elevated mean corpuscular volume (>100 fL)). It is divided into two types: megaloblastic and non-megaloblastic anemia.

1. **Megaloblastic anemia:** Megaloblastic anemia is characterized by the presence of large red blood cell precursors called megaloblasts in the bone marrow.
2. **Nonmegaloblastic anemia:** Megaloblasts are absent.

### Pathophysiology

It results from suppression of nuclear division and DNA synthesis. Defects in cytoplasmic maturation are less severe since it mostly depends on RNA and protein production. This causes the cytoplasm and nucleus of the erythroblasts to mature asynchronously, which explains why the megaloblasts are so big.

The physiological roles of these two vitamins—folic acid and vitamin B12—are related. As a result, the absence of one vitamin affects the physiological function of the other.

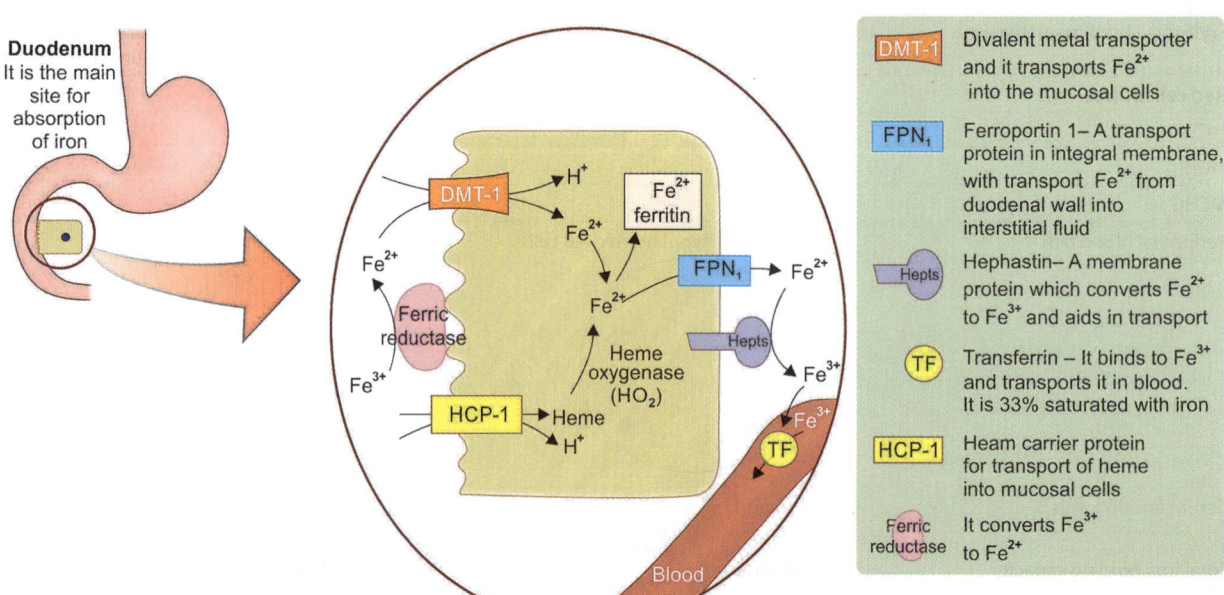

**Fig. 14.4:** Absorption of iron in GIT.

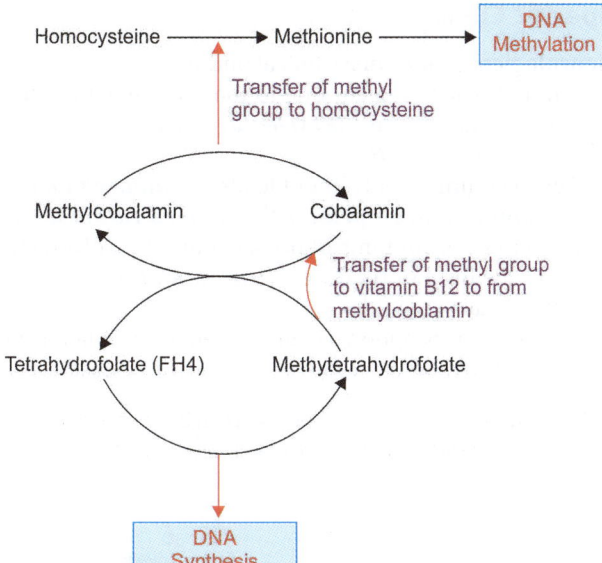

**Fig. 14.5:** Role of folic acid and vitamin B12 in DNA synthesis and maturation.

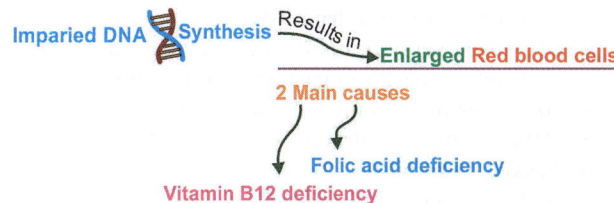

**Fig. 14.6:** Deficiency of vitamin B12 and folic acid resulting in enlarged RBCs.

As seen in **Figure 14.5**, the folic acid and vitamin B12 results in:
- Methyl group transfer for the formation of tetrahydrofolate.
- Formation of transcobalamin, which transfers the methyl group to homocysteine to form methionine. This results in DNA maturation.

In cases of vitamin B12 insufficiency, neither the methyl group transfer nor the production of tetrahydrofolate (THF) occurs. This results in nonavailability of folate resulting in the *folate trap*. Moreover, methionine is not generated.

Hence, both vitamin B12 and folic acid are required for the synthesis of DNA **(Fig. 14.6)**. This deficiency doesn't affect only red cells but all the cells in bone marrow. There is delayed maturation process in neutrophils, which is brought on by a decrease in DNA synthesis, leads to a *hypersegmented nucleus of neutrophils*.

Vitamin B12 is also necessary for the *synthesis of the myelin sheath of peripheral neurons,* because it changes methylmalonyl-CoA into succinyl-CoA. Vitamin B12 deficiency results in degeneration of dorsal columns and lateral columns of the spinal cord due to demyelination and causes neurological clinical features (peripheral neuropathy) presenting with burning sensation, paresthesia and pain in peripheral parts of body especially in lower limbs.

## Causes of Vitamin B12 and Folic Acid Deficiency (Fig. 14.7)

### Etiopathogenesis

- **Dietary deficiency**
  - Deficient folic acid/vitamin B12 in diet

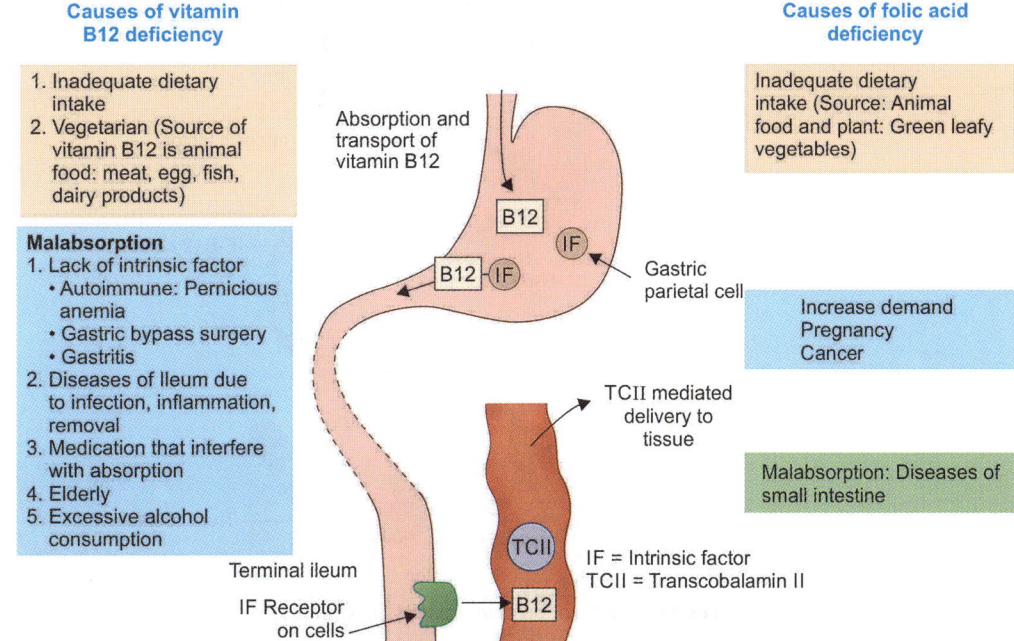

**Fig. 14.7:** Causes of folic acid and vitamin B12 deficiency.

- **Decreased absorption from GIT**
  - Decreased secretion of Castle's Intrinsic factor due to atrophic gastritis or gastrectomy for vitamin B12
  - Loss of terminal ileum for vitamin B12
  - Malabsorption syndrome
- **Increased demand**
  - Growing children
  - Pregnancy
  - Lactation
- **Pernicious anemia/autoimmune gastritis:** It is the most common cause of vitamin B12 deficiency. It is an autoimmune disorder in which auto-antibodies are formed against parietal cells and intrinsic factor.

## Absorption of Vitamin B12 from GIT (Fig. 14.8)

Normally, the intrinsic factor, is produced by the parietal cells, binds to vitamin B12 and facilitates its transport to the ileum, where it can be absorbed. Destruction of the parietal cells and subsequent intrinsic factor deficiency leads to reduced uptake of vitamin B12.

## Specific Clinical Features

**Neurological symptoms:** Clinical findings are
- Symmetrical and occur due to the involvement of the *dorsal columns, spinocerebellar tracts, and lateral corticospinal tracts*.
- Dorsal column involvement leads to *impaired tactile discrimination, proprioception, and vibration sense*.
- The earliest symptoms of dorsal column involvement are in the form of *tingling, burning, and sensory loss* of the distal extremities.
- Loss of proprioception usually presents as a difficulty in *maintaining balance in the dark* or with closed eyes.

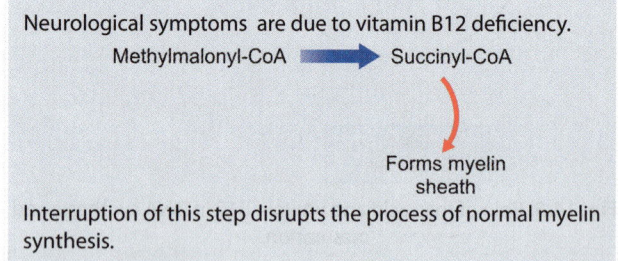

Neurological symptoms are due to vitamin B12 deficiency.
Methylmalonyl-CoA ⟶ Succinyl-CoA ⟶ Forms myelin sheath
Interruption of this step disrupts the process of normal myelin synthesis.

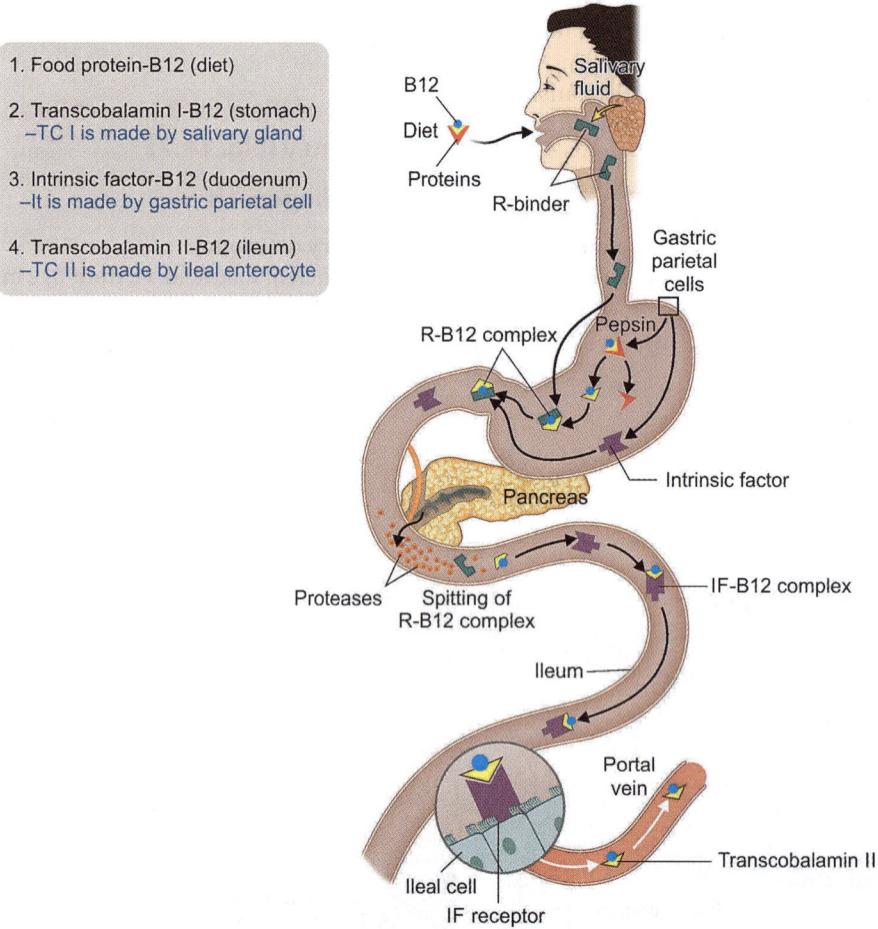

1. Food protein-B12 (diet)
2. Transcobalamin I-B12 (stomach)
   – TC I is made by salivary gland
3. Intrinsic factor-B12 (duodenum)
   – It is made by gastric parietal cell
4. Transcobalamin II-B12 (ileum)
   – TC II is made by ileal enterocyte

**Fig. 14.8:** Absorption of vitamin B12 in GIT.

- Lateral corticospinal tract dysfunction causes *muscle weakness, hyperreflexia,* and *spasticity*. Stiffness is often the initial symptom of lateral cord involvement. Spinocerebellar tract degeneration causes gait abnormalities in the form of sensory ataxia.

## Diagnosis

Laboratory findings in macrocytic anemia are tabulated in **Table 14.4**.

# HEMOLYTIC ANEMIA

Hemolytic anemia is a class of anemia that is caused by excessive the destruction of red blood cells (red blood cells have a lifespan of 120 days) resulting in decreased red cell count. It is characterized by increased hemoglobin catabolism, decreased levels of hemoglobin, and an increase in efforts of bone marrow to regenerate products.

## Pathophysiology

As seen in the etiological classification **(Table 14.2)**, there could be many reasons which result is hemolysis.

### Intracorpuscular Defects

- **Defects in red cell membrane (Figs. 14.9 and 14.10):** Hereditary spherocytosis is the defect caused by mutations in skeleton proteins resulting in membrane instability. The RBC lose their biconcave shape and become spherical due to deficiency of the *linker protein Ankyrin, α and β Spectrin and transmembrane protein band 3* in the red cell membrane.
- **Defects in red cell enzymes:** G-6-PD deficiency **(Fig. 14.11)**—It is a genetic disorder in which there is deficiency of glucose-6-phosphate dehydrogenase enzyme in the red cells.

**Table 14.4:** Laboratory findings of macrocytic anemia.

| Laboratory parameter | Macrocytic anemia | Normal values |
|---|---|---|
| Red blood cell count | ≤4 million/cc | 4–4.5 million/cc in females<br>5–5.5 million/cc in males |
| Hemoglobin content | ≤12 g% | 12–14 g% in females<br>13–15 g% in males |
| **Red cell indices** | | |
| MCV | ≥100 fL | 78–96 fL |
| MCH | ≤33 pg | 27–33 pg |
| MCHC | 33–37% | 33–37% |
| Peripheral blood film | Macrocytic normochromic red cells. Other abnormal red cells are also present.<br><br>Megaloblasts may or may not be present<br>Hypersegmented neutrophils present<br>thrombocytopenia | Normocytic normochromic red cells |
| Serum vitamin B12 level | <200 pg/mL in vitamin B12 deficiency | 300 pg/mL |
| Serum folate level | <2 µg/L in folate deficiency | 2–20 µg/L |
| Serum methylmalonic acid (MMA) | Raised in vitamin B12 deficiency | 0.07–0.27 micromoles per liter |
| Serum homocysteine | Raised in vitamin B12 deficiency | 5–15 µmoles/L |
| Autoantibodies to intrinsic factor (IF) | Present in pernicious anemia | Absent |

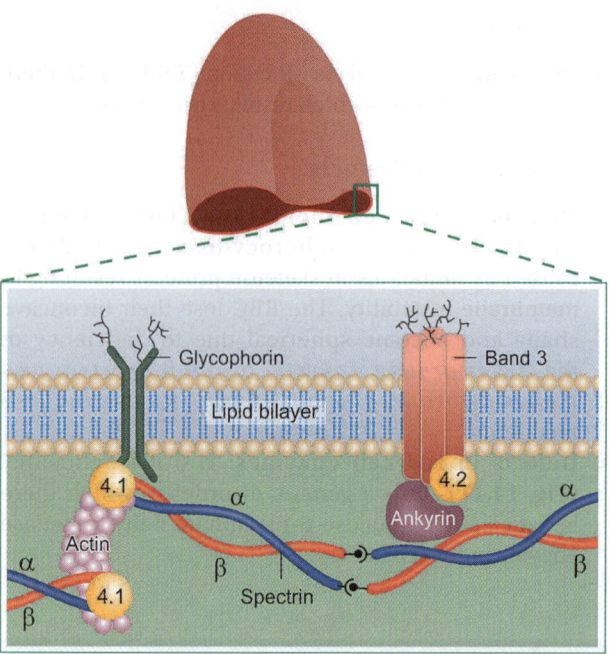

**Fig. 14.9:** Defect in red cell membrane proteins resulting in hereditary spherocytosis.

Normally, the G-6-PD keeps the glutathione in the reduced state, which is responsible for the antioxidant effect in the red blood cells. When there is a deficiency of this enzyme, level of glutathione reductase decreases. Hence, there is a compromised clearance of free oxide radicals. Incase these patients consume anything which increases the production of free oxygen radicals like fava beans, antimalarial drugs, infection, sulfa containing antibiotics; results in increased free oxygen radicals.

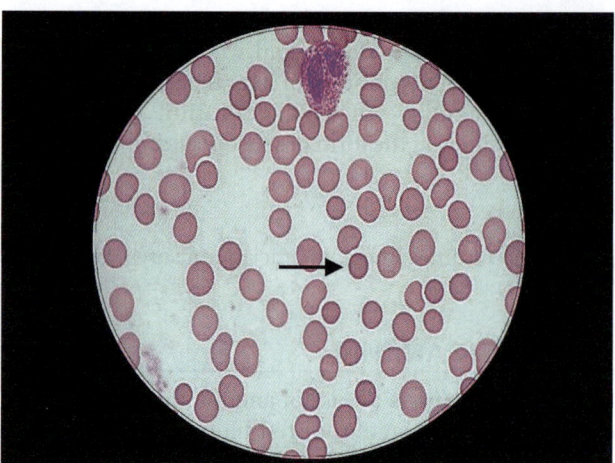

**Fig. 14.10:** Peripheral blood film showing spherocytosis.

Since the reduced glutathione is not sufficient to handle this increased load, there occurs hemolysis due to free oxide radical injury to red cells.

- **Defects in hemoglobin:**
  - *Thalassemia:* Defective/no synthesis of globin chain of hemoglobin results in the thalassemia. Depending on the type of globin chain involved, it is classified as:
    - β-thalassemia: The β-chain synthesis is affected. The fetal hemoglobin (HbF, $\alpha_2 \gamma_2$) persists after birth. The level of HbF depends upon the severity of β-thalassemia.
      - *In β-thalassemia major:* There is complete absence of synthesis of β chains
      - *In β-thalassemia minor:* There is partial absence of synthesis of β chains

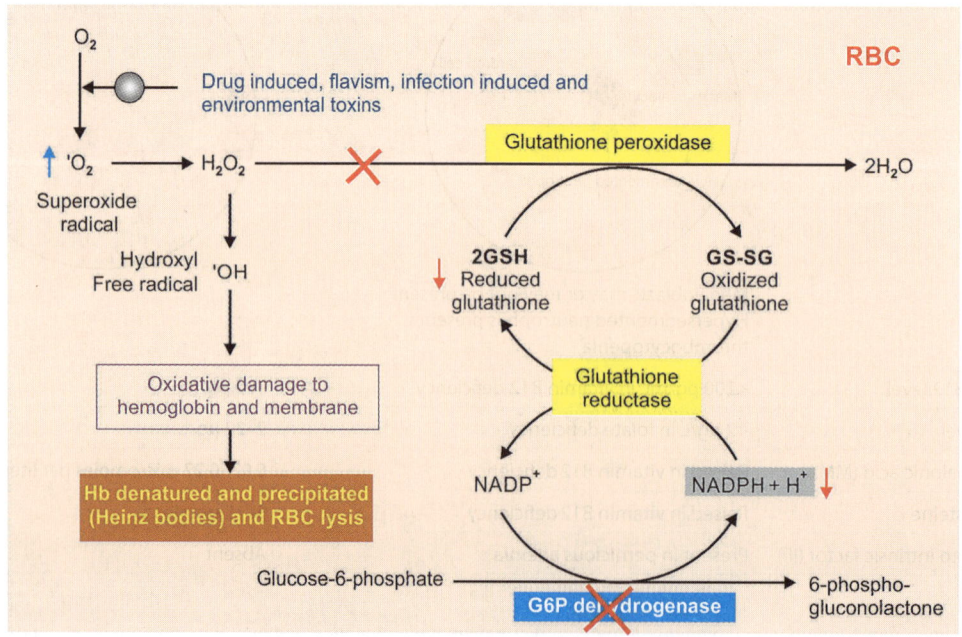

**Fig. 14.11:** Pathophysiology of G-6-PD deficiency.

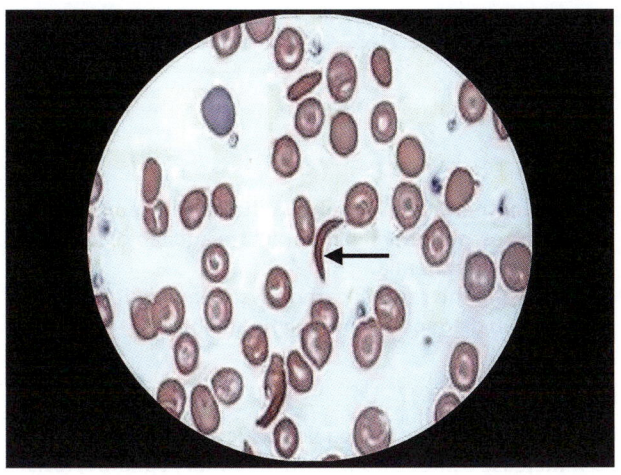

**Fig. 14.12:** Peripheral blood film showing sickle cell anemia.

glutamic acid in the beta-chain. The RBCs undergo sickling, whenever there is decrease in oxygen tension in circulating blood. The sickle cells tend to stick together, blocking small blood vessels causing painful and damaging complications.

### Extracorpuscular Defects

- **Nonimmune mediated:** These defects result in the mechanical destruction of RBCs
  - Splenomegaly
  - Chronic malaria
  - Burns
  - Drug induced
- **Immune mediated:** The antigen and antibody reaction results in hemolysis.
  - Incompatible blood transfusion
  - Hemolytic disease of newborn

## Diagnosis

Laboratory findings in macrocytic anemia are tabulated in **Table 14.5**.

- α-thalassemia: The α-chain synthesis is affected. This is less common form thalassemia.
- ***Sickle cell anemia (Fig. 14.12):*** There is a genetic defect resulting in the substitution of valine for

**Table 14.5:** Laboratory findings of hemolytic anemia.

| Laboratory parameter | Hemolytic anemia | Normal values |
|---|---|---|
| Red blood cell count | ≤4 million/cc | 4–4.5 million/cc in females<br>5–5.5 million/cc in males |
| Hemoglobin content | ≤12 g% | 12–14 g% in females<br>13–15 g% in males |
| Reticulocyte count | Increased | 1–2% |
| **Red cell indices** | | |
| MCV | Within normal limits | 78–96 fL |
| MCH | Within normal limits | 27–33 pg |
| MCHC | Within normal limits | 33–37% |
| Peripheral blood film | Normocytic normochromic red cells<br>• Spherocytosis, if there is hereditary spherocytosis **(Fig. 14.10)**<br>• Sickle cell anemia **(Fig. 14.12)** | Normocytic normochromic red cells |
| Serum bilirubin level | Raised total and unconjugated bilirubin | Total: 0.2–0.8 mg/dL<br>Unconjugated bilirubin: 0.2–0.6 mg/dL<br>Conjugated: 0–0.2 mg/dL |
| Serum LDH | Raised | 105–233 units/L |
| Free haptoglobin | Very low | 40–200 mg/dL |
| Urine hemosiderin | Present | Absent |

## SUMMARY

- Erythropoietin (EPO) stimulates the process of erythropoiesis. It is secreted by the kidneys and liver. The strongest inducer of erythropoietin release is hypoxia.
- Anemia is decrease in oxygen carrying capacity of the blood due to decrease in hemoglobin with or without decrease in red blood cell count (RBC).
- Iron, vitamin B12, and folic acid deficiencies are the main causes of nutritional anemia. Iron deficiency anemia is the most frequent type of anemia. Vegetarians are more likely to have vitamin B12 deficiency anemia. Folic acid deficiency is common during pregnancy.
- Vitamin B12 deficiency can cause neurological symptoms in addition to hematologic ones, while folic acid deficiency mostly impacts hematologic symptoms.
- In hemolytic anemia, hemolysis can take place—intravascularly or extravascularly. Hemosiderinuria and hemoglobinuria occurs in intravascular hemolysis in addition to increased LDH, Bilirubin, and hemosiderin.

# LET US SEE, HOW MUCH YOU HAVE LEARNT?

## Review Questions

### Long/Short Answer Questions

Q1. Describe the causes and blood picture of nutritional anemia.
Q2. Enumerate the red cell indices. Give its physiological and clinical significance.
Q3. Define pernicious anemia. What is the cause, clinical features, peripheral blood picture and lab diagnosis of pernicious anemia.
Q4. Describe the causes, pathophysiology, clinical features and lab diagnosis of hemolytic anemia.

### Explain Why? (Reasoning Questions)

Q1. Vitamin B12 deficiency causes neurological symptoms?
Q2. Oral vitamin B12 is of no benefit in pernicious anemia?
Q3. Vitamin B12 or folic acid deficiency leads to megaloblastic anemia?
Q4. Leukocytopenia in megaloblastic anemia?
Q5. Increase osmotic fragility in hereditary spherocytosis?
Q6. What will happen, if you give folic acid only in a patient of pernicious anemia?

### Critical Thinking Case-Based Questions

Q1. A 65-year-old woman presented with progressive fatigue and palpitations. She reported feeling dizzy and lightheaded, particularly when she stands up quickly. She also mentioned experiencing numbness and tingling in her hands and feet. The patient had been living alone since her son died in a motor vehicle collision a year ago, which has led to significant emotional distress and a poor appetite. On physical examination, she appeared pale, with a heart rate of 110 beats per minute and a blood pressure of 100/60 mm Hg. A neurological exam revealed decreased sensation in her extremities.
Based upon the clinical history, answer the following:
a. What is the probable diagnosis? Give justification.
b. Explain the pathophysiology of the diagnosed disease.
c. Give the physiological basis of all the signs and symptoms of the patient.
d. Give the physiological basis of neurological symptoms of the patient.
e. What dietary advice will you give to the patient?

### Multiple Choice Questions

Q1. The volume shows high serum ferritin and low total iron binding capacity. What is the most likely cause for this patient's anemia?
 a. Fe deficiency
 b. Anemia secondary to inflammation
 c. Thalassemia
 d. Hemoglobinopathy

Q2. Which of the following helps to differentiate between vitamin B12 deficiency and folate deficiency anemia?
 a. Serum folate level
 b. Urinary methylmalonate increase in vitamin B12 deficiency and not in folate deficiency
 c. Formiminoglutamic acid increase in vitamin B12 deficiency and not in folate deficiency
 d. Histidine increases in in vitamin B12 deficiency and not in folate deficiency

Q3. A 40-year-old female says she feels tired all the time. On examination, she is pale and has tachycardia. CBC shows: Hgb 10 g/dL (12–16), MCV 75 (80–100), Normal reticulocyte count. Which of the following is most likely?
 a. She has iron-deficiency anemia
 b. She has megaloblastic anemia, probably due to foliate deficiency
 c. She has megaloblastic anemia, probably due to B12 deficiency
 d. She has a hemolytic anemia

Q4. A patient with RA is diagnosed with anemia. What may be the likely classification of anemia?
 a. Iron deficiency anemia
 b. Megaloblastic anemia
 c. Anemia due to chronic inflammatory disease
 d. Anemia due to chronic blood loss.

Q5. A man travels to high altitude to work as a laborer in a road construction project. After two months of working in the mountains, he has to undergo some investigations and his hemoglobin is found to be 18 g/dL and RBC count is 8 million/mm$^3$. What is the clinical diagnosis along with its mechanism?
 a. Anemia due to hypoxia as a stimulus for the release of Erythropoietin from kidney
 b. Polycythemia due to hypoxia as a stimulus for the release of Erythropoietin from kidney
 c. Anemia due to hypoxia due to lung disease
 d. Polycythemia due to hypoxia due to lung disease.

Q6. A patient of anemia presents to a doctor in OPD. Auscultation reveals a flow systolic murmur. What is the physiological basis of the murmur?
 a. Increased blood flow from the stenosed valve
 b. Increased blood flow from the dilated valve
 c. Increased flow of blood from structurally normal heart valve
 d. Increased blood flow from prolapsed valve

Q7. A 43-year-old man with schizophrenia has had chronic fatigue for 6 months. He has good appetite but refuses to eat vegetables for 1 year because he hears voice saying that vegetables are poisoned. His physical and neurological examinations are normal. His Hb level is 9.1 g/dL, leukocyte count is 10,000/μL. MCV-122. What is the most likely diagnosis?
   a. Aplastic anemia
   b. Hemolytic anemia
   c. Nutritional anemia
   d. Thalassemia

Q8. A 12-year-old girl presents with fatigue for the last 2 months. She has good diet and eats regularly. She has just got her menarche 6 months back, with heavy blood flow. Physical examination reveals pallor in the palpebral conjunctiva. Lab investigations reveals Hb: 8 g/dL and a peripheral smear showing a microcytic hypochromic picture. What is the most likely cause of this patient's symptoms?
   a. Iron deficiency anemia due to increase demand
   b. Thalassemia
   c. Anemia due to chronic inflammatory disease
   d. Iron deficiency anemia due to decrease intake of iron

Q9. A 40-year-old female presents with episodic palpitations that started 6 months ago. She also reports shortness of breath, primarily during exercise and weakness. On questioning, she reveals that her hands get numb as well. Examination is significant for pallor and paresthesia. A peripheral smear shows megaloblasts. Which of the following is the most likely etiology for this patient's condition?
   a. Impaired DNA and RNA synthesis due to vitamin B12 deficiency
   b. Impaired DNA and RNA synthesis due to vitamin B9 deficiency
   c. Impaired DNA synthesis due to vitamin B12 deficiency
   d. Impaired DNA synthesis due to vitamin B9 deficiency

Q10. A 62-year-old woman presents to the outpatient department complaining of tingling and burning of both distal extremities, accompanied by unstable gait. She also complaints of not able to feel the floor when walking. Her history is notable of bariatric surgery conducted 2 months ago. She has lost 13.6 kg after the surgery and is happy about her progress. Physical examination is significant for conjunctival pallor. She also has reduced proprioceptive, vibration, and pressure sensing bilaterally in the lower limbs. The patient sways to the side when asked to stand straight with the eyes closed. Lab investigations are remarkable for Hb of 8.2 g/dL, with a mean corpuscular volume of 120 μm³. A deficiency of which of the following is responsible for the symptoms in this patient?
   a. Thiamine
   b. Cobalamin
   c. Vitamin C
   d. Folic acid

## ANSWERS

1. c   2. c   3. a   4. c   5. b   6. c   7. c   8. d   9. a   10. b

# Physiology of Jaundice

**CHAPTER 15**

### COMPETENCY ADDRESSED
**PY2.5:** Describe different types of anemia and jaundice.

### LEARNING OBJECTIVES
**At the end of this chapter, the learner should be able to:**
- Define jaundice and describe its etiology, including the role of bilirubin metabolism in its pathophysiology.
- Explain the normal physiological process of bilirubin production, transport, and metabolism in the body.
- Identify the different types of jaundice (prehepatic, hepatic, and posthepatic) based on their underlying mechanisms and clinical manifestations.
- Analyze the clinical presentation of jaundice, including signs, symptoms, and diagnostic findings, to differentiate between different types and severity levels.

## INTRODUCTION

Jaundice is defined as yellowish discoloration of skin and mucous membrane due to increased level of circulating bilirubin. It is not a disease but a clinical presentation or sign of underlying pathology either due to hemolysis or liver disease.

Since the jaundice primarily is concerned with the bilirubin levels, we must read about the fate of hemoglobin and the metabolism of bilirubin in our body **(Fig. 15.1)**.

Whenever the erythrocytes breakdown, either after completing their life span of 120 days or after any premature hemolysis, the hemoglobin is released from them. This hemoglobin breaks down into Heme part containing the tetrapyrrole rings with iron moiety and the globin chains (enter the amino acid pool, which are used for fresh globin synthesis or any other use). The heme gets broken down into a green pigment called the *biliverdin*, a green-colored pigment by the enzyme *heme oxygenase*. The enzyme biliverdin reductase further converts it to *bilirubin*, which is transported to liver bound to the albumin, to prevent its excretion in the urine.

In the albumin, the albumin-bilirubin complex dissociates to form free bilirubin (unconjugated bilirubin) and the albumin is taken up by the liver cells. The free bilirubin binds to two molecules of **UDP glucuronic acid** to form the bilirubin glucuronide (conjugated bilirubin). It is a rate limiting step. Some amount of conjugated bilirubin escapes the active conjugation process and is filtered in the kidneys and is excreted out as *urinary bilirubin*.

The conjugated bilirubin glucuronide is secreted into the duodenum through the bile, giving it the characteristic color. The bile secreted into duodenum reaches the large intestine where the bilirubin gets converted into *stercobilinogen*, giving the characteristic brown color to the feces. However some of stercobilinogen is absorbed from large intestine and forms *urobilinogen*, which gets excreted in urine, giving the characteristic yellow color to urine. If the urobilinogen is left to stand for sometime, the urobilinogen gets converted to form the *urobilin*.

*From the above discussion we draw three main conclusions:*
- The production of bilirubin, if increased due to any cause, would increase the free unconjugated and conjugated bilirubin, which would increase the urinary bilirubin excretion.
- With normal production of bilirubin, if the liver is damaged, the efficient conjugation with glucuronic acid would not take place. This would result in the insufficient conjugated bilirubin.
- However, bilirubin production is normal and the liver is also healthy, any obstruction to the flow of bile into the intestine can result in stasis of bile (cholestasis) and increases the level of conjugated bilirubin.

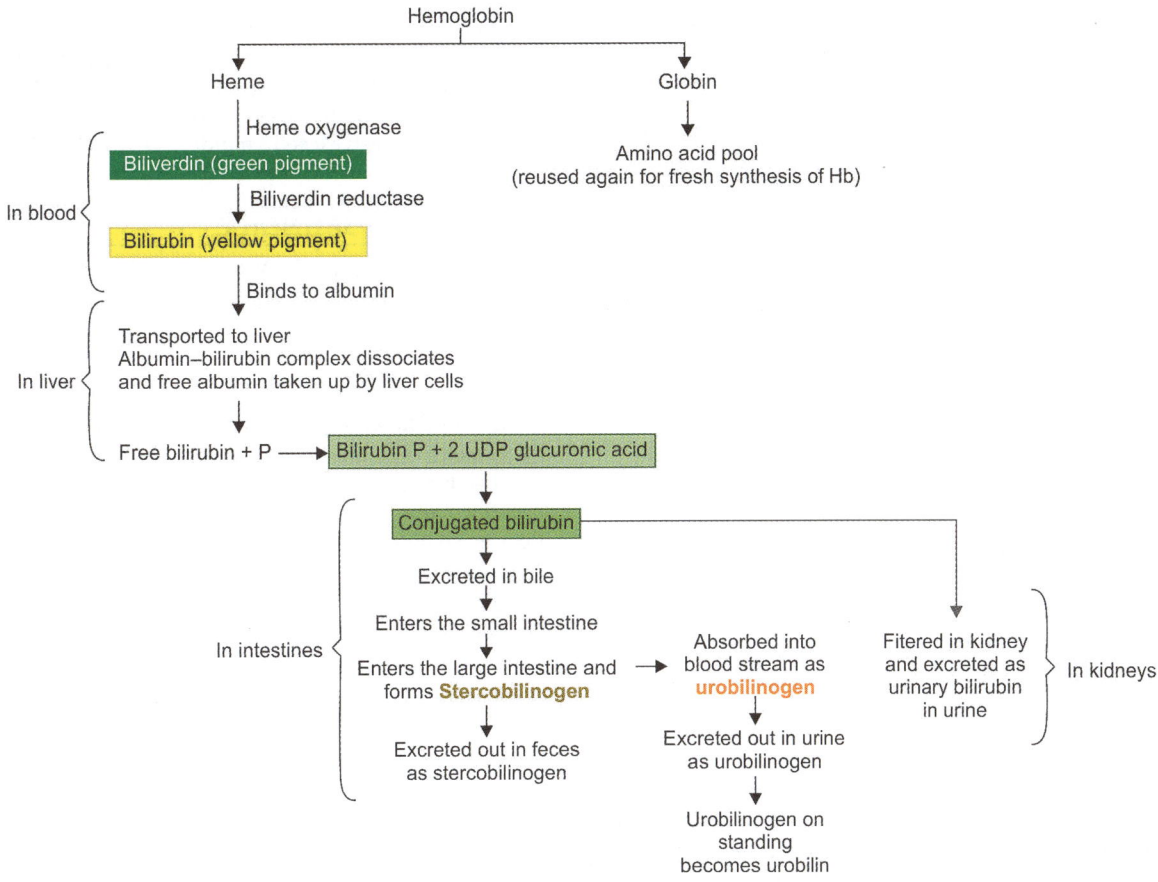

**Fig. 15.1:** Fate of hemoglobin and metabolism of bilirubin.

## CLASSIFICATION OF JAUNDICE

Based on above three observations, the jaundice is classified as **(Fig. 15.2)**:
1. Prehepatic jaundice
2. Hepatic Jaundice
3. Posthepatic/obstructive jaundice.

### Prehepatic Jaundice

As the name suggests the cause of jaundice is excessive production of bilirubin, which could occur in massive hemolysis (breakdown of RBCs) due to any of the reasons like:
- Marked hemolysis due to mismatched transfusion
- Drug induced hemolysis

The excessive bilirubin is not conjugated, hence the levels of total bilirubin and unconjugated bilirubin are high. The amount of unconjugated bilirubin in the body exceeds the amount that the liver can convert to conjugated bilirubin.

> **CLINICAL CASE SCENARIO**
>
> A 24-year-old male suffering from malaria was put on Primaquine. He developed malaise, fatigue, and yellow discoloration of sclera, and skin, dark-colored urine. Lab report showed increased total

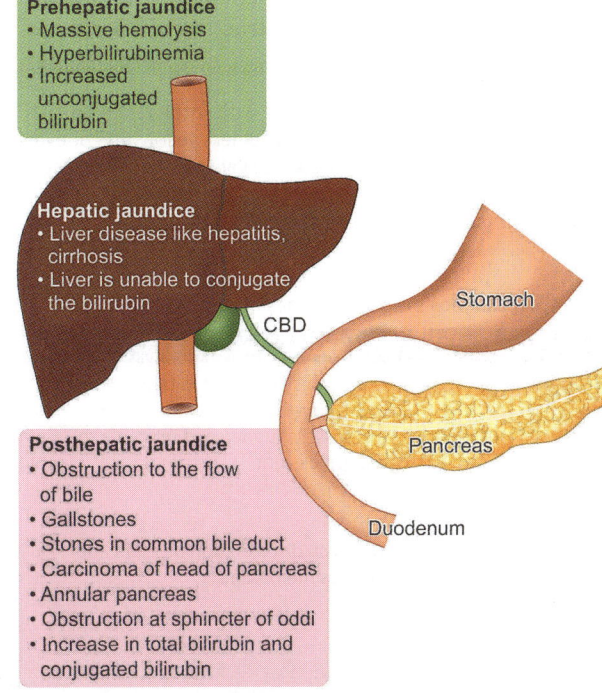

**Fig. 15.2:** Types of jaundice.
(CBD: common bile duct)

serum bilirubin and unconjugated bilirubin. Urine urobilinogen present.

This patient has probably suffered from hemolytic anemia due to consumption of Primaquine. The presence of raised serum bilirubin, unconjugated bilirubin are suggestive of hemolysis. He may be a patient of G-6-PD deficiency resulting in hemolytic anemia.

## Hepatic Jaundice

The hepatocytes get damaged as a result of:
- Viral infection called as viral hepatitis (Hepatitis A, Hepatitis B, Hepatitis C and Hepatitis E)
- Chronic alcohol consumption resulting in liver cirrhosis (fibrosis)
- Hepatotoxic drugs
- Autoimmune diseases

Hepatic jaundice is either caused due to intrahepatic bile obstruction that block the excretion of conjugated bilirubin in the bile canaliculi (cholestasis) or due to decreased liver enzymes.

In this, the total, conjugated and unconjugated bilirubin rise indicating insufficient conjugation mechanism.

## Posthepatic Jaundice

This type of jaundice is also called the ***obstructive jaundice*** as it occurs when there is an obstruction to the bile ducts, which prevents bilirubin from being excreted in the small intestine (cholestasis). The obstruction can be caused by gallstones in common bile duct, tumors involving the opening of bile duct into duodenum esp. carcinoma head of pancreas, inflammation of pancreas resulting in pancreatitis and obstruction of bile duct.

### CLINICAL CASE SCENARIO

A 35-year-old, fat female presented with intolerance to fatty food, pain in the right side of the abdomen, yellowness of eyes, and passage of clay-colored stools. Lab investigations: Increased serum total bilirubin, direct, conjugated bilirubin. Dark-colored yellow urine, stercobilinogen is absent.

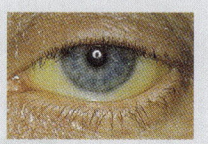

The yellowish discoloration is very clearly seen in sclera because it has high affinity for bilirubin due to their high elastin content. It is seen when serum bilirubin levels exceed 3 mg/dL.

## DIAGNOSIS OF JAUNDICE

The diagnosis of the jaundice is made on the basis of history, clinical examination and the lab diagnosis **(Table 15.1)**.

**What is the difference between Jaundice and Carotenemia?**
Carotenemia (accumulation of β-carotene in the blood). It gives a yellowish discoloration to skin. It is usually seen in patients of hypothyroidism. It can be distinguished from jaundice because the sclera is not yellow in carotenemia.

## Lab Diagnosis (Table 15.2)

Most liver functions test are conducted to diagnose the case of jaundice.

## PHYSIOLOGICAL JAUNDICE

It is the mild jaundice seen in the first few days after birth.
- It appears after 24 hours of age, peaks at around 48–96 hours, and resolves by two to three weeks in full-term infants.
- It is caused by a *lack of liver enzymes necessary for the conjugation of bilirubin* and an increase in the degradation of fetal hemoglobin. Liver is deficient in enzyme UDP-glucronyltransferase. There is an increase in serum unconjugated bilirubin.
- Very high levels of unconjugated bilirubin (>18 mg%) cause hearing loss, irreversible brain damage, and even death as they pass the blood-brain barrier and accumulate in the brain stem and basal ganglia, known as ***kernicterus.***

**Table 15.1:** Diagnosis of various types of jaundice.

| | Prehepatic | Hepatic | Posthepatic |
|---|---|---|---|
| History | There is history of blood transfusion, ingestion of hemolytic drugs. Here the onset is sudden and relatable to a specific event | The patient give a history of gradual onset. The patient might give history of chronic alcoholism or pain in right hypochondrium | There is history of dull pain in right hypochondrium radiating to right shoulder. The clay-colored stools are important finding in the history of these patients |
| Clinical examination | Yellowish discoloration of sclera and mucous membrane | • Yellowish discoloration of sclera and mucous membrane<br>• Liver may be enlarged in hepatitis and fibrosed in cirrhosis<br>• Liver enlargement may be accompanied with pain | • Yellowish discoloration of sclera and mucous membrane<br>• Liver is normal, no hepatomegaly<br>• Gallbladder may be tender or inflamed resulting in positive Murphy's sign (shoulder tip pain) |

Table 15.2: Levels of blood biochemistry in different types of jaundice.

| | Prehepatic | Hepatic | Posthepatic |
|---|---|---|---|
| **Total serum bilirubin** (0.3–1.0 mg/dL) | Mild increases | Moderate increases | Very high |
| **Conjugated/direct bilirubin** (0.1–0.3 mg/dL) | Remains near normal | Increases | Markedly increase |
| **Unconjugated/indirect bilirubin** (0.2–0.8 mg/dL) | Markedly increases | Increases | Slightly increases |
| **Van den Bergh reaction** | **Indirect** (due to marked increase in indirect/unconjugated bilirubin) | **Biphasic** (due to increase in both direct and indirect bilirubin) | **Direct** (due to marked increase in direct/conjugated bilirubin) |
| **SGOT/AST (Aspartate aminotransferase)** (10–40 IU/L) | Normal level of liver enzymes | **Elevated** | Normal level of liver enzymes initially but are elevated over long-term cholestasis |
| **SGPT/ALT (Alanine transferase)** (7–56 IU/L) | Normal level of liver enzymes | **Elevated** | Normal level of liver enzymes initially but are elevated over long-term cholestasis |
| **Alkaline phosphatase/ALP** (40–129 IU/L) | Normal level of liver enzymes | **Mild-moderate increase** | **Marked elevation** (characteristic of obstructive jaundice) |
| **Gamma glutamyl transferase (GGT)** (9–48 IU/L) | Normal level of liver enzymes | **Elevated** | Normal level of liver enzymes initially but are elevated over long-term cholestasis |
| **Fecal stercobilinogen** | **Elevated; Dark brown stool** | Normal | **Absent; pale/clay-colored stools** |
| **Urinary urobilinogen** | **Elevated** | Normal | **Absent** |
| **A:G ratio** | Normal | **Decreases** | Normal |
| **Urinary bilirubin** | Absent (acholuric jaundice) | **Present**; dark urine | **Present**; dark urine |

- Physiological jaundice of newborn is treated by **Phototherapy**. The insoluble bilirubin gets converted into water soluble *lumirubin* under the phototherapy, which is then excreted out in urine.

## SUMMARY

- Any abnormality in the metabolism of bilirubin results in hyperbilirubinemia, which is the cause of jaundice.
- The increased RBC hemolysis associated with hemolytic anemia is the cause of the hemolytic Jaundice. Increased urobilinogen, elevated unconjugated bilirubin, pale brown feces, and dark urine are its characteristic features.
- Damage to the hepatocyte that reduces bilirubin uptake and conjugation is the cause of hepatic jaundice, which is characterized by an increase in both conjugated and unconjugated bilirubin.
- Intrahepatic and extrahepatic blockage to the excretion of the conjugated bilirubin results in obstructive jaundice characterized by clay-colored stool.
- An obstruction to the excretion of conjugated bilirubin, both intrahepatic and extrahepatic, causes obstructive jaundice, which is characterized by clay-colored stools.
- Jaundice is characterized by yellowing of the skin, mucous membranes, and sclera. It may also result in pruritis or itching.

## LET US SEE, HOW MUCH YOU HAVE LEARNT?

 *Review Questions*

### Short Answer Type Questions

Q1. Describe the metabolism of bilirubin.

Q2. What is physiological jaundice?

### Explain Why? (Reasoning Questions)

Q1. Phototherapy used in the treatment of neonatal or physiological jaundice?

Q2. Dark colored urine and pale stool in obstructed jaundice?

## Critical Thinking Case-Based Questions

**Q1.** 43-year-old female complains of yellowish discoloration of eyes since 7 days, pain in right hypochondrium which is radiating to right shoulder since 7 days and fever since 2 days. On examination: yellowish discoloration of sclera and mucous membrane was observed. Laboratory investigations revealed increased serum bilirubin, conjugated bilirubin—5 mg/dL, SGOT, SGPT, and serum alkaline phosphatase.

Based on the above clinical scenario, answer the following questions:
a. What is your probable diagnosis? Give justification.
b. Describe the pathophysiology of jaundice.
c. What are the causes of different type of jaundice?
d. What is the role of liver function tests in differentiating the different types of jaundice?

## Multiple Choice Questions

**Q1.** A newborn delivered vaginally is noted to be mildly jaundiced, but no bilirubin is found in the urine. The child's symptoms are most likely attributable to a developmental delay in the expression or establishment of which of the following:
a. Colonic bacterial colonization
b. MDR2
c. UDP-glucuronyl transferase
d. Biliverdin reductase
e. Heme oxygenase

**Q2.** Which of the following is not a symptom of jaundice?
a. Yellowing of the skin and whites of the eyes
b. Dark urine
c. Pale-colored stools
d. Increased appetite

**Q3.** Which of the following is not a cause of hemolytic jaundice?
a. Sickle cell anemia
b. Gallstone
c. Blood transfusion
d. Thalassemia

**Q4.** Which of the following is not a symptom of hemolytic jaundice?
a. Dark urine
b. Yellowness of skin and whites of eyes
c. Clay-colored stool
d. Decrease appetite

**Q5.** Which of the following is not a treatment of hemolytic jaundice?
a. Phototherapy
b. Blood transfusion
c. Surgery
d. Medication

**Q6.** Which is not a cause of obstructive jaundice?
a. Gallstone
b. Carcinoma of pancreas
c. Sickle cell anemia
d. Hepatic congestion

**Q7.** A 36-year-old soldier developed a flu-like illness (fever, chills, headache, myalgia) 4 days after returning 1 year posting. He was known to have chronic hepatitis B infection. His lab investigations reported increased total bilirubin, indirect bilirubin and direct bilirubin. Urine bilirubin: Present. Increased ALT/AST. What is not included in the pathophysiology of jaundice in this case?
a. Increased production of bilirubin
b. Decrease hepatic uptake
c. Decrease hepatic conjugation
d. Decrease excretion of bilirubin into bile

### ANSWERS
1. c   2. d   3. b   4. c   5. c   6. c   7. a

# Leukocytes and their Formation

## 16 CHAPTER

**COMPETENCY ADDRESSED**

PY2.6: Describe WBC formation (granulopoiesis) and its regulation.

 **LEARNING OBJECTIVES**

**At the end of this chapter, the learner should be able to:**
- Classify the various leukocytes.
- Differentiate various leukocytes based on structural differences.
- Describe the formation of leukocytes (granulopoiesis) and the factors regulating it.
- Describe the functions of different types of leukocytes.
- Describe the physio-clinical significance of leukocytes.

## INTRODUCTION

The leukocytes are commonly called white blood cells. These cells are usually 1.5 to 2 times larger than the RBCs and are much fewer in number. The average life span of leukocytes ranges from a few hours to few days. The leukocytes are primarily concerned with the immune surveillance of our body either through the cells or by producing specific proteins called immunoglobulins or antibodies.

## GENERAL STRUCTURE OF A LEUKOCYTE

Commonly, all the leukocytes are:
- **Size:** 1.5 to 2 times larger than red blood cells except Small lymphocyte (same size as RBC) and monocyte (2–2.5 times larger than RBC).
- **Cytoplasm and granules:** Have abundant cytoplasm except small lymphocytes, filled with primary granules. The granulocytes have secondary granules in addition to primary granules. The secondary granules provide specific function to each type of cells whereas the primary granules are responsible for similar function of all leukocytes.
  - *Primary granules/Azurophilic granules:* These granules are present in all leukocytes but are best seen in neutrophils. They are believed to have the lysosomal enzymes and generalized cellular defense of the leukocytes. Even the agranulocytes (mainly monocytes due to abundant cytoplasm) have been identified with the primary granules.
  - *Secondary/specific granules:* These are responsible for assigning specific characteristics to various granulocytes. These granules are absent in agranulocytes.
- **Nucleus:** Have a large prominent nucleus which is characteristic features in each cell type.

Depending upon the types of secondary granules present in the cells, the leukocytes are classified as: Granulocytes and agranulocytes. The other differences in each of these cells are shown in **Figure 16.1**.

## LEUKOPOIESIS (FORMATION OF LEUKOCYTES)

**Site:** The leukocytes are formed in the bone marrow.

**Duration:** 10 days (5 days in mitotic pool and 5 days in maturation pool).

**Precursor cell:** Pluripotent stem cell which gives rise to committed stem cell.
- **Myeloid stem cells:** *Trilineage stem cells* give rise to three types of cell series:
  1. ***CFU-E for the formation of erythroid series*** *(RBC formation)*
  2. ***CFU-Mega for megakaryocytic series*** *(Platelet formation)*
  3. ***CFU-GM for granulocyte–monocyte series*** *(formation of neutrophils, basophils, eosinophils)*
- **Lymphoid stem cells:** Form lymphocytes.

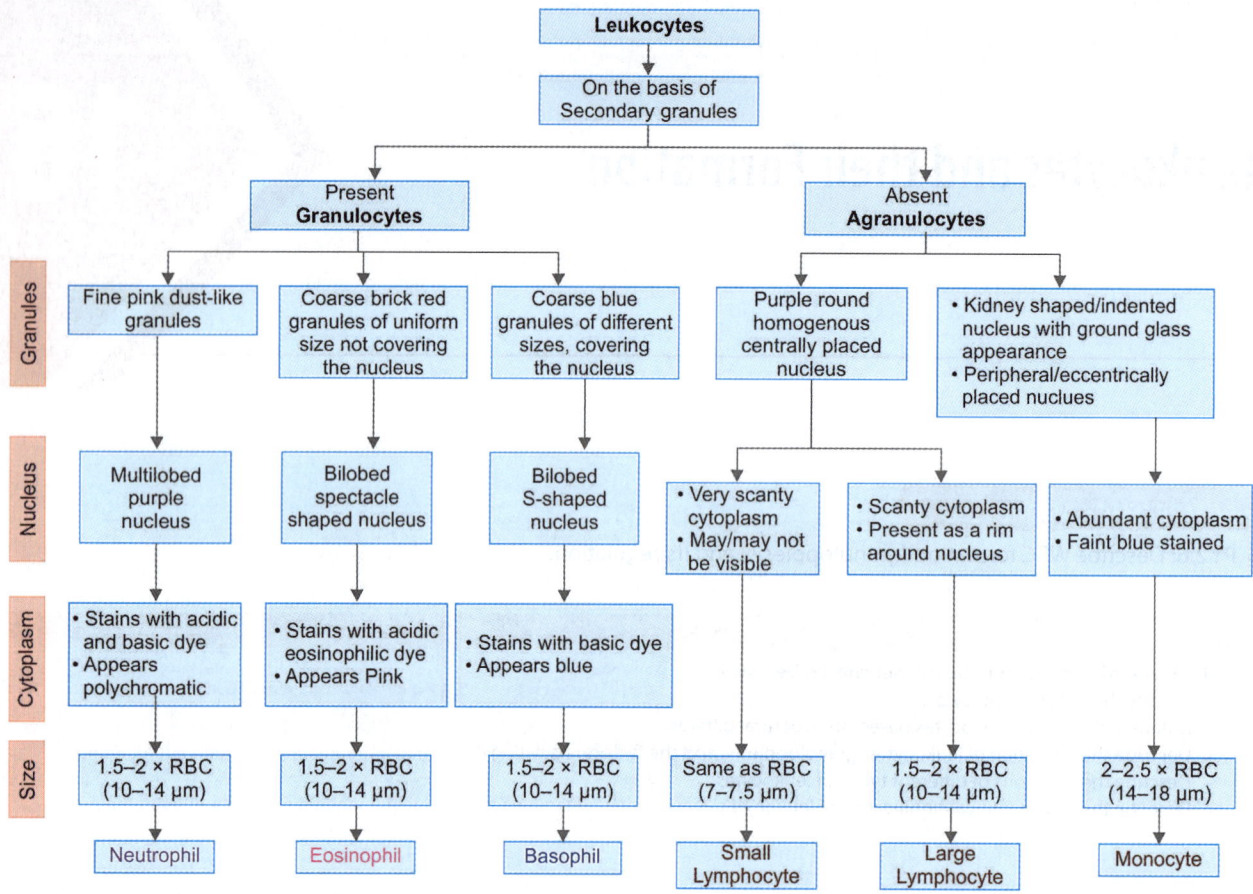

**Fig. 16.1:** Classification of leukocytes and their characteristic identification features.

## Stages and Regulation of Leukopoiesis (Fig. 16.2)

The colony-forming units (CFU) of the myeloid series are differentiated into three lineages the erythroid series, megakaryocytic series and the granulocyte-monocyte series.

- The pluripotent stem cells form the committed cells which differentiate into colony-forming units (CFU) under the influence of IL-1, IL-3 and IL-6 along with TNF (tumor necrosis factor).
- The colony-forming units further differentiate into specific series of blast cells forming various leukocytes.
  - *CFU-G* differentiates into the *neutrophils* under the influence of *G-CSF* (Colony stimulating factor—granulocyte) produced by monocytes, endothelial cells and fibroblasts.
  - *CFU-Eo* differentiates into the *eosinophils* under the influence of *GM-CSF* and *G-CSF* along with *IL-5* which is also called eosinophilic growth factor.
  - *CFU-Ba* differentiates into the *basophils* under the influence of *G-CSF* (Colony stimulating factor—granulocyte) along with *IL-3* and *IL-4*. IL-4 also stimulates the differentiation into dendritic cells.
  - *CFU-M* differentiates into the *monocytes* under the influence of *M-CSF* (Colony stimulating factor—monocyte) produced by monocytes, endothelial cells and macrophages.

> **Regulation of Leukopoiesis**
>
> *Interleukins:*
> - IL-1, IL-3, IL-6: Maturation of stem cells
> - IL-5: Eosinophilic growth factor
> - IL-3, IL-4: Maturation of basophils
> - IL-2: Inhibits myelopoiesis
>
> *Colony stimulating factors:*
> - GM-CSF: Stimulates the granulocyte monocyte series
> - G-CSF: Stimulates the granulocyte series
> - M-CSF: Stimulates the monocyte series
>
> *Tumor necrosis factor (TNF):* Proliferation and differentiation of cells

During development, all the series developed through various stages:

- **Blast stages (16–20 µm):** These are the earliest precursor cells called myeloblasts. These are morphologically indistinguishable from large nucleus. The cells have high mitotic activity with scanty cytoplasm. They are specifically called as:
  - Myeloblast for neutrophilic series
  - Eosinophilic myeloblast for eosinophils

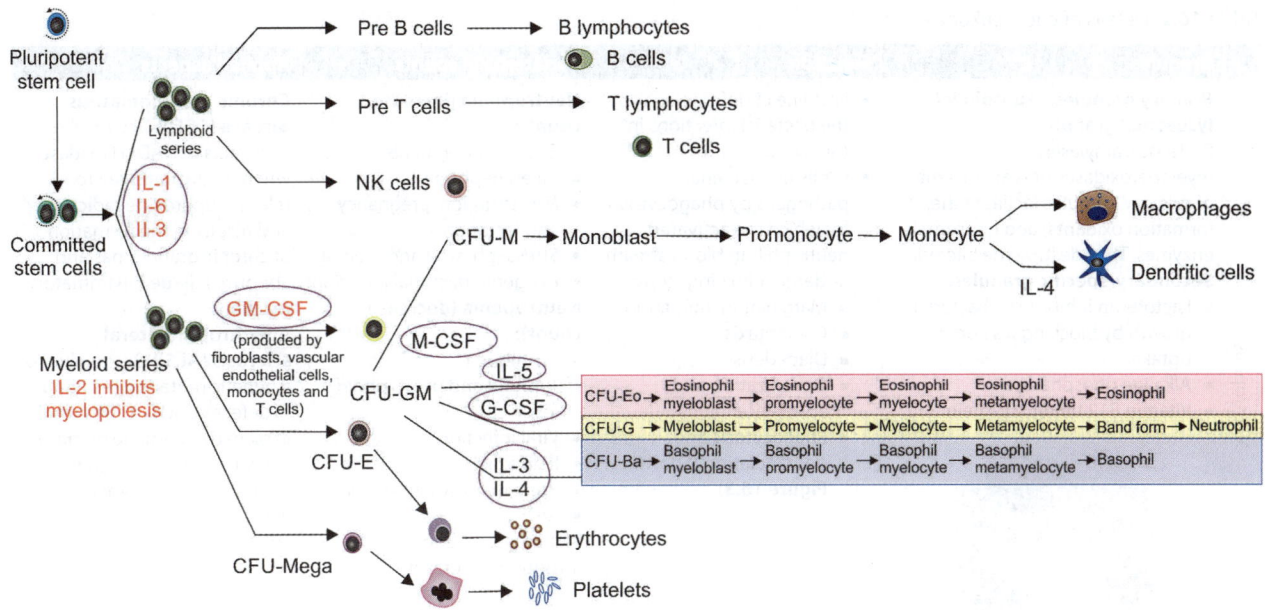

**Fig. 16.2:** Leukopoiesis—stages and regulation.

- Basophilic myeloblast for basophils
- Monoblasts for monocytic series
- Lymphoblasts for lymphocytic series
- **Promyelocytes and promonocytes:** The blast cells mature into the promyelocytes and promonocytes which have lower mitotic activity but have *abundant peroxidase positive* granules. All the cells follow the similar nomenclature.
- **Myelocytes (12–20 µm):** These cells round concentric nucleus with less mitotic activity There is an increase in *peroxidase negative granules*.
- **Metamyelocytes (12–18 µm):** These cells do not divide and have mixed granules.
- **Mature granulocytes (10–14 µm):** The mature granulocytes are formed with specific granules with specific staining character of cytoplasm and structure of nucleus.

Life cycle of leukocytes is tabulated in **Table 16.1**.

## COUNTS

Total leukocyte count is 4,000–11,000 cells/mm³ of blood.

The differential leukocyte count (Number of one type of cells counted in 100 leukocytes):

- **Neutrophils:** 50–70%
- **Lymphocytes:** 20–40%
- **Eosinophils:** 2–4%
- **Monocytes:** 2–8%
- **Basophils:** 0–1%

The variations in these counts are shown in **Table 16.2**.

After the granulopoiesis we would discuss the structure, functions counts and physiological functions of each type of leukocyte.

Neutrophils are the first line of defense in blood and are present in abundance in circulation. When the inflammatory stimulus is present anywhere, even in tissues, it sends the chemoattractant which result in migration of white blood cells towards the locus of inflammation and result in phagocytosis. It performs this activity by the following mechanisms **(Fig. 16.3)**:

- **Margination:** The neutrophils are present in the circulatory and marginal pool, adhered to endothelium in the blood vessels. Whenever there is infection resulting in tissue inflammation, there is release of various chemicals which enter the blood stream and serve as the source of neutrophilic activation. The circulating and margination pool of neutrophils start flowing along the wall of the blood vessel and begin

**Table 16.1:** Life cycle of leukocytes.

| | Marrow phase | | Circulation phase | | Tissue phase |
|---|---|---|---|---|---|
| | Mitotic pool | Maturation pool | Active circulation pool | Margination pool | Tissue pool |
| Duration | 5 days | 5 days | Few hours | | Granulocytes: few days<br>Monocytes: few weeks |
| Events | Development from myeloblasts to myelocytes. Active mitosis take place | Maturation of metamyelocytes to mature cells | Circulating in blood | Leukocytes adhering to the endothelial lining of blood vessels | The monocytes are transformed into tissue macrophages |

**Table 16.2:** Details of each leukocyte.

| | Granules | Function | Variations in counts | Applied aspects |
|---|---|---|---|---|
| **Neutrophils** | **Primary granules/azurophilic/lysosomal granules:** Proteases, amylases, myeloperoxidases (It is an enzyme of primary granules facilitate the formation oxidants) and lysosomal enzymes. They destroy the bacteria<br>**Secondary/specific granules:**<br>• Lactoferrin inhibits the bacterial growth by blocking it's iron uptake<br>• Alkaline phosphatase<br>• Vitamin B12 binding protein | • First line of defense against the bacterial infections in the blood<br>• It kills the bacterial pathogens by phagocytosis, for which the activated neutrophils in blood stream undergo following steps:<br>▪ Margination, migration<br>▪ Chemotaxis<br>▪ Diapedesis<br>▪ Opsonization and adherence<br>▪ Phagocytosis and degranulation (Shown in **Figure 16.3**) | **Neutrophilia (increase count):**<br>• Exercise after meals<br>• Inj epinephrine<br>• Menstruation, pregnancy and lactation<br>• Stress (physical and mental)<br>• Pyogenic/bacterial infection<br>**Neutropenia (decrease count):**<br>• In children<br>• Typhoid and paratyphoid fever<br>• Viral infection<br>• Kala azar<br>• Bone marrow depression<br>• AIDS<br>AI diseases (rheumatoid arthritis, purpura, etc.) | **Chronic granulomatous disease (CGD):** Occurs due to defects in NADPH oxidase, where neutrophils fail to release superoxide radicals and results in the formation of chronic granulomas and abnormal tissue inflammatory reactions<br>**Amyotrophic lateral sclerosis (ALS):** Occurs due to a genetic mutation resulting in defective SOD-1. This results in oxidative damage of motor neurons causing progressive degeneration of spinal motor neurons and skeletal muscle atrophy |
| **Eosinophils** | • **Major basic proteins:** It acts against intestinal parasites and their larvae<br>• **Eosinophil cationic proteins:** Toxic to helminthic parasites<br>• **Eosinophil peroxidase:** Toxic to adult parasites.<br>• **Cytokines:** Interleukin IL-1 to IL-6, IL-8 and IL-12, GM-CSF, TNF-α, etc.<br>• **Other chemicals:** Many proteolytic enzymes which participate in the eosinophil mediated inflammatory responses | • First line of defense against intestinal parasites especially helminthic infections<br>• It also mediates allergic reactions | **Eosinophilia (increase count):**<br>• Allergic conditions<br>• Bronchial asthma<br>• Parasitic infestations<br>• Skin diseases like urticaria, eczema, etc.<br>**Eosinopenia (decrease count):**<br>• Inj ACTH, corticoids<br>• Cushing's syndrome<br>• Acute stressful illness | • The eosinophils also secrete slow reacting substances of anaphylaxis (SRS-A) and major basic proteins (MBP) hence they cause asthma like symptoms due to bronchoconstriction in helminthic infections<br>• The eosinophil count decreases in response to glucocorticoid therapy and hence important pharmacologically |
| **Basophils** | **Specific granules of basophils contain:** Histamine, chondroitin sulfate, carboxypeptidases, cathepsins, leukotrienes, MBP | • **Allergic reactions:** Anaphylaxis due to release of histamine<br>• Chronic allergies, as they participate in late phase reactions | **Basophilia (increase count):**<br>• Chicken pox<br>• Small pox<br>• Viral infections<br>• Allergic diseases<br>**Basopenia (decrease count):**<br>• Acute pyogenic infection<br>• Glucocorticoid treatment | • In the tissues, the basophils usually function with mast cells. They mediate acute allergies resulting in anaphylaxis<br>• The **mast cells** do not circulate in blood, but are present in tissues and contain granules comprising of histamine, heparin, chondroitin sulfate, carboxypeptidase, cathepsin, ECF-A, and proteases |

*Contd...*

*Contd...*

| | Granules | Function | Variations in counts | Applied aspects |
|---|---|---|---|---|
| Monocytes | Though classified as agranulocyte due to absence of secondary granules, the monocytes have primary azurophilic granules present in them. These granules contain acid phosphatase, lysozyme, etc. but alkaline phosphatase is absent | • Phagocytosis and killing of microorganisms<br>• Acts as second line of defense against bacterial infections<br>• Act as antigen presenting cells in cell mediated immunity<br>• They release various inflammatory mediators like:<br>  ▪ IL-1 and IL-6, which result in coactivation of other immunological processes<br>  ▪ TNF-α. Interferon-γ<br>  ▪ Growth factors (GM-CSF, M-CSF, TGF, PDGF, etc.)<br>  ▪ Secretes complement factors<br>• Releases various enzymes like collagenase, protease, etc. | **Monocytosis:**<br>• TB<br>• Syphilis<br>• Leukemias<br>**Monocytopenia:** Hypoplastic bone marrow | On entering in the tissues, monocytes transform into tissue macrophages. This for the monocyte macrophage system. This provides the first line of defense in the tissues. These macrophages release the chemokines/chemoattractants for the migration of neutrophils at the site of infection |
| Lymphocytes | Usually, lymphocytes don't have any granules but very small proportion (3%) of large lymphocytes have coarse pink granules. These granular lymphocytes are usually NK cells or T cells | • T cells and NK cells mediate cellular immunity<br>• B cells proliferate into plasma cells and produce antibodies and provide humoral immunity<br>• NK cells are also responsible for non-specific immunity | **Lymphocytosis (increase count):**<br>• Children<br>• Chronic infections (TB, hepatitis)<br>• Lymphocytic leukemia<br>• Viral infections (whooping cough)<br>**Lymphopenia (decrease count):**<br>• Steroid therapy<br>• Hypoplastic bone marrow<br>• AIDS | **Lymphoblastic leukemia:**<br>• Abnormal proliferation of lymphocytes and their blast cells results in acute or chronic lymphoblastic leukemia<br>• Further details of leukemia are given in **Figure 16.4** |

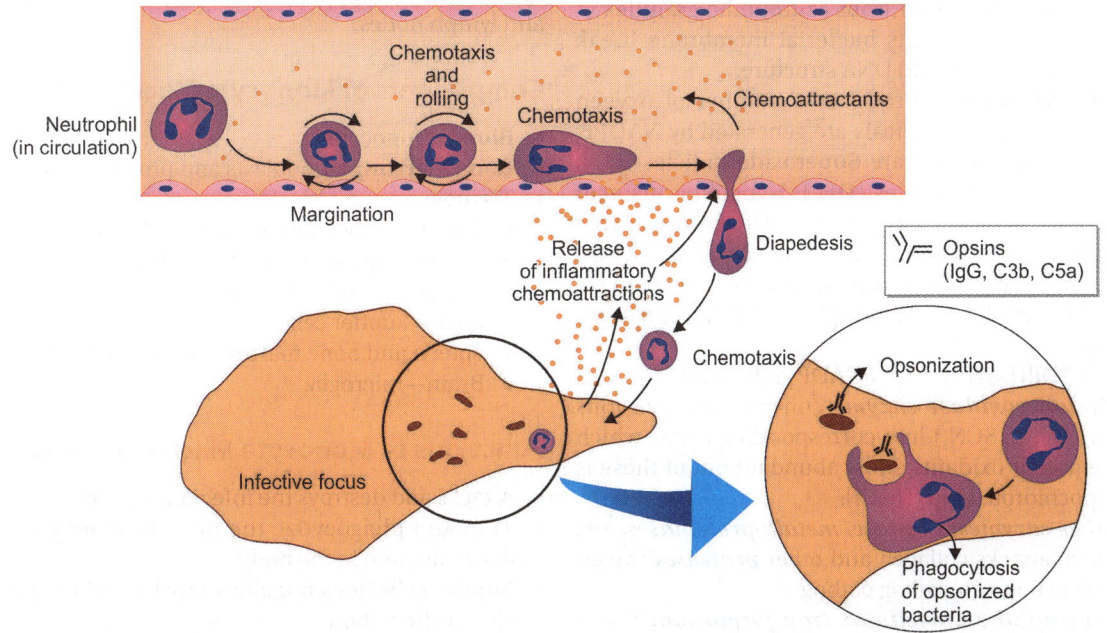

**Fig. 16.3:** Mechanism of action of neutrophils.

to migrate towards the direction of inflammatory source.

- **Chemotaxis:** Migration of neutrophils to the site of infection which releases the chemo attractants.
- **Diapedesis:** Neutrophils squeeze through capillary endothelial cells to reach the site of inflammation in the tissue.
- **Opsonization** and **adherence:** (coating of bacterial antigens with opsins).
  The *opsins* make the bacteria tasty/recognizable for neutrophils by coating them. Various opsins are *IgG, C5a, C3b*. Bacteria coated with opsins bind to receptors on neutrophil membrane. This is called as *adherence*.
- **Phagocytosis:** Neutrophils throw out their pseudopodia and ingest the opsonized and adhered bacteria. The ingested bacteria are then eliminated by the following processes.

**Why is there a sudden rise in oxygen uptake by neutrophils during phagocytic activity?**

The neutrophils kill the microorganisms by releasing the nascent oxygen species with the help of enzyme Superoxide Dismutase (SOD). Hence there is increased oxygen utilization which results in sudden increase in oxygen uptake by the neutrophils. This is called as "Respiratory Burst". It leads to activation of NADPH oxidase associated with increased oxygen uptake of neutrophil.

- **Killing of micro-organism:** This ingested bacterium then combines with lysosomes and forms phagolysosome. The bacteria get killed, broken down and digested by lysosomal enzymes.
  - *Lysozyme:* Hydrolyzes cell wall of bacteria.
  - *Lactoferrin:* Sequesters iron, required for bacterial growth.
  - *Defensins:* Released from azurophilic granules of neutrophils, disrupts bacterial membrane break down single stranded DNA structure.
  - *NADPH oxidase:* Produces a number of oxygen metabolites. The radicals are generated by NADPH dependent oxidase are Superoxide radicals ($O_2^-$), Free hydroxyl radicals ($OH^-$), Hypochlorous acid ($HOCl$), Nascent oxygen ($O^-$). Hence these free radicals hydrolyze the bacterial cell wall and DNA. It is associated with sharp increase in oxygen uptake and metabolism in neutrophils called *Respiratory Burst*.
    $$NADPH + H^+ + 2O_2 \rightarrow NADP^+ + 2H^+ + 2O_2^-$$
  - *Myeloperoxidase enzyme* converts the free ions ($Cl^-$, $Br^-$, $I^-$, $SCN^-$) into corresponding acids, which are potent oxidants. Most abundant out of these is hypochlorous acid ($HOCl$).
  - *Other enzymes: Elastase, metalloproteinases,* etc. which attacks collagen and other *proteases* causes destruction of invading pathogen.
  - *Neutrophil extracellular trap formation:* It is a mechanism by which neutrophils can trap and kill microbes extracellularly, by releasing their chromatin and granular contents. This doesn't involve phagocytosis.

**What is leukocytosis? What is its clinical importance?**

Leukocytosis refers to increase in the total leukocyte count above the normal level of 11,000 cells/mm³. with the absence of leukocyte blast cells in the peripheral blood film. In leukocytosis the TLC is always less than 50,000 cell/mm³.

**Clinical importance:**

- Leukocytosis is seen in acute inflammation and infections.
- It serves as the prognostic indicator for inflammation/infection

## How would you Differentiate Leukocytosis and Leukemia?

| | Leukocytosis | Leukemia |
|---|---|---|
| Total leukocyte count | <50,000/mm³ | >50,000/mm³ |
| Leukocytic blast cells in PBF | Absent | Present |
| Clinical condition | Inflammation/infection | Malignancy of bone marrow |

Classification of leukemia is shown in **Figure 16.4**.

## MONOCYTE MACROPHAGE SYSTEM/ RETICULOENDOTHELIAL SYSTEM (RES)

The monocyte macrophage system forms an important part of the immune system, which is a combination of monocyte, mobile macrophage, fixed tissue macrophages, specialized endothelial cells in the bone marrow, spleen and lymph nodes.

### Components of Monocyte Macrophage System

- **Blood:** Monocytes
- **Bone marrow:** Monoblasts and promonocytes
- **Tissues:**
  - Skin and subcutaneous tissue—histiocytes
  - Lymph nodes—tissue macrophages
  - Lungs—alveolar macrophages
  - Liver—kupffer cells
  - Spleen and bone marrow—tissue macrophages
  - Brain—microglia

### Functions of Monocyte Macrophage System

- Attacks and destroys the infectious agents
- Trap and phagocytize the microbes and prevents its dissemination in the body
- Kupffer cells does not allow any bacteria to pass from GIT to circulation
- Phagocytosis of old and abnormal red blood cells in spleen

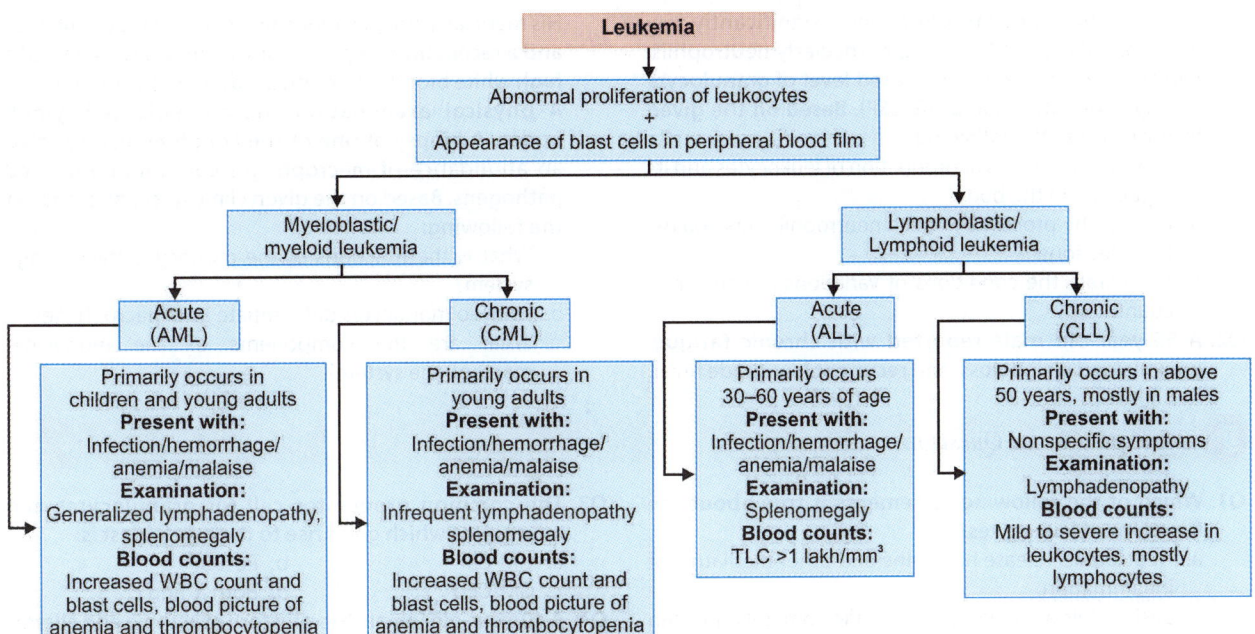

**Fig. 16.4:** Classification of leukemia.

## SUMMARY

- Leukocytes are white blood cells that are involved in the immune system and defense against pathogens. They can be classified into two main groups: granulocytes and agranulocytes, based on the presence or absence of granules in their cytoplasm.
- Granulocytes include neutrophils, eosinophils, and basophils, which have different shapes and sizes of nuclei and granules. Agranulocytes include lymphocytes and monocytes, which have round or kidney-shaped nuclei and no granules.
- The formation of leukocytes is called leukopoiesis, which occurs mainly in the bone marrow and lymphoid tissues. Leukopoiesis is regulated by various factors, such as cytokines, hormones, and feedback mechanisms. Granulopoiesis is the specific term for the production of granulocytes.
- Different types of leukocytes have different functions in the immune system. Neutrophils are the most abundant and phagocytose bacteria and other foreign particles. Eosinophils are involved in allergic reactions and parasitic infections. Basophils release histamine and other mediators of inflammation. Lymphocytes are responsible for specific immunity and can be divided into B cells, T cells, and natural killer cells. Monocytes differentiate into macrophages and dendritic cells, which present antigens to lymphocytes and secrete cytokines.
- Leukocytes have various physio-clinical significance, such as indicating the state of health, infection, inflammation, allergy, immunity, and malignancy. The number and proportion of leukocytes can be measured by a complete blood count (CBC) and a differential count (DC). Abnormalities in leukocyte count or morphology can indicate various diseases, such as leukemia, lymphoma, anemia, infection, allergy, and immunodeficiency.

## LET US SEE, HOW MUCH YOU HAVE LEARNT?

### Review Questions

#### Long/Short Answer Questions

Q1. What are leukocytes and what is their primary function?
Q2. Differentiate between the various types of leukocytes.
Q3. Explain the process of leukopoiesis.
Q4. What factors regulate leukopoiesis?
Q5. Discuss the significance of cytokines in the regulation of leukopoiesis.
Q6. Discuss the regulatory mechanisms involved in leukopoiesis, including the roles of cytokines, growth factors, and other signaling molecules.
Q7. Differentiate between acute and chronic leukemia.
Q8. Discuss the clinical presentation, diagnostic criteria, and physiological effects of different types of leukemia.

### Critical Thinking Case-Based Questions

Q1. A 40-year-old female, presented to the clinic with recurrent infections, including frequent respiratory and urinary tract infections. Her medical history revealed recent chemotherapy treatment for breast cancer. A

complete blood count (CBC) shows significantly low white blood cell (WBC) count, particularly neutrophils. Further tests indicate a decreased level of granulocyte colony-stimulating factor (G-CSF). Based on the given history answer the following:
a. Explain the process of production of leukocytes and its regulation in the body?
b. Discuss the process by which neutrophils acts against the infections.
c. Enumerate the conditions of variations in neutrophil count.

Q2. A 55-year-old male reported with chronic fatigue, unexplained weight loss, and recurrent low-grade fever. His medical history included untreated diabetes mellitus and a recent bout of pneumonia. Blood tests revealed a high white blood cell count, predominantly monocytes. A physical examination showed enlarged lymph nodes. A biopsy of one of the lymph nodes reported an abundance of macrophages containing ingested pathogens. Based on the given clinical scenario, answer the following:
a. What is the functions of the monocyte-macrophage system?
b. How do monocytes differentiate into macrophages?
c. What are the components of the monocyte-macrophage system?

## Multiple Choice Questions

Q1. Which of the following statements is true about the functions of leukocytes?
a. Neutrophils release histamine and other mediators of inflammation.
b. Eosinophils are involved in specific immunity and can be divided into B cells, T cells, and natural killer cells.
c. Basophils phagocytose bacteria and other foreign particles.
d. Lymphocytes differentiate into macrophages and dendritic cells, which present antigens to lymphocytes and secrete cytokines.

Q2. Which of the following is a process by which neutrophils can kill microbes without phagocytosis?
a. Neutrophil extracellular trap (NET) formation
b. Reactive oxygen species (ROS) production
c. Granule release
d. Diapedesis

Q3. The common progenitor cell for granulocytes and monocytes which gives rise to the myeloblast is:
a. GM-CSF        b. Eo-CSF
c. GM-CFU        d. Both a. and c.

Q4. A 40-year-old female has a history of asthma and allergic rhinitis. She reports worsening of her symptoms after exposure to dust mites. A blood smear shows increased numbers of granulocytes with bilobed nuclei and red-orange granules. What type of leukocyte is most likely to be increased in this case?
a. Neutrophil        b. Eosinophil
c. Basophil          d. Monocyte

Q5. How does leukocytosis affect the immune system?
a. Enhances          b. Impairs
c. No effect         d. Varied effect

**ANSWERS**

1. d    2. a    3. c    4. b    5. d

# Basics of Immunity

**CHAPTER 17**

### COMPETENCY ADDRESSED
PY2.10: Define and classify different types of immunity. Describe the development of immunity and its regulation.

### LEARNING OBJECTIVES
**At the end of this chapter, the learner should be able to:**
- Define immunity.
- Classify immunity with examples.
- Describe innate immunity and acquired immunity.
- Describe the mechanism of cell mediated and humoral immunity.
- Describe the various immune disorders.

The immunity is defined as the ability of the organism to defend himself against the invading organisms (bacteria, virus, fungi, etc.) and the cells expressing abnormal markers (tumor cells). The study of immune systems of body, in which the host identifies itself from nonself-antigens, are called *immunology*.

## FUNCTIONS OF IMMUNITY
- Protects against microbes
- Remove nonmicrobial foreign antigens
- Destroy cancer cells that arise in the body, hence prevents against malignancies.

## CLASSIFICATION OF IMMUNITY
See **Fig. 17.1**.

### Innate Immunity
- It is the first line of defense which is present by birth.
- It occurs due to genetic makeup of an individual.
- It provides defense against any pathogen (nonspecific).
- It acts immediately within minutes/hours and provide an immediate response to foreign invaders. It does not require previous exposure to microorganisms and activation.
- The components of innate immunity are:
  - *Anatomical barrier/physical barriers:*
    - Intact skin, mucous membranes line the respiratory, digestive, and genitourinary tracts, cilia, nasal hair, eyelashes and eyelid forms physical barrier.
    - Mucus traps pathogens and other foreign substances.
    - Cilia propel microorganisms out of the body.
  - *Physiological barriers/chemical barriers:*
    - The skin produces antimicrobial substances and has a slightly acidic pH that inhibits the growth of microbes.
    - Mucus contains antimicrobial components that help prevent infection.
    - Low pH skin (5.5), gastric acid (1.3) and vaginal pH (4.4) retards growth of organisms.
    - IgA and lysosome in saliva, tears, mucus, colostrum provide innate immunity.

> **What is the role of breast milk in providing immunity to the newborn?**
> Breast milk secreted in the first few days after delivery is called **colostrum**. It is rich in proteins and immunoglobulins (IgA type) and hence confers passive immunity to the newborn. IgA coats the gut surface and destroy bacteria. The lactoferrin and lysozymes provide immunity against pathogens. It is abundant in white blood cells that provides immunity against pathogens.

  - *Cellular defense:*
    - Cells of innate immunity include phagocytes (neutrophils, eosinophils, monocytes, macrophages, dendritic cells and reticuloendothelial system, and natural killer (NK) cells.

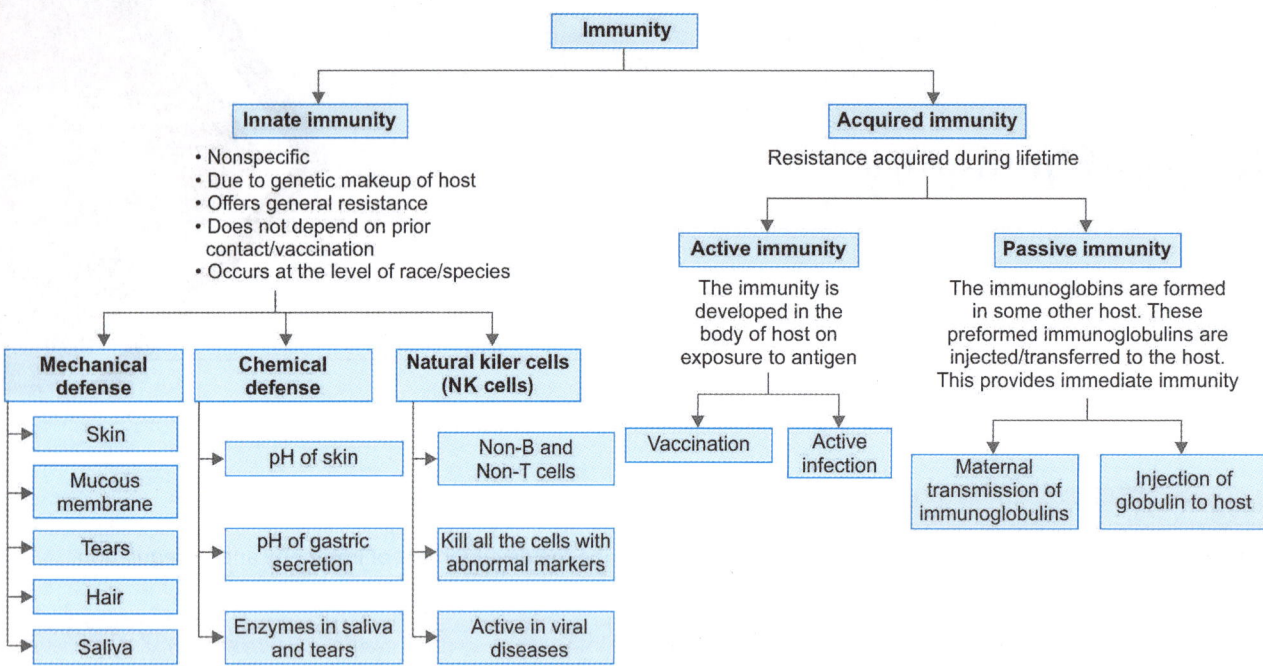

**Fig. 17.1:** Classification of immunity.

- NK cells are nonspecific, neither B cells and nor T cells. They recognize all the cells with abnormal markers and kill them.
- NK cells release interferon and cytokines to eliminate pathogens.
- Eosinophils protect against parasitic infections by releasing the content of their granules.
  - *Inflammatory immune response* and fever.
  - *The complement system:* It consists of more than 30 proteins that act in a sequence. These proteins are inactive but lead to the activation of cascade where these proteins are activated and participate in immune response.

**Limitations of innate immunity:** It is nonspecific and reacts to all infections in the same way. It provides no ongoing protection against infection in the future because it only lasts a brief time and has no memory of the foreign substance. It is unable to distinguishing between what is non-self (foreign) and what is self (lack of self-discrimination).

### Acquired/Adaptive Immunity

It is acquired during life after exposure to an antigen. It is highly specific. Cells involved in acquired immunity are T and B lymphocytes. These cells act within days (slow response). It plays a vital role in immune responses in the event of re-exposure and our utilization of vaccines as it forms memory cells to protect for future attacks.

### Formation and Maturation of Acquired Immunity

The lymphoblasts in the bone marrow develop into pre-T cells and pre-B cells. These precursor cells enter the *primary lymphoid organs* (thymus and bursa equivalent/bone marrow). T and B cells in primary lymphoid organs express antigen receptors and become mature functionally. T cells mature in the thymus, while B cells mature in the bone marrow. In *secondary lymphoid organs* (tonsils, lymph nodes, spleen) these T cells and B cells recognize antigens and develop the appropriate defense system. There are two types of acquired immunity **(Fig. 17.2)**:
1. **Cell mediated immunity:** Mediated by T cells
2. **Humoral immunity:** Mediated by B cells

## CELL MEDIATED IMMUNITY

The immunity mediated through various types of cells is called the cell mediated immunity (CMI). Various cells participating in CMI are:
- Neutrophils
- Basophils
- Eosinophils

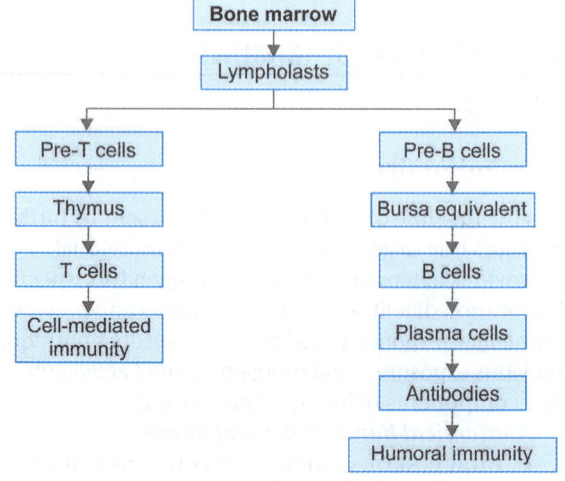

**Fig. 17.2:** Types of acquired immunity.

- Monocytes
- **Lymphocytes:**
  - *Helper T cells (T4 cells/CD4 cells)*
  - *Cytotoxic T cells (T8 cells/CD8 cells)*
- Macrophages
- Natural killer cells

## T- Lymphocytes

The specific cells for CMI are the T-lymphocytes (T cells). The T cells are classified as below:

- **Helper T cells ($T_H$ cells)/T4 cells/CD4 cells:** These cells help the $T_c$ cells in eliminating the invader. They have CD4 receptor present on their surface, hence also called as CD4 cells. They are further of two types **(Table 17.1)**:
  1. $T_{H1}$ *cells:* These cells help in cellular immunity
  2. $T_{H2}$ *cells:* These cells help in activation of humoral immunity
- **Cytotoxic T cells ($T_c$ cells)/T8 cells/CD8 cells:** These cells eliminate the invading organism.
- **Memory T cells:** These cells remain for a very long period and activates the immunological memory, whenever the antigen re-enters the body.

## Functions of T Cells

- **Cytotoxicity:** It kills the invading pathogen by the $T_c$ cells.
- **Delayed hypersensitivity:** The T cells and the macrophages, migrate to site of allergen and result in the development of delayed hypersensitivity.

**Table 17.1:** Difference between T1 and T2 cells.

|  | $T_{H1}$ | $T_{H2}$ |
| --- | --- | --- |
| Lymphokines that induce subset | IFN-γ, IL-12 | IL-4 |
| Major lymphokines/factors produced | IFN-γ, IL-12 TNF-α, GM-CSF | IL-4, IL-5, IL-6, IL-10, IL-13 |
| Major immune reactions | Macrophage activation, stimulate IgG antibody production | Stimulate IgE production, activation of mast cells and eosinophils |

(IFN: interferons, IL: interleukins, Ig: immunoglobulin, TNF: tissue necrosis factor)

- **Regulates antibody production by B cells:** The $T_{H2}$ cells stimulate the B cells to activate the humoral immunity.
- **Regulates CMI**
- **Suppresses autoimmune responses**

## Mechanism of Activation of Cell Mediated Immunity

The cell mediated immunity is activated on the initial exposure of the antigen. This antigen has to processed by the macrophages before activation of T cells. Hence, the CMI is activated in the following three steps **(Fig. 17.3)**:

1. **Antigen recognition, processing and presentation:**
   - *Recognition:* The nonself-antigen is recognized by the antigen presenting cell (APC) **Figure 17.4**, which is a macrophage in CMI.

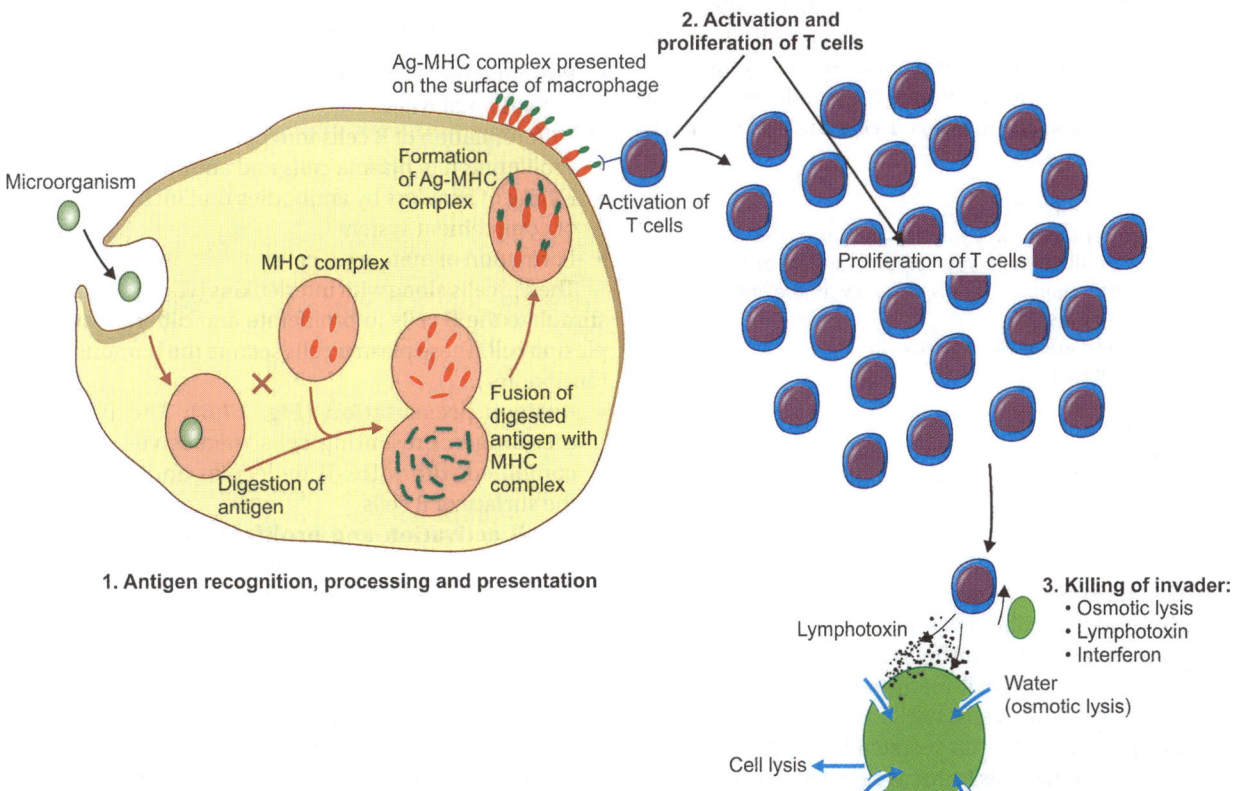

**Fig. 17.3:** Cell-mediated immune response.

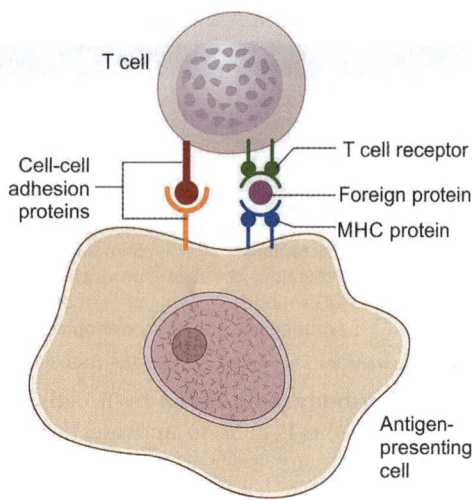

**Fig. 17.4:** Antigen presenting cell.

- *Processing:* The nonself-antigen is digested and broken down into smaller fragments. It then combines with the Major histocompatibility complex (MHC complex), secreted by the macrophages to form *Ag-MHC complex*.
- *Presentation:* The Ag-MHC complex is then presented on the surface of these APCs.

2. **Activation and proliferation of T cells:**
   - *Activation of T cells:* The T cells binds to the AG-MHC complex with its T cell receptors. This leads to the activation of T cells.
   - *Proliferation of T cells:* The activated T cells result in the proliferation of T cell population, which recognize the nonself-antigen presented by the APCs. These $T_c$ cells then eliminate the invader by different mechanisms. The memory T cells are also formed to be used in future.

---

**Natural Killer Cells (NK Cells):**
- They are neither B nor T lymphocytes.
- NK cells kill all the cells with abnormal surface antigens.
- They don't require prior sensitization with the antigen and MHC complexes.
- **The NK cells are active against:**
  - Viral antigens
  - Malignant cells
- **Mechanism of action:**
  - Osmotic lysis
  - Release interferons that activate phagocytosis
  - Possess $F_c$ receptors that allow them to kill antibody coated viruses

---

3. **Elimination of invader:** Cytotoxic T cells ($T_c$ cells) kill the invading microbes by three mechanisms:
   a. *Cytolysis:* Cells synthesize water channels and incorporate into cell membrane of invader. Water moves inside the cells, swells and undergoes lysis.
   b. *Lymphotoxin:* A toxin secreted by the lymphocytes, e.g., tumor necrosis factor, is secreted which kills the invading organism.
   c. *Interferons:* Interferons are the cytokines secreted by the lymphocytes, e.g., IF-γ, which is mainly antiviral. It increases the phagocytic activity of neutrophils.

## Functions of CMI

- Viral infections
- Fungal infections
- Tumor cells
- Chronic bacterial infections
- Parasitic infections
- Transplanted cells

## HUMORAL IMMUNITY

The immunity conferred by the circulating proteins in the blood (humor) is called the humoral immunity (HI). The circulating proteins are immunoglobulins (a type of γ globulin) or antibodies.

Hence, before moving on further, let us understand the concept of antigen and antibody:

**Antigen:** Any substance which induces the production of antibody is called as antigen
- Self-antigen—does not mount an immune response, as it belongs to the host.
- Nonself-antigen—mounts an immune response, as it is a foreign antigen.

**Antibody:** The specific gamma-globulins formed by the B lymphocytes and plasma cells on exposure to antigen.

## Mechanism of Humoral Immunity (Fig. 17.5)

- Presentation of antigen
- Activation of B cells
- Differentiation of B cells into plasma cells
- Proliferation of plasma cells and antibody production
- Killing of invaders by antibodies that include activation of complement system
- Formation of memory B cells

The $T_{H2}$ cells along with interleukins (IL-2, IL-4 and IL-5), stimulate the B cells to proliferate and differentiate into a plasma cell. These plasma cells secrete the immunoglobins (antibodies).

- **Antigen presentation (Fig. 17.6):** The B cells are the antigen presenting cells themselves. Antigen is combined with MHC-II molecules and presented on the surface of B cells
- **B cell activation and proliferation of B cells into plasma cells:** The Ag-MHC-II are presented on B cell surface; resulting in further activation of B cell activation. Activated B cells forms plasma cells and memory B cells. The plasma cells synthesize the immunoglobulins.
- **Killing of invading microorganism:** The antigen is neutralized by the antibodies resulting in antigen antibody reaction. The other modes of actions are:
  - Immobilization of microbes

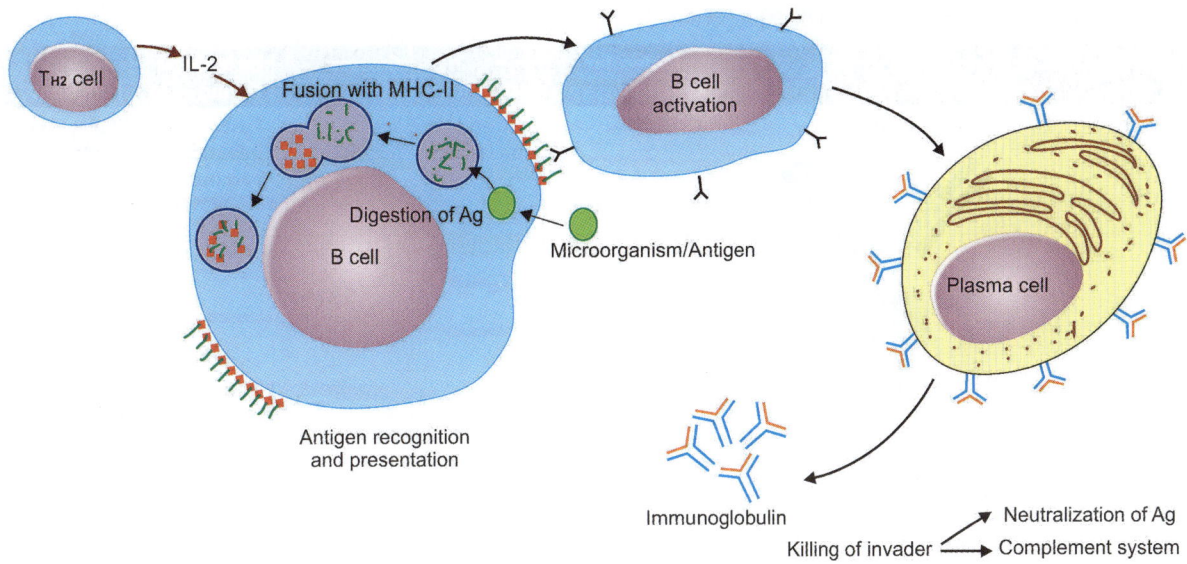

**Fig. 17.5:** Mechanism of humoral immunity.

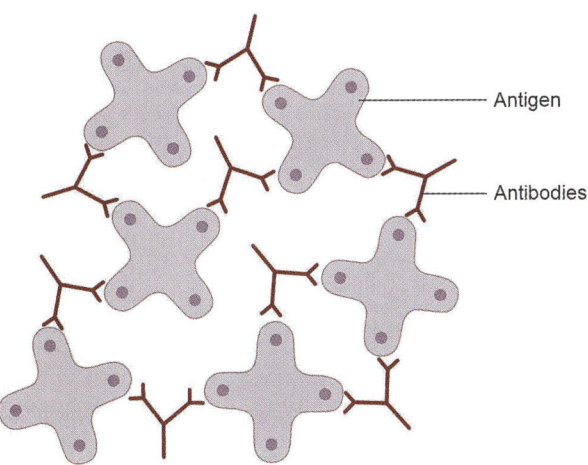

**Fig. 17.6:** Antigen antibody reaction.

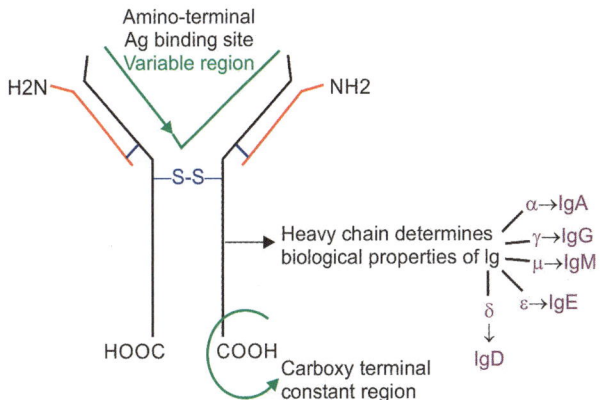

**Fig. 17.7:** Structure of immunoglobulin.

- Activation of complement system
- Precipitation of antigen
- Facilitates of phagocytosis
• **Formation of memory B cells:** The memory B cells, give a long-term immunity. On re-exposure the antibody formation is faster and much more in numbers.

## IMMUNOGLOBULIN (Ig)

It is a gamma globulin, a Y-shaped glycoprotein molecule secreted by the plasma cells, which provides the humoral immunity.

### Structure of IG (Fig. 17.7)

• Each molecule of Ig has *two light and two heavy chains*. The heavy and light chains are held by the *disulfide bonds*.

• It has two sites:
  1. **Amino terminal:** It is also called the *antigen binding site*. Since the antigens are highly variable, this site is also called as the *variable region*. The light chains are responsible for the formation of variable regions.

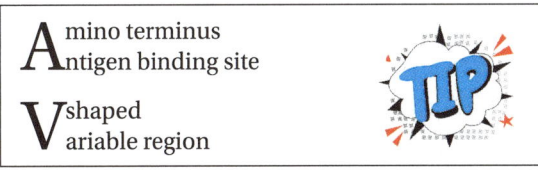

Amino terminus
Antigen binding site

V shaped
Variable region

  2. **Carboxy terminal:** It is also called the *constant region*. It is made up by the heavy chains, hence it determines the biological properties of the Ig.

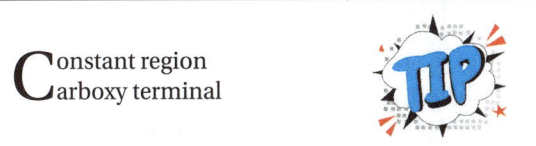

Constant region
Carboxy terminal

**Table 17.2:** Different immunoglobulins and their properties.

| | Percentage of IG | Structure | Molecular weight | Distribution | Crosses placenta | Increases during | Functions |
|---|---|---|---|---|---|---|---|
| IgG | 80% | Y-shaped monomer 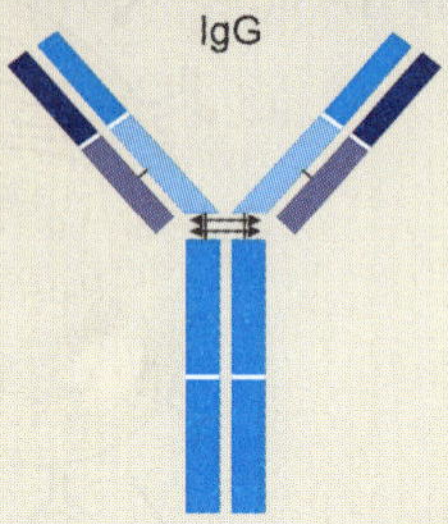 | 15,000 | Extra and Intravascular | Yes (esp. IgG₁) | Past infection/ vaccination | Protects body fluids |
| IgA | 10–13% | Dimer 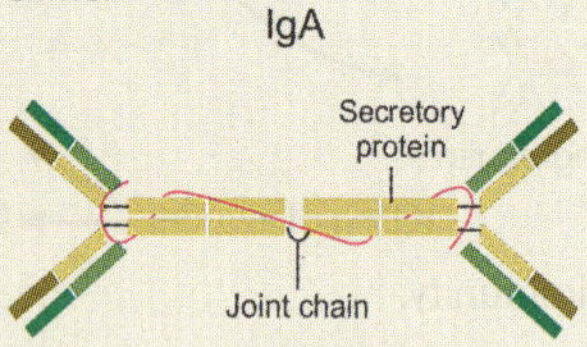 | 1,60,000 | Body secretions | No | — | Protects body surfaces |
| IgM | 5–8% | Pentamer 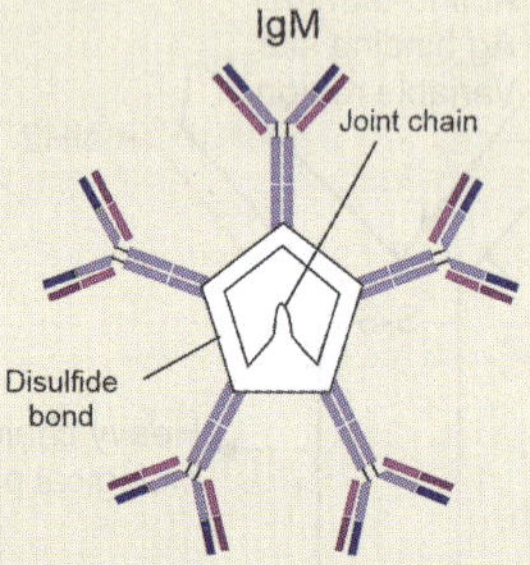 | 9,00,000 | Intravascular | No | Acute infection | Protects blood stream |
| IgD | Very less | Y-shaped monomer 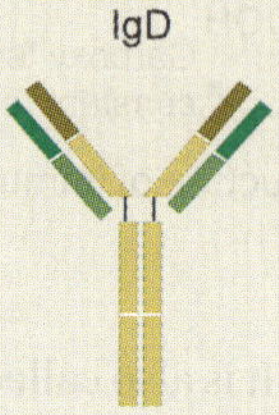 | 1,80,000 | On the surface of unstimulated B cells | No | — | Recognition of receptors |
| IgE | Very less | Y-shaped monomer 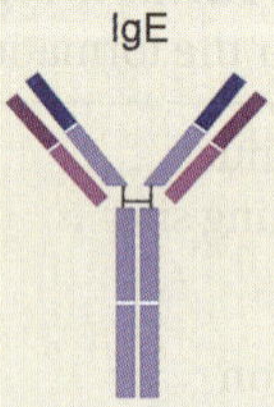 | 1,90,000 | Extra vascular | No | Allergic condition | Mediates reaginic hypersensitivity |

There are five types of heavy chains. The type of chain determines the type of Ig, shown below:
1. **IgG:** gamma ($\gamma$) heavy chain
2. **IgA:** alpha ($\alpha$) heavy chain
3. **IgM:** meu ($\mu$) heavy chain
4. **IgE:** epsilon ($\varepsilon$) heavy chain
5. **IgD:** delta ($\delta$) heavy chain

The properties of these Igs are described in **Table 17.2**.

# TYPES OF HUMORAL/IMMUNE RESPONSES

Based on the exposure of antigen and antibody titer formed, the immune response is classified as (**Fig. 17.8**):

*Primary immune response:*
- It occurs on the first exposure to antigen
- Antibodies are formed slowly after latent period of 4 days to 4 weeks

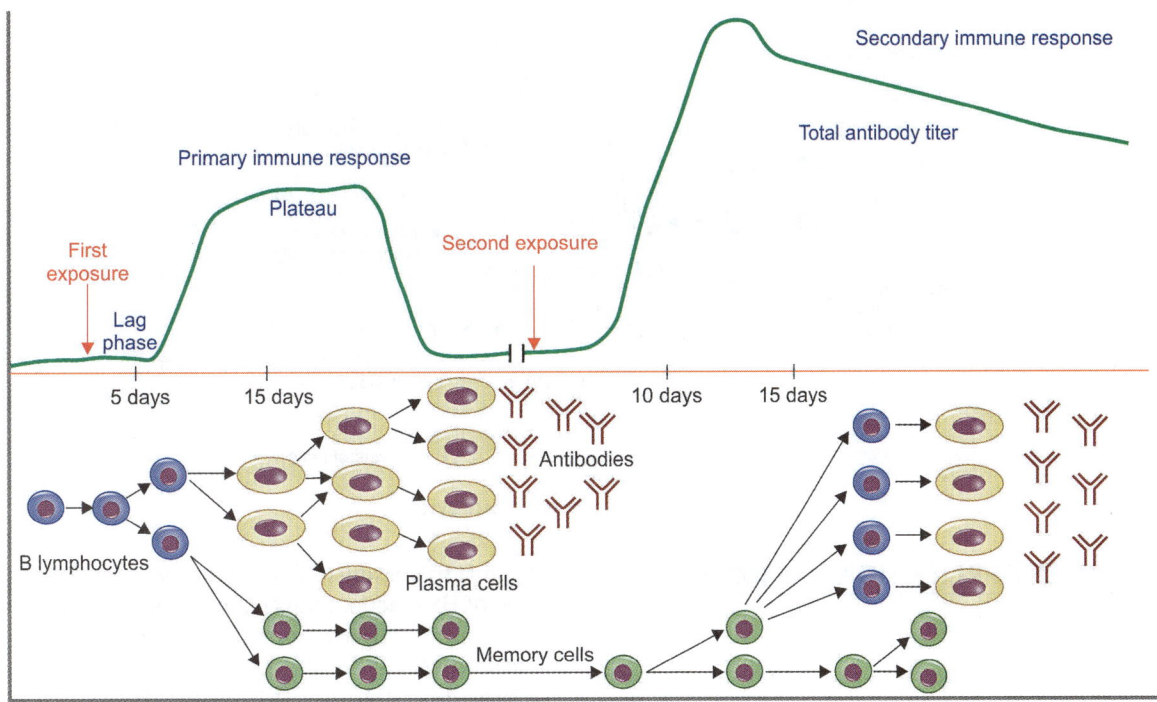

**Fig. 17.8:** Mechanism and timeline for primary and secondary immune response.

- Response is mainly due to IgM antibodies
- Antibody titer falls within few days to weeks

*Secondary immune response:*
- It occurs on re-exposure to antigen due to persistent B and T memory cells (immunological memory)
- Antibodies are formed rapidly and reach a greater peak due to higher titer of antibodies formed
- Antibody titer falls slowly and remains elevated for a long time
- This immune response occurs due to IgG type of antibodies.

Differentiating features of primary and secondary immune responses are tabulated in **Table 17.3**.

**Table 17.3:** Features of primary and secondary immune responses.

| | Primary immune response | Secondary immune response |
|---|---|---|
| Exposure to antigen | First exposure | Repeated exposure/booster dose of vaccine |
| Lag/latent phase | 4 days to 4 weeks | much less |
| Antibody titer | Rises and reaches a plateau, after which it declines to near baseline in few days to few weeks | Rises rapidly and then reaches a plateau. It doesn't come down to the base line for a very long time. This decides the time schedule for the next booster dose. |
| Type of Ig responsible | IgM type | IgG type |
| Main cells responsible | B cells get transformed into plasma cells and form Igs | Persistent B and T cells, in the form of memory cells |

## COMPLEMENT SYSTEM

- It is a group of plasma proteins called as *complement proteins* because they *complement the effects of antibodies in destroying the antigen.*
- There are total 11 complement proteins, categorized as
  - $C_1$–$C_9$
  - $C_1$ is further categorized into three subunits, $C_{1q}$, $C_{1r}$ and $C_{1s}$
- They are present in plasma in **INACTIVE** form
- They get activated by Ag-Ab complex formed during the activation of HI.
- **There are two pathways:** Classical and properdin (alternate) pathways **(Fig. 17.9)**:
  - *Classical pathway:*
    - It is activated by Ag-Ab complex, which activates $C_1$ (activated complement factors are shown with a bar on the top)
    - It results in osmotic lysis of microbes
  - *Properdin/alternate pathway:*
    - It is activated by properdin
    - The circulating Factor-1, recognizes the polysaccharides on microbial cell and interacts with it
    - It directly activates $C_3$ and the complement system instead of $C_1$

Physiological importance of complement proteins:
- It complements the humoral immunity
- $C_{3a}$, $C_{4a}$, $C_{5a}$: Promotes phagocytosis, chemotaxis, releasing histamine from mast cells and casing arteriolar dilation
- $C_{3b}$ and $C_{5a}$: Promotes opsonization
- $C_{5b}$, $C_6$, $C_7$, $C_8$ and $C_9$: Membrane attack complex (MAC), resulting in osmotic lysis of microbes

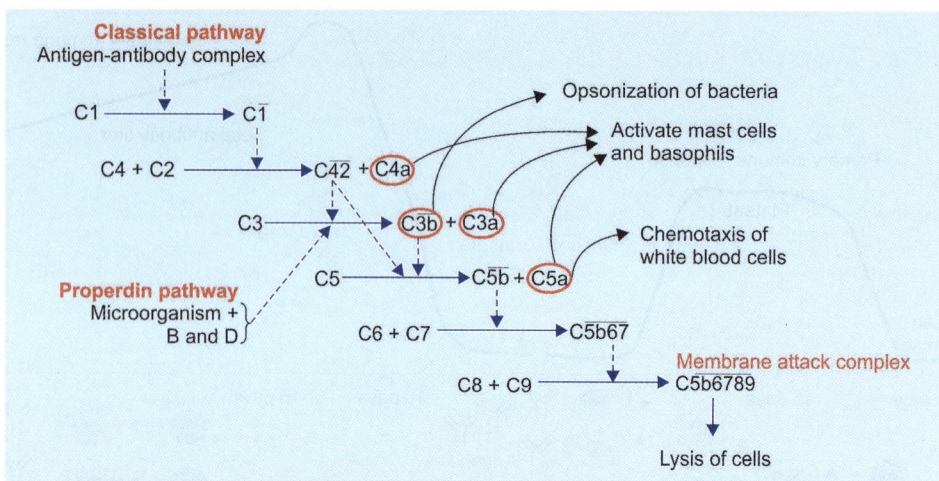

**Fig. 17.9:** Pathway of complement system.

## SOME OTHER APPLICATIONS OF IMMUNITY

### Hypersensitivity (HS)

It is defined as the exaggerated immune response to an antigen/allergen. The hypersensitivity is classified into four types:

a. **Type I hypersensitivity: Acute anaphylaxis reaction (Fig. 17.10):** The individual overreacts to particular allergen. The first exposure to the allergen doesn't cause much reaction but the subsequent exposures result in the *degranulation of mast cells*. There is release of massive amounts of *histamine*. This results in widespread vasodilation and the subsequent fall in blood pressure. This is called as *anaphylactic shock*. It is an acute medical emergency. This type of allergy is typically seen in people with *food allergies*, especially sea food allergies.
The type I HS reaction in mediated by *IgE antibodies*.

b. **Type II hypersensitivity: Cytotoxic reaction:** In this type of HS reaction, the cell lysis take place due to the antigen antibody reactions. It is mediated by ***IgG or IgM antibodies***.
**Example:** Incompatible blood transfusion, Rh incompatibility in newborn, autoimmune hemolytic anemia. The type II HS is also an acute emergency.

c. **Type III hypersensitivity: Immune complex disease:** The immune complexes (Ag-Ab complex) formed due to the antigen antibody reaction are phagocytosed and removed but if they escape phagocytosis, they get deposited in the capillary basement membrane and damages it by inducing inflammation.
**Example:** Glomerulonephrits, systemic lupus erythematosus (SLE).

d. **Type IV hypersensitivity (Delayed hypersensitivity):** It is mediated by macrophages that are activated by T cells. The APC's are presented to T cells, which result in proliferation of T cells. The activated T cells migrate to site where allergen is present and induce inflammatory response. The T cells secrete cytokines and activate macrophages, which induce delayed hypersensitivity. It is called delayed HS because it takes a couple of hours to a few days to manifest. **Example:** Mantoux test for tuberculosis.

### Autoimmunity

When the immune system fails to recognize self-antigens and triggers an immune reaction is called the autoimmunity. It occurs due to formation of autoantibodies (antibodies against self-antigens). **Example:** Myasthenia gravis, Graves' disease, etc.

Mechanism of action of autoantibodies:

- **The autoantibodies can block/digest the receptors resulting in its down regulation.** This causes the blockage of the particular physiological action. **Example:** The blockage or destruction of Acetyl choline gated sodium channels result in downregulation of

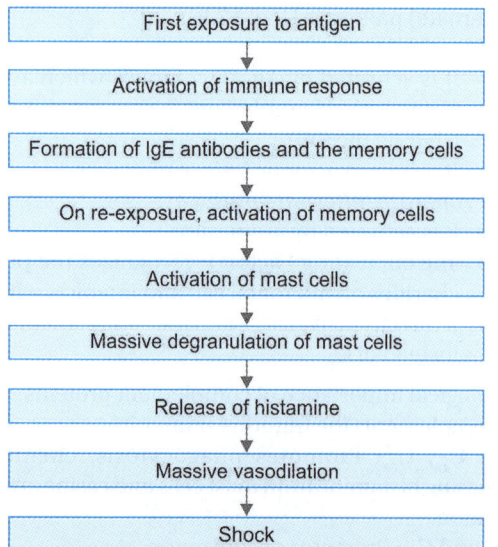

**Fig. 17.10:** Mechanism of anaphylactic shock.

these receptors. This results in the muscle weakness, as the acetyl choline receptors are not available for the excitation of muscle.
- **The autoantibodies can also stimulate the receptors acting as competitive agonist.** This causes the stimulation of the receptor producing the prolonged physiological effect of that particular receptor. **Example:** The thyroid stimulating immunoglobulin (TSI) binds to the TSH receptor on the thyroid gland and stimulates it to produce excessive thyroxine. This results thyrotoxicosis in Grave's disease.

## Immune Tolerance

It is defined as the ability of immune system to differentiate between self and nonself-antigens in order to protect healthy self-tissues. Immune tolerance arises in the thymus and bone marrow during the pre-processing of T and B cells, where the T cells and B cells develop with the self-antigens. The immune selection process takes place, depending on the:

- **Negative selection:** During the development of T cells in thymus, the TCR which do not recognize self-antigens, are destroyed by deletion or anergy
- **Positive selection:** T cells which recognize self-antigens remain active and are retained.

If there are defects in immune tolerance, it results in the development of autoimmunity.

## Immunodeficiency

It is defined as a clinical condition in which there is a failure of immune system. Based on the etiology, the immunodeficiency can be classified as:

- **Congenital immunodeficiency syndromes (Fig. 17.11):** When the immunodeficiency is present

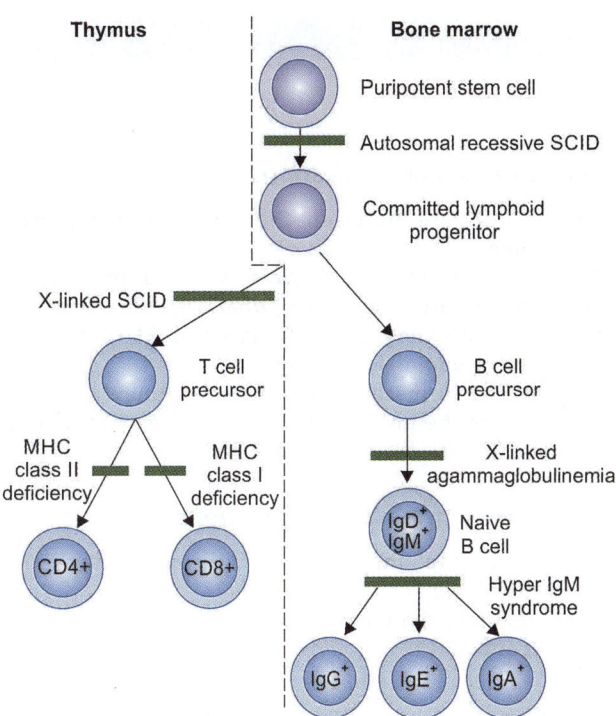

**Fig. 17.11:** Various congenital defects in development of B and T cells resulting in SCID.

since birth. **Example:** SCID (severe combined immunodeficiency). There are defects in development of either cellular or humoral immunity.
- **Acquired immunodeficiency syndrome (AIDS):** It occurs due to HIV virus, that binds to CD4 cells and decrease the number of T helper cells. It causes severe immunodeficiency which predisposes the individual to all types of serious infections and malignancies.

## SUMMARY

- Innate immune response provides immediate, nonspecific, and short-lived defense mechanisms whereas adaptive immunity provide specific responses to particular pathogens.
- Acquired cell immunity begins with the identification of antigens. MHC I and MHC II present the antigen to CD8+ cytotoxic T cells and CD4+ helper T cells.
- Natural killer cells are neither B nor T lymphocytes, they are the third category of lymphocytes and are able to kill a wide variety of organisms and tumor cells.
- Memory cells are the primary feature of acquired immunity. They are long-lasting, give the body long-term memory of the antigen, and protect it from further exposure to the same antigen.
- IgG antigen crosses placenta. Here is IgA in breast milk. In allergic situations, IgE rises. The primary immunological response is mediated by IgM, whereas the secondary immune response is mediated by IgG.
- Booster dose for the vaccines needs to be given.
- Live attenuated vaccine provide acquired artificial active immunity. It consist of a weakened form of pathogen to stimulate an immune response. The pathogen is not able to cause disease itself but can produce immune response. It usually causes long-term immunity without requiring additional dose in adulthood. *Examples:* Influenza, measles, mumps, rubella, polio.
- Autoimmune disorders result from a failure of immunological tolerance.
- Hypersensitivity reactions of types I, II, and III are categorized as humoral mediated responses because they involve antibodies, whereas Type IV hypersensitivity reactions are categorized as cell mediated responses because they involve T cells.
- Allergic transfusion reactions are associated with type I hypersensitivity reactions, while hemolytic transfusion reactions are associated with type II hypersensitivity reactions. Graft vs host is the type IV hypersensitivity reaction.

## LET US SEE, HOW MUCH YOU HAVE LEARNT?

### Review Questions

#### Long/Short Answer Questions

Q1. Differentiate between the innate and acquired immunity.
Q2. Describe the mechanism of cell mediated immunity.
Q3. What are natural killer cells? What is their function?
Q4. Write a short note on T cells. How does $TH_2$ cells help in inducing humoral immunity?
Q5. Describe the mechanism of humoral immunity.
Q6. Describe the immunoglobulin in terms of structure, classification, properties and functions.
Q7. How does the immune response behave to first and repeated exposure to the antigen? (During natural disease process/vaccination).
Q8. Why do you need to give booster dose for the vaccines? (Hint: Explain the secondary immune response here).
Q9. What is complement system? How does it augment the immune response? What is the physiological importance of the complement system?

#### Explain Why? (Reasoning Questions)

Q1. Doesn't the immune system usually attack the self-antigens.
Q2. Sometimes the immune system starts damaging the self-antigens.
Q3. A subsequent exposure to an antigen, in some individuals invoke a severe allergic reaction.
Q4. 'ABO incompatibility results in hemolysis', what is the physiological basis behind hemolysis in this case?

### Critical Thinking Case-Based Questions

Q1. A 25-year-old male presented with symptoms of fever, swollen lymph nodes, and a sore throat, recurrent over the past few months. A detailed medical history revealed that he has recently tested positive for HIV. Blood tests show a low CD4+ T cell count and elevated viral load. Despite receiving antiretroviral therapy (ART), patient's immune response seems compromised, leading to frequent infections. Based upon the given scenario, answer the following questions:
   a. Explain how HIV decreases the immune response.
   b. What are the main components and functions of the innate immune response?
   c. Tabulate the differences between 2 types of CD4 cells.

### Multiple Choice Questions

Q1. Which immunoglobulin is primarily involved in allergic reactions and defense against parasites?
   a. IgA          b. IgM
   c. IgE          d. IgD
Q2. A 45-year-old male is exposed to a bacterial infection. Which of the following cell type is responsible for the phagocytosis of bacteria in the innate immune response?
   a. T Lymphocytes     b. B Lymphocytes
   c. Neutrophil        d. Plasma cells
Q3. NK cells are known for their ability to:
   a. Produce antibodies
   b. Kill infected cells
   c. Phagocytose pathogens
   d. Activate B cells
Q4. A 28-year-old female presents with a recurrent respiratory tract infection. Upon investigations, it is found that she has low levels of immunoglobulins A (IgA). Which aspect of the immune system is primarily affected in this patient?
   a. Cellular immunity   b. Innate immunity
   c. Humoral immunity    d. Passive immunity
Q5. A person who has received a vaccine against measles is demonstrating which type of immunity?
   a. Innate immunity      b. Acquired immunity
   c. Cell mediated immunity  d. Passive immunity
Q6. Which of the following is an example of cell-mediated immunity?
   a. Production of antibodies by plasma cells
   b. Activation of cytotoxic T cells to kill infected cells
   c. Neutralization of toxins by antibodies
   d. Opsonization of pathogens for phagocytosis
Q7. A patient with decreased levels of immunoglobulins is likely to have impaired:
   a. Innate immunity
   b. Acquired immunity
   c. Both innate and acquired immunity
   d. None of the above
Q8. A patient presents with recurrent bacterial infections despite having intact skin and mucosal barriers. Which component of immunity is most likely compromised?
   a. Innate immunity
   b. Acquired immunity
   c. Cell-mediated immunity
   d. Humoral immunity
Q9. A patient receives a kidney transplant and is prescribed immunosuppressant medications to prevent rejection. Which type of immunity is primarily targeted by these medications?
   a. Innate immunity      b. Acquired immunity
   c. Cell-mediated immunity  d. Humoral immunity

Q10. A newborn baby receives maternal antibodies through breastfeeding. This is an example of:
   a. Active immunity
   b. Passive immunity
   c. Cell-mediated immunity
   d. Innate immunity

Q11. Which of the following best defines immunity?
   a. The ability of the body to maintain stable internal conditions
   b. The ability of the body to recognize and destroy foreign substances
   c. The process of blood clot formation to prevent excessive bleeding
   d. The process of nutrient absorption in the digestive system

Q12. Which component of innate immunity is responsible for engulfing and destroying pathogens?
   a. Natural killer cells    b. Macrophages
   c. B cells                 d. T cells

Q13. The process of opsonization involves:
   a. Neutralization of toxins by antibodies
   b. Coating of pathogens with antibodies to enhance phagocytosis
   c. Activation of cytotoxic T cells to kill infected cells
   d. Production of memory B cells for future immune responses

Q14. Which type of immunity is conferred through the transfer of antibodies from one individual to another?
   a. Active immunity
   b. Passive immunity
   c. Cell-mediated immunity
   d. Innate immunity

Q15. A patient presents with a severe allergic reaction after consuming peanuts. Which type of immune response is primarily responsible for this reaction?
   a. Cell-mediated immunity
   b. Humoral immunity
   c. Innate immunity
   d. Adaptive immunity

Q16. A patient with HIV/AIDS experiences frequent infections due to a weakened immune system. Which component of immunity is primarily affected by HIV?
   a. Natural killer cells    b. B cells
   c. T cells                 d. Macrophages

Q17. A patient develops an autoimmune disorder where the immune system destroys the thyroid gland. Which immune disorder does this patient likely have?
   a. Graves' disease
   b. Hashimoto's thyroiditis
   c. Myasthenia gravis
   d. Addison's disease

Q18. A patient is diagnosed with celiac disease, an autoimmune disorder triggered by gluten consumption. Which component of the immune system is primarily involved in this disorder?
   a. T cells                 b. B cells
   c. Macrophages             d. Natural killer cells

Q19. A patient is diagnosed with multiple sclerosis, a chronic inflammatory disease affecting the central nervous system. Which type of immune response is implicated in the pathogenesis of this disorder?
   a. Cell-mediated immunity
   b. Humoral immunity
   c. Innate immunity
   d. Adaptive immunity

Q20. A 55-year-old individual receives the influenza vaccine for the first time. Despite being exposed to the influenza virus in the past, the individual experiences mild symptoms of the flu after vaccination. Which of the following best explains this scenario?
   a. The individual has developed innate immunity to the influenza virus
   b. The individual is experiencing a primary immune response to the vaccine
   c. The individual's immune system has developed tolerance to the influenza virus
   d. The individual is experiencing a secondary immune response to the vaccine

Q21. A 12-year-old child receives a booster dose of the tetanus vaccine. This is the child's second vaccination against tetanus, the first dose having been administered at age 6. Which of the following accurately describes the immune response following the booster dose?
   a. The child's immune system mounts a primary response to the tetanus vaccine
   b. The child's immune system exhibits memory from the previous vaccination, leading to a secondary immune response
   c. The child's immune system becomes less responsive to the tetanus vaccine due to repeated exposure
   d. The child's immune system relies solely on innate immunity to combat tetanus infection

Q22. A 30-year-old woman develops a severe rash and difficulty breathing shortly after receiving a penicillin injection for a bacterial infection. Upon further investigation, it is discovered that she has previously received penicillin without any adverse reactions. Which type of hypersensitivity reaction is most likely responsible for her symptoms?
   a. Type I hypersensitivity reaction
   b. Type II hypersensitivity reaction
   c. Type III hypersensitivity reaction
   d. Type IV hypersensitivity reaction

Q23. A 45-year-old man presents with joint pain, swelling, and stiffness, particularly in the mornings. He also experiences dry eyes and mouth, along with occasional shortness of breath. Laboratory tests reveal the presence of antinuclear antibodies (ANA) and rheumatoid factor (RF). Which of the following autoimmune disorders is most likely affecting this patient?
   a. Rheumatoid arthritis
   b. Systemic lupus erythematosus (SLE)
   c. Sjögren's syndrome
   d. Scleroderma

## ANSWERS

1. c   2. c   3. b   4. c   5. b   6. b   7. b   8. c   9. c   10. b   11. b   12. b   13. b   14. b
15. b   16. c   17. b   18. a   19. a   20. b   21. b   22. a   23. b

# Platelets: Structure, Formation and Functions

## CHAPTER 18

### COMPETENCY ADDRESSED
PY2.7: Describe the formation of platelets, functions, and variations.

### LEARNING OBJECTIVES
**At the end of this chapter, the learner should be able to:**
- Discuss the functional structure of platelets.
- Discuss thrombopoiesis along with factors regulating it.
- Describe the functions of platelets.
- Clinical correlation:
  – Give the physiological basis of use of antiplatelet drugs.
  – Discuss physiological basis of bleeding disorders caused due to platelet defects.

Platelets are non-nucleated circulating fragments of megakaryocytes that are important mediators of hemostasis They are also called thrombocytes (Thrombus: clot; cytes: cells).

## FORMATION OF PLATELETS/THROMBOPOIESIS

Platelets are the *smallest cellular fragments* of megakaryocytes which are *1 to 4 micrometers* in diameter. They are *anucleated* cells that are derived from the megakaryocytes formed in the bone marrow. Common myeloid progenitor cells in the bone marrow differentiate into promegakaryocytes and then into megakaryocytes. Megakaryocytes while leaving and trying to squeeze through capillaries, they breakdown into pieces and each piece is a platelet. So platelets are just pieces of the membrane of megakaryocyte and a small part of its cytoplasm. The normal concentration of platelets in the blood is between 150,000 and 300,000/μL.

 **FACT CHECK**

Megakaryocytes are found in bone marrow. Platelets are seen in peripheral blood smear.

Factors stimulate thrombopoiesis are:
- The hormone *thrombopoietin (TPO)*, synthesized by liver stimulates platelet production.

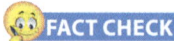 **FACT CHECK**

Severe liver disease causes thrombocytopenia.

- Interleukin (IL6) stimulate thrombopoietin.

**FACT CHECK**

Inflammation causes secondary/reactive thrombocytosis.

- Decrease platelet count stimulates thrombopoietin production (negative feedback).

**Life span of platelets:** Platelet is an active structure. It has a half-life in the blood of only *8 to 12 days*. It is eliminated from the circulation mainly by the tissue macrophage system. More than half of the platelets are removed by macrophages in the spleen.

**FACT CHECK**

In splenomegaly, there is decrease platelet count.

## FUNCTIONAL STRUCTURE OF PLATELETS (FIGS. 18.1 AND 18.2)

The outermost region of the cell contains a bilipid membrane composed of proteins and lipids. The predominant lipid is phospholipid, that helps in multiple

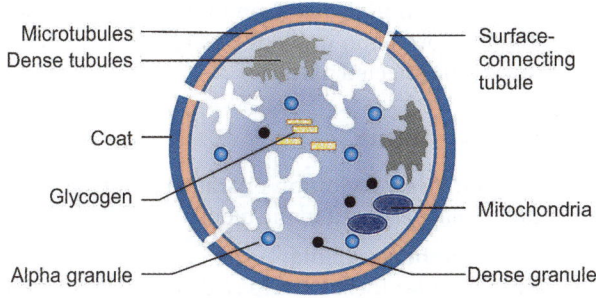

**Fig. 18.1:** Structure of platelet.

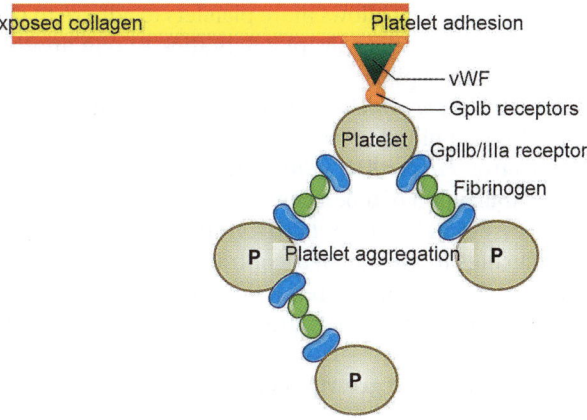

**Fig. 18.3:** Platelet adhesion and aggregation.

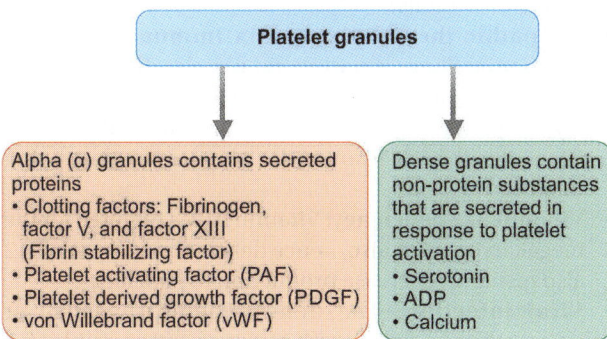

**Fig. 18.2:** Types of platelet granules.

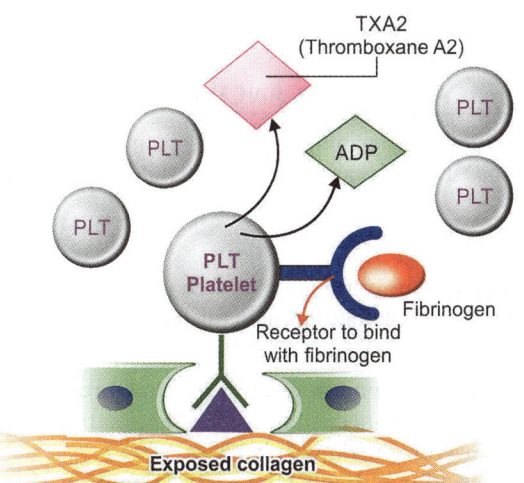

Platelets change their shape and grab other platelets. Released ADP and TXA2 results expression of receptors that bind with fibrinogen

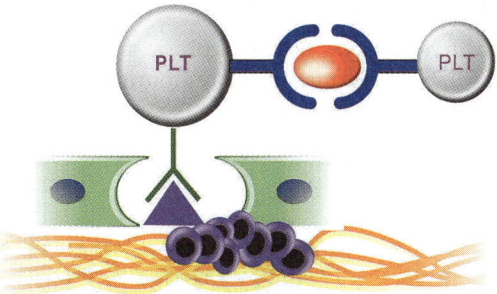

Since two platelets can adhere to a fibrinogen molecule. The platelets begin to aggregagte at the site of injury

**Fig. 18.4:** Mechanism of hemostasis by platelet aggregation.

stages of blood coagulation process. The glycoproteins present on the surface of platelet membrane serve as receptors. Glycoprotein receptors found on the platelet membrane are *GP1b and GP2b/3a*. Cytoplasm of platelets: It contains actin, myosin, glycogen, lysosomes, and two types of granules.

## FUNCTIONS OF PLATELETS (FIGS. 18.3 AND 18.4)

- **Role in hemostasis:** Platelets play an important role in hemostasis, which is the process of stopping bleeding after an injury. The primary function of platelets is to form a temporary plug at the site of injury by adhering to the damaged tissue and recruiting other platelets and blood cells to the developing clot. Platelets also activate the plasma coagulation cascade, which leads to the formation of a fibrin clot that reinforce the platelet plug.
- Platelets *releases von Willebrand factor (vWF)*, that helps in platelet adhesion and activation and also prevents the degradation of factor VIII.
- Platelets express various *glycoprotein receptors* on their surface, which play essential roles in processes such as adhesion, activation, and aggregation during hemostasis. Two important glycoproteins expressed on platelets are *GP1b and GP2b/3a*.
    - **GP1b:** This receptor *helps in platelet adhesion*. When a blood vessel is damaged, the sub-endothelial collagen fibers are exposed, which bind to von Willebrand factor(vWF) released from damaged endothelium. vWF then binds with GP1b receptor on platelets and bind platelet to exposed collagen.
    - **GP2b/3a:** This receptor *facilitates the aggregation of platelets*. It is found on the surface of platelets in an inactive form; however, it becomes active during platelet activation. This active receptor is bound by circulating fibrinogen. Fibrinogen is the linking

molecule that allows more platelets to adhere to one another. In this way, platelets stick to one another and form a plug.
- It *releases serotonin* that causes vasoconstriction of the injured blood vessels.
- It *releases Factor XIII (Fibrin stabilizing factors)* helps in stabilization of blood clot
- It is essential for *clot retraction*. The actin and myosin molecules in the platelets contract, causing the clot to decrease. During clot retraction, the injured arteries' edges come together, further sealing the blood channels.
- **Platelet derived growth factor (PDGF)** is involved in the formation of new blood vessels. It stimulates the migration and proliferation of endothelial cells, which are the building blocks of blood vessels. It facilitates *long term wound healing* after tissue damage.

## CLINICAL SIGNIFICANCE

Variations in normal count/defects in platelet results in various disorders as shown in **Fig. 18.5**.

## Thrombocytosis

**Introduction:** It is a condition characterized by a higher than normal platelet count in the blood.

**Causes:**
- **Primary thrombocytosis (Essential thrombocytosis):** It is due to abnormalities in the bone marrow, leading to an overproduction of platelets.
- **Secondary thrombocytosis (Reactive thrombocytosis):** It is usually a response to an underlying condition or stimulus due to infections, inflammatory disorders, iron-deficiency anemia, hemolytic anemia, removal of spleen, and cancer.

**Pathophysiology:** Platelets plays a crucial role in hemostasis by formation of temporary platelet plug. Elevated platelet count leads to an increase risk of blood clot/thrombus formation in blood vessels. This can block blood flow to the affected part.

## Thrombocytopenia

**Introduction:** It is a condition characterized by a lower than normal platelet count in the blood.

**Causes of thrombocytopenia:**
- **Aplastic anemia:** There is decreased platelet production in the bone marrow due to infections or sepsis, nutrient deficiencies. It also reduce production of red blood cells (white blood cells).
- **Idiopathic thrombocytopenia/immune thrombocytopenia:** There is peripheral platelet destruction by antibodies immune thrombocytopenia purpura (ITP).
- **Hypersplenism:** The enlarged, hyperfunctioning spleen decreases the life span of the platelets by destroying them early.
- **Vitamin B12 deficiency:** Vitamin B12 is required for the megakaryopoiesis also, hence deficiency of vitamin B12 also results in decrease production of platelets.
- **Viral infection:** The dengue hemorrhagic fever is commonly known viral fever responsible for thrombocytopenia.
- **Cytotoxic chemotherapy and radiation:** The toxicity of chemotherapy and radiation therapy to the blood cells and bone marrow are responsible for low platelet count.
- **Consumption of platelets in thrombi [Thrombotic thrombocytopenic purpura (TTP)]**
- Dilution of the blood from fluid resuscitation or massive transfusion.

**Pathophysiology:** Platelets plays a crucial role in hemostasis by formation of temporary platelet plug, stabilization of clot, and clot retraction. Decrease platelet count impairs blood's ability to clot, reduces clot retraction and increase risk of bleeding. The bleeding is usually from many small venules or capillaries.

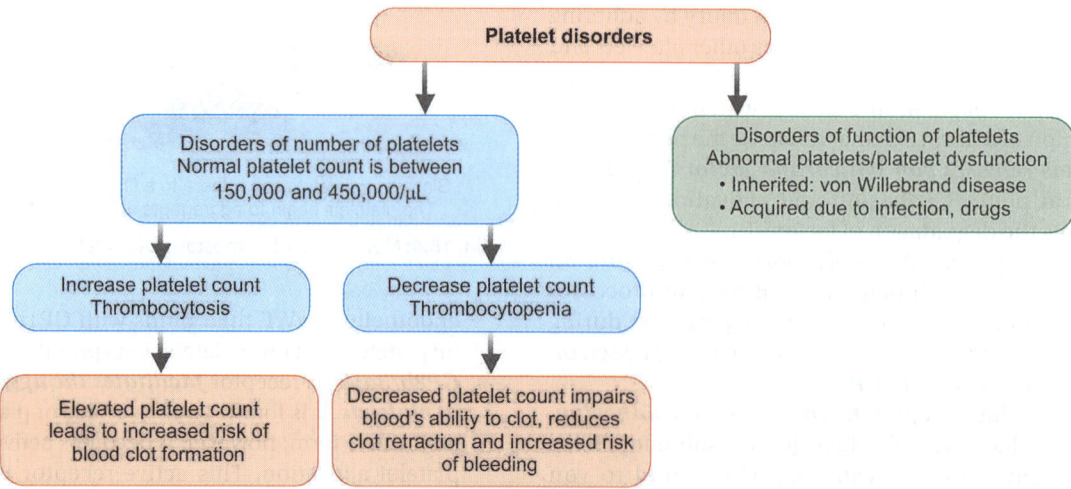

**Fig. 18.5:** Disorders of platelet.

**Table 18.1:** Symptoms associated with low platelet count.

| Platelet count | Symptoms |
|---|---|
| Above 100,000/mm³ | No clinical symptoms, bleeding is rare |
| 50,000–100,000/mm³ | Bleeding may occur after major surgery |
| 30,000–50,000/mm³ | Bleeding occurs with minor trauma |
| 10,000–30,000/mm³ | Spontaneous bleeding |

**Signs and symptoms (Table 18.1):** The decreased platelet count is characterized by increased bleeding tendencies, and easy bruisability.
- Petechiae and purpura (**Fig. 18.6**): Petechiae are small, pinpoints hemorrhages, and purpura are larger area of bleeding into the skin.
- Ecchymosis refers to large bruises.
- **Mucosal bleeding:** Nose bleeding (epistaxis), gum bleeding or gastrointestinal bleeding.
- Women may have heavier or prolonged menstrual bleeding.
- Bleeding after minor injuries.

## Diagnosis of Platelet Disorders

- Increased bleeding time
- Decreased platelet count
- Defect in platelet aggregation tests
- Defect in platelet adhesiveness tests
- Increased clot retraction time

## Purpura

Purpura is defined as the easy bruisability in a person and presence of larger area of bleeding into the skin.

**Types:** There are two kinds of purpura:
1. Thrombocytopenic purpura
2. Nonthrombocytopenic purpura

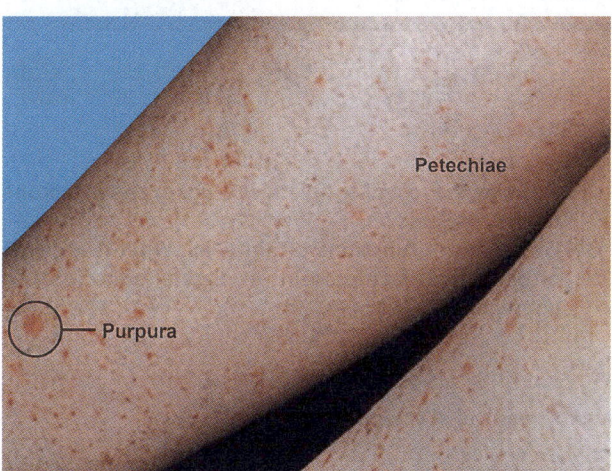

**Fig. 18.6:** Clinical difference between Petechiae and Purpura.

**Causes:**
- **Thrombocytopenic purpura** is due to decreased platelet count. The causes are:
  - Aplastic anemia
  - *Idiopathic thrombocytopenia:* Antiplatelet antibodies destroy platelets.
  - Hypersplenism
  - Vitamin B12 deficiency
  - Viral infection
  - Cytotoxic chemotherapy and radiation
  - Dilution of the blood
- **Nonthrombocytopenic purpura** is due to increased capillary fragility. The capillaries become fragile and easily get ruptured resulting in easy bruisability. It is caused by weak blood vessels, inflammation of blood vessels, vitamin C deficiency, aging, allergy, drugs and infections. There is increase bleeding time with normal platelet count.

## Platelet Function Tests

Platelet function tests are laboratory tests that assess the function of platelets, which are small blood cells responsible for blood clotting. These tests are often ordered to evaluate bleeding disorders or to assess the risk of excessive bleeding or blood clot formation.
- **Bleeding time:** This test measures the time it takes for bleeding to stop after a standardized skin puncture. It evaluates platelet function and the overall ability of blood vessels to constrict and stop bleeding.
- **Platelet aggregation test:** This test assesses the ability of platelets to clump together (aggregate) in response to certain substances, such as ADP, collagen, epinephrine, or arachidonic acid. It helps diagnose disorders of platelet function, such as von Willebrand disease or platelet dysfunction.
- **Platelet function analyzer (PFA):** This test evaluates platelet function by measuring the time it takes for blood to clot in a small tube coated with a substance that activates platelets. It's useful for detecting disorders of primary hemostasis, such as von Willebrand disease and platelet function defects.
- **Thromboelastography (TEG) and rotational thromboelastometry (ROTEM):** These tests assess the viscoelastic properties of whole blood clot formation in real-time. They provide comprehensive information about the kinetics and strength of clot formation, as well as fibrinolysis. While not specifically platelet function tests, they offer insights into overall hemostasis and can indirectly assess platelet function.
- **Clot retraction:** After a clot forms, it shrinks and releases the fluid within a few minutes. The fluid is called serum. It occurs due to contraction of actin and myosin molecule present in platelets. During clot retraction, the edges of the injured arteries are brought together, further sealing the vessels.

- **Platelet count:** While not a direct assessment of platelet function, platelet count is a basic test that measures the number of platelets in a sample of blood. Abnormally low platelet counts (thrombocytopenia) can indicate a risk of bleeding, even if platelet function is normal.

**Why the clot doesn't spread to the intact endothelium?**
Intact endothelium releases prostacyclin and nitric oxide that prevent platelet adhesion and aggregation.

**FACT CHECK**

Insufficient platelet counts lead to inadequate constriction of broken blood arteries and inadequate clot retraction.

## ANTIPLATELET DRUGS (FIG. 18.7)

Aspirin produces irreversible inhibition of cyclooxygenase. This reduces production of thromboxane and inhibits platelet aggregation. Thus, aspirin aids in preventing blood clots.

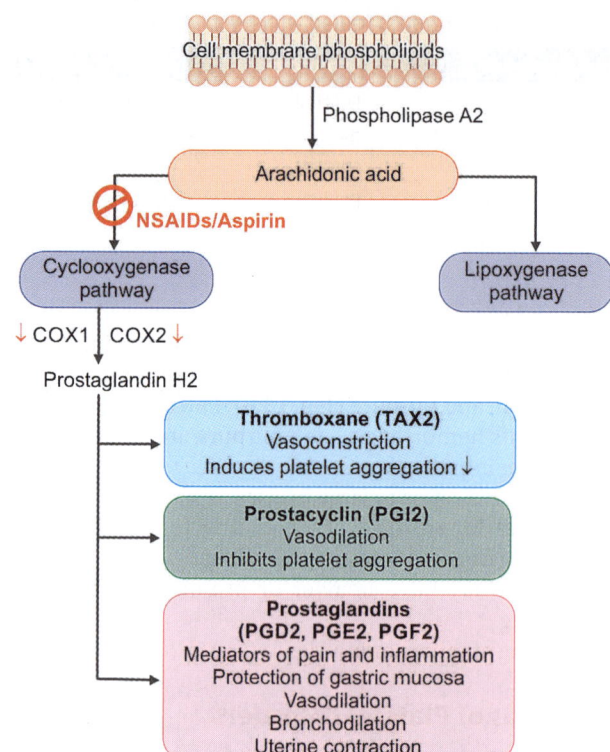

**Fig. 18.7:** Mechanism of action and role of antiplatelets drugs.

### SUMMARY

- The larger cells called megakaryocytes are disintegrated to form thrombocytes. Each megakaryocyte contains 2,000–3,000 platelets.
- Platelet adhesion, activation, and aggregation are all involved in the formation of a temporary platelet plug at the site of injury.
- Thrombocytosis causes blood clots to form in blood vessels. This can block blood flow to the affected part.
- Thrombocytopenia impairs blood's ability to clot, reduces clot retraction and increase risk of bleeding. The bleeding is usually from many small venules or capillaries.
- Immune-mediated idiopathic thrombocytopenia is characterized by the formation of antibodies against platelets, which cause purpura and easy bruisability.
- Increased bleeding time with normal platelet count is seen in Nonthrombocytopenic purpura.

### LET US SEE, HOW MUCH YOU HAVE LEARNT?

 *Review Questions*

#### Long/Short Answer Questions

Q1. Describe the function of von Willbrand factor. What will happen, if it is deficient?
Q2. Describe the idiopathic thrombocytopenic purpura in terms of pathophysiology and clinical presentation.
Q3. Describe the role of antiplatelet drugs in patients prone to atherosclerosis?
Q4. Describe the functions of platelets. What is the role of platelet surface proteins in platelet adhesion and aggregation?

#### Explain Why? (Reasoning Question)

Q1. How can a patient of thrombocytopenic purpura be benefited by removal of spleen?

## Critical Thinking Case-Based Questions

**Q1.** A 32-year-old female patient presents to the clinic with a complaint of easy bruising and petechiae on her arms and legs. She has no significant medical history. On examination, she has multiple petechiae and ecchymoses on her arms and legs. Her platelet count is 20,000/mm³.

a. What is your diagnosis? Give the justification.
b. Why is the platelet count decreased?
c. What is the physiological basis of all the clinical features of the patient?

## Multiple Choice Questions

**Q1.** Platelet transfusions are typically used to treat which of the following conditions?
a. Anemia
b. Thrombocytopenia
c. Hemophilia
d. Polycythemia

**Q2.** Platelets can adhere to damaged blood vessels by interacting with which of the following proteins?
a. Fibrinogen
b. Collagen
c. Thrombin
d. Prothrombin

**Q3.** Which of the following tests is used to evaluate platelet function?
a. Complete blood count
b. Prothrombin time
c. Platelet function assay
d. Clotting time

**Q4.** Which of the following substances can activate platelets?
a. Histamine
b. Serotonin
c. Thrombin
d. Fibrinogen

**Q5.** Which of the following conditions is associated with low platelet counts?
a. Anemias
b. Exercise
c. Hypersplenism
d. Splenectomy

**Q6.** A 35-year-old woman with a background of liver cirrhosis and portal hypertension secondary to chronic hepatitis C presented with complications of hypersplenism and thrombocytopenia. She developed severe menorrhagia requiring multiple blood transfusions. What is the cause of decrease blood count.
a. Antibodies formed against platelets
b. Sequestration of platelets due to enlarged spleen
c. Anemias
d. Consumption of platelet in thrombi.

**Q7.** A patient with a bleeding disorder is found to have normal platelet count but prolonged bleeding time. Which of the following tests would be most appropriate to further investigate the cause of the bleeding disorder?
a. Platelet count
b. Thromboelastography (TEG)
c. Platelet aggregation test
d. Platelet function analyzer (PFA)

**Q8.** A patient is diagnosed with thrombocytopenia. Which of the following factors is primarily responsible for regulating thrombopoiesis?
a. Erythropoietin
b. Interleukin-6
c. Thrombopoietin
d. Tissue factor

**Q9.** A patient is prescribed aspirin for secondary prevention of cardiovascular events. Which of the following is the primary physiological basis for using aspirin as an antiplatelet drug?
a. Inhibition of platelet aggregation via inhibition of ADP receptors
b. Inhibition of cyclooxygenase (COX) and subsequent thromboxane A2 synthesis
c. Inhibition of glycoprotein IIb/IIIa receptors
d. Enhancement of fibrinolysis

**Q10.** A patient presents with a history of easy bruising and prolonged bleeding after minor injuries. Laboratory investigations reveal normal platelet count but abnormal platelet function. Which of the following is the most likely physiological basis for the bleeding disorder in this patient?
a. Deficiency of von Willebrand factor
b. Impaired platelet adhesion
c. Decreased thromboxane A2 synthesis
d. Elevated levels of fibrinogen

**Q11.** A patient with a bleeding disorder exhibits impaired platelet aggregation in response to collagen. Which of the following tests is most likely to confirm the diagnosis of a platelet function defect?
a. Thromboelastography (TEG)
b. Platelet count
c. Platelet function analyzer (PFA)
d. Platelet aggregation test

**Q12.** A patient with a history of myocardial infarction is prescribed a P2Y12 receptor inhibitor. Which of the following best describes the physiological basis for using P2Y12 receptor inhibitors as antiplatelet therapy?
a. Inhibition of cyclooxygenase (COX)
b. Inhibition of thromboxane A2 receptors
c. Inhibition of ADP-induced platelet activation
d. Enhancement of fibrinolysis

**Q13.** A patient undergoing cardiac surgery is found to have prolonged bleeding time. Which of the following platelet function tests is most appropriate to assess platelet function in this patient?
a. Thromboelastography (TEG)
b. Bleeding time test
c. Platelet aggregation test
d. Platelet function analyzer (PFA)

**Q14.** A patient with a history of recurrent miscarriages is diagnosed with von Willebrand disease. Which of the following best describes the physiological basis for the bleeding disorder in this patient?
a. Impaired platelet aggregation
b. Deficiency of von Willebrand factor
c. Defective platelet adhesion
d. Excessive thromboxane A2 synthesis

**Q15.** A patient with a history of gastrointestinal bleeding is found to have elevated levels of thromboxane A2. Which of the following medications is most likely to reduce thromboxane A2 levels and decrease the risk of bleeding?
a. Aspirin
b. Clopidogrel
c. Prostacyclin analogs
d. Aminocaproic acid

**Q16.** A patient with a history of deep vein thrombosis is prescribed warfarin therapy. Which of the following best describes the physiological basis for using warfarin in preventing thrombosis?
a. Inhibition of platelet aggregation
b. Inhibition of vitamin K-dependent clotting factors
c. Inhibition of fibrinogen synthesis
d. Enhancement of fibrinolysis

**Q17.** A patient with a bleeding disorder exhibits normal platelet aggregation but prolonged bleeding time. Which of the following is the most likely physiological basis for the bleeding disorder in this patient?
a. Deficiency of von Willebrand factor
b. Impaired platelet adhesion
c. Decreased thromboxane A2 synthesis
d. Elevated levels of fibrinogen

**Q18.** A patient with a history of ischemic stroke is prescribed dipyridamole. Which of the following best describes the mechanism of action of dipyridamole as an antiplatelet drug?
a. Inhibition of thromboxane A2 synthesis
b. Blockade of glycoprotein IIb/IIIa receptors
c. Inhibition of ADP-induced platelet aggregation
d. Enhancement of prostacyclin production

## ANSWERS

**1.** b  **2.** b  **3.** c  **4.** c  **5.** c  **6.** b  **7.** d  **8.** c  **9.** b  **10.** b  **11.** d  **12.** c  **13.** b  **14.** b
**15.** c  **16.** b  **17.** a  **18.** d

# Hemostasis

**CHAPTER 19**

### COMPETENCY ADDRESSED
**PY2.8:** Describe the physiological basis of hemostasis and anticoagulants. Describe bleeding and clotting disorders (Hemophilia and Purpura).

### LEARNING OBJECTIVES
**At the end of this chapter, the learner should be able to:**
- Define of hemostasis.
- Discuss the mechanism of hemostasis.
- Explain how the blood is kept in liquid form in healthy cardiovascular system (Maintenance of blood liquidity in healthy cardiovascular system).
- Clinical correlation:
  - Give the physiological basis of use of anticoagulants.
  - Discuss various bleeding disorders.
  - Give the physiological basis of diagnosis of bleeding disorders.

## DEFINITION OF HEMOSTASIS

It is the *spontaneous arrest or stoppage of bleeding* from the injured/damaged blood vessels by the physiological process. Blood arteries, platelets, and clotting factors are the main components of hemostasis.

## MECHANISM OF HEMOSTASIS

Under normal circumstances, there exists a fine balance between the procoagulants and anticoagulants **(Fig. 19.1)**.

Hemostasis involves primary and secondary hemostasis **(Fig. 19.2)**.
- **Temporary/primary hemostasis (Figs. 19.3 and 19.4):** It is the first stage of hemostasis. It involves artery vasoconstriction and formation of temporary platelet plug.
- **Permanent/definitive hemostasis (Fig. 19.5):** It refers to the activation of clotting factors resulting in the formation of clot and sealing the platelet plug. The clotting factors are activated by the various factors secreted by platelets.

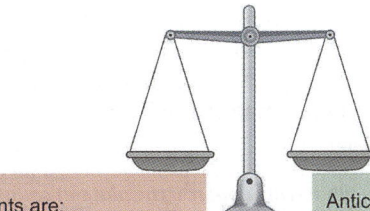

Procoagulants are:
- Damaged endothelium
- Activated platelets
- Active clotting factors
- Conversion of fibrinogen to fibrin

Anticoagulants are:
- Continuous circulation
- Smooth endothelium
- The glycocalyx layer on the endothelium
- Prostacyclin and nitric oxide generated by intact endothelium, which inhibit platelet adherence
- Thrombin-thrombomodulin complex
- Antithrombin action of antithrombin III

**Fig. 19.1:** Balance between procoagulants and anticoagulants.

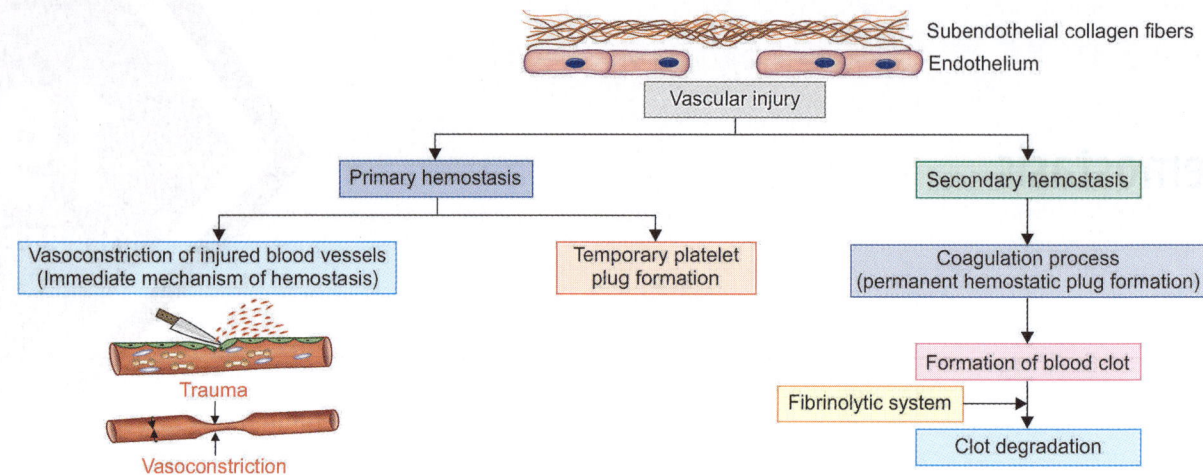

Fig. 19.2: Temporary and definitive primary hemostasis.

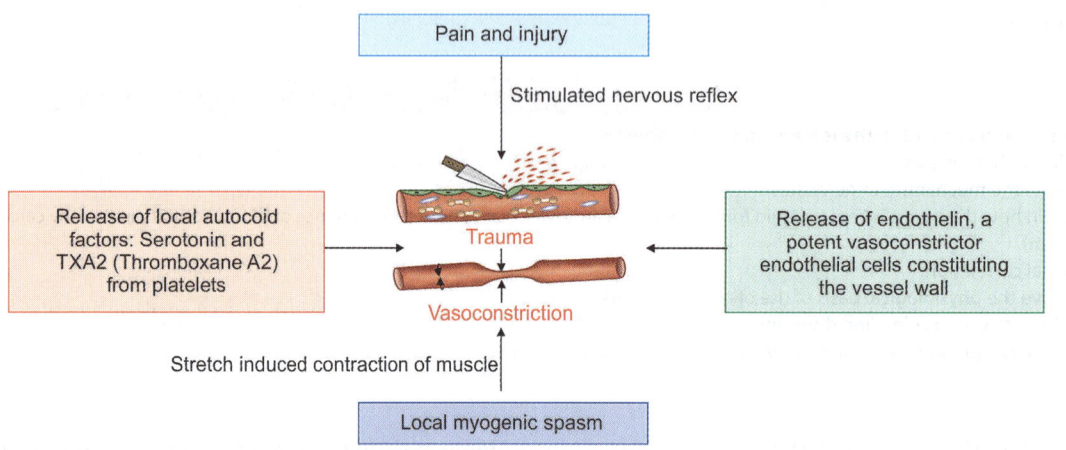

Fig. 19.3: Temporary/primary hemostasis.

## TEMPORARY HEMOSTASIS (PLATELET PLUG FORMATION) (FIGS. 19.3 AND 19.5)

- **Vasoconstriction of injured blood vessel:** Vasoconstriction is the first response to injury of a blood vessel. and subendothelial collagen is exposed where the injury has occurred.
- The mechanisms of narrowing of blood vessels include *formation of a weak platelet plug*. The phases in this process are:
  - **Platelet adhesion:** This is the initial phase where platelets adhere to the exposed collagen fibers at the site of injury in the blood vessel wall. Von Willebrand factor (vWF), a protein released by endothelial cells, helps facilitate the adhesion of platelets to the injured area.
  - **Platelet activation:** Following adhesion, platelets become activated, undergoing a series of biochemical changes. Activation triggers the release of various substances stored within the platelets, such as ADP (adenosine diphosphate) and thromboxane A2. These substances further stimulate platelet activation and recruitment.
  - **Platelet aggregation:** Activated platelets undergo a process called aggregation, where they bind together to form a loose plug at the site of injury. This aggregation is facilitated by the interaction between platelet receptors, such as glycoprotein IIb/IIIa, and adhesive proteins like fibrinogen. The formation of this weak platelet plug serves as an initial barrier to prevent excessive bleeding.

Damaged endothelium exposes subendothelial collagen, von Willebrand factor (vWF), releases ATP, and inflammatory mediators.

*What will happen, if the platelet count of a person decreases?*
The decrease in platelet count results in a condition termed as purpura. It is characterized by increased bleeding tendencies, petechial hemorrhages and easy bruisability. The platelet function tests will be deranged showing:
- Increased bleeding time
- Decreased platelet count

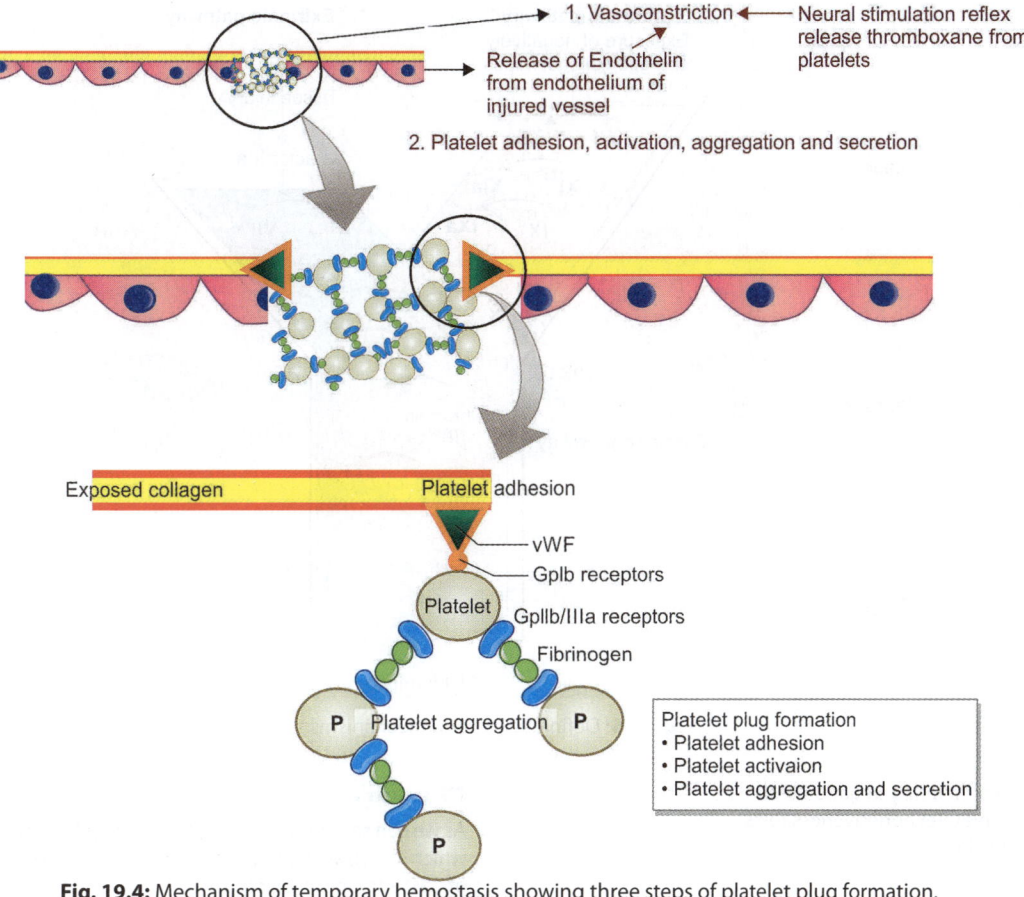

**Fig. 19.4:** Mechanism of temporary hemostasis showing three steps of platelet plug formation.

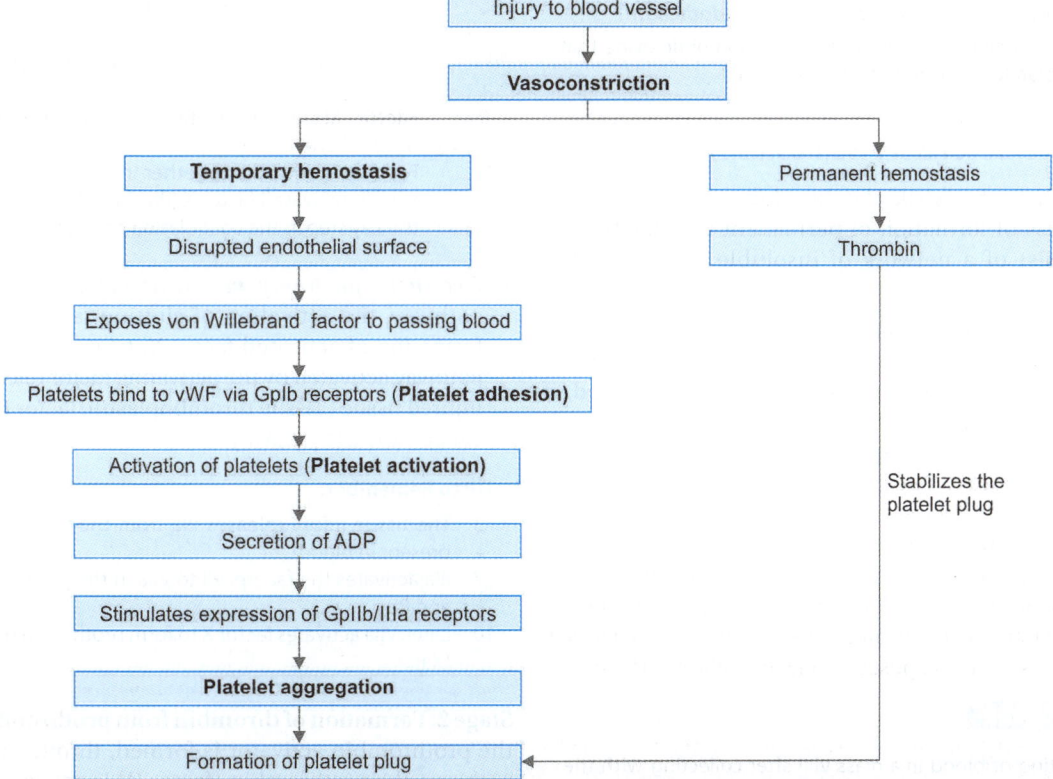

**Fig. 19.5:** Difference between temporary and permanent hemostasis.

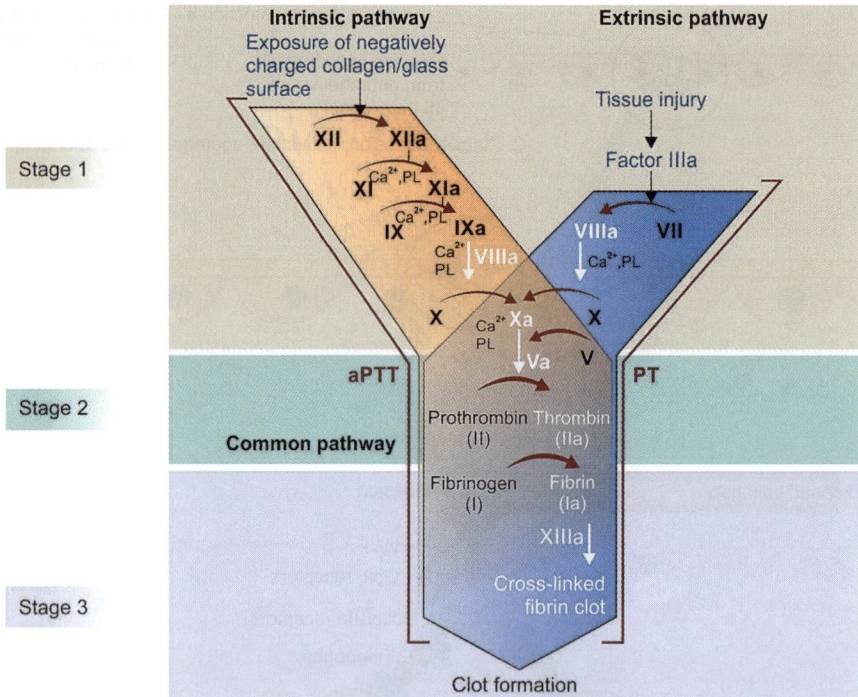

**Fig. 19.6:** Definitive clotting mechanisms.

- Defect in platelet aggregation tests
- Defect in platelet adhesiveness tests
- Increased clot retraction time

***Why the clot doesn't spread to the intact endothelium?***
Intact endothelium releases prostacyclin and nitric oxide that prevent platelet adhesion and aggregation.

## Definitive/Secondary Hemostasis/Coagulation

In this stage, the weak platelet plug is stabilized. It is the process of formation of permanent hemostatic clot that consist of a network of insoluble threads called *fibrin*.

**Definitive hemostasis has three stages (Fig. 19.6):**
**Stage 1: Formation of prothrombin activator (Factor Xa):** As seen the figure, the stage 1 is accomplished, if the factor X is activated (Xa; prothrombin activator). The Stage 1 pathways get activated depending upon the type of injury. There are two clotting pathways or cascades:
- **Intrinsic pathway/mechanism/cascade:** In this pathway, *all the clotting factors required for the activation of factor X are present inside the blood*. These factors get activated on exposure of a negatively charged surface (exposed collagen or glass surface).

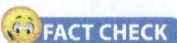

The clotting of blood in a glass vial after collecting with the needle occurs through the intrinsic mechanism.

**TIP to Remember:**
As we can see in the cascade, the clotting factors are activated, which in turn activates the other clotting factors in the presence of $Ca^{2+}$ and phospholipids (PL).

| | |
|---|---|
| 12 ↓ | Factor XII is activated to factor XIIa (activated factor XII) on coming in contact with exposed college/glass surface. |
| 11 ↓ | XIIa activates factor XI in the presence of $Ca^{2+}$ and PL |
| 9 ↓ ← 8 | Factor XIa/activates factor IX in the presence of $Ca^{2+}$, PL, and factor VIII. |
| 10 | Factor IXa and VIIIa together in the presence of $Ca^{2+}$ and PL, activated factor X (Prothrombin activator). It is the key step in the coagulation cascade. |

- ***Extrinsic pathway/mechanism/cascade:*** In this pathway, the activation of clotting factors, up to the formation of activated factor X, takes place through a pathway activated by the activating factor released from injured tissue (Tissue thromboplastin/factor III), hence called extrinsic pathway.

**TIP to Remember:**

| | |
|---|---|
| 3 ↓ | The tissue injury releases IIIa from the tissues (it is not present in blood). |
| 7 ↓ | IIIa activates the factors VII to VIIa in the presence of $Ca^{2+}$ and PL |
| 10 | Later, VIIa activates factor X to form prothrombin activator (Xa) |

**Stage 2: Formation of thrombin from prothrombin:** Once the prothrombin activator is formed, through the either pathway, the prothrombin (factor II) is activated to form thrombin in the presence of factor Va, $Ca^{2+}$ and PL.

**Table 19.1:** Clotting factors.*

| Factor | Name | Peculiarity/Specific details |
|---|---|---|
| I | Fibrinogen | It is an important factor for the formation of clot, used in step III of the clotting cascade |
| II | Prothrombin | Formed in liver, vitamin K dependent. It gets activated to form thrombin by factor Xa. Thrombin plays an important role in clotting as well as activation of thrombolytic pathways |
| III | Tissue thromboplastin | Responsible for initiating the extrinsic pathway of clotting |
| IV | Calcium | |
| V | Proaccelerin | Formed in liver |
| VII | Proconvertin | Formed in liver, vitamin K dependent |
| VIII | Antihemophilic factor | X linked recessive inheritance. Carried by vWF. It is an important component of intrinsic pathway |
| IX | Christmas factor | Formed in liver, vitamin K dependent |
| X | Stuart power factor | Formed in liver, vitamin K dependent, activation of factor X is the key step in both intrinsic and extrinsic pathways. It is also called as prothrombin activator |
| XI | Plasma thromboplastin antecedent | It is an important component of intrinsic pathway |
| XII | Hageman factor | Initiates the intrinsic pathway of clotting |
| XIII | Fibrin stabilizing factor | It converts the fibrin threads into a clot |

*There is no factor VI. Hence there are total 12 numbered clotting factor from factors I to XIII along with other specific factors.

**Stage 3: Formation of fibrin from fibrinogen and stabilization of clot:**
- The thrombin now converts fibrinogen (factor I) to a fibrin thread.
- **Stabilization of fibrin clot:** At first fibrin monomers are formed which later polymerize to form fibrin threads. These fibrin threads are then stabilized by activated factor XIII (factor XIII is activated by thrombin. Clot consist of fibrin meshwork, red cells, platelets and plasma. It acts a physical barrier that prevents further blood loss.

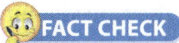 **FACT CHECK**

Plasma clots and serum cannot because serum lacks fibrinogen and other clotting factors.

**Common pathway:** Stages 2 and 3, after the formation of prothrombin activator (activated factor X) is same in both the pathways, hence termed as common pathway.

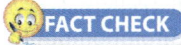 **FACT CHECK**

Clotting factors formed in liver: II, V, VII, IX, X
Vitamin K dependent factors: II, VII, IX, X

Definitive hemostasis involves the activation of clotting factors that are present in plasma in inactive form. Various clotting factors are shown in **Table 19.1**.

## CLOT RETRACTION

After a clot forms, it shrinks and releases the fluid within a few minutes. The fluid is called serum. It occurs due to thrombospondin molecule present in platelets.

Insufficient platelet counts lead to inadequate constriction of broken blood arteries and inadequate clot retraction.

## Importance of Clot Retraction Time

Clot retraction refers to shrinkage in the size of the clot to express out the serum. It results in:
- the formation of firm clot
- promotes wound healing
- strong sealing of blood vessels
- prevents thrombolysis.

Normal clot retraction time is 50% at the end of the first hour. It is said to be prolonged, if it is <50% at the end of the first hour and indicates platelet dysfunction.

## Clot Dissolution by Fibrinolytic System

This promotes lysis of the fibrin clot, and restores the flow of blood in the damaged blood vessels.

*How does the blood remain fluid in the blood vessels?*
- Dynamism of blood flow
- Role of vascular endothelium
- Heparin—antithrombin III system
- Negative feedback by thrombin
- Role of liver
- Role of platelets

- **Anticlotting mechanisms (Fig. 19.7):** These are the mechanisms that restricts clot formation to the site of injury. These are essential to maintain the fluid state the blood and prevent excessive clotting. The two major systems are the fibrinolytic systems and anticoagulants.
  - *Fibrinolytic/plasmolytic system (Fig. 19.8):* It restores the flow of blood in the damaged/obstructed blood vessels. The components of fibrinolytic system are plasminogen entrapped with fibrin in the clot and tissue plasminogen activator (t-PA) secreted by vascular endothelial cells and injured tissue.
  - Physiological anticoagulants **(Fig. 19.9)**.

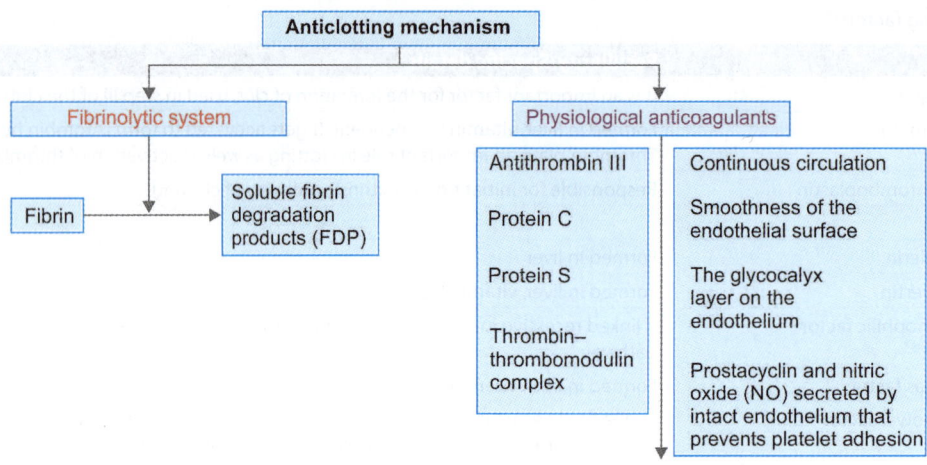

Fig. 19.7: Anticlotting mechanism.

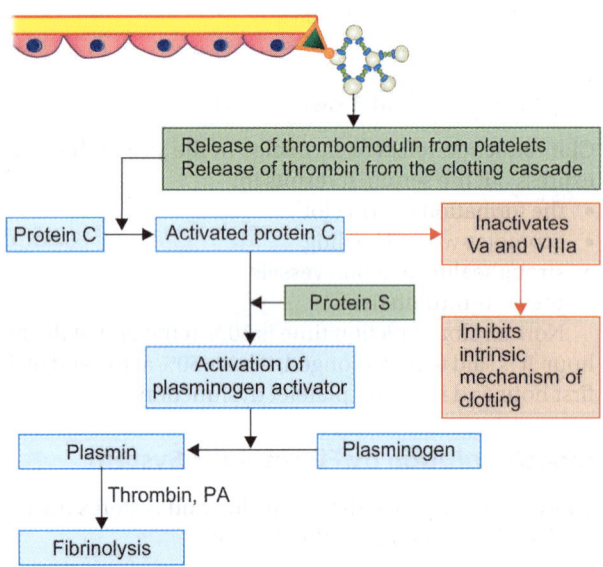

Fig. 19.8: Fibrinolytic/plasmolytic system.

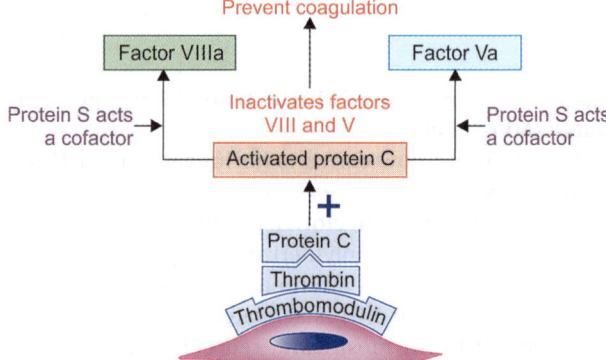

Fig. 19.9: Physiological anticoagulants.

- **Smoothness of the endothelial surface:** The nonadhesive surface of endothelial cells is maintained by endothelium smoothness, which is essential for anticoagulation. The nonadhesive surface inhibits platelet activation and the coagulation cascade, hence preventing clot formation.
- Endothelial cells produce both *prostacyclin and nitric oxide*, which are key components of anticoagulation therapy because they prevent platelet adhesion and aggregation and stimulate vasodilation.
- **Antithrombin III** is a plasma protein that is produced by liver and inactivates thrombin and other clotting factors. The activity of antithrombin is increased when it combines with heparin. Heparin is the natural anticoagulant that secreted by mast cells and basophils. The clotting factors that are inhibited are the active forms of factors IX, X, XI, and XII.
- **Protein C and protein S** are two glycoproteins that are synthesized in the liver and are important components

of natural anticoagulants in the body. They are vitamin K dependent. Protein C is activated by thrombin-thrombomodulin complex. On activation, protein C inactivates clotting factors Va and VIIa. Protein S acts a cofactor to protein C.
- **Thrombin thrombomodulin complex:** It is the complex formed between thrombin and thrombomodulin. Thrombomodulin is an integral membrane protein expressed on the surface of the endothelial cells that serve as a cofactor for thrombin. Thrombin -thrombomodulin complex activates natural anticoagulant protein C.

### Clinical correlation
Antithrombotic drugs **(Fig. 19.10)** for clinical use:
- **Antiplatelet drugs (*Refer* Fig. 18.7):** Aspirin produces irreversible inhibition of cyclooxygenase. This reduces production of thromboxane and inhibits platelet aggregation. Thus, aspirin helps in preventing blood clots.
- **Anticoagulants (Fig. 19.11):** Anticoagulants are the drugs/chemicals which prevent the clotting. They used for collection of blood samples, for anti-coagulation therapy for treatment or prevention of clot, and for preserving blood for transfusion.

**Heparin:** It is a natural anticoagulant secreted by tissue containing mast cells, lung, liver, and intestinal mucosa. Functions of heparin are:

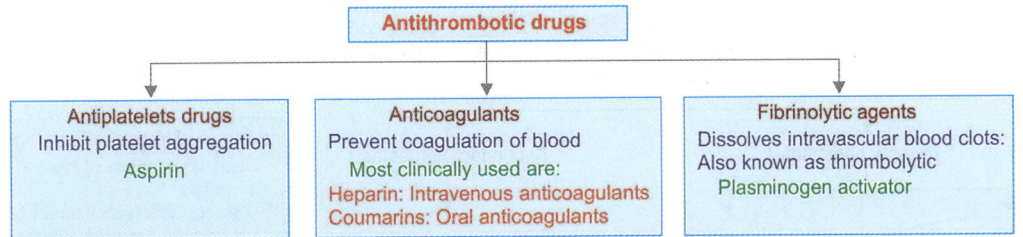

Fig. 19.10: Types of antithrombotic drugs.

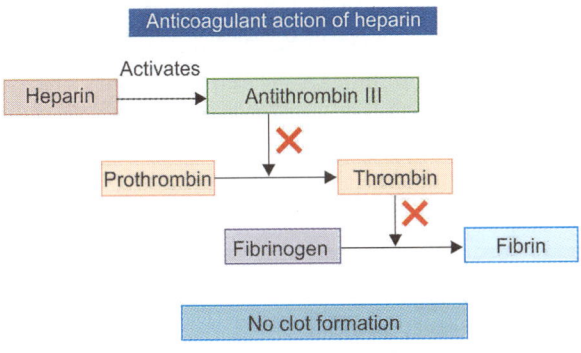

Fig. 19.11: Action of anticoagulants.

- It is used as an anticoagulant in vivo and vitro.
- It inhibits platelet aggregation and increased bleeding time (high doses)
- It helps to clear lipemia by acting as a cofactor for the enzyme lipoprotein lipase, which removes triglycerides from circulating very low-density lipoprotein (VLDL) at low dosages.

Heparin also inactivates factors IXa, Xa, XIa, XIIa, and XIIIa.

**Warfarin:** It is vitamin K antagonist. It inhibits the enzyme that converts enzyme converts the inactive, oxidized form of vitamin K to its active, reduced form. Because warfarin inhibits the enzyme that makes active vitamin K available in the tissues, it decreases the amount of vitamin K that is available for clotting, hence reducing the synthesis of prothrombin, X, VII, and IX.

**What are anticoagulants? What are the laboratory and clinical uses of anticoagulants?**

Anticoagulants are the substance which prevent/decrease the formation of clotting factors and hence inhibit the clotting mechanisms.

*Laboratory uses:*
- EDTA coated vials are used for collecting blood samples where whole blood is required for investigation such as ESR, etc.

*Therapeutic/clinical uses:*
- Tri-ammonium citrate anticoagulants are used in blood banks to preserve the collected blood.
- Low molecular weight heparin for the treatment or prophylaxis in deep vein thrombosis, myocardial infarction, thromboembolic phenomenon anywhere in body

## DISORDERS OF HEMOSTASIS

The disorders of hemostasis can be classified as (**Fig. 19.12**):
- Disorders of blood vessels
- Disorders of temporary hemostasis/platelet plug formation
- Disorders of definitive hemostasis/clot formation

### Disorders of Blood Vessels

The capillary wall is composed of a single cell thick composed of endothelium and basement membrane. In case there is any defect is vascular endothelium, it results in increased capillary fragility and increased bleeding tendency in the patient. It is called as purpura.

**What is purpura? What is etiopathogenesis, clinical features, lab findings, management of a patient with idiopathic thrombocytopenic purpura?**

Purpura is defined as the easy bruisability in a person. It occurs in two main conditions:
1. Increased capillary fragility: the capillaries become fragile and easily get ruptured resulting in easy bruisability.
2. Decreased platelet count (thrombocytopenia).

### Disorders of Temporary Hemostasis/Platelet Plug Formation

In this condition the disorder occurs due to defective platelet function tests. This results due to:
- **Decreased platelet count (thrombocytopenia):**
  - Normal platelet count id 1.5 to 3 lakh/cc.
  - ***Thrombocytopenia can occur due to:***
    - *Autoimmune origin:* Idiopathic thrombocytopenic purpura
    - *Infection:* Dengue hemorrhagic fever

**Idiopathic thrombocytopenic purpura (ITP):**

*Definition:* It is a condition in which the patient complaints of spontaneous bleeding and easy bruisability due to thrombocytopenia.
*Etiopathogenesis:* Presence of autoimmune antiplatelet antibodies.
*Clinical features:* Spontaneous bleeding in skin resulting in petechiae or ecchymosis, bleeding gums, epistaxis, etc.
*Lab findings:* Thrombocytopenia, presence of anti platelet antibodies.
*Treatment:* Immunosuppressants (corticosteroids), splenectomy.

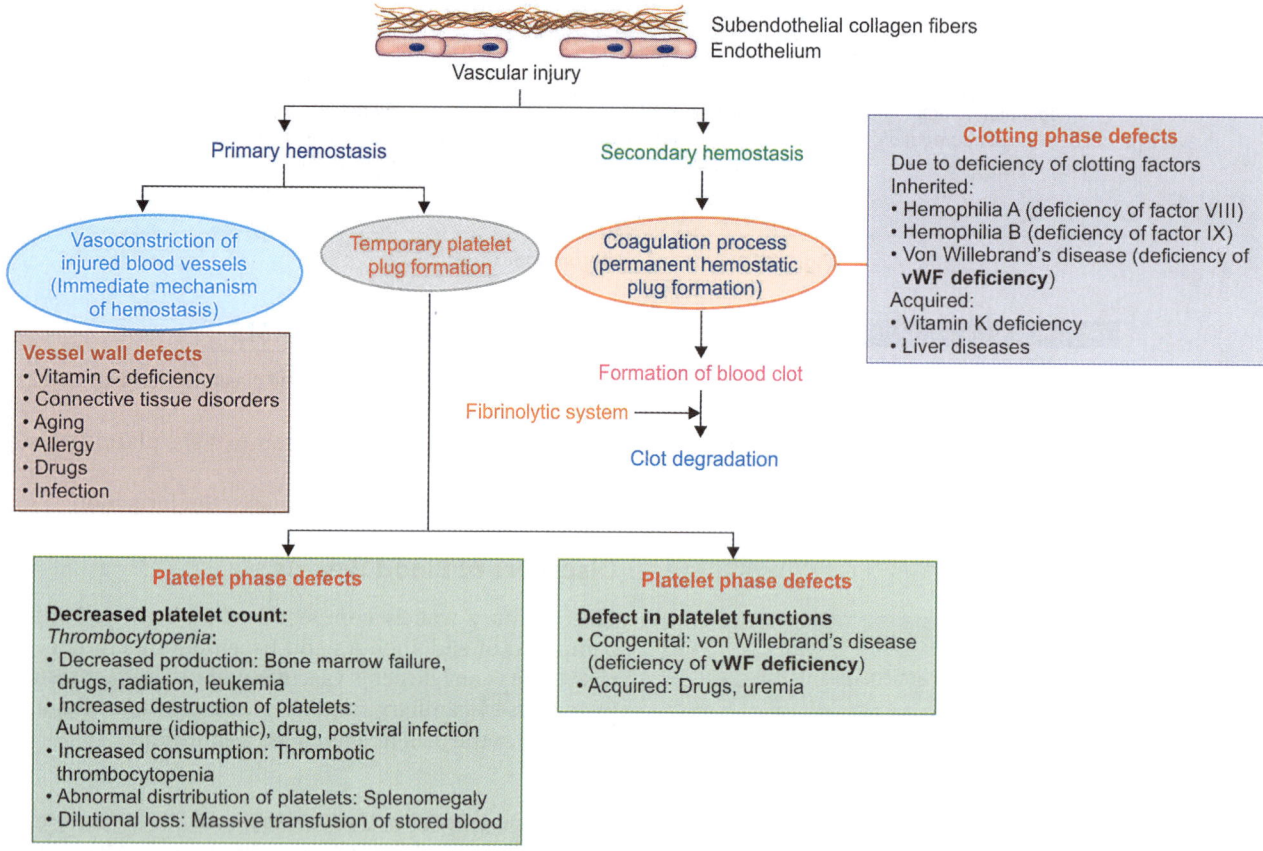

**Fig. 19.12:** Different hemostasis disorders.

- **Defective platelet function:**
  - Platelet count
  - Mean platelet volume
  - Tests for platelet aggregation
  - Bleeding time
  - Clot retraction time
  - Assay of von Willebrand factor

## Disorders of Definitive Hemostasis/Clot Formation

Any deficiency of clotting factors results in defects in formation of definitive clot and hence is responsible for bleeding disorders.

**Causes:** There are two primary types of bleeding disorders: acquired and inherited.

Hereditary bleeding illnesses are characterized by the absence or insufficiency of specific clotting proteins. The three most common hereditary bleeding disorders are:
1. von Willebrand disease,
2. hemophilia A (factor VIII deficiency),
3. hemophilia B (factor IX deficiency).

## HEMOPHILIA

- It is X-linked recessive disorder.
- The females are the carriers and it manifests in the males.

- **Clinical features:** Usually a male child, presents with prolonged bleeding even with minor injuries. Whenever the child falls on his knees, it may result in internal bleeding into his joints. These children usually present with swollen joints especially knee joint, filled with fluid. If this fluid is aspirated, it is the blood which is aspirated from it. Repeated trauma to joints and internal joint bleeds can eventually lead to crippling arthropathy and hemarthrosis. That means, the joint eventually gets damaged resulting in deformed joints.
- **Management:**
  - *Lab investigations:*
    - Clotting time is prolonged
    - Activated partial thromboplastin time (aPTT), which measures the integrity of intrinsic pathway is prolonged in hemophilia.
    - Fcator VIII assay shows deficiency of factor VIII.
  - Factor VIII replacement or transfusion of whole blood or fresh frozen plasma can show some respite in these patients.

## Laboratory Evaluation for Testing the Integrity of Definitive Hemostasis

- **Clotting time (CT):** It assess the functions of clotting factors.
- **Prothrombin time (PT):** It accesses the function of coagulation factors II, V, VII, and X which are

the hepatically synthesized vitamin K dependent factors.
- **Activated partial thromboplastin time (aPTT):** It is the measure of intrinsic pathway of coagulation.
- Clotting factor assay.
- **International normalized ratio (INR):** It is a laboratory test that measures the time it takes for blood to clot. INR is used to monitor the effectiveness of blood-thinning medications such as warfarin. The INR test is preferred over other tests because it provides a standardized result that can be compared across different laboratories. The INR value is calculated by comparing the patient's prothrombin time (PT) to a control PT standardized for the potency of the thromboplastin reagent developed by the World Health Organization (WHO). The normal INR is 0.8–1.1.

## VON WILLEBRAND DISEASE

Von Willebrand disease is a bleeding disorder caused by the deficiency of the von Willebrand factor. Affected people may complain of excessive bruising, prolonged bleeding from mucosal surfaces, and prolonged bleeding after minor trauma.

**Pathophysiology:** Von Willebrand factor is a glycoprotein that plays a part in hemostasis. It is synthesized by endothelial cells and platelets. It functions as a carrier for factor VIII and preventing its degradation. It also help in platelet adhesion. Deficiency of the factor causes a bleeding disorder by reducing platelet adhesion and by lowering plasma factor VIII. vWD is characterized by prolonged Bleeding and clotting time.

## APPROACH TO BLEEDING DISORDERS DIAGNOSIS

*See* **Table 19.2**.

*A young boy of 8 years complained of a swollen knee after he fell from the bicycle. He also complained of some bluish discoloration of the skin of his right arm. His past history is suggestive of prolonged bleeding even after minor injury. On examination he was found to have a hematoma of the knee. His lab investigations show prolonged clotting time, APTT with normal bleeding time and prothrombin time. His hemoglobin is 9.0 g%, platelet count 1.15 lakh/dL.*

a. **What is your diagnosis?**
   The patient is suffering from hemophilia A.
b. **Why is the bleeding time in this patient normal?**
   The bleeding time depends upon the platelet count, which is normal in this patient. However, raised APTT and increased clotting time indicates the clotting defect.
c. **This condition is manifested in males but women are just the carriers. Why can't women manifest this disease?**
   Hemophilia is an X linked recessive disorder in which the females are usually the carrier. The probability of a female with hemophilia is very less.

*What is von Willebrand disease? What is the function of von Willebrand factor?*

Von Willebrand factor is present in the alpha granules of platelets. It also acts as a carrier of factor VIII.
During injury to the vasculature, the vWF serves as an anchor to attach the platelets to the exposed collagen through the protein GpIIb and also activates factor VIII.

**Table 19.2:** Diagnosis of various bleeding disorders.

| Tests | Vascular disease | Platelet defects | Hemophilia A | Hemophilia B (Christmas disease) | Von Willebrand's disease |
|---|---|---|---|---|---|
| Defects | Fragile vessels | Decreased platelet counts or functions | Deficiency of factor VIII | Deficiency of factor IX | Deficiency of vWF |
| Type of bleeding | Superficial | Superficial | Deep | Deep | Superficial |
| Bleeding site | Skin and mucus membrane | Skin and mucus membrane | Deep muscle, joint | Deep muscle, joint | Skin and mucus membrane |
| BT | ↑ | ↑ | N | N | ↑ |
| CT | N | N | ↑ | ↑ | N |
| PT | N | N | N | N | N |
| aPTT | N | N | ↑ | ↑ | ↑ |
| Inheritance | – | – | X-linked recessive | X-linked recessive | Autosomal dominant |

### SUMMARY

- The three mechanisms of hemostasis are vasoconstriction, the development of a temporary plug, and blood coagulation. The two primary mechanisms of hemostasis are platelet plug formation and vasoconstriction; blood coagulation is the secondary mechanism.
- Platelet adhesion, activation, and aggregation are involved in the development of temporary plugs.
- Prostacyclin and nitric oxide are released by intact endothelium, which inhibit platelet adhesion and aggregation and stop clots from spreading to the intact endothelium.

- The breakdown of a clot in a healed artery is known as fibrinolysis.
- Chemicals known as anticoagulants stop blood from clotting.
- Insufficient synthesis of clotting factors or an insufficient number of platelets can lead to poor clotting.
- An overabundance of platelets can lead to thrombosis, or excessive clotting. A thrombus is a collection of fibrin, platelets, and erythrocytes that has accumulated along the lining of a blood vessel, whereas an embolus is a thrombus that has broken loose from the blood vessel wall and is now floating through the bloodstream.
- Increased bleeding times are used to diagnose bleeding disorders caused by vascular defects and platelet defects, whereas increased clotting times are used to identify defects in the hemostasis coagulation process.
- Clotting factors for the common and extrinsic coagulation pathways are tested by PT, while clotting factors for the intrinsic coagulation pathway are measured by aPTT.

## LET US SEE, HOW MUCH YOU HAVE LEARNT?

### Review Questions

#### Long/Short Answer Questions

**Q1.** Describe the mechanism of clotting under the following headings:
  a. Temporary hemostasis
  b. Definitive hemostasis by the intrinsic and extrinsic pathway of clotting.

**Q2.** Define hemophilia. Describe the physiological basis of the clinical features observed in the hemophilia A.

**Q3.** What is the physiological basis of von Willbrand disease?
**Q4.** Why the blood remains fluid in the blood vessels?
**Q5.** Describe the mechanism of plasmolysis.
**Q6.** Describe the role of anticoagulants in health and disease.

#### Explain Why? (Reasoning Questions)

**Q1.** Tissue plasminogen activator dissolves a clot causing an ischemic stroke?

**Q2.** Aspirin is used to prevent chest pain?

### Critical Thinking Case-Based Questions

**Q1.** An 8-year-old boy complained of swollen knee after he fell from the bicycle. He also complained of some bluish discoloration of the skin of his right arm. His past history is suggestive of prolonged bleeding even after minor injury. On examination, he was found to have a hematoma of the knee. His lab investigations show prolonged clotting time, aPPT with normal bleeding time and prothrombin time. His hemoglobin is 9.2 g%, platelet count 1.15 lakh/dL.
  a. What is your diagnosis? Give the justification.
  b. Why is the bleeding time normal in this patient?
  c. Why does this illness only affect men, with women only acting as carriers?

### Multiple Choice Questions

**Q1.** The conversion of fibrinogen to fibrin is promoted by:
  a. Factor X
  b. Thrombin
  c. Prothrombin
  d. Platelets

**Q2.** Dicumarol acts as an anticoagulant by:
  a. Precipitation of $Ca^{2+}$
  b. Inhibition of vitamin K action
  c. Inhibition of thrombin
  d. Preventing activity of factor IX

**Q3.** False about coagulation factor VII:
  a. It is synthesized in the liver
  b. It is activated by a tissue factor
  c. It is important for the intrinsic pathway of blood clotting
  d. When activated, it activates factor X

**Q4.** False about the action of anticoagulants:
  a. Dicumarol interferes with the synthesis of prothrombin in the liver
  b. Oxalates form insoluble salts with $Ca^{2+}$
  c. Citrates and other chelating agents bind $Ca^{2+}$
  d. Heparin blocks the action of antithrombin III

**Q5.** All the following about plasmin is true *except*:
  a. It is formed from plasminogen by a tissue activator (TPA)
  b. It produces fibrinogen degradation products (FDP)
  c. It can be inhibited by an antiplasmin
  d. It is responsible for the formation of fibrin

**Q6.** During a routine dental extraction procedure, a patient experiences prolonged bleeding from the extraction site. Which of the following laboratory tests would be most appropriate to assess the patient's hemostatic function?
  a. Platelet count
  b. Prothrombin time (PT)
  c. Activated partial thromboplastin time (aPTT)
  d. Fibrinogen assay

Q7. Priya, a 35-year-old woman, presents to the emergency department with signs of heavy menstrual bleeding. Which of the following conditions is most likely associated with her symptoms?
   a. Thrombocytopenia
   b. von Willebrand disease
   c. Hemophilia A
   d. Factor V Leiden mutation

Q8. Rahul, a 50-year-old man, is admitted to the hospital with chest pain suggestive of acute coronary syndrome. He is started on aspirin therapy. What is the primary mechanism of action of aspirin in preventing thrombus formation?
   a. Inhibition of platelet aggregation by blocking ADP receptors
   b. Inhibition of cyclooxygenase (COX) enzyme, reducing thromboxane A2 synthesis
   c. Enhancement of fibrinolysis by activating plasminogen
   d. Inhibition of factor Xa activity

Q9. Sunita, a 40-year-old woman, is diagnosed with hemophilia B. Which of the following clotting factors is deficient in hemophilia B?
   a. Factor VIII
   b. Factor IX
   c. Factor VII
   d. Factor XI

Q10. During a surgical procedure, a patient develops disseminated intravascular coagulation (DIC), characterized by widespread clotting and bleeding. What laboratory finding would be most consistent with DIC?
   a. Prolonged PT and aPTT
   b. Elevated platelet count
   c. Decreased levels of D-dimer
   d. Increased levels of fibrinogen

Q11. Meera, a pregnant woman, is Rh-negative, while her husband is Rh-positive. She is concerned about the risk of Rh incompatibility with her unborn baby. What intervention can prevent Rh sensitization in Meera during her pregnancy?
   a. Administering Rh immunoglobulin (RhIg) during pregnancy
   b. Recommending dietary supplementation with vitamin K
   c. Performing regular blood transfusions
   d. Prescribing anticoagulant therapy

Q12. During a trauma resuscitation, a patient requires massive blood transfusion due to hemorrhagic shock. Which blood component should be transfused first to address immediate hemostatic needs?
   a. Fresh frozen plasma (FFP)
   b. Packed red blood cells (PRBCs)
   c. Platelets
   d. Cryoprecipitate

**ANSWERS**

1. b    2. c    3. c    4. a    5. d    6. b    7. b    8. b    9. b    10. a    11. a    12. b

# Blood Groups

**CHAPTER 20**

### COMPETENCY ADDRESSED
**PY2.9:** Describe different blood groups and discuss the clinical importance of blood grouping, blood banking and transfusion.

### LEARNING OBJECTIVES
**At the end of this chapter, the learner should be able to:**
- Describe the agglutinogen, agglutinin and agglutination.
- Describe the major blood grouping systems.
- Define and describe the Landsteiner's laws.
- Describe blood group compatibility with special reference to Rh incompatibility.

Like any other cell of our body, the red cell membrane also has various antigenic proteins on it. These antigens provide the basis for blood group types of every human. There are several types of antigens identified till date, hence different types of blood groups like ABO system, Rh system, M and N system, Kell and Duffy and many more. Out of these the most widely used are the ABO and Rh system of blood grouping.

## ABO SYSTEM OF BLOOD GROUPING (TABLE 20.1)

The ABO system of blood grouping based on the presence or absence of two main *antigens A and B*. Both these antigens are complex **oligosaccharides** with a slight difference in the terminal sugar **(Fig. 20.1)**. The *H gene present universally codes for terminal fucose and forms H antigen on the cell membrane of all the RBCs.* Hence, the individuals with blood group O do not have either A or B antigen but have a basic H antigen. In the individuals with **A blood group**, the respective gene codes for **NAG transferase enzyme** which adds **N-acetylgalactosamine** (NAG) on the H antigen whereas individuals with **B blood group** have **galactosyl transferase** which adds **galactose** as the terminal sugar.

## Inheritance of ABO Blood Group

The ABO blood grouping system follows the *Mendelian inheritance* and is represented as the **dominant** gene from the parents to the off springs. It was first discovered by **Karl Landsteiner**.

### Agglutinogens and Agglutinins (Table 20.2)

The blood group *antigens* present on the surface of RBCs (discussed above) are also called as the *agglutinogens* and the corresponding *antibodies*, present in plasma are called *agglutinins*. When the corresponding agglutinogens

**Table 20.1:** Different blood groups and their properties.

| Blood group | Antigen | Enzyme | Terminal sugar |
|---|---|---|---|
| A | A and H antigen | Fucose transferase and NAG transferase | Fucose + NAG |
| B | B and H antigen | Fucose transferase and galactosyl transferase | Fucose + galactose |
| AB | A, B and H antigen | Fucose transferase, NAG transferase and galactosyl transferase | Fucose + galactose + NAG |
| O | H antigen | Fucose transferase | Fucose |
| Bombay | None | None | None |

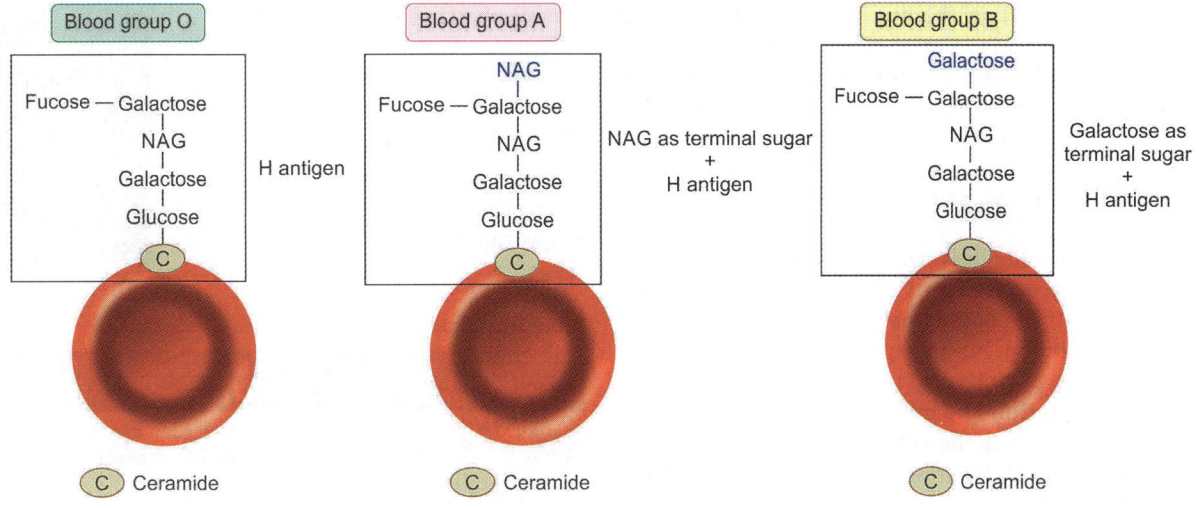

NAG (N–acetylgalactosamine)
**Fig. 20.1:** Blood group antigens on the RBC membrane.

and agglutinins react, the process is called *agglutination*. Hence, the corresponding agglutinins are absent in the plasma of the person, having the agglutinogens. This is best described by **Karl Landsteiner** in his laws regarding the blood groups:

- *If an agglutinogen is present on the RBC membrane, its corresponding agglutinin will be absent in the plasma.*
- *If an agglutinogen is absent on the RBC membrane, its corresponding agglutinin will be present in the plasma.*

Following the Landsteiner's laws and the Mendelian inheritance, the individuals with ABO Blood grouping system can have following phenotype, genotype, agglutinogens and agglutinins.

## RH BLOOD GROUPING SYSTEM

This blood grouping system was first discovered in **Rhesus** monkey by **Landsteiner** and **Weiner** in 1940; 40 years after the discovery of ABO blood grouping system. This blood grouping system is complex system following the **Mendelian inheritance** of **dominant** trait formed by six alleles; **C, D, E, c, d, e**. Out of these *D antigen is most antigenic* and hence the Rh factor is commonly referred to as D antigen and its antibody is referred to as *anti-D antibody*. If the D antigen is present on the RBC membrane, the individual is said to have blood group Rh positive and otherwise Rh negative. Hence, along with the ABO system, it becomes the second most used blood grouping system.

### Agglutinins

The various agglutinins of ABO system (**anti-A and anti-B**) are **IgM** type (**cold** agglutinin) whereas the **anti-D agglutinin** is **IgG** type (**warm** agglutinin). Since the IgM antibody is the largest antibody, it cannot cross the placenta but anti-D antibody, being *IgG type, smallest in size, can easily cross the placenta* and can adversely affect the fetus.

*What do you think should happen, if a person is transfused with any other blood group, rather than his own (mismatched/incompatible blood transfusion)?*

*Why doesn't the ABO incompatibility between mother and fetus show any effect as Rh incompatibility?*

### Rh Incompatibility

The anti-D antibody is an **exception to the second part of Landsteiner's law.** Even though the Rh antigen is absent

**Table 20.2:** Agglutinogens and agglutinins of ABO blood group system.

| Blood groups | Phenotype | Genotype | Agglutinogen | Agglutinin |
|---|---|---|---|---|
| A | A | AA, AO | A antigen | Anti-B antibody |
| B | B | BB, BO | B antigen | Anti-A antibody |
| AB | AB | AB | AB antigen | Neither A nor B antibody |
| O | O | OO | Neither A nor B antigen | Both anti-A and anti-B antibodies |
| When any individual doesn't express either of A or B gene, it is represented as O. Hence O means absence of any of these two alleles. However, these individuals do have H antigen present on their red cell membranes | | | | |
| Bombay blood group | O | OO | Neither of A, B nor H antigen | Anti-H antibody |

on the RBC membrane, the **anti-D antibody is absent in plasma**. The immune system of an individual requires exposure of the Rh antigen to form the corresponding antibody. Hence, the first exposure of the Rh antigen (blood transfusion/Rh negative mother carrying Rh positive baby) doesn't show any reactions of incompatibility. But subsequent exposures show the signs of incompatible exposure.

The Rh incompatibility is of particular **importance** in the **obstetrics** where a **Rh negative female** conceives an **Rh-positive baby**. If she doesn't have any previous exposure of Rh positive blood, her **first pregnancy is uneventful** but at the time of **delivery**, the **fetal RBCs enter the maternal circulation** and mount an **immune response** in the mother. During the **subsequent pregnancy**, the **anti-D antibodies (IgG)** present in maternal blood **cross the placenta** and adversely affect the fetus, resulting in **hemolysis** of fetal RBCs. The fetal bone marrow increases the production of the RBCs resulting in an increase in the **circulating immature erythroblasts**, hence the term **erythroblastosis fetalis** is used to describe this condition **(Fig. 20.2)**. If the mother has already had a prior exposure to Rh antigen, then even the first pregnancy is at risk of developing Rh incompatibility reaction. This is better known as *hemolytic disease of newborn (HDN)*.

## Pathophysiology of HDN

See **Figure 20.2**.

## Grades of HDN

Depending on the severity of disease, it can be classified as **(Table 20.3)**:
- Hydrops fetalis

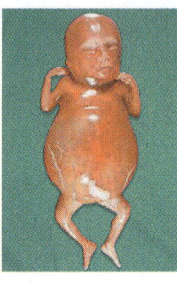

**Table 20.3:** Grades of hemolytic diseases of newborn.

| | Severity of disease | Clinical picture |
|---|---|---|
| Hydrops fetalis | Severe | Generalized edema of the fetus. The fetus can die in utero or after birth |
| Icterus gravis neonatorum | Moderate to severe | The neonate presents with severe jaundice. The bilirubin level is very high. The child can develop kernicterus. There is enlarged liver and spleen due to massive hemolysis |
| Neonatal jaundice | Mild | The bilirubin levels are high, more than physiological jaundice. Phototherapy is usually sufficient in these patients |

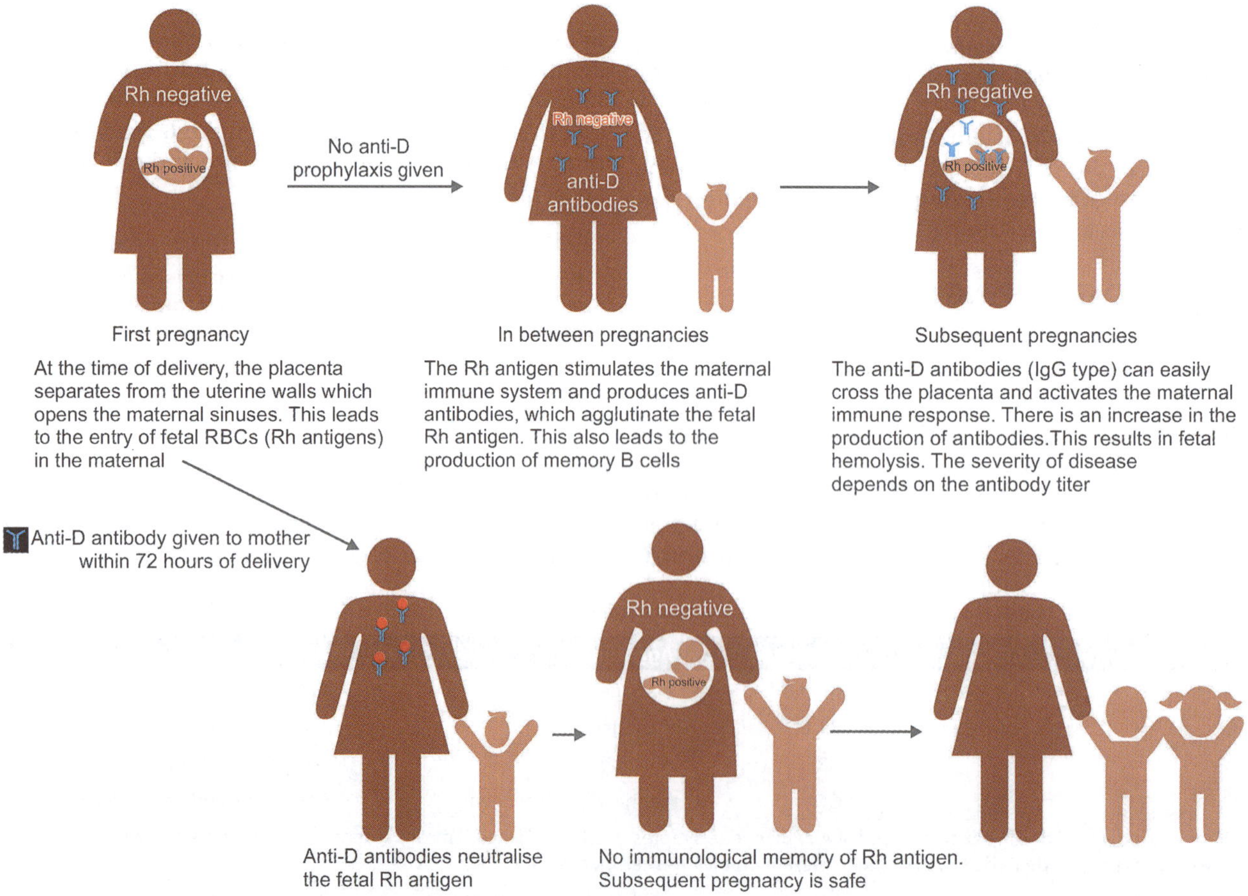

**First pregnancy**
At the time of delivery, the placenta separates from the uterine walls which opens the maternal sinuses. This leads to the entry of fetal RBCs (Rh antigens) in the maternal

**In between pregnancies**
The Rh antigen stimulates the maternal immune system and produces anti-D antibodies, which agglutinate the fetal Rh antigen. This also leads to the production of memory B cells

**Subsequent pregnancies**
The anti-D antibodies (IgG type) can easily cross the placenta and activates the maternal immune response. There is an increase in the production of antibodies. This results in fetal hemolysis. The severity of disease depends on the antibody titer

Anti-D antibody given to mother within 72 hours of delivery

Anti-D antibodies neutralise the fetal Rh antigen

No immunological memory of Rh antigen. Subsequent pregnancy is safe

**Fig. 20.2:** Pathophysiology of HDN and role of anti-D prophylaxis.

- Icterus gravis neonatorum
- Neonatal jaundice

## Clinical Presentation

The neonate has **anemia** and **jaundice** due to massive immune mediated hemolysis. The immature fetal liver is not able to handle the increased bilirubin load resulting in raised bilirubin levels. If the **bilirubin levels** are raised **above 18 mg/dL**, it can **cross** the immature **blood brain barrier** and gets deposited in the **basal ganglia**, a condition called as *kernicterus*. On examination, the neonate usually has **hepatosplenomegaly**.

## Management

- **For diagnosis of HDN:** The blood group of both the parents is determined. If father is also Rh negative, then there is no chance of Rh incompatibility. Incase father is homozygous Rh positive (DD), then the fetus will be Rh positive, however if father is heterozygous Rh positive (Dd), then there are 50% chances of the baby being Rh positive. Hence, a close watch is kept on this pregnancy by repeated ultrasonographies and blood tests of mother (antibody titer) and fetus (if necessary).
  The **Positive Indirect Coombs test** is suggestive of the presence of **active anti-D antibody** in maternal blood.
- **For prophylaxis (Fig. 20.2):** Injection of **anti-D antibody (Rhogam)**, which is a preformed immunoglobulin is given to the mother within **72 hours** of the delivery. This confers **passive immunity** to the mother and **neutralizes the fetal Rh antigen load** in the maternal circulation. It also *prevents the activation of maternal immune response to build up and formation of memory cells*. However, to cover up the accidental placental hemorrhages, an injection of anti-D is given at 28 and 34 weeks of gestation (after the antigen titer), even in first and subsequent pregnancies. It is advisable to give the inj Rhogam, even after miscarriage or medical termination of pregnancy.
- **For treatment of HDN:** Depending on the severity of disease, the various treatment modalities are suggested/being carried out:
  - *Phototherapy:* Neonate is put in the phototherapy chamber, which converts the bilirubin into water soluble **lumirubin**. This compound is easily water soluble and is excreted out through urine. Hence, it lowers the bilirubin content of the neonate.
  - *Exchange transfusion (Fig. 20.3):* The exchange transfusion can be done in utero as well as after birth. In this case the Rh positive blood of the neonate is replaced with the Rh negative blood type of the same ABO blood group as the child. This reduces hemolysis and offers some relief to the child. After some time, the antibody titer reduces, and no fresh antibodies are added into neonatal circulation. In the meanwhile, the neonatal bone marrow begins to synthesize its own RBCs, and hence the child is saved from HDN.

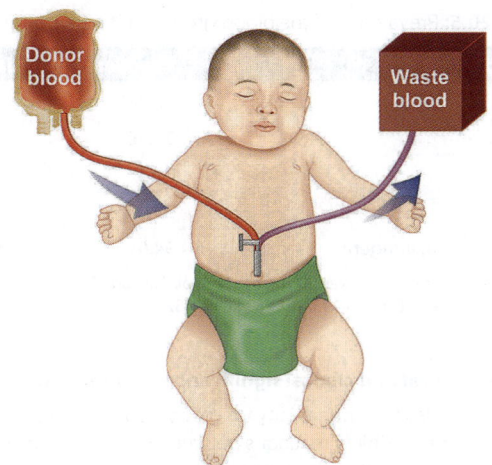

**Fig. 20.3:** Exchange transfusion.

## BLOOD GROUPS TESTING

The blood group is tested by mixing the blood in the preformed antisera containing the corresponding agglutinins called as antisera A containing anti-A antibody, antisera B containing anti-B antibody and antisera D containing anti-D antibody as shown in **Table 20.4**. the prevalence is shown in **Table 20.5**.

**Table 20.4:** Blood group testing.

| Anti-A antisera | Anti-B antisera | Anti-D antisera | Control | Blood group |
|---|---|---|---|---|
| | | | | A; Rh positive |
| | | | | A; Rh negative |
| | | | | B; Rh positive |
| | | | | B; Rh negative |
| | | | | AB; Rh positive |
| | | | | AB; Rh negative |
| | | | | O; Rh positive |
| | | | | O; Rh negative |

**Table 20.5:** Prevalence of the blood groups in Indian population.*

| Blood group | Prevalence in India (%) | Remarks |
|---|---|---|
| A | 22.88 | |
| B | 32.26 | Second most common |
| AB | 7.74 | Least common |
| O | **37.12** | Most common |
| D antigen (Rh antigen) | 94.61 | Most of Indian population is Rh positive |

*Cited from: Agrawal A, Tiwari AK, Mehta N, et al. ABO and Rh (D) group distribution and gene frequency; the first multicentric study in India. Asian J Transfus Sci. 2014;8(2):121-125. Doi:10.4103/0973-6247.137452

**Physiological and clinical significance of blood groups:**
- It provides the antigenicity for blood transfusion reactions.
- Rh incompatibility reactions between Rh negative mother and Rh positive baby.
- Due to its genetic inheritance, it can be used to solve the paternity disputes. Though it is not as confirmatory as DNA fingerprinting but, it is good for initial testing. It doesn't confirm the father but can rule out the possibility of person being father of the child.
- The H antigen present of the RBC, differentiates the human and animal blood; except in Bombay blood group.
- Some individuals secrete the blood group antigens in other body fluids like sweat, saliva and semen. These are called as *secretors*. Those who do not secrete the antigens in biological fluids are *non-secretors*. Hence, they are of medicolegal importance.

## SUMMARY

In this chapter, we have learnt that:
- The blood group antigens are present on the surface of the RBCs, and they are due to the difference of attached terminal sugar with H antigen (made by fucose terminal)
- The Landsteiner's law states that:
  - If an agglutinogen is present on the RBC membrane, its corresponding agglutinin will be absent in the plasma.
  - If an agglutinogen is absent on the RBC membrane, its corresponding agglutinin will be present in the plasma.
- There are many blood grouping systems but most commonly used are ABO system and Rh system.
- The agglutinogens of ABO system (antigen A, B) and antigen D from Rh system are present on the RBC membrane while the corresponding agglutinins (anti A, anti B and anti D) are present in plasma following the Landsteiner's law.
- Currently the most prevalent blood group in India is **O Rh-positive**.
- If an Rh-negative mother conceives and Rh-positive baby, she gets exposed to Rh antigen at the time of delivery and develops antibodies for D antigen. These antibodies are Ig G type which can cross the placenta and harm the next pregnancy. Hence, Inj. Anti-D is given to the mother at the time of delivery of first baby, preferably within 72 hours.
- The blood groups are studied to determine the antigenicity of blood, compatibility, genetic inheritance, and medicolegal aspects.

## LET US SEE, HOW MUCH YOU HAVE LEARNT?

 *Review Questions*

### Long/Short Answer Questions

Q1. Define Landsteiner's law.
Q2. Describe the physiological basis of representation of blood group antigens.
Q3. Describe the inheritance of blood groups from parents to offsprings.
Q4. What is erythroblastosis fetalis? Describe the pathophysiology of erythroblastosis fetalis.
Q5. What are the physiological and clinical significance of blood groups?

### Explain Why? (Reasoning Questions)

Q1. What will happen, if a person with blood group O Rh negative is transfused with blood group O Rh-positive?
Q2. What will happen, if again receives Rh-positive blood in future? Why?
Q3. What will happen to the second baby of an Rh-negative mother, who has not received the Inj. Anti-D at the time of delivery of first baby?
Q4. What will happen to the second baby of an Rh negative mother, who has received the Inj. Anti-D at the time of delivery of first baby?

## Critical Thinking Case-Based Questions

**Q1.** A 32-year-old female, was admitted to the hospital after a severe car accident. She had lost a significant amount of blood and required an immediate blood transfusion. Her blood type is B-negative. The hospital's blood bank was currently low on B-negative blood but had an adequate supply of O-negative blood. The medical team decided to administer O-negative blood for the transfusion.

Based upon the given case scenario, answer the following questions:
a. Explain the physiological principles behind blood group matching.
b. What are the major blood group systems?
c. Why is O-negative blood considered the universal donor?
d. Why is it important to match the Rh status of the donor and recipient?

## Multiple Choice Questions

**Q1.** Which scientist is credited with the discovery of the ABO blood group system?
a. Karl Landsteiner
b. Louis Pasteur
c. Alexander Fleming
d. Robert Koch

**Q2.** According to Landsteiner's Law, which of the following blood group combinations can safely receive blood from type O donors?
a. A$^+$
b. B$^-$
c. AB$^+$
d. O$^-$

**Q3.** Which component of blood determines the ABO blood group system?
a. Agglutinogens
b. Agglutinins
c. Plasma
d. Platelets

**Q4.** Which of the following is an example of an agglutinin in blood?
a. Antibodies
b. Red blood cells
c. White blood cells
d. Plasma

**Q5.** What is the term used for the presence of Rh antigen on the surface of red blood cells?
a. Rh factor
b. Rh antibody
c. Rh agglutinin
d. Rh plasma

**Q6.** Rh incompatibility can occur during pregnancy when:
a. The mother is Rh-negative and the fetus is Rh-positive
b. The mother is Rh-positive and the fetus is Rh-negative
c. Both the mother and fetus are Rh-negative
d. Both the mother and fetus are Rh-positive

**Q7.** Which blood type is considered the universal recipient?
a. O$^+$
b. AB$^+$
c. A$^+$
d. B$^+$

**Q8.** Which blood type is considered the universal donor?
a. AB$^-$
b. O$^-$
c. B$^-$
d. A$^-$

**Q9.** What is one of the practical applications of understanding blood groups?
a. Organ transplant compatibility
b. Predicting hair color
c. Determining IQ
d. Assessing muscle strength

**Q10.** A hospital laboratory technician is preparing blood samples for a patient who requires a transfusion. The patient's blood type is A$^+$, and the available blood types in the blood bank are O$^-$, A$^+$, B$^-$, and AB$^+$. Which blood type(s) can safely be transfused to the patient?
a. O$^-$ and A$^+$
b. A$^+$ only
c. O$^-$ and B$^-$
d. A$^+$ and B$^-$

**Q11.** Sarah, a pregnant woman, is Rh-negative. Their first child is healthy with no complications after the delivery. Now Sarah is expecting her second child. What precautionary measures should Sarah's obstetrician take to prevent Rh incompatibility during her second pregnancy?
a. Administer Rh immunoglobulin (RhIg) to Sarah during pregnancy and after childbirth
b. Test the father's blood type to confirm Rh compatibility
c. Encourage Sarah to consume a diet rich in folic acid
d. Recommend genetic counseling to determine the likelihood of Rh incompatibility

**Q12.** Dev, who is blood type O$^-$, was involved in a severe car accident and urgently requires a blood transfusion. His best friend, Mahesh, wants to donate blood to help Dev. However, Mahesh does not know his blood type. What should Mahesh do to ensure he can safely donate blood to Dev?
a. Request a blood type test from the hospital
b. Assume he can donate blood since David is type O$^-$
c. Refrain from donating blood due to potential risks
d. Proceed with the donation and monitor David's reaction closely

**Q13.** Meera and Jai are expecting their first child. Meera is blood type AB$^+$ while Jai is blood type O$^-$. What blood types could their child possibly inherit, and what implications does this have for potential blood transfusions?
a. The child could be A$^+$, B$^+$, AB$^+$, or O$^+$. Blood transfusions may be complicated due to potential ABO incompatibility
b. The child could only be AB$^+$ or O$^+$. Blood transfusions may be straightforward as both parents cover the full range of blood types
c. The child could be A$^+$, B$^+$, or AB$^+$. Blood transfusions may be complicated due to potential Rh incompatibility
d. The child could be A$^+$, B$^+$, AB$^+$, or O$^-$. Blood transfusions may be straightforward due to the child's universal donor status

Q14. Ema is preparing a blood transfusion for a patient whose blood type is A$^+$. However, she mistakenly grabs a bag of blood labeled B$^-$. What immediate action should Ema take to rectify the situation?
   a. Proceed with the transfusion since both blood types are compatible
   b. Inform the attending physician and discard the bag of blood
   c. Double-check the patient's blood type to confirm compatibility
   d. Administer the blood but monitor the patient closely for adverse reactions

**ANSWERS**
1. a   2. d   3. a   4. a   5. a   6. a   7. b   8. b   9. a   10. a   11. b   12. a   13. a   14. b

# Blood Banking and Blood Transfusion

**CHAPTER 21**

### COMPETENCY ADDRESSED
**PY2.9:** Describe different blood groups and discuss the clinical importance of blood grouping, blood banking and transfusion.

### LEARNING OBJECTIVES
**At the end of this chapter, the learner should be able to:**
- Describe the process of blood banking, including blood typing, screening for diseases, and proper storage procedures to ensure blood safety and availability.
- Recognize the importance of blood transfusions in treating conditions like anemia and injuries, while being aware of potential risks and complications.
- Discuss the ethical and legal considerations involved in blood transfusion, including consent and donor screening, to maintain patient safety and uphold medical standards.

Blood banking is the process of collecting, typing, screening, and storing blood components for transfusion. It ensures the availability of safe blood products for medical treatments, such as for surgery, trauma, and managing blood disorders. We must adhere to strict protocols, as blood banking aims to maintain patient safety and minimize risks associated with blood transfusions.

The blood is stored in the blood banks, which follows a specific process which will be subsequently discussed in this chapter.

## BLOOD COLLECTION

The blood is collected from the voluntary donors for which the donor recruitment is done.
- **Donor recruitment:** Donors are invited to give blood through community drives, blood donation centers, or mobile units. They may volunteer or be called upon during emergencies.
- **Donation process:**
  - *Registration of donors:* Donors provide personal information and medical history to assess eligibility.
  - *Pre-donation screening:* Donors undergo a brief physical examination and answer questions about their health and recent activities to determine eligibility.
  - *Blood donation:* A trained nurse inserts a wide bore sterile needle into a vein in the donor's arm to collect blood into a specialized blood collection bag. This blood collection bag collects about 350 mL of blood, which is called 1 unit of blood. The bag has:
    - Anticoagulant solution which prevents clotting during storage and processing of blood. The usual anticoagulant used in citrate-phosphate-dextrose (CPD)
    - An additive solution is also added to increase the viability of cells. The commonly used additives are Glucose, adenine and mannitol.
    - Most of the blood collection bags contain a sampling diversion port for collection of small blood samples for testing before transfusion.
  - *Post-donation care:* Donors receive refreshments and rest to recover from the donation process.
  - *Labeling and identification (Fig. 21.1):* Each blood donation is labeled with a unique identifier and the donor's information for traceability.
  - *Transportation:* Collected blood is transported to a blood bank or processing facility for further testing and processing.

## BLOOD TYPING AND CROSSMATCHING

The collected blood is then typed and crossmatched for the following grouping system:
- **ABO blood group system:** The blood is grouped as per the ABO blood grouping system and segregated.

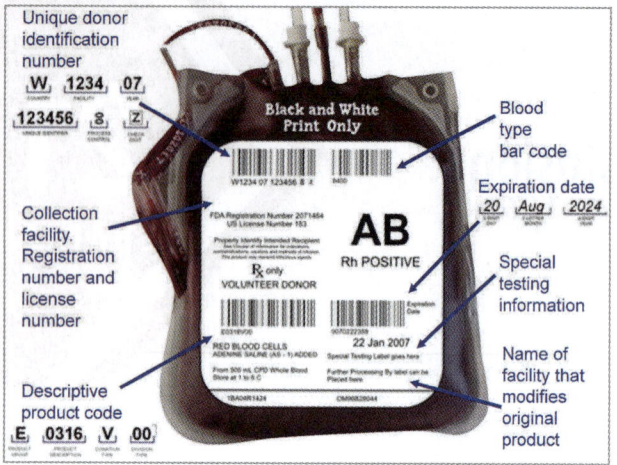

**Fig. 21.1:** Labeling and information on blood bag.

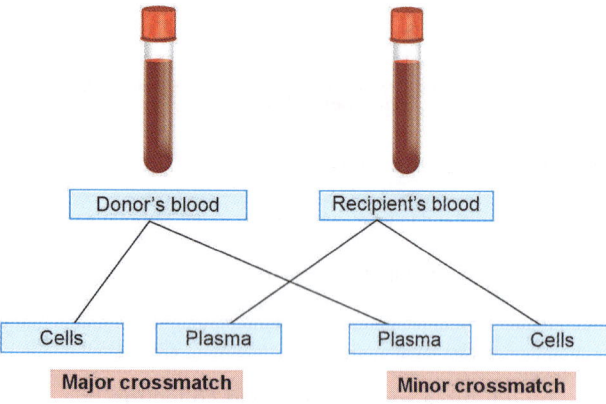

**Fig. 21.2:** Major and minor cross matching.

- **Rh factor:** The Rh factor typing is also done for the donor blood.
- *Crossmatching procedures:* Before issuing the blood for transfusion, the major and minor crossmatching is done for both the donor and recipient. This ensures complete matching before the transfusion.
    - *Major crossmatching:* Donor cells are mixed in recipient's plasma. It is then observed for any agglutination or precipitation. The volume of recipient's plasma will be major having different types of agglutinins, hence called as major crossmatch.
    - *Minor crossmatching:* Recipient cells are mixed in donor's plasma. It is then observed for any agglutination or precipitation. The volume of donor's plasma will be small having different types of agglutinins, hence called as minor crossmatch.

## SCREENING FOR DISEASES

- **Infectious disease testing:** It is mandatory to do the screening of the transfused blood transmissible diseases like hepatitis, HIV, etc.
- **Blood-borne pathogen screening:** The screening is also done for the presence of any blood borne pathogens to prevent the transmission to the recipient. The blood is screened for pathogens of malaria, syphilis, etc.

## PROPER STORAGE PROCEDURES

- **Refrigeration and freezing:**
    - *Whole blood:* Stored at temperatures between 1 and 6°C in refrigerators to preserve the viability of red blood cells (RBCs) and prevent bacterial growth. Refrigeration helps slow down the metabolic processes within the blood components, extending their shelf life.
    - *Plasma and platelets:* Plasma and platelets are typically stored at temperatures below freezing (−20 to −30°C) to maintain their clotting factor activity and cell viability. Freezing halts metabolic processes and prevents degradation of labile components.
    - *Cryopreservation:* Some specialized blood components, such as cryoprecipitate and certain stem cell products, require storage in ultra-low temperatures (below −65°C) to maintain their therapeutic efficacy.
- **Shelf life and expiry dates:**
    - *Whole blood:* Typically stored for up to 21 days under refrigeration.
    - *Red blood cells (RBCs):* Stored for up to 42 to 49 days under refrigeration.
    - *Platelets:* Stored for up to 5 to 7 days under continuous agitation at room temperature between 22 and 25°C.
    - *Plasma:* Frozen plasma can be stored for up to 1 year if maintained at appropriate temperatures.

## Changes in Cells in Stored Blood

- **Red blood cells (RBCs):**
    - *Decreased viability:* Over time, stored RBCs undergo cellular aging and metabolic changes, leading to decreased viability and structural integrity. The activity of $Na^+K^+$-ATPase pump also decreases.
    - *Reduced oxygen-carrying capacity:* The levels of 2,3-diphosphoglycerate (2,3-DPG), a compound that facilitates oxygen release from hemoglobin, decline during storage, resulting in reduced oxygen-carrying capacity of RBCs.
    - *Increased hemolysis:* Prolonged storage can lead to hemolysis, the breakdown of RBCs, resulting in the release of intracellular components such as potassium and free hemoglobin into the plasma. The RBCs lose their biconcave shape and become spherical. Hence, they become more fragile than the fresh RBCs.
- **Platelets:**
    - *Loss of viability:* Platelets stored at room temperature undergo activation and progressive loss of viability, resulting in reduced platelet function and aggregation capacity.
    - *Morphological changes:* Stored platelets may undergo shape changes, including pseudopodia formation and membrane vesiculation, which can affect their ability to adhere to injured blood vessels and participate in hemostasis.

- ***Decreased response to agonists:*** Stored platelets exhibit decreased response to agonists such as adenosine diphosphate (ADP) and thrombin, impairing their ability to initiate and propagate clot formation.
- **Leukocytes:**
  - ***Leukocyte accumulation:*** Leukocytes in stored blood undergo activation and aggregation, leading to the formation of leukocyte aggregates and microaggregates.
  - ***Release of inflammatory mediators:*** Activated leukocytes release pro-inflammatory cytokines, chemokines, and reactive oxygen species, which can contribute to transfusion-related inflammatory responses and adverse effects.
  - ***Immunomodulatory effects:*** Leukocyte-derived factors in stored blood may modulate the recipient's immune response, potentially influencing post-transfusion outcomes and alloimmunization.

## IMPORTANCE OF BLOOD TRANSFUSIONS

### Treatment of Anemia

The blood transfusion/packed red cells are used for the treatment of severe anemia, thalassemia and other causes of chronic anemia.

### Management of Injuries and Surgical Procedures

- **Trauma and blood loss:** Blood transfusion helps in preventing the hypovolemic shock in patients with massive blood loss. However, there is an upper limit to volume of blood transfusion, that can be done in 24 hours. Transfusion of 5 L of whole blood in 24 hours is called ***massive transfusion*** and can result in coagulopathy, electrolyte imbalances and transfusion-related acute lung injury (TRALI). Hence, in patients, where massive transfusion would be required, the blood components are used.
- **Surgical procedures requiring blood transfusion:** The planned surgeries in which a large blood loss is expected, the blood transfusion may be indicated. These patients can donate their own blood which can be reinfused after surgery. It is called as the *autologous transfusion*.

### Role of Transfusion in Hemostatic Disorders

The blood transfusion or component transfusion can help in restoration of blood volume, replenish the deficient clotting factors and hence plays an important role in the management of coagulopathies.

### Transfusion of Blood Components

- **Packed red blood cells (PRBCs):**
  *Indications:* PRBC transfusion is indicated to increase oxygen-carrying capacity and correct anemia due to acute or chronic blood loss, hemolysis, or decreased red cell production. Common indications include:
  - Acute hemorrhage or trauma
  - Anemia due to chronic conditions such as kidney disease or cancer
  - Surgical procedures with significant blood loss
  - Hemoglobinopathies such as sickle cell disease or thalassemia
- **Fresh frozen plasma (FFP):**
  *Indications:* FFP contains clotting factors and is used to correct coagulation factor deficiencies or to manage bleeding disorders. Indications for FFP transfusion include:
  - Coagulopathy due to liver disease or vitamin K deficiency
  - Massive transfusion or hemorrhage with prolonged clotting times
  - Reversal of warfarin anticoagulation in cases of bleeding or urgent surgery
  - Treatment of coagulation factor deficiencies such as hemophilia or disseminated intravascular coagulation (DIC)
- **Platelets:**
  *Indications:* Platelet transfusion is indicated to prevent or treat bleeding due to thrombocytopenia or platelet dysfunction. Common indications include:
  - Thrombocytopenia due to bone marrow suppression (e.g., chemotherapy, radiation therapy)
  - Platelet disorders such as idiopathic thrombocytopenic purpura (ITP) or thrombotic thrombocytopenic purpura (TTP)
  - Prophylaxis or treatment of bleeding in patients with platelet dysfunction or qualitative platelet disorders
- **Cryoprecipitate:**
  *Indications:* Cryoprecipitate is rich in clotting factors, fibrinogen, and von Willebrand factor, making it useful in managing bleeding disorders associated with specific factor deficiencies. Common indications include:
  - Hypofibrinogenemia or dysfibrinogenemia
  - Hemophilia A with inhibitors
  - von Willebrand disease with significant bleeding or prior to surgery
  - Massive transfusion or DIC with low fibrinogen levels
- **Albumin:**
  *Indications:* Albumin transfusion is indicated for volume expansion in patients with hypovolemia or hypoalbuminemia. Common indications include:
  - Hypovolemic shock due to acute hemorrhage or fluid loss
  - Hypoalbuminemia in patients with liver disease, nephrotic syndrome, or burns
  - Plasma volume expansion in critically ill patients or during major surgery

## RISKS AND COMPLICATIONS OF BLOOD TRANSFUSIONS

- **Hemolytic reactions:** The mismatched blood transfusion can result in the serious ABO Rh incompatibility or even with the other blood grouping systems.

**Immediate symptoms:**
- *Fever:* A sudden rise in body temperature may occur shortly after the transfusion begins.
- *Chills:* Patients may experience shaking chills or feel cold during or shortly after the transfusion.
- *Flushed skin:* Some individuals may develop flushed or reddened skin, particularly in the face and neck.
- *Hypotension:* A drop in blood pressure may occur, leading to dizziness, lightheadedness, or fainting.
- *Tachycardia:* Rapid heart rate may be observed as the body responds to the transfusion reaction.
- *Respiratory symptoms:*
  - *Dyspnea*: Shortness of breath or difficulty breathing may develop, indicating a potential respiratory reaction.
  - *Cough*: Some individuals may develop a cough, wheezing, or chest tightness during the transfusion.
- *Hemolytic reaction:*
  - *Back pain*: Severe pain in the lower back or flank area may indicate a hemolytic transfusion reaction, which occurs when the recipient's antibodies attack donor red blood cells.
  - *Dark urine*: Hemoglobinuria, characterized by the presence of hemoglobin in the urine, may result in dark-colored urine.
- *Anaphylactic reaction:*
  - *Hives*: Itchy, raised welts on the skin (urticaria) may develop as a result of an allergic reaction to components in the transfused blood.
  - *Swelling*: Facial swelling, particularly around the eyes and lips, may occur in severe allergic reactions.

**Delayed symptoms (may occur hours to days after transfusion):**
- *Delayed hemolytic reaction:* Patients may experience fatigue, jaundice (yellowing of the skin and eyes), and dark urine due to delayed destruction of red blood cells.
- *Acute lung injury (TRALI):* Symptoms may include shortness of breath, cough, and respiratory distress within hours of the transfusion.

- **Transfusion-transmitted infections:** Various transfusion transmitted infections can be transmitted, if the donor blood is not screened properly.
- **Allergic reactions:** The recipient can show the allergic reaction to the
  - Components of blood additives like anticoagulants, etc.
  - Immediate hypersensitivity reaction like urticaria, anaphylaxis, etc.
  - *Thrombophlebitis:* Infection of the vein where the blood transfusion was done.
- **Transfusion-associated circulatory overload (TACO):** It results in dyspnea, orthopnea (difficulty breathing while lying flat), cough, pulmonary edema (fluid accumulation in the lungs), and signs of congestive heart failure such as peripheral edema and jugular venous distention.

  Patients may also experience hypertension, tachycardia, and elevated central venous pressure (CVP) due to fluid overload. It can be prevented by adhering to transfusion guidelines and administering blood products at a controlled rate appropriate for the patient's clinical condition.
- **Graft-versus-host disease (GVHD):** Though rare but a serious adverse reaction of blood transfusion occurs when the antibodies in the donor's plasma react with the cells of the recipient resulting in the hemolysis. It can be minimized by minor crossmatching.

## ETHICAL AND LEGAL CONSIDERATIONS

Ethical and legal considerations play a crucial role in blood transfusion practices to ensure patient safety, uphold ethical standards, and comply with regulatory requirements.

- **Informed consent:**
  - Patients have the right to receive comprehensive information about the risks, benefits, and alternatives of blood transfusion before giving consent.
  - Informed consent ensures that patients understand the potential risks associated with transfusion, including allergic reactions, transfusion-transmitted infections, and transfusion-related complications.
  - Healthcare providers must obtain informed consent from competent patients or their authorized representatives before initiating transfusion, except in emergency situations where obtaining consent may not be feasible.
- **Donor screening and testing:**
  - Blood donors undergo thorough screening to assess their eligibility and ensure the safety of donated blood.
  - Donor screening includes medical history assessment, physical examination, and laboratory testing for infectious diseases such as HIV, hepatitis B and C, syphilis, and other transfusion-transmissible infections.
  - Donor deferral criteria are established to exclude individuals at higher risk of transmitting infectious diseases or other contraindications to donation.
- **Blood product management and traceability:**
  - Blood product management involves proper handling, storage, labeling, and traceability of blood components to ensure their integrity and safety.
  - Each unit of blood or blood product is labeled with a unique identifier, donor information, expiration date, and other relevant details for traceability.
- **Regulatory compliance and quality assurance:**
  - Blood transfusion services must adhere to regulatory standards and quality assurance practices to maintain the safety and effectiveness of transfusion therapy.
  - Regulatory requirements may include licensure, accreditation, and adherence to guidelines established by regulatory agencies.

## SUMMARY

- Blood banking encompasses a meticulous process starting from donor recruitment, where eligible donors are identified and invited to donate blood. The donation process involves thorough screening of donors to assess eligibility, followed by the collection of blood samples. Blood typing is performed to determine the blood group and Rh factor of donated blood, ensuring compatibility with the recipient. Screening for diseases, including infectious pathogens such as HIV, hepatitis B and C, syphilis, and malaria, is crucial to prevent transfusion-transmitted infections.
- Proper storage procedures, such as refrigeration and freezing, are implemented to maintain the integrity and viability of blood components, ensuring their availability for transfusion when needed.
- Blood transfusions are indispensable in the treatment of various medical conditions, including anemia, hemorrhage, and coagulation disorders. Transfusions replenish blood volume, restore oxygen-carrying capacity, and provide essential blood components such as red blood cells, platelets, and clotting factors.
- While transfusions are life-saving interventions, healthcare professionals must be vigilant about potential risks and complications, including transfusion reactions, infections, and immunological sensitization.
- Ethical principles such as informed consent, patient confidentiality, and autonomy are paramount in blood transfusion practices.

## LET US SEE, HOW MUCH YOU HAVE LEARNT?

### Review Questions

Q1. Describe the hazards of matched and mismatched blood transfusion.
Q2. What are the indications of blood transfusion? How can we minimize the risks of transfusion?
Q3. What changes occur in the cells during storage of the blood?
Q4. Enumerate the blood components that can be transfused in a patient. Give their indications.
Q5. What is major and minor crossmatching. What is its significance?
Q6. What is autologous transfusion?
Q7. What are the risks of massive transfusion?

### Multiple Choice Questions

Q1. Which of the following blood components is primarily indicated for correcting coagulation factor deficiencies?
   a. Packed red blood cells (PRBCs)
   b. Fresh frozen plasma (FFP)
   c. Platelets
   d. Cryoprecipitate

Q2. What is the primary indication for transfusing platelets?
   a. Correcting anemia
   b. Preventing or treating bleeding due to thrombocytopenia or platelet dysfunction
   c. Reversing warfarin anticoagulation
   d. Treating coagulopathy due to liver disease

Q3. A patient with sickle cell disease presents with acute anemia following a vaso-occlusive crisis. Which blood component is most appropriate for transfusion in this scenario?
   a. Packed red blood cells (PRBCs)
   b. Fresh frozen plasma (FFP)
   c. Platelets
   d. Cryoprecipitate

Q4. Which blood product is indicated for patients with hypofibrinogenemia or dysfibrinogenemia?
   a. Packed red blood cells (PRBCs)
   b. Fresh frozen plasma (FFP)
   c. Platelets
   d. Cryoprecipitate

Q5. A patient with chronic liver disease presents with coagulopathy and prolonged clotting time. Which blood component is most appropriate for correcting this coagulopathy?
   a. Packed red blood cells (PRBCs)
   b. Fresh frozen plasma (FFP)
   c. Platelets
   d. Cryoprecipitate

Q6. A patient with idiopathic thrombocytopenic purpura (ITP) is experiencing severe bleeding. Which blood component is most appropriate for transfusion in this scenario?
   a. Packed red blood cells (PRBCs)
   b. Fresh frozen plasma (FFP)
   c. Platelets
   d. Cryoprecipitate

Q7. A patient undergoing major surgery develops hypovolemic shock due to acute hemorrhage. Which blood component is most appropriate for volume expansion in this scenario?
   a. Packed red blood cells (PRBCs)
   b. Fresh frozen plasma (FFP)
   c. Platelets
   d. Albumin

Q8. Which blood component is primarily indicated for increasing oxygen-carrying capacity and correcting anemia?
   a. Packed red blood cells (PRBCs)
   b. Fresh frozen plasma (FFP)
   c. Platelets
   d. Albumin

**Q9.** A patient with severe liver disease develops hypoalbuminemia. Which blood component is most appropriate for volume expansion in this scenario?
a. Packed red blood cells (PRBCs)
b. Fresh frozen plasma (FFP)
c. Platelets
d. Albumin

**Q10.** Which blood product is indicated for the reversal of warfarin anticoagulation in cases of bleeding or urgent surgery?
a. Packed red blood cells (PRBCs)
b. Fresh frozen plasma (FFP)
c. Platelets
d. Cryoprecipitate

**ANSWERS**

1. b  2. b  3. a  4. d  5. b  6. c  7. d  8. a  9. d  10. b

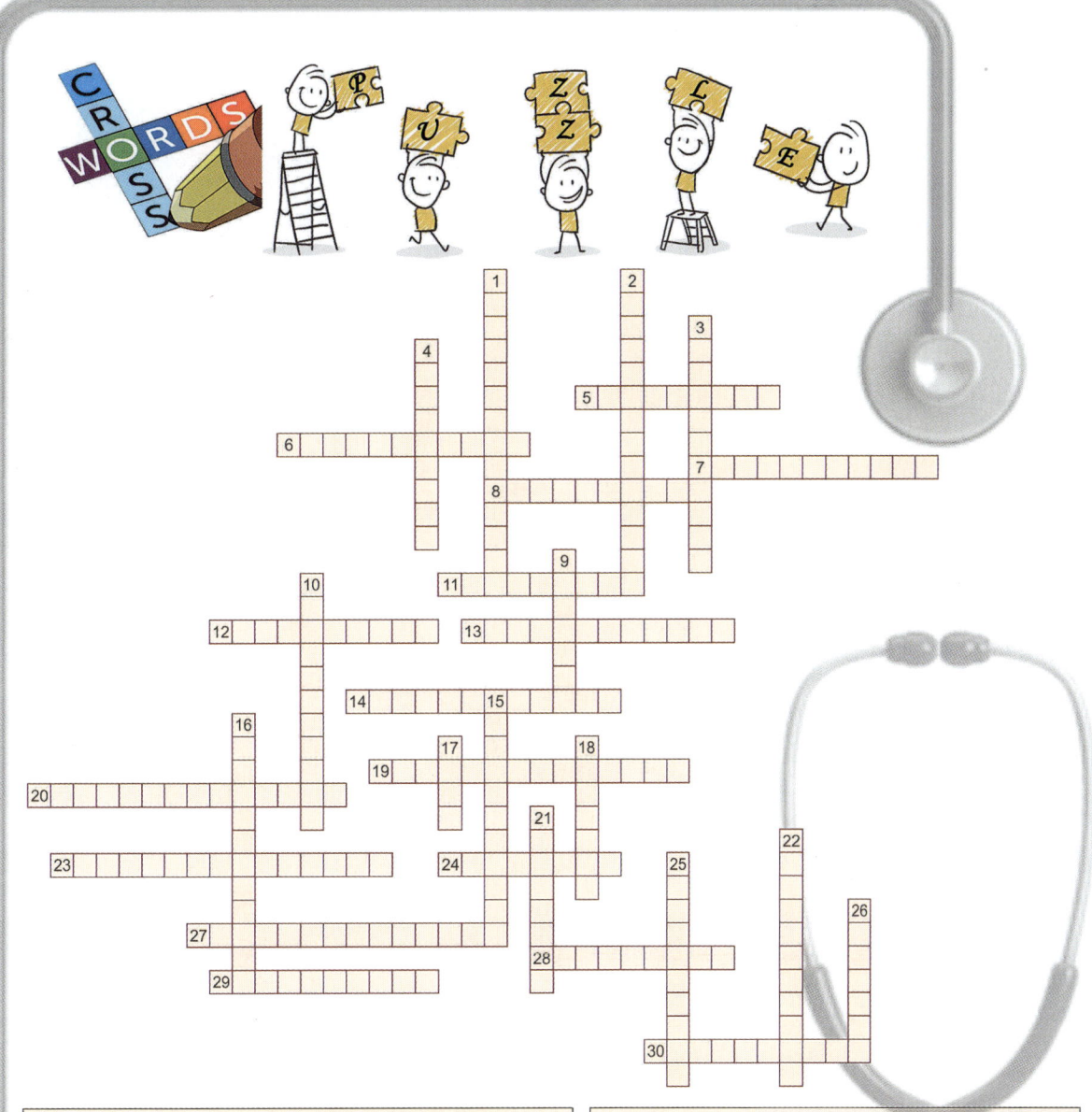

### Across

5. Cell fragments involved in prevention of excessive bleeding
6. Granulocytes with more than 2 lobes (polymorphonuclear)
7. Cytokines secreted by the lymphocytes which is mainly antiviral
8. Breakdown green color product of heme by heme oxygenase
11. Agranulocytes that transform intomacrophage system
12. Membrane protein that converts $Fe^{2+}$ to $Fe^{3+}$
13. Formation of leukocytes in the bone marrow
14. Insoluble bilirubin gets converted into water soluble lumirubin
19. Drugs/chemicals which prevent the clotting
20. Hormone synthesized by liver that stimulates platelet production
23. Pigment giving the characteristic brown color to the feces
24. One of the structural proteins of RBC membrane responsible for biconcave structure
27. Glycoprotein hormone secreted by kidneys due to activation of HIF-1
28. Released from azurophilic granules of neutrophils for breakdown of bacterial DNA
29. Complex conjugated blood element necessary for oxygen transport
30. X-linked recessive bleeding disorder affecting primarily males only

### Down

1. A Y-shaped glycoprotein molecule secreted by the plasma cells
2. Therapeutic separation of plasma from the blood removed from body
3. Antibodies present in plasma for RBC surface antigens
4. Main granulocytes involved in allergic reactions
9. Condition that is prime regulator of erythropoiesis
10. Disease characterized by decreased or no synthesis of either of the globin chain
15. Form of ferritin that may be present in lysosomal membrane
16. Nucleus gets extruded out at this stage of erythropoiesis
17. Craving to eat non-food items
18. Plasma protein whose levels increases in acute dehydration
21. Specific gama globulins formed by the B lymphocytes and plasma cells
22. Accumulation of β-carotene in the blood
25. Type I clotting factor
26. Easy bruisability and presence of larger area of bleeding into the skin

# SECTION 3

# NERVE AND MUSCLE PHYSIOLOGY

## Section Outline

- **Chapter 22:** Neurons and Neuroglia
- **Chapter 23:** Nerve Growth Factor and Cytokines
- **Chapter 24:** Nerve Fibers and their Properties
- **Chapter 25:** Degeneration and Regeneration of Peripheral Nerves
- **Chapter 26:** Neuromuscular Junction
- **Chapter 27:** Muscle: Structure, Properties and Physiology of Muscle Contraction

# Neurons and Neuroglia

## CHAPTER 22

**COMPETENCY ADDRESSED**

PY3.1: Describe the structure and functions of a neuron and neuroglia. Discuss nerve growth factor and other growth factors/cytokines.

**LEARNING OBJECTIVES**

At the end of this chapter, the learner should be able to:
- Describe the structure, types and functions of neurons.
- Describe the structure, types and functions of neuroglia.

The structural and functional unit of the nervous system is called as a neuron/nerve cell.

## STRUCTURE OF A NEURON

The basic prototype structure of neuron comprises of (**Fig. 22.1**):
- A *cell body or soma*, which contains nucleus, organelles, dendrites and axon. The soma does not have centrioles as the *neurons do not divide after birth*. The cell organelles present in soma are responsible for the synthesis of various neurotransmitters and neurotrophic factors, required for propagation of signal and nerve growth. It contains specific granules, which stain with basophilic dyes and are present in neurons with high activity of protein synthesis.
- The soma has many processes called *dendrites*, that branch extensively to form multiple extensions. These dendrites receive the signals from other neurons and hence play an important role in signal transmission across the neurons. Since the dendrites doesn't have the synaptic vesicles, they do not send/transmit the signal to other neurons. Each cell body/soma receives the input from thousands of neurons.
- *Axon is the longest process* arising from soma. At the origin of axon, the segment of cell body is thickened, called *axon hillock*. Then the axon starts from axon hillock and first part of axon is called the *initial segment*, which has *plenty of Na⁺ channels*. Hence, the initial segment is the place from where the *impulse is initiated*.

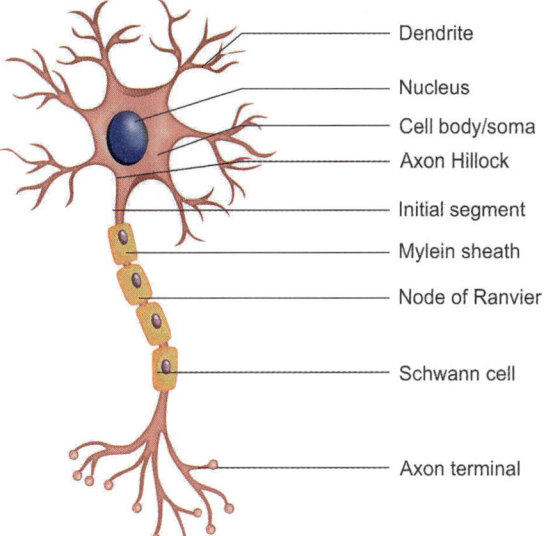

**Fig. 22.1:** Structure of a neuron.

The axon divides into the presynaptic terminals before ending and forms the dilated knobs called the *synaptic knobs/terminal buttons*. These synaptic knobs *store the neurotransmitter* in them, in the form of *synaptic vesicles*. The axons are usually insulated by the covering of myelin sheath, which is done by the Schwann cells in the peripheral nervous system and oligodendrocytes in central nervous system.

## CLASSIFICATION OF NEURONS

There are many classifications of the neurons.
- The most basic classification is **based on the number of processes arising from the cell body**, based on which the neurons are classified as:
  - *Multipolar neurons:* These have multiple dendrites and one axon. These types of neurons are most abundant. A few examples of multipolar neurons are shown in **Figure 22.2**.
  - *Bipolar neurons (Fig. 22.3B):* These neurons have two processes, one dendrite and one axon. These are present in retinal bipolar cells.
  - *Unipolar neurons (Fig. 22.3A):* These neurons have one process arising from soma. The different segments of this process serve as receptive surface and releasing terminal. They are present in embryo, invertebrates.
  - *Pseudounipolar neurons (Fig. 22.3C):* A single process emerges out of the cell body, which divides into two processes and forms the dendrite and axon. It is present in dorsal root ganglia of posterior root of spinal cord.
- Depending on the length of axons:
  - *Golgi Type I neurons:* They have long axons and can project at long distances. They are also called as projection neurons. Example: Pyramidal cells, Purkinje cells
  - *Golgi Type II neurons:* Have short axons. They discharge in the vicinity of the cell body. Example: Basket cells, Granule cells etc.
- Depending on the function of the neurons:
  - *Sensory neurons:* They carry the sensations from the receptor to the central nervous system.

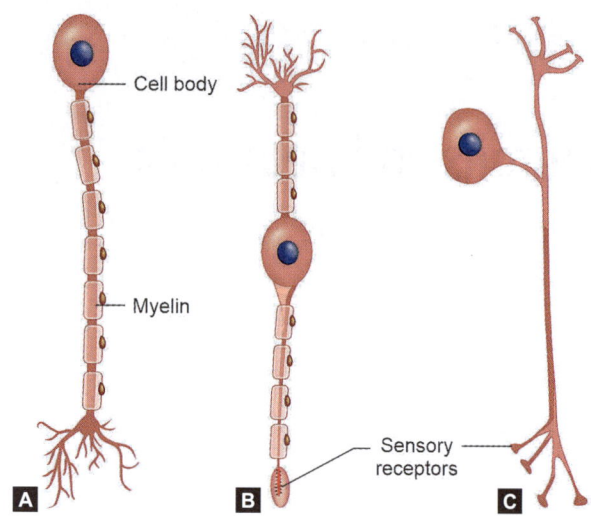

**Figs. 22.3A to C:** (A) Unipolar neuron; (B) Bipolar neuron; (C) Pseudounipolar neuron.

- *Motor neurons:* These neurons carry the motor impulses from cerebrum to the muscles for meaningful muscular contractions.
- *Interneurons:* These are small neurons present in the spinal cord which modulate the signals of sensory and motor neurons.

## NEUROGLIA

These are the supporting cells of the central and peripheral nervous system. The various types of neuroglial cells along with their function are described below:
- Astrocytes
- Microglia

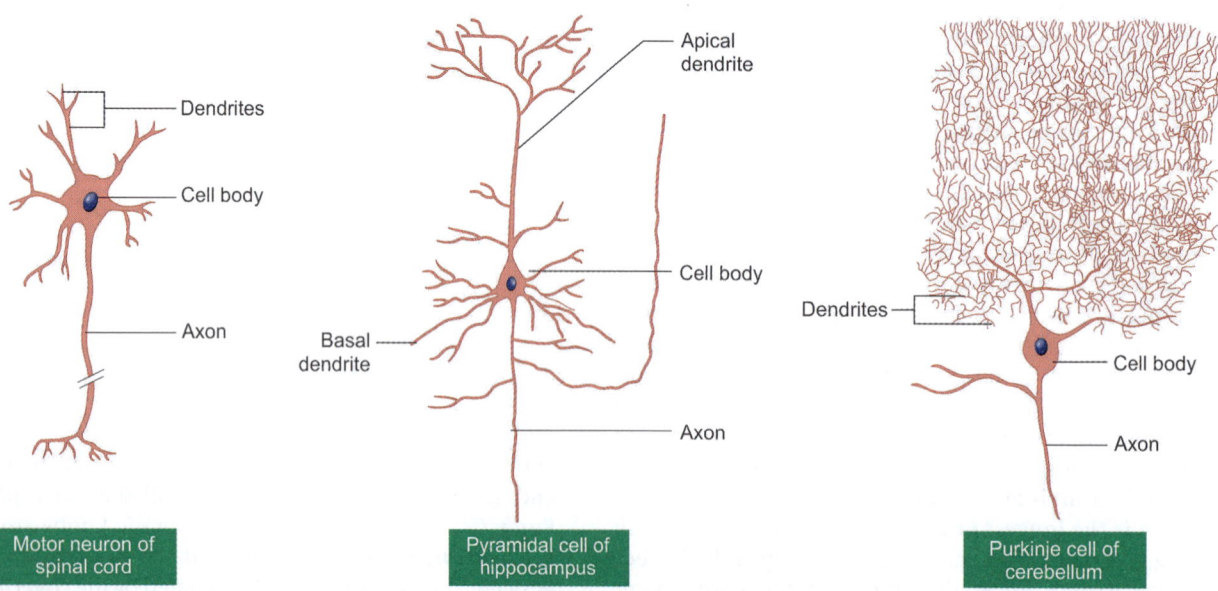

**Fig. 22.2:** Various multipolar neurons.

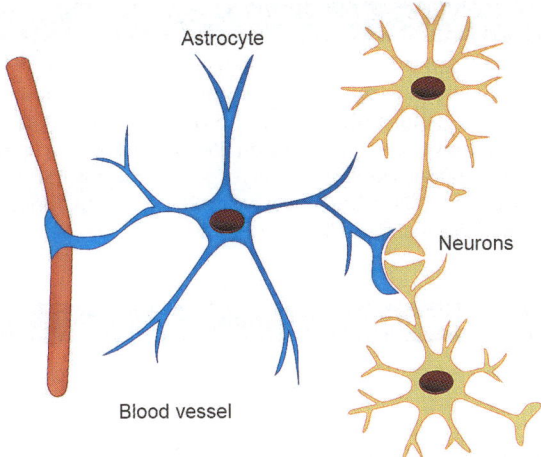

**Fig. 22.4:** Astrocytes showing the formation of blood-brain barrier (BBB) and synaptic insulation.

- Oligodendrocytes
- Ependymal cells

## Astrocytes

These cells are most abundant glial cells and are star shaped, present throughout the brain. They are of two types:
1. **Protoplasmic astrocytes:** Found in gray matter with granular cytoplasm
2. **Fibrous astrocytes:** Found in white matter and contain intermediate filaments.

*Functions of astrocytes:*
- The processes of astrocytes for the tight junctions are participate in the *formation of blood-brain barrier* (**Fig. 22.4**).
- They *insulate/envelope the synapses* to prevent the leakage of the neurotransmitter from the synaptic cleft.
- They produce *neurotropic substances*.
- They *absorb excessive neurotransmitters* like glutamate and GABA, released by the neurons and prevent the prolongation of the action of neurotransmitter.
- They maintain the *ionic balance around the neurons*, by absorbing excessive $K^+$ ions.

## Microglia

These cells are the part of *immune system* and act as the scavengers of the central nervous system. They are analogous to tissue macrophages in rest of body. They

> Various diseases neurodegenerative diseases like multiple sclerosis, Parkinson's disease, Alzheimer's disease occur due increased activity of microglia in removing the neural debris and hence resulting in disease progression.

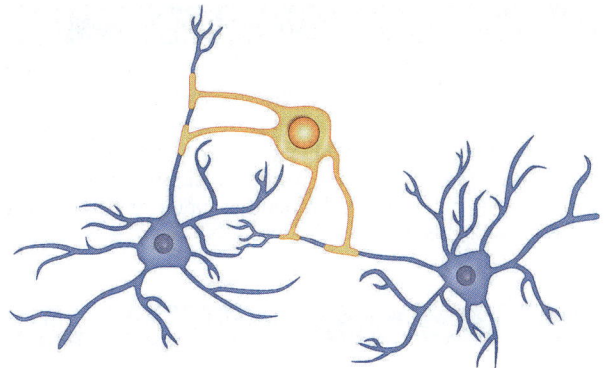

**Fig. 22.5:** An oligodendrocyte, myelinating multiple fibers.

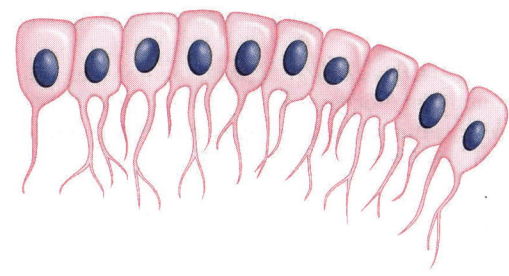

**Fig. 22.6:** Ependymal cells.

remove tissue debris resulting from injury, infection and other diseases. Since the neural tissue, once damaged, doesn't regenerate, it gets replaced by the fibrous tissue.

## Oligodendrocytes

They are a type of macroglia, responsible for the *myelination of neurons of central nervous system*. A single oligodendrocyte is capable of myelinating hundreds of axons together (**Fig. 22.5**). In the peripheral nervous system, the myelination is done by the *Schwann cells*.

> Loss of myelin sheath results in delayed or blocked conduction. An autoimmune peripheral demyelinating disease called *Guillain-Barré syndrome*, occurs when the **autoantibodies** are formed against the protein components myelin **protein zero (P0)** and **PMP22**; resulting in sudden muscle weakness. Another disease *Charcot-Marie-Tooth disease* occurs due to **mutation** in the **genes coding for myelin sheath**, which disrupts the myelination and cause axonal degeneration.

## Ependymal Cells

They are a type of *glial cells* that forms a membrane that lines the ventricles of the brain and the spinal cord (ependyma) (**Fig. 22.6**). They are columnar or cuboidal in shape, with microvilli and cilia. These cells are involved in the secretion, circulation, and homeostasis of the cerebrospinal fluid that fills the central nervous system.

## SUMMARY

- **Neurons** are the structural and functional unit of the nervous system that transmit nerve impulses. They generate electrical signals called action potentials that allow them to communicate over long distances. Neurons are classified into 4 types based on their processes arising from the soma: multipolar neurons, bipolar neurons, unipolar neurons and pseudounipolar neurons.

- **Neuroglia** are the supporting cells that facilitate the functioning of the neurons. They provide physical and metabolic support, insulation, and protection to the neurons. Neuroglia are classified into two types based on their shape and function. In CNS neuroglia include astrocytes, oligodendrocytes, microglia, and ependymal cells. However, in PNS neuroglia include Schwann cells and satellite cells.

## LET US SEE, HOW MUCH YOU HAVE LEARNT?

### Review Questions

Q1. Describe the structure of neuron with the help of a diagram.
Q2. What are the different types of neurons, based on the number of processes arising from soma?
Q3. What is the role of astrocytes in the CNS? How do they support the neurons?
Q4. What is the role of microglia in the pathogenesis of neurodegenerative diseases such as Alzheimer's disease (AD), Parkinson's disease (PD), and multiple sclerosis (MS)?
Q5. What is the function of ependymal cells in the CNS?
Q6. How does astrocytes prevent the excitotoxicity?

### Multiple Choice Questions

Q1. Which part of the neuron acts as a "trigger zone" for generating action potentials?
   a. Axon           b. Dendrite
   c. Cell body    d. Axon hillock

Q2. Which part of the neuron releases chemical neurotransmitters?
   a. Axon           b. Dendrite
   c. Cell body    d. Axon terminus

Q3. Which neurons have long axons that can move signals over long distances?
   a. Golgi type I neurons    b. Golgi type II neurons
   c. Bipolar neurons       d. Unipolar neurons

Q4. Which neurons generally have shorter axons?
   a. Golgi type I neurons    b. Golgi type II neurons
   c. Bipolar neurons       d. Unipolar neurons

Q5. Which type of neuroglia forms the myelin sheath in the peripheral nervous system?
   a. Astrocytes       b. Oligodendrocytes
   c. Microglia        d. Schwann cells

Q6. A patient presents with a history of visual disturbances, headache, and seizures. MRI of the brain reveals a tumor in the brainstem. Which type of neuroglia is most likely involved in this patient?
   a. Astrocytes       b. Oligodendrocytes
   c. Microglia        d. Schwann cells

Q7. The impulse normally travels from _____ to the _____ of a neuron.
   a. dendrite, dendrite    b. dendrite, axon
   c. axon, axon         d. axon, dendrite

**ANSWERS**

  **1.** d    **2.** d    **3.** a    **4.** b    **5.** d    **6.** a    **7.** b

# Nerve Growth Factor and Cytokines

## CHAPTER 23

### COMPETENCY ADDRESSED
PY3.1: Describe the structure and functions of a neuron and neuroglia. Discuss nerve growth factor and other growth factors/cytokines.

### LEARNING OBJECTIVES
At the end of this chapter, the learner should be able to:
- Describe the functions of various nerve growth factors/cytokines.

Neurotrophins are the specific proteins which *regulate the function, growth and differentiation and survival of various neurons*.

The neurotrophins can be secreted by the target tissue (like muscle) and transported in retrograde manner upto the neuronal cell body where they influence the synthesis of proteins required for neuronal function. They can also be synthesized in the cell body, from where they are transported anterogradely and maintains the integrity of post synaptic neuron.

These are four main types of neurotrophins identified so far:
1. Nerve growth factor (NGF)
2. Brain-derived neurotrophic factor (BDNF)
3. Neurotrophin-3 (NT-3)
4. Neutrophin-4/5 (NT-4/5)

## NERVE GROWTH FACTOR

Nerve growth factor is a protein growth factor, which was the first to be identified. It is required for *growth and maintenance of sympathetic and sensory neurons*. It has six subunits ($2\alpha$, $2\beta$ and $2\gamma$ subunits).
- The $\beta$ subunits have nerve growth promoting activity. It is similar to insulin.
- The $\alpha$ subunit has trypsin like activity
- The $\gamma$ subunit are serine proteases.

They act on *tyrosine kinase A (Trk A) receptors and p75 receptors*.

**Functions:**
- NGF is picked up by the neuron terminals and transported in a retrograde fashion from nerve endings to cell body.
- The NGF increases the survival of neurons by suppressing the apoptosis, i.e., it suppresses the programmed cell death.
- It is responsible for cholinergic neurons in basal forebrain and the striatum.

## BRAIN-DERIVED NEUROTROPHIC FACTOR

Brain-derived neurotrophic factor is neurotrophic factor which is also associated with neural survival, maturation and differentiation. It acts on *Tyrosine kinase B receptors (Trk B)*. It rapidly depolarizes the cells. BDNF provides *neuroprotective effect under stressful conditions* like cerebral ischemia, hypoglycemia, neurotoxicity, etc. BDNF has a role to play in energy homeostasis. Administration of BDNF suppresses energy intake and result in weight loss.

**Functions:**
- Synaptic plasticity
- Promote angiogenesis, vascular smooth muscle cells and cardiomyocytes.
- BDNF show neuroprotective activity against multiple sclerosis and other neuroinflammatory diseases.
- It facilitates synaptic transmission and regulates gene expression by increasing levels of synapsin I.

## NEUROTROPIN-3, NEUROTROPIN-4/5

NT-3 is required for *proprioceptor neurons, muscle spindle and mechanoreceptors*. Even the *sympathetic neurons* require NT-3. They act through the tyrosine kinase receptor C and B *(Trk C, Trk B)*.

NT-4/5 are required for the neurons innervating *hair follicle*. They act through the tyrosine kinase receptor B (Trk B).

## OTHER FACTORS AFFECTING NEURONAL GROWTH

These growth factors are produced by Schwann cells and astrocytes. Various growth factors are as follows:

- **Ciliary neurotrophic factor (CNTF):** For survival of damaged and embryonic spinal cord neurons. They can be useful for treating degenerative motor diseases.
- **Glial cell line-derived neurotrophic factors (GDNF):** They are responsible for survival of midbrain dopaminergic neurons. They also prevent apoptosis of spinal motor neurons.
- **Leukemia inhibitory factor (LIF):** It enhances the growth of neurons
- Insulin-like growth factor (IGF-1)
- Transforming growth factor (TGF)
- Fibroblast growth factor (FGF)
- Platelet growth factor (PDGF).

### SUMMARY

Neurotrophins are a family of proteins that induce the survival, development, and function of neurons. They belong to a class of growth factors, secreted proteins that can signal particular cells to survive, differentiate, or grow. Neurotrophins promote the survival of neurons and are known as neurotrophic factors. The four types of neurotrophins are NGF, BDNF, NT-3, and NT-4. Neurotrophins are important regulators for survival, differentiation, and maintenance of nerve cells in the peripheral and central nervous systems.

### LET US SEE, HOW MUCH YOU HAVE LEARNT?

 *Review Questions*

Q1. What are neurotrophins? Enumerate its types.

Q2. Write a short note on nerve growth factors.

 *Multiple Choice Questions*

Q1. Neurotrophins foster the production of proteins associated with neuronal development, growth, and survival. Which of the following statement about nerve growth factor (NGF) is true?
   a. NGF is made up of one α, two β, and one γ polypeptide subunits
   b. NGF is responsible for the growth and maintenance of adrenergic neurons in the basal forebrain and the striatum
   c. NGF is important for the growth of sensory neurons that innervate the muscle spindle
   d. NGF binds to both p75 receptor and Trk B receptors

Q2. What is the function of neurotrophins?
   a. Induce the survival, development, and function of neurons
   b. Regulate the size of neuronal populations during development
   c. Support the growth, survival, and maintenance of neurons
   d. All of the above

Q3. Which of the following is not a type of neurotrophin?
   a. Nerve growth factor (NGF)
   b. Brain-derived neurotrophic factor (BDNF)
   c. Neurotrophin-3 (NT-3)
   d. Neurotrophin-5 (NT-5)

Q4. Which neurotrophin is involved in the survival and differentiation of sympathetic and embryonic sensory neurons?
   a. Nerve growth factor (NGF)
   b. Brain-derived neurotrophic factor (BDNF)
   c. Neurotrophin-3 (NT-3)
   d. Neurotrophin-4 (NT-4)

Q5. Which of the following is not a function of brain-derived neurotrophic factor (BDNF)?
   a. Regulates neuron survival, differentiation, and function
   b. Involved in synaptic transmission, apoptosis, and memory
   c. Promotes the growth and differentiation of sympathetic and embryonic sensory neurons
   d. Involved in nerve growth

Q6. Which of the following is not a type of neuroglia?
   a. Astrocytes
   b. Oligodendrocytes
   c. Macrophages
   d. Schwann cells

### ANSWERS
1. b    2. d    3. d    4. a    5. c    6. c

# Nerve Fibers and their Properties

**CHAPTER 24**

### COMPETENCY ADDRESSED
PY3.2: Describe the types, functions and properties of nerve fibers.

### LEARNING OBJECTIVES
**At the end of this chapter, the learner should be able to:**
- Classify the different types of nerve fibers based on their structure and function.
- Describe the properties of myelinated and non-myelinated nerve fibers.
- Describe the process of nerve impulse transmission in myelinated and non-myelinated nerve fibers.

The axons of the neurons form the nerve fibers. A typical mixed nerve is formed by the multiple nerve fibers with different functions like the motor, sensory, autonomic neurons.

A typical mixed nerve has many bundles/fascicles of nerve fibers. All these bundles are enclosed in perineurium (Fig. 24.1). Each of these axons are also individually covered by endoneurium.

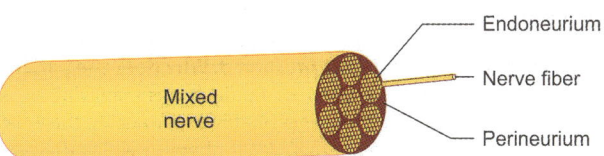

**Fig. 24.1:** Organization of mixed nerve.

## STRUCTURE OF AN AXON

The axon is the longest extension of the neuron, which carries the impulses away from the cell body toward the terminal buttons of the axon. Depending upon the myelination, they are of two types:
- **Myelinated fibers (Fig. 24.2):** These fibers are covered by the myelin sheath which act as insulation covering the axons. The axons are myelinated by the Schwann cells in peripheral nervous system and by oligodendrocytes in central nervous system. The myelinated nerve fibers are thicker and have faster conduction velocity.
- **Unmyelinated fibers:** These fibers lack the myelin sheath. Hence, these fibers are thinner and slower as compared to myelinated fibers.

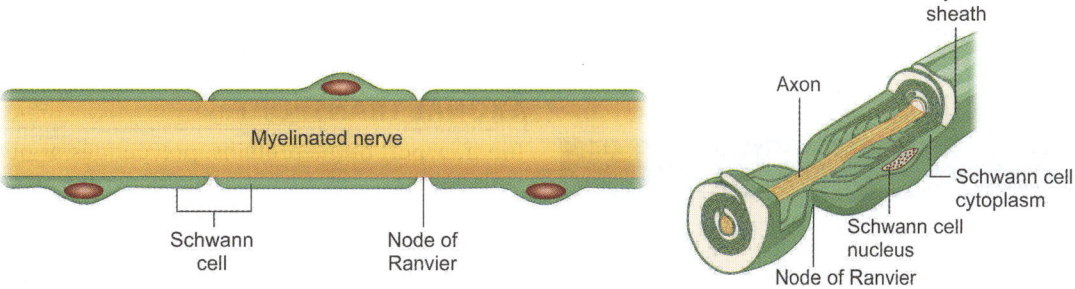

**Fig. 24.2:** A myelinated nerve fiber.

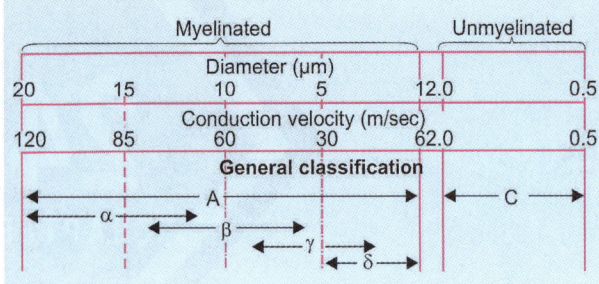

**Fig. 24.3:** Erlanger Gasser's classification of nerve fiber.

**Table 24.1:** Erlanger Gasser's classification of nerve fibers.

| Type of nerve fiber | Diameter | CV | Function |
|---|---|---|---|
| Aα | 12–20 | 70–120 | **P**roprioception, **m**otor |
| Aβ | 5–12 | 30–70 | **P**ressure, **t**ouch |
| Aγ | 3–6 | 15–30 | Muscle **s**pindle |
| Aδ | 2–5 | 12–30 | **T**ouch, **c**old, **f**ast pain |
| B | <3 | 3–15 | Autonomic |
| C | 0.5–2.0 | 0.7–2.5 | Autonomic, slow pain |

**Note:** Mneumonic "**P**rime **M**inister **P**ressurised **T**o **S**ign **T**he **C**ontract **F**ast".

## CLASSIFICATION OF NERVE FIBERS

Before learning further about the properties of nerve fibers, lets quickly go through the classification of nerve fibers.

- In the *Erlanger Gasser classification*, the nerve fibers are classified based on their diameter and conduction velocity **(Fig. 24.3 and Table 24.1)**.
  
  *To remember this classification, remember the diameters of the nerve fibers, which can be written in the multiples of 5, starting from right for the myelinated fibers (1, 5, 10, 15, 20). Add the conduction velocity (CV) below each diameter, which is roughly 6 times the diameter of nerve fiber (**CV = 6 times diameter**). The unmyelinated fibers however don't follow this rule. All the myelinated fibers, with diameters between 1 and 20 μm are classified as Type A fibers and unmyelinated fibers are Type C fibers. Type A fibers are further classified as Aα, Aβ, Aγ and Aδ fibers. The type B fibers (autonomic sympathetic fibers are having the diameter of <3 μm and a conduction speed of 3–15 m/sec).*

- The other classification of nerve fibers is based on their susceptibility to hypoxia, pressure and local anesthetics. Hence, it is called the **Physioclinical classification** (Table 24.2).

**Table 24.2:** Physioclinical classification of nerve fibers.

| | Most susceptible | Intermediate susceptible | Least susceptible |
|---|---|---|---|
| Hypoxia | B | A | C |
| Pressure | A | B | C |
| Local anesthetics | C | B | A |

**Table 24.3:** Numerical classification of nerve fibers.

| Numerical classification | Fiber type | Origin |
|---|---|---|
| Ia | Aα | Muscle spindle: Annulospiral ending |
| Ib | Aα | Golgi tendon organ |
| II | Aβ | Muscle spindle: Flower spray ending, touch, pressure |
| III | Aδ | Pain and cold receptors, some touch receptors |
| IV | C | Pain, temperature and other receptors |

- **Numerical classification of nerve fibers (Table 24.3):** This classification specifically describes the sensory fibers, hence also called classification of sensory fibers. In this the fibers are named as Type Ia, Ib, II, III and IV fibers. It is also based on their diameter and conduction velocity.

*Why a patient feels the touch and not the pain, when given local anesthetics?*

The type C fibers carrying pain are most sensitive to local anesthetics whereas Type A, the large sensory fibers are least sensitive to local anesthetics. Hence, after the administration of local anesthetics, the touch sensation persists but the pain is blocked.

### CLINICAL CASE SCENARIO

A 24-year-old male was brought to orthopedics OPD with wrist drop in right arm. History reveals that he was normal at the last night, before he slept. On waking up in the morning he noticed the wrist drop. He doesn't recall any significant incident during night but on further enquiry, he said that went to sleep in his chair itself where he was reading his book. He got up somewhere near morning and went to his bed. He did not notice anything abnormal but there was a tingling sensation in his right arm. Later, in morning he observed wrist drop in the same arm. Sensory examination of the radial nerve reveals loss of touch but the pain is preserved. Why does the patient have loss of touch and presence of pain in this scenario?

The patient in above scenario is probably experiencing the wrist drop due to compression of the Type A fibers, to which they are most sensitive. The unmyelinated C type fibers are not easily affected by the pressure; hence they escape the compression resulting in the preservation of pain sensation. As this type of compressions had been reported in people who got intoxicated by alcohol on Saturdays and got up on Sunday mornings with compression of nerves of upper limbs, it had been named as Saturday night palsy or Sunday morning Palsy.

## AXONAL TRANSPORT

The transport of the proteins, polypetides or other molecules in the axons are described under the axonal transport. Depending on the direction of flow, it classified as:

- **Orthograde transport:**
  - The flow takes place from the cell body toward the axonal terminals.

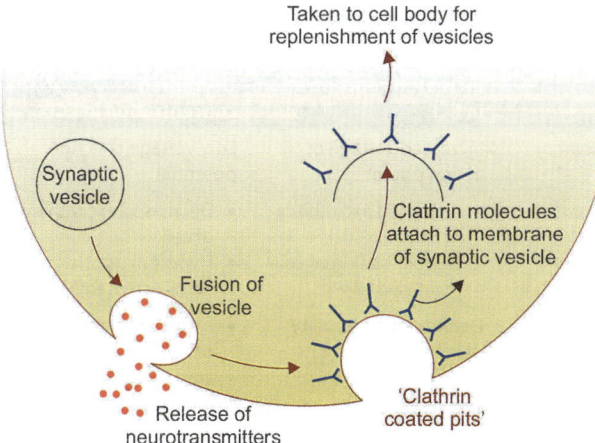

**Fig. 24.4:** Clathrin-mediated vesicular transport for recycling of synaptic vesicles.

- It leads to transport of many proteins and polypeptides synthesized in the cell body.
- These molecules are carried by two molecular motors viz. dynein and kinesin.
- It has two components:
  i. *Fast axonal transport:* Occurs at the rate of 400 mm/day
  ii. *Slow axonal transport:* Occurs at the rate of 0.5–10 mm/day
- **Retrograde transport:**
  - This flow takes place from nerve terminal to cell body
  - Occurs at the rate of 200 mm/day
  - Used for:
    ◆ *Recycling of synaptic vesicles:* The membrane of the vesicles is taken back into presynaptic terminal by the clathrin-mediated endocytosis and transported to the cell body **(Fig. 24.4)**. Fresh neurotransmitter is synthesized in the cell body and transported to nerve terminals with the axoplasmic flow.
    ◆ Absorption of the nerve growth factors by the nerve terminals, which are then transported back to the cell body.
    ◆ Some viruses (e.g., poliovirus) are also transported through the retrograde transport.

## PROPERTIES OF NERVE FIBERS

The nerve fibers act as the electrical conduits in our body. Hence, the main properties of the nerve fibers could be classified on the basis of their electrical properties (excitability). Hence, it will not be wrong if classify the properties as:

### Excitability

The neurons exhibit electrical changes, whenever they are stimulated with electrical current, chemical or mechanical stimuli. These electrical changes can occur locally (called non-propagated/local/electrotonic potentials). If these potential changes are strong enough to raise the intracellular voltage above the threshold potential, it can be propagated resulting in the action potential. We have studied the genesis of resting and action potential in Chapter 8 in detail. We had learnt that the resting membrane potential is formed due to the unequal distribution of the ions in the unstimulated cell whereas the stimulation of the tissue results in the genesis of action potential.

### Conductivity

Once the action potential is generated, it is conducted/transmitted along the axon, in both the directions. Hence, conduction refers to self-propagation of impulse at a constant amplitude and velocity. The conduction of action potential (AP) depends on many factors:

- **Diameter of nerve fiber:** The conduction velocity is roughly 6 times of the diameter of the nerve fibers. Hence, it is maximum in thickest nerve fibers (Aα fibers) followed by others. The conduction velocity of nerve fibers follows the following order:

  $A\alpha > A\beta > A\gamma > A\delta >$ Type B > Type C (Unmyelinated fibers)

> *What will happen to nerve conduction studies, if there is decrease in the nerve diameter due to destruction of axons in it (axonal loss)?*
>
> In the axonal loss, the nerve conduction velocity remains normal due to the normal axons but the amplitude of the current decreases.

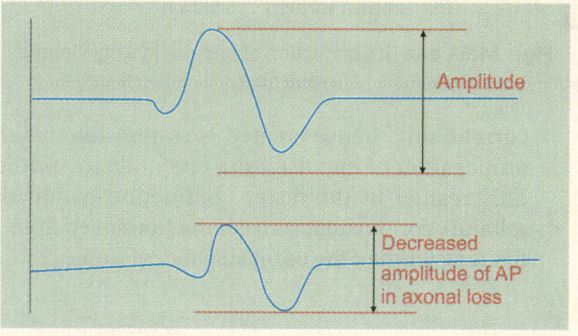

- **Myelination:** The myelinated fibers have higher velocity of conduction as compared to the unmyelinated nerve fibers. The physiological difference in transmission of impulse is shown below:
  - *Transmission of impulse in an unmyelinated nerve fiber:* See **Figs. 24.5A to C**
  - *Transmission of impulse in a myelinated nerve fiber (Figs. 24.6A and B):* The myelinated fibers have the myelin sheath covering the nerve fiber. This myelin sheath is not continuous, resulting in the small areas which are not myelinated called the nodes of Ranvier. *The $Na^+$ channels are concentrated in the nodes of Ranvier* and the initial segment of the neuron. The

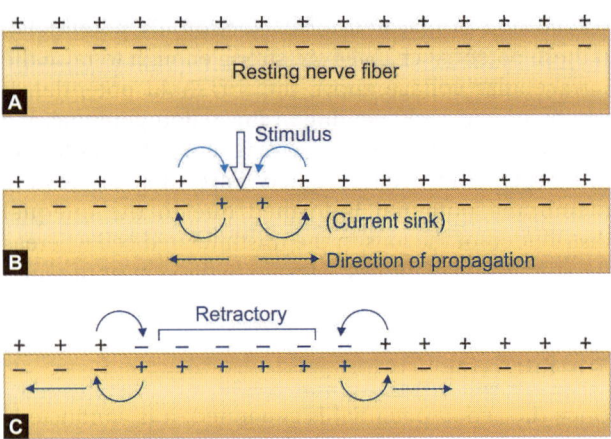

**Figs. 24.5A to C:** Conduction of impulse in unmyelinated nerve fiber.

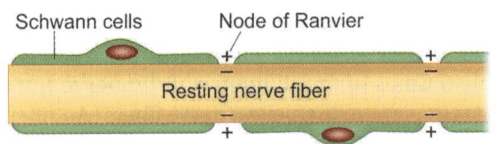

**A** In myelinated nerve fiber, only the nodes of Ranvier are polarized, showing the electrical activity

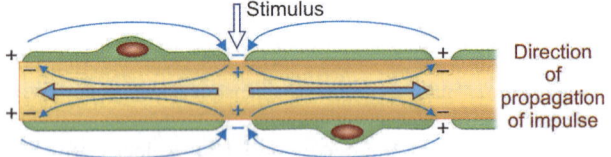

Only the nodes of Ranvier polarize.
This results in jumping of the impulse from one node to another.
**B** This is called saltatory conduction

**Figs. 24.6A and B:** Conduction of impulse in a myelinated nerve fiber.

current sink, hence created is responsible for the propagation of impulse from one node to another. This results in the faster conduction called the saltatory conduction, with conduction speed upto 50 times faster than the unmyelinated neurons.

*What happens to conduction velocity of nerves in demyelinating disorders like multiple sclerosis or Guillain–Barré syndrome?*

In the demyelinating disorders, the continuity of myelin sheath is broken resulting in slowing of conduction and hence reduces the nerve conduction velocity.

- **Ionic composition of extracellular fluid (Table 24.4):** The ionic composition of the extracellular fluid affects the resting membrane potential of the nerve, hence affecting the excitation and conduction of the nerve impulse. Let us study the variations of some important electrolytes in ECF.
- **Temperature:** The increase in the ambient/body temperature increases the conduction velocity whereas the decrease in temperature decreases the conduction

**Table 24.4:** Effect of extracellular fluid ionic changes on excitability and conductivity of nerve.

| | Increased concentration in ECF | Decreased concentration in ECF |
|---|---|---|
| Sodium | Increased voltage of action potential | Low voltage of action potential |
| Potassium | • Increased excitability of cell<br>• Depolarization of cell/Increased RMP | • Decreased excitability of cell<br>• Hyperpolarization of cell/Decreased RMP |
| Calcium | Decreased excitability of cell | • Increased excitability of cell<br>• Depolarisation of cell/increased RMP |

speed due to its affect on ionic pumps, viscosity of the tissue fluid and enzymatic kinetics. *For this reason, the nerve conduction studies especially for myasthenia gravis are best done at 18°C.*

- **All or none principle:** If a nerve is stimulated at its threshold potential, it will get excited and result in the generation of propagated potential. Below the threshold potential it will result in non-propagated local electrical changes in the nerve. But the conduction will happen only if the threshold excitation has taken place.

## Strength-Duration Relationship (Fig. 24.7)

The strength of the current, with which the nerve is stimulated for a sufficient period of time to result in the action potential is explained by the strength-duration relationship.

- The minimum strength of current required to stimulate a nerve is called a *Rheobase*. The time for which this current is applied is called *Utilization time*. Rheobase is measured in Milliampere (mA).
- Another way to express the excitability of the nerve is *Chronaxie*, which is the time taken by the nerve to respond, if a current of double the rheobase is applied to it. It is expressed in millisecond (msec).

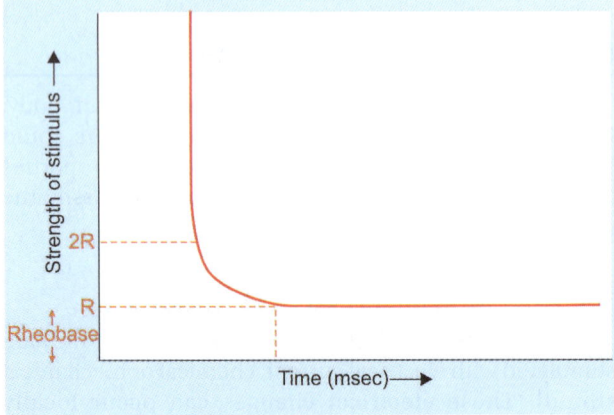

**Fig. 24.7:** Strength-Duration curve.

## Compound Action Potential (Fig. 24.8)

It is the property of mixed nerve, having all types of nerve fibers [fast conducting Type A (Aα, Aβ, Aγ, Aδ), Type B and unmyelinated slow conducting Type C fibers]. When a nerve is stimulated at one end the recording electrode, placed at the other end of nerve, picks up different action potentials due to difference in the conduction velocity of different types of the nerve fibers.

Here, the first peak of action potential is obtained due to type A fibers in the order of their conduction velocity Aα, Aβ, Aγ, Aδ, followed by type B fibers and then Type C fibers in the end.

## Regeneration after Injury

Though the nerve cells cannot divide after birth, but the injured axons can regenerate. The nerve injury and regeneration is discussed in detail, in Chapter 25.

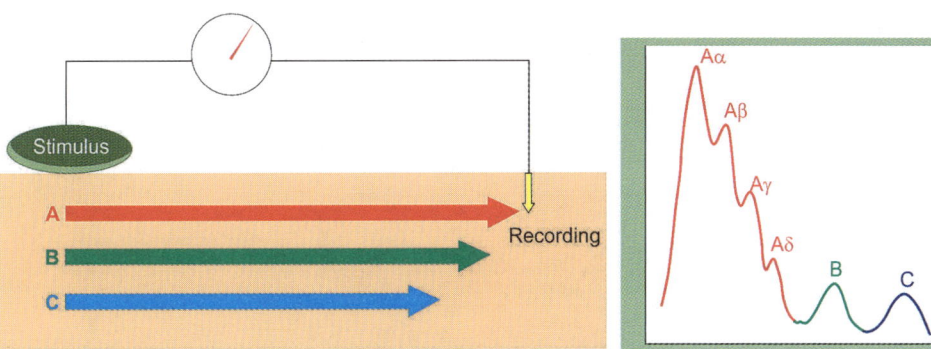

**Fig. 24.8:** Compound action potential.

### SUMMARY

- According the diameter of the nerve fibers, the nerve fibers are classified by Erlanger Gasser's classification into three types: Type A (Aα, Aβ, Aγ, Aδ), Type B and Type C fibers. Due to myelination status, the fibers are classified as myelinated and unmyelinated fibers. Also, the fibers are classified as their susceptibility to local anesthetics, hypoxia and pressure. This helps us in understanding the response of nerves to various physical and clinical scenarios. The third type of classification is numerical or sensory classification in which the fibers are classified as (Type Ia, Ib, II, III and IV).
- The main properties of the nerves are excitation and conduction, which can be affected by various factors like diameter of nerve, myelination, ionic composition of extracellular fluid, temperature, compound action potential, etc.

### LET US SEE, HOW MUCH YOU HAVE LEARNT?

#### Review Questions

Q1. Describe the Erlanger Gasser's classification of nerve fiber. What are other classification systems?
Q2. How is the impulse propagated in a myelinated and unmyelinated nerve fiber?
Q3. What will happen to the excitability of nerves in patients of advanced renal failure/adrenal insufficiency/distal tubular acidosis/type 1 diabetes mellitus/dehydration/administration of angiotensin II receptor blockers/angiotensin-converting enzyme inhibitors/potassium sparing diuretics? (All these conditions lead to impaired ability of kidney to excrete potassium resulting in hyperkalemia).
Q4. What will happen in a patient in patient of hypokalemia (increased excretion of $K^+$) due to Barter syndrome/Gitelman syndrome/diabetic ketoacidosis?

#### Multiple Choice Questions

Q1. A patient presents with a loss of sensation of pain and temperature in the left leg. The physician suspects that the patient has a nerve injury. Which of the following nerve fibers is most likely to be affected?
   a. A alpha fibers
   b. A beta fibers
   c. A delta fibers
   d. B fibers

Q2. Tarun was undergoing the incision and drainage of the abscess on the gluteal region. The surgeon gave him the local anesthesia. Doctor counseled him that he would continue to feel the touch but will not feel the pain after local anesthesia. What is the physiological basis behind this statement of the doctor?
   a. The touch sensation is carried by type C fibers which are least susceptible to local anesthetics

b. The pain sensation is carried by type A fibers which are most susceptible to local anesthetics
c. The touch sensation is carried by type A fibers which are most susceptible to local anesthetics
d. The pain sensation is carried by type C fibers which are most susceptible to local anesthetics

Q3. A patient with chronic renal failure is brought to emergency with muscle pain and weakness, numbness, cardiac arrhythmias, and nausea. Her laboratory findings show serum potassium levels of 6.2 mEq/L. What could be the changes in the excitability and electrical properties of her neural tissue?
a. Increased neuromuscular excitability
b. Hyperpolarization of neurons
c. The resting membrane potential shifts from −70 mV to −80 mV
d. The threshold potential is raised.

## ANSWERS

1. c    2. d    3. a

# Degeneration and Regeneration of Peripheral Nerves

## 25 CHAPTER

**COMPETENCY ADDRESSED**

**PY3.3:** Describe the degeneration and regeneration in peripheral nerves.

**LEARNING OBJECTIVES**

**At the end of this chapter, the learner should be able to:**
- Describe the different types of peripheral nerve injuries.
- Classify the nerve injuries.
- Describe the changes in an injured nerve.
- Describe the mechanism of regeneration in nerve.

The peripheral nerves are usually very well protected from the factors which can result in nerve injury. But it is not uncommon to come across the patients with injuries of peripheral nerves occurring due to pressure or complete/partial transection. Hence, to diagnose the severity of nerve injury, it is classified by *Sunderland's classification (5 grades) and Seddon's classification (3 grades)*.

## GRADING OF NERVE INJURY

As per Seddon's and Sunderland's classification the nerve injury is graded into three grades (**Fig. 25.1**):
1. **Neuropraxia:** It is similar to **Grade I** injury of Sudderland's classification. The nerve fiber is affected by the pressure. The nerve damage is minimal as the axon and endoneurial tube is intact. The nerve recovers in about two weeks.
2. **Axonotemesis:** It is similar to **Grade II** injury of Sudderland's classification. The nerve fiber is affected by the *prolonged pressure*. The endoneurial tube is intact. The nerve recovers completely but takes a little more time than grade I injury.
3. **Neurotemesis:** It refers to when there is structural damage of the nerve. Hence Grades III, IV and V of Sunderland classification describes the neurotemesis.
   a. **Grade III:** There is disruption or damage to the endoneural tube.
   b. **Grade IV:** The endoneurial tube and the nerve fascicles are disrupted.
   c. **Grade V:** There is complete transection of nerve fiber. It is the most severe form of the nerve injury.

## CHANGES IN THE NERVE AFTER THE INJURY

Since the injury usually happens in the axon (**Fig. 25.2**), the changes in the axon are described in both the ends separately. These two stumps are (especially in Grade V injury):
1. **Proximal end/stump:** Toward the cell body of neuron
2. **Distal end/stumps:** Toward the nerve terminal.

Changes in the injured neuron are hence described as:
- Changes in the cell body of neuron
- Changes in proximal end
- Changes in distal end

## CHANGES IN THE CELL BODY OF NEURON

Changes that occurs in cell body are (**Fig. 25.3**):
- The cell body swells up
- The nucleus is pushed to one side and becomes eccentric
- The cell organelles disintegrate
- The ribosomes become disorganized
- The nissl granules disintegrate and stain weakly with basic dye called chromatolysis.

## CHANGES IN PROXIMAL AND DISTAL STUMPS (FIG. 25.4)

The proximal stump is degenerated *only upto the nearest node of Ranvier*, from the site of injury. The myelin breaks and cleared by macrophages. The neurotrophins secreted by the soma, makes the growth cone, from which many neurofibers sprout out.

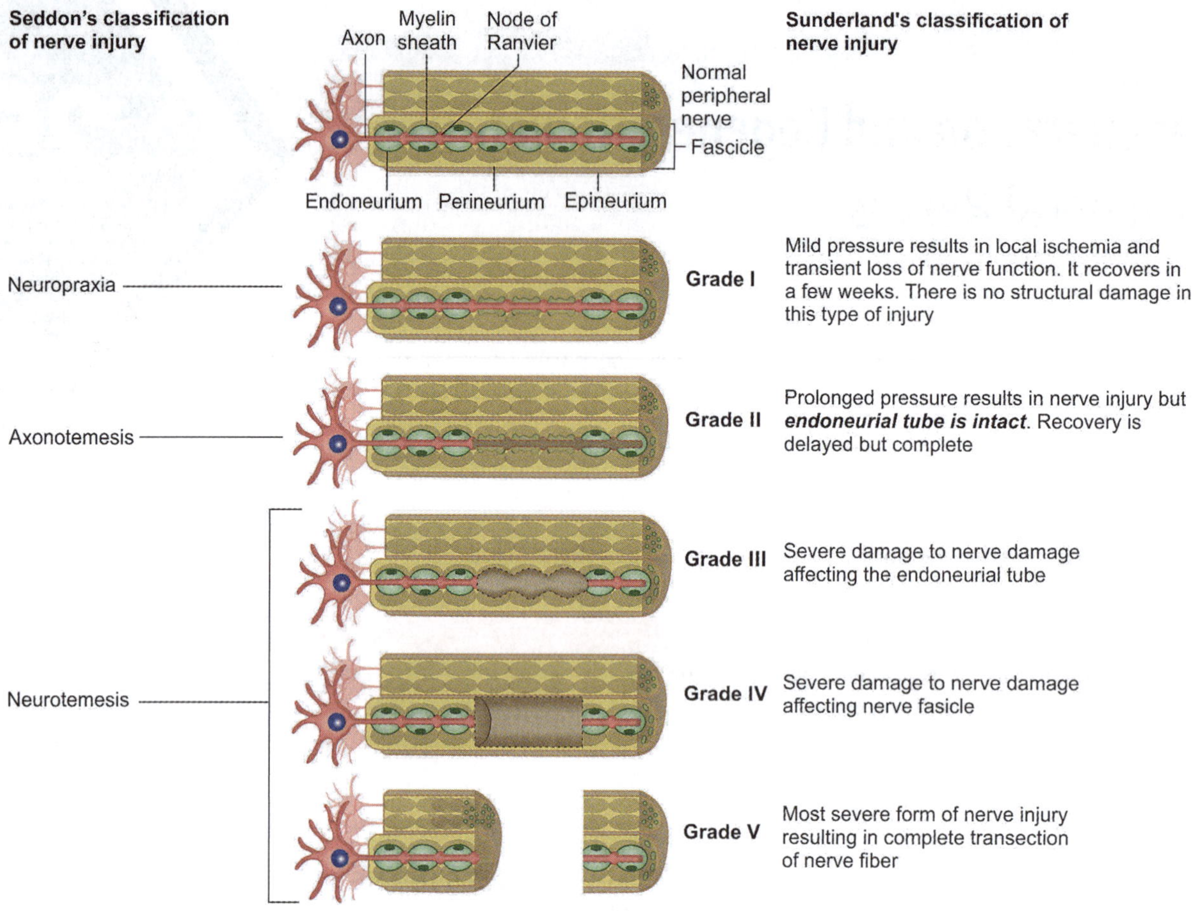

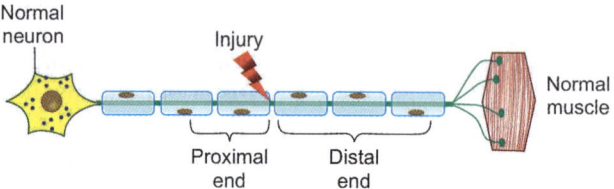

**Fig. 25.1:** Grades of nerve injury.

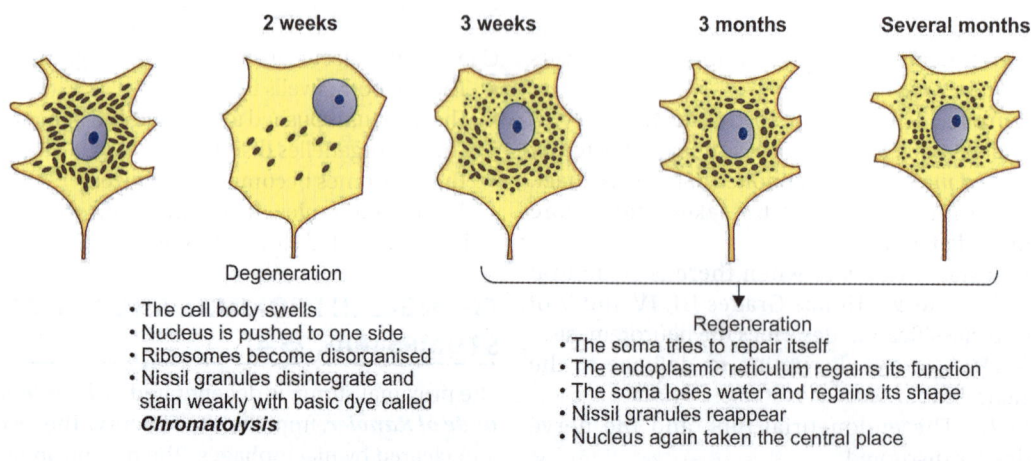

**Fig. 25.2:** The proximal and distal stump of neuron.

**2 weeks** — **3 weeks** — **3 months** — **Several months**

**Degeneration**
- The cell body swells
- Nucleus is pushed to one side
- Ribosomes become disorganised
- Nissil granules disintegrate and stain weakly with basic dye called **Chromatolysis**

**Regeneration**
- The soma tries to repair itself
- The endoplasmic reticulum regains its function
- The soma loses water and regains its shape
- Nissil granules reappear
- Nucleus again taken the central place

**Fig. 25.3:** Changes in the cell body of the injured neuron.

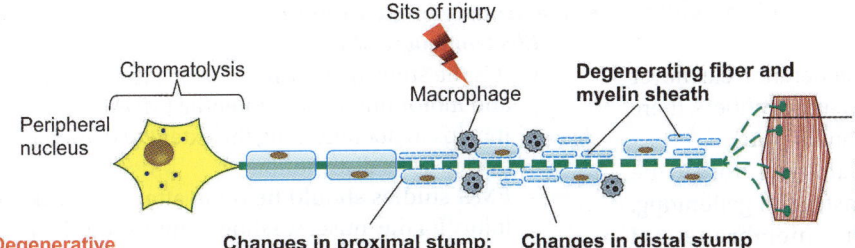

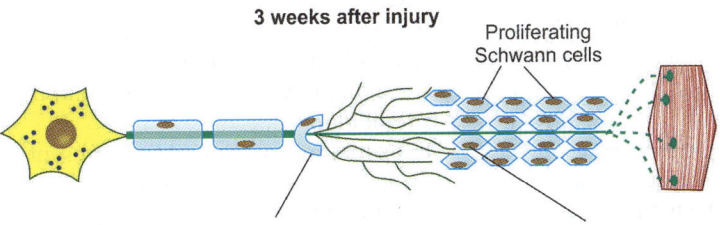

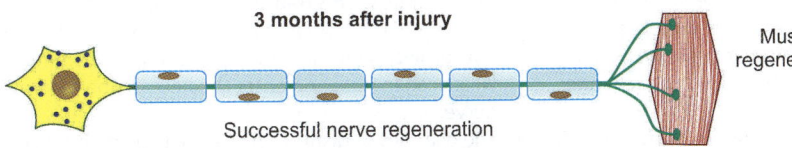

**Fig. 25.4:** Changes in proximal and distal stumps.
(PNS: peripheral nervous system, CNS: central nervous system)

The changes in the *distal stump* are specifically called as the *Wallerian Degeneration*, as it was first described by Dr August Waller.

The axon swells up and results in the break down of the axon cylinder and the myelin sheath. The macrophages infiltrate the entire degenerating axon and phagocytose the debris to clear up the area. The Schwann cells remain viable. These Schwann cells, then grow to form the endoneurial tubes. The distal stump regenerates under the effect of nerve growth factors-released by target tissue and Schwann cells. Most commonly identified neurotrophin is NGF and Glial cell line-derived neurotrophic factor (GDNF).

One of the growing sprouts enters the endoneurial tube and develops into the nerve fiber which innervates the target tissue.

## Effect on the Target Tissue

The nerve terminal retract from the post synaptic target. Due to the absence of innervation, there is increase in number of receptors on the target tissue (*upregulation of receptors*). This results in the hypersensitivity of target tissue to even small amount of neurotransmitter, if present is called *Denervation hypersensitivity*.

## FACTORS INFLUENCING REGENERATION OF NERVE

The nerve regeneration happens successfully, if the following factors are providing the favorable environment:

1. **Severity of injury:** If the gap between the proximal and distal parts is more than 3 mm, the multiple outgrowths

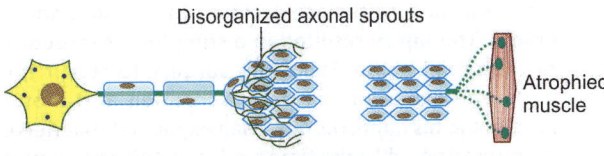

**Fig. 25.5:** Formation of neuroma in the growing axon from the proximal stump.

intermesh and form a tumor like swelling called *neuroma* (Fig. 25.5).

If neuroma is formed, successful regeneration can never occur. In case, the neuroma involves sensory fibers, there is hyperalgesia at the site (Touch causes pain).

2. **Condition of soma:** If the axonal damage is close to the cell body, the neuron often dies instead of generating. This occurs due to loss of neural membrane and cytoplasm. Hence, the injuries closer to cell body have poor recovery as compared to the ones away from soma.
3. **Location of injury:** The nerve injuries in peripheral nerves regenerate better than in the central nervous system.
4. **Neurotrophins:** The neurotrophins are secreted by the target tissue and Schwann cells. Clinically also, application of neurotrophins to the site, promotes healthy regeneration of nerve fibers.

## DIAGNOSIS OF NERVE INJURY

- **Clinical examination:** A thorough clinical examination of motor and sensory functions of the affected nerves.
- **Electrodiagnostic studies:**
  - *Electromyography:*
    - It is the study of muscles in which the contraction and motor unit action potential (MUAP).
    - It helps in documenting the extent of denervation as well as its distribution.
    - EMG studies should be done after 2–3 weeks of injury for the muscle to show denervation changes.
    - Complete denervation is characterized by low amplitude *sharp waves or fibrillation potential* with muscle at rest and absent evoked motor unit action potential (MUAP).
    - With reinnervation these changes begin to reverse.
  - *Nerve conduction studies:*
    - They play an important role in identifying the type and age of peripheral nerve injury.
    - In neuropraxia compound muscle action potential (CMAP) amplitude remains normal distal to the site of injury and drops to zero with proximal site stimulation.
    - In axonal injury the CAMP is present in the first week and thereafter falls rapidly after Wallerian degeneration has occurred.

### SUMMARY

In this chapter we had learnt about the 5 grades of nerve injury, which is used clinically for treatment of various nerve injuries. Various changes in different parts of neuron were discussed:
- **Cell body:** Shows swelling of soma, chromatolysis and pushing of nucleus to one side. During regeneration, all these changes are reversed.
- **Axon:** Axon shows swelling. The proximal stump shows demyelination and break down only till the nearest node of Ranvier. But the myelin sheath of entire distal distal stump disintegrates. The debris is cleared by macrophages. The Schwann cells grow in distal stump to for endoneurial tube. The growth cone in proximal stump gives neural sprouts which regenerate and enter the neural tube to form a normal nerve.
- The changes in distal stump in particular are called Wallerian degeneration.

### LET US SEE, HOW MUCH YOU HAVE LEARNT?

*Review Questions*

**Q1.** Discuss various gradings of nerve injury based upon Seddon's and Sunderland's classification.
**Q2.** Describe the degenerative changes that occur in axonal injury, including degenerative changes at the proximal and distal ends, anterograde degeneration (Wallerian degeneration), and transneuronal degeneration.
**Q3.** Define Wallerian degeneration and explain the process that results when a nerve fiber is cut or crushed, in which the part of the axon separated from the neuron's cell body degenerates.

*Critical Thinking Case-Based Questions*

**Q1.** A 45-year-old male, suffered with severe injury to his right arm in a workplace accident involving a sharp object. The injury resulted in a complete transection of the radial nerve. Following surgery to repair the nerve, he experiences loss of sensation and motor function in his hand. His physician explained that nerve regeneration will take time and that full recovery is uncertain.

Based upon the given scenario, answer the following questions:
a. Explain the physiological processes involved in the degeneration of peripheral nerve in this condition.
b. Discuss the factors that influence the success of nerve regeneration in this case.
c. What are the various methods of diagnosis of nerve injury?

## Multiple Choice Questions

**Q1.** Which part of the neuron undergoes Wallerian degeneration after injury?
   a. Soma
   b. Axon hillock
   c. Distal axon segment
   d. Dendrites

**Q2.** What happens to the myelin sheath during Wallerian degeneration?
   a. Remains intact
   b. Rapidly regenerates
   c. Breaks down and disintegrates
   d. Transforms into scar tissue

**Q3.** Which type of nerve fibers exhibit Wallerian degeneration more prominently?
   a. Afferent fibers
   b. Motor fibers
   c. Sensory fibers
   d. Mixed fibers

**Q4.** What cellular process is responsible for the removal of debris during Wallerian degeneration?
   a. Phagocytosis by microglia
   b. Mitosis of neurons
   c. Proliferation of astrocytes
   d. Apoptosis of damaged cells

**Q5.** What is the primary function of Wallerian degeneration in the nervous system?
   a. Preventing further injury
   b. Facilitating neuronal repair and regeneration
   c. Initiating inflammation
   d. Isolating damaged neurons

**Q6.** Which of the following statements about Wallerian degeneration is true?
   a. It occurs only in the central nervous system
   b. It is a reversible process
   c. It is independent of the type and severity of the nerve injury
   d. It involves retrograde degeneration of the proximal axon

**Q7.** What role do Schwann cells play in Wallerian degeneration?
   a. They inhibit the process
   b. They promote axonal growth
   c. They phagocytose myelin debris
   d. They form a barrier to prevent degeneration

**Q8.** Which neurological disorders are associated with abnormal Wallerian degeneration?
   a. Alzheimer's disease
   b. Parkinson's disease
   c. Amyotrophic lateral sclerosis
   d. Multiple sclerosis

## ANSWERS

**1.** c    **2.** c    **3.** b    **4.** a    **5.** b    **6.** d    **7.** c    **8.** c

# Neuromuscular Junction

## CHAPTER 26

### COMPETENCY ADDRESSED
PY3.4: Describe the structure of neuromuscular junction and transmission of impulses.
PY3.5: Discuss the action of neuromuscular blocking agents.
PY3.6: Describe the pathophysiology of myasthenia gravis.

### LEARNING OBJECTIVES
**At the end of this chapter, the learner should be able to:**
- Describe the physiological anatomy of neuromuscular junction (NMJ).
- Describe the transmission of impulse across the NMJ.
- Describe the action of various neuromuscular blocking agents.
- Describe the pathophysiology and physiological basis of clinical features of the disorders of NMJ.

## PHYSIOLOGICAL ANATOMY OF THE NEUROMUSCULAR JUNCTION

The neuromuscular junction (NMJ) is located at the belly of the skeletal muscle between the synaptic knob of the large myelinated motor nerve (alpha motor neurons, originating from the anterior horns of the spinal cord) and the sarcolemma of the skeletal muscle (**Fig. 26.1**). The entire NMJ is called as *motor end plate*. The NMJ is divided into three main components:

1. **The presynaptic membrane**—formed by the neural component, i.e., the **synaptic knob** containing the **synaptic vesicles**, filled with the neurotransmitter acetylcholine (ACh).

2. **The synaptic cleft**—is the space between the pre- and postsynaptic membrane. It is around *20–30 nm wide* and contains the extracellular fluid and the enzyme acetylcholinesterase (AChE), which is embedded in the basal lamina of the postsynaptic membrane.

3. **The postsynaptic membrane**—is formed by the **sarcolemma** of the muscle. The region, just below the nerve terminal, form a depression called as *synaptic gutter*. The membrane of the synaptic gutter is thrown into *junctional folds or palisade*.

Let us now discuss, each of these three components in detail (**Fig. 26.2**).

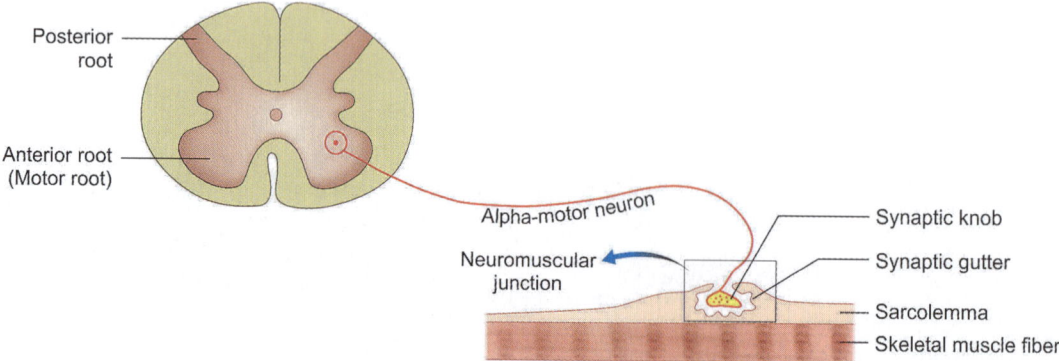

**Fig. 26.1:** Site of neuromuscular junction.

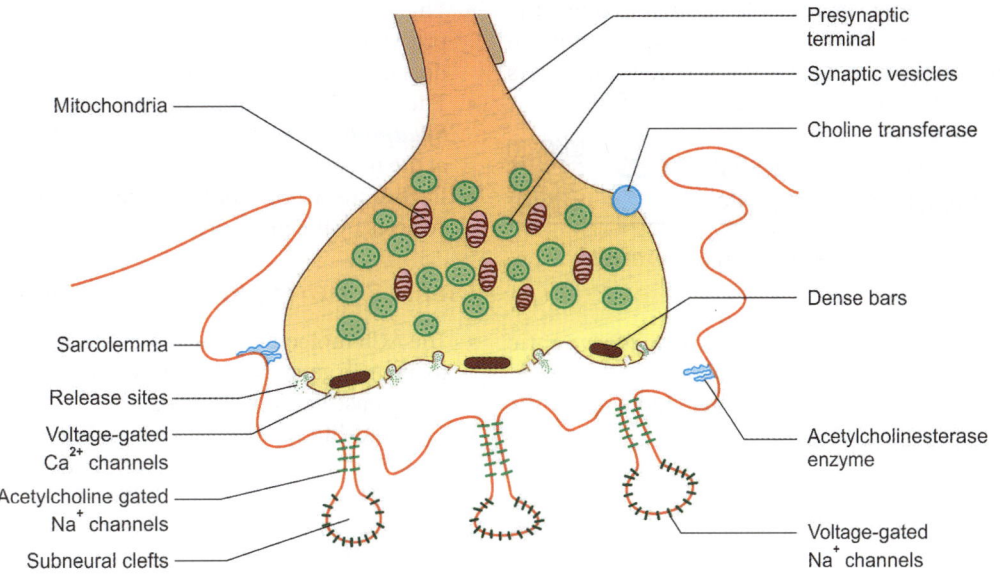

**Fig. 26.2:** Structure of neuromuscular junction.

## The Presynaptic Terminal

This terminal contains 300,000 synaptic vesicles, each containing around 10,000 molecules of ACh. These synaptic vesicles, are synthesized as shown in **Figure 26.3**.

Apart from the synaptic vesicles, it contains a large amount of mitochondria for the resynthesis of ACh. The presynaptic membrane consists of *voltage-gated calcium channels (VGCC)*, located adjacent to the dense bars. There are active sites, next to the VGCCs, which contain the docking proteins, t-SNARE proteins, called as *Syntaxin*.

## The Postsynaptic Terminal

The postsynaptic membrane, is thrown into many junctional folds/palisades. Just below the dense bars, the sarcolemma forms the *subneural cleft* which has *ACh-gated Na⁺ channels* (Nicotinic, $N_M$ receptors) and the *voltage-gated Na⁺ channels (VGNC)*, as shown in the **Figure 26.2**.

The acetylcholine gated sodium channels **(Fig. 26.3)**, are the ion channels with **5 subunits [2α, β, γ (in fetal)/ε (in adults) and δ]**. These channels have a pore size of 0.65 nm which increases when the ACh molecules bind

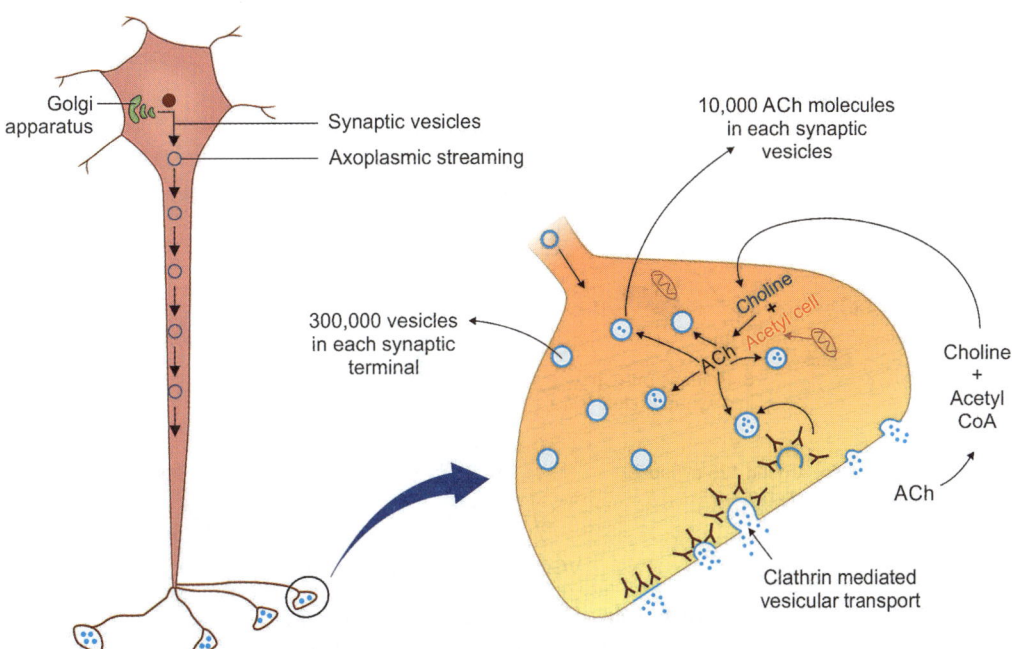

**Fig. 26.3:** Synthesis of synaptic vesicles.

to both the α subunits. This is wide enough to allow the movement of Na⁺, K⁺ and Ca²⁺ ions through it. But the electrochemical gradient across the sarcolemma favors only the *Na⁺ influx* and does not allow the K⁺ efflux.

## TRANSMISSION OF IMPULSE ACROSS NEUROMUSCULAR JUNCTION

### Events Occurring in Presynaptic Terminal (Fig. 26.4)

- Impulse/action potential reaches the presynaptic terminal
- Depolarization of the axon terminal (increase in the voltage)
- Opening off the VGCC
- Calcium influx
- Activation of calcium calmodulin dependent protein kinase
- Phosphorylation of protein *Synapsin*. (Synapsin anchors the synaptic vesicles with the cytoskeleton of the axon terminal)
- Release of the synaptic vesicles from cytoskeleton
- The vesicles move toward the release sites on the presynaptic membrane. These release sites have the docking protein called as **Syntaxin**
- The v-SNARE protein on the vesicular membrane, *Synaptobrevin*, with the help of *SNAP* proteins, docks at the release site.
- Each action potential releases around 125 synaptic vesicles by the process of exocytosis

### Events Occurring in Synaptic Cleft (Fig. 26.5)

- The ACh molecules released in the synaptic cleft, binds to the ACh gated Na⁺ channels resulting in the Na⁺ influx in the postsynaptic terminal
- The half-life of ACh is a few milliseconds, which is broken down into acetyl CoA and choline in the synaptic cleft by the enzyme acetylcholinesterase present in the basal membrane of the postsynaptic membrane
- The choline formed after the breakdown in transported inside the presynaptic terminal. Fresh ACh is synthesized from this choline and acetyl CoA, formed in the mitochondria, present in the presynaptic terminal.

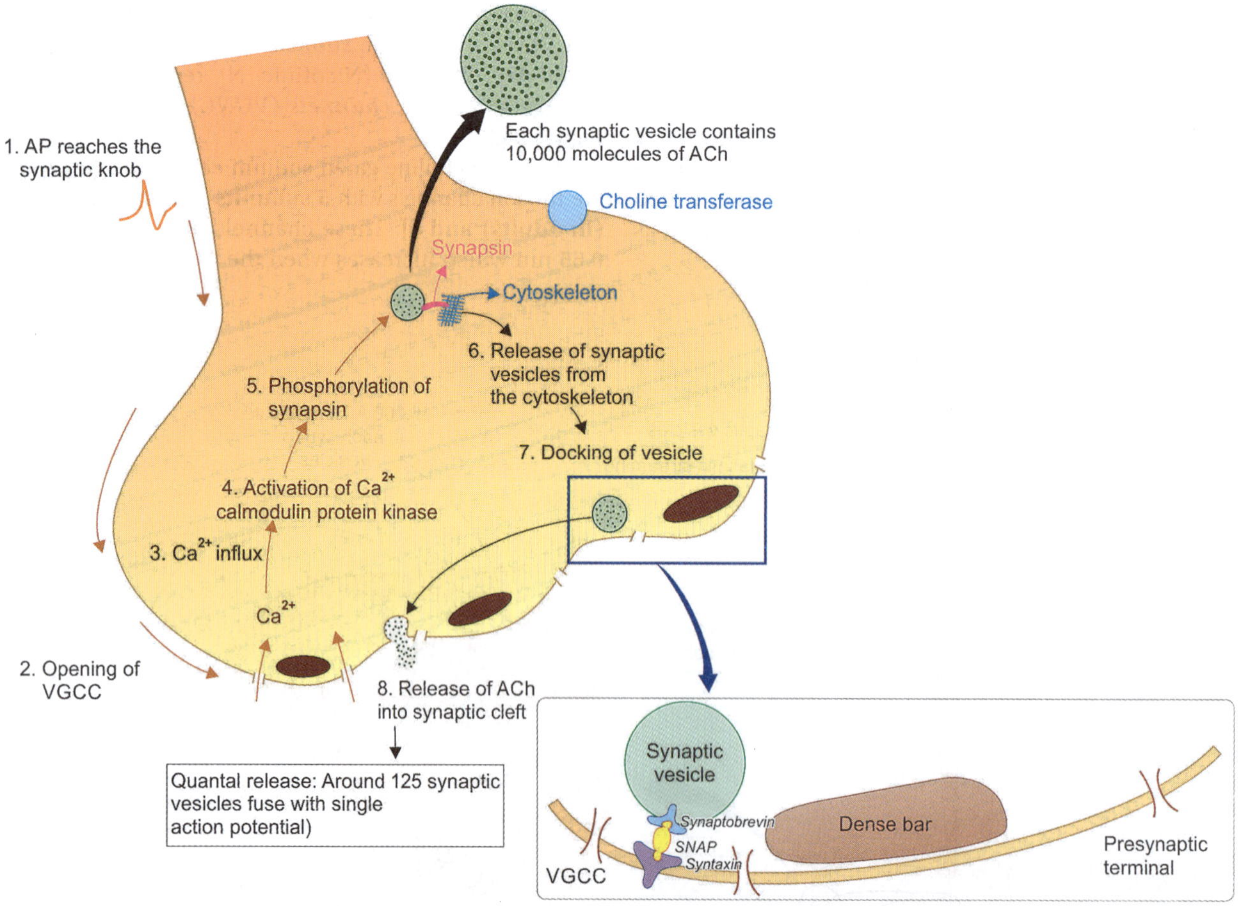

**Fig. 26.4:** Events occurring at presynaptic terminal.
(AP: action potential, VGCC: voltage-gated calcium channel)

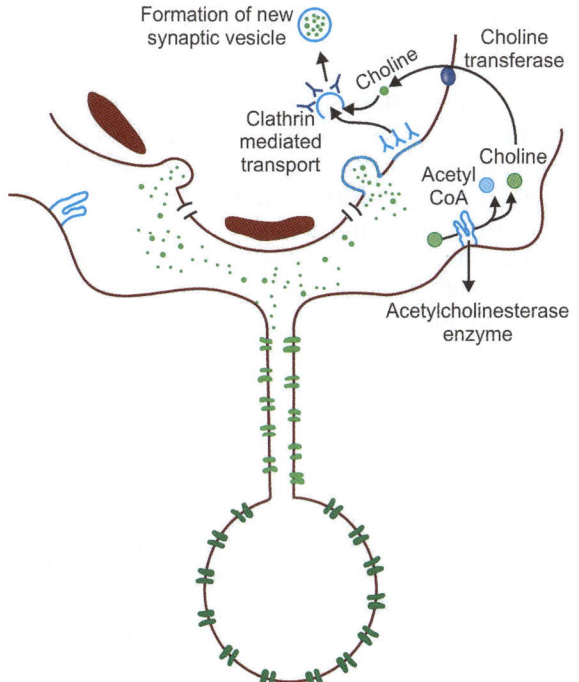

Fig. 26.5: Events occurring in synaptic cleft.

- This ACh is concentrated in the empty synaptic vesicles, either formed in the Golgi bodies present in the cell body of the neurons and transported to the nerve terminal or recycled by the clathrin mediated vesicular transport.

## Events Occurring in the Postsynaptic Membrane (Fig. 26.6)

- Binding of ACh molecules to the ACh gated $Na^+$ channels results in the $Na^+$ influx in the postsynaptic terminal
- This raises the voltage of the postsynaptic membrane/sarcolemma, to the firing/threshold level
- Opening of VGNC
- Further increase in the voltage resulting in the depolarization of the muscle and generation of action potential in the muscle.
- Hence, the action potential is transmitted to the muscle from nerve.
- The action potential generated in the muscle is called as motor end plate potential.
- Even at rest, a few synaptic vesicles keep on fusing with the presynaptic membrane resulting in the release of some ACh molecules and minimal voltage changes in

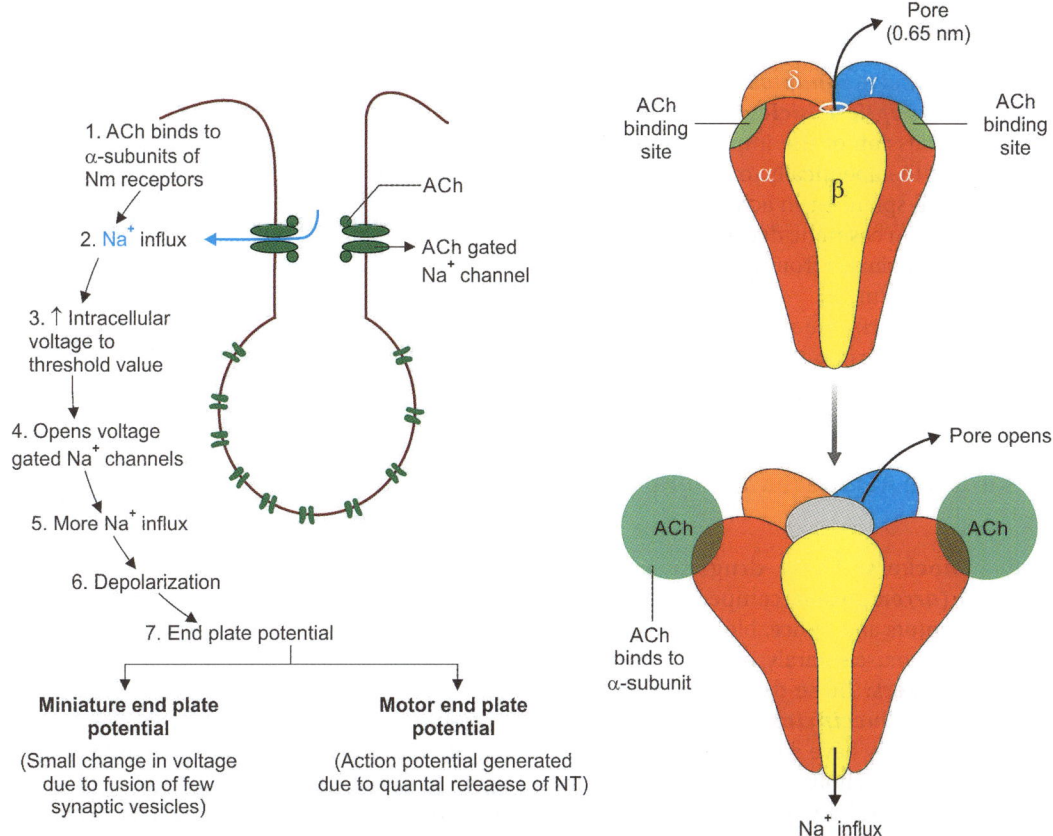

Fig. 26.6: Events occurring at postsynaptic membrane.
(NT: neurotransmitter)

postsynaptic membrane, called as the miniature end plate potential.

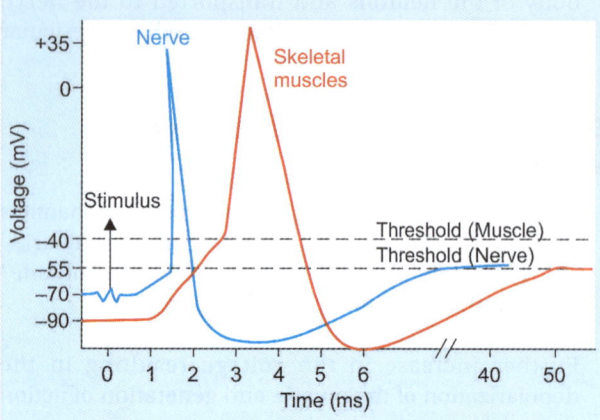

The above graph shows the difference in the action potentials of the nerve and the skeletal muscle. The duration of AP of nerve is 1–2 ms while that of skeletal muscle is 2–4 ms and it begins after a delay of around 0.5 seconds due to transmission of impulse across the NMJ.

## DRUGS ACTING ON NEUROMUSCULAR JUNCTION (FIG. 26.7)

### Drugs Blocking the Release of Neurotransmitter

- **Botulinum toxin:** Bind to *synaptobrevin* and *inhibits the docking of synaptic vesicles*. It results in the blockage of transmission of the impulse and muscle paralysis. It is used therapeutically to relieve the spasm of lower esophageal sphincter in achalasia cardia. It is also used now a day in cosmetic dermatology to get rid of the fine line and wrinkles from the face, commonly called as the botox treatment.
- **Hemicholinium:** It blocks the reuptake of the choline into the presynaptic terminal. This diminishes the renewal rate of the synaptic vesicles affecting the ACh release and hence the motor activity.

### Drugs Blocking the ACh-gated Sodium Receptors

- **Competitive blockers:** These drugs, curare and *d-tubocurarine (arrow poison)* competitively binds to the nicotinic receptors and hence, blocks the action of ACh resulting in the muscle paralysis.
- **Depolarizing blockers:** These drugs like *carbachol, methacholine and succinylcholine* binds to the nicotinic receptors. They have a longer half life as they are resistant to the acetylcholinesterase once they bind to the receptors, they result in the depolarization of the muscle. As these drugs stay attached to the receptors, they block the further action of the ACh, resulting in the muscle paralysis. Succinylcholine is used as an inducing agent for the general anesthesia.

### Acetylcholinesterase Inhibitors (Anti-acetylcholinesterase)

- **Reversible inhibitors:** These inhibitors (*neostigmine and physostigmine*) block the degradation of ACh and increases its half life. These drugs are used, whenever there is a requirement to increase the availability of ACh, as in treatment of myasthenia gravis (MG).
- **Irreversible inhibitors:** These drugs, *organophosphorus* compounds (OPC poisoning) bind irreversibly with the AChE inhibitors and result in the over exposure to the ACh in both the $N_M$ and $N_N$ receptors, resulting in increased muscular twitching, increased secretions, salivation, lacrimation, vomiting and diarrhea, etc.

> **Tetrodotoxin (TTX)** is a potent neurotoxin primarily found in certain species of pufferfish, as well as other marine organisms such as some species of newts, frogs, and octopuses. Its mechanism of action involves the *disruption of voltage-gated sodium channels*, which play a crucial role in the generation and propagation of action potentials in neurons and muscle cells.

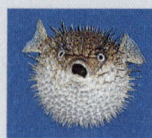

## DISORDERS OF NEUROMUSCULAR JUNCTION

The NMJ is an important conduit for passage of nerve impulse to the muscle for a useful activity. If there is any gap in the presynaptic and postsynaptic terminal, this transmission will be seriously hampered resulting in the muscular weakness. Though there are many such neuromuscular disorders which can be discussed in this heading, the most important pertaining to your current syllabus are MG and Lambert-Eaton Myasthenic syndrome (LEMS).

> **CLINICAL CASE SCENARIO**
>
> We will learn about the MG and LEMS, with this case study:
>
> **Patient presentation:**
>
> Mr Shastri, a 52-year-old male, presents to the neurology clinic with complaints of **muscle weakness** and **fatigue** that have been **progressively worsening over the past several months**. He reports experiencing **difficulty with activities such as climbing stairs, holding his arms up for extended periods, and speaking for prolonged periods**.
>
> **History of present illness:**
>
> Mr Shastri reports that his symptoms tend to **worsen as the day progresses**, particularly after physical exertion or prolonged periods of activity. He notes **intermittent double vision**, especially when looking to the sides, and **drooping of his eyelids (ptosis), which improves temporarily after resting**. He also mentions **difficulty swallowing**, particularly with solid foods.
>
> **Physical examination:**
>
> Upon examination, Mr Shastri is found to have **bilateral ptosis**, with the right eyelid drooping more prominently than the left. He also demonstrates **weakness in his extraocular muscles**, particularly evident when attempting to look laterally. His speech is **slurred and effortful**. Examination of his limb muscles reveals **generalized**

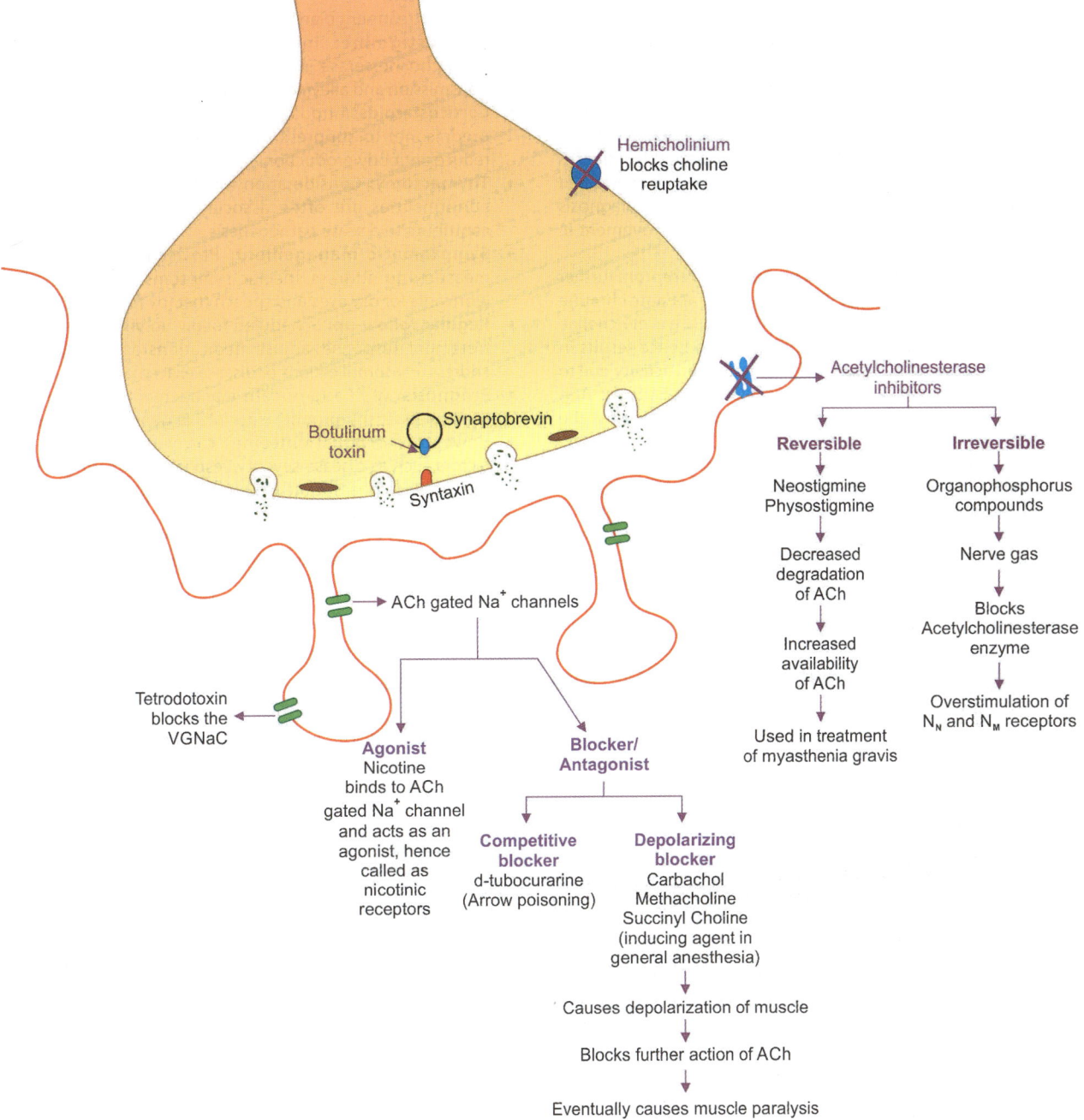

**Fig. 26.7:** Drugs acting on neuromuscular junction.

weakness, with greater involvement of the proximal muscles compared to distal ones. **Deep tendon reflexes are diminished throughout.**

Here, the presenting complaint of the patient is progressive muscle weakness, in which he has difficulty in doing the activities which require either the repetition or prolonged activity. Further, his history of present illness suggests that he is having the weakness of proximal muscles of the body resulting in weakness of extraocular muscles, which is causing diplopia and ptosis. He also finds difficulty in swallowing.

***Probable diagnosis***: All these clinical features are suggestive of neuromuscular disorder, where the initial motor activity is good but it becomes difficult for the patient to sustain the activity. It occurs due to depletion of the neurotransmitter at the NMJ. Hence our provisional diagnosis is neuromuscular disorder, which could be MG or LEMS. Hence to further strengthen our provisional diagnosis, we would conduct some diagnostic tests, shown below:

***Diagnostic workup:***
Based on the clinical suspicion of a NMJ disorder, Mr Shastri undergoes several diagnostic tests, including:

- **Edrophonium (tensilon) test:** Administration of edrophonium results in **temporary improvement of ptosis and muscle strength**

- ***Serum acetylcholine receptor antibody test:*** *Elevated levels of acetylcholine receptor antibodies*
- ***Electrodiagnostic test:*** *Demonstrates **decremental responses** on repetitive nerve stimulation.*
- Here the **edrophonium test/tensilon test** results in the improvement of the muscle strength and ptosis. Edrophonium is an anti-acetylcholinesterase, which inhibits the breakdown of the ACh in the synaptic cleft. This increases the half life of acetylcholine and its availability for sustained muscular activity. This supports our provisional diagnosis of MG. Edrophonium tests does not show improvement in LEMS.
- **Elevated levels of antibodies against ACh receptors** further strengthens our diagnosis and confirms its autoimmune nature. These antibodies block or damage the acetylcholine receptors on postsynaptic membrane and hence results in the muscle weakness especially on prolonged activity due to exhaustion of neurotransmitter. However, in LEMS, the ACh receptors are normal but there are antibodies against the VGCC on the presynaptic membrane.
- The **electrodiagnostic test** also shows a decremental response on repetitive nerve stimulation **(Fig. 26.8)**, which is suggestive of neurotransmitter exhaustion and hence MG. Whereas the LEMS shows exactly opposite, i.e., the incremental response on the repetitive nerve stimulation **(Fig. 26.9)**.

Hence, Mr Shastri is diagnosed with MG, an autoimmune disorder characterized by antibodies targeting the ACh receptors at the NMJ, leading to muscle weakness and fatigue.

*Treatment plan:*
Mr Shastri's treatment plan includes:
- **Pyridostigmine:** Initiation of pyridostigmine, an acetylcholinesterase inhibitor, to enhance neuromuscular transmission and alleviate symptoms.
- **Corticosteroids:** Introduction of corticosteroid therapy (e.g., prednisone) to suppress the autoimmune response and reduce antibody production.
- **Thymectomy:** Consideration for thymectomy, as thymic abnormalities are often associated with MG and may contribute to disease pathogenesis.
- **Symptomatic management:** Provision of supportive measures to address specific symptoms, such as ocular lubricants for dry eyes and speech therapy for dysarthria.
- **Regular follow-up:** Scheduled follow-up visits to monitor treatment response, adjust medications as needed, and address any complications or disease exacerbations.
- **Prognosis:** With appropriate management and ongoing medical care, the prognosis for MG is generally favorable. However, individual outcomes can vary depending on factors such as disease severity, response to treatment, and the presence of associated comorbidities. Close monitoring and collaboration between the patient, neurologist, and multidisciplinary healthcare team are essential for optimizing long-term outcomes and maintaining quality of life.

To sum up, both these clinical conditions.

## Myasthenia Gravis

It is an autoimmune disorder characterized by muscle weakness and fatigue due to antibodies attacking the ACh receptors at the NMJ. This interference disrupts the transmission of nerve impulses to muscles, leading to weakness that worsens with activity and improves with rest.

### Key Features

- **Muscle weakness:** MG commonly presents with proximal muscle weakness, i.e., muscles controlling eye movement (resulting in ptosis and diplopia), facial muscles, swallowing muscles, and limb muscles, nasal twang in speech.
- **Fatigability:** Symptoms worsen with exertion and typically improve with rest.
- **Thymus involvement:** Many patients with MG have an abnormal thymus gland, which plays a role in the immune system. Thymectomy may improve symptoms in certain cases.

### Diagnosis

Clinical evaluation, including physical examination and specialized tests such as the edrophonium (Tensilon) test, serum ACh receptor antibody test, and electrodiagnostic studies aids in diagnosis.

### Treatment

- **Acetylcholinesterase inhibitors:** Medications such as pyridostigmine enhance neuromuscular transmission, improving muscle strength.

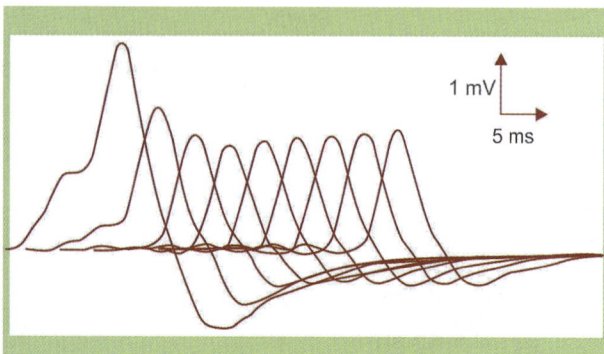

**Fig. 26.8:** Decremental response on repetitive nerve stimulation (RNS) in MG.

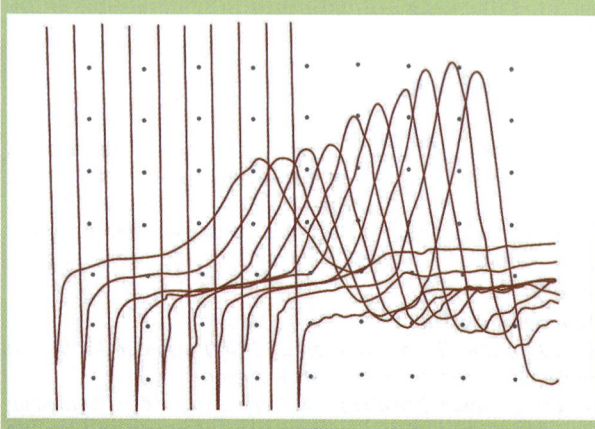

**Fig. 26.9:** Incremental response on RNS in LEMS.

- **Immunosuppressive therapy:** Corticosteroids, immunosuppressants, and other medications help suppress the autoimmune response.
- **Thymectomy:** Surgical removal of the thymus gland may be beneficial, especially in younger patients or those with thymoma.
- **Supportive measures:** Symptomatic treatments include ocular lubricants, speech therapy, and physical therapy to manage specific symptoms.

## Complication

Myasthenic crisis is a potentially life-threatening complication of MG. Myasthenic crisis occurs when muscle weakness becomes severe and affects vital muscles involved in breathing and swallowing, leading to respiratory failure or dysphagia with the risk of aspiration pneumonia.

## Lambert–Eaton Myasthenic Syndrome

It is a rare autoimmune disorder characterized by muscle weakness and fatigability resulting from antibodies targeting **VGCC at the presynaptic membrane of NMJ**. This leads to impaired release of ACh and subsequent muscle weakness **(Fig. 26.10)**.

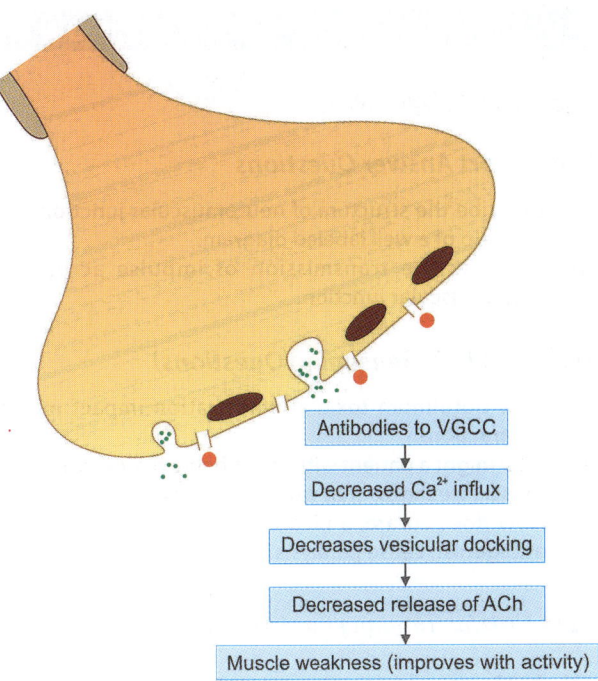

**Fig. 26.10:** Pathogenesis of Lambert–Eaton myasthenic syndrome.

### Key Features

- **Proximal muscle weakness:** LEMS typically affects the proximal muscles of the limbs, causing difficulty with activities such as climbing stairs, rising from a seated position, and lifting objects.
- **Autonomic symptoms:** Patients may experience symptoms related to autonomic dysfunction, such as dry mouth, constipation, and erectile dysfunction.
- **Characteristic electrophysiological findings:** Electromyography (EMG) typically reveals a characteristic pattern of low-amplitude compound muscle action potentials (CMAPs) with incremental response following rapid nerve stimulation.

### Treatment

- **Symptomatic therapy:** 3,4-diaminopyridine (3,4-DAP) improves neuromuscular transmission by prolonging the action potential, leading to increased ACh release.
- **Immunosuppressive therapy:** Corticosteroids, immunosuppressants, and intravenous immunoglobulin (IVIG) may be used to modulate the autoimmune response.

---

### SUMMARY

- The chapter begins by elucidating the intricate anatomy of the NMJ, where motor neurons innervate skeletal muscle fibers. Detailed descriptions of presynaptic terminals, synaptic vesicles containing ACh, postsynaptic membrane with ACh receptors, and synaptic cleft structure are provided. Emphasis is placed on the crucial role of ACh in neurotransmission and muscle contraction.
- The process of neuromuscular transmission is explored, highlighting the sequential events leading to muscle contraction. This includes depolarization of the presynaptic terminal, calcium influx, vesicle fusion, ACh release, binding of ACh to receptors, generation of end plate potentials, propagation of action potentials along the muscle membrane, and release of calcium from sarcoplasmic reticulum leading to muscle contraction.
- The chapter delves into the mechanisms of action of neuromuscular blocking agents (NMBAs), including depolarizing and nondepolarizing agents. Detailed explanations are provided regarding how these agents interfere with neuromuscular transmission, leading to muscle paralysis.
- The chapter concludes with an in-depth exploration of disorders affecting the NMJ, such as MG and LEMS. The pathophysiology underlying these disorders, including autoimmune dysfunction, antibody-mediated destruction of ACh receptors, VGCC dysfunction, and genetic mutations affecting neuromuscular transmission, is elucidated. Clinical manifestations of these disorders, including muscle weakness, fatigue, ptosis, diplopia, and respiratory compromise, are explained in relation to the underlying pathophysiological mechanisms.
- In summary, this chapter provides a comprehensive understanding of the NMJ physiological anatomy, transmission mechanisms, pharmacological modulation, and the pathophysiology of disorders affecting its function.

# LET US SEE, HOW MUCH YOU HAVE LEARNT?

## Review Questions

### Long/Short Answer Questions

Q1. Describe the structure of neuromuscular junction with the help of a well labeled diagram.
Q2. Describe the transmission of impulse across the neuromuscular junction.
Q3. Describe the physiological basis of various neuromuscular blocking agents.
Q4. Describe the physiological basis of clinical features of myasthenia gravis.

### Explain Why? (Reasoning Questions)

Q1. How botulinum toxin administration impact muscle contraction?
Q2. Why might a patient with myasthenia gravis experience muscle weakness that worsens with activity?
Q3. How does curare, a nicotinic acetyl choline receptor antagonist, cause paralysis?
Q4. Why might a patient with botulism present with flaccid paralysis?
Q5. Why succinyl choline is used as inducer in general anesthesia?

## Critical Thinking Case-Based Questions

Q1. A 28-year-old female, presented to the OPD with muscle weakness, especially in her arms and legs, which worsens with activity and improves with rest. She also reports difficulty swallowing and occasional drooping of her eyelids. After a series of tests, she is diagnosed with an autoimmune disorder affecting the neuromuscular junction.

Based on the given scenario, answer following questions:
a. What is the probable diagnosis in this case?
b. Explain the physiological mechanisms of the neuromuscular junction in this condition.
c. What are the physiological consequences of impaired neuromuscular transmission on muscle function?
d. Describe the treatment for this patient.

## Multiple Choice Questions

Q1. Which of the following components is primarily responsible for the release of acetylcholine at the neuromuscular junction?
   a. Synaptic cleft
   b. Presynaptic terminal
   c. Postsynaptic membrane
   d. Motor end plate

Q2. Which of the following events occurs first during neuromuscular transmission?
   a. Release of acetylcholine
   b. Depolarization of the motor end plate
   c. Calcium influx into the presynaptic terminal
   d. Generation of end plate potentials

Q3. Which class of neuromuscular blocking agents acts by depolarizing the motor end plate and causing sustained muscle depolarization?
   a. Nondepolarizing agents
   b. Competitive inhibitors
   c. Depolarizing agents
   d. Nicotinic antagonists

Q4. Myasthenia gravis is primarily characterized by the production of antibodies against which of the following targets at the neuromuscular junction?
   a. Acetylcholinesterase
   b. Voltage-gated sodium channels
   c. Acetylcholine receptors
   d. GABA receptors

Q5. A patient presents with drooping eyelids, double vision, and difficulty swallowing that worsens with activity. Which disorder of the neuromuscular junction is most likely responsible for these symptoms?
   a. Lambert–Eaton myasthenic syndrome (LEMS)
   b. Botulism
   c. Myasthenia gravis
   d. Congenital myasthenic syndrome

Q6. A patient undergoing surgery receives succinylcholine as part of their anesthesia induction. This medication acts as a neuromuscular blocking agent by:
   a. Blocking acetylcholine receptors
   b. Stimulating acetylcholine release
   c. Blocking voltage-gated sodium channels
   d. Depolarizing the motor end plate

Q7. A patient with Lambert–Eaton myasthenic syndrome (LEMS) experiences transient improvement in muscle strength after vigorous physical activity. This phenomenon is most likely due to:
   a. Increased acetylcholine release
   b. Enhanced neuromuscular transmission
   c. Augmented calcium influx into the presynaptic terminal
   d. Potentiation of voltage-gated sodium channels

Q8. A patient presents with muscle weakness and autonomic symptoms, such as dry mouth and constipation. Electromyography (EMG) reveals characteristic low-amplitude compound muscle action

potentials (CMAPs) with incremental response following rapid nerve stimulation. Which disorder of the neuromuscular junction is most likely responsible?
a. Myasthenia gravis
b. Lambert–Eaton myasthenic syndrome (LEMS)
c. Botulism
d. Congenital myasthenic syndrome

Q9. Which of the following medications is commonly used as an acetylcholinesterase inhibitor in the treatment of myasthenia gravis to enhance neuromuscular transmission?
a. Rocuronium
b. Vecuronium
c. Pyridostigmine
d. Succinylcholine

Q10. In the context of neuromuscular junction disorders, which of the following diagnostic tests is most specific for confirming the presence of acetylcholine receptor antibodies?
a. Electromyography (EMG)
b. Serum acetylcholinesterase levels
c. Edrophonium (Tensilon) test
d. Serum acetylcholine receptor antibody test

Q11. Which of the following is a potential complication of myasthenia gravis that may require urgent intervention?
a. Bradycardia
b. Hypertension
c. Myocardial infarction
d. Myasthenic crisis

Q12. What is the primary mechanism of action of botulinum toxin, the causative agent of botulism, at the neuromuscular junction?
a. Inhibition of acetylcholine release
b. Blockade of acetylcholine receptors
c. Stimulation of neuromuscular transmission
d. Enhancement of voltage-gated sodium channels

## ANSWERS

1. b    2. c    3. c    4. c    5. c    6. d    7. b    8. b    9. c    10. d    11. d    12. a

# Muscle: Structure, Properties and Physiology of Muscle Contraction

## 27 CHAPTER

### COMPETENCY ADDRESSED

**PY3.7:** Describe the different types of muscle fibers and their structure.
**PY3.8:** Describe action potential and its properties in different muscle types.
**PY3.9:** Describe the molecular basis of muscle contraction in skeletal and in smooth muscles.
**PY3.17:** Describe strength-duration curve.
**PY3.10:** Describe the mode of muscle contraction (isometric and isotonic).
**PY3.11:** Explain energy source and muscle metabolism.
**PY3.12:** Explain the gradation of muscular activity.
**PY3.13:** Describe muscular dystrophy: Myopathies.

### LEARNING OBJECTIVES

**At the end of this chapter, the learner should be able to:**
- Describe the structure of different types of muscle fibers (skeletal, cardiac and smooth muscle).
- Describe the electrical properties (action potential) of different types of muscle fibers.
- Describe the molecular basis of the muscle contraction using excitation contraction coupling mechanism, sliding filament theory and walk along theory.
- Describe the different types of muscle contractions and differentiate between them.
- Describe the energy sources and metabolism for muscle contraction.
- Describe the motor unit and grades of muscle power.
- Describe the muscular dystrophy: Pathophysiology of clinic laboratory findings.

The muscular tissue is the excitable tissue which shows the contractile response when stimulated by electrical, chemical or mechanical stimuli. The muscular tissue is broadly classified as **Table 27.1**:
- **Skeletal muscle:** The muscles which are attached to the skeleton and are responsible for the voluntary activity/locomotion/physical work.
- **Cardiac muscle:** This muscle is present in the heart
- **Smooth muscle:** This muscle is present in the hollow viscera like gastrointestinal system, blood vessels etc.

## STRUCTURE OF THE MUSCLE

### SKELETAL MUSCLE

The skeletal muscle is present attached to skeleton and serves the main function arranged in fascicles/bundles. These fascicles are formed of parallelly arranged muscle fibers which are connected by layers of connective tissue layers.

- The connective tissue layers are *epimysium* (present around the muscle), *perimysium* (present around each fascicle) and *endomysium* (surrounding each muscle fiber).
- These layers are made up of *collagen* and *elastin* which increases the efficiency of these muscles.
- The *perimysium contains blood vessels* and *nerves* supplying the muscle fibers.
- Skeletal muscles are attached to bones by collagen fibers called tendons.

The basic molecular structure of these three muscles is same but has few structural peculiarities which differentiates one type of muscle from other.

### MUSCLE PROTEINS

The muscle proteins form the basic building blocks of all types of muscles. These are contractile proteins: actin, myosin, and regulatory proteins: troponin and tropomyosin and various attachment proteins.

Table 27.1: Different types of muscles.

| | Skeletal muscle | Cardiac muscle | Smooth muscle |
|---|---|---|---|
| Location | Attached to skeleton | Present in heart | • **Single unit smooth muscle:** Present in hollow viscera, e.g., GIT, uterus, etc.<br>• **Multiunit smooth muscle:** Blood vessels, piloerector muscle, Iris in eye |
| Shape | Cylindrical, non-branched (1–40 mm long and 50–100 μ in diameter) | Short cylindrical, branching present (100 μ long and 15 μ in diameter) | Spindle shaped with variable size |
| Nucleus | Multinucleated | Single nucleus | Single nucleus |
| Striations | Present | Present | Unclear, almost appear smooth |
| Light microscopic structure | | | |
| Intercalated discs | Absent | Present at the point of contact of two muscle fibers | Absent |
| Gap junctions | Absent | Gap junctions present in intercalated discs | Gap junctions present |
| Syncytial structure | Absent | Functional syncitium due to gap juctions. The ionic movement across the various cells result in spread of impulse across the entire muscle | Functional syncitium due to gap juctions. The ionic movement across the various cells result in spread of impulse across the entire muscle |

## Actin

The actin filament is formed by two F-actin filaments, coiled around each other. Each F-actin is formed by the globular G-actin molecules **(Fig. 27.1)**.

- The actin molecules have myosin binding sites called the *active sites of actin filaments*. These sites are actually the ADP binding sites present on the G-actin molecule. These active sites are 2.7 nm apart.

> Metaphorically, the G-actin molecules, if considered as a pearl then the F-actin filaments appear as pearl strings. The actin filament appears as two pearl strings coiled around each other.

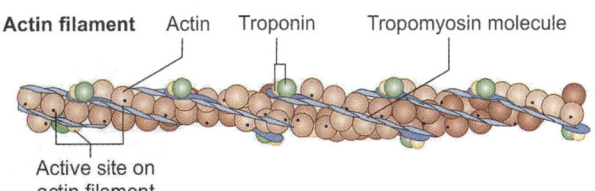

**Fig. 27.1:** The molecular structure of actin filament, tropomyosin and troponin.

- The actin filaments has a *troponin binding site* which binds to troponin I.
- It also has a *tropomyosin binding site*.

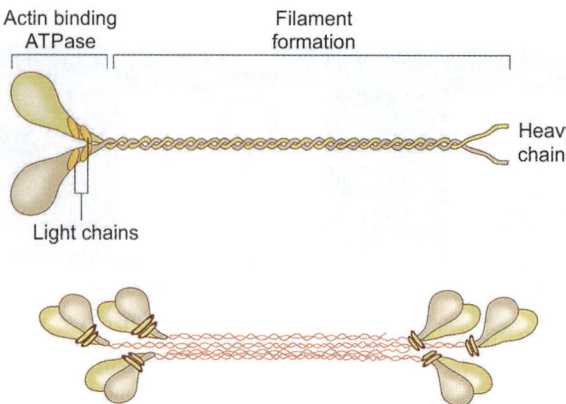

Fig. 27.2: The molecular structure of myosin filament.

## Myosin

The myosin is made up of bundles of polymers of myosin II molecules (M.wt. 480,000). The length of the myosin molecule is 1.6 μm. These myosin filaments are composed of six polypeptide chains **(Fig. 27.2)**:

- **Heavy chains:** The two heavy chains (M.wt. 200,000) intertwine to form the tail of the myosin filament. One end of each of these chains is folded to form the globular myosin head.
- **Light chains:** There are four light chains (M.wt. 20,000). The four light chains also form the part of myosin head. The light chains control the function of head during muscle contraction.

## Organization of Myosin Filaments (Fig. 27.3)

Each myosin filament is a bundle of myosin >200 myosin filaments. The tails of the myosin filaments are bundled up forming the body of the myosin filament while the heads of myosin filaments hang outwards with the arm. The protruding arms and heads together are called as *crossbridges*. These crossbridges are flexible at two points, called hinges (at the place where the filament leaves the body of filament and other at the attachment of head). If we put up all these polymers of myosin molecules together, we get a myosin filament, which is twisted in a way so that every myosin head/crossbridge is located at an angle of 120° from the previous pair. This twisting further ensures that the crossbridges are present in all the directions around the filament. The ends of the myosin filaments are inserted on the M line. The myosin filaments from both sides are inserted in the midline, forming a bulge in the middle of myosin filament. Myosin heads on either side of M-line have opposite polarity. The myosin filaments are held in place by the attachment proteins.

*Each myosin head has:*
- At ATP binding site which has the ATPase activity which results in the cleavage of ATP to energize the contraction process.
- Actin binding site.

## Regulatory Proteins (Fig. 27.4)

- **Troponin:** It is a globular protein, which is formed by three components: Troponin I, troponin C and troponin T.
    - *Troponin T:* This component (M.wt. 30,000) of Troponin complex to tropomyosin.
    - *Troponin I:* Troponin I binds the troponin complex to actin.
    - *Troponin C:* This component of troponin complex (M.wt. 18,000) has a binding site for calcium.
- **Tropomyosin:** It is a filamentous protein, which is coiled around the actin filament in the groove of the actin helix. The tropomyosin covers the active site of actin filament. It does not allow the actin filaments to interact with myosin filaments and hence maintains a resting phase of the muscle.

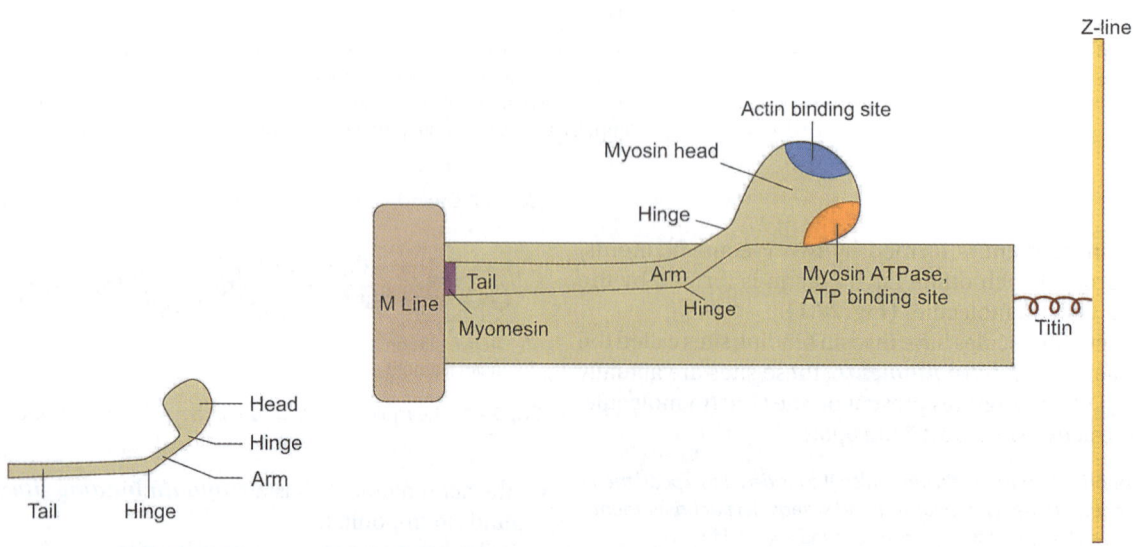

Fig. 27.3: Organization of myosin filament.

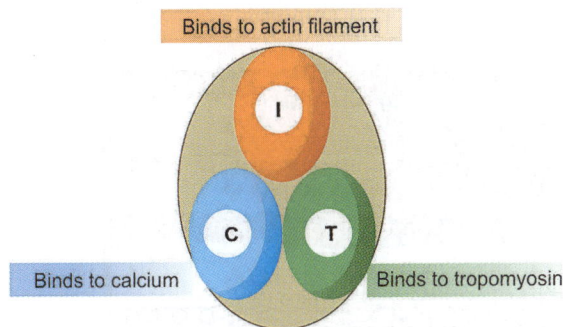

**Fig. 27.4:** Regulatory proteins.

## Attachment Proteins (Fig. 27.5)

- **Titin:** It is filamentous cytoskeletal protein extending from Z to M line. It maintains the length of A band. It prevents the extension of myosin filaments at the time of contraction.
- **Nebulin:** It stabilises the length of actin filaments. This protein is present along the length of actin filaments.
- **Desmin:** It connects Z line to sarcolemma. It also connects the myofibrils to each other.
- **Alpha actinin:** This protein anchors the actin filaments to the Z line.
- **Dystrophin:** It is a rod like cytoskeletal muscle protein which binds actin filaments to a membrane protein β-dystroglycan. It is also connected to dystrophin through another protein laminin present in extracellular matrix. The synthesis of these proteins is controlled by dystrophin gene. In the partial or complete absence of this gene, the child develops muscular dystrophy. We will study later about muscular dystrophy in detail.
- **Myomesin:** This protein binds the tail end of myosin polymer molecule to the M line in the middle.

## Sarcomere (Fig. 27.6)

It is the *structural and the functional unit of the muscle*/ myofibril. It is located *between two Z lines*. It is the basic contractile unit of muscle. The average length of the sarcomere is *2 μm*. A single myofibril is composed of thousands of sarcomeres, which are placed end to end.

The microscopic picture of sarcomere shows a zig-zag *Z line* (Zwischen line, a German word which means 'in between'), to which the actin filaments are attached by the protein alpha actinin. The thin filaments (composed of F actin, tropomyosin and troponin molecules) don't meet in the center and leave gap between two thin filaments. These thin filaments are arranged parallel to each other. These thin filaments are seen as light bands on light microscopy. They are also called as *I bands*.

The myosin filaments are thick and located in the middle of sarcomere, in between the parallel actin fibers. The thick filaments are held in place by titin and attached in the middle M line with myomesin. *The thick filament is 1.6 μm long and 10 nm thick.* They appear dark on light microscopy and hence form the A band. Typically, an A band comprise of myosin filaments and the ends of thin filaments. The A band shows a lighter colored band in the middle of A band called **H band**; which is formed by only thick filaments in the center. The thin filaments are not present in this area. However, in the middle of H band, there is dark line, **M line**, where the ends of myosin filaments are inserted.

## Arrangement of Thin and Thick Filaments in a Sarcomere (Fig. 27.7)

The thick and thin filaments follow a strict *hexagonal pattern*. Each thick filament is surrounded by six thin

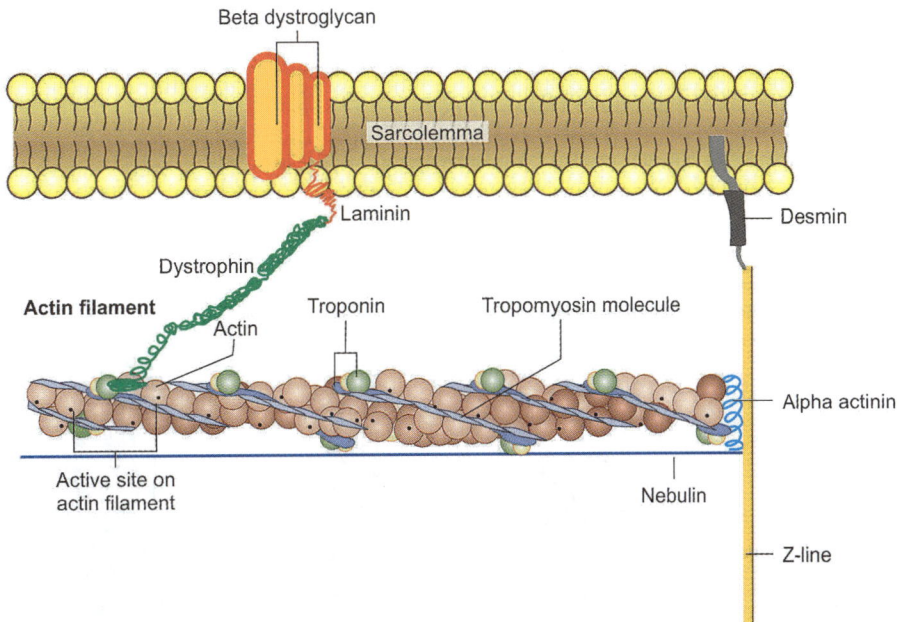

**Fig. 27.5:** Attachment proteins.

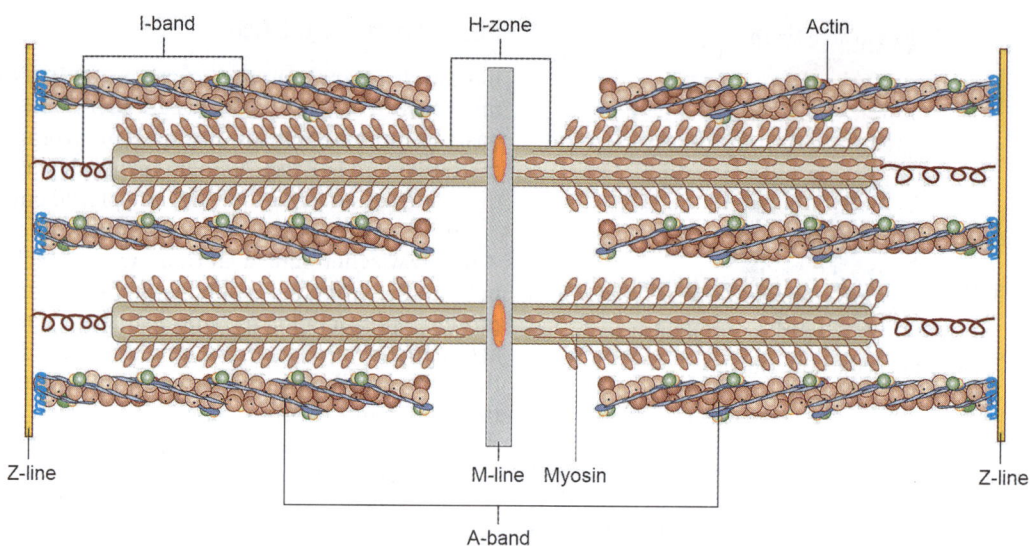

**Fig. 27.6:** Structure of sarcomere.

filaments and vice versa (**Fig. 27.7**). It is clearly seen in the cross section of the muscle fiber.

The heads of the myosin filaments are also projected out in all directions forming the maximum interactions between thick and thin filaments. These myosin heads are called crossbridges.

### Types of Muscle Fibers in Skeletal Muscle

The skeletal muscle has two types of fibers classified on the basis of their color, twitch duration and metabolism:
- Type I fibers/slow oxidative fibers/red muscle fibers
- Type II fibers/fast glycolytic fibers/white muscle fibers

The difference in these fibers is tabulated in **Table 27.2**.

## MYOFILAMENTS IN SMOOTH MUSCLES

There are three types of myofilaments (**Fig. 27.8**):
1. **Thick filaments:** Composed of myosin molecules, interspersed among thin filaments
2. **Thin filaments:** They are composed of actin and tropomyosin filaments. *Troponin is absent.*
3. **Intermediate filaments/dense bodies:** These are present in between the thick and thin filaments. The thin filaments are inserted on the dense bodies with the help of protein *α-actinin, hence are analogous to Z lines.*

These filaments are *arranged obliquely* to the long-axis of muscle and lack the organized arrangement present in skeletal muscle. The smooth muscle cells have the *gap junctions* present between them.

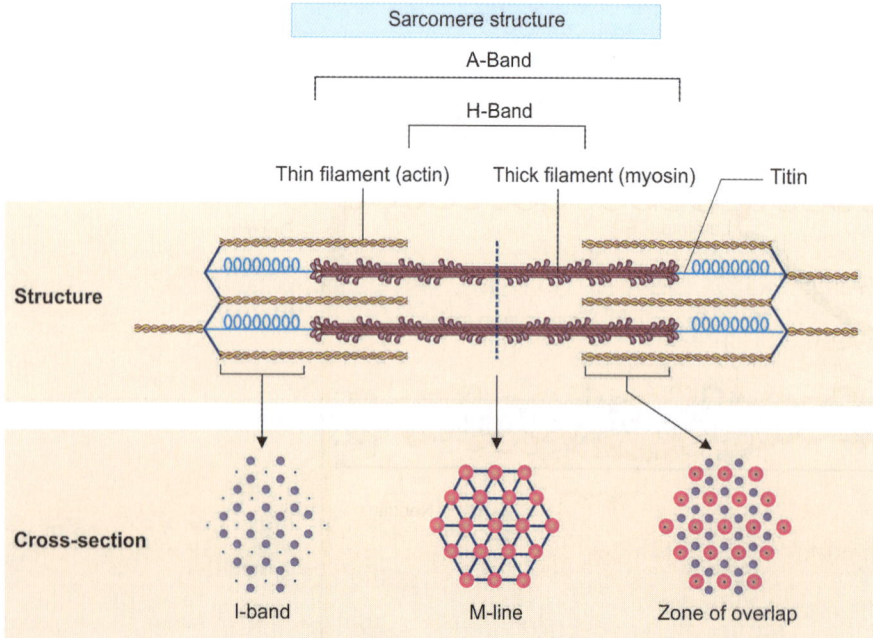

**Fig. 27.7:** Arrangement of thick and thin filaments.

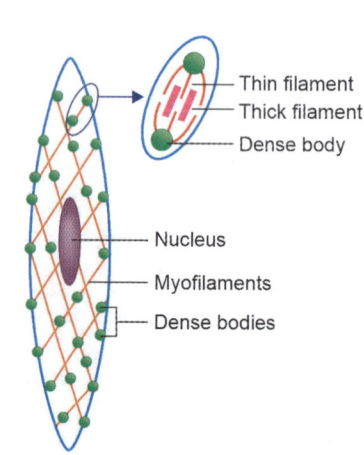

**Fig. 27.8:** Structure of myofilaments.

**Table 27.2:** Differences between type I and type II skeletal muscle fibers.

|  | Type I | Type II |
|---|---|---|
| Contraction velocity | Slow | Fast |
| Twitch duration | Less | More |
| Myosin ATPase activity | Low | High |
| $Ca^{2+}$ pumping capacity of SER | Low | High |
| Rate of fatigue | Slow | Fast |
| Diameter of muscle fiber | Moderate | Large |
| Mitochondria | Numerous | Less |
| Myoglobin content | High | Low |
| Glycogen content | Small | Large |
| Glycolytic capacity | Low | High |
| Oxidative capacity | High | Low |
| Source of ATP production | Oxidative phosphorylation | Glycolysis |
| Size of motor unit | Small | Large |
| Sites, where they are present | Postural muscles of back, limbs, etc. | Muscles of hand. Ciliary muscles. Extraocular muscles, etc. |

The differences in structure of different muscles are tabulated in **Table 27.3**.

Before we study the molecular mechanism of the muscle contraction, we should learn about the sarcotubular system.

## SARCOTUBULAR SYSTEM OF THE MUSCLE

The sarcotubular system is also called the sarcoplasmic reticulum, which is homologous to the endoplasmic reticulum of other cells. The sarcotubular system is well developed in skeletal muscle and has a typical arrangement. Differences with other muscles are mentioned in **Table 27.4**.

### SKELETAL MUSCLE

- They form longitudinal sarcoplasmic reticulum (LSR) and transverse tubules (T-tubules).
- The LSR forms the dilated sacs at the ends called terminal cisterns, which are present of either side of T tubules, as seen in **Figure 27.9**. It is the main site which stores the calcium for muscle contraction.
- The T tubules are the invaginations of cell membrane (sarcolemma) which extend deep down into the muscle, which take the electrical changes into the muscle fiber. These T tubules also communicate with the extracellular fluid.
- Hence, two terminal cisterns and one T tubule forms a triad.

### CARDIAC MUSCLE

Though the basic structure of the sarcotubular system in cardiac muscle is quite similar to skeletal muscle, but it is not so well organized.

**Table 27.3:** Structural differences between various types of muscles.

|  | Skeletal muscle | Cardiac muscle | Smooth muscle |
|---|---|---|---|
| Basic functional unit | Sarcomere | Sarcomere | Sarcomere |
| Contractile muscle proteins | Actin and myosin | Actin and myosin | Actin and myosin |
| Regulatory muscle proteins | Troponin and tropomyosin | Troponin and tropomyosin | Tropomyosin |
| Z-line | Present | Present | The dense bodies are present instead of the Z-lines. The actin filaments are inserted on the dense bodies |
| Direction of the sarcomere | Present along the length of the muscle fiber | Present along the length of the muscle fiber | Present obliquely |
| Result of contraction | Results in the longitudinal shortening of the muscle | Results in the longitudinal shortening of the muscle | Results in the oblique shortening of the muscle |

**Table 27.4:** Sarcotubular system of different type of muscles.

|  | Skeletal muscle | Cardiac muscle | Smooth muscle |
|---|---|---|---|
| Sarcoplasmic reticulum | Well developed, highly organized | Well developed, less organized | Poorly developed and rudimentary |
| T tubules | Well developed. Present at the junction of A and I bands | Well developed, present at the Z lines | Not present. Only small pits are present called caveolae |
| Source of calcium for muscle contraction | The calcium is stored in the terminal cisterns | Calcium stored in the T tubules. It communicates with the extracellular fluid | It is stored in the smooth muscle bound to the calmodulin |

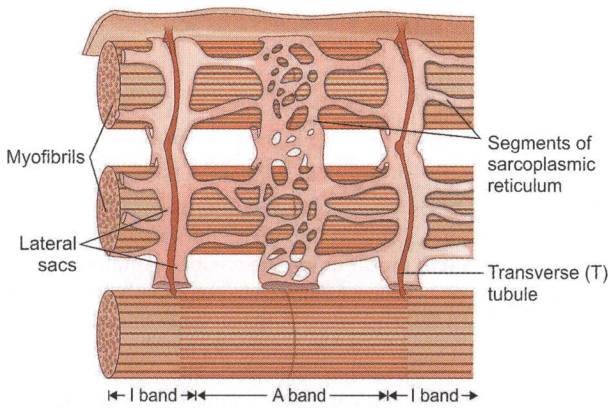

**Fig. 27.9:** Surface membrane of skeletal muscle fiber.

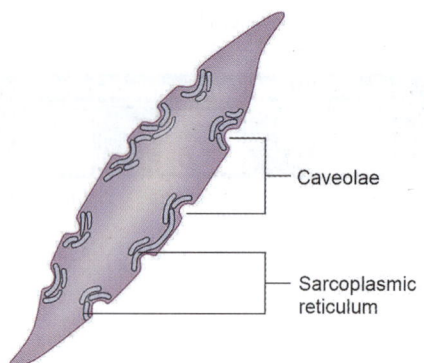

**Fig. 27.10:** Caveolae system in smooth muscle.

- The T-tubules are five times wide and has 25 times more volume as compared to skeletal muscle. In contrast to skeletal muscle, the T-tubules are the main site for storage of calcium. Since these T-tubules communicate with the extracellular fluid, the changes in serum calcium levels directly affect the cardiac muscle.

- The terminal cisterns and LSR is not well in cardiac muscle, so there are diads present instead of triads (as seen in skeletal muscle).

## SMOOTH MUSCLE

The sarcotubular system in smooth muscle is poorly developed and rudimentary.

- There are caveolae present in the cell membrane instead of T tubules **(Fig. 27.10)**.

## EXCITABILITY (ELECTRICAL PROPERTIES OF THE MUSCLES)

The muscular tissue is an electrically excitable tissue, which responds to the stimulation by contraction. Like the nervous tissue, the muscles also have the resting membrane potential due to the unequal distribution of the ions.

- The *resting membrane potential* of *skeletal and cardiac muscle* is nearly *–90 mV*.
- There as the *resting membrane potential* of the *smooth muscle* is not stable but varies between *–40 and –65 mV*.

---

**Motor Unit**

It is defined as a single alpha motor neuron arising from the anterior horn cell of spinal cord, innervating all the muscle fibers by it.

**Properties of motor unit:**
- **Size of motor unit:** The number of muscle fibers innervated by the alpha motor neuron, determines the *size of the motor unit,* as small or large motor unit.
- **Asynchronous discharge:** Usually the motor units discharge **Asynchronously**, i.e., they do not get activated together, rather the motor units get stimulated one after the other resulting in continuous and smooth activity The stimulation of one motor unit results in a sub tetanic contraction of the muscle fibers, resulting in a jerky movement. However the asynchronous discharge, results in fusion of these sub tetanic contractions resulting in a smooth, nonjerky contraction. But this contraction is not spasmodic, as it allows the muscle fibers to relax in between.

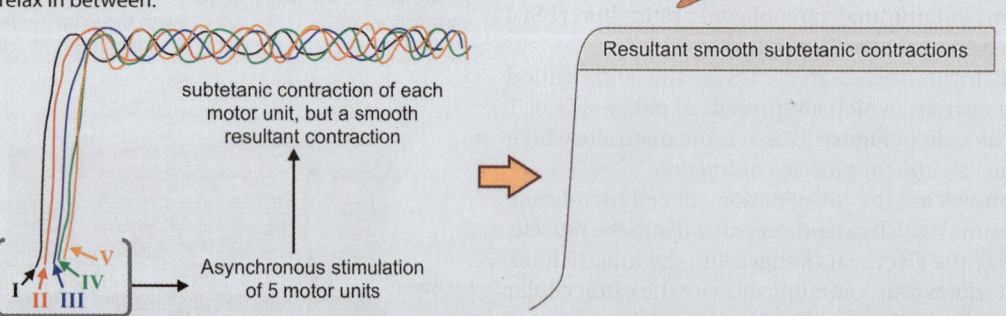

If we stimulate just 5–6 motor units also, it would result in a resultant smooth sub tetanic contraction. Whereas in reality, there are thousands of motor units resulting in the muscle contraction.

- **Recruitment of motor units:** The number of motor units activated during a muscular contraction depends upon the force required to accomplish that task, **e.g.** What do you think is the difference between pat and slap, when both require a same action?
*A pat requires less force; hence a smaller number of motor units are stimulated whereas slap requires larger force, which activates a greater number of motor units.* The increase in activation of a greater number of motor units, depending upon the intended action is called *recruitment of motor units*.

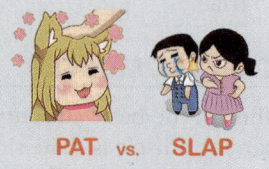

- **Grading of muscle power:** The muscular power is graded on the bases of number of recruited motor units. Hence, a normal muscular power is graded as Grade 5. The various other grades of power are mentioned below:
  1. *Grade 5:* Person is able to contract his muscles against resistance and gravity with normal muscular power.
  2. *Grade 4:* Person is able to contract his muscles against resistance and gravity, with slightly less power than the normal.
  3. *Grade 3:* Person is able to contract his muscles against gravity but not against resistance.
  4. *Grade 2:* Person is not able to contract his muscles against either gravity or resistance.
  5. *Grade 1:* No contraction seen, only a flicker is seen as an attempt to contract.
  6. *Grade 0:* No contraction is seen.

The action potential generated in each of these muscles is different because of the difference in the functional requirement of these muscles. Let's discuss the action potentials of these muscles one by one.

## ACTION POTENTIAL OF SKELETAL MUSCLE

We have read in the chapter 3, that the impulse is transmitted from the nerve to the muscle through the neuromuscular junction. Hence, the action potential is generated in the skeletal muscle. The action potential is quite similar to the action potential of the nerve except that the duration here is almost double, i.e., 2 to 4 ms and the resting membrane potential is –90 mV, **Figure 27.11** compares the action potential of nerve and skeletal muscle on the time and voltage scale. The action potential of nerve is discussed earlier in chapter.

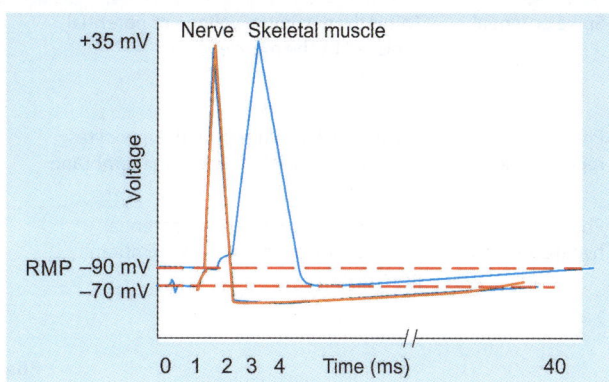

**Fig. 27.11:** Comparison of action potential of nerve with that of skeletal muscle.

### Phases of the Action Potential of Skeletal Muscle

There are five phases of the action potential in skeletal muscles. They are shown in **Figure 27.12** and their description is tabulated in **Table 27.5**.

## ACTION POTENTIAL OF THE CARDIAC MUSCLE

There are five phases of the action potential in cardiac muscles as seen in skeletal muscles but the graph and phases are different. They are shown in **Figure 27.13** and their description is tabulated in **Table 27.6**.

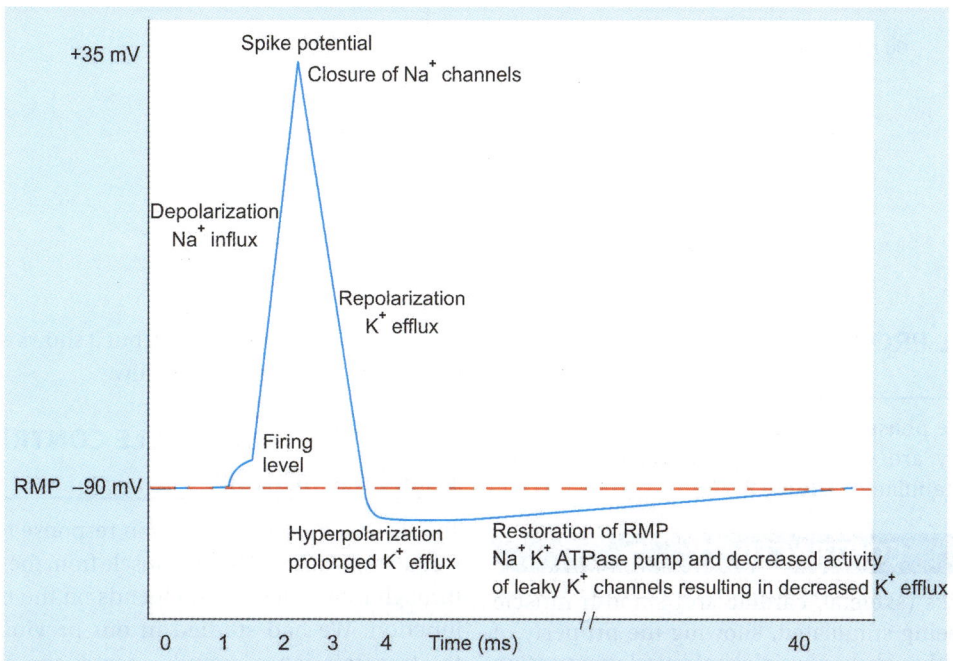

**Fig. 27.12:** Action potential phases and graph in skeletal muscle.

**Table 27.5:** Phases of action potential in skeletal muscle.

| Phase | Event | Physiological basis |
|---|---|---|
| Latent phase | It is the time taken by the muscle to show the electrical changes after this stimulation of nerve | It occurs due to the following reasons:<br>• Transmission of impulse from nerve to the neuromuscular junction<br>• Transmission of impulse across the neuromuscular junction to the sarcolemma |
| Phase of depolarization | Increase in the voltage (potential) of the muscle from the resting membrane potential due to the influx of positively charged $Na^+$ ions | $Na^+$ influx |
| Spike potential | This is the maximum voltage or potential achieved by the muscle | All the voltage-gated sodium channels are open resulting in the maximum sodium in flux. After this potential is achieved the sodium channels begin to close reducing the voltage. Also the potassium channels begin to open which result in potassium efflux |
| Phase of repolarization | The intracellular voltage of the myocytes begin to fall back to the resting membrane potential | The potassium efflux results in loss of positive ions from the muscle into the extracellular fluid which brings down the voltage back to the resting membrane potential |
| Phase of hyperpolarization | In this phase the voltage or potential decreases below the resting membrane potential | The continuous potassium a flux results in loss of positive ion from the cell into the ECF. This decreases the intracellular voltage below the resting membrane potential |

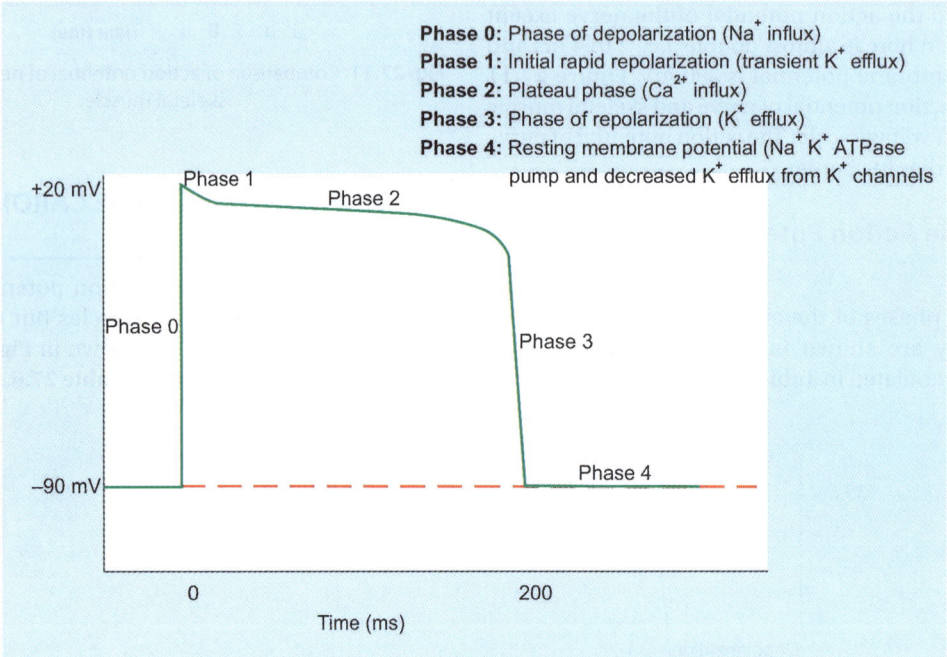

**Fig. 27.13:** Action potential phases and graph in cardiac muscle.

## ELECTRICAL PROPERTIES OF SMOOTH MUSCLE

There are three phases of the action potential in smooth muscles. They are shown in **Figure 27.14** and their description is tabulated in **Table 27.7**.

## CONTRACTILITY

All the muscles (skeletal, cardiac and smooth muscle contract on being stimulated, showing the property of contractility. Although the physiology of muscle contraction for all these muscles is similar, but it shows a little variation in each of them, discussed below.

## PHYSIOLOGY OF MUSCLE CONTRACTION IN SKELETAL MUSCLE

The skeletal muscle contracts in response to the electrical stimulation received by the muscle from the cerebral cortex through motor nerve, which ends on the neuromuscular junction. We had studied in our previous chapter 26, the transmission of impulse across the neuromuscular

**Table 27.6:** Phases of action potential in cardiac muscle.

| Phase | Event | Physiological basis |
|---|---|---|
| Phase of depolarization | Increase in the voltage (potential) of the muscle from the resting membrane potential due to the influx of positively charged Na⁺ ions | Na⁺ influx results in the increased concentration of positive ions in the cell resulting in depolarization |
| Initial rapid repolarization | After reaching the peak depolarization, the cardiac muscle begins to repolarize because of opening of transient potassium channels which results in transient potassium efflux | The opening up of transient potassium channels results in some fall in the intracellular voltage or potential of the cardiac myocyte |
| Plateau phase | In this phase, the voltage of the cell remains constant or shows no change for few hundred milliseconds | The slow calcium channels open and result in slow calcium influx. This maintains a positive intracellular voltage, i.e., in a depolarized stage. This stage is responsible for a prolonged phase of depolarization of few hundred milliseconds (100–150 ms in atria and 250–300 ms for ventricles) |
| Phase of repolarization | The intracellular voltage of the myocytes begin to fall back to the resting membrane potential | The potassium efflux results in loss of positive ions from the muscle into the extracellular fluid which brings down the voltage back to the resting membrane potential |
| Phase of hyperpolarization | In this phase the voltage or potential decreases below the resting membrane potential | The continuous potassium efflux results in loss of positive ion from the cell into the ECF. This decreases the intracellular voltage below the resting membrane potential |

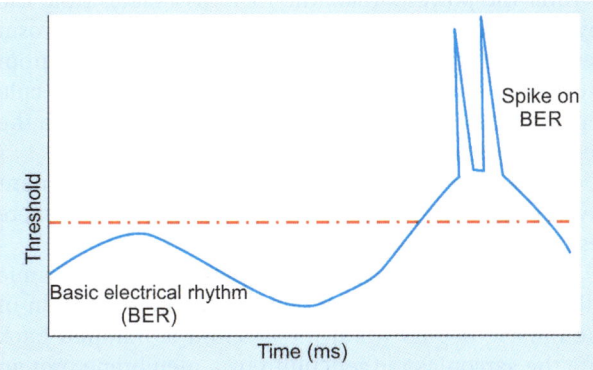

**Fig. 27.14:** Action potential graph in smooth muscle.

**Table 27.7:** Phases of action potential in smooth muscle.

| Phase | Event | Physiological basis |
|---|---|---|
| Resting membrane potential | Ranges from –30 to –70 mV with an average of –50 mV | Spontaneous wave like pattern |
| Basic electrical rhythm (BER) | • It is similar to pacemaker potentials<br>• The upstroke of BER is considered as depolarization with low amplitude of around 60 mV and prolonged duration of around 100 ms<br>• The repolarization phase is the downstroke of BER, which is also slow to take place | • Depolarization is caused by Ca²⁺ influx due to opening of voltage-gated Ca²⁺ channels<br>• Repolarization is caused by closure of voltage-gated Ca²⁺ channels and opening of K⁺ channels resulting in K⁺ efflux |
| Spike on plateau | The spike potential are seen overlapping on the BER, having depolarization and repolarization phase similar to the other spike potentials | |

junction. The impulse transmitted to muscle results in the excitation of skeletal muscle resulting in the action potential, which brings about the muscle contraction.

## Sliding Filament Theory (Fig. 27.15)

When the muscle contracts, it leads to the shortening of the sarcomere. A length of resting sarcomere is 2 μ, while maximally shortened sarcomere is around 1 μ and stretched sarcomere is around 3.5 μ. During the muscular contraction the thin filaments move toward the center of the sarcomere, pulling the two Z lines together, thus shortening the length of the sarcomere.

If we observe a contracting muscle under a light microscope, we will observe that the *I band shortens* due to the movement of thin filaments toward each other, while the *length of a band remains constant*. This mechanism of contraction has been called as *sliding filament theory* based on the appearance of muscle during the contraction,

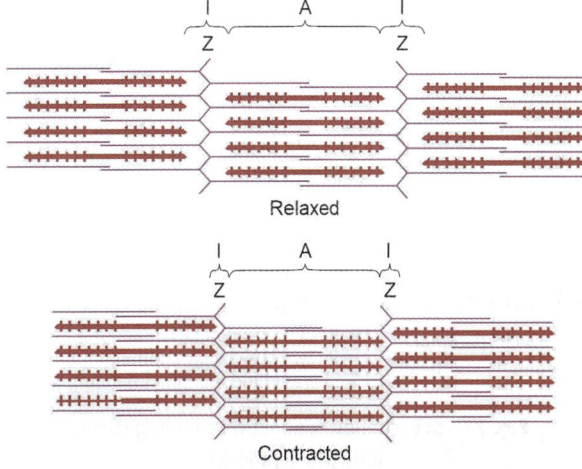

**Fig. 27.15:** Sliding filament theory.

in which the thin filaments appear to be sliding over the thick filaments. This theory was proposed by *Sir AF Huxley in 1957*.

## Molecular Mechanism of Muscle Contraction

The muscle contraction is explained by the walk along theory of contraction, where the myosin head binds to the actin filament and appear to be walking on the actin filaments. Before we discuss the molecular walk along theory, lets learn about the excitation contraction coupling theory.

## Excitation Contraction Coupling Theory (Fig. 27.16, Flowchart 27.1)

This theory explains the mechanism of contraction after the electrical stimulation of the muscle.

**Excitation:** The excitation of muscle (action potential) spreads into the muscle through the T tubules. The T tubules have *voltage-gated calcium channels [The dihydropyridine receptors (DHP receptors)]*. These channels, when activated, open up the *ryanodine receptors* present on the terminal cisterns.

**Coupler:** Opening of DHP and ryanodine receptors opens the calcium channels in terminal cisterns. The calcium stored in lateral cisterns bound to *calsequestrin*. The calcium released from the terminal cisterns through the ryanodine receptor channels and entry of extracellular calcium through the DHP receptor channels result in *calcium spark* in cytoplasm. The calcium, thus binds to the troponin C subunit of troponin molecule and initiates the muscle contraction. *Hence, the calcium acts as the coupler; converting the excitation into contraction*.

**Contraction (Walk along theory/crossbridge theory/ratchet theory) (Fig. 27.17):** In the relaxed state, when the actin filaments are covered by tropomyosin, the myosin heads are energized by the hydrolysis of ATP. The myosin heads is cocked up and are held perpendicular to the tail of myosin filament. The myosin filament is ready to bind with the actin filament, as soon as actin filament is uncovered.

The calcium ions bind to troponin C subunit of troponin molecule. There is confirmational change in the troponin and tropomyosin molecules. The tropomyosin filaments slide away from its attachment on the actin filaments, uncovering its active sites (myosin binding sites). These sites are usually kept covered by tropomyosin, preventing the interaction between the actin and myosin filaments. Now, when these sites are uncovered, the myosin heads bind with actin filament, forming the *actomyosin complex or a crossbridge*.

The attached myosin head bend forward at an angle of 45°, pulling the actin filament along with it toward the center of the sarcomere by 11 nm. The movement of myosin head toward midline is called *crossbridge cycling* (Fig. 27.18). Sudden tilting of myosin head is called *power stroke*.

After the power stroke, the ADP dissociates from the myosin head and fresh ATP molecule binds to the myosin head leading to the detachment of the myosin head from the actin filament. The hydrolysis of fresh ATP molecule repeats the cycle, but now the myosin head binds to the next actin molecule.

Each crossbridge cycling moves the actin filament toward the center, which shortens the length of sarcomere resulting in the contraction.

The crossbridge cycling continues till the sarcoplasmic calcium concentration remains high. The relaxation of the muscle begins when the calcium is pumped back into the sarcoplasmic reticulum by a membrane protein called *sarcoplasmic endoplasmic reticulum calcium ATPase (SERCA)*. This pump relocates two molecules of calcium ions for one molecule of ATP into the terminal cisterns, where the calcium is stored bound to calsequestrin, until next contraction.

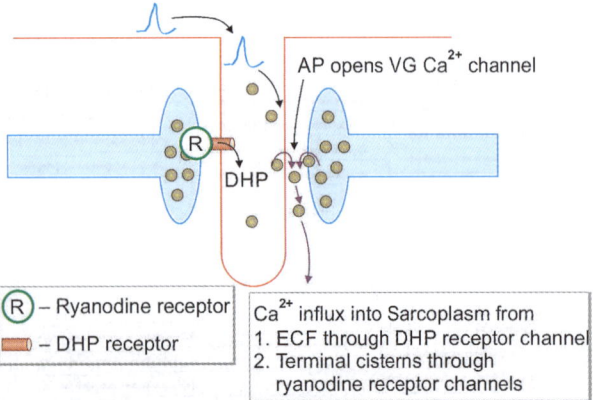

**Fig. 27.16:** Excitation contraction coupling theory.
(DHP: dihydropyridine)

---

### Rigor Mortis

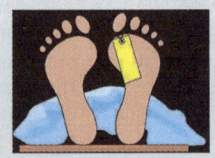

Rigor means 'stiffness' and mortis means 'death'; hence the muscular stiffness occurring in the body after death is called rigor mortis. We have read above that ATP is required for:

- Detaching the myosin head from the actin filaments during muscle contraction.
- Pumping out calcium from the muscle cell into the terminal cisterns.

Hence, the depletion of ATP after death results in failure to detach the crossbridges and the muscle remains in the state of contraction resulting in postmortem rigidity/rigor mortis. This rigidity sets in 3–6 hours after death and completes in about 12 hours. However, it disappears after 40–60 hours due to disintegration of muscle proteins.

The forensic experts use the rigor mortis to determine the time of death.

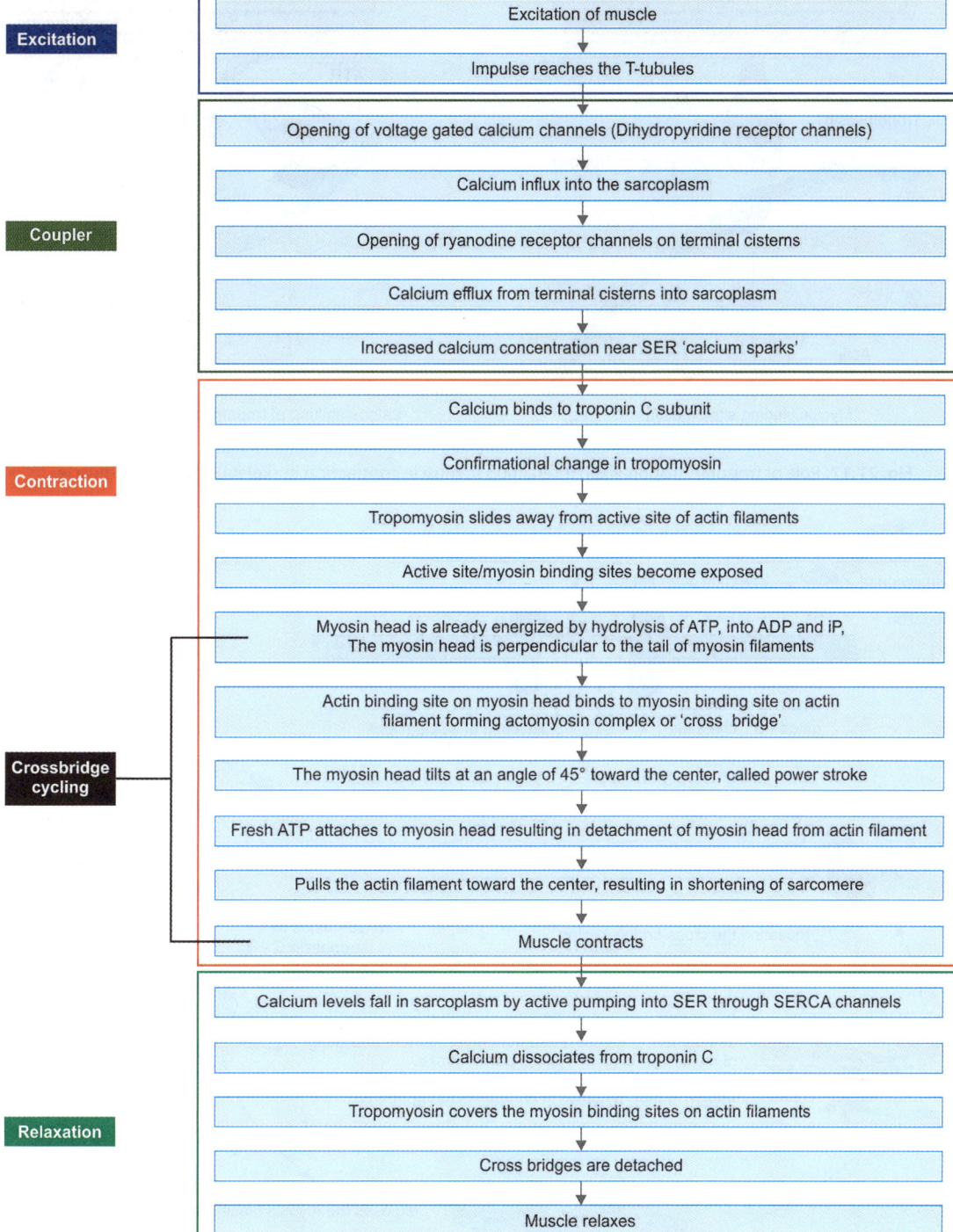

**Flowchart 27.1:** Excitation contraction coupling theory.

(SERCA: sarcoplasmic endoplasmic reticulum calcium ATPase)

## CONTRACTION IN CARDIAC MUSCLE

The mechanism of contraction in cardiac muscle is very similar to the skeletal muscle contraction. However, the differences are listed below:

- The T tubules are wider in cardiac muscle storing around 25 times more calcium as compared to the skeletal muscle. Hence, the T tubules are the main source of calcium instead of terminal cisterns.
- When the impulse, generated from SA node, reaches the T tubule, the DHP receptor channels open resulting in calcium influx into the sarcoplasm from the ECF. This results in the opening of the ryanodine receptor channels in terminal cisterns causing calcium efflux

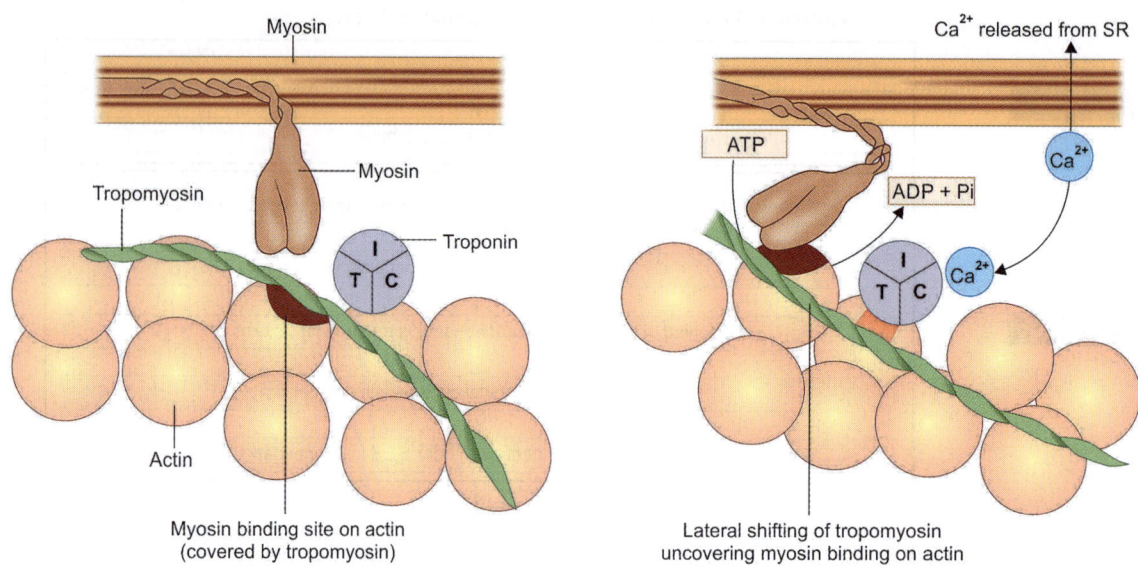

**Fig. 27.17:** Role of troponin-tropomyosin interaction in muscle contraction in skeletal and cardiac muscle.

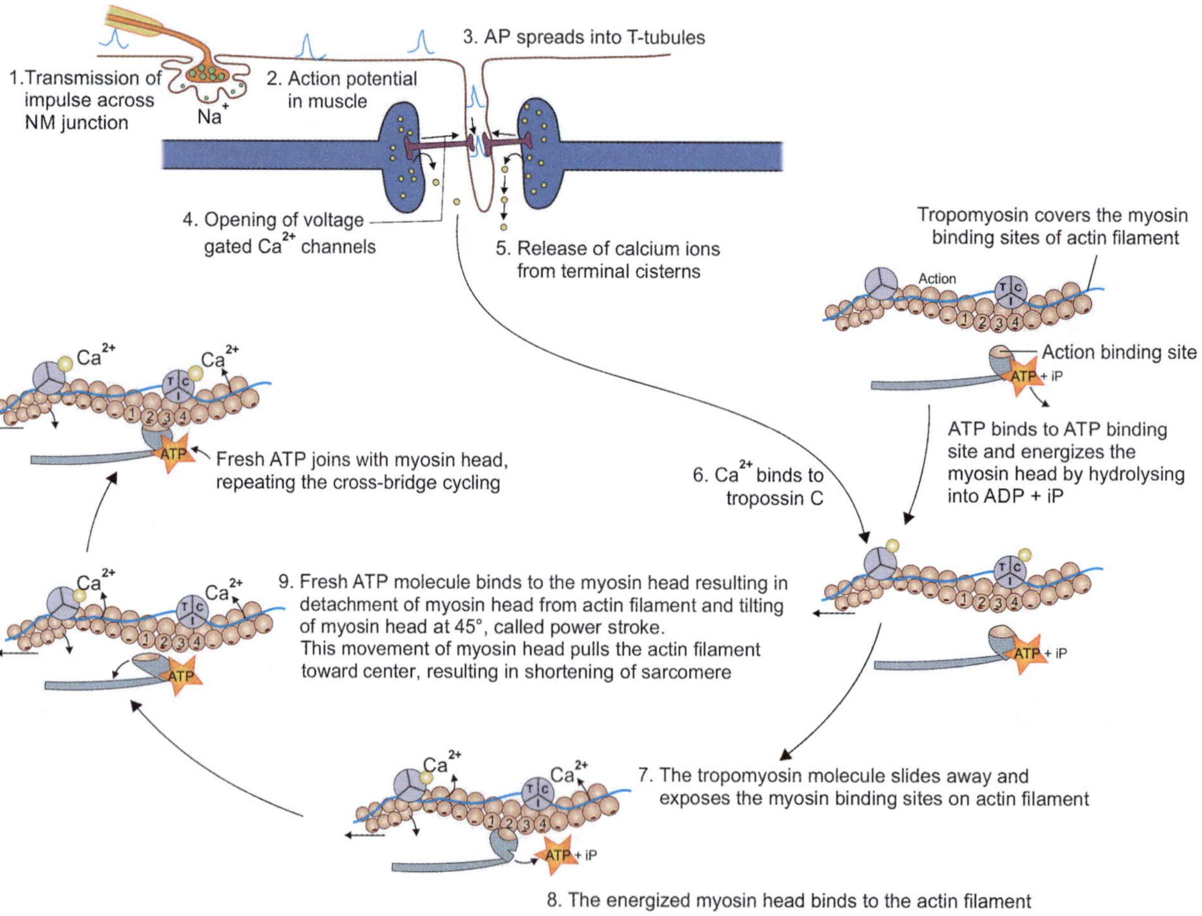

**Fig. 27.18:** Mechanism of crossbridge cycling.

from SR into sarcoplasm. Unlike skeletal muscle, the main source of calcium is ECF. This is called *calcium induced calcium release (CICR)*

- The rest of molecular mechanism of contraction is same as the skeletal muscle.

## CONTRACTION IN SMOOTH MUSCLE

Unlike the skeletal and cardiac muscle, the smooth muscle can get stimulated by the stretching of muscle, hormone, neurotransmitter or chemical changes in vicinity of

smooth muscle. Whatever, may be source of stimulation, the smooth muscle also shows contractile activity due to changes in sarcoplasmic calcium levels. The levels of calcium in the smooth muscle sarcoplasm increase by following mechanisms:
- **Calcium influx from the interstitial fluid** through the voltage-gated calcium channels and ligand gated calcium channels.
- **Calcium release from SR:**
  - *Calcium induced calcium release:* Calcium influx from interstitial fluid stimulates the release of calcium from SR.
  - Through *IP$_3$ mediated pathway*, which releases calcium from SR.

## Molecular Mechanism of Smooth Muscle Contraction (Flowchart 27.2)

- The four molecules of cytosolic calcium binds to one molecule calmodulin forming the *calcium calmodulin complex*, which activates the *myosin light chain kinase (MLCK)*, a Ca$^{2+}$ calmodulin dependent kinase.
- Activated MLCK *phosphorylates the myosin head*.
- It stimulates the *myosin ATPase activity*. It is a key step in the smooth muscle contraction.

- Increased myosin ATPase activity results in actin myosin crossbridge formation and crossbridge cycling occurs and shortening of muscle.
- The molecular mechanism of contraction remains same as the skeletal muscle.
- In the skeletal muscle, the contraction is regulated by the actin filaments *(actin linked regulation), i.e., actin filaments need to be activated by bringing* changes in regulatory proteins by calcium. Whereas, calcium ions need to activate the myosin head for smooth muscle contraction *(myosin-linked contraction)*.

For relaxation of smooth muscle, the *dephosphorylation of myosin chain* is brought about by *myosin light chain phosphatase (MLCP)*. The enzyme MLCP is active throughout the contraction and relaxation but in the presence of activated MLCK, the phosphorylation of myosin head is more than dephosphorylation, hence results in contraction. The decrease in cytosolic calcium reduces the MLCK activity and the myosin head dephosphorylates resulting in relaxation.

## RELATIONSHIP OF ELECTRICAL AND CONTRACTILE/MECHANICAL RESPONSE OF MUSCLES

### SKELETAL MUSCLE

We have discussed the action potential of skeletal muscle in section 3.7.3, the RMP of skeletal muscle is −90 mV, and duration of AP is 2–4 ms. The absolute refractory period (ARP) of skeletal muscle is 1–3 ms. The brief period of contraction followed by relaxation after the skeletal muscle stimulation is called a *simple muscle twitch (SMT)*.

**Figure 27.19** shows the AP and SMT on the same scale, which shows that the SMT begins after around 2 ms after the beginning of depolarization phase of AP. This delay is onset of SMT is called *latent period*. The physiological basis of latent period can be explained as:
- Transmission of impulse from NM junction to T tubules
- Release of calcium from SR
- Initiation of crossbridge cycling resulting in contraction

The other phases of SMT are:
- **Contraction phase:** The contractile process begins due to crossbridge cycling. The tension develops in the muscle. The contraction time is denoted from onset of contraction to peak of contraction.
- **Relaxation phase:** The relation phase is marked from peak to the end of the SMT.

*The total twitch duration ranges from 7.5 ms in fast muscles to 100 ms in slow muscle fibers.*

### CARDIAC MUSCLE

The cardiac muscle begins to contract *2 ms after the phase of depolarization* and completes its muscle twitch *in 200–300 ms*. Unlike AP of skeletal muscle, the ARP of cardiac muscle is very long which coincides with most of the contraction phase **(Fig. 27.20)**. This makes the cardiac

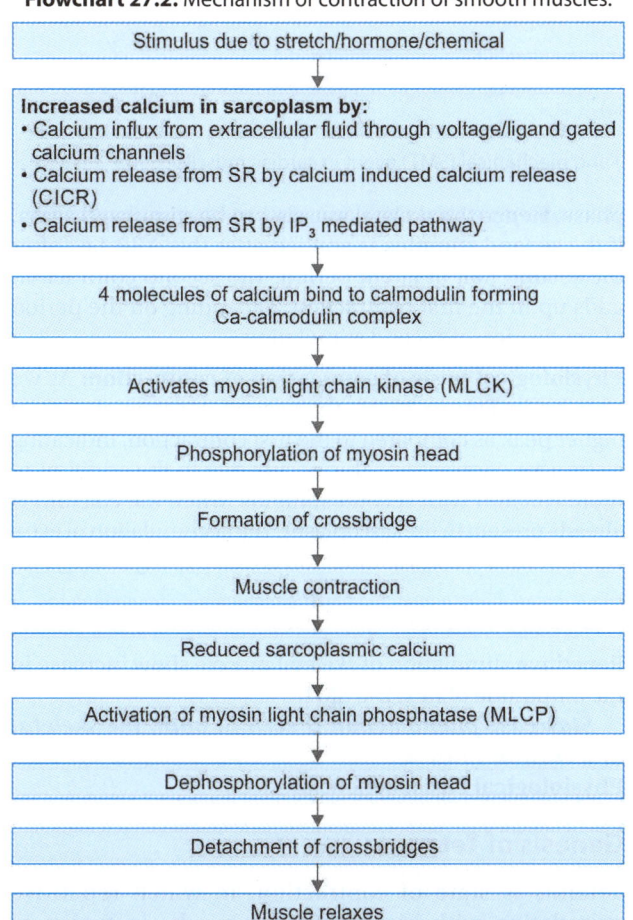

**Flowchart 27.2:** Mechanism of contraction of smooth muscles.

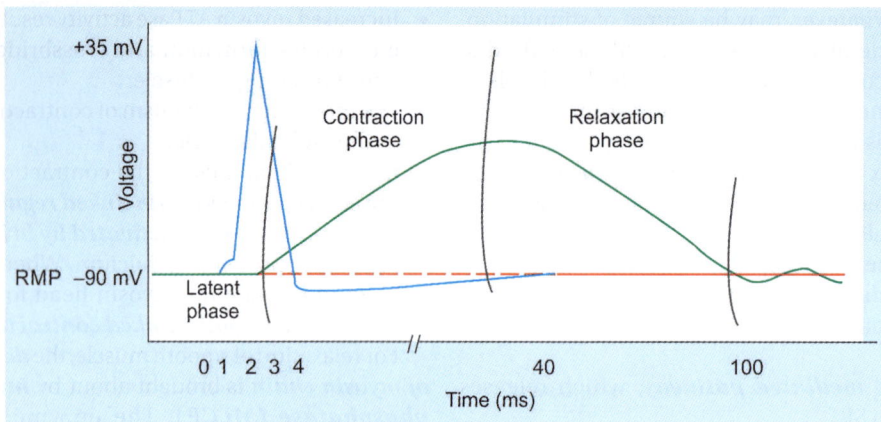

**Fig. 27.19:** Correlation of electrical (action potential) and mechanical (SMT) event in skeletal muscle.

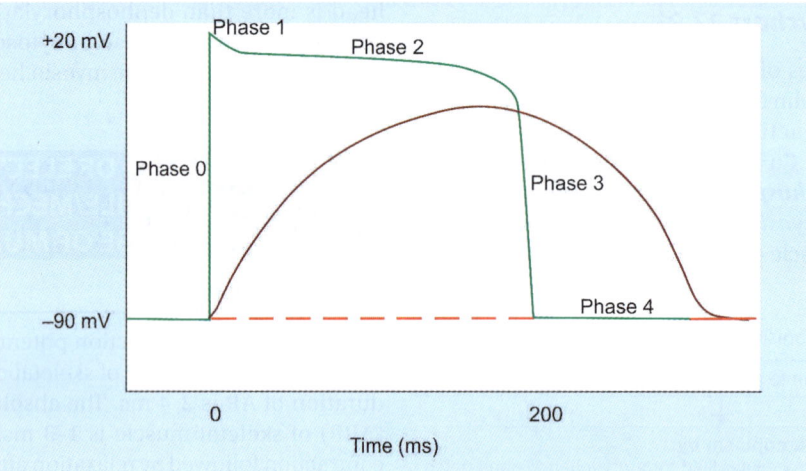

**Fig. 27.20:** Correlation of electrical (action potential) and mechanical (SMT) event in cardiac muscle.

muscle refractory to subsequent stimulations during systole and hence prevents it from getting tetanized.

## SMOOTH MUSCLE

The smooth muscles have a prolonged twitch time with slow latent phase of around 100–200 ms and contraction time of 200–500 ms. The relaxation phase can take few more 100 ms.

### CONTRACTILE PROPERTIES OF DIFFERENT TYPES OF MUSCLES

The contractile properties of three different types of muscles are shown in **Table 27.8**.

After the comparative chart, we will discuss all these properties one by one.

## PROPERTIES OF SKELETAL AND CARDIAC MUSCLES

### Summation of Contraction

As seen in **Figure 27.21**, the ARP of the action potential of the skeletal muscle coincides with the first half of the latent phase. Hence the skeletal muscle can be stimulated again, if the second stimulus is applied after this ARP, i.e., after the second half of latent period. The second contraction adds up in the first contraction, depending on the period of application of second stimulation.

**Physiological basis of summation of contraction:** As we observe in **Figure 27.21**, the second contraction shows higher peak as compared to the first contraction, indicating a stronger contraction. This occurs due to the addition of more calcium with second stimulus, when the calcium is already present in the sarcoplasm. The accumulation of extra calcium with second stimulation is called *beneficial effect*.

### Staircase Effect (Fig. 27.22)

Repetitive stimulation of skeletal muscle show increase in the amplitude of next 2–3 SMT.

*Staircase phenomenon is seen in both, the skeletal and cardiac muscle.*

**Physiological basis:** Beneficial effect.

### Genesis of Tetanus

Tetanus is state of contraction, in which repetitive stimulation with high frequency results in fusion of

Table 27.8: Contractile properties of different types of muscles.

| | Skeletal muscle | Cardiac muscle | Smooth muscle |
|---|---|---|---|
| Summation of contraction | Seen in skeletal muscle due to repetitive stimulation in contraction phase | Cannot be stimulated during contraction phase. Hence can't be seen | Very slow contractile process. May be present |
| Staircase phenomenon | Repetitive stimulation shows increase force of contraction due to beneficial effect | Repetitive stimulation shows increase force of contraction due to beneficial effect | Not seen |
| All or none law | Not present in the motor unit, but observed in a single muscle fiber | Observed in atria or ventricle because the cardiac muscle has gap junction and it behaves like syncytium | Observed due to gap junctions |
| Genesis of tetanus | Skeletal muscle can be tetanized | Cardiac muscle cannot be tetanized due to long refractory period. It can also be demonstrated by the extrasystole and compensatory pause | Cannot be demonstrated |
| Genesis of fatigue | When the nerve is repeatedly stimulated, it shows a phenomenon of fatigue due to exhaustion of neurotransmitter at neuromuscular junction | Cardiac muscle is not fatigued because it relaxes more (0.7 s for atria and 0.5 s for ventricles) than the contraction phase (0.1 s for atria and 0.3 s for ventricles) | Cannot be demonstrated |
| Post tetanic potentiation | Present | Not seen | Not seen |
| Length tension relationship | Maximum tension is developed in the muscle at the optimal length | Maximum tension is developed in the muscle at the optimal length | Shows plasticity |
| Load velocity relationship/force velocity relationship | Load velocity relationship is seen | Load velocity relationship is seen | Force velocity relationship is seen |
| Plasticity | Not seen | Not seen | Present, occurs due to latch bridge mechanism |
| Muscle hypertrophy | Seen | Seen | Seen |

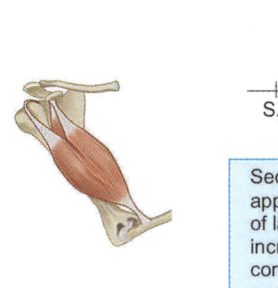
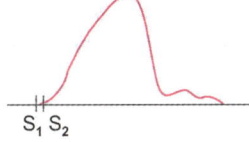
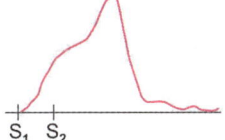
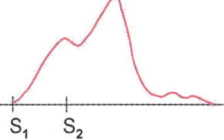

Second stimulus ($S_2$) is applied during second half of latent period resulting in increased amplitude of contraction, 'summation of contraction'

$S_2$ given during contraction phase gives a second, higher peak as compared to the first peak

$S_2$ applied during relaxation phase results in a second contraction with higher peak than the first contraction

Fig. 27.21: Summation of contraction in skeletal muscle.

contraction. *This property is seen only in the skeletal muscle due to very short ARP.*

**Physiological basis:** When the muscle is repeatedly stimulated during the contraction period, it doesn't allow the muscle to relax in between the contractions, resulting in the fusion of contractions, called tetanus. The frequency of stimulations at which the tetanus occurs is called as the *tetanizing frequency*. The tetanizing frequency is calculated as 1/duration of SMT (seconds).

$$\text{Tetanizing frequency} = \frac{1}{\text{Twitch duration (seconds)}}$$

*Calculate the tetanizing frequency of a SMT, if its duration is 100 ms.*

**Solution:** Twitch duration of 100 ms = 0.1 seconds

$$\text{Tetanizing frequency} = \frac{1}{0.1} = 10 \text{ stimuli/second}$$

**Figure 27.23A** shows that in when we stimulated with a frequency of five stimulations per second, it resulted in staircase effect. Also observe that the muscle is allowed to completely relax before the next contraction. Whereas

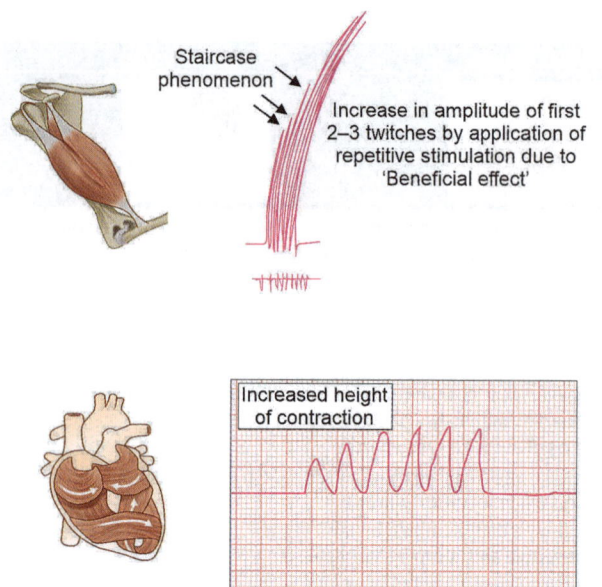

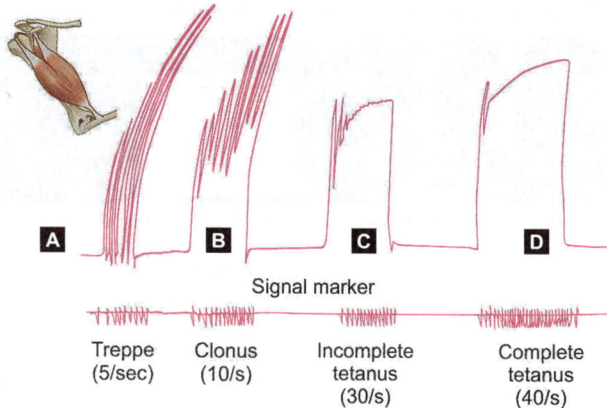

**Figs. 27.23A to D:** Types of tetanus.

**Fig. 27.22:** Staircase effect in skeletal muscle and cardiac muscle.

the **Figures 27.23B to D** show that on increasing the frequency of stimulation, the muscle does not relax, rather the contraction fuses and the tension is generated in the muscle.

**Physiological significance of tetanus:** The fusion of contraction/tetanus in the skeletal muscle results in increased tension in the muscle and helps in maintaining sustained contractions for useful work in our body. Since the complete tetanus actually result in muscular spasms, as it occludes the blood supply to the muscles. The incomplete or subtetanic contractions are responsible for work done in muscular contractions.

It is quite surprising that our muscular contractions are smooth instead of jerky, if the subtetanic contractions are responsible for muscular activity. Wonder why? *It is due to the asynchronous discharge of motor units (discussed above).*

**Why the cardiac muscle cannot be tetanized?**

The cardiac muscle has a long ARP, which coincides with most of the contraction period of the cardiac muscle. Hence the cardiac muscle cannot be tetanized. It is a safety factor for the cardiac muscle, as it is an important muscle, and its function is to pump the blood continuously to the body.

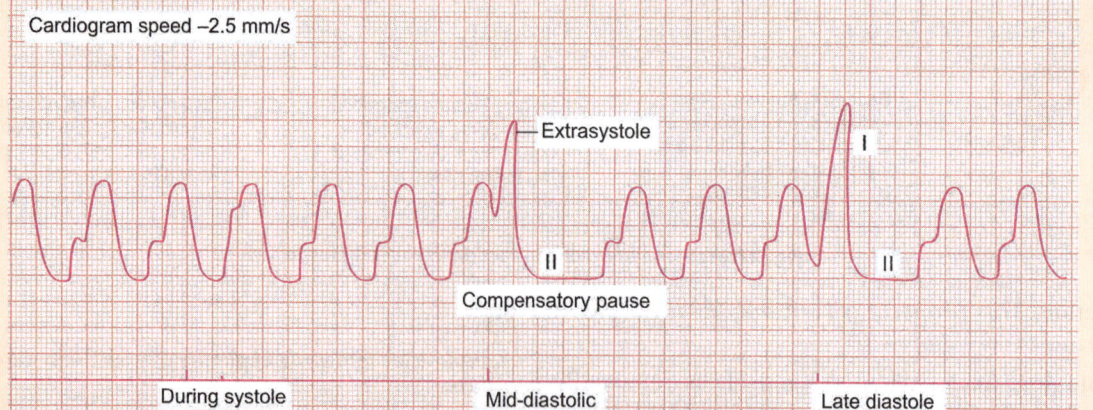

Experimentally, when the beating heart is stimulated during systole, it doesn't result in any extra contraction/extrasystole. But when stimulated during diastole (Relaxation phase), it produces an extrasystole followed by the compensatory pause.

The compensatory pause occurs due to nonconductance of the normal impulse, originating from SA node, due to the absolute refractory period of extrasystole. This event of extrasystole and compensatory pause also demonstrates that the cardiac muscle has a long refractory period and cannot be stimulated during contraction phase. Hence, cardiac muscle cannot be tetanized.

## Length Tension Relationship in both Skeletal and Cardiac Muscles

Both the muscles, skeletal and cardiac muscles generate maximum tension in muscle, when the muscle is stretched to its optimum length before contraction. As per the Frank Starling's law, which states that, **"Within physiological limits, the force of contraction of muscle is directly proportional to the initial length of the muscle fiber"**. Before we learn further about the L-T relationship, please refer to the **Box 27.1** to learn about the different type of muscle lengths.

**Physiological basis:** The tension developed in the muscle depends on the number of crossbridges formed during the contraction. According to the Frank Starling's Law **(Figs. 27.24 and 27.25)**:

- *"Within the physiological limits",* means that the length of sarcomere is optimum, neither overlapping nor overstretched. Hence the number of crossbridges formed are adequate. Let us see, what will happen, if the length of sarcomere changes.
- *"Force of contraction/tension generated in muscle is directly proportional to initial length of muscle fiber."*

In cardiac muscle, the initial length of the muscle fiber is determined by the amount of blood in the ventricle, before systole, i.e., end diastolic volume (EDV) **(Fig. 27.26)**.

Hence, the Frank Starling Law is restated as *"Within physiological limits, the force of contraction of muscle is directly proportional to the initial length of the muscle fiber/EDV".*

Physiological basis remains same as the skeletal muscle.

The **smooth muscles** do not show the length tension relationship, but they have a peculiar property of *plasticity*. The smooth muscles, when stretched initially show the contractile response, similar to skeletal muscle, i.e., it follows the length tension relationship. But if stretch is maintained, the pressure/tension in the smooth muscle decreases because of its adaptability/plasticity.

### Box 27.1:
**Lengths of muscles.**

> **Initial length:** It is the length of the muscle, at which the contraction begins. It can be any length from resting length to optimum length and stretched beyond optimum length
>
> **Optimum length:** This is the length of muscle, which generates the maximum tension, when stimulated as initial length. Our skeletal muscles are attached to bones at the optimum length (they are slightly stretched), hence yield maximum response to stimulation
>
> **Resting length:** It is the length of muscle, when it is detached from its bony attachments. It is less than the optimum length. It is 2 μ for a resting sarcomere

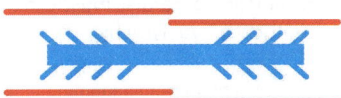

a. When the length of sarcomere is very less. The actin filaments overlap, resulting in less number of crossbridge formation

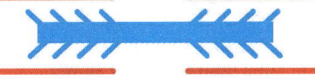

b. The length of sarcomere is optimum, where maximum number of crossbridges are formed

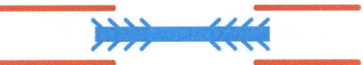

c. The sarcomere is overstretched reducing the number of crossbridges, hence reducing the tension generated in the muscle

**Fig. 27.24:** Mechanism of Frank Starling's law.

**Physiological basis of plasticity:** This property of smooth muscle is due to a special mechanism called *'Latch bridge mechanism'* **(Fig. 27.27)**.

In this mechanism the actin and myosin filaments, remain latched to each other, due to slow crossbridge

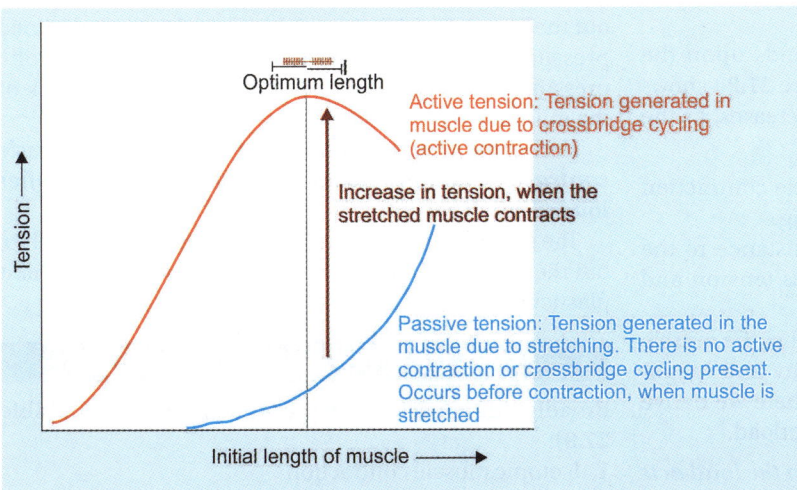
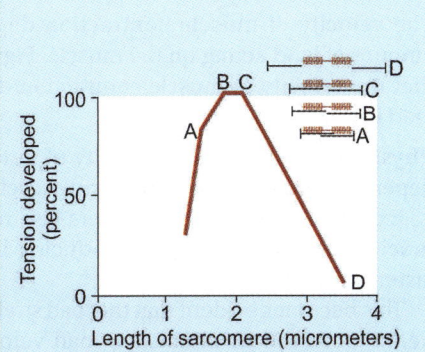

The tension generated in the muscle is maximum in B & C, i.e., at optimum length. However, the tension decreases at A and D (beyond the physiological limits)

**Fig. 27.25:** Graphs showing length of muscle during active and passive tension.

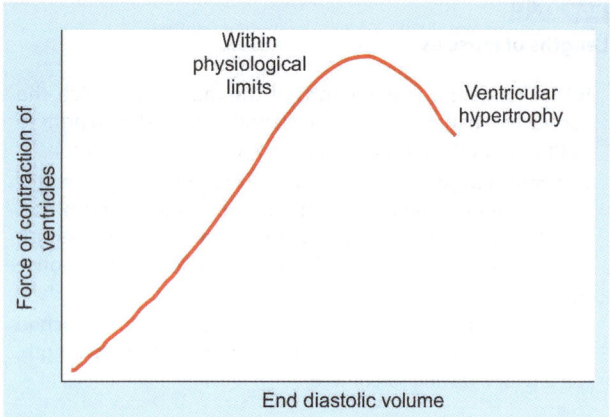

**Fig. 27.26:** Force of contraction of cardiac muscle in normal and ventricular hypertrophy.

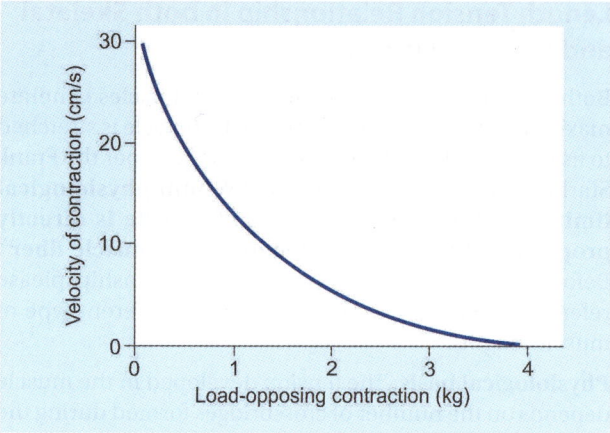

**Fig. 27.28:** Relationship between velocity of contraction and load on muscle.

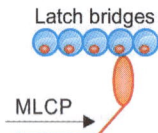

**Fig. 27.27:** Latch bridge mechanism.

cycling, maintaining the tension in the smooth muscle. If the smooth muscle is stretched, the tension increases in it. After sometime, the actomyosin complex breaks and the myosin head attaches to a new actin molecule. The new site of attachment reduced the tension in the muscle.
- In blood vessels, this property is called as *stress relaxation* of vasculature
- In GIT, it is called as the *receptive relaxation*.

### Load-Velocity Relationship

The velocity of muscle contraction depends upon the amount of load acting on the muscle. **Figure 27.28** shows that the velocity of muscle contraction decreases, as the load increases on the muscle.

**Physiological basis:** The velocity of muscle contraction depends upon the rate of crossbridge cycling.

**Example:** A lighter load offers less resistance to the movement of crossbridges, producing less tension and faster contraction.

This becomes evident that the load stretches the muscle hence both the mechanisms, load velocity and length tension relationship work together. From here we derive two new terminologies, the preload and afterload.

**Preload:** By definition, it means that *"When the load acts on the muscle before it begins to contract."*

**Explanation:** The load is stretching the muscle to its optimum length before the contraction. When this stretched muscle is stimulated, the active tension generated in the muscle will be higher than resting length.

**Example:** If a person is holding a bucket full of water in his hand, the weight of bucket is stretching the muscles of his arm. This is called a preloaded muscle.

Preloaded condition is also seen in the cardiac muscle. The EDV in ventricles acts as the preload, as it stretches the resting ventricular muscles before systole.

**Afterload:** It is a condition, when *"the load acts on the muscle after the muscle begins to contract".*

**Explanation:** The load doesn't act on the resting muscle. It begins to act after the muscle begins to contract.

**Example:** The person has started flexing is elbow and he is asked to fill the bucket with water from tap, holding it in his hand. This is the after loaded condition.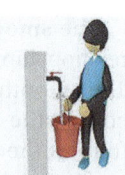

Afterload in the cardiac muscle refers to the pressure in the circulation, against which the ventricles have to pump out the blood. For right ventricle, it is pulmonary diastolic pressure and for left ventricle, it is systemic diastolic pressure. An increase in afterload, increases the work of the muscle.

Hence, *the preloaded muscle results in efficient muscle contraction and generates more tension than the after loaded condition*.

The smooth muscle show the force velocity relationship, but the velocity of smooth muscle is very slow and exhibit plasticity.

## TYPES OF MUSCLE CONTRACTIONS

Broadly, the muscle contraction is of two types (**Table 27.9**):
1. Isotonic muscle contraction
2. Isometric muscle contraction

**Table 27.9:** Isometric versus isotonic contractions.

|  | Isometric contraction | Isotonic contraction |
|---|---|---|
| Length of muscle | Remains same | Shortens |
| Tension in muscle | Increases | Remains same |
| Work done (Force x displacement) | No work done, since displacement is zero | Work done present |
| Heat dissipation | More | Less |
| Mechanical efficiency | Less | More |
| Fatigue | Fatigue sets up quickly | Fatigue sets up slowly as compared to isometric contractions |

The isotonic muscle contractions can further be classified as:
- **Concentric contractions:** In this type of contraction, the muscle shortens while generating the force. Example: raising the weight toward shoulder. These contractions result in positive work and are helpful in building muscle mass.
- **Eccentric contractions:** When the muscle lengthens while generating force is called eccentric contraction. This results whenever the muscle is performing the negative work, e.g., lowering of the weight or walking down the stairs. These contractions slow down the movement and are also called, the braking contractions.

## RECORDING OF ISOTONIC AND ISOMETRIC CONTRACTIONS (FIGS. 27.29A AND B)

The isotonic contractions can be recorded by stimulating the nerve in a nerve muscle preparation, where one end on muscle is fixed on the board and other end is free. The shortening of muscle is recorded by the isotonic muscle lever.

The isometric exercise is recorded by fixing the muscle between two fixed points, which doesn't allow the muscle to shorten. Using the isometric lever, the tension generated in the muscle is recorded.

*If there is no change in length during isometric muscle contraction, why it is called as contraction?*

The isometric muscle contraction is called so because of the generation of tension during the muscle contraction. The tension generated can be described as:
- The crossbridge cycling occurs between same actin and myosin molecules resulting in increased muscle tension with no change in the muscle length.
- Some of the sarcomeres tend to shorten while others are stretched, keeping the length of the muscle constant.
- Stretching of series elastic elements like tendons and connective tissue, which stretches to compensate for any muscular shortening, keeping the net length constant during the isometric contraction.

## SERIES ELASTIC COMPONENT (FIG. 27.30)

The series elastic components (SECs) are noncontractile structures within skeletal muscle fibers that play a vital role in muscle contraction and force generation. These are *tendons and structural proteins* within the muscle fibers themselves.

When a muscle contracts, the SECs are stretched due to the force generated by the muscle fibers. This stretching of the SECs *stores potential energy*, similar to a spring being stretched, which can be released during subsequent muscle activity. This stored energy within the SECs *helps to enhance the efficiency and effectiveness of muscle contractions*.

Hence, the primary function of the SECs is to *transmit the force generated by the muscle fibers* to the bones, resulting in movement at the joints. Additionally, they protect the muscle fibers from damage by acting as *shock absorbers, dampening the impact of sudden or rapid movements*.

The series elastic components play a crucial role in the biomechanics of muscle function, allowing for efficient force transmission, energy storage, and protection of muscle fibers during contraction and movement.

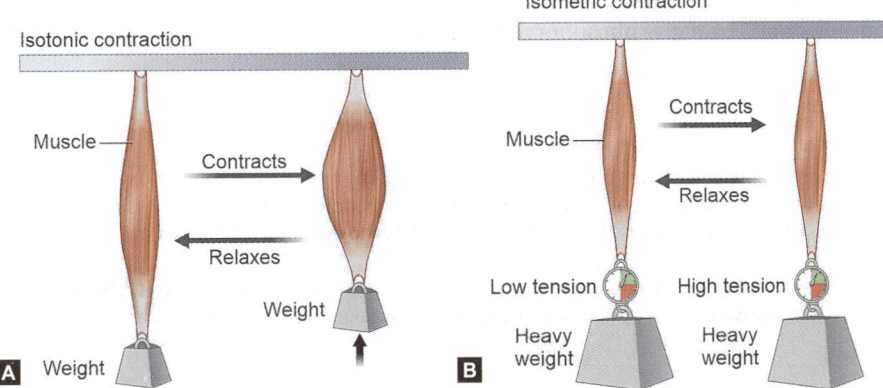

**Figs. 27.29A and B:** Recording of isotonic and isometric contractions.

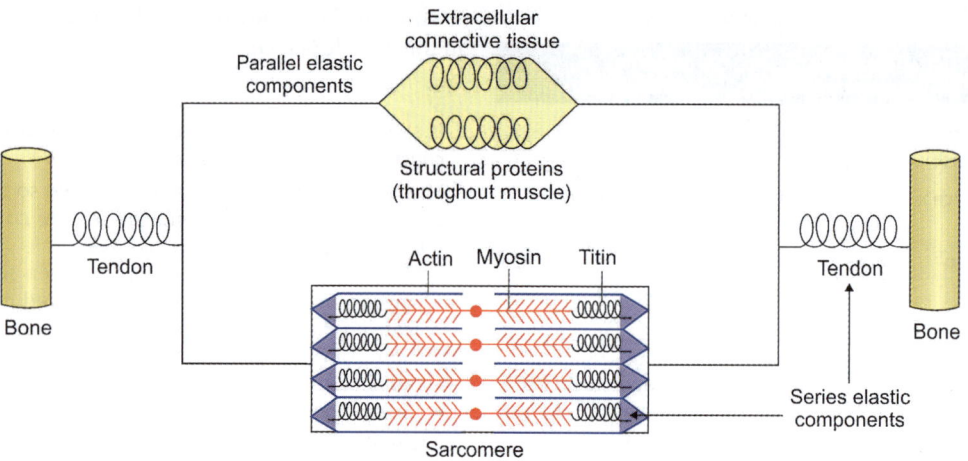

**Fig. 27.30:** Series elastic component.

## ENERGY SOURCES OF MUSCLE CONTRACTION

*"Muscle is a machine which converts chemical energy to mechanical work."*\*

The muscles require energy for contraction and relaxation. This energy is provided by various sources, depending upon the duration of muscle contraction. Various chemicals providing energy for muscle contraction are:
a. Adenosine triphosphate
b. Creatine phosphate
c. Oxidative phosphorylation

## ADENOSINE TRIPHOSPHATE

- It provides immediate source of energy for muscle contraction.
- Each molecule of ATP releases 7.3 kcal/mole
- ATP is required for:
  - Formation of crossbridges
  - Crossbridge cycling
  - Activation of SERCA for pumping of $Ca^{2+}$ into SER
- Stored ATP provides energy for maintaining the contraction for initial 1–2 seconds only.
- In longer/sustained contractions, the ATP are replenished by glycolysis and oxidative phosphorylation.

## CREATINE PHOSPHATE

- It is also called as phosphocreatine.
- The concentration of creatine phosphate is five times the concentration of ATP in the muscle.
- The creatine phosphate converts ADP into creatine and ATP by the enzyme creatine kinase (an enzyme present in the muscle)

  Creatine phosphate + ADP $\xrightarrow{CKinase}$ creatine + ATP

- The stores of CP is replenished after the contraction, during the relaxation phase.
- ATP and CP provides the energy for total 5–8 seconds.

## OXIDATIVE PHOSPHORYLATION

In longer contractions the ATP are constantly formed by the glycolytic pathway and oxidative phosphorylation depending upon the availability of oxygen.
- In anaerobic metabolism, the glycolytic pathway result in lactic acid formation, releasing two moles of ATP. It maintains the contraction for 1–2 minutes.
- In aerobic metabolism, the oxidative phosphorylation of free fatty acids, metabolism of glucose and glycogen. It releases 38 moles of ATP. More than 95% of all energy used by muscles is derived from oxidative phosphorylation.
- It provides energy of sustained contraction for 2–4 hours.

**Why there is increase in respiratory rate after exercise?**
During exercise the blood flow to the active muscle increases. During strenuous exercise, the oxygen consumption increases which increases the anaerobic glycolysis, depleting the oxygen stores in myoglobin. It is called the ***Oxygen debt/excess postexercise oxygen consumption (EPOC)***, which occurs due to depletion of oxygen stores for replenishing ATP stores.
After the exercise is over, the respiratory rate increases to replenish the depleted oxygen stores. The oxygen debt is measured as difference is excessive oxygen uptake and basal oxygen uptake. This can be as high as six times the basal consumption.

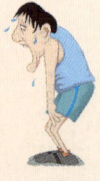

---
\*Barret KE, Barman SM, Brooks HL, Yuan JX. Ganong's Review of Medical Physiology. Lange McGraw HIll Education. 26th edition,2019:269.

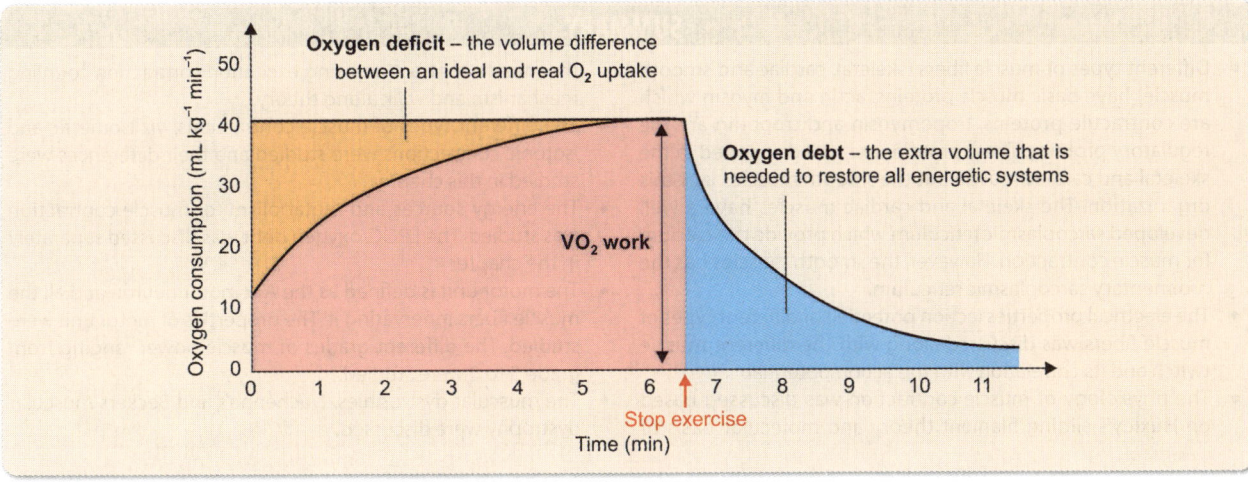

## DISORDERS OF MUSCLES/MUSCULAR DYSTROPHY

Muscular dystrophy is defined as the progressive weakness of skeletal muscle. These diseases can occur due to many causes, as shown in the **Table 27.10**.

**Table 27.10:** Summary of different disorders of muscles.

| Muscular dystrophy | Cause | Clinical features | Lab diagnosis |
|---|---|---|---|
| **Duchenne muscular dystrophy** | Absence of dystrophin protein. X-linked disorder | • Progressive muscular weakness, which is fatal by the age of 30 years<br>• Delayed motor milestones<br>• Difficulty in running, climbing stairs and getting up from ground<br>• Muscle pain and stiffness<br>• There is pseudohypertrophy of calf muscles (enlarged calf muscle)<br>• Increased curvature of spine<br>• Positive Gower's sign indicating the proximal limb weakness. In this the patient uses his hands to walk up on his own body to stand up from the sitting position | • Elevated creatinine kinase, indicating muscle damage. The CK enzyme leaks from the muscle<br>• Genetic testing indicating absence of gene coding for dystrophin protein<br>• Muscle biopsy showing disruption of muscle and absence of dystrophin<br>• Electromyography shows changes in muscle function and nerve conduction |
| **Becker muscular dystrophy** | Altered or reduced amount of dystrophin protein | It is similar to Duchenne's muscular dystrophy but it is less severe | Same as above |
| **Dilated cardiomyopathy** | Shorter titin in cardiac muscle | Increased risk of heart failure, arrhythmias and sudden cardiac death | • Blood test shows raised CK<br>• Genetic test shown mutation in TTN gene coding for titin protein<br>• Echocardiogram to evaluate the size, shape and function of cardiac chambers and valves |
| **McArdle syndrome** | Metabolic myopathy due to *PYGM* gene coding for enzyme myophosphorylase | • Exercise intolerance<br>• Episodes of rhabdomyolysis leading to dark urine and kidney damage<br>• Second wind phenomenon: improvement in exercise tolerance due to availability of glucose after some time | • Raised CK enzyme in blood<br>• Genetic testing shows mutation of *PYGM* gene<br>• Muscle biopsy<br>• Exercise testing shows absence of lactate productions and oxygen uptake during exercise. Impaired glycogenolysis |

(CK: creatine kinase; TTN: titin; PYGM: Glycogen Phosphorylase, Muscle Associated)

## SUMMARY

- Different types of muscle fibers (skeletal, cardiac and smooth muscle) have basic muscle proteins, actin and myosin which are contractile proteins, tropomyosin and troponin are the regulatory proteins. These proteins are well developed in the skeletal and cardiac muscle but the smooth muscles lack this organization. The skeletal and cardiac muscles have a well developed sarcoplasmic reticulum which provide the calcium for muscle contraction. However, the smooth muscles has the rudimentary sarcoplasmic reticulum.
- The electrical properties (action potential) of different types of muscle fibers was discussed along with the different muscle twitch and its correlation with the action potential.
- The physiology of muscle contraction was discussed based on Huxley's sliding filament theory and molecular basis of the muscle contraction using excitation contraction coupling mechanism and walk along theory.
- The different types of muscle contractions, viz Isometric and Isotonic contractions were studied and their differences were studied in this chapter.
- The energy sources and metabolism for muscle contraction was studied. The EPOC/oxygen debt was discussed separately in the chapter
- The motor unit is defined as the A α motor neuron and all the muscle fibers innervating it. The properties of motor unit were studied. The different grades of muscle power ranging from grade 5 to 0 were studied.
- The muscular dystrophies, Duchenne's and Beckers muscular dystrophy were discussed.

## LET US SEE, HOW MUCH YOU HAVE LEARNT?

 **Review Questions**

### Long/Short Answer Questions

**Q1.** Describe the excitation contraction theory under the following headings:
  a. Definition
  b. Transmission of impulse from nerve to muscle
  c. Excitation of muscle
  d. Conversion of excitation to contraction (role of calcium)
  e. Physiology of muscle contraction.

**Q2.** Differentiate between:
  a. Type I and type II muscle fibers
  b. Isometric and isotonic contractions
  c. Skeletal, cardiac and smooth muscles

**Q3.** Justify the statement "Muscle is a machine which converts chemical energy to mechanical work".

**Q4.** Define motor unit. Describe the properties of motor unit.

### Explain Why? (Reasoning Questions)

**Q1.** Identify the type of muscle contraction, shown in figure. Describe the physiology of contraction in it.

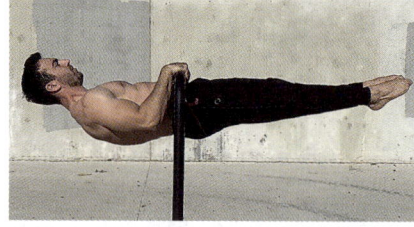

**Q2.** What is the role of isometric and isotonic contractions in our daily life activities?

**Q3.** What are isometric and isotonic exercises? What is their importance?

**Q4.** What is the effect of 100 m dash on respiration and why?

**Q5.** Why a person becomes stiff after death?

**Q6.** How does the isometric contraction generate tension in the muscle, even though the length remains constant?

**Q7.** Why does creatinine kinase increase in the blood during the muscle injury?

**Q8.** What will happen to muscle contraction, if a person:
  a. Lifts a heavy lead from the ground?
  b. Holds a bucket full of water and then lifts it up?
  c. Lowers the bucket full of water and keeps on ground?

 **Critical Thinking Case-Based Questions**

**Q1.** A 50-year-old male, presented to the OPD with complaints of intermittent chest pain and difficulty swallowing. He reported that the chest pain sometimes occurs at rest and is accompanied by a feeling of tightness. Additionally, he experienced episodes of cramping and spasms in his calf muscles after mild exercise. Physical examination and diagnostic tests revealed esophageal spasms and peripheral arterial disease.

Based on the given scenario, answer the following questions:
  a. Compare the structural properties of skeletal and smooth muscle.
  b. How do the mechanisms of contraction differ between skeletal and smooth muscle, particularly in terms of calcium handling and regulation?

## Multiple Choice Questions

Q1. Calculate the tetanizing frequency for the skeletal muscle with the twitch duration of 10 ms:
  a. 10/s
  b. 20/s
  c. 50/s
  d. 100/s

Q2. What will happen to contractility of cardiac muscle if serum calcium levels are >12 mg/dL?
  a. Decreased excitability of cardiac muscle
  b. No effect on cardiac muscle as it stores its own calcium
  c. The heart can stop in systole
  d. The cardiac muscle responds only to hypocalcemia.

Q3. The increased blood pressure in the blood vessels stretches the smooth muscles. But the pressure drops in blood vessels after some time due to which property of smooth muscles?
  a. Receptive relaxation
  b. Plasticity
  c. Length tension relationship
  d. Force velocity relationship

Q4. The series elastic elements are responsible for:
  a. Maintaining the contraction of the muscle
  b. Stretching during the muscular contraction
  c. Maintaining the viscous resistance of muscle
  d. Transmitting the force to the joints during contraction.

Q5. A 5-year-old boy presents with a history of delayed motor milestones and frequent falls. On examination, he has a waddling gait and difficulty climbing stairs. He also has calf hypertrophy and a positive Gower's sign. His serum creatinine kinase is markedly elevated. What is the most likely diagnosis?
  a. Duchenne muscular dystrophy
  b. McArdle's Syndrome
  c. Limb-Girdle muscular dystrophy
  d. Spinal muscular atrophy

Q6. Which theory describes the process where myosin heads bind to actin and pull them towards the center of the sarcomere, causing muscle contraction?
  a. Excitation-contraction coupling mechanism
  b. Sliding filament theory
  c. Walk-along theory
  d. Cross bridge cycling theory

Q7. Which type of muscle contraction occurs when the muscle shortens while generating force?
  a. Concentric contraction
  b. Eccentric contraction
  c. Isometric contraction
  d. Isotonic contraction

Q8. Which energy source is primarily used during short bursts of high-intensity muscle contractions?
  a. Glycolysis
  b. Oxidative phosphorylation
  c. Lipolysis
  d. ATP-PCr system

Q9. Which term refers to the smallest functional unit of a muscle composed of a motor neuron and all the muscle fibers it innervates?
  a. Sarcomere
  b. Myofibril
  c. Motor unit
  d. Neuromuscular junction

Q10. Which grade of muscle power describes muscle contraction against gravity with full range of motion and without resistance?
  a. Grade 0
  b. Grade 1
  c. Grade 2
  d. Grade 3

Q11. Which type of muscular dystrophy is characterized by progressive muscle weakness and degeneration primarily affecting skeletal muscles?
  a. Duchenne muscular dystrophy
  b. Becker muscular dystrophy
  c. Limb-Girdle muscular dystrophy
  d. Myotonic dystrophy

Q12. Which type of muscle fiber would be most likely affected in a patient with hypertension due to its role in regulating blood vessel diameter?
  a. Skeletal muscle fibers
  b. Cardiac muscle fibers
  c. Smooth muscle fibers
  d. Striated muscle fibers

Q13. During intense exercise, which metabolic pathway is predominantly utilized by skeletal muscle fibers to generate ATP?
  a. Aerobic respiration
  b. Anaerobic glycolysis
  c. Krebs cycle
  d. Electron transport chain

Q14. Which muscle contraction type would be most effective in lowering a heavy object slowly and under control?
  a. Concentric contraction
  b. Eccentric contraction
  c. Isometric contraction
  d. Isotonic contraction

Q15. A patient presents with muscle weakness and difficulty walking. EMG reveals abnormal electrical activity in the muscles. Which neuromuscular disorder is most likely present?
  a. Myasthenia gravis
  b. Amyotrophic lateral sclerosis (ALS)
  c. Polymyositis
  d. Charcot-Marie-Tooth disease

Q16. Which neurotransmitter is released at the neuromuscular junction to initiate muscle contraction?
  a. Acetylcholine
  b. Dopamine
  c. Serotonin
  d. Norepinephrine

Q17. Which factor contributes to the increased strength and endurance of cardiac muscle fibers compared to skeletal muscle fibers?
  a. Presence of intercalated discs
  b. Higher concentration of myoglobin
  c. Greater reliance on anaerobic metabolism
  d. Lack of multinucleation

Q18. A patient with skeletal muscle weakness undergoes a muscle biopsy revealing the absence of dystrophin protein. Which type of muscular dystrophy is most likely present?
  a. Duchenne muscular dystrophy
  b. Becker muscular dystrophy
  c. Limb-Girdle muscular dystrophy
  d. Myotonic dystrophy

Q19. Which type of muscle fiber would be most resistant to fatigue and able to sustain prolonged contractions?
  a. Type I skeletal muscle fibers
  b. Type II skeletal muscle fibers
  c. Type I cardiac muscle fibers
  d. Type II cardiac muscle fibers

Q20. A patient with a heart condition experiences irregular contractions of the heart muscle. Which type of muscle contraction is occurring?
  a. Isometric contraction
  b. Tetanic contraction
  c. Fibrillation
  d. Twitch contraction

Q21. Which enzyme plays a key role in the conversion of ATP to ADP, providing energy for muscle contraction?
  a. Creatine kinase
  b. Adenylate kinase
  c. Phosphofructokinase
  d. Myosin ATPase

## ANSWERS

1. d   2. c   3. b   4. b   5. a   6. b   7. a   8. d   9. c   10. d   11. a   12. c   13. b   14. b
15. a   16. a   17. a   18. a   19. a   20. c   21. d

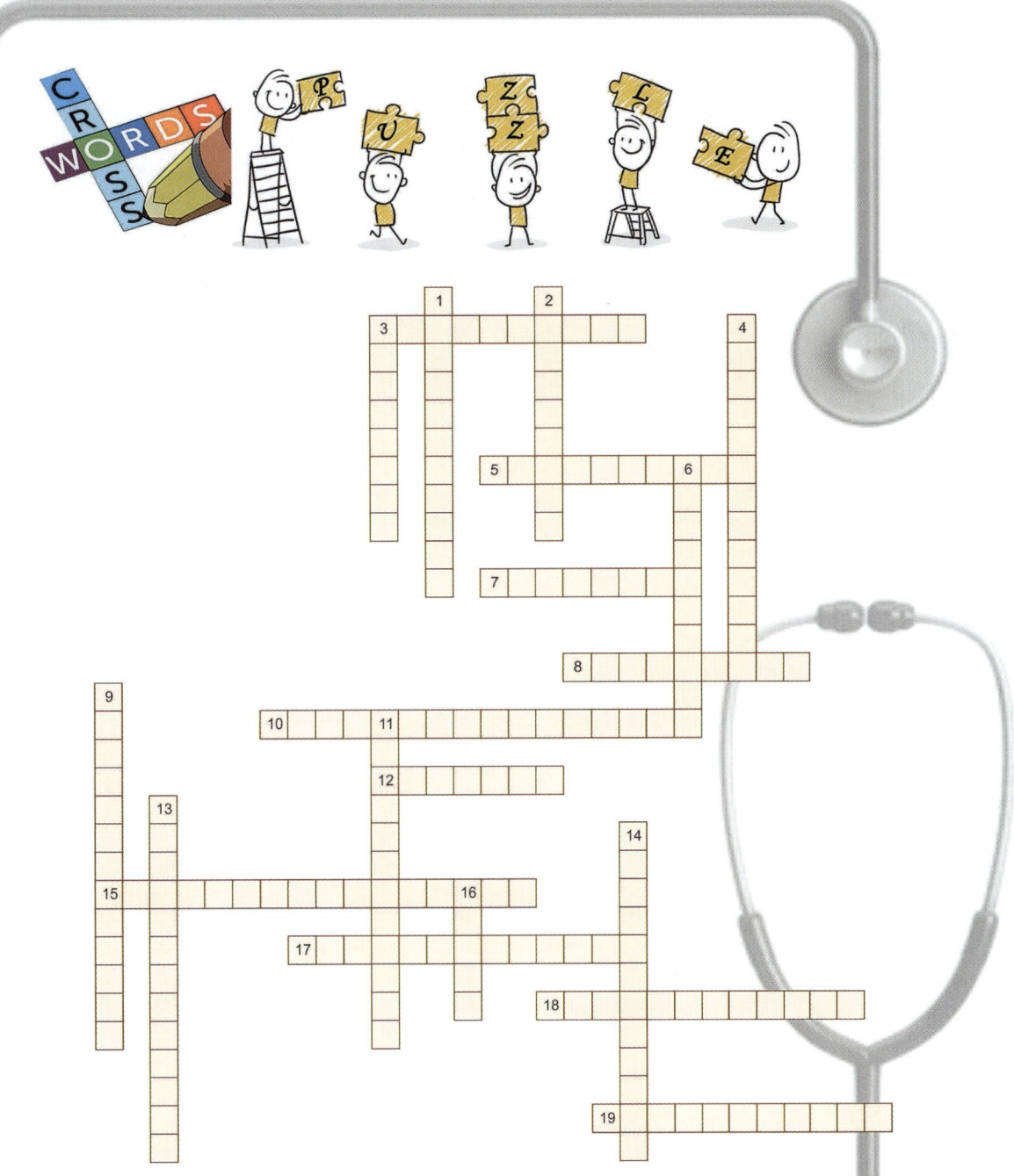

### Across

3. Cell membrane of the muscle fiber
5. Abundant star shaped glial cells forming blood brain barrier
7. Depressions present in the cell membrane of smooth muscles in place of T tubules
8. Structural and the functional unit of the myofibril
10. Study of contraction of muscle sand motor unit action potential
12. State of contraction, in which repetitive stimulation with high frequency results in fusion of contraction
15. Responsible for the myelination of neurons of CNS
17. Disintegration of Nissil's granules which stain weakly with basic dye
18. It refers to when there is structural damage of the nerve
19. Nerve damage is minimal as the axon and endoneurial tube is intact

### Down

1. Filamentous protein, coiled around the actin filament
2. Branches of soma forming extensions
3. These anchors the synaptic vesicles with the cytoskeleton of axon terminal
4. Reversible inhibitor that block degradation of ACh and increases half-life
6. Surgical removal of the thymus gland
9. Proteins released by Schwann cells regulating regeneration of neurons
11. Potent neurotoxin primarily found in certain marine organisms
13. Blocks the reuptake of the choline into the presynaptic terminal
14. The protruding arms and heads of myosin filament together
16. Filamentous cytoskeletal protein extending from Z to M line

# SECTION 4

# GASTROINTESTINAL SYSTEM

## Section Outline

- **Chapter 28:** Organization of Gastrointestinal System
- **Chapter 29:** Digestion in Oral Cavity and Esophagus
- **Chapter 30:** Physiology of Digestion in Stomach
- **Chapter 31:** Physiology of Digestion in Small Intestine (Including Pancreas)
- **Chapter 32:** Physiology of Hepatobiliary System
- **Chapter 33:** Physiology of Digestion in the Large Intestine
- **Chapter 34:** Physiology of Digestion and Absorption of Nutrients

# Organization of Gastrointestinal System

## 28 CHAPTER

**COMPETENCY ADDRESSED**

**PY4.1:** Describe the structure and functions of digestive system.
**PY4.6:** Describe the gut-brain axis.

### LEARNING OBJECTIVES

**At the end of this chapter, the learner should be able to:**
- Describe the physiologic anatomy of the gastrointestinal system.
- Describe the electrical activities in GIT.
- Describe the contractile properties of GIT.
- Describe the regulation of GI functions (neural and hormonal).
- Describe the splanchnic circulation.
- Describe the immune apparatus of gut.
- Describe the gut microflora and its significance.
- Describe the concept of the gut-brain axis and its significance in physiological and psychological health.

## PHYSIOLOGICAL ANATOMY OF GI SYSTEM

The gastrointestinal system, commonly called as digestive system constitutes of a continuous tubular structure extending between mouth to the anal canal. It serves specific functions at specific points, which are due to difference in the secretory glands, musculature and motility. Anatomically, the various parts of the gastrointestinal tracts can be enumerated as below, from oral cavity to anal canal.
- Mouth
- Esophagus
- Stomach
- Small intestine: Duodenum, jejunum and ilium
- Large intestine: Ascending colon, transverse colon, descending colon and sigmoid colon
- Anus

Apart from these structures in the gastrointestinal system, there are few important but additional secretory organs, which pour their secretions into the gastrointestinal system and aids in its functioning organs:
- Salivary glands: Parotid, submandibular, sublingual
- Liver
- Gallbladder
- Pancreas

These structures and organs help to absorb nutrients and water into the body. The gastrointestinal tract is responsible for variety of secretions for the digestion of ingested food, movement of the food through the gut by variety of motility patterns and absorption through lining of the intestine at various levels.

### Histology of GI Wall

The gastrointestinal (GIT) wall is composed of four distinct layers, proceeding from the outer to the inner:
1. **Serosa** is the outer most layer of the intestine. It consists of mesothelial cells.
2. **Layer of muscularis propria:**
   a. *Longitudinal smooth muscles* helps in peristalsis, mixing and propulsive contractions.
   b. *Layer of circular smooth muscles* helps in mixing of the digesting food with the secretions and segmentation movements of the intestine. Helps in mixing and propulsive movements along with longitudinal muscles.

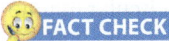

Muscularis propria is helps in peristalsis (GIT motility) whereas muscularis mucosa is the part of the mucosal layer and does not have any role in motility.

3. **Submucosa** is present just beneath muscularis mucosa.
4. **Mucosa** is the innermost layer. In its deeper layers sparse bundles of smooth muscle are present known as

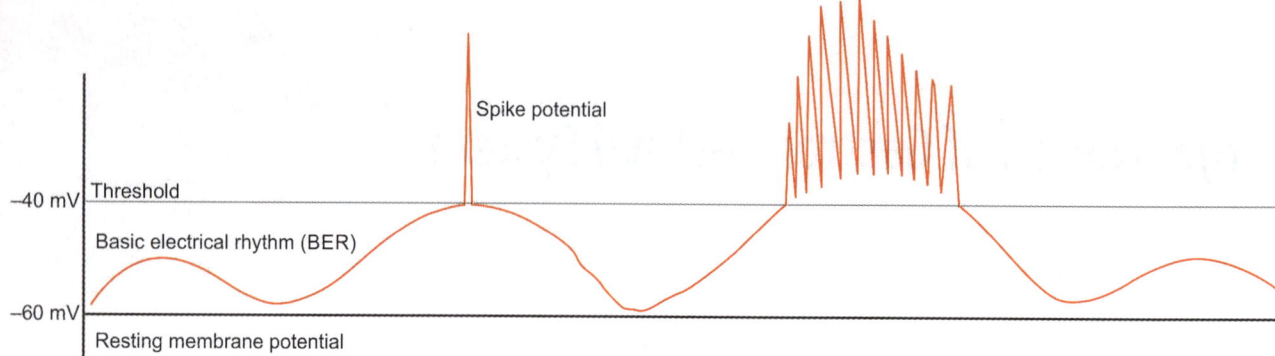

**Fig. 28.1:** BER and spike potential in GIT smooth muscles.

muscularis mucosa. Muscularis mucosa causes short folds to appear in the intestinal mucosa and also extends into the intestinal villi that cause their intermittent contraction. It is the layer where secretion of mucous and variety of digestive juices occurs. It is also responsible for absorption of digested food nutrients and water.

## SMOOTH MUSCLES OF GIT

As seen in the histology of gut, the smooth muscles of GIT are present throughout the tract. Their function is movement of GIT, e.g., mixing, propulsive or segmentation. These variety of movements help in breakdown of the digesting food into smaller particles, mixing of food with digestive juices and after absorption of nutrients, propulsion of the product of digestion towards the anal canal.

> **FACT CHECK**
>
> Basic electrical rhythm (BER) starts from greater curvature of body of stomach and goes till the colon.

The smooth muscles of GIT are unique as they are innervated by enteric nervous system and function as syncytium. Each smooth muscle fiber is connected to each other by *Gap Junctions*. Gap junctions offer low resistant movement of ions from one muscle fiber to another. Due to this there is rapid transmission of electrical impulses through large number gap junctions placed in-between muscle fibers. The muscle bundles although separated by loose connective tissue fuse at many points, thus action potential once generated travels in all directions.

The distance travelled by the electrical impulse can vary from mm, cm or entire length. It depends upon excitation of muscle. As many as 1000 parallel fibers of smooth muscles are arranged in bundles. In longitudinal muscle layers smooth muscle fibers are arranged longitudinally and in circular muscle layer they extend in circular manner around the alimentary tract. Their *length* being 200–500 μm and *diameter* = 2–10 μm.

## Electrical Activity of GIT Smooth Muscles

GIT smooth muscles shows intrinsic electrical activity which causes slow and continuous membrane excitation. The resting membrane potential (RMP) can vary to different levels which can affect motor activity of the tract. The normal RMP of GIT smooth muscle is **–50 to –60 millivolts, and** averages to **–56 millivolts.**

There are 2 types of electrical activity shown by GIT smooth muscle which are slow waves and spike potentials (Fig. 28.1).

> **FACT CHECK**
>
> BER also called as slow wave seen during resting state and whenever there is stimulus (eating food), spike potentials will be generated to cause muscle contraction.

### Slow Waves

These are the electrical waves which determine the rhythmical contractions of GIT smooth muscles. They are slow undulating changes in RMP. Their intensity is **5–15 millivolts.** and frequency is **3 to 12/min.** In body of stomach they are 3/min, in duodenum and in terminal ileum about 8–9/min. They are caused by electrical pacemakers of smooth muscle which are interstitial cells interposed between layers of smooth muscle cells called, *Interstitial cells of Cajal*. They are responsible for cyclic changes of membrane potential.

> **BER:**
> - 5–15 mV, 3–12/minute
> - Caused by electrical pacemakers, *Interstitial cells of Cajal*
> - Stomach: 3/min
> - Duodenum and Ileum: 8–9/min
> - Cecum: 2/min

- BER is due to ion channels that periodically open and produce inward (pacemaker) currents that cause slow entry of sodium ions.
- They do not cause muscle contraction except in stomach.
- They are responsible for the appearance of spike potentials.

Note: *Spike potentials causes muscle contraction and not slow waves.*

### Spike Potential

They are also the *true action potential of smooth muscles*. Spike potential automatically occurs *when RMP rises more positively above –40 millivolts*. They depend on slow waves, when the peak of the slow wave reaches –40 millivolts spike potentials appear over slow waves. The higher the slow waves rises, the greater is the frequency of spike potentials.

- Normal frequency of the spike potentials is 1–10 spikes/second with the duration of 10–20 milliseconds.
- The spike potential of GIT have *10–40 times longer duration* than of large nerve.
- Spike potentials are generated by *Calcium-sodium channels*. These channels are slow channels and allow large number of calcium ions to enter along with sodium. This causes *long action potential*. Calcium influx also helps in GIT smooth muscle contraction by calmodulin control mechanism. It is also responsible for the tonic contraction of the GIT.

### Tonic Contraction

It is produced by continuous repetitive spike potentials. Thus greater the frequency of spike potentials more will be the tonic contraction, due to continuous entry of calcium inside the cell. It can also be caused by hormones (hormone induced tonic contraction).

### Factors Causing Depolarization/Hyperpolarization of RMP

#### Depolarization

- **Stretching:** Stretching of smooth muscles
- **Acetylcholine:** Stimulation of parasympathetic nervous system
- Gastrointestinal hormones

#### Hyperpolarization

- Norepinephrine
- Epinephrine
- Sympathetic nerves stimulation

These rhythms are produced by *pacemaker cells known as Interstitial Cells of Cajal*, located in the inner circular muscle layer, as mentioned above.

> BER begins in the stomach's greater curvature, peaks in the duodenum and jejunum, and is lowest in the ileum.
>
> The frequency of these waves varies, with around 3/min in the stomach, and about 8–9/min in the duodenum and terminal ileum. They do not directly cause muscle contractions, except in the stomach where they trigger slow waves with spike potential, leading to contractions when stimulated.

## MIGRATING MOTOR COMPLEXES (MMC)

During the fasting period between bouts of digestion, there is a noticeable alteration in the electrical and motor

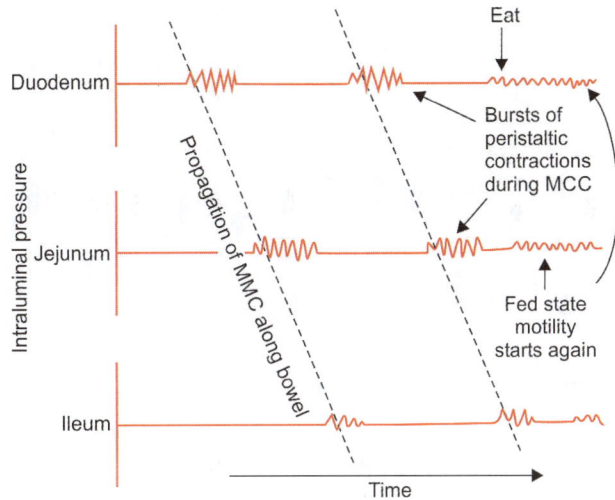

**Fig. 28.2:** Intraluminal pressure in various parts of small intestine.

activity within the smooth muscles of the gastrointestinal tract. This alteration prompts cycles of motor activity to shift from the stomach towards the distal ileum. Each cycle, termed a migrating motor complex (MMC), follows a distinct pattern consisting of several phases:

- **Phase I:** A quiet phase
- **Phase II:** A phase characterized by irregular electrical and mechanical activity
- **Phase III:** A phase marked by a burst of regular activity

The initiation of MMCs is attributed to motilin, a hormone. During the interdigestive phase, the levels of motilin in circulation rise approximately every 100 minutes, coinciding with the contractile phases of the MMC. These contractions progress downward through the digestive tract at a pace of around 5 cm/min and recur at similar intervals of approximately 100 minutes **(Fig. 28.2)**. *(These MMCs are metaphorically viewed as broom, which swipes clean the gut between the meals).*

Moreover, gastric secretion, bile flow, and pancreatic secretion experience augmentation during each MMC. These physiological responses likely facilitate the clearance of luminal contents from the stomach and small intestine in anticipation of the forthcoming meal. However, the motilin is supressed after the ingestion of food. This abolishes the MMCs until the digestion and absorption is complete.

## GENERAL PRINCIPLES OF GASTROINTESTINAL SECRETIONS

The gastrointestinal system is primarily concerned with the digestion and absorption of food and hence is fully equipped with the secretory glands throughout the gut. These glands however, secrete the fluids which have different composition, pH and enzymes, required to suit the digestive process in that particular area of the gut. Here, we will become familiar with certain general principles, followed by all type of secretions from all these glands in terms of mechanisms of secretion, phases and regulation in the respective chapters.

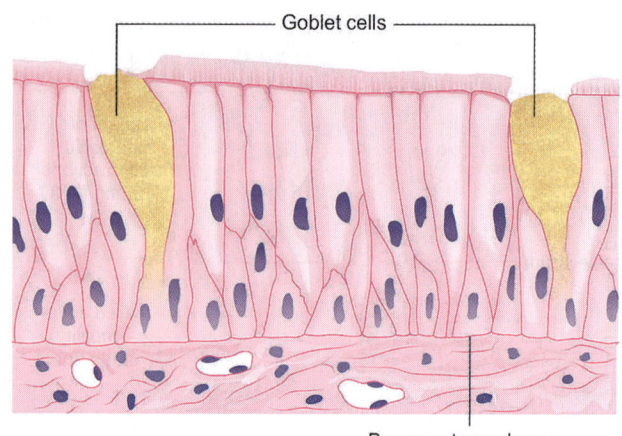

**Fig. 28.3:** Goblets cells.

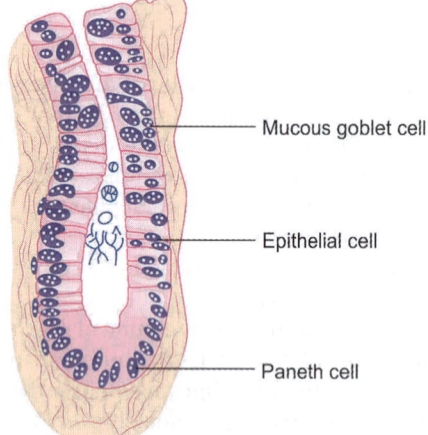

**Fig. 28.4:** Crypts of Lieberkühn.

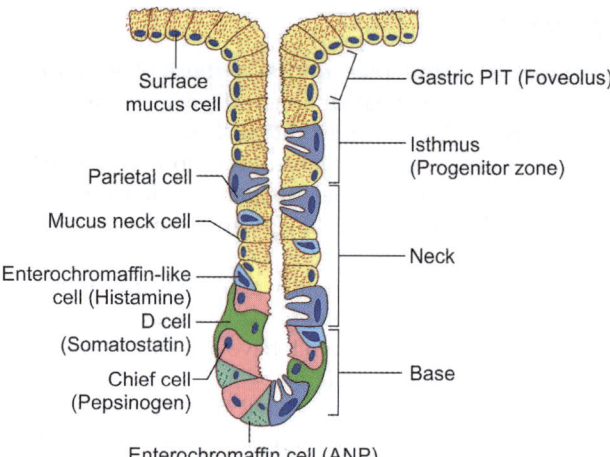

**Fig. 28.5:** Oxyntic glands of stomach.
(ANP: atrial natriuretic peptide)

## Types of Glands Present in GIT

- **Single cell mucous glands/goblet cells (Fig. 28.3):** Secrete mucous which act as lubricant and prevents the mucous membrane of GIT from digestion and excoriation.
- **Pits:** They are invaginations of epithelium into submucosa. These pits have specialized cells.
  - Crypts of Lieberkühn in small intestine **(Fig. 28.4)**
- **Tubular glands:** They are present in stomach and upper duodenum:
  - Oxyntic gland in the stomach which secrete pepsinogen and hydrochloric acid **(Fig. 28.5)**
- **Complex glands:** They provide secretions to digest food.
  - *Salivary glands:* Acinous glands
  - *Liver:* Specialized structure
  - *Pancreas:* Acinous glands

The presence of food directly stimulates these glands to release their secretions. The tactile stimulation, chemical irritation and distension of gut wall stimulates the enteric nervous system.

The parasympathetic nervous system stimulates these glands to produce copious secretions whereas the sympathetic stimulation results in vasoconstriction and hence reduces the GI secretions.

## Phases of GI Secretions

Gastrointestinal (GI) secretions play a crucial role in the digestive process, breaking down food and aiding in nutrient absorption. These secretions originate from various glands along the GI tract and can be categorized into different phases. Here are the main phases of GI secretions:

- **Cephalic phase:** This phase occurs before food enters the stomach, typically triggered by the sight, smell, or even the thought of food. It involves the stimulation of the vagus nerve, leading to the secretion of saliva by the salivary glands. Saliva contains enzymes like salivary amylase, which begins the breakdown of carbohydrates. This phase also stimulates the gastric secretion.
- **Gastric phase:** Once food enters the stomach, the gastric phase begins. This phase is primarily initiated by the presence of food in the stomach, which triggers the release of gastrin, a hormone that stimulates gastric gland secretion. Gastric glands secrete gastric juice, which consists of hydrochloric acid (HCl), pepsinogen (the precursor to pepsin, an enzyme that breaks down proteins), and intrinsic factor (necessary for vitamin B12 absorption). About 90% of gastric secretions occur during this phase. It remains active, till the food remains in the stomach.
- **Intestinal phase:** As partially digested food moves into the duodenum, the intestinal phase begins. This phase is triggered by the presence of food in the duodenum and is regulated by hormones such as secretin, cholecystokinin (CCK), and gastric inhibitory peptide (GIP). These hormones stimulate the secretion of bile from the liver and enzyme rich pancreatic secretion from the pancreas. When this phase begins, the gastric phase is inhibited and there is stimulation of intestinal secretions. The crypts of Lieberkühn in small intestine also increase their secretory activity for proper digestion and absorption of food.

# GENERAL PRINCIPLES OF GASTROINTESTINAL MOTILITY

The gastrointestinal tract shows the typical movements resulting in the propulsion of food from esophagus to anus. These movements are generally called the peristaltic movements. Though the peristaltic movements can result in the movement in forward and backward direction, there is a fixed direction (from oral to caudal), in which the peristalsis occur. This is called the *'Law of gut'*.

The peristaltic movements are of two types:
1. Propulsive peristaltic movements
2. Segmentation peristaltic movements

> **Law of gut:** The peristaltic reflex results in the movement of food from the orad to caudad.
>
> The myenteric plexus is polarized from the orad (mouth) to caudad (anus) resulting in the peristaltic movement toward the anus. Once the food bolus is pushed, there is a wave of constriction which squeezes the food bolus forward. However, the segment of gut preceding the bolus relaxes to receive the it (receptive relaxation). This phenomenon is seen only when the myenteric plexus is normal. In patients with defects in myenteric plexus (aganglionic segments), the peristaltic reflex is not seen resulting in absence of gut motility.

## Propulsive Peristaltic Movements (Fig. 28.6)

As the name suggests, the movements propel the food forward toward the caudal end of the gut. These movements follow the peristaltic reflex according to the law of the gut.

The contractile ring appears in the gut due to contraction of circular muscles of GIT, which squeezes the bolus

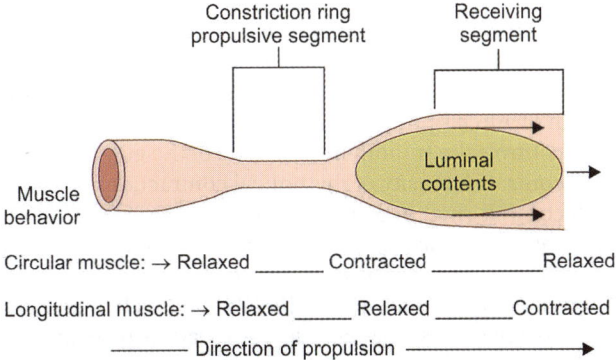

**Fig. 28.6:** Propulsive peristaltic movements.

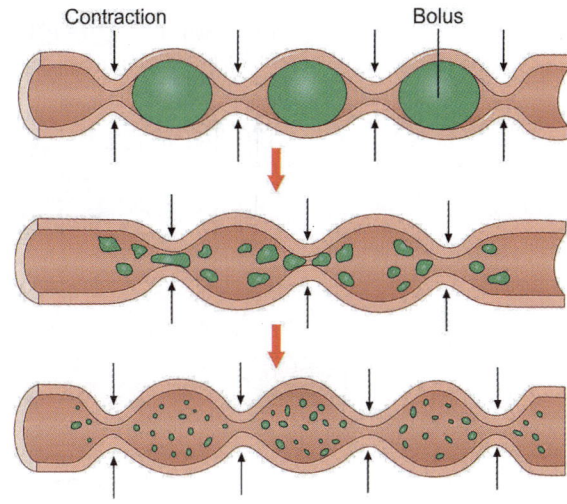

**Fig. 28.7:** Segmentation peristaltic movements.

of food forward. This movement is usually stimulated by distension of gut, which can occur due to:
- Presence of food resulting in stretching of walls of gut
- Physical or chemical irritation of epithelial lining of gut
- Parasympathetic stimulation of gut.

## Segmentation Peristaltic Movements (Fig. 28.7)

These movements do not propel the food, but the gut wall show repetitive contraction and relaxation in small areas resulting in churning, mixing and breaking the down the food bolus. Hence, these are also called the mixing movements.

# REGULATION OF GI FUNCTIONS (SECRETIONS AND MOTILITY)

The GI functions are regulated by nervous systema and hormonal control, which can be classified as:
- **Nervous regulation:**
  - *Intrinsic innervation:* By enteric nervous system
  - *Extrinsic innervation:* The sympathetic and parasympathetic nervous system (**Fig. 28.8**)
- Hormonal control discussed below in **Table 28.1**.
- Local control due to stretching of muscle.

## Nervous Regulation (Fig. 28.9)

### Enteric Nervous System (ENS)

As discussed above, the enteric nervous system forms the intrinsic innervation of GIT. It is composed of two kinds of neural plexuses extending from esophagus to anus with more than 100 million neurons. Enteric nervous system is directly connected to extrinsic sympathetic and parasympathetic fibers that can highly influence its functioning. However, enteric nervous system can also function independently.

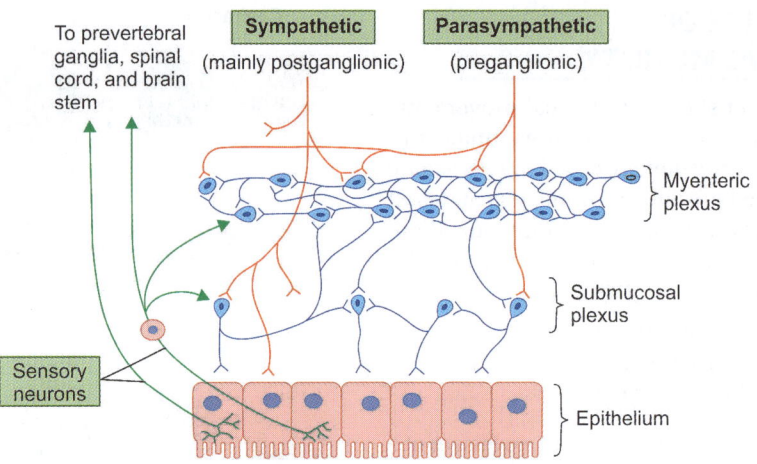

**Fig. 28.8:** Extrinsic innervation.

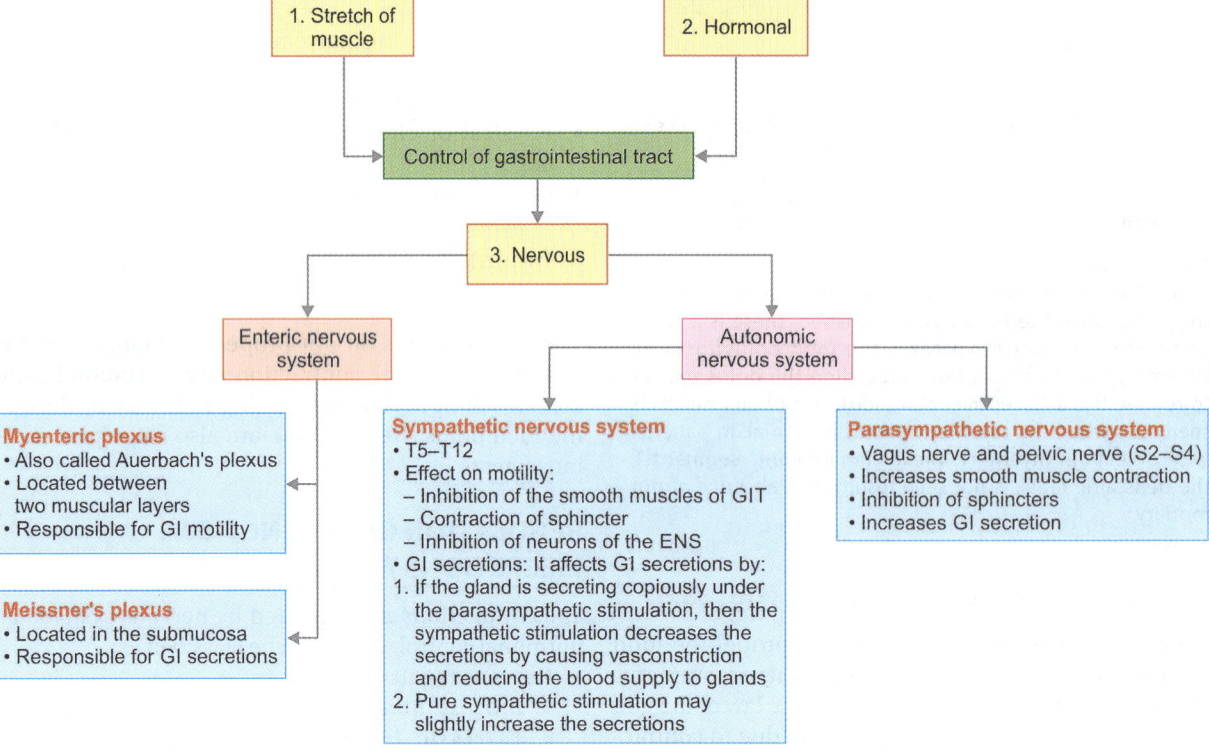

**Fig. 28.9:** Nervous control of GI system.

There are 2 neural plexus are embedded in the wall of GIT:
- *Myenteric plexus or Auerbach's plexus:* This plexus present between the outer longitudinal and inner circular muscle layer. Hence, it is concerned motility of gut.
- *Submucosal or Meissner's plexus:* It is present in the submucosal layer of GIT. Hence, it is responsible for GI secretions.

Sensory nerve endings originate from inside of the gut wall and send afferent fibers to the areas like myenteric plexus, Meissner's plexus, prevertebral ganglia of sympathetic nervous system, spinal cord, vagus nerve and all the way to brain stem either to initiate local reflexes or reflexes relayed from prevertebral ganglia or basal regions of the brain.

## Myenteric Plexus

Myenteric or Auerbach plexus is mainly responsible for control of GIT movements. It is a linear chain of neurons present between two muscle layers, that runs an entire length of gut. It's principal functions are as follows:
- It controls the smooth muscle tone of the gut,
- It controls intensity of rhythmical contractions,
- It controls rhythm of the contractions,
- It causes increase in conduction of the excitatory waves resulting in peristaltic movements.
- Inhibitory control on intestinal sphincters by releasing vasoactive intestinal peptides. This causes relaxation of sphincters like pyloric sphincter and ileocecal valve, and propulsion of the chyme forward.

**What would happen if ENS isn't functioning?**

Failure of neural crest migration to GIT causes absence of Myenteric and Meissner's plexus (aganglionic) in a particular segment called "**Hirschsprung**" disease. The most common region is rectosigmoid region. There is absence of GI motility. So, all the food accumulated in the proximal segment. The proximal segment contracts forcefully to push the food forward and thus become hypertrophied.

### Meissner's/Submucosal Plexus

Submucosal or Meissner's plexus mainly controls GIT secretions and local blood flow. It functions in controlling each minute segment of inner intestinal wall. It is called the *"second brain"* due of its 100 million neurons, and is derived from the neural crest cells.

### Sensory (afferent) nerves arising from GIT

Sensory nerves arising from GIT either have cell bodies in both the plexus of enteric nervous system or in the dorsal root of ganglia in spinal cord. The afferents are stimulated on irritation of mucosa, distention of the gut and chemical substances. This can either excite, inhibit the movements or can cause increase in secretions. For example, 80% of vagus fibers are afferents which carry sensory signals to medulla and brain causing vagal reflexes.

## Autonomic Nervous System

The extrinsic innervation is done by both the divisions of autonomic nervous system.

### Parasympathetic Stimulation

Parasympathetic postganglionic neurons innervates Myenteric and Meissner's plexus of GIT and causes increase in the activity of enteric nervous system, increasing the GI motility and secretions.

- Cranial division of PNS is supplied through vagus nerve. It innervates regions of pharynx, esophagus, stomach, pancreas, small intestines and first half of large intestines up to the splenic flexure.
- Sacral PNS originates from pelvic nerves (S2,3 and 4) and innervates second half of large intestine till anus.

### Sympathetic Stimulation

Sympathetic fibers that innervate GIT arises from $T_5$–$L_2$ and the preganglionic fibers enter *celiac and mesenteric ganglions*, from where postganglionic fibers arises and spreads to whole of the gut. There innervations is more extensive towards oral and anal ends. Sympathetic fibers release norepinephrine which causes inhibition of the GI motility and secretions.

## Hormonal Control of GIT Functions (Table 28.1)

Gastrointestinal hormones (GI Hormones) are chemicals mediators produced and secreted by specialized epithelial of the GI tract mucosa known as enteroendocrine cells.

- **Local control due to stretching of muscle:** Whenever the food stretches the gut walls, it stimulates the secretions of the GI glands and peristalsis.

## GASTROINTESTINAL REFLEXES

The gastrointestinal system regulates many functions of motility and secretion due to various gastrointestinal reflexes. These reflexes are a result of enteric nervous system and the autonomic nervous system. Various reflexes can be classified as:

### Short Loop Reflexes

These reflexes are integrated within the gut wall enteric nervous system. They control GI secretion, peristalsis, mixing contraction, etc.

Example:
- **Deglutition reflex:** The swallowing of food from the oral cavity to the esophagus is called swallowing/deglutition reflex.
- **Colonoileal reflex:** Reflexes from the colon inhibits the emptying of ileal contents into the colon.

### Long Loop Reflexes

Long loop reflexes in the gastrointestinal (GI) tract involve communication between the GI tract and the central nervous system (CNS), including the brain and spinal cord. Unlike short loop reflexes, which are entirely contained within the enteric nervous system (ENS) of the GI tract, long loop reflexes involve afferent (sensory) and efferent (motor) pathways that connect the GI tract to higher centers in the CNS. These reflexes are crucial for coordinating GI functions with other physiological processes and environmental stimuli. Here are some examples of long loop reflexes:

- **Gastrocolic reflex:** This reflex involves the stimulation of colonic motility by the presence of food in the stomach. When food enters the stomach, stretch receptors in the stomach wall are activated, sending sensory signals via afferent nerves to the CNS. The CNS then sends efferent signals back to the colon, triggering an increase in colonic motility and promoting the movement of fecal material toward the rectum.

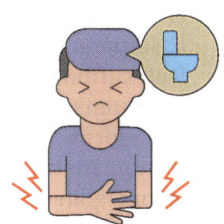

**Why does a baby defecate just after feeding?**

The gastrocolic reflex causes the baby to defecate immediately after feeding.

- **Enterogastric reflex:** The enterogastric reflex helps regulate gastric emptying by inhibiting gastric motility and secretion in response to the presence of chyme in the duodenum. When the duodenum becomes

**Table 28.1:** The various GI hormones regulating the GI functions.

| Name of the hormone | Source | Regulation of secretion | Target organs and functions |
|---|---|---|---|
| Gastrin | G cells in the antrum of the stomach and duodenum | Stimulated by:<br>• Breakdown products of protein digestion (Such as amino acids and peptides)<br>• Distention by food<br>• Vagus nerve<br>Inhibited by:<br>• Acid (H$^+$) | • Parietal cells in the stomach: Stimulates H$^+$ (acid) secretion<br>• **Mucosa of the small intestine, colon, and stomach:** Trophic (growth) effects<br>• Inhibits the actions of secretin and GIP |
| Cholecystokinin | I-cells in the duodenum and jejunum | • Acid<br>• Fat<br>• Breakdown products of protein digestion (Such as amino acids and peptides) | • **Pancreas:** Stimulates the secretion of bicarbonate and pancreatic enzymes, lipases, amylase, and proteases. Also, causes growth of the exocrine pancreas (Trophic effect)<br>• **Gallbladder:** Contraction of the gallbladder with simultaneous relaxation of the sphincter of Oddi and growth of gallbladder (Trophic effect)<br>• **Stomach:** Inhibits gastric emptying |
| Secretin | S cells in the duodenum | • Acid (H$^+$) in the lumen (less than 4.5)<br>• Fatty acids in the lumen | • **Stomach:** Inhibits gastrin, H$^+$ secretion, and growth of stomach mucosa (Trophic effect)<br>• **Pancreas:** Stimulates secretion of bicarbonate and growth of exocrine pancreas (Trophic effect)<br>• **Bile:** Stimulates biliary secretion of bicarbonate and fluid |
| Motilin | M cells of the duodenum and jejunum | • Fat<br>• Acid<br>• Vagus nerve | • Stimulate gastric motility by stimulating the "migratory motility"<br>• Stimulate intestinal motility |
| Gastric inhibitory peptide (GIP) | K cells of the duodenum and jejunum | • Protein<br>• Fat<br>• Carbohydrate | • Stimulate insulin release<br>• Inhibits gastric acid secretion |
| Vasoactive intestinal peptide (VIP) | • Pancreas<br>• Intestine<br>• Brain | Distension | • Induce secretion of pancreatic juice and bile<br>• Inhibits gastric acid secretion<br>• Stimulates the intestinal secretion of water and electrolytes<br>• Relaxation of smooth muscle including relaxation of sphincters |

distended or acidic due to the presence of food, sensory signals are sent to the CNS, which then sends inhibitory signals to the stomach via efferent nerves, slowing gastric emptying and allowing for more efficient digestion and absorption in the small intestine.
- **Defecation reflex:** The defecation reflex is initiated by distension of the rectum, which activates stretch receptors in the rectal wall. Sensory signals from the rectum are transmitted to the spinal cord, where they are integrated with higher CNS centers. If defecation is appropriate, efferent signals are sent back to the colon and rectum, promoting relaxation of the internal anal sphincter and contraction of the rectal muscles to facilitate bowel movements.
- **Vomiting reflex (Fig. 28.10):** The vomiting reflex, is a protective mechanism triggered by various stimuli, including ingested toxins, excessive distension of the stomach, or stimulation of the chemoreceptor trigger zone in the brain. Afferent signals from the GI tract, vestibular system, or higher brain centers are integrated in the vomiting center located in the brainstem, which then sends efferent signals to the GI tract and abdominal muscles, leading to forceful expulsion of stomach contents.

## PHYSIOLOGY OF SPLANCHNIC CIRCULATION

It is the circulation of blood from heart to visceral organs (intestines, spleen, pancreas and liver) and from visceral organs to liver through portal vein and from liver back to heart through (hepatic vein).

## FUNCTIONS OF SPLANCHNIC CIRCULATION

- Blood supply to the submucosal glands for the production of GI secretions.
- Blood supply to the muscular layers for the proper GI motility.
- The proper blood flow to intestines ensure proper digestion and absorption of nutrients in gut.
- The absorbed nutrients pass through the hepatic sinusoids, which have reticuloendothelial cells, which ensure that the harmful microorganisms, from gut do not enter the blood stream.

### Anatomy of GI Blood Supply

GI blood supply is shown in **Figures 28.11 and 28.12**.

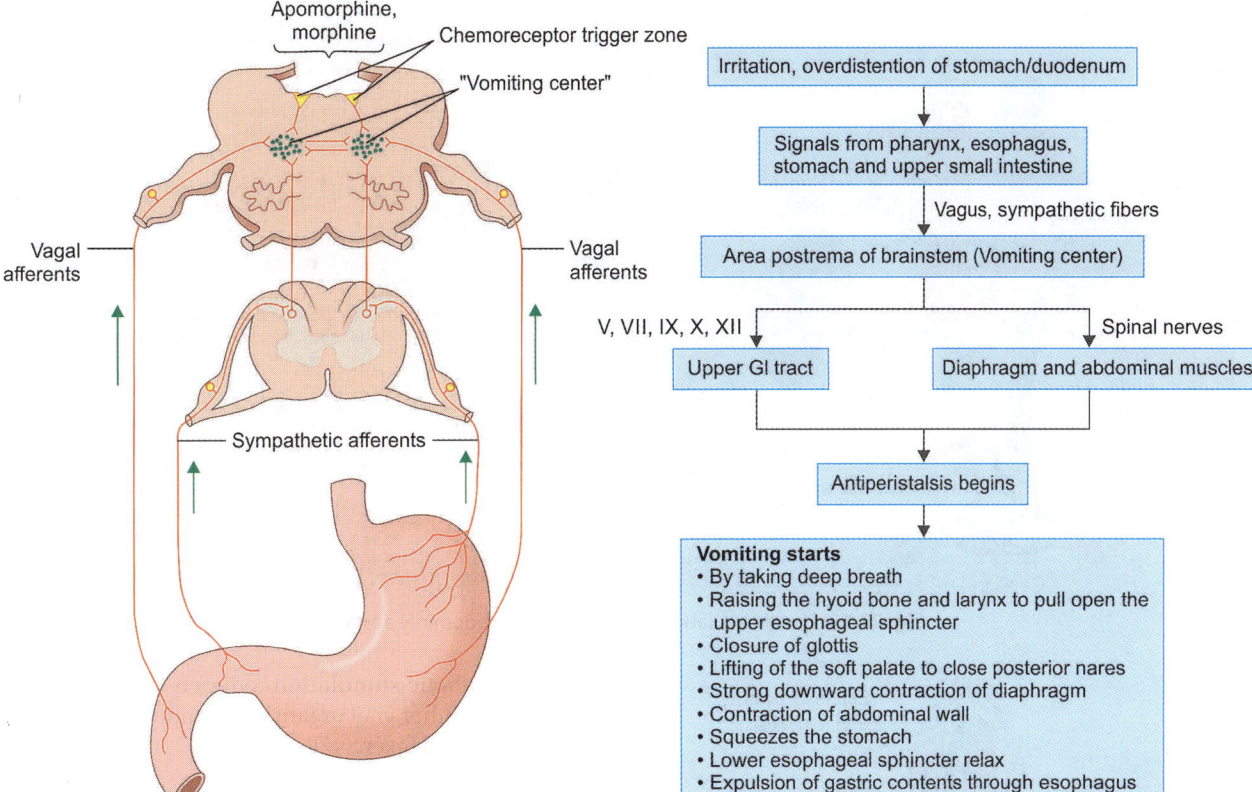

**Fig. 28.10:** Vomiting reflex.

## Blood Supply in Intestinal Microvilli (Counter-Current Flow)

By definition, the counter-current mechanism means, where the outflow is parallel to, close to and opposite to the inflow (hairpin bend flow). In the intestinal villi, the counter-current flow results in shunting the oxygen from artery to vein. **Figure 28.13** shows a typical arrangement of blood vessel in an intestinal villi. About 80% of oxygen, directly enters the venules, without reaching the tip of villi.

Under usual circumstances, the transfer of oxygen from arterioles to venules poses no harm to the villi. However, in disease states where blood flow to the gut is severely reduced, such as in circulatory shock, the oxygen deficiency in the villi's tips can reach critical levels, resulting in ischemic necrosis and subsequent disintegration of either the villus tip or the entire villus. Consequently, in numerous gastrointestinal disorders, including other factors, the villi undergo significant blunting, resulting in a considerable reduction in intestinal absorptive capability.

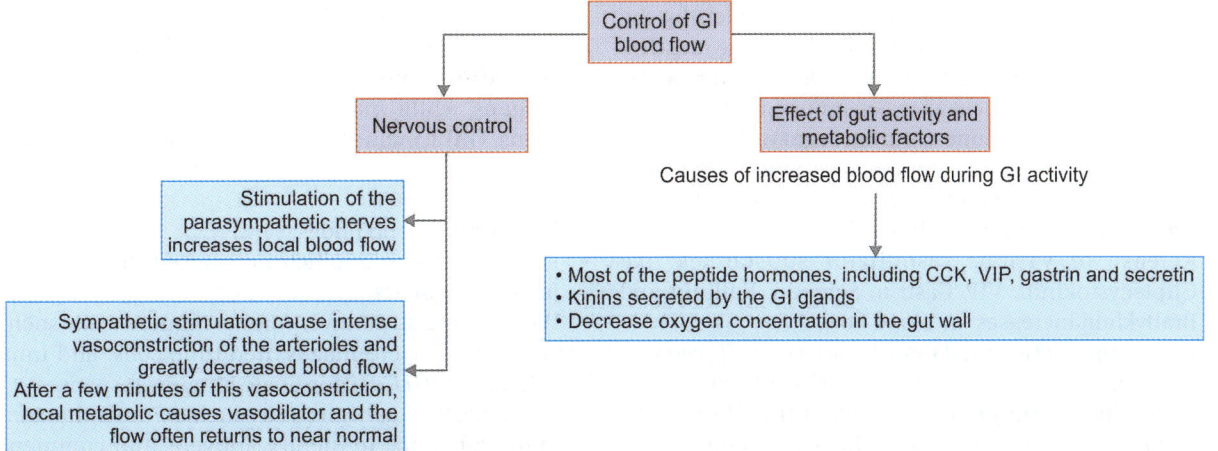

**Fig. 28.11:** Control of blood flow to GI system.
(CCK: cholecystokinin; VIP: vasoactive intestinal peptide)

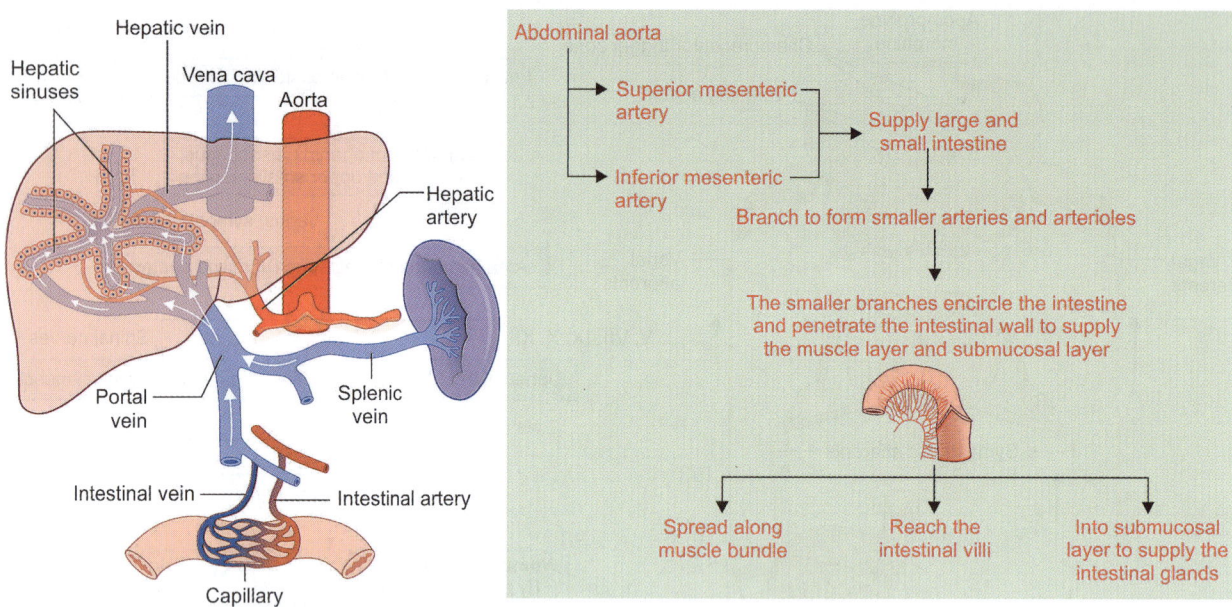

Fig. 28.12: Portal circulation and branches of abdominal aorta.

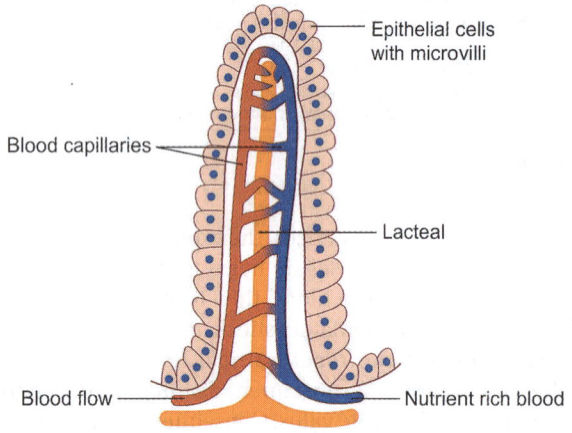

Fig. 28.13: Counter current flow in intestinal microvilli.

## Factors Affecting the Blood Flow to Gut

The blood flow to the gut is primarily regulated by the metabolic demand of the intestinal glands and the muscles. Hence, it is primarily regulated by the local factors along with various neural mechanisms, mentioned below:
- **Decreased oxygen concentration in gut wall:** Increased metabolism in the gut, after the meals due to increased activity, results in increased blood flow to the gut.
- **Adenosine:** Increases the blood flow.
- Release of various vasodilator substances like Cholecystokinin, VIP, Gastrin, Secretin, Kallidin and Bradykinin increases the blood flow.
- **Parasympathetic stimulation:** Increases the GI secretion and motility, hence increasing the GI blood flow.
- **Sympathetic stimulation:** Decreases the GI secretion and motility, hence decreasing the GI blood flow.
  The GI blood blow recovers from the prolonged sympathetic inhibition by the override mechanism under the influence of local factors called the 'autoregulatory escape'.

The sympathetic stimulation redirects the blood flow form GIT to other vital organs at the time of emergency (shock) or need (exercise).

**What happens to GI blood flow when other parts of the body need extra blood flow like during heavy exercise or in state of low blood volume (shock)?**

**Physiological importance of GI blood flow:**
- Sympathetic vasoconstriction of GI blood vessels decreases the GI blood flow for short period to supply blood flow to the active muscles or vital organs.
- Sympathetic stimulation of veins decreases volume of these veins and displaces large volume of blood onto the general circulation.

## IMMUNE APPARATUS OF GUT

The immune apparatus of the gut, often referred to as *gut-associated lymphoid tissue (GALT)*, constitutes a sophisticated network of immune cells and structures dedicated to protecting the gastrointestinal tract from pathogens while maintaining tolerance to harmless antigens. GALT includes specialized lymphoid structures such as:
- Peyer's patches
- Mesenteric lymph nodes
- Isolated lymphoid follicles dispersed throughout the intestinal mucosa.

Within these structures, various immune cells such as lymphocytes, macrophages, dendritic cells, and innate lymphoid cells (ILCs) coordinate immune responses.

Key aspects of gut immunity include the induction of immune tolerance to dietary antigens and commensal microbes, the production of secretory IgA antibodies to neutralize pathogens, and the regulation of immune responses by regulatory T cells (Tregs).

Interactions between the gut microbiota and the immune system play a crucial role in shaping immune responses and maintaining gut homeostasis.

Dysregulation of gut immunity can lead to inflammatory bowel diseases (IBD) and other gastrointestinal disorders, highlighting the importance of understanding and supporting the immune apparatus of the gut for overall health.

## INTESTINAL FLORA/GUT MICROBIOTA

Our gastrointestinal system is loaded with normal commensal gut commensals/intestinal flora/microbiota. Various organisms, which are found in our gut are:
- **Bacteria:** The majority of gut microbiota consists of bacteria, including various species such as Firmicutes, Bacteroidetes, Actinobacteria, and Proteobacteria.
- **Viruses:** Though less studied compared to bacteria, viruses, predominantly bacteriophages, are also part of the gut microbiota and can influence bacterial populations and functions.
- **Fungi:** While less abundant than bacteria, fungi such as *Candida* species can inhabit the gastrointestinal tract and impact gut health.
- **Other microbes:** Archaea and protists are present in smaller quantities in the gut microbiota, contributing to its overall diversity.

This gut flora is quite essential for normal functioning of our GI system. Some of their functions are summed up below:
- **Digestion and nutrient metabolism:** Gut microbiota aid in the digestion of dietary fibers, complex carbohydrates, and other indigestible compounds, producing short-chain fatty acids and vitamins such as vitamin B and vitamin K.
- **Immune regulation:** Intestinal flora plays a crucial role in modulating the immune system, helping to maintain immune homeostasis, promoting tolerance to harmless antigens, and protecting against pathogens.
- **Barrier function:** Gut microbiota contributes to the integrity of the intestinal barrier, preventing the invasion of harmful pathogens and toxins into the bloodstream.
- **Metabolic function:** Gut microbiota influence host metabolism, including energy harvest, lipid metabolism, and regulation of appetite, and are implicated in metabolic disorders such as obesity and diabetes.
- **Synthesis of bioactive compounds:** It produces various bioactive compounds, including neurotransmitters, bile acids, and secondary metabolites, which can impact host physiology and metabolism.
- **Protection against pathogens:** By competing for resources and producing antimicrobial compounds, gut microbiota helps to inhibit the colonization and growth of pathogenic bacteria in the gastrointestinal tract.
- **Gut-brain axis:** Emerging evidence suggests a bidirectional communication pathway between the gut and the brain, known as the gut-brain axis, in which gut microbiota play a significant role in influencing mood, behavior, and cognitive function.

## GUT-BRAIN AXIS (FIG. 28.14)

Gut brain axis or GBA is a bidirectional communication between neural plexus of enteric nervous system and

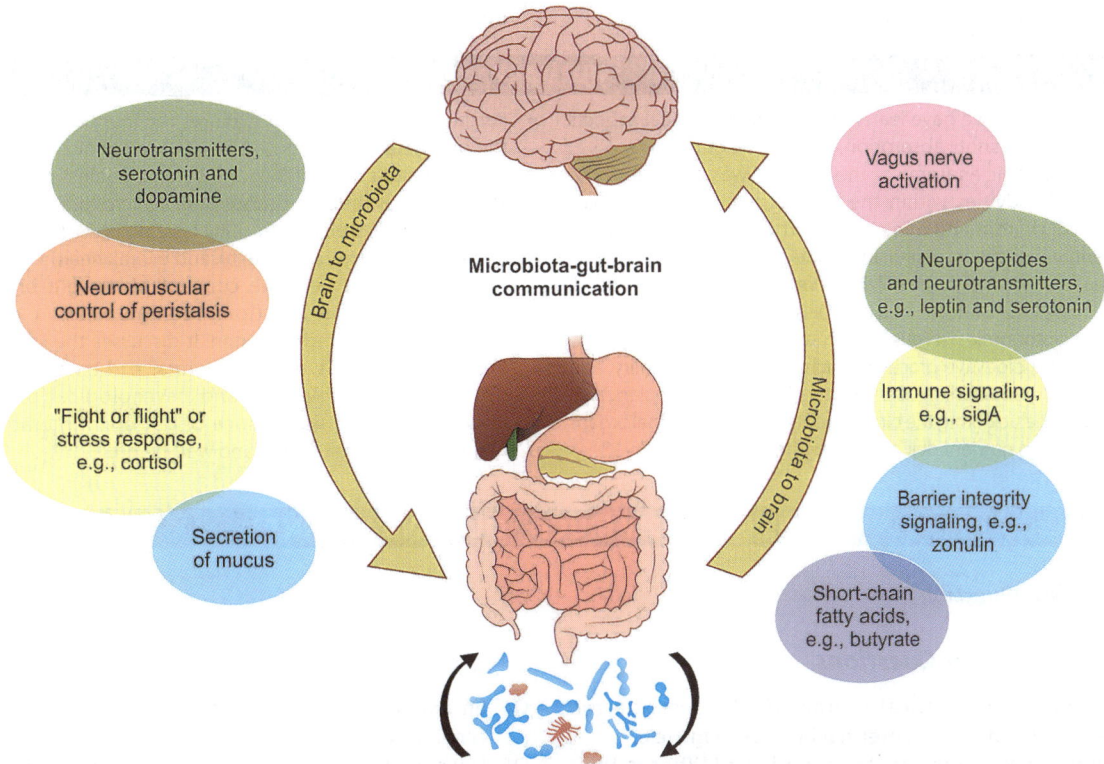

**Fig. 28.14:** Gut brain axis.

central nervous system. It is a complex communication system between central nervous system (CNS), autonomic nervous system (ANS), enteric nervous system (ENS) and hypothalamic pituitary axis (HPA) and enteric microbiota, which is responsible for the gastrointestinal homeostasis. The enteric microbiota which mainly consists of *Firmicutes* and *Bacteroides* interact locally and with CNS through neuroendocrine and metabolic pathways.

## Functions of the Gut Brain Axis

- **Digestion:** The gut-brain axis plays a crucial role in **regulating digestion** by coordinating processes such as peristalsis, secretion of digestive enzymes, and absorption of nutrients. Signals from the brain can influence gut motility and secretion, while gut hormones and neurotransmitters can affect brain function related to appetite and satiety.
- **Regulation of mood and emotion:** It leads to linking of peripheral intestinal functions with emotional and cognitive centers of the brain.
- There is a strong connection between the gut and emotions, with the gut often referred to as the "second brain." The gut microbiota produces neurotransmitters such as *serotonin* and *gamma-aminobutyric acid (GABA), brain-derived neurotrophic factor (BDNF)* which can influence mood and emotional states. *Dysbiosis of the gut microbiota* has been linked to neurological conditions such as *depression, anxiety*, and neurodegenerative diseases like *Alzheimer's and Parkinson's disease*.
  Conversely, stress and emotions can impact gut function and microbial composition.
- **Stress response:** The gut-brain axis is involved in the regulation of the stress response, with stress affecting gut function and vice versa. Chronic stress can lead to alterations in gut motility, permeability, and microbial composition, contributing to gastrointestinal disorders such as irritable bowel syndrome (IBS).
- **Regulation of appetite:** Gut hormones such as ghrelin and leptin, as well as signals from the gut microbiota, can influence appetite regulation and food intake. Changes in gut-brain signaling can contribute to obesity and metabolic disorders.
- **Modulates immune function:** The gut-brain axis plays a role in regulating immune function, with the gut-associated lymphoid tissue (GALT) serving as a key interface between the immune system and the gut. Communication between the gut and the brain can influence immune responses in the gut and other parts of the body. It maintains integrity of tight junction and intestinal barrier, enteric sensory efferent modulation, mucosal immunity.

## Applied Physiology

- Clinically altered microbiota is seen in patients of autism, mood disorders, anxiety and depression.
- Dysbiosis and irritable bowel disease is closely associated with microbiota.
- It is seen that normal gut microbiota is closely associated with maturation of CNS and ENS.
- The absence of microbial colonies is associated with abnormal release of neurotransmitters like serotonin, GABA and BDNF, gut sensory-motor function, reduced migratory motor complexes, delayed gastric emptying and intestinal transit with enlargement of cecum.

---

### SUMMARY

- In this chapter, we have learnt various physiological aspects crucial for digestion, absorption, and overall gut health.
- The physiologic anatomy of the GI tract, was discussed. The electrical activities within the GI tract, including the basic electrical rhythm and generation and propagation of action potentials essential for peristalsis and gut motility.
- We had also studied the neural and hormonal control mechanisms. It discusses the intricate interplay between the enteric nervous system, autonomic nervous system, and various GI hormones in modulating digestive processes such as secretion, motility, and absorption. Additionally, the chapter sheds light on splanchnic circulation, elucidating the blood supply to the abdominal organs and its role in nutrient delivery and waste removal.
- Furthermore, the chapter explores the immune apparatus of the gut, detailing the gut-associated lymphoid tissue and its role in immune surveillance and defense against pathogens. It also discusses the significance of gut microflora, highlighting the diverse microbial community residing in the GI tract and its impact on digestion, immunity, and overall health.
- We had also studied, the concept of the gut-brain axis, elucidating the bidirectional communication pathway between the gut and the brain. It discusses the influence of gut-derived signals, gut microbiota, and emotional states on various physiological and psychological processes, underscoring the significance of gut-brain interactions in maintaining overall health and well-being.

---

### LET US SEE, HOW MUCH YOU HAVE LEARNT?

 *Review Questions*

#### Long/Short Answer Questions

Q1. Define basal electrical rhythm (BER). Describe the generation of action potential in smooth muscle.
Q2. What are migrating motor complexes? What is their physiological significance?
Q3. Describe the functions of enteric nervous system.
Q4. Enumerate the gastrointestinal hormones and give their functions.
Q5. Describe the role of gut brain axis in maintaining good health in a person.

## Explain Why (Reasoning Questions)

**Q1.** There is increase blood flow in splanchnic circulation after meals.

**Q2.** The person feels happy after having a good meal.

## Multiple Choice Questions

**Q1.** Which of the following accurately describes the physiologic anatomy of the gastrointestinal (GI) system?
  a. The stomach primarily functions in nutrient absorption
  b. The small intestine is responsible for the majority of water reabsorption
  c. The large intestine is where most enzymatic digestion occurs
  d. The esophagus has smooth muscle for peristaltic movement

**Q2.** What electrical activities are essential for gut motility?
  a. Action potentials propagate only in the longitudinal muscles
  b. Slow wave potentials initiate peristalsis in the stomach
  c. High-frequency spikes are characteristic of relaxed smooth muscle
  d. Tonic contractions occur without involvement of electrical activity

**Q3.** What contractile properties contribute to gastrointestinal (GIT) function?
  a. The tonic contraction of circular muscles helps mix and propel food
  b. Phasic contractions occur independently of neural input
  c. Relaxation of longitudinal muscles aids in food absorption
  d. Slow wave potentials inhibit smooth muscle contraction

**Q4.** Which of the following accurately describes the regulation of GI functions?
  a. Hormonal control plays a minor role in modulating digestive processes
  b. The enteric nervous system solely regulates motility and secretion
  c. Parasympathetic stimulation inhibits gastric acid secretion
  d. Cholecystokinin stimulates pancreatic enzyme secretion

**Q5.** A patient with a severe stress response experiences altered GI function due to:
  a. Increased parasympathetic activity leading to enhanced peristalsis
  b. Elevated levels of serotonin resulting in decreased gut motility
  c. Dysregulation of gut microbiota impacting digestive processes
  d. Reduced sympathetic activity leading to enhanced gastric acid secretion

**Q6.** Which of the following factors contribute to the regulation of GI functions?
  a. Activation of sympathetic nervous system inhibiting gut motility
  b. Release of gastrin promoting gastric acid secretion
  c. Presence of tight junctions facilitating paracellular absorption
  d. Inhibition of somatostatin promoting pancreatic enzyme release

**Q7.** A patient presents with impaired nutrient absorption. Which aspect of splanchnic circulation is likely affected?
  a. Increased blood flow to the liver via the portal vein
  b. Reduced arterial supply to the stomach from the celiac trunk
  c. Impaired venous drainage from the intestines through the hepatic portal vein
  d. Enhanced blood flow to the small intestine through the superior mesenteric artery

**Q8.** Which immune apparatus plays a crucial role in immune surveillance and defense against pathogens in the gut?
  a. The thymus gland
  b. Gut-associated lymphoid tissue (GALT)
  c. Spleen
  d. Bone marrow

**Q9.** A patient with prolonged antibiotic use develops diarrhea due to:
  a. Overgrowth of beneficial gut bacteria
  b. Increased production of short-chain fatty acids
  c. Disruption of gut microbiota leading to *Clostridium difficile* infection
  d. Enhanced immune surveillance by gut-associated lymphoid tissue

**Q10.** How do gut microbiota contribute to gastrointestinal health?
  a. By producing bile acids essential for digestion
  b. By competing with pathogens for colonization sites and nutrients
  c. By inhibiting peristalsis and gastric acid secretion
  d. By enhancing immune tolerance to dietary antigens

**Q11.** A patient with irritable bowel syndrome (IBS) experiences altered gut-brain axis signaling leading to:
  a. Increased serotonin production by gut microbiota
  b. Dysregulation of gut hormone secretion
  c. Enhanced sympathetic activity reducing gut motility
  d. Disruption of communication between the enteric nervous system and the central nervous system

**Q12.** Which aspect of the gut-brain axis influences emotional states and cognitive function?
  a. Regulation of gut motility by the autonomic nervous system
  b. Production of neurotransmitters by gut microbiota
  c. Synthesis of bile acids by the liver
  d. Activation of the hypothalamic-pituitary-adrenal (HPA) axis by gut-derived signals

## ANSWERS

**1.** d    **2.** b    **3.** a    **4.** d    **5.** d    **6.** a    **7.** c    **8.** b    **9.** c    **10.** b    **11.** d    **12.** b

# Digestion in Oral Cavity and Esophagus

**29**
CHAPTER

### COMPETENCY ADDRESSED
**PY4.2:** Describe the composition, mechanism of secretion, functions, and regulation of saliva, gastric, pancreatic, intestinal juices and bile secretion.
**PY4.3:** Describe GIT movements, regulation and functions. Describe defecation reflex. Explain the role of dietary fiber.
**PY4.4:** Describe the physiology of digestion and absorption of nutrients.

### LEARNING OBJECTIVES
**At the end of this chapter, the learner should be able to:**
- Describe the general principles, basic mechanisms of salivary secretion.
- Describe the composition and functions of salivary secretions.
- Describe the general regulation of salivary secretions.
- Describe the process of chewing in the mouth.
- Discuss the physiology of swallowing (deglutition)/deglutition reflex.
- Describe the relevant applied physiology related to salivary secretion and deglutition.

Digestion of food begins in the oral cavity after it has been ingested. Food is mechanically processed by the tongue, teeth, and palatal surfaces of the mouth. It is mixed with saliva and mucus and propelled from the pharynx to the esophagus and finally into the stomach via the esophagus. Peristalsis in the esophagus move the food into the stomach.

**An overview:**
Let's us consider that you are eating your favorite food, say a slice of Pizza...

**How would you eat it?**
- While you open the box of freshly baked pizza, the aroma stimulates your salivary secretion *(cephalic phase of salivary and other GI secretions)*.
- The first bite of that scrumptious pizza stimulates further salivation. This pizza is broken down into smaller pieces by chewing/mastication by the teeth. The tongue rolls the food into the mouth and it is mixed with the saliva. The digestion begins right from the oral cavity.
- This chewed bolus of food (no longer a pizza) is swallowed with the help of tongue and pharyngeal muscles into the esophagus. It takes the food bolus to stomach.
- In the stomach, the food is mixed with hydrochloric acid and enzymes further churning the food into partially digested chyme. Food stays there 3–4 hours.
- This partially digested chyme is released in small batches into the duodenum, where it is further mixed with pancreatic juice and bile required for the digestion of nutrients.
- The digested chyme enters the small intestine, from where the nutrients are absorbed into the blood stream and the lymph for the utilization in body. The unabsorbed part then passes to the large intestine.
- In the large intestine, the colon absorbs the water and solidifies the fecal matter.
- The fecal matter is then expelled from the body through the anal opening.
- After this brief overview, let us discuss the secretions and motility in each part of the gut, starting from the oral cavity. The processes in various other partes will be discussed in subsequent chapters.

## ORAL CAVITY/MOUTH

The oral cavity, commonly known as the mouth, is a crucial anatomical structure that serves several essential functions in the human body. It is the initial part of the digestive system and plays a significant role in mastication, sense of taste and the speech production.

## Parts of Oral Cavity (Fig. 29.1)

- **Lips:** The lips form the anterior boundary of the oral cavity. They are composed of soft, movable tissue and are involved in functions such as speech articulation, eating, and facial expression.
- **Cheeks:** The cheeks are the fleshy sides of the face that form the lateral walls of the oral cavity. They contain muscles and glands and help to keep food within the mouth during chewing.
- **Teeth:** Teeth are hard structures embedded in the jawbones (maxilla and mandible) and are used for biting, tearing, and grinding food during the process of mastication (chewing). They also play a crucial role in speech production.
- **Gums (gingiva):** The gums are the soft tissues that surround and support the teeth. They help to anchor the teeth in place and protect the underlying bone and tissues.
- **Hard palate:** The hard palate is the bony structure that forms the roof of the mouth. It separates the oral cavity from the nasal cavity and provides a rigid surface for the tongue to push against during swallowing.
- **Soft palate:** The soft palate is a muscular structure located behind the hard palate. It helps to close off the nasal cavity during swallowing to prevent food and liquid from entering the nose.
- **Uvula:** The uvula is a small, fleshy structure that hangs down from the back of the soft palate. It plays a role in speech articulation and helps to prevent food from entering the nasal cavity during swallowing.
- **Tongue:** The tongue is a muscular organ located on the floor of the oral cavity. It is involved in various functions, including tasting, chewing, swallowing, and speech production. The surface of the tongue contains taste buds that detect different tastes.
- **Salivary glands:** Salivary glands are located within and around the oral cavity and produce saliva, which helps to moisten food, facilitate chewing and swallowing, and initiate the digestion of carbohydrates.

## SALIVARY SECRETION

### Physiology of Salivary Secretion

Salivary glands are essential structures in the human body responsible for producing saliva, a fluid crucial for digestion and oral health.

There are three main types of salivary glands: parotid glands, submandibular glands, and sublingual glands. These glands secrete saliva into the oral cavity through specific ducts (**Fig. 29.2**):

1. The parotid glands, located near the ears, produce a watery secretion rich in enzymes like *amylase* for initiating carbohydrate digestion.
2. Submandibular glands, positioned beneath the lower jaw, produce a mix of *serous and mucous secretions*.
3. Sublingual glands, situated beneath the tongue, produce predominantly *mucous secretions*.

Together, these glands and their secretions play a vital role in lubricating food, initiating digestion, and maintaining oral health.

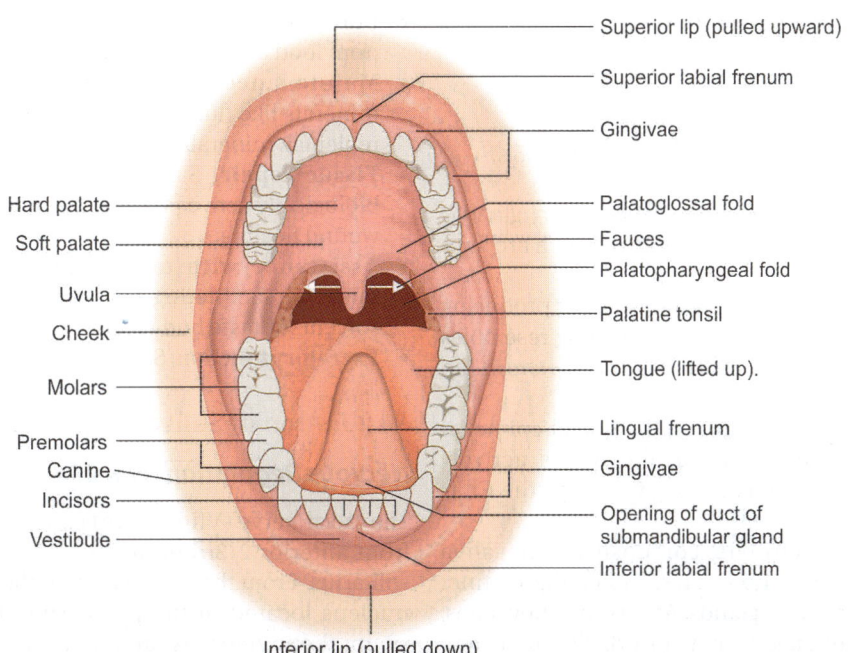

**Fig. 29.1:** Parts of oral cavity.

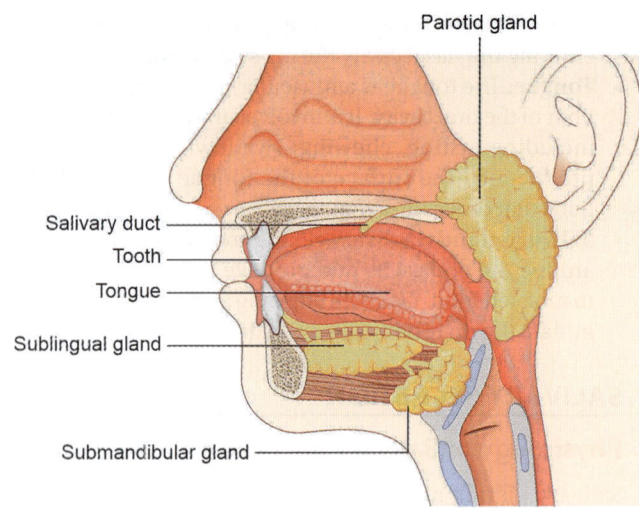

**Fig. 29.2:** Salivary glands anatomy.

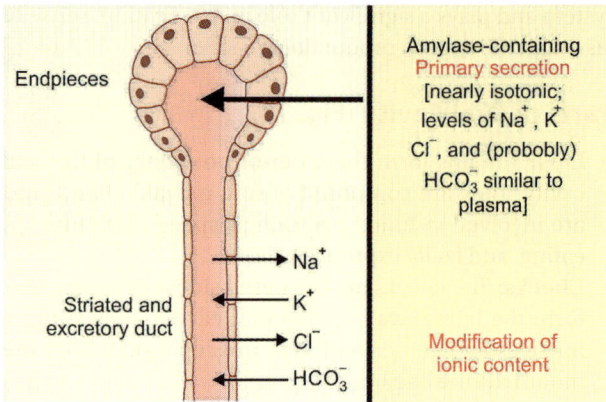

**Fig. 29.3:** Secretion of saliva.

## Secretion of Saliva

**Composition:** Saliva is the initial digestive fluid released upon food entry into the mouth, possesses a *hypotonic nature*, meaning it has a lower osmolality than plasma.

Saliva has a pH between 6.0 and 7.0, which is a favorable range for the digestive action of ptyalin.

**Daily secretion:** Each day, *the body secretes about 5 L of saliva*, highlighting its crucial role in the early stages of digestion.

**Composition of Saliva**
- Water (99.5%)
- Inorganic solids
  - $Na^+$, $K^+$, $Ca^{++}$, $Mg^{++}$, $Cl^-$, $HCO_3^-$, $PO_4^{2-}$, $SO_4^{2-}$
- Organic solids
  - Enzymes (Ptyalin)
  - Lysozyme
  - Lactoferrin
  - Carbonic anhydrase
  - Lingual lipase
  - Nuclease
- Others (Blood group factors, IgA, nerve growth factors)

**Formation and secretion of saliva:** Each salivary gland is composed of an acinus and a duct, both of which are lines by epithelial cells.

The acinar epithelial cells are responsible for producing the *primary salivary secretion*, which closely resembles plasma in composition **(Fig. 29.3)**. It is rich is *ptyalin* (an enzyme), mucus and extracellular fluid.

As this secretion travels through the ductal epithelial cells, modifications occur. Here, the $Na^+$ is actively reabsorbed and $K^+$ is secreted. Along with that, the $Cl^-$ is absorbed and $HCO_3^-$ secreted.

Differences in electrolyte composition in saliva are observed at varying flow rates, indicating distinct stimulations of the salivary glands. At very high flow rates, ductal cells may not effectively reabsorb $Na^+$ or secrete $K^+$ into saliva, with bicarbonate being an exception.

Stimulating the glands and ductal cells also triggers bicarbonate secretion, resulting in an increasingly alkaline salivary secretion at high flow rates. ***Hence, the saliva tastes salty, at high flow rates.***

Saliva production is influenced by autonomic nerves, food flavors, odors, and auditory stimuli, while fear, sleep, and fatigue decrease it.

**Functions of saliva:**
- **Lubrication:** Mucin in saliva aids in the formation of boluses, facilitating the movement of food between oral segments.
- **Digestion:** Saliva contains salivary amylase (Ptyalin) and lingual lipase, aiding in carbohydrate and fat digestion. Salivary amylase is deactivated by stomach acid and does not digest proteins.
- **Protection:** IgA antibodies, lactoferrin, and lysozyme in saliva help eliminate bacteria and prevent infections. Mucin coats the oral mucosa, protecting it from toxins and injuries.
- **Buffering:** Bicarbonate buffers in saliva neutralize acids from food and oral bacteria, preventing dental caries.
- **Maintenance of tooth integrity:** Saliva contains minerals like fluoride, calcium, and phosphate, which replenish minerals lost due to tooth decay.
- **Tissue repair:** Saliva contains growth factors and biologically active proteins that aid in tissue repair and wound healing.
- **Assistance with taste:** Saliva dissolves ingested material, facilitating taste perception by acting as a solvent for taste bud receptors.
- **Excretory function:** Saliva excretes certain heavy metals.

## Regulation of Salivary Secretion

### Nervous Regulation (Fig. 29.4)

The facial nerve (VIIth nerve) carries the taste sensations from anterior 2/3rd of tongue to the nucleus of tractus solitarius. From there it relays into the superior salivatory nucleus located in the pons. The preganglionic parasympathetic neurons, arising from superior salivatory nucleus synapses in submandibular ganglia, from where

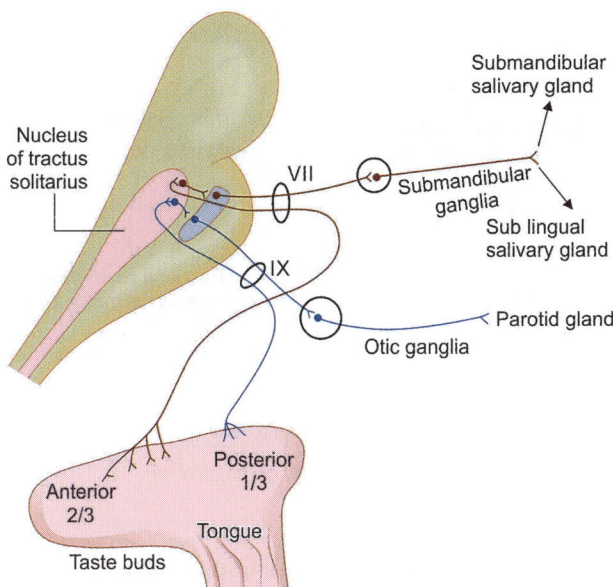

Fig. 29.4: Nervous regulation of salivary secretion.

the post ganglionic parasympathetic neurons innervate the submandibular and sublingual salivary glands.

However, the taste sensation from posterior 1/3rd of tongue is carried by glossopharyngeal nerve (IXth nerve), which relays in nucleus of tractus solitarius, relaying into inferior salivatory nucleus. The parasympathetic fibers arise from the inferior salivatory nucleus and synapse in Otic ganglia. The post ganglionic parasympathetic fibers arising from otic ganglia innervates the parotid gland.

Other factors are shown in **Figure 29.5**.

## Clinical Correlation

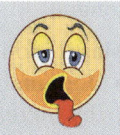

- Autoimmune destruction of salivary glands produces dry mouth. One condition called Sjögren syndrome.
- Destruction of salivary and lacrimal gland causes dry mouth and dry eyes.

- ***Sialorrhea***, or excessive salivation, can occur due to either increased production and stimulation of salivary glands or weakened muscles that impede the flow of saliva from the mouth. Additionally, it can manifest as a side effect of various medications.
- ***Xerostomia,*** or dry mouth, refers to reduced salivary secretion. This condition may arise from adverse reactions to medications, infections, radiation therapy targeting the head and neck, autoimmune reactions against the salivary glands (such as Sjögren's syndrome), or age-related alterations.

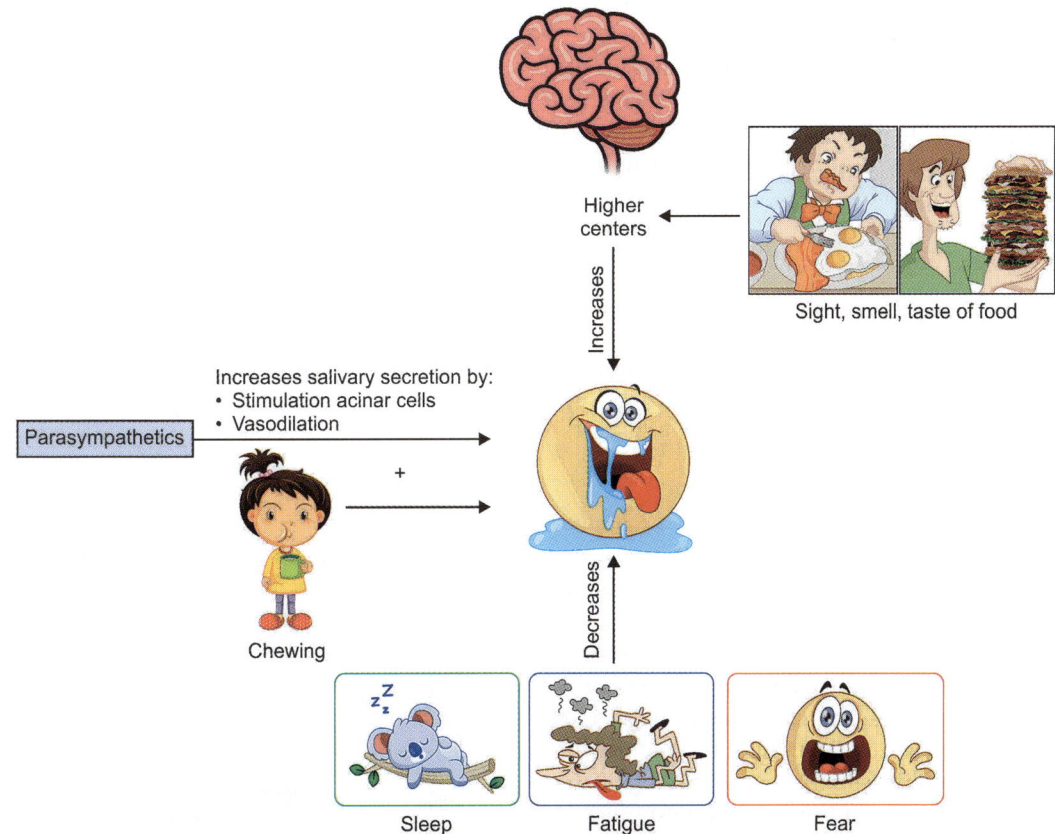

Fig. 29.5: Various factors affecting salivary secretions.

## PHYSIOLOGY OF MASTICATION (CHEWING)

Chewing, known as mastication, marks the beginning of the digestive process by crushing and blending food with saliva to create a bolus suitable for swallowing. This physiological process involves the synchronized movement of the jaw, the cutting and grinding actions of the teeth on food, saliva secretion, and the thorough mixing of food particles with saliva by the tongue.

Mastication serves various functions:
- **Enhancing digestion:** Chewing aids in food digestion by increasing the exposed surface area for digestive enzymes to act upon. By grinding food into smaller particles, digestion becomes more efficient as enzymes can access the surfaces more effectively.
- **Facilitating swallowing:** Breaking down food into smaller pieces through chewing makes it easier to swallow, facilitating the movement of food through the esophagus and into the digestive system.
- **Mixing saliva with food:** Through mastication, food gets thoroughly mixed with saliva, which contains digestive enzymes initiating chemical digestion and helps lubricate the food bolus for easier swallowing.
- **Minimizing gastrointestinal irritation:** By grinding food into finer particles, mastication reduces the risk of irritation or damage to the gastrointestinal tract that larger food particles might cause during digestion.
- **Digesting fibrous foods:** Mastication assists in the digestion of fibrous foods like fruits and raw vegetables by breaking down their tough cellulose membranes, enabling better nutrient absorption and promoting overall digestive health.

### Chewing Reflex (Fig. 29.6)

- **Afferent:** Sensory nerves from V, VII and IX nerves
- **Centre:** Specific reticular areas in brainstem (Higher centres: Hypothalamus, amygdala, cerebral cortex)
- **Efferent:** Motor branch of Vth nerve

## PHYSIOLOGY OF SWALLOWING/ DEGLUTITION

Swallowing, also known as deglutition, encompasses the process of moving food from the mouth (oral cavity) to the stomach via the pharynx and esophagus. This physiological act holds immense significance as the pharynx serves as a common pathway for both food and air, posing the risk of food entering the trachea. Therefore, swallowing serves to safeguard the airway from aspiration by pushing the bolus back into the mouth with the tongue, closing off the nasopharynx and airway, and opening the esophageal pathway.

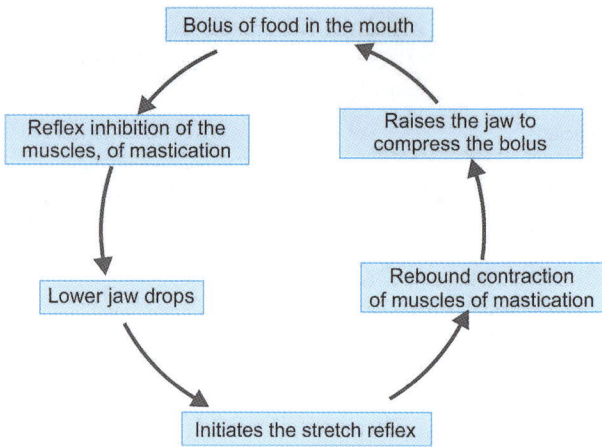

**Fig. 29.6:** Physiology of mastication.

### Functional Anatomy of the Esophagus

It is a muscular tube measuring between 18 and 25 centimeters in length, comprises three distinct sections: the upper esophageal sphincter (UES), middle esophageal body, and lower esophageal sphincter (LES), also referred to as the Gastroesophageal Sphincter or Cardiac Sphincter. The UES, composed of striated muscle, remains tonically contracted to prevent air from entering the esophagus, while the LES, comprising smooth muscle, maintains tonic constriction at rest to prevent reflux from the stomach.

### Deglutition Occurs in Three Phases

The oral phase which is voluntary, followed by the involuntary pharyngeal and esophageal phases.
1. During the *oral/buccal phase* (**Fig. 29.7**), the tongue elevates to propel the bolus posteriorly into the oropharynx, where it is temporarily retained until the initiation of the pharyngeal phase.
2. In the *pharyngeal phase* (**Figs. 29.8 and 29.9**), triggered by the bolus contacting the oropharyngeal wall, a reflex response stimulates sensory receptors, leading

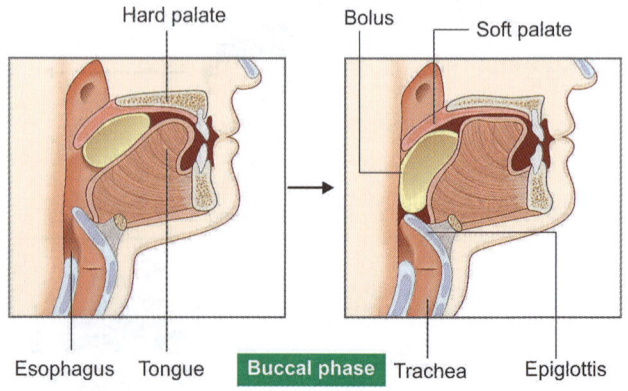

**Fig. 29.7:** Buccal phase of deglutition.

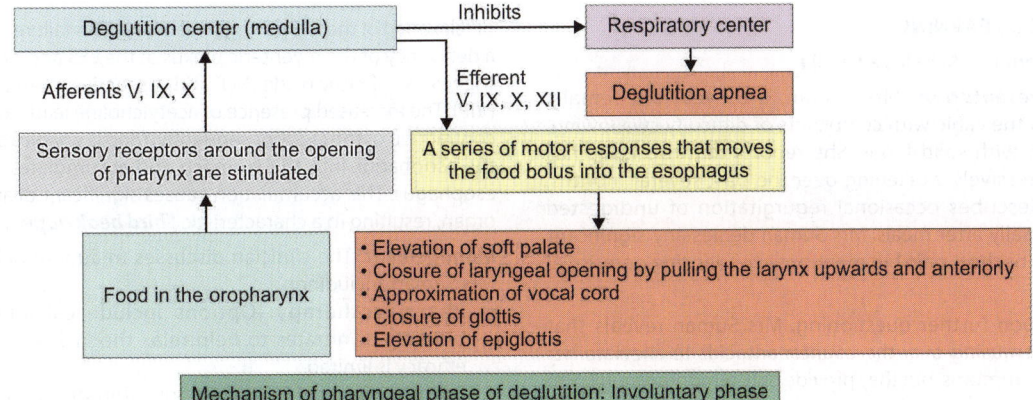

Fig. 29.8: Involuntary phase of deglutition.

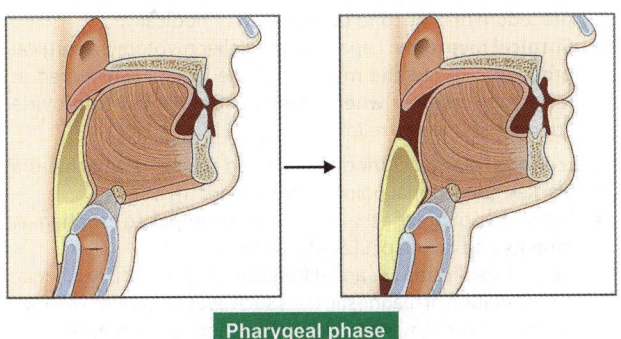

Fig. 29.9: Pharyngeal phase of deglutition.

to involuntary contraction of pharyngeal muscles that propel the bolus into the esophagus. Concurrently, *the soft palate elevates to close off the nasopharynx, the larynx is pulled upward and anteriorly to close the laryngeal opening, vocal cords approximate, the glottis closes, and the epiglottis elevates to prevent food from entering the respiratory passage.* There is **deglutition apnea**, a momentary cessation of respiration induced by the swallowing center inhibiting the respiratory center, lasting less than one second. Finally, relaxation of the upper esophageal sphincter allows the bolus to enter the esophagus, concluding the pharyngeal phase.

3. During the *esophageal phase* (**Fig. 29.10**), the food moves from the pharynx to stomach. It is done by two waves of peristalsis:
   - *Primary peristalsis:* As food traverses the esophagus, a peristaltic wave is initiated. It occurs as a continuation of the peristaltic wave initiated in the pharynx. This wave pushes the bolus down into the stomach through the lower esophageal sphincter.
   - *Secondary peristalsis:* Usually, all the food is pushed into stomach by primary peristaltic wave but if there is some remnant food, the secondary wave gets initiated when the food causes distension and results in reflex constriction, emptying the entire esophageal contents through the LES. The LES relaxes, when the food reaches the caudal end of the esophagus. Failure to relax LES results in achalasia cardia (mentioned further).

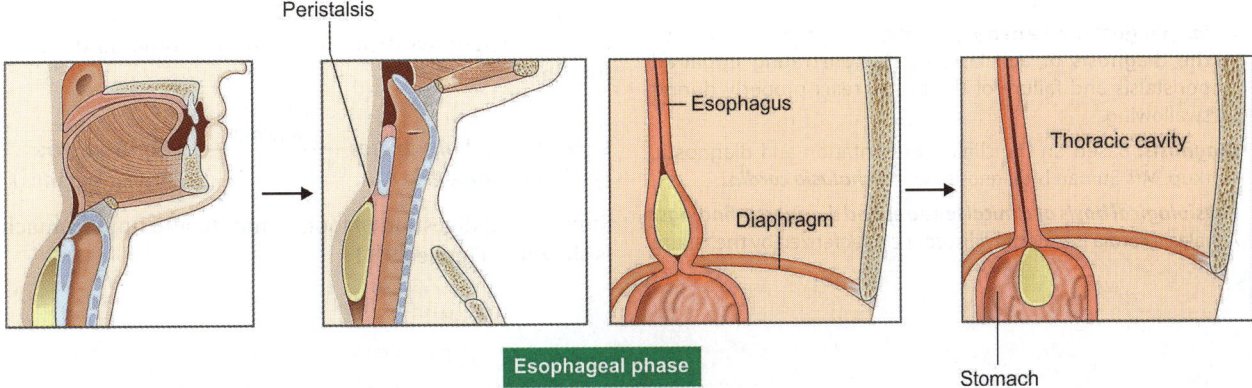

Fig. 29.10: Esophageal phase of deglutition.

## CASE BASED LEARNING
### Clinical Scenario: Achalasia Cardia

***Patient presentation:*** Mrs Suman, a 55-year-old female, presents to the clinic with complaints of difficulty swallowing, particularly with solid foods. She reports that this issue has been progressively worsening over the past several months. She also describes occasional regurgitation of undigested food, especially after meals. Mrs Suman denies any significant weight loss or chest pain but mentions experiencing occasional heartburn.

***History:*** Upon further questioning, Mrs Suman reveals that she has been using over-the-counter antacids to alleviate her heartburn symptoms, but they provide only temporary relief. She has no significant medical history apart from occasional episodes of heartburn. There is no family history of gastrointestinal disorders.

***Physical examination:*** On physical examination, Mrs Suman appears generally well-nourished with no signs of distress. Vital signs are within normal limits. Examination of the oral cavity and neck reveals no abnormalities. Auscultation of the chest is unremarkable.

***Diagnostic workup:*** Based on her symptoms, the clinician decides to pursue further evaluation. Mrs Suman undergoes the following diagnostic tests:

- **Esophagogastroduodenoscopy (EGD):** EGD reveals dilation of the esophagus with retained food particles and fluid. No evidence of mucosal ulceration or masses is noted. Biopsies are obtained for histological examination.
- **Barium swallow study:** Barium swallow demonstrates a dilated esophagus with a narrowed lower esophageal sphincter (LES) and a characteristic "bird's beak" appearance. There is delayed emptying of the contrast material into the stomach.

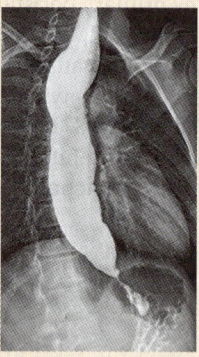

- **Esophageal manometry:** Esophageal manometry confirms the diagnosis of achalasia by demonstrating impaired peristalsis and failure of the LES to relax properly during swallowing.

***Diagnosis:*** Based on the clinical presentation and diagnostic workup, Mrs Suman is diagnosed with ***achalasia cardia.***

***Physiological basis of clinical features and diagnostic findings:*** Achalasia cardia is a motility disorder characterized by the failure of relaxation of the LES during swallowing. This failure results from a deficiency of the myenteric plexus at the LES and a decrease in the release of nitric oxide (NO) and vasoactive intestinal peptide (VIP). The increased presence of acetylcholine leads to sustained contraction of the LES. Consequently, food is unable to pass from the esophagus into the stomach and accumulates within the esophagus. This accumulation causes significant dilation of the organ, resulting in a characteristic ***"bird beak appearance."***

***Management:*** The clinician discusses treatment options with Mrs Suman, including:

- **Pharmacotherapy:** Options include calcium channel blockers or nitrates to help relax the LES, although their efficacy is limited.
- **Botulinum toxin injection:** Injection of botulinum toxin into the LES can provide temporary relief of symptoms by inducing muscle relaxation.
- **Pneumatic dilation:** Widening of the LES using a balloon catheter can help improve esophageal emptying. This procedure may need to be repeated periodically.
- **Surgical myotomy:** Laparoscopic Heller myotomy, a surgical procedure to cut the muscles of the LES, is considered in refractory cases or when other treatments fail to provide adequate symptom relief.

***Educational points:*** During case-based teaching on achalasia cardia, key educational points may include:

- Pathophysiology of achalasia, including impaired esophageal motility and failure of LES relaxation.
- Clinical manifestations and differential diagnosis of dysphagia.
- Interpretation of diagnostic tests such as EGD, barium swallow, and esophageal manometry in the diagnosis of achalasia.
- Treatment options for achalasia, including pharmacotherapy, endoscopic interventions, and surgical management.
- Prognosis and potential complications of achalasia if left untreated or undertreated.

## DIGESTION OF FOOD IN ORAL CAVITY

The food bolus primarily undergoes mechanical digestion in the mouth being subjected to chewing and mixing with saliva. However, the chemical digestion takes place for complex carbohydrates. The main enzyme involved in carbohydrate digestion in the mouth is **salivary amylase**, secreted by the salivary glands. Salivary amylase begins the breakdown of complex carbohydrates (such as starch) into simpler sugars, such as maltose. This enzymatic action initiates the process of carbohydrate digestion. However, there is insignificant/no digestion of protein and fats in mouth.

*Complex carbohydrates* $\xrightarrow{\text{salivary amylase}}$ *Simple sugars*
*(polysaccharides)* *(disaccharides)*

Summary of digestion of food in mouth and upto stomach is shown in **Figure 29.11**.

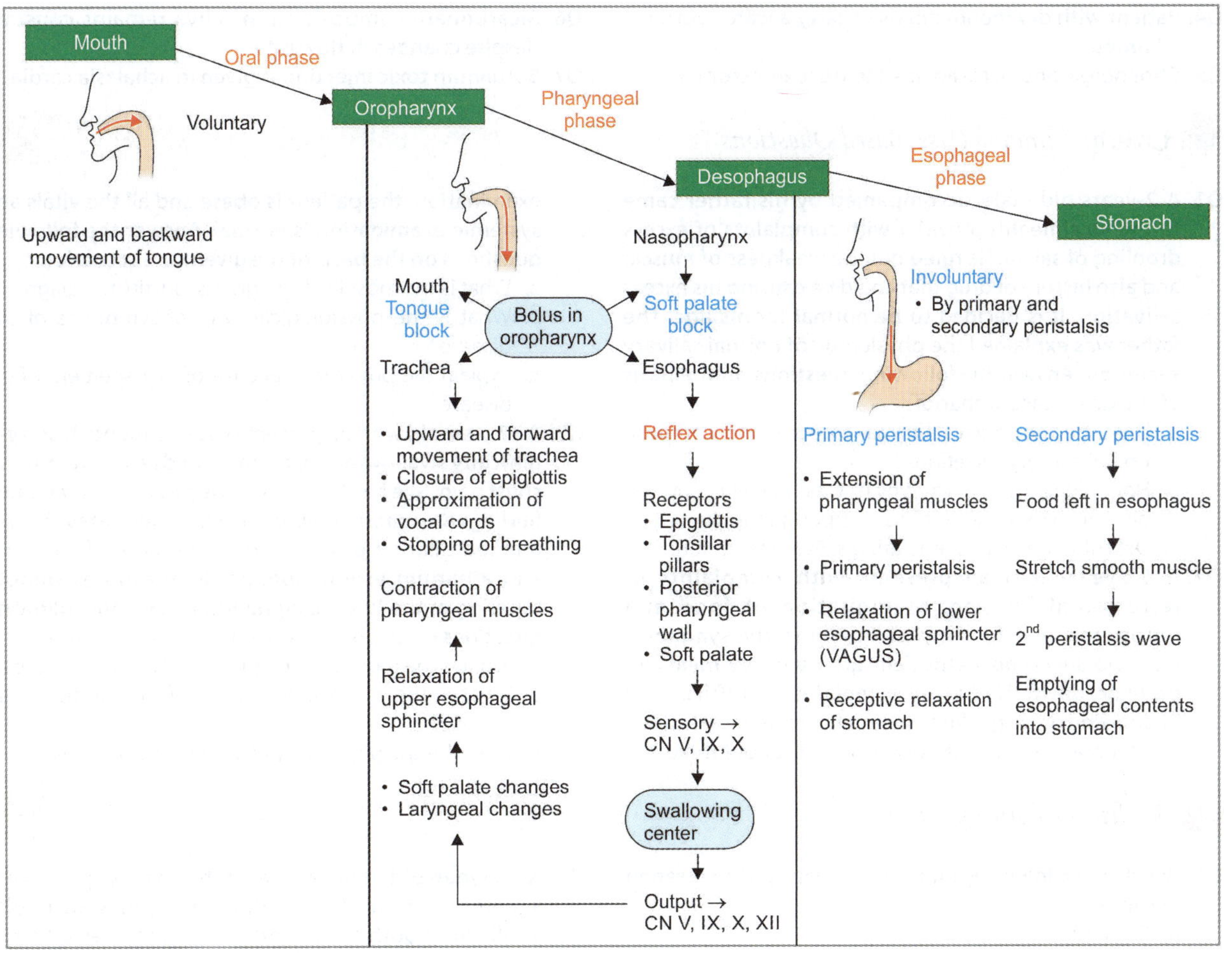

**Fig. 29.11:** Summary of digestion in mouth to stomach.
(*Courtesy:* Credit to Ms Muskan Singh.)

## SUMMARY

- About 1.5 L/day of saliva is secreted. It's pH is 7 and is hypotonic to plasma. Major source is submandibular gland. Saliva has highest potassium secretion per day. Both parasympathetic and sympathetic nervous system increases saliva. PNS produces thin watery saliva whereas SNS produces thick saliva.
- In sialorrhea, saliva is rich in sodium, potassium, chloride and bicarbonate because there is no ductal modification.
- Swallowing is triggered centrally and is coordinated with a peristaltic wave along the length of the esophagus that drives the food bolus to the stomach, even against gravity.
- Failure of relaxation of LES causes motility disorder called achalasia cardia.

## LET US SEE, HOW MUCH YOU HAVE LEARNT?

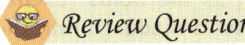Review Questions

### Long/Short Answer Questions

Q1. Write the functions of saliva.
Q2. Describe the composition, mechanism of secretion, functions and regulation of salivary secretion.
Q3. Describe the mechanism of deglutition reflex.
Q4. Write a note on achalasia cardia.

### Explain Why? (Reasoning Questions)

Q1. A patient with dry mouth is more susceptible to dental caries.
Q2. Anticholinergic drugs cause dry mouth.
Q3. Swallowing and speech is affected in xerostomia.

Q4. Patient with dry mouth needs to carry a water bottle at all times.
Q5. Cholinergic agonist is advised to treat xerostomia.
Q6. Bicarbonate composition in saliva remains constant despite changes in flow rate.
Q7. Botulinum toxic injection is given in achalasia cardia.

## Critical Thinking Case-Based Questions

Q1. A 2-years old male, accompanied by his father came to the local health provider with complaints of excess drooling of salvia. He ruled out the weakness of muscle and also history of drug that could be causing his excess salivation. It is decided to be normal for his age. The father was explained the physiology of normal salivary secretion. Answer the following questions on the basis of the given case scenario:
   a. Describe the sources, normal amount, and composition of salivary secretion.
   b. How does the saliva which was initially isotonic, become hypotonic as it passes through the ducts?
   c. Describe the factors regulating salivary secretion.

Q2. A 52-year-old man presents with complaints of retrosternal burning, regurgitation of food and retrosternal pain for the past 4 months. The symptoms have worsened now especially after a heavy meal and on lying down. He has no complaints of difficulty in swallowing or weight loss. No significant medical history. He is a non-smoker with occasional alcohol intake. On examination, the patient is obese and all the vitals and systemic examination is normal. Answer the following questions on the basis of the given case scenario:
   a. What is the most likely diagnosis? Justify the diagnosis.
   b. What is the physiological basis of symptoms of this disease?
   c. Explain the physiological basis of management of the disease.

Q3. A 32-year-old woman presents with a 3-month history of difficulty swallowing solids and liquids and intermittent chest pain. She has lost 4.5 kg. The physical examination findings are unremarkable. A Lateral chest X-ray showed marked dilation of esophagus with an air-fluid level, and a barium esophagogram demonstrates smooth tapering of the lower esophagus. Answer the following questions on the basis of the given case scenario:
   a. What is the most likely diagnosis? Justify the diagnosis.
   b. What is the physiological basis of symptoms of this disease?
   c. Describe the physiology of swallowing in detail.

## Multiple Choice Questions

Q1. Which of the following molecules enhances the secretion of saliva:
   a. Dopamine
   b. Secretin
   c. Vasoactive intestinal peptide
   d. Acetylcholine

Q2. A 40-year-old female concerned about her 18-month-old son because of excess drooling. Her friend explained her that sialorrhea is normal in young children until around the age of 3 years. Which of the following is most accurate about an increase in secretion of saliva?
   a. Epinephrine stimulation of muscarinic receptors increases salivation
   b. Norepinephrine stimulation of muscarinic receptors increases salivation
   c. Acetylcholine stimulation of cholinergic receptors increases salivation
   d. Epinephrine stimulation of cholinergic receptors increases salivation

Q3. A 34-year-old man presents for a swallowing study. History of present illness reveals that he has had dysphagia along with weight loss for the past few months. His vital signs are normal. The patient was given a bolus of food and asked to swallow. At what point in a swallow does the first involuntary phase begins?
   a. Oral preparatory     b. Oral phase
   c. Pharyngeal phase     d. Esophageal phase

Q4. A 40-year-old man presents to the hospital with a complaint of dysphagia. He reports difficulty swallowing both solids and liquids that started a few months ago and is progressively getting worse. The patient also complains of bad breath and regurgitation of food particles. The provider suspects an esophageal motility disorder. Further investigations revealed absent peristalsis in the lower esophagus. Which of the following abnormalities in esophageal physiology is most likely to be seen?
   a. Failure of lower esophageal sphincter (LES) to relax
   b. Decreased lower esophageal sphincter (LES) tone
   c. Abnormal spasms in the upper esophageal sphincter (UES)
   d. Irregular, uncoordinated esophageal contraction

Q5. A patient is referred to a gastroenterologist because of persistent difficulties with swallowing. Endoscopic examination reveals that the lower esophageal sphincter fails to fully open as the bolus reaches it, and a diagnosis of achalasia is made. During the examination, or in biopsies taken from the sphincter region, a decrease would be expected in which of the following?
   a. Esophageal peristalsis
   b. Acetylcholine receptors
   c. Deficiency of neuronal NO
   d. Substance P release

### ANSWERS

**1.** d  **2.** c  **3.** d  **4.** a  **5.** c

# Physiology of Digestion in Stomach

**30**
CHAPTER

### COMPETENCY ADDRESSED

**PY4.2:** Describe the composition, mechanism of secretion, functions, and regulation of saliva, gastric, pancreatic, intestinal juices and bile secretion.
**PY4.3:** Describe GIT movements, regulation and functions. Describe defecation reflex. Explain the role of dietary fiber.
**PY4.8:** Describe and discuss gastric function tests.
**PY4.9:** Discuss the physiology aspects of: Peptic ulcer, gastroesophageal reflux disease, vomiting, diarrhea, constipation, adynamic ileus, Hirschsprung's disease.

### LEARNING OBJECTIVES

**At the end of this chapter, the learner should be able to:**
- Describe the functional anatomy of stomach.
- Describe the functions of stomach.
- Describe the composition, mechanism of secretion, phases and regulation of gastric juice.
- Discuss the physiology of gastric motility.
- Describe the physiological basis of various disorders related to stomach.
- Enumerate the gastric function tests (physiology integrated with biochemistry).

## FUNCTIONAL ANATOMY OF STOMACH

The stomach is an expandable muscular sac which receives bolus of food from esophagus and converts into chyme, a semiliquid mass of partially digestive food. The stomach has a volume from 50 mL to 1 to 1.5 L. However, it still be stretched to 4 L. The interior of stomach has many folds called rugae, which increases its surface area. Anatomically and physiologically, it is divided into four regions: fundus of stomach, cardiac end, body of stomach, pyloric end of stomach (**Fig. 30.1**).

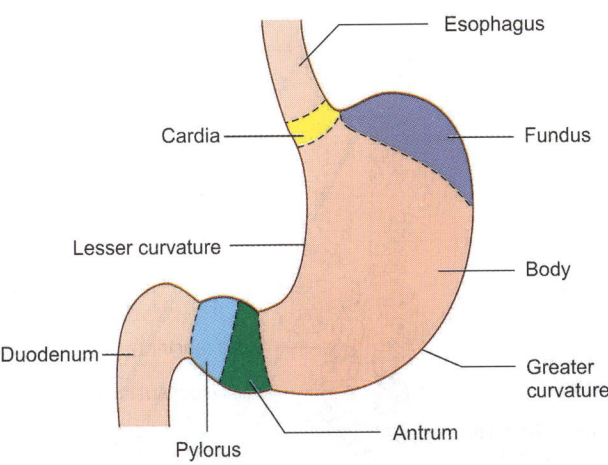

**Fig. 30.1:** Regions of stomach.

## Histology of Stomach (Fig. 30.2)

Like the basic organization of walls of GIT, the wall of stomach consists of four layers:

1. **Mucosa:** The mucosa is lined with the surface epithelium which falls into the underlying connective tissue. There are two main types of the tubular glands present in the stomach mucosa:
    i. *Oxyntic glands/gastric glands (Fig. 30.3A):* They are located in mucosa of fundus and body of stomach (proximal 80% of stomach). They have cells as mentioned below:
        - *Mucus cells/goblet cells:* Secrete thick mucus, which coats the surface of stomach mucosa,

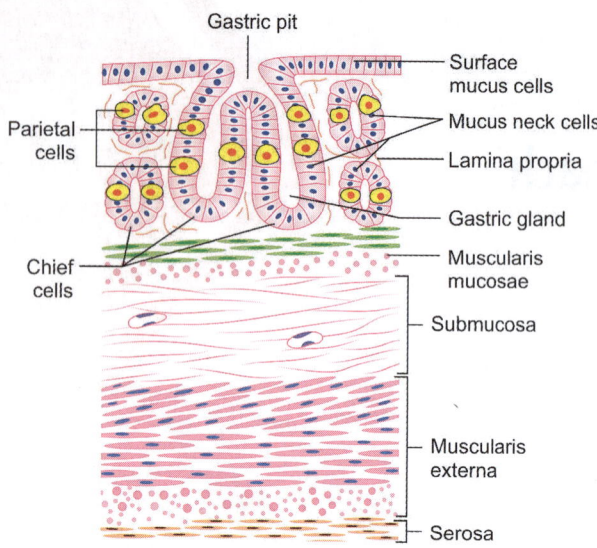

**Fig. 30.2:** Histological layers of stomach.

preventing it from digestion by the hydrochloric acid (HCl).
- *Parietal cells:* These cells secrete HCl and Castle's intrinsic factor, required for the absorption of vitamin B12.
- *Chief cells:* These calls secrete pepsinogen, an enzyme required to digestion of proteins.
- *Enteroendocrine cells:* Secrete somatostatin D from D-cells
- *Enterochromaffin-like cells (ECL cells):* Secretes Histamine

ii. **Pyloric glands (Fig. 30.3B):** They are located in mucosa of pylorus of stomach (distal 20% of stomach). They have cells as mentioned below:
- *Mucus cells/goblet cells:* Secrete thick mucus, which coats the surface of stomach mucosa, preventing it from digestion by the HCl.
- *Enteroendocrine cells:* Secrete Somatostatin D from D-cells, and gastrin from G-cells
- *Enterochromaffin cells (ECL cells):* Secretes Histamine

2. **Submucosa:** The gastric submucosa supports the stomach's architecture, housing essential blood vessels, nerve fibers, and lymphatic channels.
3. **Muscularis mucosa/externa:** The muscularis externa comprises of three layers of muscles which are required for the proper mixing, churning and breakdown of food. The food is converted to a semisolid chyme in stomach by various stomach contractions. The muscles responsible for the same are mentioned below:
    - *Longitudinal muscle:* Having the muscles oriented in the longitudinal direction, from cardiac to pyloric end.
    - *Circular muscle:* Having the muscles oriented in circular fashion, performs the circular constricting movements.
    - *Oblique layer:* Oblique muscle is unique to the stomach. It enables the churning motions required for mechanical digestion.
4. **Serosa:** It is the outermost covering of the stomach, closely attached with visceral peritoneum. It provides smooth surface to stomach on outside, which minimizes friction between the abdominal contents and stomach.

## FUNCTIONS OF STOMACH

- The *motor functions* of the stomach include storage, mixing food with gastric juice, and facilitating progressive duodenal emptying.
- *Digestive functions* of the stomach primarily involve protein digestion.
- The stomach *absorbs alcohol and water*.
- **Secretory function (Fig. 30.4):**
    - Parietal cells *secrete intrinsic factor*, which is crucial for the absorption of vitamin B12 in the distal part

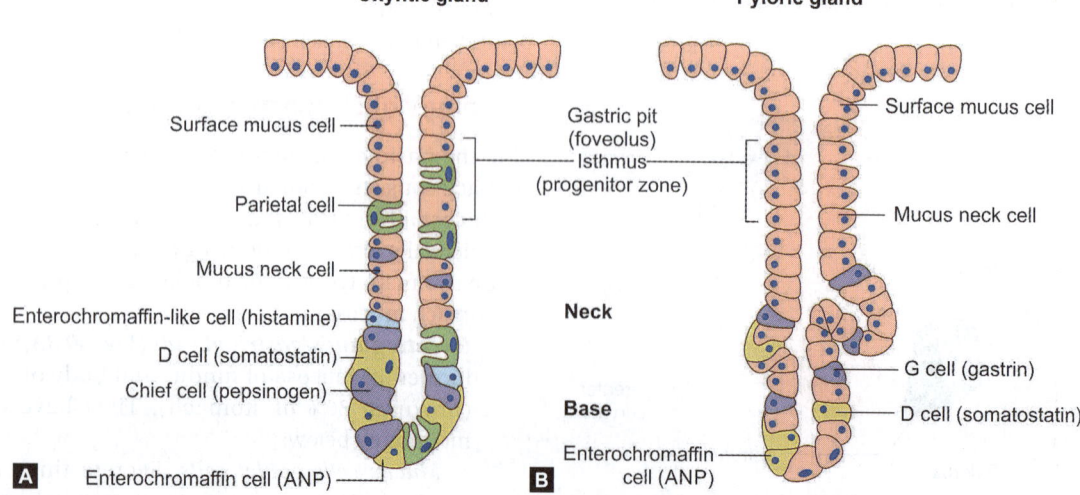

**Figs. 30.3A and B:** (A) Oxyntic gland anatomy and secretions; (B) Pyloric gland anatomy and secretions.
(ANP: atrial natriuretic peptide)

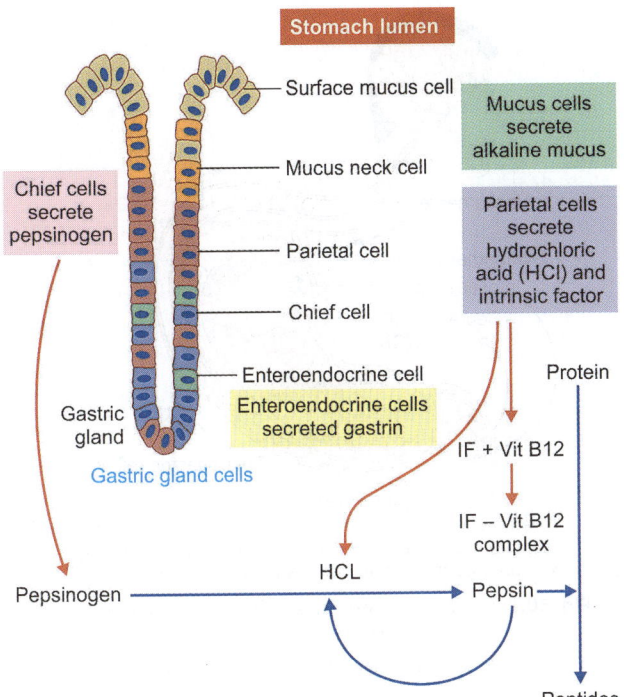

**Fig. 30.4:** Secretions from stomach.

**Composition of gastric secretion/juice**
- Water (99.5%)
- Inorganic solids
  - $H^+$, $Na^+$, $K^+$, $Ca^{2+}$, $Mg^{2+}$, $Cl^-$, $HCO_3^-$, $PO_4^{2-}$, $SO_4^{2-}$
- Organic solids
  - Enzymes (pepsinogen, rennin)
  - Intrinsic factor
  - Mucin
  - Gastric lipase
  - Carbonic anhydrase
  - Lysozyme

of the digestive tract by enterocytes of the terminal ileum.
- Parietal cells also *secrete HCl* which plays a role in digestion by activating pepsinogen, destroys microorganisms and possesses antiseptic properties. The HCl converts the $Fe^{3+}$ form into the absorbable $Fe^{2+}$ form. Hence, the patients with damage to parietal cells can present with iron deficiency anemia.
- **Excretory function:** Some alkaloids and toxins are expelled from the body through the stomach.
- **Endocrine function:** The stomach secretes a few GI hormones like
  - Gastrin which controls the secretion of HCl from stomach.
  - Somatostatin D
  - Histamine from ECL cells
- **Reflex action:** Various reflexes are integrated by the stomach are the gastro-salivary reflex, gastroileal reflex, and gastrocolic reflex.
- **Regulation of secretion from other parts of intestine:** The presence of food in the stomach also triggers the secretion of pancreatic juice and bile.

## GASTRIC SECRETION

The stomach secretes around 1,200–1,500 mL/day of acidic gastric juice having pH 3. It is secreted from the glands in the wall of the stomach and also from the surface cells.

## Phases of Gastric Secretion

As we have read in Chapter 28, the phases of GI secretion are divided into 3 phases, the gastric secretions are characteristically explained in these phases. So, as we have read, the gastric secretions are also divided into 3 phases:

### Cephalic Phase (Fig. 30.5)

- The smell/thought of the food stimulates the parasympathetic center in the cerebral cortex and appetite center of amygdala and hypothalamus.
- These signals are carried by the vagus nerve, arising from dorsal median nucleus of vagus, to influence the submucosal plexus of enteric nervous system of stomach.
- There is secretion of gastric juice from the gastric glands amounting to about *30% of the gastric juice*.

Hence, the cephalic phase occurs even before gastric secretion even before the food enters the stomach.

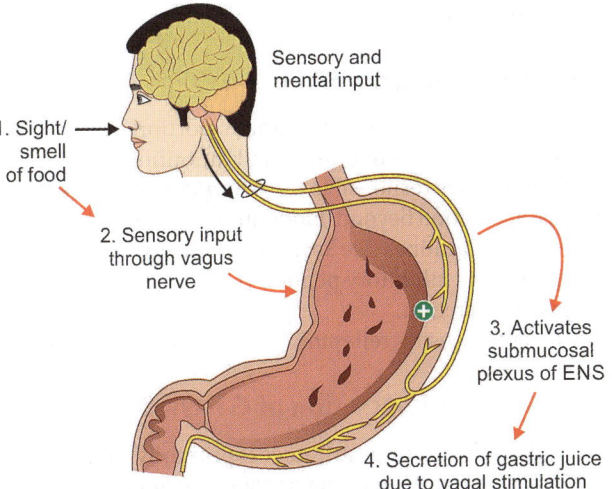

**Phase 1: Cephalic Phase**
Gastric secretion begins to be secreted even before actually eating the food

**Fig. 30.5:** Cephalic phase: Gastric secretion begins even before eating the food.
(ENS: enteric nervous system)

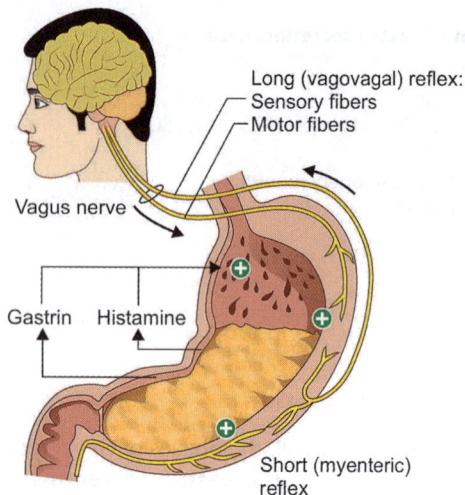

**Phase 2: Gastric Phase**
When the food reaches the stomach, it stretches its walls activating the myenteric and vagovagal reflexes. These reflexes stimulates gastric secretion. The hormones, Histamine and Gastrin further stimulates secretion of gastric juice

Fig. 30.6: Gastric phase: Starts when food reaches stomach.

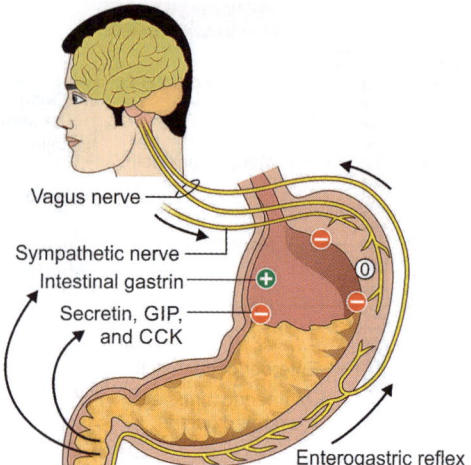

**Phase 3: Intestinal Phase:**
When the food enters the intestines, there is secretion of hormones Secretin, GIP, CCK. These hormones, along with enterogastric reflex inhibits the gastric secretion

Fig. 30.7: Intestinal phase: Starts when food reaches/enters upper portion of intestine.

(CCK: cholecystokinin; GIP: gastric inhibitory peptide)

## Gastric Phase (Fig. 30.6)

- The food enters the stomach and stretches the walls of stomach.
- It excites following reflexes, responsible for gastric secretion for 3–4 hours till the food remains in stomach:
  - Long vagovagal reflex from stomach to brain and back to stomach
  - Local enteric reflexes
  - Secretion of hormone gastrin and histamine
- Gastric phase is responsible for *secretion of 60% of gastric juice*.

## Intestinal Phase (Fig. 30.7)

- When the food enters the upper portion of intestine, especially in duodenum, small amounts of gastrin is secreted. It is responsible for *10% of gastric secretion*.
- Passage of food beyond duodenum results in secretion of various hormones like Secretin, cholecystokinin (CCK) and gastric inhibitory peptide (GIP) which inhibits the gastric secretion.
- The enterogastric reflex inhibits the gastric secretion.

## Mechanism of Secretion of Gastric Juice

As studied above, the gastric juice is primarily composed of HCl, mucus and the enzyme pepsinogen along with other constituents **(Fig. 30.8)**.

- The surface mucus cells secrete primarily mucus and bicarbonate making it alkaline. It also secretes substances known as trefoil peptides that stabilize the *mucus-bicarbonate layer*. This thick layer of mucus prevents the direct exposure of the stomach wall to highly acidic proteolytic gastric secretions. Even the slightest irritation of gastric mucosa stimulates the secretion of mucus.

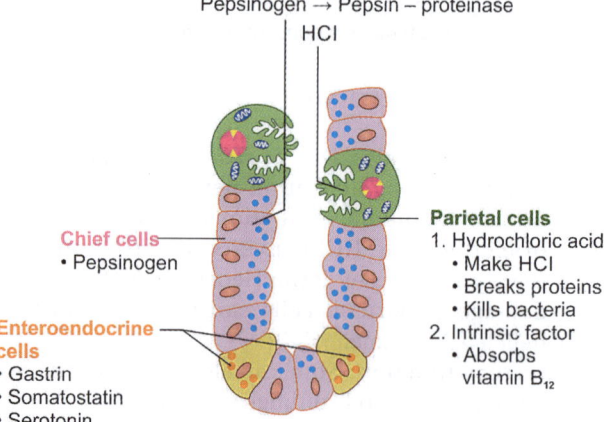

Fig. 30.8: Gastric secretions from different cells.

*If the pH of gastric juice is 3, why the stomach walls are not auto-digested?*

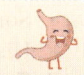

- The chief cells secrete pepsinogen and gastric lipase. The secretion of pepsinogen occurs either due to the parasympathetic stimulation (acetyl choline) or due to release of acid in the stomach. The acid sets up the local enteric reflexes for the release of pepsinogen.
- The parietal cells in the fundus or body of stomach secrete HCl and intrinsic factor (IF).

**Role of Castle's Intrinsic Factor (CIF):** It combines with the ingested vitamin B12 to for a complex CIF-vitamin B12. This complex is required for the binding and absorption to the enterocytes at the terminal ileum.
The patients of atrophic gastritis or partial gastrectomy where the secretion of CIF is affected, present with vitamin B12 deficiency called the *Pernicious anemia*. These patients present with features of megaloblastic anemia and peripheral neuropathy.

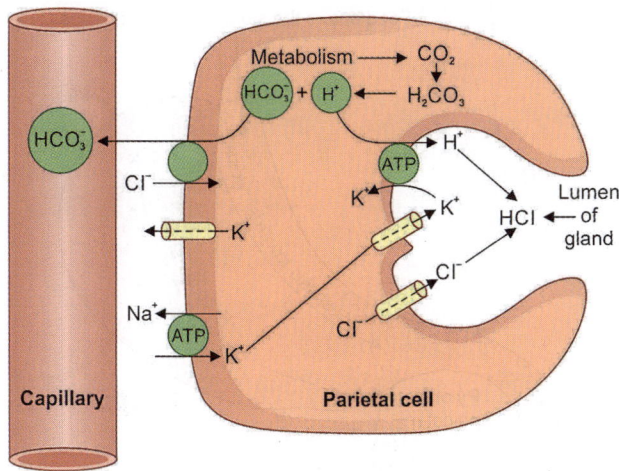

**Fig. 30.9:** Mechanism of HCl secretion.

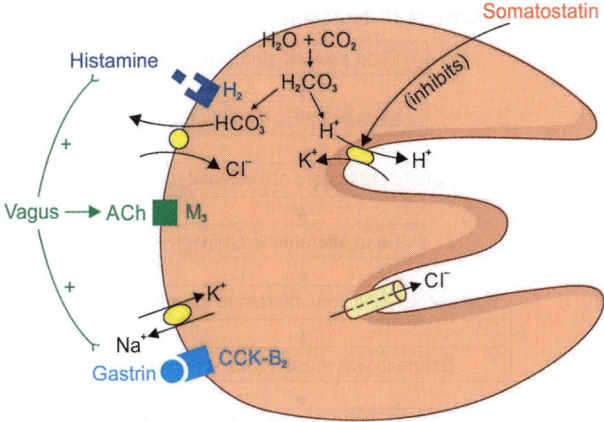

**Fig. 30.10:** Regulation of secretion of HCl.

Since the main constituent of gastric juice is HCl, we will primarily focus on the same.

## Mechanism of Secretion of HCl (Fig. 30.9)

- The $CO_2$ produced from the cellular metabolism combines with the water to produce carbonic acid ($H_2CO_3$) in the presence of enzyme carbonic anhydrase. This $H_2CO_3$ readily dissociates into $HCO_3^-$ and $H^+$.
- The $HCO_3^-$ formed in this reaction enters the blood capillaries in exchange with $Cl^-$, increasing the pH of the blood and urine, called as the *postprandial alkaline tide* (*Postprandial* means after the meals; *alkaline tide* means raised pH of blood). The $Cl^-$ thus entering the parietal cells diffuses into the canalicular lumen.
- The $H^+$ formed in the above reaction is actively exchanged for $K^+$ at the apical membrane of the canalicular cell by the $H^+$-$K^+$ ATPase pump.
- The concentration of $K^+$ is maintained in the lumen of the gland by the continuous diffusion of $K^+$ from the parietal cell, owing to the $Na^+$-$K^+$ ATPase pump.
- The $H^+$ and the $Cl^-$ entering the canaliculi, combines to form HCl. Water enters the canaliculi through osmosis. Hence the final secretion of HCl takes place with concentration of HCl at 150–160 mEq/L.

## REGULATION OF GASTRIC SECRETION (FIG. 30.10)

There are many factors which influence the secretion of gastric juice, they are tabulated in **Table 30.1**.

## GASTRIC MOTILITY

Once the food enters the stomach from the esophagus through the LES/gastroesophageal sphincter. *The intraluminal pressure at LES is 30 mm Hg.* As we have learnt above, the gastric contents are highly acidic, hence the tonic constriction of LES prevents the reflux of gastric secretions into esophagus. The mucosa of lower 1/8th of esophagus is resistant to digestive action of gastric juice.

As we have discussed earlier in the general principles of GI motility, the stomach also shows the phenomenon of receptive relaxation, peristaltic waves and migratory motor complexes. Let's discuss each one of these in detail, in the section below.

## Receptive Relaxation

When food enters the stomach, the fundus and upper portion of the body relaxes and accommodates food without much increase in pressure and tension in its wall. When empty, the stomach has a capacity of 50 mL; when full, it can expand to accommodate 1–1.5 L. The process that relaxes the stomach is known as receptive and adaptive relaxation (**Flowchart 30.1 and Fig. 30.11**). *Receptive*

**Table 30.1:** Factors influencing gastric secretion.

| | Factors increasing gastric secretion | Factors decreasing gastric secretion |
|---|---|---|
| **Food** | • Smell, sight, taste of food<br>• Food in the stomach | Food/chyme in the intestines |
| **Hormones** | Gastrin, acetylcholine, histamine | GIP, secretin CCK |
| **Nervous factors** | Parasympathetic stimulation | Sympathetic stimulation |
| **Reflexes** | | **Reverse enterogastric reflex** slows down gastric emptying. It gets activated when there is:<br>• Distension of small bowel<br>• Acid in duodenum<br>• Protein breakdown products<br>• Irritation of mucosa |
| **Emotional stimulus** | Increases gastric secretion in inter-digestive period, which is primarily comprising of mucus and little pepsin with no acid | |

**Flowchart 30.1:** Storage of food in stomach.

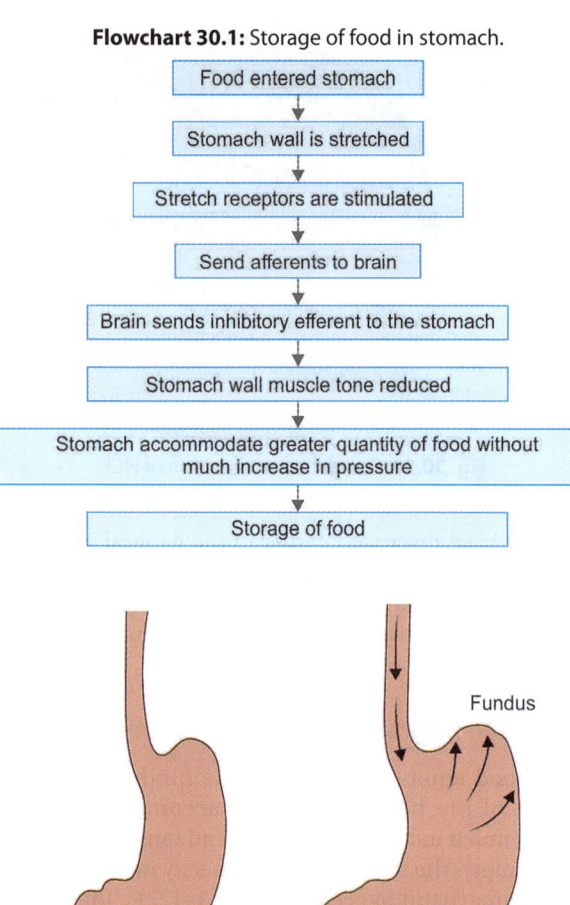

Fig. 30.11: Receptive relaxation.

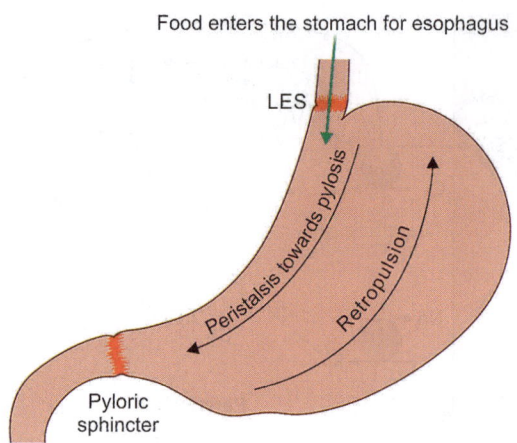

Fig. 30.12: Peristalsis and retropulsion.
(LES: lower esophageal sphincter)

relaxation is the dilatation of the stomach on seeing the food or by keeping the food in the mouth to accommodate food. *Adaptive relaxation* is the dilatation of stomach when the food reaches stomach.

## Motility in Fasting State/Interdigestive Phase is the Migration Migratory Complex (MMC)

$M_o$ cells of the stomach secretes hormone, *Motilin* that *causes motility in the fasting state to propel the food* that is stuck up in the GIT. These complexes are referred to as the broom of the GIT. These occur 90–120 minutes after meals. During this movement, gastric juice is also secreted that washes the food remnants. The MMCs are discussed in detail in Chapter 28.

## Peristalsis (Fig. 30.12)

The mixing peristaltic waves originate in the middle section of the stomach and are most prominent in the distal portion of the stomach. These result from rhythmic alterations in the basal electric rhythm. Peristaltic waves move the food particles toward the pylorus, where they strike the closed pylorus sphincter that force most of the stomach's contents back into the stomach cavity (a process referred to as retropulsion). The food is once again propelled toward the pylorus by the contraction of peristalsis. This backward and forward motion facilitates the food's mixing with the stomach's contents. Additionally, it aids in churning and the preparation of a semi-liquid food called *chyme*. Various factors like distention, vagal stimulation, sympathetic stimulation, hormones like acetylcholine and gastrin increase force of peristalsis.

## Gastric Emptying (Fig. 30.13)

It is the process by which the stomach gradually empties its contents into the duodenum. *The normal gastric emptying time after a normal meal is 3–4 hours*. The mechanism of stomach emptying involves pyloric sphincter relaxation and strong antral peristalsis, also known as *pyloric pump action*. Antral peristalsis is the powerful, ring-like contractions that begin in the center of the stomach and extend distally. These strong contractions push the meal in the direction of the duodenum. The more peristalsis there is in the antrum, the faster the stomach empties **(Fig. 30.14)**. The duodenal inhibitory forces ensure that the amount of chyme that leaves the stomach is just right for the intestine's capacity to absorb and digest nutrients. The contents of the duodenum cannot become extremely osmolar or acidic.

> **Gastric Emptying Time**
> Carbohydrate rich food: Rapid
> Protein rich food: Slow
> Fat rich food: Slowest

> **Hunger Pangs**
> These are intense contractions occurring in stomach causing tetanic contractions lasting for 2–3 minutes. They are also called hunger contractions, which begins 12–24 hours of last meal. If a person is starving for 3–4 days and gradually weakens in a few days.

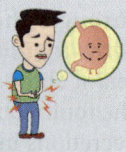

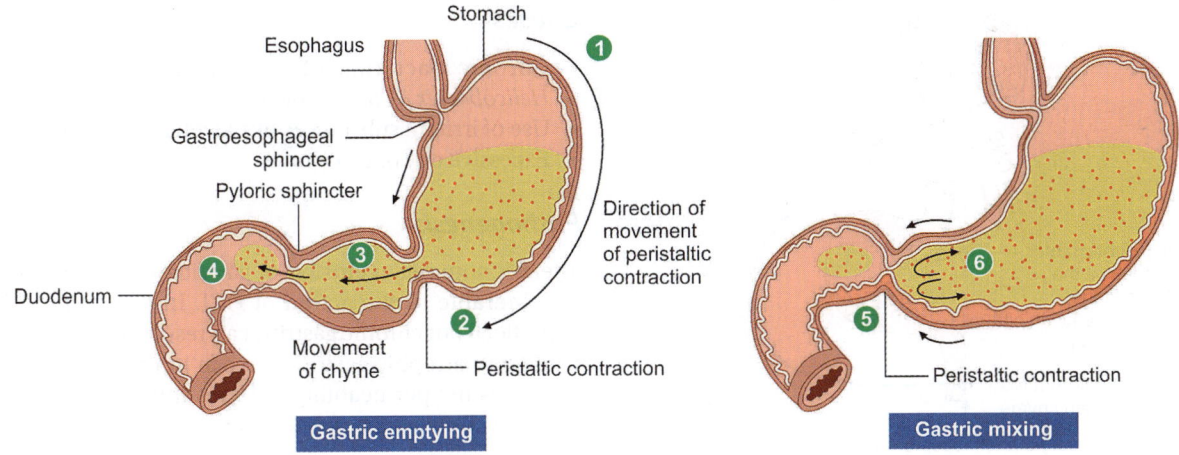

**Fig. 30.13:** Process of gastric emptying.

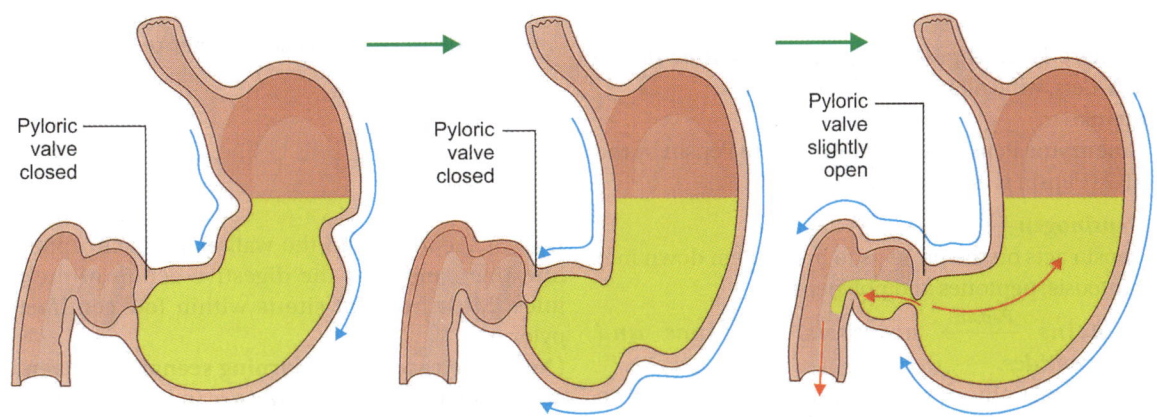

**Fig. 30.14:** Propulsion and grinding.

## REGULATION OF GASTRIC EMPTYING

As discussed earlier, the gastric emptying is affected by many factors, classified as neurohormonal, and local factors, mentioned below:

- **Neural regulation:** The myenteric plexus of enteric nervous system, play an important role in gastric motility and emptying. However, the parasympathetic nervous system, stimulates the motility.
- **Hormonal regulation:**
  - **Gastrin** has a mild-to-moderate stimulatory effects on motor functions of the stomach. It enhances the activity of pyloric pump, hence promotes the gastric emptying.
  - **Cholecystokinin, GIP and secretin** inhibits the gastric emptying. It controls the amount of acidic chyme entering into the duodenum. It is protective for duodenum, as it allows enough chyme to enter the duodenum, which can be neutralized and processed. Till then the stomach stores the chyme and releases in small batches.
- **Local factors:** Various factors in the stomach and upper small intestine closely regulate the gastric motility.
- **Gastric volume:** Higher food volume in stomach promotes gastric emptying due to stretching of gastric walls and stimulating the myenteric plexus to initiate local reflexes.

### Enterogastric Inhibitory Reflex/Reverse Enterogastric Reflex (Fig. 30.15)

It is the nervous reflex in which stimulation of the stretch receptors in the wall of duodenum results in inhibition of gastric motility and reduces gastric emptying. The duodenal factors that can initiate enterogastric reflex includes duodenal distention, duodenal irritation, duodenal acidity, osmolarity of the duodenum's chyme, and protein content of the duodenum's chyme. It is significant as it inhibits excessive amount of chyme entering the duodenum. It reduces intestinal erosion by limiting inflow of gastric acid, and also increases duration of digestion of chyme before it is moved to the small intestine.

## DIGESTION AND ABSORPTION IN STOMACH

The stomach secretes the abundant quantity of pepsinogen, a protein digesting enzyme and some amount of gastric

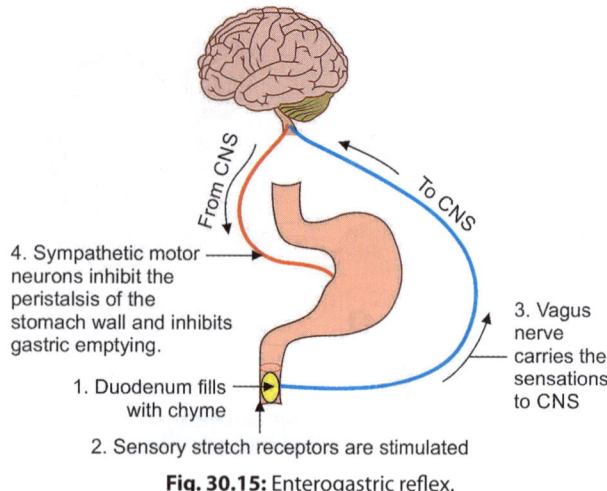

**Fig. 30.15:** Enterogastric reflex.
(CNS: central nervous system)

lipase. There is *no digestion of carbohydrates in the stomach*. Lets, what all happens in stomach.
- **Proteins:**
  - Proenzyme Pepsinogen is converted to Pepsin by the HCl (Pepsin is activated at pH 2.0–3.0)
  
  *Pepsinogen* $\xrightarrow{\text{pH 2.0–3.0 by HCl}}$ *Pepsin*
  
  - Pepsin acts on the proteins to break them down into proteosis, peptones and polypeptides.
  
  *Proteins* $\xrightarrow{\text{Pepsin}}$ *proteosis, peptones and polypeptides.*
  
  - These partially digested proteins pass down to intestine, where they are further digested.
- **Fats:** Most of the digestion occurs in small intestine but very little amount of *triglycerides* are digested by lingual lipase, which is present in saliva but swallowed with food. It result in digestion of around 10% of fats.

## Absorption in Stomach

The stomach has a poor absorptive capacity because of:
- Lack of absorptive surface
- Presence of gastric barrier, i.e., the presence of tight junctions in epithelial cells.

But highly lipid soluble substances like *alcohol and some drugs like aspirin are absorbed from stomach*.

## DISORDERS OF STOMACH

- Gastritis
- Peptic ulcer
- Physiology of gastroesophageal reflex disease (GERD)
- Zollinger-Ellison Syndrome (ZES)
- Dumping Syndrome

## Gastritis

It is the superficial inflammation of gastric mucosa.

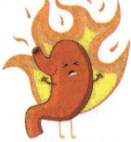

### Causes
- Chronic bacterial infection of gastric mucosa by *Helicobacter pylori (H. pylori)*
- Use of irritant substances like alcohol or aspirin.
- Excessive oily or spicy food.

### Pathogenesis

There is superficial erosion of gastric mucosa, rendering it vulnerable to the action of HCl. In acute cases, it is superficial but chronic gastritis can result in deep erosions leading to atrophic gastritis. Breach in the gastric barrier increases the permeability of $H^+$ resulting in digestion of gastric wall called the peptic ulcer.

### Complications
- **Hypochlorhydria/achlorhydria:** Decreased or no secretion of HCl. This can further result in pernicious anemia.
- Peptic ulcer
- Gastric carcinoma.

## Peptic Ulcer

It is an excoriation in the wall of stomach/upper small intestine caused by the digestive action of the gastric juice. Most frequent site is within few centimeters of pylorus.
(Note: The case-based learning scenario is given in the author's Early Clinical Exposure in Clinical physiology)

### Causes
- Damage to gastroduodenal mucosal barrier by *H. pylori*, alcohol or drugs (NSAIDS: nonsteroidal anti-inflammatory drugs/pain killers)
- Inefficient neutralization of gastric acidic contents in the duodenum

## GERD

(Note: The case–based learning scenario is given in the author's Early Clinical Exposure in Clinical physiology)
It is defined as a clinical condition that arises due to the backflow or regurgitation of the gastric contents into the esophagus which is anatomically not designed to withstand the acidic contents leading to local inflammation of the esophagus, i.e., esophagitis due to loss of tone of the lower esophageal sphincter (LES).

### Pathophysiology
- Decreased low esophageal sphincter pressure
- Disruption of anatomical barrier
- Esophageal clearance
- Decrease in normal mucosal defenses
- Delayed gastric emptying

## Zollinger–Ellison Syndrome

Zollinger–Ellison Syndrome (ZES) is a rare disorder characterized by the excessive production of gastric acid, leading to recurrent peptic ulcers in the stomach, duodenum, and occasionally, the jejunum. It is caused by gastrin-secreting tumors known as gastrinomas, which are typically located in the pancreas or duodenum.

### Causes

- **Gastrinomas:** The primary cause of ZES is the presence of gastrin-secreting tumors called gastrinomas. These tumors are usually found in the pancreas or duodenum, although they can occur in other areas of the gastrointestinal tract (GIT).
- **Genetic factors:** While most cases of ZES occur sporadically, a small percentage may be associated with inherited genetic syndromes such as multiple endocrine neoplasia type 1 (MEN1), which predisposes individuals to develop tumors of the endocrine glands, including gastrinomas.

### Pathogenesis

- **Gastrin overproduction:** Gastrinomas produce excessive amounts of gastrin, a hormone that stimulates the secretion of gastric acid from parietal cells in the stomach. Elevated levels of gastrin lead to hyperchlorhydria, resulting in increased gastric acid secretion and a reduction in the pH of the gastric contents.
- **Peptic ulcer formation:** The increased acidity of the gastric contents damages the mucosal lining of the stomach and duodenum, leading to the formation of peptic ulcers. These ulcers are typically recurrent, deep, and refractory to conventional ulcer treatment.

### Complications

ZES can lead to severe complications such as:
- Gastrointestinal bleeding
- Perforation of ulcers
- Obstruction of the GIT
- Additionally, long-term exposure to high levels of gastric acid increases the risk of developing GERD
- Barrett's esophagus
- Esophageal adenocarcinoma.

## Dumping Syndrome

Dumping syndrome refers to a set of symptoms that occur when stomach contents are rapidly emptied into the small intestine.

### Causes

- **Gastric surgery:** Dumping syndrome commonly occurs as a complication of gastric surgeries, such as gastric bypass or gastrectomy, where alterations in the stomach anatomy result in accelerated gastric emptying.
- **Functional disorders:** Certain conditions affecting stomach function, such as diabetic gastroparesis, can also lead to dumping syndrome due to impaired gastric emptying.
- **Postprandial hypoglycemia:** In some cases, rapid transit of glucose-containing food into the small intestine can cause a surge in insulin release, leading to hypoglycemia, which contributes to the symptoms of dumping syndrome.

### Pathogenesis

- **Early dumping syndrome:** Rapid emptying of hyperosmolar gastric contents into the small intestine triggers an osmotic shift, drawing water into the intestinal lumen. This leads to abdominal distension, cramping, and diarrhea. Additionally, the release of vasoactive peptides, such as serotonin and substance P, can cause vasomotor symptoms like flushing, palpitations, and sweating.
- **Late dumping syndrome:** The rapid absorption of carbohydrates into the small intestine stimulates an exaggerated insulin response, leading to a subsequent drop in blood glucose levels (reactive hypoglycemia). This hypoglycemia triggers the release of counterregulatory hormones, such as adrenaline and glucagon, resulting in symptoms like weakness, sweating, tremors, and palpitations.

# GASTRIC FUNCTION TESTS

Gastric function tests are diagnostic procedures used to evaluate the physiological functioning of the stomach. These tests provide valuable information about gastric motility, acid secretion, and mucosal integrity. Some common gastric function tests include:

## Gastric Emptying Study

This test measures the rate at which food empties from the stomach into the small intestine. It involves ingesting a meal or a radiolabeled substance followed by imaging studies (such as scintigraphy) to track the movement of the ingested material through the GIT.

## Gastric Acid Secretion Tests

These tests assess the production of gastric acid by the stomach. They include methods such as the gastric acid stimulation test, where the patient is given a substance (such as histamine or pentagastrin) to stimulate acid secretion, and gastric pH monitoring, which measures the acidity of the gastric contents using a pH probe placed in the stomach.

- **Pentagastrin test**: The Pentagastrin Test/Pentagastrin Stimulation Test, is a diagnostic procedure used to *assess gastric acid secretion in the stomach*. It involves the administration of pentagastrin, a synthetic peptide that stimulates the release of gastric acid by acting on the gastrin receptors of the stomach.

During the test, the patient is typically asked to fast for a certain period before the procedure. Then, a baseline measurement of gastric acid secretion may be obtained by collecting gastric fluid through a nasogastric tube or performing gastric aspiration. After the baseline measurement, the patient receives an intravenous injection of pentagastrin.

Following the administration of pentagastrin, gastric acid secretion is stimulated, leading to an increase in the acidity of the gastric fluid. Serial samples of gastric fluid may be collected at intervals after pentagastrin injection to measure the acid output and assess the response to stimulation.

It is primarily used to evaluate gastric acid secretion in patients suspected of having disorders related to gastric acid hypersecretion, such as ZES or gastrinoma.

- *BAO (Basal Acid Output) and MAO (Maximal Acid Output)* are parameters used to measure gastric acid secretion in the stomach, providing valuable information about the functioning of the gastric mucosa and its ability to produce acid.
  - *Basal acid output:* BAO refers to the amount of acid secreted by the stomach under basal or resting conditions, typically over an hour-long period during fasting. It reflects the intrinsic acid secretion capacity of the gastric mucosa in the absence of external stimuli or food intake. It is measured in milliequivalents per hour (mEq/h) or millimoles per hour (mmol/h) and serves as a baseline for assessing gastric acid secretion.
  - *Maximal acid output:* MAO represents the maximum acid secretion capacity of the stomach in response to a stimulant, such as pentagastrin or histamine. It reflects the maximal acid secretory capacity of the gastric mucosa when stimulated by pharmacological agents. MAO is typically measured during a gastric acid stimulation test, where a stimulant is administered intravenously, and gastric acid output is measured at regular intervals to determine the peak acid secretion response. MAO is also expressed in milliequivalents per hour (mEq/h) or millimoles per hour (mmol/h).

Both BAO and MAO are important parameters in the *evaluation of gastric acid secretion* and are used in diagnosing and monitoring acid-related disorders, such as peptic ulcer disease, GERD, and ZES. Abnormalities in BAO and MAO levels can indicate underlying gastric mucosal abnormalities or disorders affecting acid secretion, guiding appropriate management and treatment strategies.

### Gastric Motility Studies

These tests evaluate the muscular contractions and movement of food within the stomach. Techniques such as *gastric manometry measure intragastric pressure changes and motility patterns* to assess gastric function.

### Gastric Mucosal Biopsy

This procedure involves obtaining tissue samples from the lining of the stomach (gastric mucosa) for histological examination. Gastric mucosal biopsies can provide information about the *presence of inflammation, infection (such as H. pylori), or other abnormalities* affecting the stomach.

### Gastric pH Capsule Monitoring

This test involves the placement of a wireless pH capsule in the stomach to continuously monitor gastric acidity over a period of time. It is used to assess acid reflux, evaluate gastric acid suppression therapy, and diagnose conditions such as GERD and gastric ulcer disease.

---

### SUMMARY

- The stomach is the initial site of protein digestion. 10–20% of protein digestion occurs in stomach. Pepsin secreted by chief cells, is active at pH 2–3 in stomach and inactive at pH 5 in intestine.
- Stomach is a poor absorptive area of GIT, due to lack of villi, and presence of tight junctions between epithelial cells. Only a few highly-lipid soluble substances can be absorbed such as alcohol and aspirin.
- The stomach accommodates the meal by a process of receptive relaxation. This permits an increase in volume without a significant increase in pressure.
- Mixing of food with gastric secretions occurs in three stages: propulsion, grinding, and retropulsion.
- Gastrin is a stimulatory hormone, whereas secretin, CCK, and GIP are inhibitory hormones.
- After a gastrectomy, anemia is commonly observed due to the body's reduced ability to absorb vitamin B12 caused by a lack of intrinsic factor.
- Stress increases acid production, slowed digestion, altered gut motility, and alters the composition of intestinal bacteria.

---

### LET US SEE, HOW MUCH YOU HAVE LEARNT?

 *Review Questions*

#### Long/Short Answer Questions

Q1. Mention the gastric glands and their cell types and secretions.
Q2. Gastric emptying.
Q3. Write short notes on gastrin.
Q4. Physiological basis of management of peptic ulcer.

## Explain Why? (Reasoning Questions)

Q1. High fat meal takes a longer time to digest.
Q2. Stomach is protected from self-digestion and why this is necessary.
Q3. Presence of HCl in stomach is necessary for the process of digestion.
Q4. Fatty food is taken with alcohol consumption.
Q5. Chronic use of pain killers (NSAIDs) causes ulcers in stomach.
Q6. Stomach has poor absorptive function.

## Critical Thinking Case-Based Questions

Q1. 45-year-old male patient complaints of epigastric pain for the past 3 days which increases after taking food. History reveals taking on and off pain killers over the counter. Answer the following questions on the basis of the given case scenario:
  a. What is your provisional diagnosis?
  b. What are the probable causes of his problem?
  c. Explain the mechanism of hydrochloric acid (HCl) secretion.
  d. What is postprandial alkaline tide?
  e. What is the rational for managing this case?

## Multiple Choice Questions

Q1. A 57-year-old man presents with a history of fatigue. His surgical history is significant for a gastric bypass 2 years ago. On physical examination, he has a conjunctival pallor that indicates anemia. His surgery will result in decreased absorption of which of the following compound that leads to anemia:
  a. Iron
  b. Vitamin C
  c. Vitamin B
  d. Calcium

Q2. Which is true of the rate of gastric emptying?
  a. It is not affected by the force and frequency of gastric peristalsis
  b. It is independent of the nervous regulation
  c. It is decreased by the presence of fats and acids in the duodenum
  d. It is directly proportional to the volume introduced into the stomach

Q3. The proenzyme pepsinogen is secreted mainly from which of the following structure?
  a. Acinar cells of the pancreas
  b. Ductal cells of the pancreas
  c. Epithelial cells of the duodenum
  d. Gastric glands of the stomach

Q4. The gastric motility is stimulated by:
  a. Cholecystokinin
  b. Distension of the stomach
  c. Secretin
  d. Peptide YY

Q5. Histamine stimulates acid secretion by binding with which of the following receptor on parietal cells:
  a. CCK-B receptors
  b. $H_2$ receptors
  c. $H_1$ receptors
  d. $M_3$ receptors

Q6. In which phase, gastric secretion involves distension of the stomach through vasovagal reflexes?
  a. Large intestinal phase
  b. Cephalic phase
  c. Gastric phase
  d. Small Intestinal phase

Q7. Mechanism of HCL production depends on:
  a. $H^+/K^+$ ATPase Pump
  b. $Na^+/K^+$ ATPase Pump
  c. $H/HCO_3$ exchanges
  d. $H/Cl^-$ ATPase Pump

Q8. In case of hormonal feedback, CCK, Secretin, and gastric inhibitory peptide released, the result will be:
  a. Inhibition of pyloric sphincter
  b. Facilitation of pyloric pump
  c. Increased gastric secretion
  d. Strongly contraction of pyloric sphincter

Q9. What is the primary function of the stomach?
  a. Absorption of nutrients
  b. Storage of food
  c. Production of bile
  d. Regulation of blood glucose levels

Q10. Which region of the stomach is responsible for the secretion of gastric juice?
  a. Fundus
  b. Body
  c. Antrum
  d. Pylorus

Q11. Which enzyme is primarily responsible for protein digestion in the stomach?
  a. Amylase
  b. Lipase
  c. Pepsin
  d. Trypsin

Q12. During which phase of gastric secretion does the sight, smell, or thought of food stimulate gastric juice secretion?
  a. Cephalic phase
  b. Gastric phase
  c. Intestinal phase
  d. Postprandial phase

Q13. What initiates the receptive relaxation of the stomach to accommodate food intake?
  a. Gastrin release
  b. Cholecystokinin (CCK)
  c. Vagus nerve stimulation
  d. Secretin release

Q14. A patient presents with symptoms of epigastric pain and discomfort after meals. Which physiological process may be impaired in this patient?
  a. Gastric emptying
  b. Gastric acid secretion
  c. Gastric motility
  d. Gastric mucosal barrier function

Q15. A patient is diagnosed with peptic ulcer disease. Which factor is most likely contributing to the pathophysiology of this condition?
  a. Increased gastric motility
  b. Excessive gastric acid secretion
  c. Impaired gastric emptying
  d. Deficient mucosal blood flow

Q16. A patient with diabetes mellitus complains of bloating and early satiety. Which gastric function test may help diagnose the underlying condition?
   a. Gastric emptying study
   b. Gastric acid secretion test
   c. Gastric motility study
   d. Gastric mucosal biopsy

Q17. A patient is suspected of having gastrinoma. Which gastric function test can assess the maximal acid secretory capacity of the stomach?
   a. Gastric emptying study
   b. Basal acid output (BAO) measurement
   c. Maximal acid output (MAO) measurement
   d. Gastric pH monitoring

Q18. A patient presents with symptoms of GERD. Which physiological mechanism is likely impaired in this patient?
   a. Lower esophageal sphincter tone
   b. Gastric acid secretion
   c. Gastric motility
   d. Gastric emptying

## ANSWERS

1. a    2. c    3. d    4. b    5. b    6. c    7. a    8. d    9. b    10. b    11. c    12. a    13. c    14. c
15. b   16. a   17. c   18. a

# Physiology of Digestion in Small Intestine
## (Including Pancreas)

**CHAPTER 31**

### COMPETENCY ADDRESSED

**PY4.2:** Describe the composition, mechanism of secretion, functions, and regulation of saliva, gastric, pancreatic, intestinal juices and bile secretion.
**PY4.3:** Describe GIT movements, regulation and functions. Describe defecation reflex. Explain the role of dietary fiber.
**PY4.9:** Discuss the physiology aspects of: Peptic ulcer, gastroesophageal reflux disease, vomiting, diarrhea, constipation, adynamic ileus, Hirschsprung's disease.

### LEARNING OBJECTIVES

**At the end of this chapter, the learner should be able to:**
- Describe the functional anatomy of small intestine and pancreas.
- Describe functions of pancreatic juice and secretions of small intestine.
- Describe the mechanism of secretions pancreas and small intestine.
- Describe the types of small intestinal motility.
- Describe the role of small intestine in digestion and absorption of nutrients.
- Describe the physiological basis of various disorders of pancreas and small intestine.

## ANATOMY OF SMALL INTESTINE AND PANCREAS

Small intestine begins from the end of pylorus of stomach and extends upto the ileocecal junction. Anatomically, the small intestine is 6–7 meters long and divided into three parts:

1. **Duodenum:** It is the proximal/upper part of small intestine. It is the shortest segment with a length of 10–12 inches. It is curved in the C shape to accommodate the pancreas. It is the site where pancreas and liver pour their secretions and result in digestion of food. We have discussed the biliary secretion separately in Chapter 32, but we will discuss the pancreatic secretions in this chapter itself, as majority of digestion in duodenum and upper jejunum occurs due to pancreatic enzymes. Pancreas is a large compound gland having both exocrine and exocrine function. The exocrine pancreas assists in food digestion by secrete alkaline pancreatic juice. This endocrine gland produces ghrelin, pancreatic polypeptide, glucagon, somatostatin, and insulin.

2. **Jejunum:** It is the middle portion of small intestine measuring 2.5 meters. It is responsible for both digestion and absorption. The jejunal mucosa has numerous fingers like projections (villi). The walls have abundant blood vessels and lacteals.

3. **Ileum:** It is the last part of small intestine which measures 3.5 meters long. It is primarily responsible for absorption of bile salts, vitamin B12 and remaining nutrients due to the presence of intense brush border in its mucosa.

Since, we are going to study the small intestine and pancreas together in this chapter we will study both these under all the sections described below:

1. **Functional anatomy of pancreas (Fig. 31.1):** Pancreas consist of acini (exocrine part) and islet of Langerhans (endocrine part). *Acini forms 99% of gland whereas islet of Langerhans forms 1% of the gland.* Pancreas is an accessory gland, and lie outside the walls of GIT. There are many acini with secretory cells. The acini drain their contents (containing sodium bicarbonate and enzymes) into the ducts, which drain into the long pancreatic duct. This pancreatic duct joins common bile duct before emptying into through papilla of Vater into duodenum. It is guarded by Sphincter of Oddi.

2. **Functional anatomy of small intestine (Fig. 31.2):**
   - *Mucosa:* The innermost layer that is in direct contact with the food. It contains the villi and microvilli, which

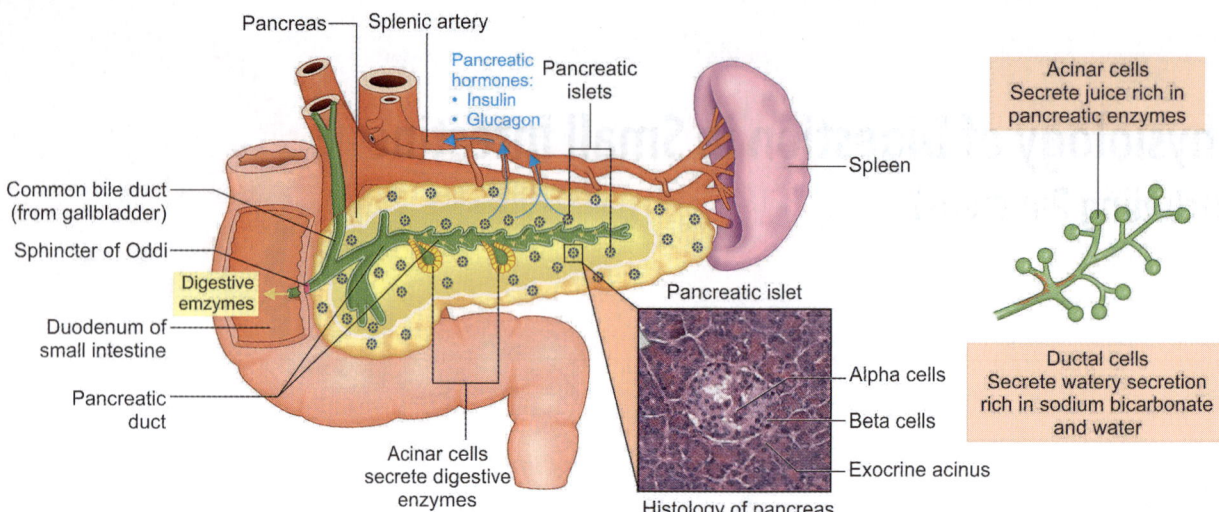

**Fig. 31.1:** Functional anatomy of pancreas.

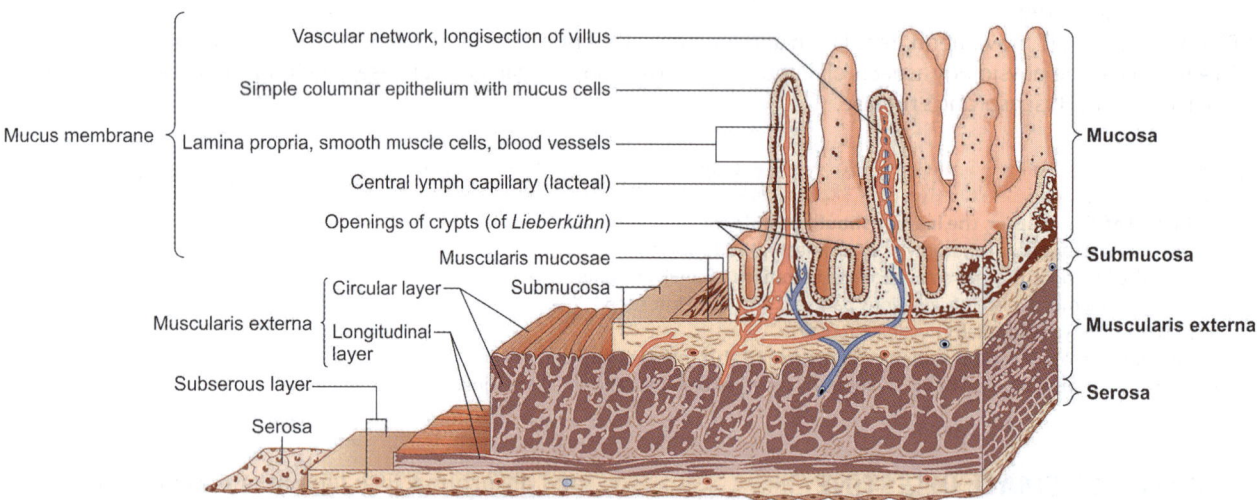

**Fig. 31.2:** Layers of small intestine.

greatly increase the absorptive surface area. The mucosa also contains glands (Crypts of Lieberkühn) that secrete digestive enzymes and mucus.
- **Submucosa:** This layer contains blood vessels, lymphatic vessels, and nerves that support the mucosa.
- **Muscularis externa:** Consists of smooth muscle layers responsible for peristalsis, the rhythmic contractions that propel food through the intestine.
- **Serosa:** The outermost layer, which is a serous membrane that provides protection and support.

## SECRETIONS OF PANCREAS AND SMALL INTESTINE

### PANCREATIC SECRETION

Pancreatic acini and ducts secrete digestive pancreatic juice rich in enzymes and bicarbonate ions. It is secreted in response to the presence of chyme in the upper portion of the small intestine. The juice then flows through a long pancreatic duct. Pancreatic duct joins the common bile duct to form hepatopancreatic ampulla that empties its content tin the 2nd part of duodenum.

### Pancreatic Juice

It is a *colorless, odorless, isotonic alkaline fluid. The pH of pancreatic juice is 8.3*.

### Composition

**Composition of Pancreatic Juice:**
- Water: 90–95%
- Pancreatic enzymes:
  - Amylase: 2–5%
  - Lipase: 2–5%
  - Proteases (including trypsin, chymotrypsin, and carboxypeptidase): 10–20%
- Electrolytes:
  - Bicarbonate ions ($HCO_3^-$): 80–85%
- Other substances (including mucus): Minimal, typically less than 5%

It is composed of water, digestive enzymes, and sodium bicarbonate solution. The acinar cells secretes digestive juice rich in digestive enzymes and ductal cells secreted watery secretions rich in sodium bicarbonate and water. The combined product of enzymes and bicarbonate then flows through a long pancreatic duct and empties into the duodenum.

## Mechanism of Formation of Pancreatic Juice (Figs. 31.3A and B)

- Carbon dioxide diffuses to the interior of the ductal cells from the blood and combines with water to form carbonic acid in the presence of carbonic anhydrase.
- The carbonic acid in turns dissociates into bicarbonate ions and hydrogen ions.
- Then the hydrogen ions are counter transported in in exchange with sodium ions through $Na^+$-$H^+$ counter transport at the luminal brush border of the cell. This results in acidification of the venous blood.
- The bicarbonate ions formed by dissociation of carbonic acid inside the cell are exchanged into the lumen against chloride ions.
- Sodium ions are then transported across the *luminal border* into the lumen of pancreatic ducts. The negative voltage of the lumen pulls the positively charged $Na^+$ across the tight junctions between the cells.
- The overall movement of $Na^+$, $Cl^-$ and $HCO_3^-$ from the blood into the duct lumen creates an osmotic pressure gradient that causes osmosis of water also into the pancreatic duct, thus forming an almost completely isosmotic bicarbonate solution.

- The enzymes secreted by the pancreatic cells are in inactive proenzymes are stored in zymogen granules until needed for digestion.

## Functions of Pancreatic Juice (Secreted from Exocrine Pancreas)

- **Digestive function:** The components of meal which need to be digested are carbohydrate, proteins and peptides and fats, nucleic acids (DNA and RNA). Pancreatic acinar secretions consist of digestive enzymes to digest each of these components.
  - ■ *Digestion of proteins (Fig. 31.4):* There are two categories of enzymes: endopeptidases and exopeptidases.
    - ♦ *Exopeptidases* cleave the terminal amino acid residues of proteins. Example: *trypsin (most abundant) and chymotrypsin*
    - ♦ *Endopeptidases* work within the protein chain. Example: *carboxypeptidase and aminopeptidase.*
    - ♦ Initially released as inactive forms including trypsinogen, chymotrypsinogen, and procarboxypeptidase, these proteases are activated once they are secreted by acinar cells and reach the duodenum. In the duodenum, trypsinogen is converted into its active form, trypsin, by the duodenal enzyme enterokinase.
    - ♦ Subsequently, activated trypsin initiates the activation of other proteases.
    - ♦ It is critical that these proteases are only activated upon entering the duodenum, where they act on ingested food components.

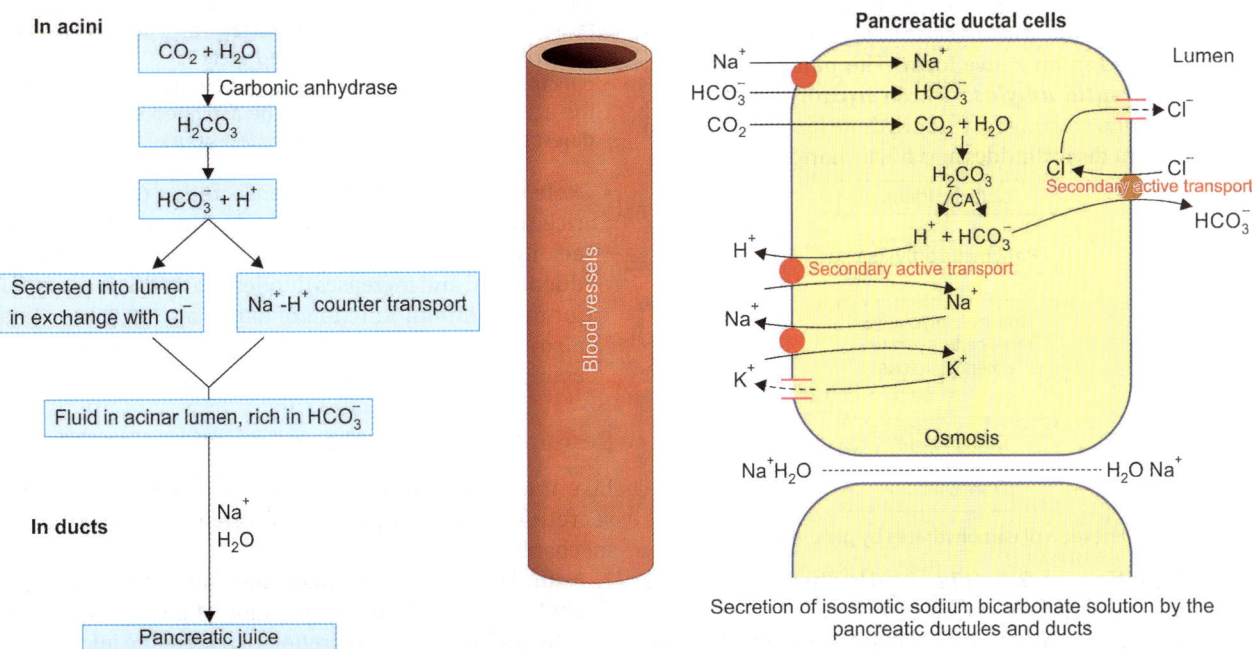

**Figs. 31.3A and B:** Formation of pancreatic juice: (A) Schematic; (B) Ductal cells.
(ATP: adenosine triphosphate; CA: carbonic anhydrase)

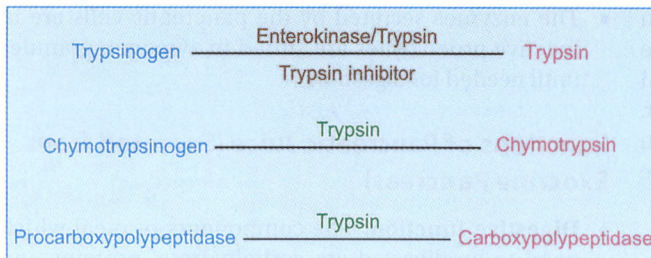
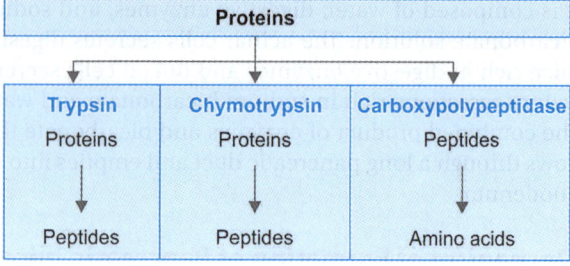

Activation of trypsin by enterokinase which activates other proteases

Digestion of protein by proteolytic enzymes

**Fig. 31.4:** Activation of pancreatic enzymes and their action of proteins.

- Activation prior to reaching the duodenum could result in the digestion of pancreatic tissue and blood vessels, leading to pancreatitis.

**What protects the pancreas from being autodigested by its own enzymes?**
- Proteolytic pancreatic enzymes are secreted in their *inactive form*: Trypsinogen, chymotrypsinogen, and procarboxypolypetidase.
- Activation of trypsin occurs only in duodenum by duodenal enzyme *enterokinase* and not earlier. Trypsin activates other inactive pancreatic enzymes involved in protein digestion.
- The acinar cells also secrete *trypsin inhibitor* along with these enzymes. The trypsin inhibitor prevents activation of trypsin both inside the secretory cells (acini) and ducts of the pancreas. Because it is trypsin that activates the other pancreatic proteolytic enzymes, trypsin inhibitor prevents activation of the proteases in the pancreas.

- **Digestion of carbohydrates (Fig. 31.5):** Pancreatic enzymes for the digestion of carbohydrate are secreted in an active form. The pancreas secretes *pancreatic amylase* which hydrolyzes starches, glycogen and most of carbohydrate (except cellulose) to form disaccharides and trisaccharides.

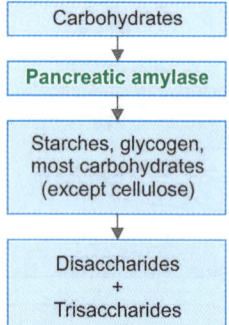

**Fig. 31.5:** Digestion of carbohydrates by pancreatic enzymes.

- **Digestion of fats (Fig. 31.6):** The fat digesting enzymes produces by pancreas are:
  - *Pancreatic lipase:* It hydrolyses the neutral fats into fatty acids and glycerol.
  - *Cholesterol esterase:* It hydrolyzes the cholesterol esters.

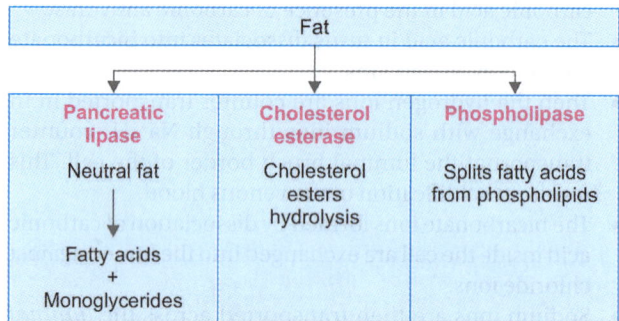

**Fig. 31.6:** Digestion of lipids by pancreatic enzymes.

- *Phospholipase:* It splits the fatty acids from phospholipids.

**What happens when the pancreas is damaged or the duct is blocked?**

When the pancreas becomes severely damaged or when a duct becomes blocked, large quantities of pancreatic enzymes get accumulated in the damaged area of pancreas. The trypsin inhibitor cannot inhibit activation of the accumulated enzymes and the activated enzymes will digest the entire pancreas within a few hours.

- **Role of sodium bicarbonate:** Secretion of ductal cells rich in sodium bicarbonate and water neutralizes the acidity of the chyme empties from the stomach into the duodenum and increases duodenal pH. This is essential for the optimum function of pancreatic enzymes. This also prevents damage to duodenal mucosa by acid coming from stomach.

## Regulation of Pancreatic Secretion (Fig. 31.7)

Like the regulation of any other secretion, pancreatic secretion is also regulated by three basic regulatory mechanisms:
1. **Neural regulation:** The vagal stimulation, through acetyl choline, results in the stimulation of pancreatic acinar cells and increase in secretion of pancreatic juice.
2. **Hormonal regulation:**
   - *Cholecystokinin (CCK or CCK-PZ):* Which is secreted by the "I-cells" of duodenal and upper

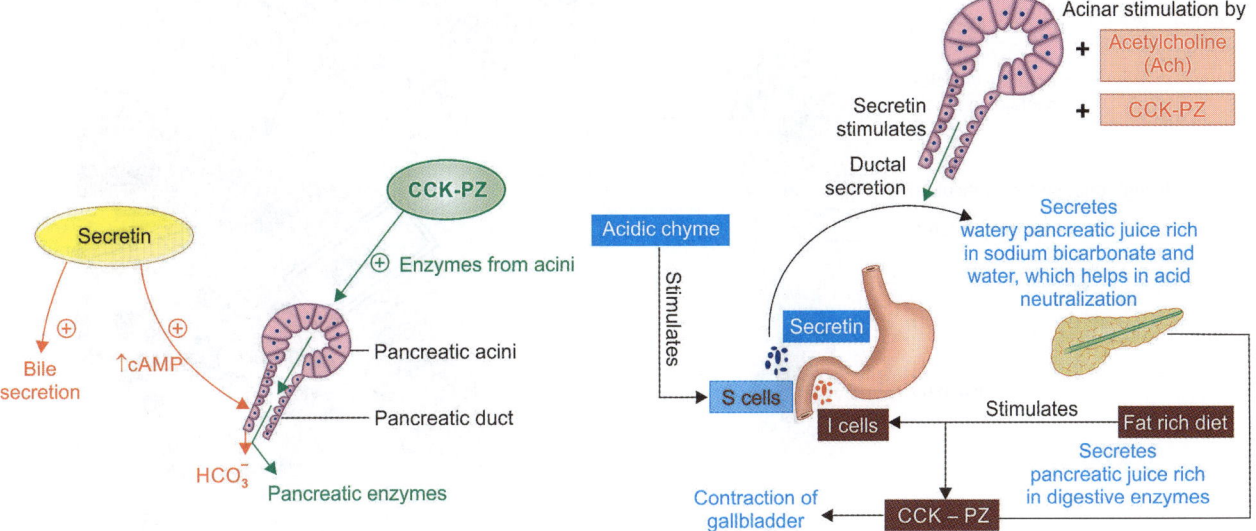

**Fig. 31.7:** Regulation of pancreatic secretion.
(CCK-PZ: cholecystokinin-pancreozymin)

jejunal mucosa when fat rich food enters the small intestine. *(ACh and CCK stimulate the acinar cells of the pancreas, causing production of large quantities of pancreatic digestive enzymes but relatively small quantities of water and electrolytes)*

- *Secretin* is secreted from the "S Cells" of the duodenum in response to the entry of acidic chyme in the duodenum and stimulates secretion of large quantities of water solution of sodium bicarbonate by the pancreatic ductal epithelium.

3. **Local changes:**
   - *pH of chyme in the duodenum:* The entry of acidic chyme in the duodenum stimulates the pancreas to produce alkaline pancreatic juice to neutralize the acidic chyme.
   - *Feedback from duodenum:* The entry of partially digested chyme in the duodenum stretches the duodenal walls sending the local and short loop reflexes to pancreas for secretion of pancreatic juice.

**What happens when secretin is not secreted in sufficient amount?**
In the absence of secretin, pancreatic secretion mainly composed of digestive enzymes with relatively small quantities of water and bicarbonate. Then without water, most of enzymes remain temporarily stored in acini or ducts and are not released into duodenum in sufficient quantity.

### Phases of Pancreatic Secretion

Pancreatic secretion also occurs in three phases, as we have read earlier: cephalic, gastric, and intestinal phase.

1. **Cephalic phase:** This phase is responsible for *20% of secretions*. The neural signal from the brain via the *vagus nerve endings* in the pancreas releases ACh. This causes the secretion of moderate amount of enzymes secretion with only small amount of water and electrolytes.

2. **Gastric phase:** There is continuous secretion of enzymes under the influence of nervous stimulation. This phase is responsible for *5–10% of pancreatic secretion*. Even though the secretion of enzymes occurs in both, cephalic and gastric phase still there is very small amount of secretion reach the duodenum due to low lack of water and electrolyte secretions.

3. **Intestinal phase:** When the chyme leaves the stomach and reaches small intestine, pancreatic secretion becomes copious. This phase is called intestinal phase of pancreatic secretion. The main regulator of pancreatic secretion in intestinal phase is the GI hormone, Secretin. It is responsible for watery and alkaline pancreatic secretion. When acidic chyme with pH <4.5 to 5.0, reaches duodenum, the secretin is released from duodenal mucosal. Secretin in turn causes the pancreas to secrete large quantities of fluid containing a high concentration of $HCO_3^-$ (up to 145 mEq/L) but a low concentration of $Cl^-$. Another GI hormone, cholecystokinin-pancreozymin *(CCK-PZ) is secreted by "I cells" of duodenal mucosa* in response to the presence of products of partial protein digestion and fatty acids in the chyme. It causes the secretion of digestive enzymes from the acinar cells, accounting for *the 70–80% of total pancreatic secretion*.

## SECRETIONS OF SMALL INTESTINE

### Secretions in Duodenum from Brunner's Glands (Fig. 31.8)

As mentioned above the first part of small intestine, receives the partially digested acidic chyme from stomach. Apart from neutralizing this acidic chyme, the duodenal mucosa has to be protected from the action of the acid

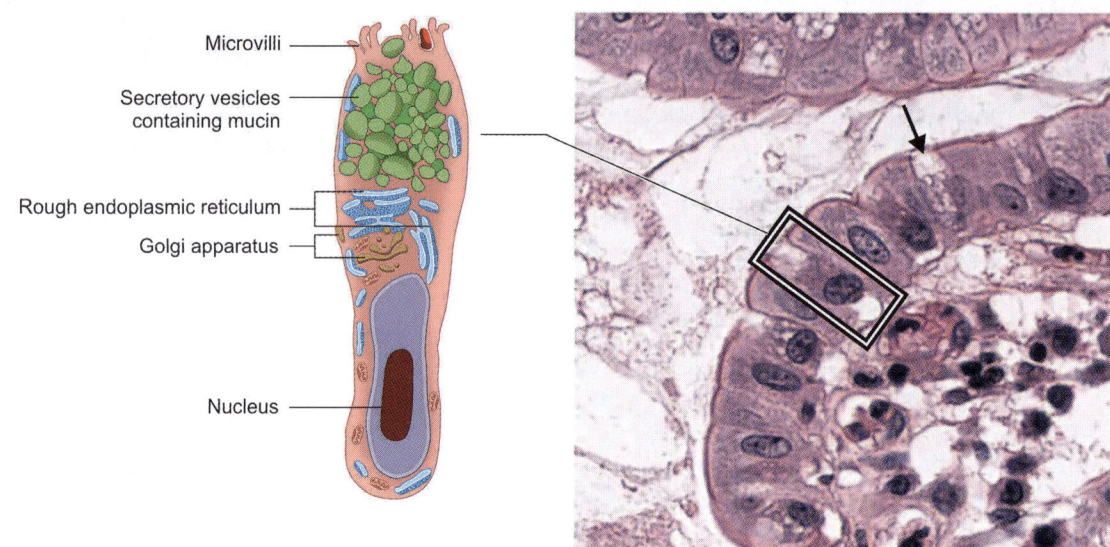

**Fig. 31.8:** Histology of Brunner's gland.

at least till the Ampulla of Vater. Hence the duodenum is coated with thick coat of alkaline mucus from pylorus to Ampulla of Vater, which is secreted from the mucous secreting *Brunner's glands*.

The Brunner's glands are stimulated by:
- Irritation of duodenal mucosa
- Vagal stimulation
- GI hormone, secretin

## Secretions from Crypts of Lieberkühn (Fig. 31.9)

The crypts of Lieberkühn lie between the intestinal villi of all the segments of the small intestine. These crypts and the intestinal villi are covered with epithelium which have two types of cells:
- **Goblet cells:** They secrete mucus which lubricates and protects the intestinal surface.
- **Enterocytes:** They form the majority of cells. They secrete water, electrolytes.

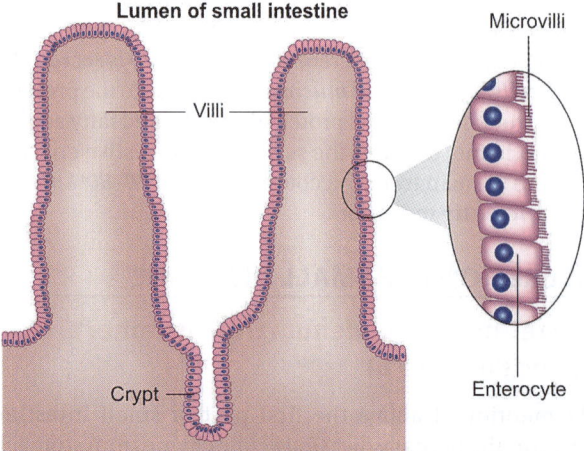

**Fig. 31.9:** Crypts of Lieberkühn.

**Daily secretion:** The intestinal secretion are formed by the enterocytes of the crypts at a rate of *1,800 mL/day*.

**Composition of Intestinal Secretion**
- pH: 7.5–8.0
- Water: 90–95%
- Electrolytes: (1–2%): $Na^+$, $K^+$, $HCO_3^-$, $Cl^-$
- Mucus: 1–2%
- Bruch border enzymes: 1%
  - Lactase, sucrase, maltase, isomaltase
  - Peptidases
  - Intestinal lipase

## Mechanism of Secretion of Intestinal Juice

The intestinal juice is primarily secreted enterocytes of crypts of Lieberkühn of small intestine by:
- Active secretion of chloride ions into crypts
- Active secretion of bicarbonate ions into crypts
- This results in movement of $Na^+$ into the fluid
- Water moves into the crypts through osmosis
- *These secretions have no enzymes*. The enzymes are present in the enterocytes covering the intestinal villi. The digestion takes place on the absorbed nutrients, instead of the intestinal lumen. These *epithelial cells undergo continuous renewal with a life span of enterocyte of 5 days*.

## Regulation of Small Bowel Secretions

The secretions of the small bowel are regulated by the neurohormonal regulatory factors:
- **Neural control:** The neural control is exhibited by the *Meissner's plexus* of enteric nervous system, which initiates short loop reflexes which modulate the intestinal secretion, blood flow and the hormonal secretion.

Further the extrinsic influence of parasympathetic nervous system on enteric nervous system also increases the intestinal secretion.
- **Hormonal control:** The intestinal secretions are influences by the GI hormones:
  - *CCK:* The fats and partially digested proteins in the chyme present in the duodenum and jejunum results in the release of CCK, which result in secretion of mucus from the intestinal glands.
  - *Secretin:* Stimulates the pancreatic and intestinal secretion, maintaining optimum pH for intestinal enzymes.
  - *Gastric inhibitory peptide (GIP):* When the chyme enters the duodenum, the GIP inhibits the gastric emptying, controlling the amount of chyme entering the duodenum.
- **Local control:**
  - *Luminal pH:* The luminal pH, particularly in duodenum, plays an important role in regulation of intestinal secretion.
  - Local stretching of the intestinal wall.

## MOTILITY OF SMALL INTESTINE

As discussed in Chapter 28, the small bowel shows typical peristaltic movements. These peristaltic movements are of two types; propulsive and mixing (segmentation) contractions.

*Although we have discussed these movements previously, we will do a small recap of the same.*
- **Mixing/segmentation contraction:**
  - Distention of small intestine with chyme
  - Stretching of intestinal wall
  - Elicits local concentric contractions
  - These contractions are spaced along the length of intestine
  - They divide the into segments like a chain of sausages.
  - These contractions chop the chyme 2–3 times/min.
- **Propulsive contractions:**
  - Chyme is propelled forward through the small intestine by peristaltic wave
  - Velocity of peristaltic wave: 0.5–2.0 cm/sec
  - Takes 3–5 hours for chyme to pass from pylorus to ileocecal valve.
  - *Peristaltic rush:* if any irritation of small bowel mucosa occurs, the parasympathetic nervous system and brainstem, stimulates the myenteric plexus resulting in the powerful and rapid peristalsis. It sweeps the intestine into colon within a few minutes. *It relieves the small bowel of irritation and distention*.

## Regulation of Intestinal Motility

The factors regulating the motility of intestine are almost same as the factors regulating the secretions. But still, lets quickly go through them:

- **Nervous factors:**
  - The myenteric plexus of enteric nervous system
  - Extrinsic influence through vagus increases motility
- **Hormonal factors increasing the motility:**
  - Motilin
  - ACh
- **Local factors:**
  - Presence of chyme in duodenum
  - Irritation of mucosa.
  - Stretching of the bowel wall.

## DIGESTION AND ABSORPTION IN SMALL INTESTINE

In small intestine, the digestion of all the nutrients occurs due to enzymes secreted by the exocrine pancreas because the intestinal juices do not have any enzymes. All the enzymes are present inside the enterocytes. Hence, the majority of digestion takes place in duodenum and upper part of jejunum due to action of pancreatic juice and bile. Hence, we will study the digestion of all the nutrients as a joint effort of intestinal and pancreatic juice along with the bile. In this section, we will outline the digestion and absorption of all nutrients however, the detail are discussed in Chapter 34.

- **Carbohydrates:** The starch/carbohydrate are partially digested in the mouth by the action of salivary amylase. After reaching the duodenum, these starches are acted upon by a stronger α-amylase, secreted by the pancreas called the **pancreatic amylase**. *Around 50–80% digestion of starch occurs due to the action of pancreatic amylase in duodenum*. The pancreatic amylase completes the digestion of carbohydrates in duodenum within 15–30 minutes, after being thoroughly mixed with the chyme. The digested carbohydrates form the glucose (mainly), galactose and fructose which are absorbed by the microvilli from the intestinal brush border.
- **Fats:** The ingested fats are *primarily digested in the first part of small intestine*. In the oral cavity, lingual lipase digests around 10% of triglycerides. The digestion of fats is aided by the biliary secretion into the duodenum, which emulsifies the fats and makes it soluble in water.
  - The **Pancreatic lipase** breaks down the emulsified fats into fatty acids and monoglycerides.
  - The other fat digesting enzymes like *cholesteryl ester hydrolase* and *phospholipase $A_2$*, results in further digestion of cholesterol esters and phospholipids.
- **Proteins:** The digestion of proteins begins in the stomach where the pepsin breaks the proteins into smaller peptone and peptides. On reaching the duodenum, *these partially digested proteins are acted upon by the trypsin, chymotrypsin, carboxypeptidases, elastases to form polypeptides and amino acids*. The peptidases further break down

the polypeptides to amino acids, which are absorbed by the intestinal villi.

## DISORDERS OF PANCREAS AND SMALL INTESTINE

### Pancreatitis

It is the inflammation of the pancreas. Depending on the duration of disease, it is classified into two types: acute and chronic pancreatitis.

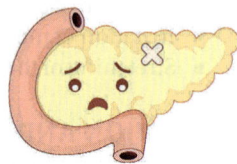

1. **Acute pancreatitis** occurs in the inflammation of short duration. It can be associated with viral infection, gallstones or excessive alcohol consumption.
2. **Chronic pancreatitis** results from repeated episodes of acute pancreatitis or a long-standing disease. It can result from long term alcohol abuse, autoimmune disorders or genetic factors. It can lead to pancreatic insufficiency.

#### Pathophysiology

- **Acute pancreatitis:**
  - *Premature activation of enzymes:* There is accumulation of pancreatic enzymes in the duct and acini of the pancreas. Trypsinogen accumulates and overcomes Trypsin inhibitors. Trypsinogen becomes activated to form Trypsin and the activated Trypsin activates other enzymes.
  - *Autodigestion of pancreas and tissue damage:* These enzymes rapidly digest pancreatic tissue and blood vessels. This causes inflammation, edema and necrosis.
- **Chronic pancreatitis:**
  - Chronic exposure to various factors causing injury to pancreas like
    - long-term alcohol consumption,
    - obstruction of pancreatic duct by gallstones,
    - genetic factors like mutations in genes (*PRSS1* for trypsinogen, *CFTR* gene for Cystic fibrosis transmembrane regulator),
    - causes unknown
  - This chronic exposure triggers inflammatory response within pancreas. There is release of pro-inflammatory substances, cytokines and activation of fibroblasts.
  - Persistent inflammation leads to deposition of collagen, resulting in fibrosis and scarring of pancreas, which replaces the functional tissue.
  - This results in the narrowing of pancreatic ducts and impairing the pancreatic secretions, resulting in *Pancreatic insufficiency*.
  - Chronic pancreatitis is associated recurrent severe abdominal pain.

**Cystic fibrosis**: A Genetic disorder caused by mutations in *CFTR* gene, affecting lungs and pancreas with thick mucus production. Symptoms include chronic respiratory infections, malabsorption, pancreatic insufficiency, and intestinal obstruction, and poor growth. Requires lifelong management for symptom relief and improved quality of life.

### Steatorrhea

It is defined as an increase in fat excretion in the stools. Fecal fat contents increases up to 40–50 g/day (Normal fecal fat content is <7 g/d). *It is the clinical feature of fat malabsorption due to pancreatic or biliary insufficiency*.

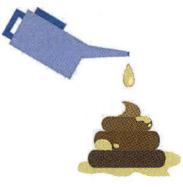

#### Pathophysiology

There is decrease digestion and absorption of fats due to *deficiency of bile acids, digestive enzymes*, and a normally functioning small intestinal mucosa. Therefore, any defects in the availability or function of bile acids, pancreatic digestive enzymes, or absorptive villi will lead to poor digestion and absorption of fat.

#### Clinical Features

- There is production of pale (in case of biliary obstruction), large volume, fowl smelling oily stools due to an increase in the fat content of stools.
- Signs and symptoms due to deficiency of fat soluble vitamins (A, D, E, and K)
- Weight loss
- Increase chances of infection

## PANCREATIC FUNCTION TESTS

Pancreatic function tests are a group of diagnostic tests used to assess the exocrine and endocrine functions of the pancreas. These tests help evaluate pancreatic enzyme secretion, pancreatic ductal function, and insulin secretion.
- **Serum amylase and lipase:** Serum amylase and lipase levels are commonly measured to assess pancreatic enzyme activity. Elevated levels of these enzymes in the blood are indicative of pancreatic injury or inflammation, such as acute pancreatitis. Lipase levels are considered more specific for pancreatic disorders than amylase levels.
- **Pancreatic enzyme stimulation tests:**
  - *Secretin-cerulein test:* In this test, synthetic secretin and cerulein (synthetic analog of CCK) are administered intravenously to stimulate pancreatic secretion. Duodenal fluid samples are collected through a nasogastric tube at specific time intervals, and the concentrations of bicarbonate and enzymes (such as amylase and lipase) are measured. Abnormal results may indicate pancreatic exocrine insufficiency.

- **Lundh test:** Similar to the secretin-cerulein test, this test assesses pancreatic enzyme secretion by stimulating the pancreas with secretin and monitoring the concentration of bicarbonate in duodenal fluid samples.
- **Fecal elastase-1:** It is a pancreatic enzyme that is stable in stool samples and serves as a marker of pancreatic exocrine function. Measurement of fecal elastase-1 levels can help diagnose pancreatic insufficiency, as reduced levels indicate inadequate pancreatic enzyme secretion.
- **Endoscopic retrograde cholangiopancreatography (ERCP):** ERCP is a procedure used to visualize the pancreatic duct and bile ducts using an endoscope. Contrast dye is injected into the ducts, and X-ray images are obtained to evaluate for abnormalities such as *strictures, stones, or ductal dilatation*. ERCP can help diagnose conditions such as *chronic pancreatitis, pancreatic ductal obstruction, or pancreatic cancer*.
- **Pancreatic function imaging:**
  - ***Secretin-enhanced magnetic resonance cholangiopancreatography (MRCP):*** This imaging technique involves administering secretin intravenously to stimulate pancreatic secretion, followed by magnetic resonance imaging (MRI) to visualize the pancreatic ducts and assess pancreatic function.
  - ***Endoscopic ultrasound (EUS):*** EUS combines endoscopy with ultrasound imaging to visualize the pancreas and surrounding structures. It can help *assess pancreatic size, morphology, and the presence of lesions or abnormalities*.
- **Glucose tolerance test (GTT):** GTT is used to assess pancreatic endocrine function, specifically insulin secretion and glucose metabolism. Patients ingest a standardized glucose solution, and blood glucose levels are measured at specific time intervals to evaluate insulin secretion and glucose clearance. Abnormal results may indicate impaired glucose tolerance or diabetes mellitus, which can be associated with pancreatic dysfunction.

## SUMMARY

- About 1200–1500 mL of pancreatic digestive juice is secreted in response to the presence of chyme in the upper portion of small intestine.
- Enterokinase activates trypsin and trypsin activates other inactive pancreatic enzymes involved in protein digestion. Trypsin inhibitor prevent the autodigestion of pancreas.
- Trypsin, chymotrypsin, and elastase are endopeptidase, while carboxypeptidase and aminopeptidase are exopeptidase.
- The major digestion takes place in duodenum and jejunum of small intestine, while absorption takes place in jejunum and ileum.
- The Brunner's glands protect the duodenal mucosa from acidic chyme till the ampulla of Vater, where the alkaline contents from pancreas and liver enter to neutralize the acid.
- Severe damage of pancreas in acute pancreatitis causes accumulation and activation of digestive enzymes which causes autodigestion of pancreas results in pancreatitis insufficiency.
- Secretin, CCK, ACh increases pancreatic and small intestinal secretion. ACh and CCK increase the secretion of pancreatic digestive enzymes from the acinar cells. Secretin in contract stimulates secretion of large quantity of water solution of sodium bicarbonate by the pancreatic ductal cells. Both these GI hormones also stimulate the secretions from Crypts of Lieberkühn.
- Alcohol is the most common cause of chronic pancreatitis. Increase serum amylase is seen in acute pancreatitis.
- Steatorrhea is the presence of large amount of fat in the stool. The stools are pale, large in volume, fowl smelling, and float on the water.

## LET US SEE, HOW MUCH YOU HAVE LEARNT?

### Review Questions

Q1. Describe the pancreatic juice under the following headings:
  a. Composition
  b. Mechanism of secretion
  c. Functions

Q2. Describe the functions of crypts of Lieberkühn in small intestine.

Q3. Why pancreatic enzymes enzymes don't cause autodigestion of pancreas?

Q4. Why secretin is important for pancreatic secretion?

Q5. Why the secretions of small intestine are devoid of enzymes?

Q6. Why there are Bulky foul-smelling stools (Steatorrhea) in pancreatic insufficiency?

### Critical Thinking Case-Based Questions

Q1. A 35-year-old male patient was admitted in the male ward with the chief complaints of pain in the epigastric region for 2 days associated with nausea and vomiting. He is a chronic alcoholic and smoker. His lab investigation showed increase serum amylase and lipase. Answer the following questions on the basis of the given case scenario:
  a. What is the probable diagnosis of the constipation?

b. What is the physiological basis of the disease?
c. How can the pancreas be prevented from self-auto-digestion?

Q2. Manoj, a 42-year-old man, presents to a physician with complaints of recurrent abdominal pain, diarrhea, and unintended weight loss over the past several months. He has a history of heavy alcohol consumption for the past 10 years. Physical examination reveals tenderness in the epigastric region, and laboratory tests show elevated serum amylase and lipase levels. A subsequent abdominal ultrasound reveals pancreatic fibrosis, calcification and dilated pancreatic ducts. Based on these findings, answer the following questions:
a. What is your probable diagnosis?
b. What is physiological basis of his disease?
c. How will pancreatic insufficiency affect the digestion of various nutrients?

## Multiple Choice Questions

**Q1.** Which of the following has minimal effects on pancreatic secretions?
a. Glucagon
b. Secretin
c. Gastrin
d. Acetylcholine

**Q2.** Which of the following is NOT a feature, when the exocrine function of pancreas is affected:
a. Increase blood glucose level
b. Fat in stool
c. Weight loss
d. Abdominal pain

**Q3.** A 16-year-old girl presents with diarrhea, tiredness, and abdominal pain. Quantitative estimation of fat in stools was 8 g/24 hours Which one of the following should be considered in the differential diagnosis:
a. Deranged renal physiology
b. Deranged exocrine pancreatic physiology
c. Deranged endocrine pancreatic physiology
d. Deranged intestinal physiology

**Q4.** Secretion of pancreatic juice rich in bicarbonate ion is stimulated by:
a. Gastrin
b. Secretin
c. CCK-PZ
d. Enterogastrone

**Q5.** True regarding pancreatic secretion:
a. When acid enters the duodenum, it releases CCK-PZ which stimulates pancreatic secretion rich in digestive enzymes.
b. When acid enters the duodenum, it releases gastrin which inhibits pancreatic secretion rich in bicarbonate ions.
c. When acid enters the duodenum, it releases secretin which stimulates pancreatic secretion rich in bicarbonate ions.
d. When acid enters the duodenum, it releases CCK-PZ which stimulates pancreatic secretion rich in bicarbonate ions.

**Q6.** Secretion of vagus nerve produces:
a. Enzyme rich pancreatic secretion
b. Alkaline watery secretion
c. Both a and b
d. No effect on pancreatic secretion

**Q7.** Secretin does not cause:
a. Bicarbonate rich secretion
b. Augments the action of CCK-PZ
c. Contraction of pyloric sphincter
d. Increase in gastric secretion

**Q8.** What is NOT TRUE in pancreatic juice in pancreatitis:
a. Volume decreases
b. Bicarbonate level decreases
c. Enzyme level is normal or low
d. Serum amylase decreases

**Q9.** A gallstone lodged in which location increases the risk of pancreatitis:
a. Left hepatic artery
b. Right hepatic artery
c. Common bile duct
d. Sphincter of oddi

**Q10.** Which of the following is not expected in patients with removal of pancreas?
a. Weight gain
b. Steatorrhea
c. Decreased absorption of amino acids
d. Hyperglycemia

**Q11.** Which of the following is NOT a function of intestinal motility?
a. Mixing and propulsion of luminal contents
b. Facilitation of nutrient absorption
c. Clearance of undigested material
d. Regulation of hormone secretion

**Q12.** Esha, a 25-year-old woman, undergoes a secretin-pancreatic function test to assess her pancreatic exocrine function. After administration of secretin, duodenal fluid samples are collected at specific intervals. Which of the following substances would be expected to increase in concentration in the duodenal fluid samples following secretin administration?
a. Bicarbonate ions
b. Gastrin
c. Pepsin
d. Glucagon

### ANSWERS
1. a   2. a   3. b   4. b   5. c   6. a   7. d   8. d   9. d   10. a   11. d   12. a

# Physiology of Hepatobiliary System

**CHAPTER 32**

> **COMPETENCY ADDRESSED**
> **PY4.2:** Describe the composition, mechanism of secretion, functions, and regulation of saliva, gastric, pancreatic, intestinal juices and bile secretion.
> **PY4.7:** Describe and discuss the structure and function of liver and gallbladder.
> **PY4.8:** Describe and discuss gastric function tests, pancreatic exocrine function tests and liver function tests.

**LEARNING OBJECTIVES**

At the end of this chapter, the learner should be able to:
- Describe the physiological anatomy and functions of liver.
- Describe the physiology of biliary secretion, composition, mechanism and regulation.
- Describe the formation and circulation of bile salts through the enterohepatic circulation.
- Describe the physiological basis of various liver disorders.

## FUNCTIONAL ANATOMY OF LIVER

Liver is the largest organ in the body, weighing around 1.4–1.6 kg in an adult human. The functional unit of the liver is the hexagon shaped lobule, that contains functional cells called hepatocytes. Every lobule contains the central vein in the center and portal triad (hepatic artery, bile duct, and portal vein) at the corners **(Fig. 32.1)**. It consists capillaries called sinusoids. So, the blood flows from portal vein and hepatic artery flows to the hepatic sinusoids. There is large space between the hepatocytes and a sinusoid called perisinusoidal space. This space lymphatics and cells like *Ito cells (stellate cells) and Kupffer cells (macrophages)*. The Ito cells serve as storage for fat and fat-soluble products such as vitamin A.

### Special Features of Liver

- The Liver has high blood flow total averaging about *1,350 mL/min, which is 25% of the resting cardiac output*. It has dual blood supply, receives *75% of blood from portal vein and 25% from hepatic artery*.
- The liver sinusoid has a larger diameter than other types of capillaries and is lined by fenestrated epithelium. The capillary epithelium has large pores that make them highly permeable. They are also known as discontinuous capillaries.

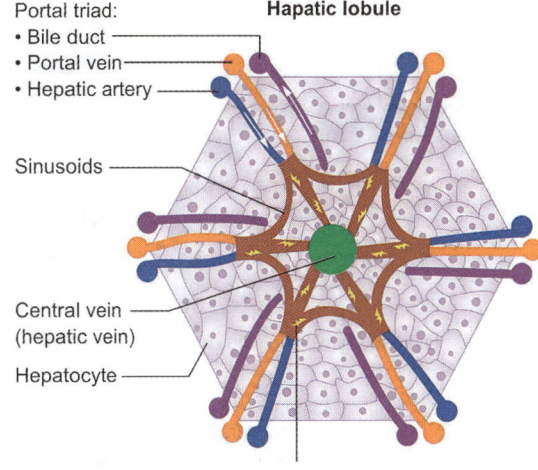

**Fig. 32.1:** Hepatic architecture showing portal triad.

- The liver has a very high lymph flow. The liver sinusoid epithelium is very permeable and produces a large amount of lymph. In addition, the diameter of the liver lymphatics is larger than that of other capillaries.
- Blood, bile, and lymphatic flow all flow in the opposite directions. *Blood flows to the liver and bile and lymph flows out of the liver*

**Why the lymph draining from the liver has a high protein concentration?**

Because the hepatic sinusoid is type of fenestrated capillary that are lined by endothelium cells having large pores. This allows ready passage of proteins and tissue fluid into the perisinusoidal space.

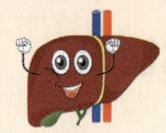

- **Regeneration of liver:** The liver has a capacity to regenerate (repair) itself after severe hepatic tissue loss. *If seventy percent of the liver is removed, the remaining lobes enlarge to restore the liver to its original size*

## FUNCTIONS OF LIVER

### Metabolic Function of Liver (Fig. 32.2)

- **Carbohydrate metabolism:** It maintains blood glucose levels within normal ranges by performing glycogenesis and gluconeogenesis activities related to the metabolism of carbohydrates.
- **Protein metabolism:** The most important functions of the liver in protein metabolism are:
  - *Deamination* of amino acids
  - Formation of plasma proteins, clotting factors, hormones, carrier proteins, and formation of other compounds.
  - *Liver is the source of all the clotting factors except vWF.*
  - *Vitamin K is* required by the metabolic processes of the liver for the formation of *II, VII, IX, and X*.
  - Large amount of ammonia is formed by the deamination process.

*Why a patient with liver disease has increased bleeding tendencies/prolonged clotting time?*

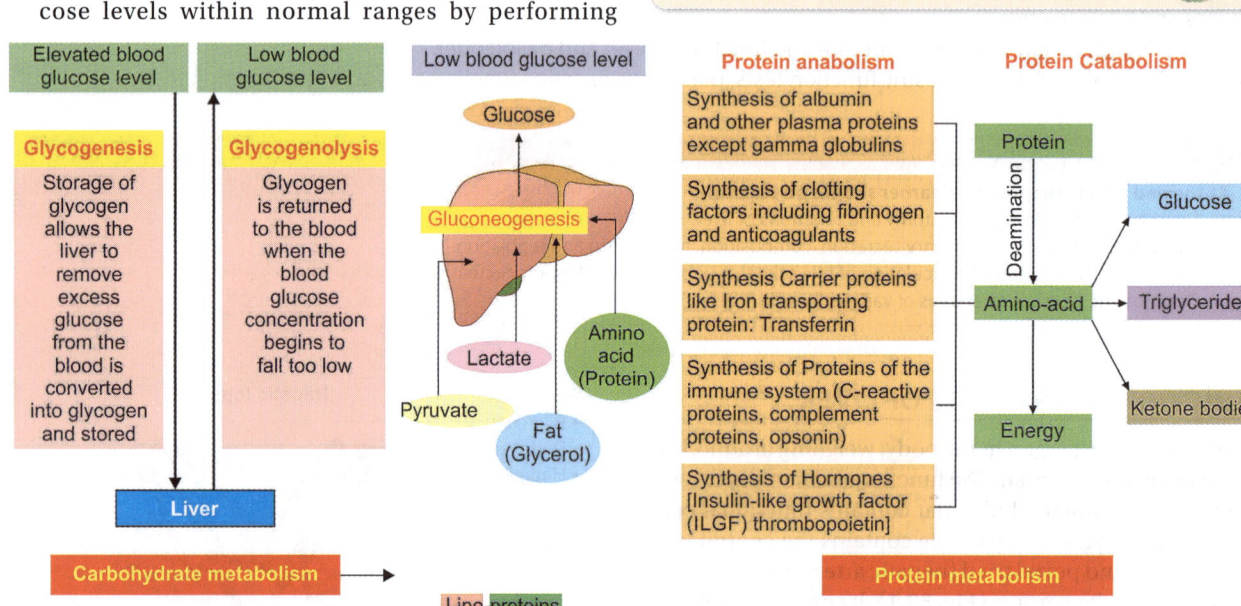

**Fig. 32.2:** Metabolism of different macro-nutrients in liver.

(VLDL: very low density lipoproteins; LDL: low density lipoproteins; HDL: high density lipoproteins; IDL: intermediate density lipoproteins)

- **Lipid metabolism:** The functions of liver in lipid metabolism are β-*Oxidation of fatty acids* to supply energy for other body functions, synthesis of large quantities of cholesterol, phospholipids, and most lipoproteins, and synthesis of fat from proteins and carbohydrates. *In conditions, where body is starving or not getting enough calories, the liver starts using fats as the substrate for energy production by β-oxidation of fatty acids resulting in production of ketone bodies.*

> **Why a patient with uncontrolled diabetes mellitus, who is not able to use glucose for energy, is more prone to have high ketone bodies (ketonemia)?**

- **Bilirubin metabolism:** When RBC dies, it is phagocyted by macrophages and hemoglobin is broken down into its components: Heme and globin. The fate of heme and globin is mentioned in the chapter (jaundice)
- **Excretory function:** The liver metabolizes and excretes ammonia, drugs, hormones and calcium.
    - The ammonia is converted into urea and excreted in urine (Urea cycle). *Hence, a patient of liver failure presents with high levels of ammonia in blood causing hepatic encephalopathy* (altered mental functions due to high levels of ammonia).
    - Thyroxine and several steroidal hormones like estrogen, cortisol, etc. are also metabolized and excreted by the liver.

> **Why a male patient with liver failure, presents with gynecomastia?**
>
> Liver failure leads to hormonal imbalances in the body, specifically a decrease in the breakdown of estrogen and an increase in the conversion of testosterone to estrogen. As a result, there is a relative excess of estrogen compared to testosterone in the body, leading to gynecomastia.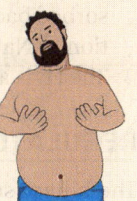

## Storage Function

Liver is the storage site of vitamins. Large quantity of Vitamin A, D3 and B12 are normally in liver. It stores iron in the form of ferritin. Hepatic cells contain large amount of apoferritin. Iron combines with it to form ferritin.

## Filtration of Blood (Cleansing Function)

The large phagocytic cells known as Kupffer cells, which are found in the perisinusoidal space between sinusoids and hepatocytes, remove unnecessary or pathologic material from the circulation.

## Detoxification of Drugs

Liver makes the fat-soluble drugs into water soluble substances, which are excreted through bile or urine.

## Endocrine Function of Liver

It is the site for:
- The deiodination of T4 to T3 (Conversion of T4 to T3).
- Vitamin D3 is also converted to 25-hydroxyvitamin D3 in liver before its final conversion into its active form in kidney.

### Functions of Liver
- Reservoir of blood
- Blood cleansing through liver macrophage system
- Metabolic functions
    - Carbohydrate metabolism: (glucose buffer)
        - Storage of glycogen
        - Conversion of galactose and fructose to glucose
        - Gluconeogenesis
    - Fat metabolism:
        - β-oxidation of fatty acids to provide energy
        - Synthesis of cholesterol, phospholipids and lipoproteins
        - Synthesis of fats from carbohydrates and proteins
    - Protein metabolism:
        - Deamination of amino acids
        - Formation of urea for removal of ammonia.
        - Formation of plasma proteins.
        - Interconversion of amino acids
        - Synthesis of other compounds from proteins.
    - Other products:
        - Metabolism of iron, urea and alcohol
    - Storage:
        - Vitamins (Vitamin A, D and B12)
        - Iron as ferritin (apoferritin-ferritin system acts as blood iron buffer)
        - Storage of glycogen, fats and proteins.
    - Synthetic functions:
        - Clotting factors (II, V, VII, IX, X)
        - Acute phase reactant proteins.
        - Bile pigments
    - Secretory functions:
        - Secretion of bile (600–1,000 mL/day)
    - Detoxification of chemicals, drugs and toxins
    - Excretory functions:
        - Bile salts, cholesterol and some metals
    - Endocrine functions:
        - Converts Vitamin D3 to 25-hydroxycholecalciferol
        - Peripheral conversion of T4 to T3
        - Secretion of IGF-I (somatomedin)
        - Degradation of steroid hormones (estradiol, etc.)

## BILIARY SECRETION

The bile is the main secretion of the liver with a daily rate of secretion between **600 to 1000 mL**.

It is a *yellow-green alkaline* (pH: *8–8.6*) fluid formed in liver and is important for digestion of fat.

### Composition of Bile
- Water
- Bile acids
- Bile pigments
- Cholesterol
- Electrolytes (Na$^+$, K$^+$, Ca$^{2+}$, Cl$^-$, HCO$_3^-$)

**Table 32.1:** Difference in composition of bile secreted from liver and gallbladder.

| Composition | Liver bile | Gallbladder bile |
|---|---|---|
| Water content | 95% | 85% |
| pH | Alkaline | Acidic (due to high $H^+$) |
| Solids (cholesterol, lecithin, bilirubin) | 2 g% | 10–15 g% |
| Bile salts and bile pigments | Less | More |
| $Na^+$, $Cl^-$, $HCO_3^-$ | More | Less |
| $K^+$, $Ca^{2+}$ | Less | More |

Bile is secreted by the liver and *concentrated 5–6 times in gallbladder by absorption of fluid and electrolytes*. Gallbladder also secretes mucin that makes the bile thick **(Table 32.1)**.

## Functions of Bile

- Aids in the digestion of fat via fat emulsification (Bile converts large lipid droplets into small droplets/micelle)
- Absorption of fat and fat-soluble vitamins
- Excretion of bilirubin (Bile pigments)
- Excretion of excess cholesterol
- Neutralization of gastric acid: Provides an alkaline fluid in the duodenum to neutralize the acidic pH of the chyme that comes from the stomach.
- Activates pancreatic lipase.
- It provides bactericidal activity against microorganisms present in the ingested food.

**Functions of Bile**
- Bile helps in absorption of lipids from intestines by forming micelles.
- Bile salts in bile are important choleretics (Increase bile secretion).
- Absorption of fat-soluble vitamins
- Activate pancreatic lipase
- Bile pigments (bilirubin and biliverdin) provide greenish yellow coloration

## MECHANISM OF BILIARY SECRETION

- Site of formation: Hepatocytes → initial secretion
  - Contains bile acids, cholesterol, other organic constituents.
  - Secreted into bile canaliculi → terminal bile ducts → hepatic duct → common bile duct → duodenum
- Liver adds watery solution of $Na^+$ and $HCO_3^-$ under the effect of **Secretin**, while passing through the bile duct (second secretion).
- This increases the volume of bile.

The biliary secretion is synthesized in two stages **(Fig. 32.3)**:
- **Stage I/initial secretion:** It is secreted by liver cells (hepatocytes). It contains large amounts of bile acids, cholesterol and other organic substances. It is secreted into bile canaliculi.
- **Stage II/second secretion:** In the interlobular septa, the canaliculi empty into the bile ducts, then to hepatic ducts and common bile duct. Here the bile either flows into duodenum or gets diverted into the gallbladder. In these bile ducts, second portion of liver secretion is added into bile, which is composed of Water, $Na^+$, $HCO_3^-$. The second secretion is stimulated by the hormone *Secretin*.

## Changes in Bile in the Gallbladder

In the gallbladder, following changes occur in the bile:
- **Storage of bile:** Volume of gallbladder is 30–60 mL.
- **Concentration of bile:** It stores the concentrated bile by absorption of water from the bile from 5- to 20-folds
- **Acidification of bile (Fig. 32.4):** The $HCO_3^-$ is reabsorbed back from the gallbladder along with the absorption of $Na^+$ and $Cl^-$ resulting in the acidification of bile. The $H^+$ is added by the $Na^+$-$H^+$ counter transport.

## REGULATION OF BILE SECRETION (FIG. 32.5)

The biliary secretion is affected by mainly the following factors:

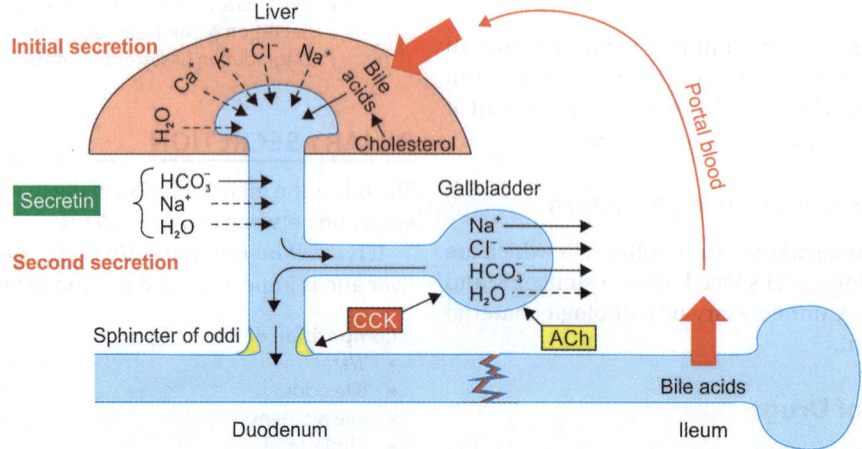

**Fig. 32.3:** Secretion of bile from liver and storage in gallbladder.

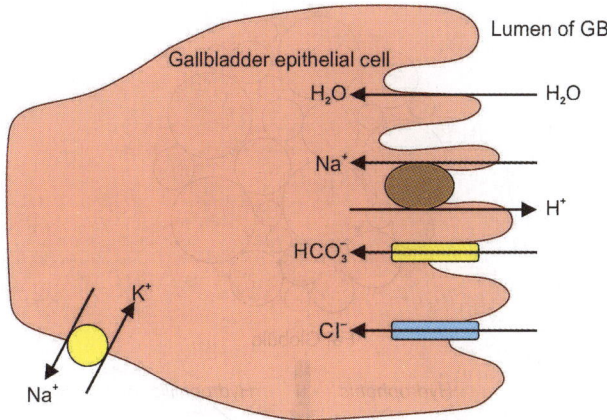

**Fig. 32.4:** Acidification of bile in gallbladder.

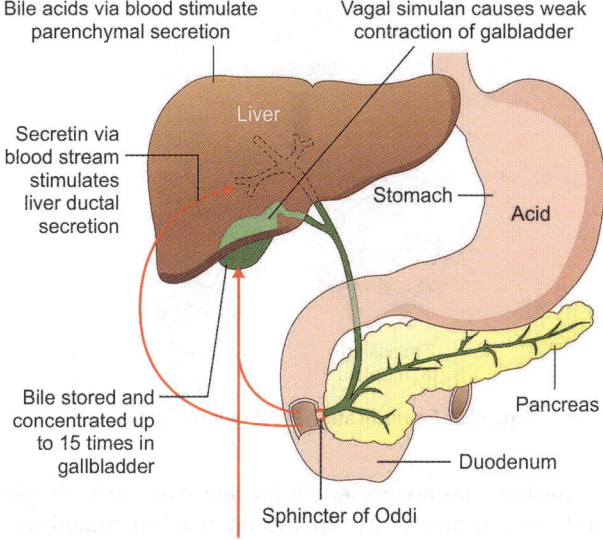

**Fig. 32.5:** Regulation of bile secretion.

## Neural Regulation

The vagal stimulation increases the biliary secretion by causing the contraction of gallbladder.

## Hormonal Regulation

Many hormones are responsible for influencing the biliary secretion, mentioned below:
- **Acetyl choline:** Similar to vagal stimulation, the ACh contracts the gallbladder and releases the stored bile into the duodenum.
- **Secretin:** Acts on the second secretion and increases the biliary secretion by 100%. It increases the volume of biliary secretion.
- **Cholecystokinin:** CCK is the most potent hormone resulting in the contraction of the gallbladder and releases the stored bile into the duodenum by relaxing the sphincter of Oddi.

## Local Regulation

Many local factors in the duodenum, influences the biliary secretion like
- Presence of fats in the duodenum/fatty meal.

## BILE SALTS

The bile salts form the main constituent of the bile juice. These bile salts are made from the bile acids, which are actually made from the *Cholesterol (the precursor) (Flowchart 32.1). Liver synthesizes around 6 g of bile salts daily.*

In the liver, the cholesterol forms the **primary bile acids**:
- Cholic acid
- Chenodeoxycholic acid

Further, when the bile is released into the duodenum, it passes through the intestine, where the intestinal bacteria convert them into the *secondary bile acids*:
- Deoxycholic acid
- Lithocholic acid.

These bile acids get conjugated with the amino acids forming their $Na^+$ or $K^+$ salts, as shown in **Flowchart 32.2**.

### Functions of Bile Salts

- Absorption of fats
- Emulsification of fats
- Source of bile acids
- Bile secretion (choleretics)
- Absorption of fat soluble vitamins
- Activation of pancreatic enzymes
- Prevention of gallstone formation

*Deficiency of bile → Steatorrhea (passage of greasy and fatty stools)*

**Flowchart 32.1:** Bile salts production.

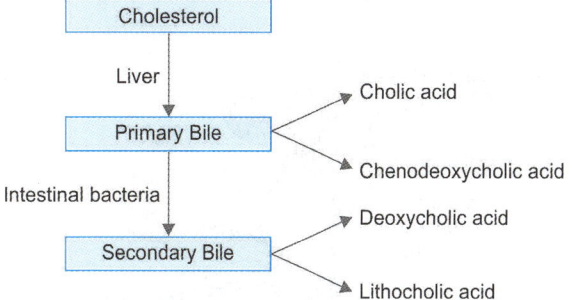

**Flowchart 32.2:** Conjugation of amino acids.

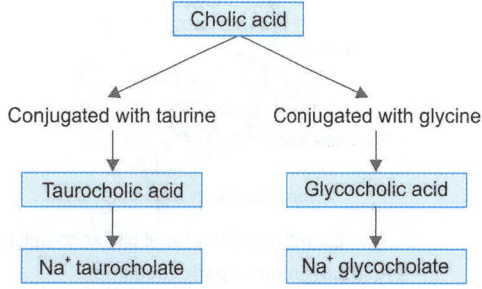

## ENTEROHEPATIC CIRCULATION (FIG. 32.6)

> **Importance of Enterohepatic Circulation**
> - Absorbed bile salts act as a choleretic agent (agents that increases the production of bile)
> - This recirculation is important because of limited pool of bile salts. The same bile salts are utilizing and reutilized for the digestive function.

It is the recirculation of bile salts from the intestine to the liver and then back to the intestine. Bile salts are transported from liver to small intestine by common bile duct during digestion. Bile salts are reabsorbed into the blood from small intestine. The absorbed bile salts are returned via portal vein to the liver, where they are once again secreted into the bile. *Around 94% of bile salts is recirculated. A small amount of bile salts (5%) escapes this recycling and lost in feces*. Each molecule is approximately recirculated for *17 times*, before being lost in feces.

## CHOLERETICS AND CHOLAGOGUES

- **Choleretics:** They are the substances that *enhance the bile secretion*. Important choleretics are:
  - Bile salts
  - Secretin
  - ACh
- **Cholagogues** are the substances that *cause contraction of the gallbladder*. Important cholagogues are:
  - Cholecystokinin (CCK)—the most potent stimulus
  - Fatty acids

## ROLE OF BILE IN DIGESTION OF FATS

As we have seen earlier, the bile is an important secretion for the emulsification of bile, which is then digested by pancreatic lipase **(Fig. 32.7)**.

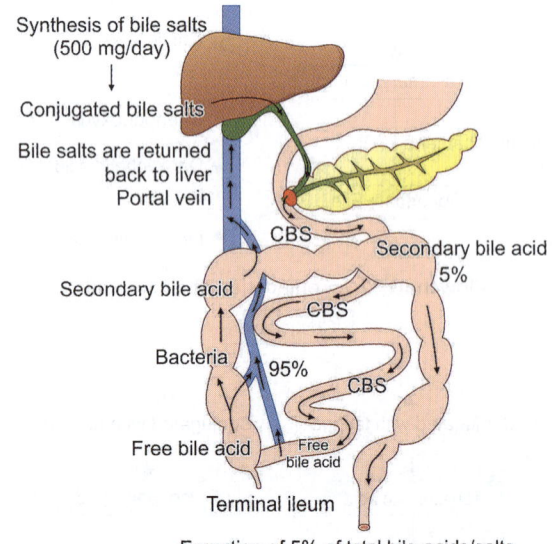

**Fig. 32.6:** Enterohepatic circulation.

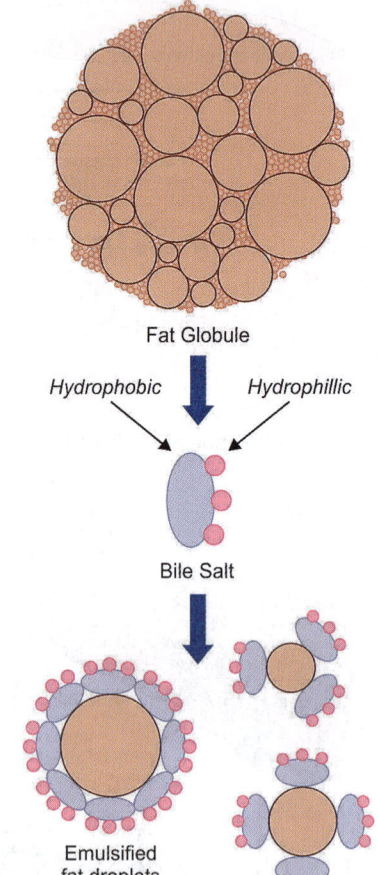

**Fig. 32.7:** Emulsification of fat globule by bile salt.

The bile salts are present in the bile, coat the fat droplet and break it down into smaller fat droplets coated with the bile salts called the micelles. The bile salts have the hydrophobic ends which binds to the fat molecule while the other hydrophilic end makes the micelle water soluble.

## DISORDERS OF LIVER AND GALLBLADDER

- Nonalcoholic steatohepatitis (NASH)
- Jaundice
- Cholelithiasis

### Nonalcoholic Steatohepatitis (NASH)

It is a progressive form of nonalcoholic fatty liver disease (NAFLD) characterized by liver inflammation and damage resembling alcoholic hepatitis but occurs in individuals who consume little or no alcohol. NASH can progress to advanced liver disease, including cirrhosis and liver failure.

### Causes

The exact cause of NASH is not fully understood, but it's believed to be multifactorial, involving a combination of genetic, environmental, and metabolic factors. Risk factors for NASH include **obesity, insulin resistance, type 2**

**diabetes, dyslipidemia (abnormal lipid levels), and metabolic syndrome**. Sedentary lifestyle and poor dietary habits, such as excessive intake of refined carbohydrates and saturated fats, also contribute to its development. Hence, NASH is emerging as a common lifestyle disorder.

## Pathophysiology

In individuals predisposed to NASH, excess fat accumulates in liver cells (hepatocytes), leading to hepatic steatosis (fatty liver). This fat accumulation can trigger inflammatory responses and oxidative stress within the liver, resulting in the activation of immune cells and release of proinflammatory cytokines. Chronic inflammation and oxidative stress promote liver cell injury and apoptosis (cell death), leading to fibrosis and scarring of the liver tissue. Over time, progressive fibrosis can lead to cirrhosis and its associated complications, such as liver failure and hepatocellular carcinoma.

## Clinical Features

Clinical manifestations of NASH can vary widely, ranging from asymptomatic to advanced liver disease. Common clinical features include:
- Fatigue
- Right upper abdominal discomfort or pain
- Elevated liver enzymes (SGOT and SGPT) on blood tests
- Hepatomegaly (enlarged liver)
- Elevated levels of serum markers of inflammation and fibrosis
- Advanced stages may present with symptoms of cirrhosis, such as jaundice, ascites, and hepatic encephalopathy.

# Jaundice

It has been covered in Chapter 15.

# Cholelithiasis (Gallstones)

Cholelithiasis refers to the presence of gallstones in the gallbladder or bile ducts. Gallstones can vary in size and composition, ranging from small, sand-like particles to larger, crystalline structures. These stones can obstruct the flow of bile and cause various symptoms and complications.

## Causes

The exact cause of gallstone formation is not fully understood, but several factors can contribute to their development, including:
- Imbalance in the composition of bile, such as high cholesterol or bilirubin levels.
- Reduced gallbladder motility, leading to stasis of bile.
- Obesity and rapid weight loss.
- Pregnancy, hormonal therapy, or estrogen replacement therapy.
- Certain medical conditions, such as cirrhosis, diabetes, and Crohn's disease.
- Genetic predisposition.
- Diet high in fat and cholesterol.

## Pathophysiology (Fig. 32.8)

Gallstones form when substances in bile, such as cholesterol, bilirubin, and calcium salts, become supersaturated and precipitate out of solution. The exact mechanism of stone formation may vary depending on the type of stone (cholesterol, pigment, or mixed).

Cholesterol stones are the most common and typically form due to an imbalance between cholesterol and bile salts in bile.

Pigment stones, on the other hand, form primarily from bilirubin and are associated with conditions such as cirrhosis and hemolytic disorders.

Once formed, gallstones may remain in the gallbladder or migrate into the bile ducts, leading to obstruction and inflammation.

## Clinical Features

The clinical presentation of cholelithiasis can vary widely, ranging from asymptomatic to severe complications.

Common clinical features include:
- **Biliary colic:** Intermittent, severe pain in the upper right or middle abdomen, often radiating to the back or right shoulder, typically triggered by fatty meals.
- Nausea and vomiting.
- Jaundice (yellowing of the skin and eyes) if the stone obstructs the common bile duct.
- Fever and chills if associated with cholecystitis (inflammation of the gallbladder).

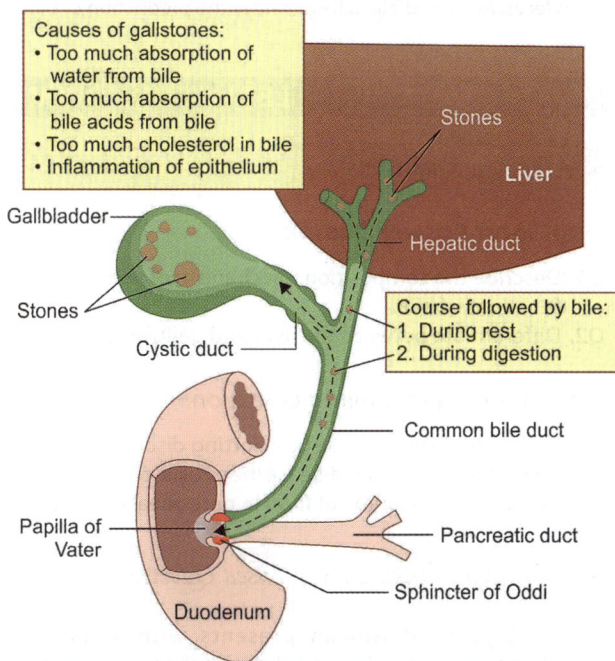

**Fig. 32.8:** Pathophysiology of gallstones.

- Complications such as cholecystitis, cholangitis (infection of the bile ducts), pancreatitis (inflammation of the pancreas), and gallstone ileus (obstruction of the small intestine by a gallstone).

## LIVER FUNCTION TESTS

Liver function tests (LFTs) are a group of blood tests commonly performed to assess the health and function of the liver. They provide valuable information about the liver's ability to perform its various functions, including metabolism, detoxification, and synthesis of proteins.

### Components of Liver Function Tests

Liver function tests typically include several blood markers that evaluate different aspects of liver function:
- **S. Bilirubin:** A breakdown product of red blood cells. Elevated levels of bilirubin may indicate liver disease or obstruction of bile flow.
- **Alanine aminotransferase (ALT) and aspartate aminotransferase (AST):** Enzymes released into the bloodstream when liver cells are damaged or inflamed. Elevated levels of ALT and AST indicate liver injury, though ALT is more specific to liver damage.
- **Alkaline phosphatase (ALP):** An enzyme found in bile ducts and bone. Elevated ALP levels may indicate liver or bile duct obstruction, bone disorders, or certain medications.
- **Gamma-glutamyl transferase (GGT):** An enzyme found in the liver, bile ducts, and kidneys. Elevated GGT levels are associated with liver disease, alcohol consumption, and certain medications.
- **Albumin and total protein:** Proteins are synthesized by the liver. Hence, low levels may indicate impaired liver function or malnutrition.
- **Prothrombin time (PT) and international normalized ratio (INR):** Measures of blood clotting function, which are affected by liver synthesis of clotting factors.

### SUMMARY

- The liver is the largest organ and has a high lymphatic and blood flow. It performs storage, filtration, excretion, metabolic, detoxification, and synthesis functions.
- Liver can store vitamin A for up to 10 months to prevent vitamin A insufficiency. Vitamin D deficiency can be avoided for 3–4 months if sufficient stores are kept, while sufficient amounts of vitamin B12 can last for at least 1 year.
- The liver produces all of the plasma proteins, with the exception of gamma-globulins. Liver diseases can cause bleeding because the liver produces clotting factors.
- The fluid needed for the digestion of fat, called bile, is formed, concentrated, and stored in the biliary system. 95% of bile acid is reabsorbed by enterohepatic circulation and 5% excreted in feces. Absorbed bile salts increases the production of bile.
- CCK-PZ increases gallbladder emptying and secretin increases bile production.
- Heme metabolism produces the bile pigments seen in bile. Jaundice results from a defect in the heme metabolism pathway.
- The physiological basis of gallbladder stones is explained by the overproduction of cholesterol by the liver, an excess of bilirubin, and hypomotility, or impeded gallbladder emptying.
- Bile is concentrated and stored in the gallbladder. The removal of the gallbladder results in the continuous discharge of hepatic bile into the intestine. The patient finds it challenging to digest large and fatty meals.

### LET US SEE, HOW MUCH YOU HAVE LEARNT?

 *Review Questions*

#### Long/Short Answer Questions

Q1. Describe the composition, mechanism of secretion and functions of bile.
Q2. Differentiate between the liver and gallbladder bile.
Q3. Write a short note on enterohepatic circulation.
Q4. Enumerate the metabolic functions of liver.
Q5. What are the factors affecting gallbladder emptying?

#### Explain Why? (Reasoning Questions)

Q1. A patient of liver disease has clotting disorders.
Q2. The patient of liver disease/hepatitis presents with ascites (Accumulation of fluid in peritoneal cavity).
Q3. There is itching in a patient of liver disease.
Q4. There is confusion and delirium in liver disorder (Hint: think about hepatic encephalopathy).

 *Critical Thinking Case-Based Questions*

Q1. A 65-year-old woman presents with worsening abdominal distension and abdominal pain. His medical history includes alcohol use liver disorder. On physical examination, his eyes appear yellow. The abdominal examination shows a positive fluid wave showing massive ascites. Laboratory test results are albumin

2.1 g/dL. Answer the following questions on the basis of the given case scenario.
a. What are the functions of liver?
b. What is the physiological basis of yellowness of the eyes of the patient?
c. Why do you think is the cause of massive ascites in this patient?
*(ascites in patients with liver failure is primarily attributed to portal hypertension, hypoalbuminemia, sodium and water retention, activation of the renin–angiotensin–aldosterone system, and peritoneal inflammation)*
d. What is the physiological basis of decrease albumin of the patient?
e. What kind of preventive guidance should a physician give a patient?

Q2. A 35-year-old female, weight 76 kg came to OPD with pain in abdomen and vomiting. Pain increases after fatty meals. Following examination, they suspected the presence of stones in one of the gastrointestinal organs, which a USG verified. The physician recommended that the affected organ be removed. Answer the following questions on the basis of the given case scenario.
a. Which part of the digestive system is affected?
b. Which digestive organ is involved?
c. What are the functions of the involved organ?
d. Explain the physiological basis of signs and symptoms of the patient.
e. What kind of advice about prevention should a doctor give a patient following the removal of the problematic organ?
*(For description, refer to the early clinical exposure in clinical physiology)*

## Multiple Choice Questions

Q1. Bile is produced in liver is associated with which of the following?
a. Activates pancreatic amylase
b. Emulsification of fat
c. Actives pancreatic lipase
d. Actives stomach pepsinogen

Q2. What is the most common clinical manifestation of symptomatic gallstones?
a. Recurrent left upper quadrant pain
b. Recurrent right upper quadrant pain
c. Recurrent lower abdominal pain
d. Recurrent upper back pain

Q3. What happens if bile duct gets blocked
a. Feces become dry
b. Acidic chyme will not be neutralized
c. There will be little digestion in intestine
d. Little absorption of fat will occur

Q4. Fat in the duodenum lumen
a. Stimulates gallbladder contraction
b. Inhibits gallbladder contraction
c. Inhibits CCK secretion
d. Release secretin

Q5. Which juice secreted by the organ in the alimentary canal plays an important role in the digestion of fat?
a. Pancreatic juice, saliva
b. Hydrochloric acid, mucus
c. Bile juice, pancreatic juice
d. Saliva, hydrochloric acid

Q6. A patient presents with jaundice, abdominal pain, and fever. Laboratory investigations reveal elevated levels of alkaline phosphatase and bilirubin. What is the most likely cause of these symptoms?
a. Cholelithiasis     b. Cirrhosis
c. Viral hepatitis    d. Pancreatitis

Q7. A patient with a history of chronic liver disease develops ascites. Which of the following mechanisms is most likely responsible for the development of ascites in this patient?
a. Decreased albumin synthesis
b. Increased bile secretion
c. Activation of pancreatic enzymes
d. Intestinal obstruction

Q8. A patient with liver failure develops hepatic encephalopathy. Which of the following physiological changes contributes to the development of hepatic encephalopathy?
a. Decreased bile production
b. Increased ammonia levels in the bloodstream
c. Increased synthesis of clotting factors
d. Decreased levels of serum bilirubin

Q9. A patient undergoes a liver biopsy, and histological examination reveals extensive fibrosis and nodular regeneration of liver tissue. Which of the following conditions is most likely associated with this histological finding?
a. Cirrhosis
b. Hepatitis A
c. Nonalcoholic fatty liver disease (NAFLD)
d. Cholecystitis

Q10. Which of the following liver function tests would be most useful in assessing liver injury in a patient with suspected hepatitis?
a. Serum albumin
b. Serum bilirubin
c. Alanine aminotransferase (ALT)
d. Gamma-glutamyl transferase (GGT)

Q11. A patient with chronic liver disease experiences spontaneous bleeding. Which of the following laboratory tests would be most indicative of impaired liver function contributing to the bleeding tendency?
a. Prothrombin time (PT) and international normalized ratio (INR)
b. Serum albumin
c. Serum bilirubin
d. Serum creatinine

## ANSWERS

1. b    2. b    3. d    4. a    5. c    6. c    7. a    8. b    9. a    10. c    11. a

# Physiology of Digestion in the Large Intestine

**33 CHAPTER**

### COMPETENCY ADDRESSED

**PY4.2:** Describe the composition, mechanism of secretion, functions, and regulation of saliva, gastric, pancreatic, intestinal juices and bile secretion.
**PY4.3:** Describe GIT movements, regulation and functions. Describe defecation reflex. Explain the role of dietary fiber.
**PY4.9:** Discuss the physiological aspects of: Peptic ulcer, gastroesophageal reflux disease, vomiting, diarrhea, constipation, adynamic ileus, Hirschsprung's disease.

###  LEARNING OBJECTIVES

**At the end of this chapter, the learner should be able to:**
- Describe the functional anatomy of large intestine.
- Describe functions of large intestine.
- Describe the secretions large intestinal.
- Describe the types of large intestinal motility.
- Describe the mechanism of defecation and defecation reflex.
- Describe the role of large intestine in digestion and absorption.
- Describe the physiological basis of various disorders of secretion and motility of large intestine.

## FUNCTIONAL ANATOMY OF LARGE INTESTINE (FIG. 33.1)

The length of the last portion of the gastrointestinal tract is **1.5 m**. It consists of cecum, colon (ascending, transverse, and descending colon), rectum and the anal canal. The cecum receives liquid chyme from the ileum via the ileocecal valve. *The proximal colon is the absorptive colon, and the distal colon is the storage colon.* Hence, the consistency of the chyme changes from fluid in cecum, semifluid in ascending colon, mushy in transverse colon, semi mush in upper descending colon, semisolid in descending colon and finally becoming solid fecal matter in rectum. Rectosigmoid region, and anal canal, and pelvic floor musculature maintains fecal continence.

### Histology of Large Intestine

The wall of the large intestine is composed of four layers:

#### Mucosa

The mucosa is the innermost layer of the large intestine and is directly in contact with the contents of the intestinal lumen. The innermost layer composed of simple columnar epithelial cells, which absorb water and electrolytes from the fecal material. It has many crypts of Lieberkühn but has no intestinal villi. It has abundant mucus secreting glands.

#### Submucosa

The submucosa is a layer of connective tissue that lies beneath the mucosa.

It contains blood vessels, lymphatic vessels, and nerves, including the submucosal plexus (Meissner's plexus), which controls secretory functions and blood flow in the intestines.

#### Muscularis Externa

The muscularis externa is composed of two layers of smooth muscle:
- **Inner circular layer:** Smooth muscle fibers oriented circumferentially around the intestine, which contract to produce segmentation movements and aid in mixing and propelling fecal material.
- **Outer longitudinal layer:** Specialized three strips of smooth muscle fibers oriented longitudinally along

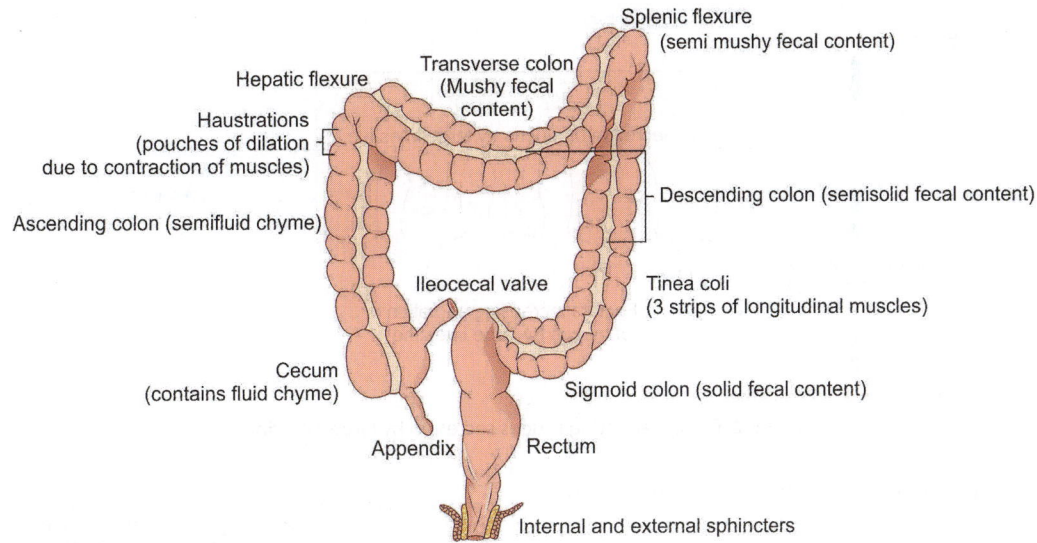

**Fig. 33.1:** Anatomical parts of large intestine and last section of GIT.

the length of the intestine are present in large intestine called *taenia coli*. Taenia is not present around whole circumference of large intestine. Hence, its contraction causes bulging of large intestinal wall called *haustrations*.

### Serosa (or Adventitia in Some Areas)

The serosa is the outermost layer of the large intestine and consists of a thin layer of connective tissue covered by a layer of mesothelial cells.

The serosa helps to provide support and protection to the large intestine and allows it to move freely within the abdominal cavity.

## FUNCTIONS OF LARGE INTESTINE

The large intestine, also known as the colon, plays several important functions in the digestive system.
- **Absorption of water and electrolytes:** One of the primary functions of the large intestine is to absorb water and electrolytes (such as sodium and chloride) from the undigested material (chyme) that enters it from the small intestine. This absorption process converts the liquid contents into a semisolid form, which ultimately forms feces.
- **Storage of fecal material:** The large intestine serves as a reservoir for fecal material until it is ready to be eliminated from the body. By storing feces temporarily, the colon allows for controlled defecation, preventing the immediate and involuntary expulsion of waste.
- **Fermentation and production of short-chain fatty acids:** Bacteria residing in the large intestine ferment undigested carbohydrates and fibers that reach the colon. This fermentation process produces short-chain fatty acids (SCFAs), such as acetate, propionate, and butyrate. SCFAs serve as an energy source for the cells lining the colon and have various health benefits, including promoting colon health and regulating metabolism.
- **Production of vitamins:** Intestinal bacteria also play a role in synthesizing certain vitamins, such as vitamin K and some B vitamins (e.g., biotin and vitamin B12). These vitamins are absorbed in the large intestine and contribute to overall health.
- **Formation of feces:** As the undigested material moves through the large intestine, water is progressively absorbed, and the remaining waste material becomes more compacted and formed into feces. The feces consist of water, undigested food particles, bacteria, cellular debris, and bile pigments.
- **Defecation:** The large intestine is responsible for initiating and coordinating the process of defecation, which involves the expulsion of fecal material from the rectum through the anus. This process is regulated by reflexes involving the nervous system and coordinated contractions of the muscles in the colon and rectum.

## SECRETION OF LARGE INTESTINE

Large intestinal secretion is a watery fluid with pH 8.0.

**Composition**
- It contains 99.5% water and 0.5% solids
- Digestive enzymes are absent
- High concentration of bicarbonate
- Mucus forms the main component of large intestinal secretion.

Mucus is secreted by the mucus cells of crypts of Lieberkühn (Fig. 33.2). The functions of mucus are:
- It lubricates the mucosa of large intestine and bowel contents, so that, the movement of bowel is facilitated.
- The mucin protects mucus membrane of large intestine by preventing the damage caused by mechanical injury or chemical substances.

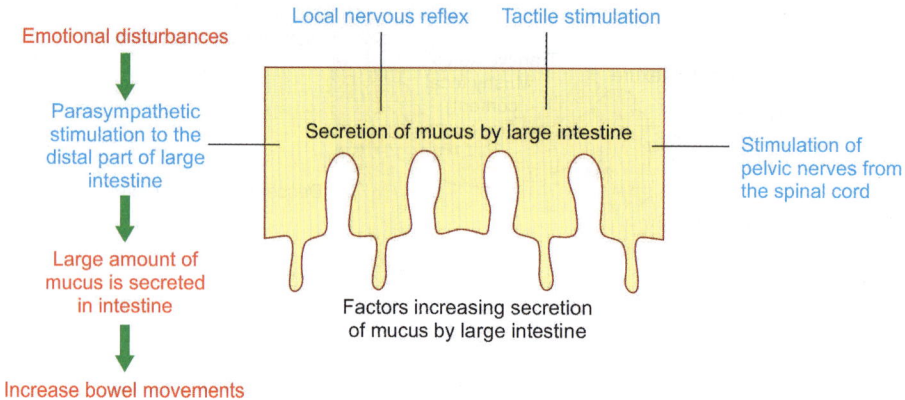

**Fig. 33.2:** Factors affecting mucus secretion by large intestine.

- It acts as an adherent medium for holding fecal matter together.
- The alkaline mucus $NaHCO_3$ neutralizes the fecal acid produced by the intestinal gut microbes.

**Inflammation of the large intestine causes diarrhea**

Irritation of inflammation of large intestine is called *enteritis*. The mucosa of the inflamed and irritated large intestine secretes water, electrolytes and normal viscid alkaline mucosa. This causes the dilution of irritating factors and increases the bowel movements to wash them out of the body, thus causes diarrhea.

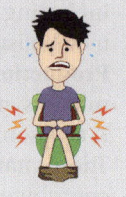

## COLONIC MOTILITY

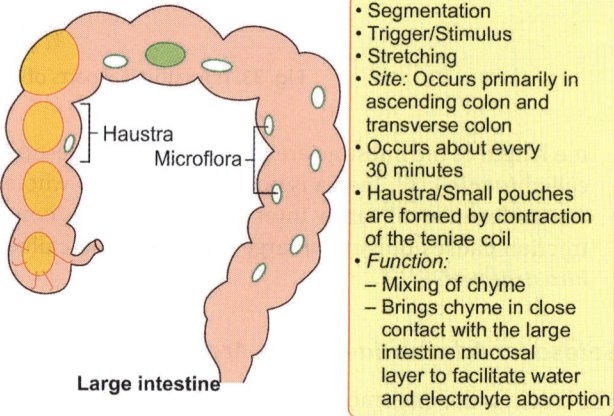

**Fig. 33.3:** Mechanism of haustral contractions.

The principal functions of the colon are:
- Absorption of water and electrolytes from the chyme, leading to the formation of solid feces,
- Storage of fecal matter until expulsion becomes viable.

Unlike the small intestine, where vigorous contractions are seen, the movements of the colon typically sluggish due to its roles in absorption and storage.

### Mixing Movements (Haustrations)

Similar to segmentation movements in the small intestine, the large intestine experiences large circular constrictions known as *haustrations* **(Fig. 33.3)**. These constrictions involve approximately 2.5 cm of circular muscle contracting, sometimes nearly occluding the colon's lumen. The three strips of longitudinal muscle, called the teniae coli, contracts. This coordinated effort results in the formation of bulging sacs termed haustrations, allowing the unstimulated portions of the large intestine to extend outward.

*Each haustration peaks in intensity within about 30 seconds before dissipating over the subsequent 60 seconds.* They exhibit slow movement toward the anus during contraction, particularly in the cecum and ascending colon, thereby contributing to minor forward propulsion of colonic contents. The new haustral contractions begin in adjacent areas, gradually exposing all fecal material to the mucosal surface for progressive absorption, ultimately resulting in the expulsion of 80 to 200 mL of feces daily.

### Propulsive Movements (Mass Movements) (Fig. 33.4)

While haustral contractions facilitate propulsion in the cecum and ascending colon over several hours, mass movements take over from the cecum to the sigmoid colon. These mass movements, occur one to three times daily, typically peak within the first hour post-breakfast and lasts for about 15 minutes.

These movements result in a modified type of peristalsis, characterized by a constrictive ring forming in response to distension or irritation in the colon, usually in the transverse colon. Subsequently, a segment of the colon distal to the constriction loses its haustrations, contracting as a unit to propel fecal material further down the colon.

This contraction increases progressively over about 30 seconds before relaxation sets in during the next 2 to 3 minutes. The cycle repeats, with a series of mass movements persisting for 10 to 30 minutes before ceasing temporarily and resuming later, culminating in the urge for defecation upon the accumulation of feces in the rectum.

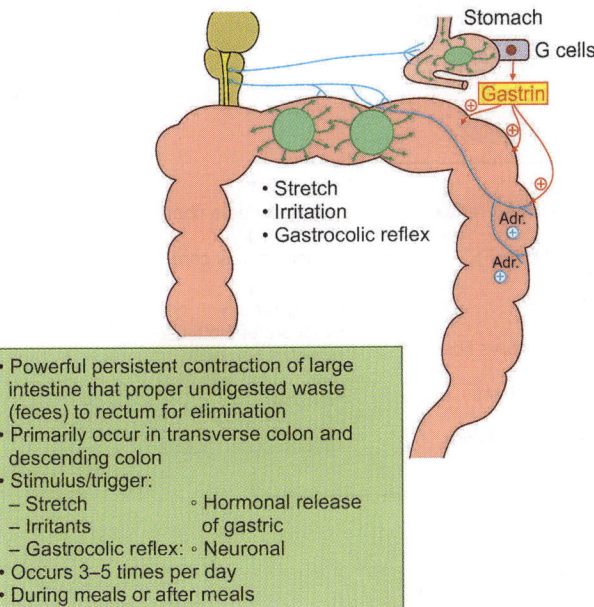

**Fig. 33.4:** Mechanism of mass movements (peristalsis).

- Powerful persistent contraction of large intestine that proper undigested waste (feces) to rectum for elimination
- Primarily occur in transverse colon and descending colon
- Stimulus/trigger:
  – Stretch
  – Irritants
  – Gastrocolic reflex:
  ○ Hormonal release of gastric
  ○ Neuronal
- Occurs 3–5 times per day
- During meals or after meals

After eating, the mass movements are facilitated by *gastrocolic and duodenocolic reflexes*, triggered by stomach and duodenal distension, respectively. These reflexes are likely transmitted via the autonomic nervous system, given their dependence on intact extrinsic autonomic nerves to the colon. Furthermore, irritation within the colon, such as in ulcerative colitis, can incite intense and persistent mass movements.

## DEFECATION

It is the process of expulsion of the fecal matter through the anal canal. As we have learnt above, the large intestine stores the fecal matter until it's the time to defecate. The rectum remains typically devoid of fecal matter due to a weak functional sphincter which is located 20 cm from the anus. There is a sharp angulation at the junction of the sigmoid colon and rectum, further impeding fecal accumulation.

The mass movement pushes the feces into the rectum producing the urge for defecation occurs, characterized by reflex contraction of the rectum and relaxation of the anal sphincters. The continuous dribbling of fecal matter is prevented by tonic constriction of both the internal and external anal sphincters (the external anal sphincter is under voluntary control via the pudendal nerve).

### Defecation Reflexes

Defecation is chiefly initiated by intrinsic and parasympathetic defecation reflexes (**Table 33.1, Flowchart 33.1 and Fig. 33.5**). The intrinsic reflex, mediated by the enteric nervous system in the rectal wall, induces peristaltic waves upon distension of the rectum. The *internal defecation reflex* occurring through the enteric nervous system is weak, hence, it is reinforced by the parasympathetic defecation reflexes, involving the sacral segments of the spinal cord which intensify peristaltic waves and relax the internal anal sphincter, enhancing the process of defecation.

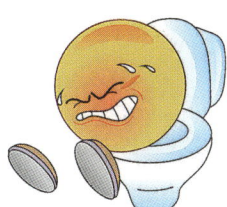

These reflexes, reinforced by actions such as taking a deep breath and contracting abdominal muscles, facilitate fecal expulsion. However, conscious inhibition of these reflexes may lead to severe constipation, emphasizing the importance of allowing natural defecation reflexes to function unimpeded.

- People who too often inhibits their natural reflexes are likely to become constipated
- In newborn or transected spinal cords, there is loss of conscious control of sphincter. Defecation reflex cause automatic emptying of the lower bowel at inconvenient time during the day. This is called *fecal incontinence*.

**Table 33.1:** Defecation reflexes.

|  | **Intrinsic defecation reflex** | **Parasympathetic defecation reflex** |
|---|---|---|
| **Stimulus** | Distension of the rectal wall due to the entry of fecal material | Distension of the rectal wall due to the entry of fecal material |
| **Receptor** | Sensory stretch receptors within the rectal wall | Sensory stretch receptors within the rectal wall |
| **Afferent** | Sensory fibers terminating in myenteric plexus | Pelvic parasympathetic nerves terminating in S2–S4 |
| **Center** | S2–S4 spinal cord segment | S2–S4 spinal cord segment |
| **Efferent** | Motor fibers from myenteric plexus | Pelvic parasympathetic nerves |
| **Effector** | Smooth muscles of the rectum and the internal and external anal sphincters. The external sphincter is inhibited by pudendal nerve and relaxes it | Smooth muscles of the rectum and the internal and external anal sphincters. The external sphincter is inhibited by pudendal nerve and relaxes it |
| **Response** | Peristaltic waves forcing feces toward rectum. Relaxation of internal sphincter | • The smooth muscles of the rectum contract, propelling fecal material toward the anus. Simultaneously, the internal anal sphincter relaxes<br>• Deep breath, closure of the glottis, and contraction of the abdominal wall muscles to force the fecal contents of the colon downward, and simultaneous relaxation of the pelvic floor and pull outward on the anal ring to evaginate the feces |

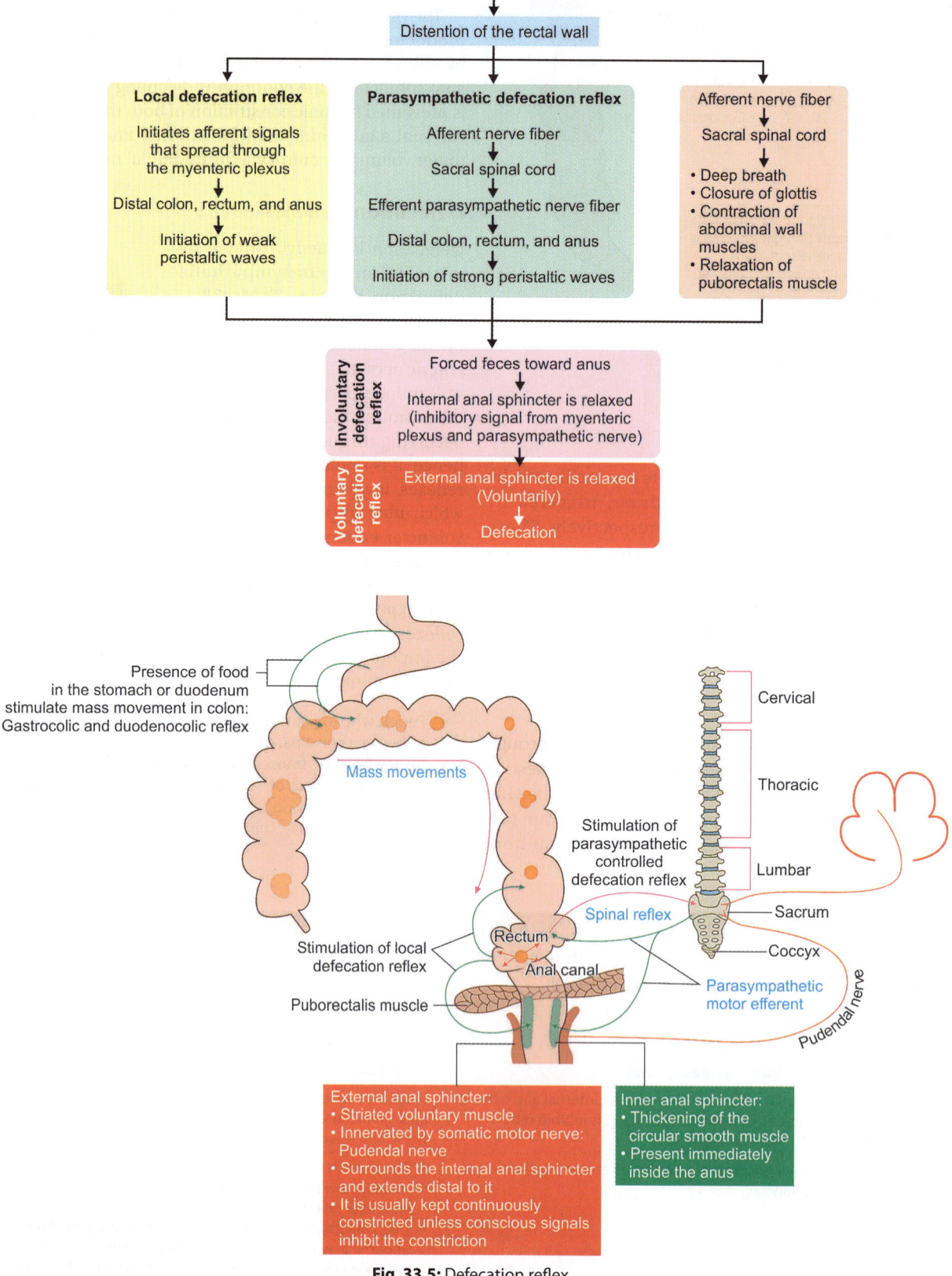

**Flowchart 33.1:** Process of defecation reflex.

**Fig. 33.5:** Defecation reflex.

- **Peritoneointestinal reflex:** Irritation of peritoneum causes strong inhibition of excitatory enteric nerves and intestinal inhibition.
- **Renointestinal reflex:** Kidney irritation causes inhibition of intestinal activity.
- **Vesicointestinal reflex:** Bladder irritation causes inhibition of intestinal activity.

## DIGESTION AND ABSORPTION IN LARGE INTESTINE

Since, the large intestine has no digestive enzymes, the primary function is absorption.

- Around 1500 mL of chyme enters the large intestine through the ileocecal valve, from which the water and electrolytes are absorbed. Only 100 mL of fluid is lost in feces every day.
- The proximal half of colon is called the absorbing colon. It is responsible for most of the absorption in large intestine (distal colon stores the feces and hence called the storage colon).
- Active absorption of $Na^+$ resulting in passive absorption of $Cl^-$
- Aldosterone greatly increases the $Na^+$ absorption.
- Secretion of $HCO_3^-$ by distal colon, in exchange with absorption of $Cl^-$.
- The osmotic gradient created by $Na^+$ and $Cl^-$ results in $H_2O$ absorption.
- Hence, large intestine absorbs around 5–8 L of fluid and electrolyte per day.

### Role of Bacteria in Colon

The commensal bacteria form the normal colonic flora are capable of:

- Digestion of small amount of cellulose
- Formation of vitamin K, vitamin B12, riboflavin and thiamine
- Formation of various gases like methane, $CO_2$, $H_2$ gas responsible for production of flatus.

## COMPOSITION OF FECES

- Water: 70–75%
- Solid matter: 25–30%
    - Dead bacteria (30%)
    - Fat (10–20%)
    - Inorganic matter (10–20%)
    - Protein (2–3%)
    - Undigested roughage (30%)
    - Pigments: Stercobilin and urobilin, responsible for brown color of feces.
    - Odor is produced by bacterial action, produced due to indole, skatole, mercaptans, $H_2S$.

## PHYSIOLOGICAL IMPORTANCE OF DIETARY FIBERS

Dietary fibers are nondigestible carbohydrates found in plant-based foods, including fruits, vegetables, whole grains, nuts, seeds, and legumes. They are classified into soluble and insoluble fibers based on their solubility in water.

- **Digestive health:** Dietary fibers play a crucial role in maintaining digestive health by promoting regular bowel movements and preventing constipation. Insoluble fibers add bulk to stool, which helps to stimulate bowel movements and prevent fecal stagnation. Soluble fibers absorb water in the digestive tract, forming a gel-like substance that softens stool and facilitates its passage through the intestines.
- **Prevention of digestive disorders:** Adequate intake of dietary fibers is associated with a reduced risk of various digestive disorders, including diverticulosis, diverticulitis, hemorrhoids, and colorectal cancer. Fiber-rich diets promote the health of the gastrointestinal tract, prevent inflammation, and support the growth of beneficial gut bacteria.
- **Regulation of blood sugar levels:** Soluble fibers, such as pectins, gums, and mucilages, can help regulate blood sugar levels by slowing down the absorption of glucose from the small intestine. This can help prevent rapid spikes in blood sugar levels after meals, making dietary fibers beneficial for individuals with diabetes or insulin resistance.
- **Management of cholesterol levels:** Soluble fibers have been shown to reduce levels of low-density lipoprotein (LDL) cholesterol, also known as "bad" cholesterol, in the blood. By binding to cholesterol in the digestive tract and promoting its excretion, soluble fibers help lower LDL cholesterol levels, thereby reducing the risk of cardiovascular diseases.
- **Weight management:** Dietary fibers contribute to satiety and fullness, which can help control appetite and reduce calorie intake. Foods high in dietary fibers require more chewing and take longer to digest, leading to a prolonged feeling of satisfaction after meals. This can be beneficial for weight management and preventing overeating.
- **Regulation of gut microbiota:** Dietary fibers serve as prebiotics, providing nourishment for beneficial bacteria in the gut microbiota. By fermenting dietary fibers, gut bacteria produce short-chain fatty acids (SCFAs) that support intestinal health, strengthen the gut barrier, and modulate immune function.

## CLINICAL CORRELATION: LARGE INTESTINAL DISORDERS

### Constipation

It is a common gastrointestinal condition characterized by infrequent bowel movements, difficulty passing stools, or the passage of hard and dry stools. It may also involve a sense of incomplete evacuation or straining during bowel movements.

#### Causes

Several factors can contribute to constipation, including:

- Inadequate fiber intake
- Insufficient fluid intake

- Sedentary lifestyle
- Certain medications (e.g., opioids, anticholinergics)
- Neurological disorders (e.g., Parkinson's disease)
- Hormonal imbalances (e.g., hypothyroidism)
- Structural abnormalities (e.g., colorectal cancer, pelvic floor dysfunction)

### Physiological Basis

Normal bowel movements result from coordinated contractions of the colon and relaxation of the pelvic floor muscles, allowing the passage of stool. This process is regulated by the enteric nervous system, hormones, and reflex pathways. Constipation occurs when there is a disruption in this process, leading to decreased motility, increased water absorption in the colon, or dysfunction in the defecation reflex.

> When colonic motility is slower or if defecation is delayed, the large intestine will absorb more water and constipation may result. On the other hand, if colonic motility is fast due to ingested toxin/pathogen, the large intestine will absorb less water and diarrhea may result.

### Pathophysiology

- **Decreased motility:** Reduced contraction of the colon muscles can slow down the transit of stool through the intestines, leading to increased water absorption and the formation of hard stools.
- **Pelvic floor dysfunction:** Impaired relaxation of the pelvic floor muscles during defecation can result in difficulty expelling stool from the rectum.
- **Delayed transit time:** Prolonged transit time allows for excessive water absorption, resulting in dry and hard stools.
- **Obstruction:** Structural abnormalities or impacted feces can obstruct the passage of stool, leading to symptoms of constipation.

### Clinical Features

- Infrequent bowel movements (fewer than three times per week)
- Difficulty passing stools or straining during bowel movements
- Sensation of incomplete evacuation
- Hard or lumpy stools
- Abdominal discomfort or bloating
- Rectal bleeding or hemorrhoids due to straining

### Treatment

Constipation can significantly impact quality of life and may lead to complications such as fecal impaction, hemorrhoids, or rectal prolapse if left untreated. Management typically involves dietary and lifestyle modifications, increased fluid intake, fiber supplementation, and, in some cases, medications or biofeedback therapy to improve bowel function. Persistent or severe constipation warrants evaluation by a healthcare professional to rule out underlying causes and determine appropriate management strategies.

## Diarrhea

It is a common gastrointestinal condition characterized by frequent, loose, and watery bowel movements. It often accompanies abdominal cramps, urgency, and may be associated with other symptoms such as nausea, vomiting, or fever.

### Causes

- Infections (e.g., viral, bacterial, parasitic)
- Foodborne illnesses (e.g., food poisoning)
- Intestinal disorders (e.g., inflammatory bowel disease, celiac disease)
- Medications (e.g., antibiotics, laxatives)
- Dietary factors (e.g., excessive intake of certain foods or beverages)
- Stress or anxiety (also called as psychological/emotional diarrhea)
- Travel-related factors (e.g., traveler's diarrhea)
- Irritable bowel syndrome (IBS)
- Malabsorption syndromes

### Physiological Basis

Normal bowel function involves the coordinated absorption of water and electrolytes in the intestines, resulting in formed stools. Diarrhea occurs when there is an imbalance in this process, leading to increased secretion of fluids into the intestine, decreased absorption of water, or rapid transit of stool through the intestines.

### Pathophysiology

- **Increased intestinal secretion:** Infections, inflammatory conditions, or certain medications can stimulate the secretion of fluids into the intestine, resulting in watery stools.
- **Decreased absorption:** Conditions that impair the absorption of water and electrolytes, such as malabsorption syndromes or certain medications, can lead to diarrhea.
- **Altered intestinal motility:** Rapid transit of stool through the intestines, as seen in conditions like irritable bowel syndrome (IBS), can result in diarrhea.
- **Disruption of intestinal microbiota:** Imbalance in the gut microbiota, often due to infections or antibiotics, can lead to diarrhea by affecting normal intestinal function.

In cholera; cholera toxin directly stimulates excessive secretion of electrolytes and fluid from the crypts of Lieberkühn in the distal ileum and colon. There can be secretion of around 10 to 12 L/day. Although the colon can reabsorb a maximum of only 6 to 8 L/day; yet there is a loss of fluid and electrolytes can be so severe that can prove to be fatal.

**Psychogenic diarrhea:** Most people are familiar with the diarrhea that accompanies periods of nervous tension, such as during examination time or when a soldier is about to go into battle. This type of diarrhea, called psychogenic emotional diarrhea, is caused by excessive stimulation of the parasympathetic nervous system, which greatly excites both (1) motility and (2) excess secretion of mucus in the distal colon. These two effects added together can cause marked diarrhea.

## Clinical Features

- Frequent, loose, and watery bowel movements
- Abdominal cramps or pain
- Urgency to have bowel movements
- Bloating or gas
- Nausea and vomiting
- Fever, if diarrhea is due to an infection
- Dehydration, especially in severe or prolonged cases, characterized by thirst, dry mouth, decreased urine output, and lethargy.

## Treatment

Treatment of diarrhea depends on the underlying cause and severity of symptoms. Management may include dietary modifications, fluid and electrolyte replacement, medications (e.g., antimotility agents, antibiotics for infections), and addressing any underlying conditions contributing to diarrhea. Severe or persistent diarrhea should be evaluated by a healthcare professional to determine the appropriate treatment and to prevent complications such as dehydration.

# Irritable Bowel Syndrome

Irritable Bowel Syndrome (IBS) is a common gastrointestinal disorder characterized by a group of symptoms including abdominal pain or discomfort, changes in bowel habits, and bloating. IBS is considered a functional disorder, meaning there is no structural abnormality or specific biomarker associated with the condition.

## Causes

The exact cause of IBS is not fully understood, but it is believed to involve a combination of factors including:
- Abnormalities in the gut-brain axis, which controls intestinal motility and sensation
- Altered gastrointestinal motility or sensitivity
- Abnormalities in the gut microbiota
- Inflammation or immune system dysfunction
- Psychological factors such as stress, anxiety, or depression

## Physiological Basis

In individuals with IBS, there may be abnormalities in the way the brain and gut communicate, leading to alterations in intestinal motility, sensation, and secretion. These abnormalities can result in symptoms such as abdominal pain, diarrhea, constipation, or a mix of both.

## Pathophysiology

- **Altered motility:** Some individuals with IBS may experience abnormal contractions of the intestinal muscles, leading to changes in bowel habits such as diarrhea or constipation.
- **Visceral hypersensitivity:** Heightened sensitivity to normal bowel sensations, such as gas or stool movement, can lead to abdominal discomfort or pain.
- **Gut microbiota dysbiosis:** Imbalance in the gut microbiota, characterized by changes in the composition or function of gut bacteria, may play a role in the development of IBS symptoms.
- **Brain-gut axis dysfunction:** Abnormalities in the bidirectional communication between the brain and the gut may contribute to symptoms of IBS, particularly in response to stress or emotional triggers.

## Clinical Features

- Abdominal pain or discomfort, often relieved by bowel movements
- Changes in bowel habits, including diarrhea, constipation, or alternating between the two
- Bloating or abdominal distention
- Excessive gas or flatulence
- Urgency to have bowel movements
- Feeling of incomplete evacuation after bowel movements
- Symptoms may fluctuate over time, with periods of exacerbation and remission

## Treatment

Management of IBS typically involves a combination of dietary modifications, lifestyle changes, stress management techniques, and medications to alleviate symptoms and improve quality of life. Treatment is often tailored to individual symptoms and may require a multidisciplinary approach involving healthcare professionals such as gastroenterologists, dietitians, and mental health specialists.

# Hirschsprung Disease

It is a congenital condition characterized by the *absence of ganglion cells in the distal portion of the colon*, resulting in functional obstruction and impaired peristalsis. This leads to difficulty passing stool and chronic constipation.

## Causes

Hirschsprung disease occurs due to a failure of neural crest cells to migrate properly during fetal development, resulting in a lack of ganglion cells in the affected segment of the colon. The exact cause of this migration failure is not fully understood, but genetic factors are believed to play a role.

## Physiological Basis

Ganglion cells are essential for coordinating smooth muscle contractions in the colon, allowing for the coordinated movement of stool through the intestines. In Hirschsprung disease, the absence of ganglion cells leads to uncoordinated contractions and functional obstruction, resulting in symptoms of constipation.

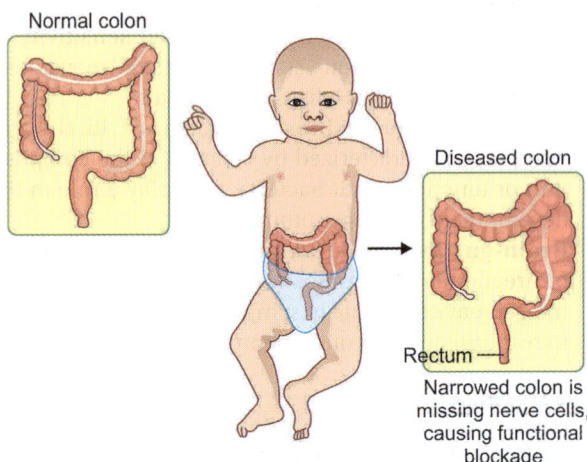

## Pathophysiology

In Hirschsprung disease, the affected segment of the colon lacks the normal nerve cells (ganglion cells) that control peristalsis. As a result, the affected portion of the colon remains contracted and unable to relax, leading to functional obstruction and accumulation of stool proximal to the affected area. This causes dilation of the colon and chronic constipation.

## Clinical Features

- Failure to pass meconium (first stool) within 48 hours of birth
- Chronic constipation, often with abdominal distention
- Failure to thrive or poor weight gain
- Foul-smelling, ribbon-like stools
- Abdominal pain or bloating
- Vomiting, particularly in severe cases
- Delayed growth and development

## Treatment

Management of Hirschsprung disease typically involves surgical removal of the affected portion of the colon (pull-through procedure) to restore normal bowel function. In some cases, temporary measures such as colostomy may be necessary before definitive surgery. Early diagnosis and intervention are important to prevent complications and improve long-term outcomes for individuals with Hirschsprung disease.

For case-based learning, refer to author's early clinical exposure for clinical physiology.

### SUMMARY

- *Taenia coli* and haustra are characteristics to the colon. The mucous membrane of the colon lacks villi.
- The ileocecal valve prevents backflow of contents from colon.
- The role of the ascending colon is to absorb the remaining water and other key nutrients from the indigestible material, solidifying it to form stool.
- Most of absorption occurs in the proximal half of the colon. The descending colon stores feces that will eventually be emptied into the rectum.
- The mucus produced by Lieberkühn's crypts can be utilized as an adhesive medium to hold feces together. When there are emotional problems, the activation of the parasympathetic nervous system increases its secretion. Its production is elevated when a certain segment of the large intestine is severely irritated.
- Three movements of large intestine are mixing movements (haustration), propulsive movements (mass movements), and antiperistalsis. Mass movements is mainly initiated by gastrocolic reflex.
- Defecation is a spinal reflex which is influenced by higher center. Distension of the rectum causes reflex contraction of the internal anal sphincter and the desire to defecate. After toilet training, defecation can be delayed until a convenient time via voluntary contraction of the external anal sphincter. Person with spinal cord injury have fetal incontinence.
- Reflexes initiated just by contracting abdominal muscles are almost never as effective as those arise naturally.
- When a patient has spinal cord damage, intentional mass reflexes like stroking or squeezing the thighs can cause them to defecate.
- The gut-brain axis facilitates communication between the gut flora and the brain. It affects our thinking processes, emotions, and behavior.

### LET US SEE, HOW MUCH YOU HAVE LEARNT?

 *Review Questions*

#### Long/Short Answer Questions

Q1. Describe defecation reflex with the help of a well labeled diagram/flowchart.

Q2. Describe the movements of large intestine.

Q3. What is the physiological role of gut microflora.

## Explain Why? (Reasoning Questions)

**Q1.** The infants defecate immediately after meals.

**Q2.** There is diarrhea while the patient is on antibiotics.

 *Critical Thinking Case-Based Questions*

**Q1.** A 32-year-old female patient has complaints of recurrent abdominal pain, bloating, and distention. She has loose stools occurring approximately 2 to 3 times per day. The pain worsens just before defecation and reliefs after passing stool.

Answer the following questions on the basis of the given case scenario:
a. What is your provisional diagnosis?
b. Explain the mechanism of defecation?
c. Why infants defecate after meals?

 *Multiple Choice Questions*

**Q1.** In defecation reflex, the short reflex stimulates:
a. Myenteric reflex
b. Submucosal reflex
c. Vagus
d. Pelvic plexus

**Q2.** Ring like contractions (about 2.5 cm) of the circular muscle divide the colon into pockets:
a. Propulsive movements
b. Mixing contractions (Haustration)
c. Antiperistalsis movement
d. Rush movement

**Q3.** Which of the following is NOT a function of large intestine:
a. Absorption of water and electrolytes
b. Formation of feces
c. Producing and absorbing vitamins
d. Absorption of digestive products of nutrients

**Q4.** Which part of the gastrointestinal tract has the main function of reabsorption of water and electrolytes?
a. Sigmoid colon
b. Rectum
c. Proximal part of colon
d. Distal part of colon

**Q5.** Which of the following is involved in the mechanism of defecation?
a. Reduced intrarectal pressure
b. Contraction of internal anal sphincter
c. Relaxation of external anal sphincter
d. Increased activity of colonic bacteria

**Q6.** An 80-year-old female patient presents to the clinic with constipation and increased straining in bowel movements. Which of the following nerves innervated the pelvic muscles most involved in this process?
a. Sciatic nerve
b. Obturator nerve
c. Pudendal nerve
d. Superior gluteal nerve

**Q7.** Following a natural disaster in a town, there is an outbreak of cholera in the refugees. The affected individuals display severe diarrheal symptoms because of which of the following changes in intestinal transport?
a. Increased $Na^+$–$K^+$ cotransport in the small intestine
b. Reduced $K^+$ absorption in the crypts of Lieberkühn
c. Increased $Na^+$ absorption in the small intestine
d. Increased $Cl^-$ secretion into the intestinal lumen

**ANSWERS**

**1.** a    **2.** b    **3.** d    **4.** c    **5.** c    **6.** c    **7.** d

# Physiology of Digestion and Absorption of Nutrients

**34**
CHAPTER

> **COMPETENCY ADDRESSED**
> PY4.4: Describe the physiology of digestion and absorption of nutrients.

> **LEARNING OBJECTIVES**
> At the end of this chapter, the learner should be able to:
> - Describe the digestion of all the nutrients in different parts of the digestive system.
> - Describe the absorption of digested nutrients from the small intestine.
> - Describe the physiology of malabsorption syndrome.

## DIGESTION AND ABSORPTION

**Digestion** is a process of breaking down of large insoluble nutrients in ingested food into substances that can be absorbed by the gastrointestinal tract. The food contains three macronutrients: carbohydrates, proteins, and fats. These nutrients are broken down both mechanically and enzymatically (chemical digestion) before being absorbed. Chemical digestion is dependent upon the secretions of enzymes from the oral cavity, stomach, small intestine, and accessory digestive organs such as the pancreas, liver, and gallbladder. Polysaccharides and disaccharides are broken down into monosaccharides, proteins into amino acids, and lipids into glycerol and triglycerides. In this chapter, we will learn about the digestion of each nutrient separately in different parts of digestive system.

## Absorption of Nutrients

The digestive system absorbs around 8–9 L of fluid everyday, out of which most of the fluid (about 8–8.5 L) is absorbed in the small intestine and 1.5 L is passed to the large intestine. Hence, the small intestine has some special feature for the absorption of fluids and other nutrients, which are discussed in detail here. The small intestine has enormous absorptive area which is made by:
- The extensive mucosal folding called *valvulae conniventes (Folds of Kerckring)* **(Fig. 34.1)**. This increases the mucosal surface area by 3-folds. They are well developed in duodenum and jejunum.
- The epithelial cells of small intestine have numerous finger like projections called the *villi*. These project about 1 mm from surface of mucosa. These villi are dense in upper small intestine and less dense in distal small intestine. These villi increase the surface area by another 10-folds. The intestinal villi has a typical organization of the blood vessels, as shown in the **Figure 34.2**.

In the center, there is a central lacteal, a lymph vessel, for the absorption of lymph. It is surrounded by the blood vessels, in a typical counter current system.
- Each intestinal villi further have the brush border, consisting of 1,000 microvilli of 1 μm length and 0.1 μm in diameter. The brush border increases the absorptive surface area by 20-folds. The microvilli of brush border have multiple actin filaments that contract rhythmically to cause continuous movement of microvilli.

Hence, all the three, folds of Kerckring, Intestinal villi and brush border, increases the absorptive area by

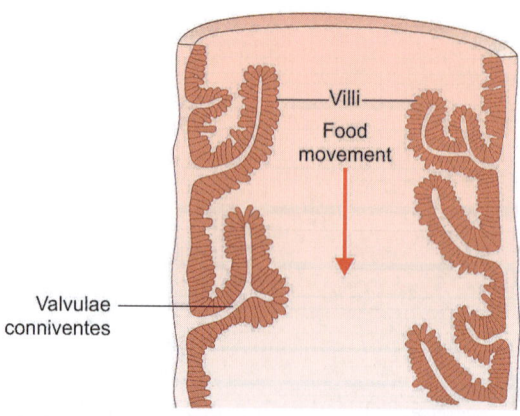

**Fig. 34.1:** Extensive mucosal foldings (Folds of Kerckring).

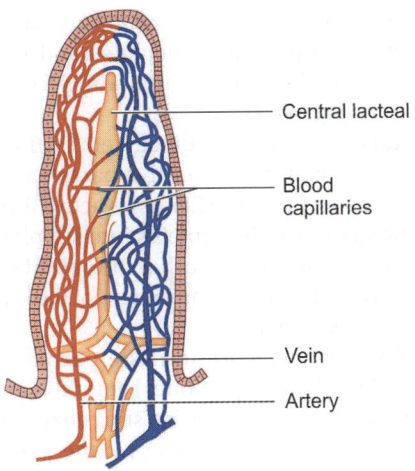

Fig. 34.2: Organization of blood vessels in villi.

1,000-folds making the total small intestinal area of 250 m². As a point not to miss, *the gastric mucosa does not have any such absorptive villi and hence has a poor absorptive surface*. However, alcohol and aspirin are absorbed from stomach.

## DIGESTION AND ABSORPTION OF CARBOHYDRATES

Carbohydrates are an essential part of any nutrient-rich diet. The digestion of carbohydrates/starch occurs in mouth and small intestine **(Fig. 34.3)**. There is no digestion of carbohydrate in stomach.

- **In oral cavity:** The digestion of carbohydrate begins in the mouth, where salivary amylase starts the breakdown. The salivary amylase is weak and is responsible for digestion of 20–40% of starch. The salivary amylase is inactivated in the stomach due to its acidic contents.

- **In duodenum:** The pancreatic amylase secreted in the pancreatic juice is responsible for digesting 50–80% of starch. It is the similar to salivary amylase but is more potent than it.

After break down, the starch (polysaccharides) forms the maltose (disaccharide), ingested disaccharides (lactose and fructose) are further digested to form monosaccharides, as shown in the **Figure 34.6**. These monosaccharides are absorbed into the bloodstream by secondary active transport. Undigested carbohydrates like cellulose are not absorbed in the gut but remain in the colon and undergo fermentation by colonic bacteria. In a healthy adult's diet, the amount of carbohydrates consumed should be between 200 and 300 g, or 45–65% of total calories. Carbohydrates have about 4 kcal/g (17 kJ/g).

## Absorption of Carbohydrates (Fig. 34.4)

The most abundant form of monosaccharide, absorbed in Glucose (80%). The remaining 20% is absorbed as galactose and fructose. These monosaccharides are absorbed by the secondary active transport along with Na⁺ through the *Sodium-glucose cotransporter-1 (SGLT-1)*. Hence the *Na⁺ is required for the absorption of glucose* though the apical membrane. Once inside the epithelial cell, the the glucose is transported through the *Glucose transporter (GLUT)* across the basolateral membrane. The undigested disaccharides (maltose, lactose, etc.) in the small intestine are absorbed into the epithelial cells and digested inside the epithelial cells by the specific enzymes like maltase and lactase to form the monosaccharides, which are further absorbed through the basolateral membrane. The figure below shows the mechanism of absorption of glucose. The glucose and galactose are transported by SGLT

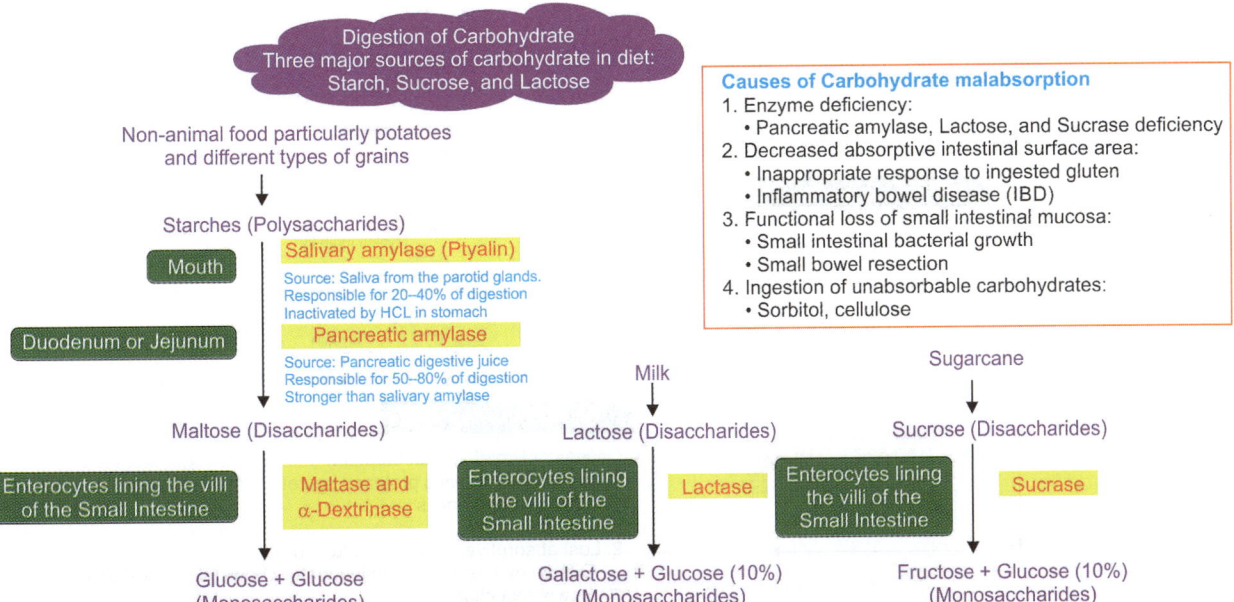

Fig. 34.3: Summary of digestion and absorption of carbohydrates and their malabsorption causes.

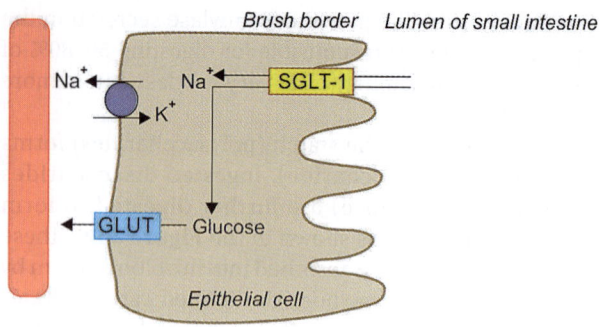

**Fig. 34.4:** Absorption of carbohydrates from intestinal lumen.

and GLUT-2. Fructose is not absorbed through SGLT-1 rather it is transported by facilitated diffusion. Inside the cell, it is converted into glucose and absorbed through the basolateral membrane by GLUT-2 while, unbroken fructose is absorbed through GLUT-5.

## DIGESTION AND ABSORPTION OF PROTEINS

Dietary proteins are composed of chemically long sequences of amino acids bound together by peptide bonds. Chemical digestion of proteins begins in the stomach and continues in the jejunum. The stomach, pancreas, and intestinal brush border release peptidases, which are the enzymes responsible for breaking down of polypeptides into tripeptides, dipeptides, and amino acids. Protein is absorbed in the jejunum and proximal ileum after digestion **(Fig. 34.5)**.

- **In stomach:** As we have discussed in the previous chapter, the stomach secretes the inactive Pepsinogen, which is activated by the HCl into its active form Pepsin. Pepsin breaks down the Proteins into simpler Peptides and Peptones. Pepsin also has the ability to digest collagen, which is a major constituent of the intercellular connective tissue of meats.
- **In duodenum and jejunum:** The partially digested proteins (Peptides and peptones) enter the duodenum, where the pancreatic protein digesting enzymes (trypsin, Chymotrypsin) further break down the peptones and peptides into polypeptides.

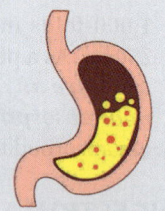

People with low pepsin digest meat less effectively. Collagen is one of the primary constituents of the intracellular connective tissue in meat. Breaking down collagen fibers is a prerequisite for the digestive enzymes to reach and break down other animal proteins. Pepsin is the enzyme that digests collagen. The meat is therefore not as thoroughly digested when pepsin levels are low since the digestive enzymes are unable to completely penetrate it.

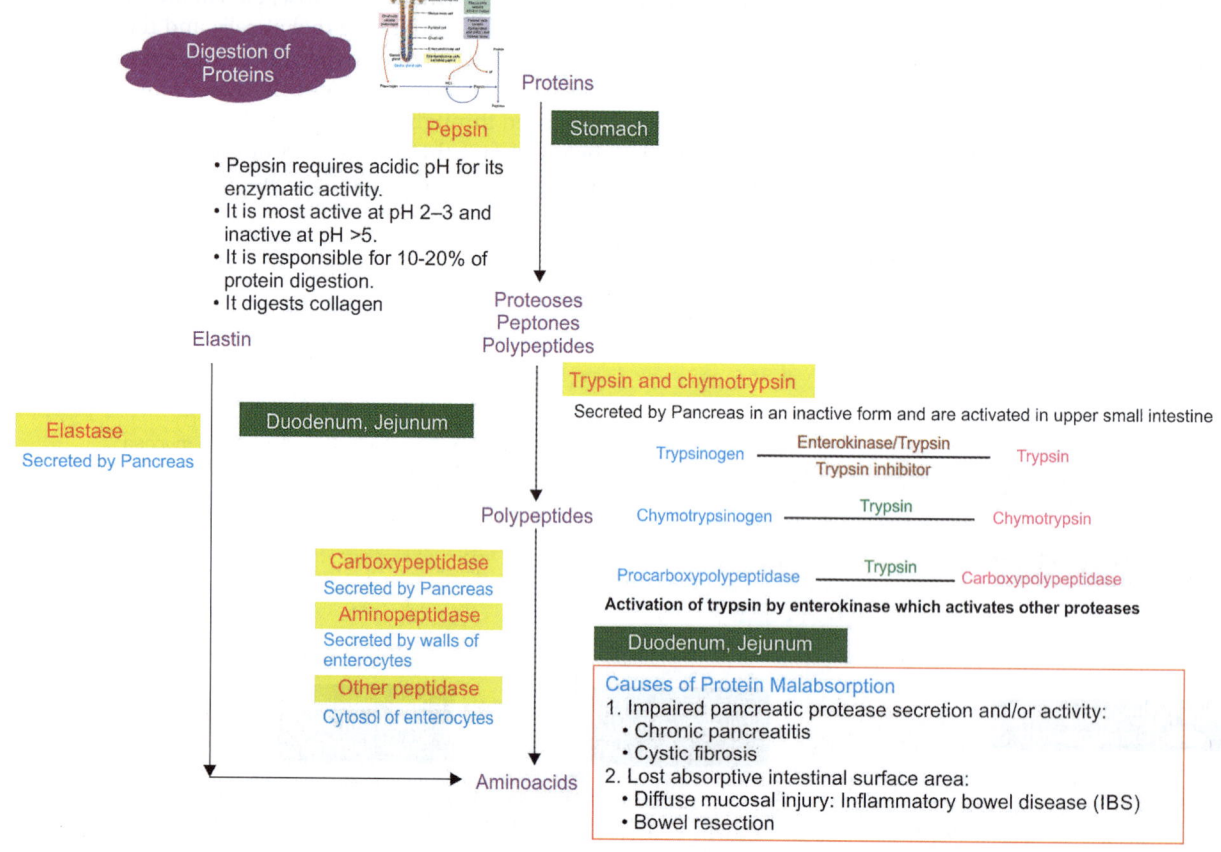

**Fig. 34.5:** Summary of digestion and absorption of proteins and their malabsorption causes.

The undigested polypeptides are further digested by peptidases to form amino acids.

## Absorption of Proteins

Most of the proteins are absorbed as tripeptides, dipeptides and amino acids. Like the glucose absorption,
- They are also absorbed by the *sodium linked cotransport* from the luminal brush border.
- A few amino acids are absorbed by the facilitated diffusion by *specific carrier proteins*.

## DIGESTION AND ABSORPTION OF FATS

The lipids in the diet are mostly neutral fats, abundant in triglycerides containing a glycerol molecule and three fatty acid chains. However, phospholipids and cholesterol esters are also considered as fats **(Fig. 34.6)**.
- **Digestion in oral cavity:** The digestion of fats due to lingual lipase secreted by lingual glands and ingested with saliva. It is responsible for 10% digestion of fats in the stomach.
- **Digestion in small intestine:** In small intestine, the fat digestion begins with emulsification of fats by the bile salts. The steps of fact digestion are described below:

1. **Emulsification of fats:** The first step in fat digestion is to physically break the fat globules into small sizes, allowing water-soluble digestive enzymes to act effectively. This process, known as *emulsification*, involves agitation in the stomach and is predominantly facilitated in the duodenum under the influence of bile, a secretion from the liver containing bile salts and lecithin.

2. **Role of bile:** Bile salts and lecithin in bile play a crucial role in emulsification by reducing the interfacial tension of fat globules. They dissolve in the surface layer of fat globules, with their polar portions projecting outward, thereby making the fat more soluble in surrounding watery fluids.

3. **Function of emulsification:** Emulsification decreases the interfacial tension of fat, facilitating fragmentation of fat globules upon agitation in the small intestine. This *detergent-like action of bile salts and lecithin* enables the fat globules to be readily broken up into tiny particles, increasing the total surface area of fats manyfold.

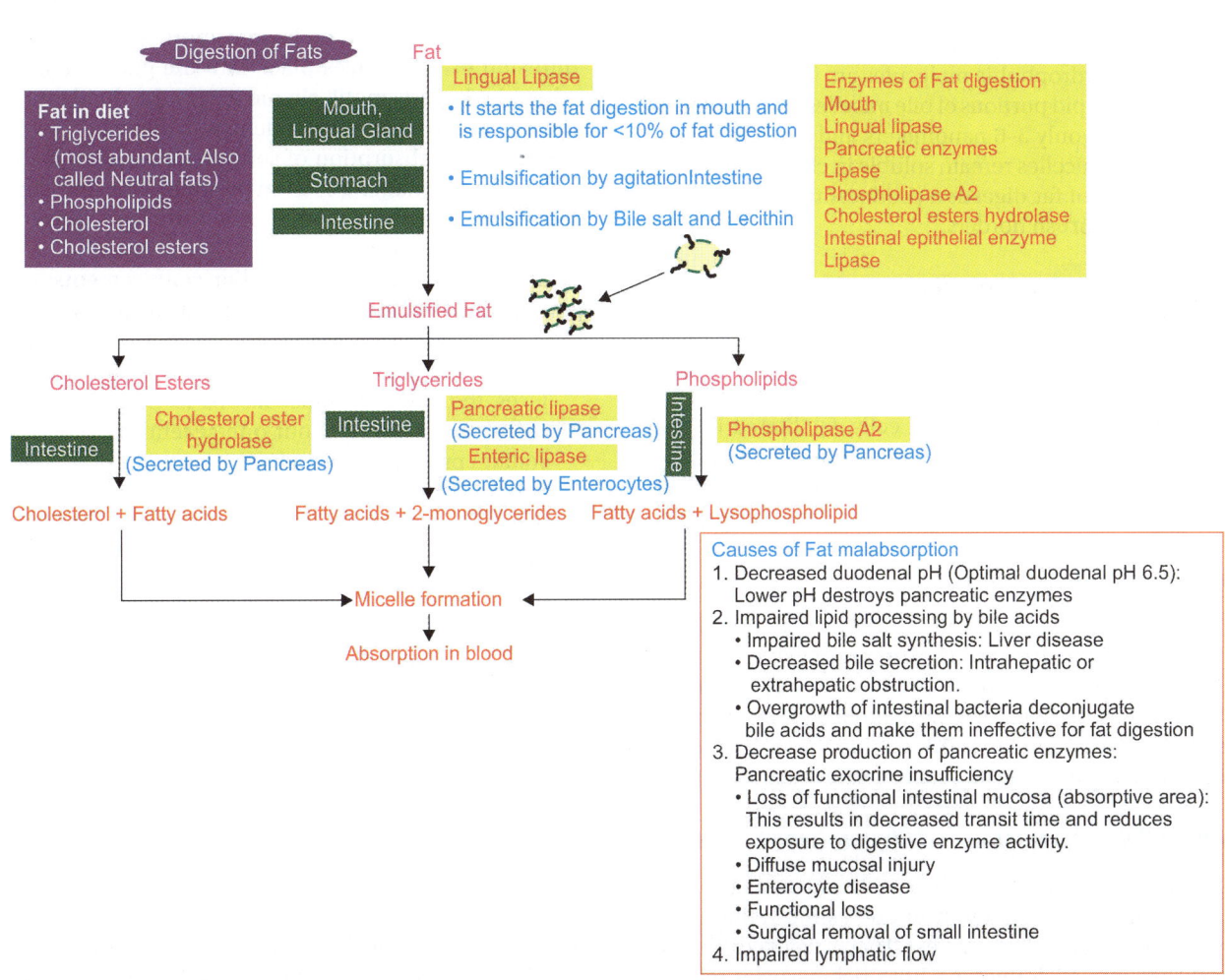

**Fig. 34.6:** Summary of digestion and absorption of fats/lipids and their malabsorption causes.

4. ***Digestion of triglycerides:*** Triglycerides, the main constituents of dietary fats, are primarily digested by pancreatic lipase into free fatty acids and 2-monoglycerides. Pancreatic lipase, abundant in pancreatic juice, is essential for triglyceride digestion, while enteric lipase in enterocytes plays a supplementary role.
5. ***Formation of micelles:*** Bile salts form *micelles* in the presence of water, which encompass the fat digestion, including monoglycerides and free fatty acids. These micelles serve as a transport medium, carrying the relatively insoluble end products of fat digestion to the brush borders of intestinal epithelial cells for absorption into the bloodstream.
6. ***Digestion of cholesterol esters and phospholipids:*** Cholesterol esters and phospholipids in the diet are hydrolyzed by pancreatic lipases—cholesterol ester hydrolase and phospholipase A2, respectively. Bile salt micelles also aid in the absorption of free cholesterol and phospholipids by ferrying them to the intestinal epithelial cells for absorption into the bloodstream.

## Absorption of Fats

When fats are digested into monoglycerides and free fatty acids, these hydrophobic molecules are initially dissolved in the central lipid portions of bile micelles. With molecular dimensions of only 3–6 nanometers and a highly charged exterior, bile micelles remain soluble in chyme, facilitating the transport of fat digestion products to the surfaces of intestinal cell brush borders.

### *Micelle-assisted Absorption*

At the brush border, monoglycerides and fatty acids diffuse out of the micelles and penetrate into the recesses among the microvilli of intestinal epithelial cells. The lipids then enter the interior of epithelial cells, facilitated by their solubility in the epithelial cell membrane. Bile micelles, remaining in the chyme, continue to function repeatedly, aiding in the absorption of additional fat digestion products.

### *Importance of Micelles*

The ferrying function of bile micelles is crucial for fat absorption. In their presence, approximately 97% of fat is absorbed, while their absence reduces absorption to only 40–50%. Micelles enhance the solubility and transport of fatty acids and monoglycerides across the epithelial cell membrane, optimizing fat absorption efficiency.

### *Intracellular Processing and Chylomicron Formation*

Once inside epithelial cells, fatty acids and monoglycerides are utilized by the smooth endoplasmic reticulum to synthesize new triglycerides. These triglycerides are packaged into chylomicrons, lipid-rich particles released from the base of epithelial cells. Chylomicrons enter the lymphatic system, eventually reaching the bloodstream to transport dietary fats to various tissues throughout the body.

## Direct Absorption of Short-chain Fatty Acids into Portal Blood

Unlike long-chain fatty acids, which are predominantly absorbed as triglycerides via the lymphatic system, short- and medium-chain fatty acids, such as those found in butterfat, exhibit a unique absorption pathway. These fatty acids are directly absorbed into the portal blood, bypassing conversion into triglycerides and lymphatic transport. It provides an efficient pathway for their delivery to the liver, where they can be utilized for energy production or undergo metabolic processes.

## ABSORPTION OF WATER, MINERALS AND TRACE ELEMENTS (SODIUM, CHLORIDE, CALCIUM, BICARBONATE) (FIGS. 34.7 AND 34.8)

- **Absorption of water:** Iso-osmotic water absorption takes place by the diffusion. The water from the liquid chyme is absorbed through the intestinal mucosa into the blood. If a person consumes the hyperosmotic solutions, the diffusion of water takes place into the gut. Similarly, when the hyperosmotic chyme enters the duodenum, the water moves into the duodenum to dilute it.
- **Sodium:** The absorption of sodium in the intestine is crucial for maintaining sodium balance in the body and facilitating the absorption of other nutrients, such as sugars and amino acids.
  - **Sodium balance and absorption requirements:** The intestines secrete approximately 20–30 g of sodium each day, while the average person consumes 5–8 g of sodium daily. To prevent net loss of sodium into the feces, the intestines must absorb 25–35 g of sodium daily, representing about one-seventh of the total sodium present in the body.
  
    Sodium absorption is also facilitated by cotransport with $Cl^-$, sodium-glucose cotransporter, sodium-amino acid cotransporters, and the sodium-hydrogen exchanger. The active transport of sodium ions into the interstitial fluid and paracellular spaces is powered by the sodium-potassium $Na^+$–$K^+$ ATPase pump located on the basolateral membrane of epithelial cells. This pump maintains the sodium concentration gradient necessary for efficient sodium absorption and facilitates secondary active absorption of glucose and amino acids.
    
    The $Na^+$ when depleted are restored by aldosterone. Aldosterone increases the activity of $Na^+$–$K^+$ ATPase pump and hence results in increased absorption of $Na^+$.
- **Chloride:** The chloride ions are absorbed through the brush border membrane mainly by diffusion, following the electrical gradient by the movement of $Na^+$. The $Cl^-$

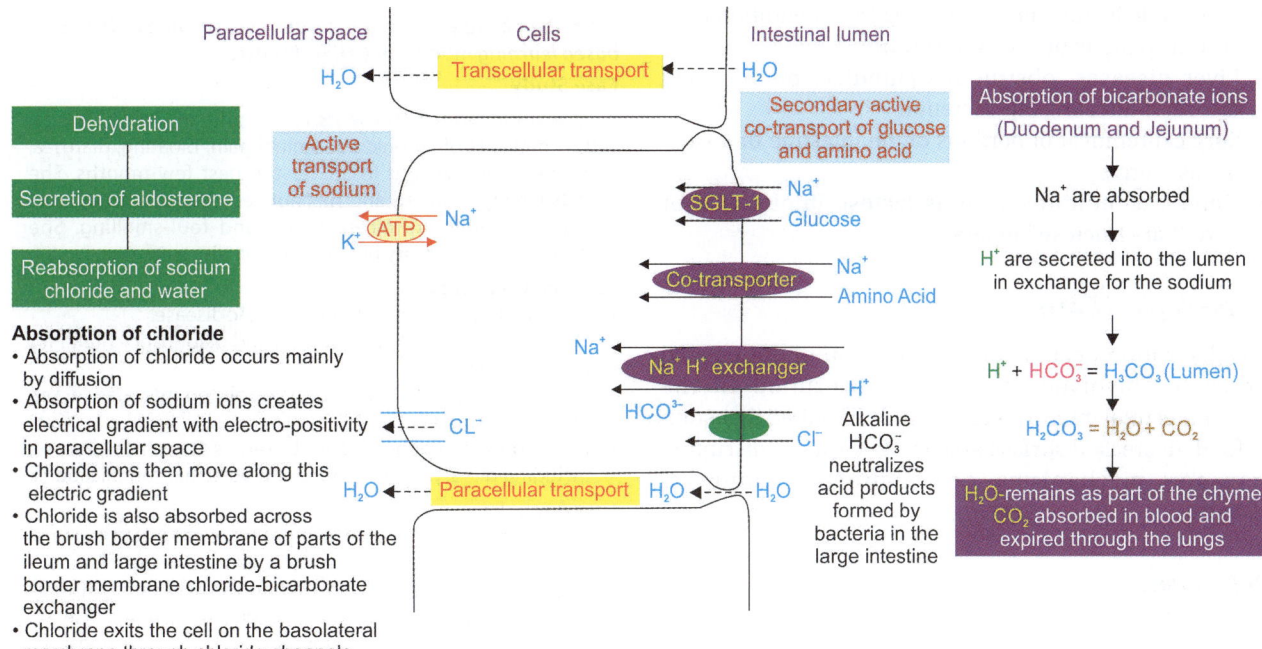

**Fig. 34.7:** Summary of digestion and absorption of minerals from GIT.

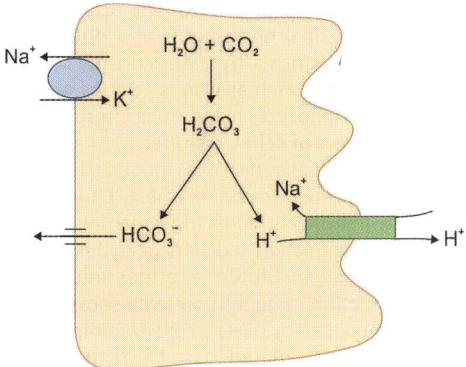

**Fig. 34.8:** Exchange of ions in intestinal cells.

crosses the basolateral membrane through the chloride channels.
- **Calcium:** Calcium ions are actively absorbed into the blood from the duodenum. Parathyroid hormone and Vitamin D increases the intestinal absorption of calcium. Parathyroid hormone activates vitamin D and activated vitamin D in turn enhances calcium absorption.
- **Bicarbonate:** The bicarbonate ions are absorbed from the small intestine as shown in the **Figure 34.8**.

## DISORDERS OF DIGESTION AND ABSORPTION

### Cholera (Flowchart 34.1)

Cholera and other diarrheal bacteria stimulate more secretions than the body can reabsorb, resulting in the increased loss of water in the stools.

### Malabsorption Syndrome

Malabsorption syndrome refers to a group of disorders characterized by impaired absorption of nutrients from the gastrointestinal tract, leading to deficiencies in essential vitamins, minerals, and macronutrients.

### Causes of Malabsorption Syndrome Include

- Intestinal disorders such as celiac disease, Crohn's disease, and intestinal infections.

**Flowchart 34.1:** Cholera infection resulting in dehydration.

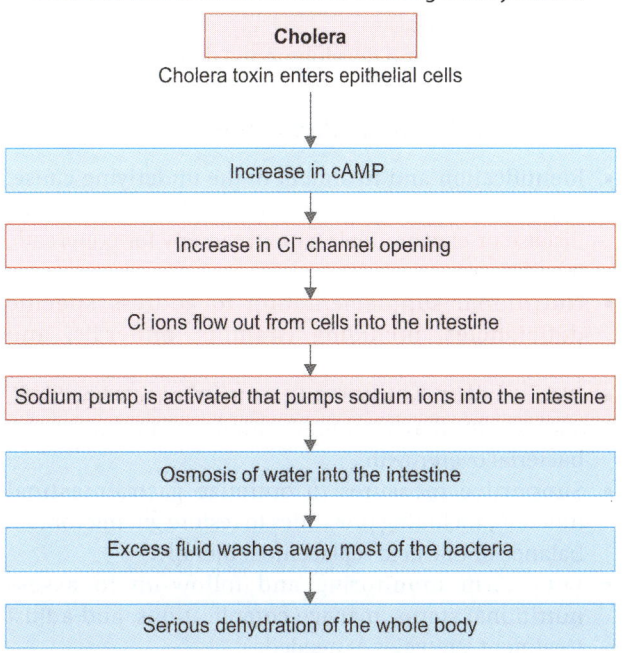

- Pancreatic insufficiency, resulting from conditions like chronic pancreatitis or cystic fibrosis.
- Liver diseases, obstructive jaundice, or bile acid disorders affecting bile secretion.
- Surgical removal of portions of the intestine or gastric bypass surgery.
- Genetic conditions such as lactose intolerance or hereditary fructose intolerance.

## Physiological Basis

Malabsorption occurs due to disruption of the normal processes involved in nutrient absorption in the gastrointestinal tract. This can include impaired digestion of food, decreased surface area for absorption, disrupted transport mechanisms, or compromised mucosal integrity.

## Pathogenesis

The pathogenesis of malabsorption syndrome varies depending on the underlying cause. It may involve inflammation and damage to the intestinal mucosa, enzyme deficiencies affecting digestion, disruption of bile secretion and micelle formation, or alterations in the gut microbiota.

## Clinical Features

- Chronic diarrhea, steatorrhea (fatty stools), and weight loss.
- Abdominal bloating, cramping, and flatulence.
- Nutrient deficiencies leading to symptoms such as anemia, vitamin deficiencies (e.g., vitamin D, B12), and osteoporosis.
- Fat-soluble vitamin deficiencies causing night blindness or easy bruising.
- Growth failure and developmental delays in children.

## Physiological Basis of Management

- Identification and treatment of the underlying cause, such as dietary modifications for conditions like celiac disease or enzyme replacement therapy for pancreatic insufficiency.
- Nutritional supplementation to address specific deficiencies, including vitamins, minerals, and macronutrients.
- Pharmacological interventions to manage symptoms, such as antidiarrheal medications or antibiotics for bacterial overgrowth.
- Supportive measures to optimize gastrointestinal function, including probiotics to restore gut microbiota balance or bile acid replacement therapy.
- Long-term monitoring and follow-up to assess nutritional status, manage complications, and adjust treatment strategies as needed.

*From the above discussed disorder, lets see one of the case-based learning module of Celiac disease:*

### Case Study

A 35-year-old woman, presents to her primary care physician with complaints of chronic abdominal pain, bloating, diarrhea, and unintended weight loss over the past few months. She reports feeling fatigued and has noticed changes in her stool consistency, which is often greasy and foul-smelling. She mentions a family history of autoimmune diseases.

*Learning Objectives:*
- Describe the pathophysiology of celiac disease.
- Describe the clinical presentation and diagnostic criteria for celiac disease.
- Describe the physiological basis of gluten intolerance and intestinal damage.
- Prescribe the management strategies for celiac disease, including dietary modifications and potential complications.

*Case Analysis:*
- **Clinical presentation:** Her symptoms of chronic abdominal pain, bloating, diarrhea, and unintended weight loss are suggestive of malabsorption syndrome. Her family history of autoimmune diseases raises suspicion for celiac disease, an immune-mediated disorder triggered by gluten ingestion.
- **Diagnostic evaluation:** The patient undergoes serological testing for celiac disease, including immunoglobulin A anti-tissue transglutaminase antibodies (IgA-TTG) and anti-endomysial antibodies (EMA-IgA). She also undergoes an upper gastrointestinal endoscopy with duodenal biopsy to confirm the diagnosis by assessing for characteristic histological changes, such as villous atrophy and increased intraepithelial lymphocytes in the small intestinal mucosa.
- **Physiological basis of celiac disease:**
    - *Gluten sensitivity:* Celiac disease is triggered by the ingestion of gluten, a protein found in wheat, barley, and rye. In susceptible individuals, gluten triggers an immune response, leading to inflammation and damage to the small intestine.
    - *Intestinal damage:* Gluten peptides initiate an autoimmune reaction in genetically predisposed individuals, primarily mediated by CD4+ T cells. This immune response targets tissue transglutaminase (TG2) and results in the production of autoantibodies, leading to villous atrophy, crypt hyperplasia, and intestinal inflammation.
    - *Malabsorption:* Villous atrophy reduces the absorptive surface area of the small intestine, impairing nutrient absorption. This leads to malabsorption of essential nutrients, including vitamins, minerals, and macronutrients, resulting in symptoms such as diarrhea, weight loss, and nutritional deficiencies.
- **Management strategies:**
    - *Gluten-free diet:* The cornerstone of celiac disease management is strict adherence to a gluten-free diet, eliminating all sources of gluten from the diet, including wheat, barley, and rye. She is referred to a registered dietitian for education and guidance on gluten-free meal planning.
    - *Nutritional support:* She may require nutritional supplementation to address existing deficiencies, such as iron, calcium, vitamin D, and B vitamins. Close monitoring of nutritional status and regular follow-up with healthcare providers are essential.
    - *Follow-up and monitoring:* She will undergo regular follow-up evaluations to assess response to treatment, monitor symptoms, and evaluate for potential complications, such as refractory celiac disease or associated autoimmune conditions.

## SUMMARY

- Digestion is a process that involves both chemical and mechanical breakdown of food and nutrients. Chemical digestion is accomplished by the hydrolytic activity of enzymes.
- The passage of nutrients through the GI tract's lining and into circulation is known as absorption.
- Nutrient absorption occurs via four mechanisms: Primary active transport, secondary active transport, facilitated diffusion, and passive diffusion.
- The small intestine is the site of chemical digestion and absorption.
- Nutrients absorption occurs via four mechanisms: Primary active transport, secondary active transport, facilitated diffusion, and passive diffusion.
- Food and saliva combine to start the process of digestion in the mouth. But the main site for digestion of fat and carbohydrate is small intestine, though minor digestion takes place by the action of salivary enzymes. The protein digestion takes place in the stomach and duodenum.
- The failure to absorb the nutrients due to any cause, results in malabsorption syndrome
- Dietary fibers are essential components of a healthy diet, supporting digestive health, blood sugar control, cholesterol management, weight management, and overall well-being. Incorporating a variety of fiber-rich foods into the diet is key to reaping the benefits of these important nutrients.

## LET US SEE, HOW MUCH YOU HAVE LEARNT?

### Review Questions

#### Long/Short Answer Questions

Q1. Describe the digestion and absorption of carbohydrates.
Q2. Describe the digestion and absorption of fats.
Q3. Describe the digestion and absorption of Proteins.
Q4. Write a short note on Lactose intolerance.
Q5. Write a short note on pancreatic insufficiency.
Q6. Write a short note on Malabsorption syndrome.
Q7. Describe the role of pancreatic enzymes in digestion.

#### Explain Why? (Reasoning Questions)

Q1. Why does absence of HCl or pepsin causes edema in a patient?
Q2. Why the consumption of dairy products cause diarrhea in some patients?
Q3. Why the consumption of wheat causes bloating, diarrhea and irritable bowel syndrome in some patients?
Q4. What will happen if 100 cm of terminal ileum is resected? (Malabsorption of Bile Salts, Vitamin B12 Deficiency, Malabsorption of Fat-soluble Vitamins, Diarrhea and Malabsorption, Bacterial Overgrowth).

### Critical Thinking Case-Based Questions

Q1. A 12-years old boy presents to the clinic with loose stools, flatulence, and bloating approximately 1 hour after drinking cow's milk. His symptoms have developed over the past month. Physical examination reveals a mildly distended abdomen in an otherwise well-developed child. A fecal occult blood test is negative and stool pH is low. Answer the following questions on the basis of the given case scenario.
   a. What is your provisional diagnosis? Support with the evidence (hint: lactose intolerance).
   b. Explain the pathophysiology of the diagnosed disease.
   c. What is the preventive measures to be taken?

### Multiple Choice Questions

Q1. Which of the following does not produce digestive enzymes:
   a. Acini of pancreas
   b. Liver
   c. Stomach
   d. Duodenum

Q2. Which statement about nutrient absorption by the enterocyte is true?
   a. Carbohydrates are absorbed as disaccharides
   b. Fats are absorbed as fatty acid and monoglycerides
   c. Amino acids move across the plasma membrane only by diffusion
   d. Fructose is absorbed by facilitated transport

Q3. Jejunum is the major site for absorption of the following, *except*:
   a. Amino Acid
   b. Fatty acid
   c. Water
   d. Bile salts

Q4. Which of the following vitamins is commonly deficient in celiac disease due to malabsorption?
   a. Vitamin B12
   b. Vitamin D
   c. Vitamin K
   d. Vitamin E

Q5. A 72-years-old woman presents to the emergency department with worsening abdominal pain. His vitals are normal. Physical examination reveals bilateral lower extremity edema and tenderness to palpation in the epigastric region. A biopsy of the gastric mucosa reveals defective oxyntic glands. Which of the following findings can be expected in this patient?

a. Excessive gastrin production resulting in overstimulation of parietal cells
b. A defect in mucous production
c. Interrupted propulsive movements and hindered mechanical digestion
d. Undigested and unabsorbed protein

**ANSWERS**

1. d   2. d   3. d   4. a   5. d

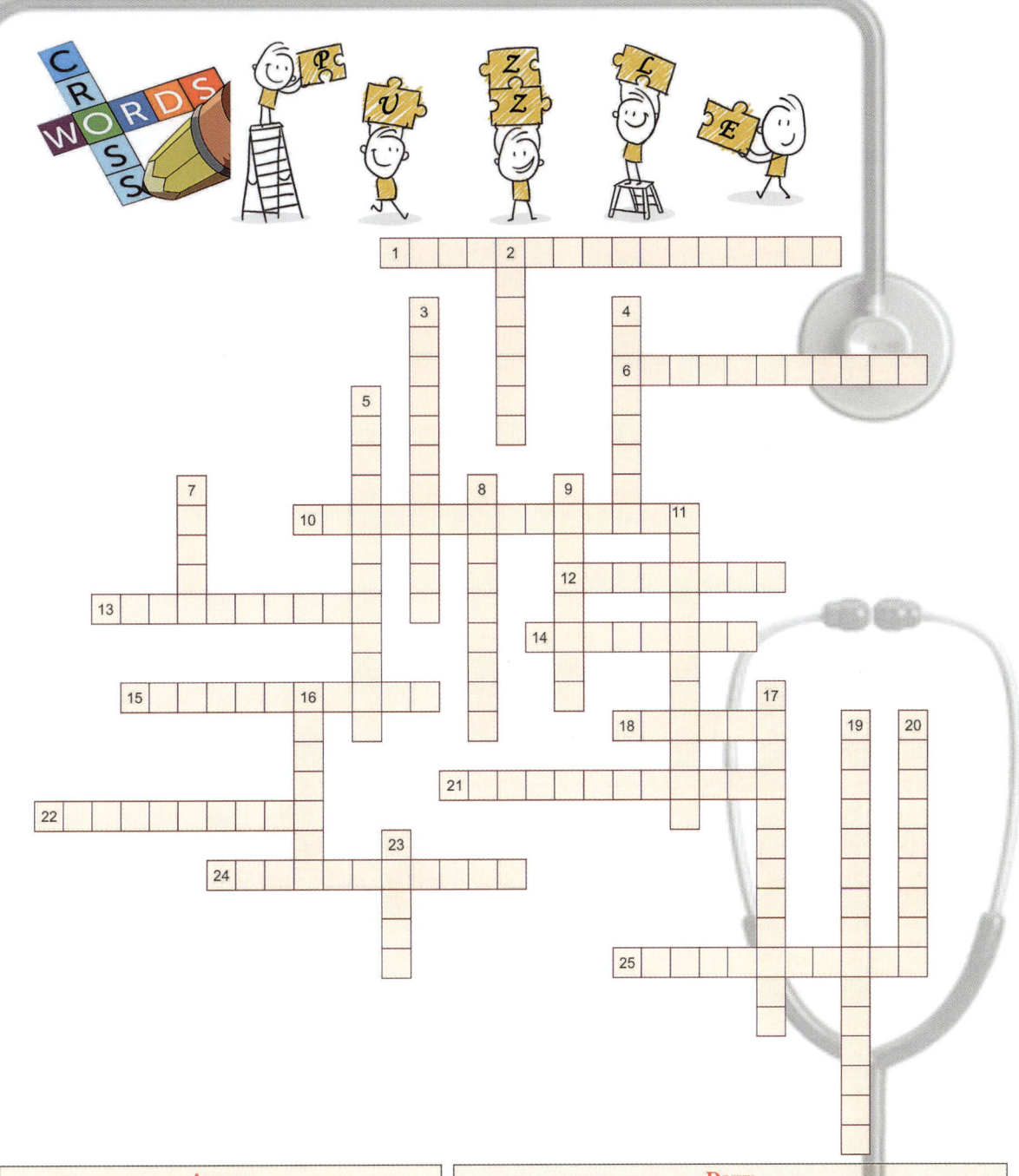

### Across
1. Type of proteases that works within the protein chain
6. Substances that enhance the bile secretion
10. Presence of stones in the gallbladder or bile ducts
12. C-shaped shortest part of small intestine
13. Process of expulsion of the fecal matter through the anal canal
14. This hormone inhibits the gastric emptying
15. By this process amino acids releases ammonia
18. Outermost covering of the stomach, closely attached with visceral peritoneum
21. Large phagocytic cells of the liver
22. Term for excessive salivation
24. Type of epithelial cells covering villi and secrete water, electrolytes
25. Functional units of the liver

### Down
2. Glands in the stomach which secrete pepsinogen and hydrochloric acid
3. One of the solid constituents of bile composition
4. These are formed by bile salts in presence of water and helps in fat digestion
5. Storage of excess glucose in form of glycogen in liver
7. Semi liquid food in stomach after churning
8. Secreted by enterochromaffin like cells in pyloric glands
9. Appearance of achalasia cardia on barium swallow study
11. Clinical feature of fat malabsorption due to pancreatic insufficiency
16. Enzyme that starts digestion in mouth
17. Pouches of dilation due to large circular constrictions of large intestine
19. GI hormone causes contraction of the gallbladder
20. Superficial inflammation of gastric mucosa
23. These constitute 90% of structure of pancreas

# SECTION 5

# CARDIOVASCULAR SYSTEM

## Section Outline

**Chapter 35:** Functional Anatomy of Heart
**Chapter 36:** Cardiac Cycle
**Chapter 37:** Basics of Electrocardiography
**Chapter 38:** Physiological Basis of Abnormalities of Electrocardiogram
**Chapter 39:** Circulation and Hemodynamics
**Chapter 40:** Cardiovascular Regulatory Mechanisms
**Chapter 41:** Heart Rate and Regulation
**Chapter 42:** Cardiac Output
**Chapter 43:** Venous Return and its Regulation
**Chapter 44:** Blood Pressure and its Regulation
**Chapter 45:** Coronary Circulation
**Chapter 46:** Blood Flow in Systemic Circulation: Arterial, Capillary, Venous and Lymphatic Circulation
**Chapter 47:** Physiological Basis of Cardiovascular Diseases

# Functional Anatomy of Heart

**35 CHAPTER**

> **COMPETENCY ADDRESSED**
>
> **PY5.1:** Describe the functional anatomy of heart including chambers, sounds; and Pacemaker tissue and conducting system.

> **LEARNING OBJECTIVES**
>
> **At the end of this chapter, the learner should be able to:**
> - Describe the external and internal anatomy of the heart, including its location within the thoracic cavity, surface features, and the four chambers.
> - Enumerate the major structures associated with each cardiac chamber, such as valves and major blood vessels and describe their function.

The human heart is a remarkable organ responsible for **pumping blood throughout the body**, delivering essential nutrients and oxygen while removing waste products. Understanding the functional anatomy of the heart is paramount for medical students, particularly those studying physiology, as it forms the basis for comprehending the complex processes involved in cardiovascular function. By grasping the intricate structures and mechanisms of the heart, students can gain insights into normal cardiac physiology and pathophysiology, enabling them to diagnose and manage various cardiovascular disorders effectively. Moreover, a sound understanding of cardiac anatomy lays the foundation for future studies in cardiology, surgery, and other medical specialties, empowering students to become competent healthcare professionals capable of delivering high-quality patient care.

## EXTERNAL ANATOMY

The external anatomy of the heart encompasses its positioning within the thoracic cavity and surface features that are visible externally.

- **Location and orientation:** The heart is situated within the mediastinum, a central compartment of the thoracic cavity located between the lungs. It rests upon the diaphragm and is tilted slightly to the left, with its apex pointing downwards and to the left.
- **Surface features (Fig. 35.1):**
  - *Apex:* The apex of the heart is the blunt, conical tip located at the inferior aspect. It is formed primarily by the left ventricle and is palpable at the fifth intercostal space along the midclavicular line.
  - *Base:* The base of the heart is the broad, superior aspect where major blood vessels enter and exit. It is primarily formed by the atria and is located opposite the apex.
  - *Borders:* The borders of the heart are formed by the interactions of its various chambers and structures. They include the superior (base), inferior (apex), right, and left borders, each demarcating the external extent of the heart from different angles.

## INTERNAL ANATOMY

### Atria and Ventricles

**Atria:** The atria are thin-walled chambers located at the top of the heart. They receive blood returning to the heart from the body (via the superior and inferior vena cava into the right atrium) and from the lungs (via the pulmonary veins into the left atrium). The atria contract to push blood into the ventricles during ventricular diastole, contributing to the filling of the ventricles.

Both the atria are separated by the inter atrial septum, which contains several structures, including the fossa

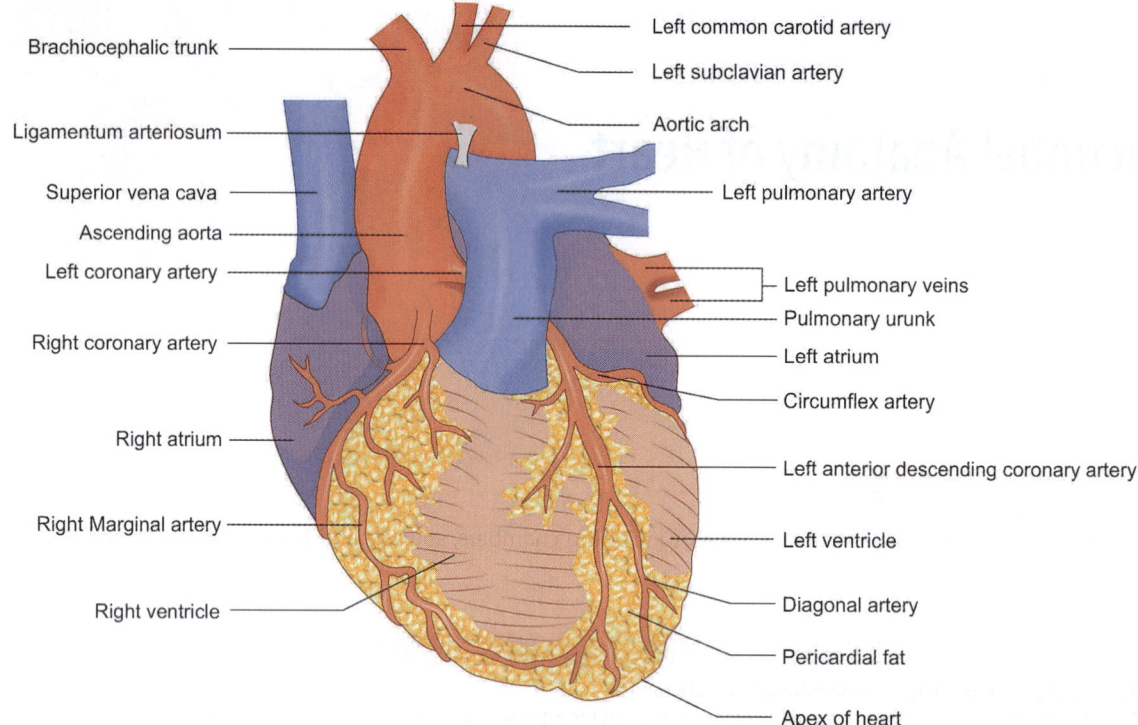

**Fig. 35.1:** Surface features of heart anatomy.

ovalis, a depression that marks the location of the fetal foramen ovale, which allowed blood to bypass the lungs before birth. If this foramen persists after birth, causes the atrial septal defect (ASD).

**Ventricles:** The ventricles are the two lower chambers of the heart and are responsible for pumping blood out of the heart. The right ventricle pumps deoxygenated blood to the lungs for oxygenation, while the left ventricle pumps oxygenated blood to the rest of the body. The walls of the ventricles are much thicker and more muscular than those of the atria, allowing them to generate the force necessary to propel blood through the circulatory system.

The interventricular septum is the thick wall that separates the right ventricle from the left ventricle. It is largely composed of myocardium and plays a crucial role in preventing the mixing of oxygenated and deoxygenated blood between the two ventricles.

The atrial and the ventricular muscles act as separate syncytial masses having gap junctions; but there are no such intercellular junctions between atria and ventricles. The only means of communication between these two muscle masses is through the conducting system, discussed later.

## Walls of Heart (Fig. 35.2)

- **Pericardium:** It is the outermost covering of the heart. It is of two types: Fibrous pericardium and Serous pericardium. The space between these two layers is filled with fluid called the pericardial fluid.
- **Myocardium:** It forms the main muscle bulk of heart. It is the specialized cardiac muscle.
- **Endocardium:** It is the innermost glistening lining of heart. It continues as endothelium of great vessels (pulmonary trunk and aorta).

## Heart Valves

The atria communicates with the ventricles through the *atrioventricular valve (AVV)* and ventricles push the blood forward through the *semilunar valves (SLV)*. Depending on the location, there are four valves: two AV valves and two semilunar valves (**Fig. 35.3** and **Table 35.1**).

### Atrioventricular Valves

- **Tricuspid valve:** The tricuspid valve is located between the right atrium and the right ventricle. It consists of three cusps (flaps) and prevents the backflow of blood from the right ventricle into the right atrium during ventricular systole.
- **Mitral valve (bicuspid valve):** The mitral valve is situated between the left atrium and the left ventricle. It consists of two cusps and prevents the backflow of blood from the left ventricle into the left atrium during ventricular systole.

### Semilunar Valve

- **Pulmonary valve:** The pulmonary valve is positioned at the entrance of the pulmonary trunk from the right ventricle. It consists of three semilunar cusps and prevents the backflow of blood from the pulmonary trunk into the right ventricle during ventricular diastole.

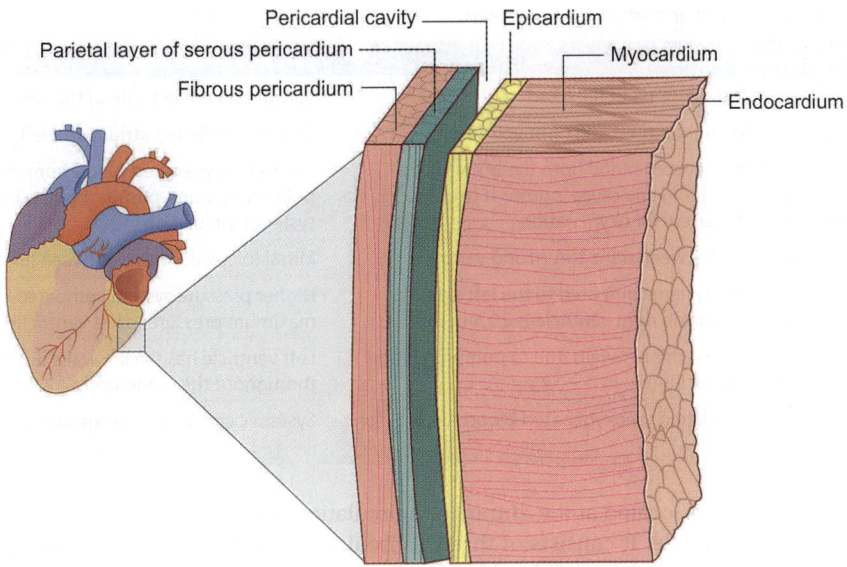

**Fig. 35.2:** Layers of the heart and pericardium.

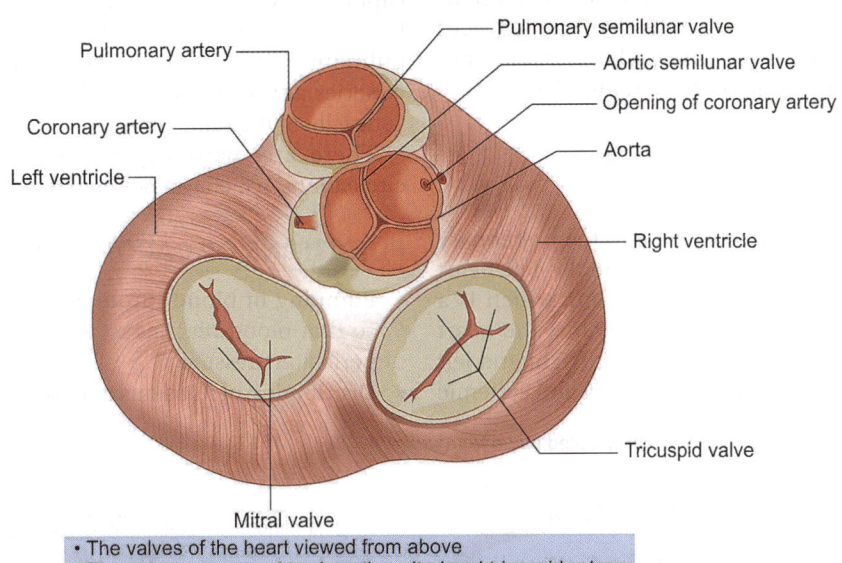

- The valves of the heart viewed from above
- The atria are removed to show the mitral and tricuspid valves

**Fig. 35.3:** Valves of heart.

**Table 35.1:** Differences between atrioventricular (AV) and semilunar valves.

| Aspect | Atrioventricular valves | Semilunar valves |
| --- | --- | --- |
| Location | Between the atria and ventricles | Between the ventricles and great arteries |
| Structure | Consist of tricuspid valve and mitral valve | Consist of pulmonary valve and aortic valve |
| Leaflets | Typically have three leaflets or two leaflets. These are *thin and flexible* | Consist of three pocket-like cusps. These are *thick and fleshy* as they have to with stand higher pressures in the ventricles. |
| Mechanism | Connected to papillary muscles via chordae tendineae | Free-floating, supported by the sinuses of Valsalva |
| Function | Prevents backflow of blood from ventricles to atria during ventricular contraction | Prevents backflow of blood from arteries to ventricles during ventricular relaxation |
| Opening/closing | Open during ventricular diastole, closed during ventricular systole. | Open during ventricular systole, closed during ventricular diastole |
| Heart sounds | Its closure sets in the vibrations in the blood and results in first heart sound *(S1)* | Its closure sets in the vibrations in the blood and results in second heart sound *(S2)* |
| Abnormal heart sounds (murmurs) | The AV regurgitation produces the murmur during systole (systolic murmur) The AV stenosis produces the murmur during diastole (diastolic murmur) | The SLV regurgitation produces the murmur during diastole (diastolic murmur) The SLV stenosis produces the murmur during systole (systolic murmur) |

**Table 35.2:** Differences between right and left side of the heart.

| Aspect | Right side of the heart | Left side of the heart |
|---|---|---|
| Location | Located on the right side of the heart | Located on the left side of the heart |
| Chambers | Consists of the right atrium and right ventricle | Consists of the left atrium and left ventricle |
| Blood flow | Receives deoxygenated blood from the body via the superior and inferior vena cavae, pumps it to the lungs via the pulmonary artery for oxygenation | Receives oxygenated blood from the lungs via the pulmonary veins, pumps it to the body via the aorta for systemic circulation |
| Valves | Tricuspid valve between right atrium and ventricle | Mitral (bicuspid) valve between left atrium and ventricle |
| Pressure | Lower pressure system compared to the left side. The maximum pressure in right ventricle is 25 mm Hg | Higher pressure system compared to the right side. The maximum pressure in left ventricle is 120 mm Hg |
| Thickness of walls | Right ventricle has thinner walls due to pumping blood only to the nearby lungs | Left ventricle has thicker walls due to pumping blood throughout the entire body |
| Function | Pulmonary circulation (deoxygenated blood to lungs for oxygenation) | Systemic circulation (oxygenated blood to body tissues) |

- **Aortic valve:** The aortic valve is located at the entrance of the aorta from the left ventricle. It consists of three semilunar cusps and prevents the backflow of blood from the aorta into the left ventricle during ventricular diastole.

It is interesting to point out that the right and left sides of heart do not communicate with each other and have some differences that are tabulated in **Table 35.2**.

## Pulmonary and Systemic Circulation (Figs. 35.4 and 35.5)

The right side of heart pumps blood into the pulmonary circulation, a low pressure system, while the left heart pumps the blood into systemic circulation, which is a high pressure system. Hence, we can say that the heart consists of two pumps connected in series (right and left halves); which are connected by pulmonary and systemic circulation. However, there are parallel circuits in systemic circulation which provides same composition and arterial pressure. These parallel circulatory systems are different capillary beds like splanchnic circulation, muscle blood flow, renal circulation, etc. But it must be noted that the pulmonary and systemic circulations are connected in series and same amount of blood is pumped by both ventricles at the same time.

There are many other differences in both these circulations, which can be seen in the **Table 35.3**.

## FUNCTIONS OF CARDIOVASCULAR SYSTEM

- Pumping of blood through various circulatory beds so that blood reaches to all the parts with sufficient perfusion pressure
- Distribution of nutrients and oxygen to all body cells

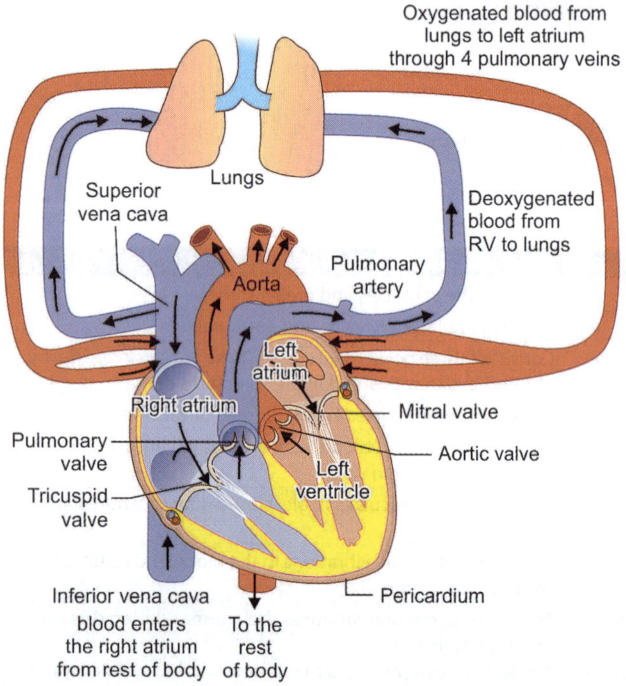

**Fig. 35.4:** Blood flow through the heart.

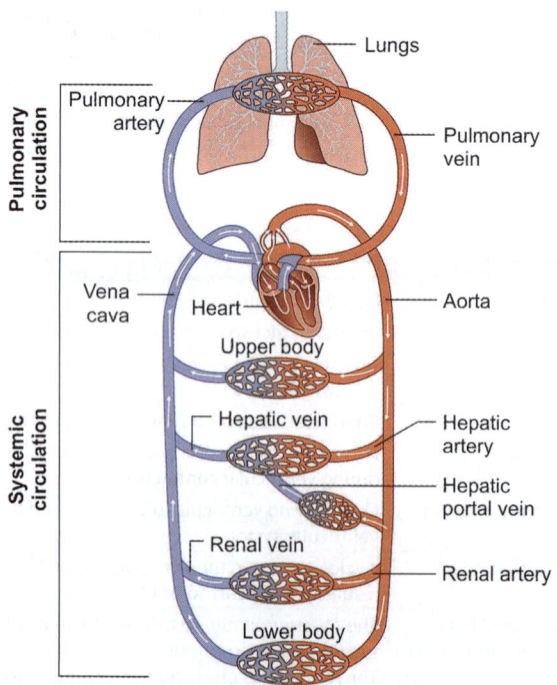

**Fig. 35.5:** Pulmonary circulation and systemic circulation.

- Collection of waste products and $CO_2$ from all body cells to excretory system
- Thermoregulation
- Distribution of hormones to the target tissues
- Delivery of antibodies, platelets and leucocytes to aid body defense mechanisms

**Table 35.3:** Pulmonary circulation versus systemic circulation.

| Aspect | Pulmonary circulation | Systemic circulation |
| --- | --- | --- |
| Function | Transports deoxygenated blood from the heart to the lungs for oxygenation, and returns oxygenated blood back to the heart | Transports oxygenated blood from the heart to the body tissues and returns deoxygenated blood back to the heart |
| Starting point | Begins at the right ventricle, where deoxygenated blood is pumped out of the heart through the pulmonary artery | Begins at the left ventricle, where oxygenated blood is pumped out of the heart through the aorta |
| Ending point | Ends at the left atrium, where oxygenated blood returns to the heart through the pulmonary veins | Ends at the right atrium, where deoxygenated blood returns to the heart through the superior and inferior vena cavae |
| Vessels involved | Involves the pulmonary artery, pulmonary capillaries in the lungs, and pulmonary veins | Involves the aorta, systemic arteries, systemic capillaries in various body tissues, and systemic veins |
| Gas exchange | Facilitates the exchange of carbon dioxide for oxygen in the lungs | Facilitates the exchange of oxygen for carbon dioxide in the body tissues |
| Pressure | Generally lower pressure system compared to systemic circulation:<br>• Systolic pressure: 25 mm Hg<br>• Diastolic pressure: 8 mm Hg | Generally higher pressure system compared to pulmonary circulation:<br>• Systolic pressure: 120 mm Hg<br>• Diastolic pressure: 80 mm Hg |
| Distance traveled | Short distance traveled from heart to lungs and back | Longer distance traveled from heart to body tissues and back |
| Blood oxygenation | Deoxygenated blood becomes oxygenated in the lungs | Oxygenated blood becomes deoxygenated in the body tissues |

## SUMMARY

- The cardiovascular system is composed of two main subunits: the heart and the vascular (circulatory system).
- The heart is a hollow muscular organ located in the mediastinum. Its main function is to pump blood.
- The right heart is connected to the left heart through the pulmonary circulation while the left is connected to right heart via systemic circulation. Both these pumps are connected in series.
- There are two atria and two ventricles, separated by the interatrial and interventricular septum respectively.
- The atria open into respective ventricles though the atrioventricular valves. While the ventricles open into great arteries though the semilunar valves.
- The wall of heart has three main layers: pericardium, myocardium and endocardium.

## LET US SEE, HOW MUCH YOU HAVE LEARNT?

###  Review Questions

**Q1.** Enumerate the functions of cardiovascular system.
**Q2.** Differentiate between:
  a. AV valves and SL valves
  b. Low pressure and high pressure heart
  c. Systemic and pulmonary circulation.

### Multiple Choice Questions

**Q1.** What is the location of the heart within the thoracic cavity?
  a. Left side, beneath the diaphragm
  b. Right side, near the liver
  c. Central, between the lungs, slightly to the left
  d. Upper chest, above the sternum

**Q2.** Which of the following accurately describes the surface features of the heart?
  a. Smooth and uniform texture
  b. Rough and irregular appearance
  c. Divided into four lobes
  d. Marked by grooves called sulci

**Q3.** How many chambers does the human heart have?
  a. Two
  b. Three
  c. Four
  d. Five

**Q4.** Which chamber of the heart receives deoxygenated blood from the body?
  a. Right atrium
  b. Left atrium
  c. Right ventricle
  d. Left ventricle

Q5. What is the function of the valves associated with the cardiac chambers?
   a. To regulate blood pressure
   b. To produce blood cells
   c. To prevent backflow of blood
   d. To synthesize hormones

Q6. Which valve separates the right atrium from the right ventricle?
   a. Mitral valve
   b. Aortic valve
   c. Tricuspid valve
   d. Pulmonary valve

Q7. Blood is pumped from the right ventricle to the:
   a. Lungs
   b. Brain
   c. Liver
   d. Kidneys

Q8. Which blood vessel carries deoxygenated blood from the heart to the lungs?
   a. Aorta
   b. Pulmonary artery
   c. Pulmonary vein
   d. Superior vena cava

Q9. The major artery that carries oxygenated blood away from the heart is the:
   a. Pulmonary artery
   b. Aorta
   c. Pulmonary vein
   d. Inferior vena cava

Q10. Which chamber of the heart pumps oxygenated blood to the body?
   a. Right atrium
   b. Left atrium
   c. Right ventricle
   d. Left ventricle

Q11. Which valve separates the left atrium from the left ventricle?
   a. Mitral valve
   b. Aortic valve
   c. Tricuspid valve
   d. Pulmonary valve

Q12. What is the primary function of the atria in the heart?
   a. To pump blood to the body and lungs
   b. To receive blood from the body and lungs
   c. To regulate blood pressure
   d. To filter waste products from the blood

Q13. The heart is supplied with oxygenated blood by the:
   a. Coronary arteries
   b. Pulmonary veins
   c. Coronary sinus
   d. Aortic arch

Q14. Which chamber of the heart has the thickest muscular wall?
   a. Right atrium
   b. Left atrium
   c. Right ventricle
   d. Left ventricle

**ANSWERS**

1 c   2. a   3. c   4. a   5. c   6. c   7. a   8. b   9. b   10. d   11. a   12. b   13. b   14. d

# Cardiac Cycle

**36 CHAPTER**

### COMPETENCY ADDRESSED
**PY5.3:** Discuss the events occurring during the cardiac cycle.

### LEARNING OBJECTIVES
At the end of this chapter, the learner should be able to:
- Define cardiac cycle.
- Describe the phases of cardiac cycle.
- Describe the correlation of various events like ECG, JVP and phonocardiography with different phases of cardiac cycle.

## DEFINITION

It is defined as sequence of events occurring in the heart between two heart beats.

## CARDIAC CYCLE TIME

It is the time required for one complete cardiac cycle. At heart rate (HR) of 75 bpm, CCT is 60/75 = 0.8 seconds

*The cardiac cycle time (CCT) is inversely proportional to heart rate.* Hence, for a HR of 75 beats per minute, CCT is 0.8 seconds. Since, it primarily describes the mechanical events in the cardiac cycle, it describes the various events happening in atria and ventricles during systole and diastole. The atria and ventricles remain in diastole for much longer duration, than it does in systole **(Table 36.1)**.

## METHODS TO STUDY CARDIAC CYCLE

There are many direct and indirect methods to study the cardiac cycle. To understand it better we will briefly discuss all these method:

**Noninvasive methods:**
- Electrocardiography
- Jugular venous pulse
- Phonocardiogram

**Table 36.1:** Timings of systole and diastole.

|  | Atria | Ventricles |
|---|---|---|
| Systole | 0.1 sec | 0.3 sec |
| Diastole | 0.7 sec | 0.5 sec |
|  | Joint diastole: 0.4 sec | |

- Cine radiography
- Echocardiography

**Invasive method:** Cardiac catheterization

## Electrocardiography

It is an *indirect method* of measurement of the cardiac cycle. It studies the electrical changes occurring between any two fixed points. Conventionally, we study the changes between 2 R peaks, i.e., during one RR interval. Any change in the duration of magnitude of any of the ECG waves, intervals or segments is indicative of some changes in the cardiac cycle.
- P wave appears just prior to atrial systole
- QRS complex appears prior to ventricular systole (end of atrial systole)
- T wave appears during ventricular systole and ends just before incisura of aortic pressure curve

## Jugular Venous Pulse

It is also an indirect method to study the cardiac cycle. It is a *direct reflection of right atrial pressure*, indicating various phases of the cardiac cycle. It gives a rough idea about the right heart pressures on physical examination.

The JVP has three waves:

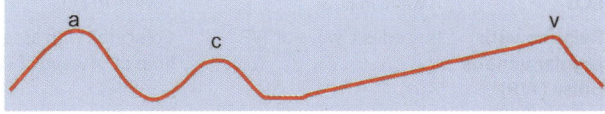

- *'a' wave* coincides with atrial systole (last rapid filling)

- *'c' wave* occurs due to bulging of AV valves into atria during isovolumetric contraction
- *'v' wave* coincides with the filling of atria during atrial diastole

## Phonocardiogram

It is the recording of heart sounds during various phases of the cardiac cycle. There are four heart sounds that can be recorded using a sophisticated electronic phonocardiogram but a stethoscope can clearly auscultate two heart sounds (S1 and S2).

The difference in all four heart sounds is tabulated in **Table 36.2**.

### Significance of S1 and S2 (audible sounds)
**S1:** indicates onset of clinical systole of ventricles
- Clear S1 indicates healthy AV valves
- Duration and intensity of S1 indicates condition of myocardium

**S2:** indicates end of systole and beginning of diastole
- Its pitch is directly proportional to blood pressure
- Clear sound indicates healthy semilunar valves

The interval between S1 and S2 is ventricular systole and interval between S2 and S1 is ventricular diastole.

## Cineradiography

It is also called as cine imaging, cine sequencing or cine MRI. In this repeated images of heart through various points of the cardiac cycle along with synchronization with ECG. It constructs a 3D picture of the cardiac cycle.

## Echocardiography

It is clinically the most commonly used most reliable non-invasive method for the study of cardiac cycle. It is based on the Doppler principle, similar to the ultrasonography. It tells us about the condition of cardiac walls and valves along with the measurement of intracardiac pressures and volumes during each phase of cardiac cycle.

## Cardiac Catheterization

It is the most reliable method for the measurement of cardiac cycle. In this, a catheter is inserted into the right atrium through right arm or into left heart, through aorta from femoral artery The pressures inside the cardiac chambers can be measured through this.

## MECHANICAL EVENTS IN THE CARDIAC CYCLE

*Atrial events*: Atrial systole and diastole
*Ventricular events:*
- **Ventricular systole:** → **"EJECTS AND PUSHES THE BLOOD FORWARDS"**
  - Isovolumetric contraction phase
  - Rapid ejection phase
  - Slow ejection phase
- **Ventricular diastole → "FILLING"**
  - Protodiastole
  - Isovolumetric relaxation phase
  - First rapid filling phase
  - Diastasis (longest phase with minimal/no blood flow)
  - Last rapid filling phase (corresponds with atrial systole)

## DESCRIPTION OF EVENTS IN CARDIAC CYCLE

During the cardiac cycle, the heart undergoes a series of events to pump blood efficiently. This includes atrial and ventricular contraction (systole) followed by relaxation (diastole), allowing blood to fill the chambers. The sequential opening and closing of heart valves ensure unidirectional blood flow, facilitating oxygenation and nutrient delivery to tissues throughout the body. Different events occurring in one cardiac cycle are described in **Table 36.3**.

**Table 36.2:** Features of four types of heart sounds.

|  | First heart sound (S1) | Second heart sound (S2) | Third heart sound (S3) | Fourth heart sound (S4) |
|---|---|---|---|---|
| Cause of sound | Vibrations set in by closure of atrioventricular valves | Vibrations caused by the sudden closure of semilunar valves | Vibrations set up in the cardiac wall by an inrush of blood during first rapid filling phase | Vibrations set up by inrush of blood during atrial systole |
| Character of sound | Long, Loud, LUBB | Short, Loud and High pitched, DUPP | Short, soft, low pitched | Normally not audible Short, low pitched |
| Duration | 0.15 sec | 0.12 sec | 0.1 sec | 0.03 sec |
| Frequency | 25–40/sec | 50 Hz |  | 3 Hz |
| Relation to cardiac cycle | Correspond to Isovolumetric contraction phase and early ejection phase | Corresponds with onset of ventricular diastole | It indicates the beginning of ventricular filling | Indicates the end of ventricular filling |
| Relation with ECG | Coincides with peak of R wave in ECG | Coincides with end of T wave in ECG | Appears between T and P wave of ECG | Appears at the end of P wave and onset of Q wave |
| Relation with jugular venous pulse (JVP) | Precedes 'c' wave of JVP | Coincides with ascending limb of 'v' wave of JVP | Coincides with the end of descending limb of 'v' wave of JVP | Coincides with 'a' wave of JVP |

**Table 36.3:** Events in cardiac cycle (To study this graph try to interlink the changes in atria, ventricle and arteries in each phase of cardiac cycle).

| | Atrial systole/Last rapid filling | Isovolumetric contraction | Rapid ejection | Slow ejection | Isovolumetric relaxation | First rapid filling | Diastasis | Last rapid filling/AS |
|---|---|---|---|---|---|---|---|---|
| Atrium | Pressure increases due to atrial systole. Remaining 25% of blood pushed into ventricles. Results in 'a' wave | Small increase in atrial pressure due to bulging AV valves into atria. Results in 'c' wave | • Atria relaxes in diastole and receive blood from veins. RA receives blood from IVC and SVC whereas LA receives blood from pulmonary veins<br>• Volume and pressure gradually rises in the atria due to increasing volume of blood | | | Atrial pressure becomes higher than the ventricular pressure and forces open the AV Valves | Pressure in atria and ventricles become almost equal resulting in minimal or no flow and hence, the term "dia-diastolic, Stasis- no flow". It is the longest period in ventricular diastole. When HR increases upto 180 bpm, this period shortens without affecting the efficiency of heart. | Same as discussed in column 1 |
| Ventricle | Small increase in ventricular pressure due to filling | Both the valves; AV and SL valves are closed. Ventricles contract resulting in tremendous increase in the pressure and opening of SLV when ventricular pressure becomes equal to diastolic pressure | On opening of SLV, blood is rapidly and forcefully ejected out into the arteries (75%). The contraction continues and the ventricular pressure becomes as high as systolic pressure of arteries | The pressure in the ventricles drop and decreases in the force of ejection of blood. Remaining 25% of EF is pumped out | Closure of SLV. Ventricles begin to relax, dropping the pressure tremendously | Rapid filling of ventricles take place due to pressure gradient | | Same as discussed in column 1 |
| Great arteries | Equivalent to diastolic pressure in arteries<br>Pulmonary trunk: 8 mm Hg;<br>Aorta: 80 mm Hg | Equivalent to diastolic pressure in arteries | Pressure increases due to ejection of blood from ventricles | Pressure slowly becomes higher than the ventricular pressure | Higher pressure in arteries, as compared to ventricles, result in backflow of blood into ventricles. This results in sudden *closure of SLV* and reflection of blood back into arteries and hence, the *dicrotic notch* | Pressure slowly decreases to DBP | Pressure slowly decreases to DBP | |
| Valve status and heart sounds | AV valves open, SLV are closed | AV valves and SLV Closed | AV valves close. SLV open when pressure rises to diastolic pressure. Produces *First Heart Sound (S1)* | AV valves close. SLV open | AV valves and SLV Closes suddenly and produce *Second Heart Sound (S2)* | SLV Closed. AV valves open when ventricular pressure becomes less than atrial pressure and produces *Third Heart Sound (S3)* | AV valves open. SLV Closed | AV valves open. SLV Closed.<br>Last rapid filling produces *Fourth heart sound (S4)* |
| Correlation with ECG | Atrial systole occurs at the end of P wave | R wave coincides with beginning of isovolumetric contraction | | | T wave begins in the middle of ventricular systole and ends with the end of isovolumetric relaxation phase | | | |

## PRESSURE AND VOLUME CHANGES IN LEFT AND RIGHT HEART (FIGS. 36.1 AND 36.2)

The pressure and the volume changes in the atria, ventricles and the arteries are discussed in detail in the **Table 36.4**. For the better understanding, lets summarize all these changes here and refer to the Wigger's diagram for the same:

- During the atrial systole, the ventricles are in the last phase of diastole.
  - *Pressure:* During this phase the pressure in atria is highest, forcing the remaining amount of blood into the ventricles. There is small rise in ventricular pressure.
  - *Volume:* The ventricular volume is increased to the end diastolic volume (120–130 mL).
- Once the atrial systole is over, the ventricular systole begins. The ventricles begin to contract, which tends to cause the back flow of blood into atria. There is sudden closure of the AV valves. At this point, the ventricular pressure begins to rise above the atrial pressure.
  - *Pressure:* The ventricular pressure increases most rapidly in the isovolumetric contraction period. Hence, the rate of change of pressure (dp/dt) is highest. When the intraventricular pressure just crosses the diastolic pressure of arteries (8 mm Hg for right ventricle and 80 mm Hg for left ventricle), the semilunar valves open. The continued contraction of the ventricles raises the intraventricular pressure up to the systolic pressure of arteries (25 mm Hg for right ventricle and 120 mm Hg for left ventricle). The high ventricular pressure results in rapid ejection. Once, most of the stroke volume is pumped out (about 70%), the ejection volume and pressure decreases. At this point, the ventricular pressure decreases below the arterial pressure. The blood tries to fall back into the ventricle due to pressure gradient, which results in closure of the semilunar valves. The closure of SLV, results in second heart

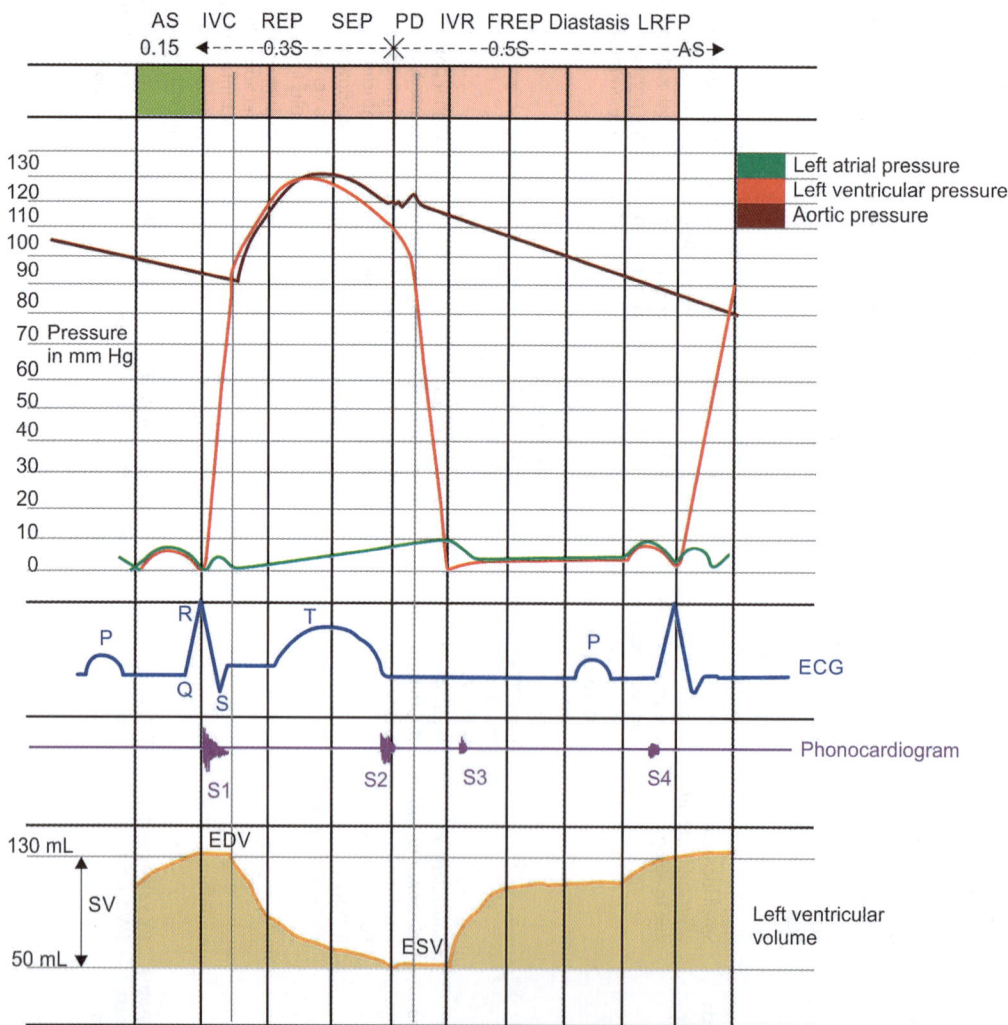

**Fig. 36.1:** Wiggers diagram showing pressure and volume changes with correlation to ECG and heart sounds.
(EDV: end diastolic volume, ESV: end systolic volume)

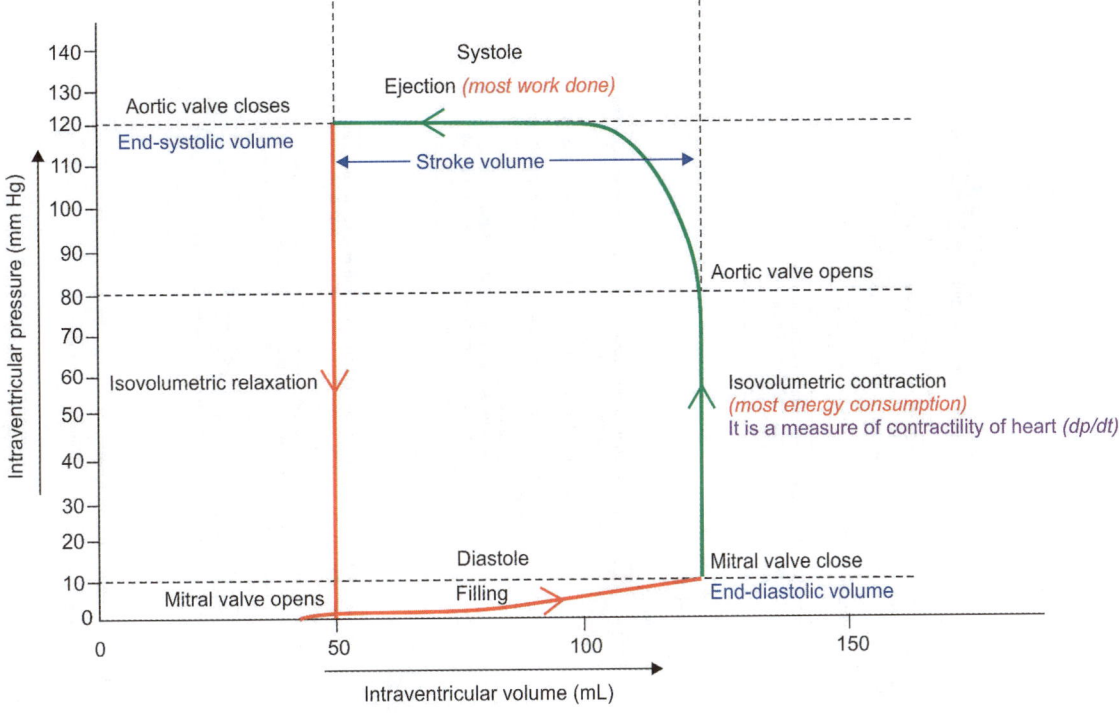

**Fig. 36.2:** Left ventricular volume pressure loop.

**Table 36.4:** Pressure and volume in the left side and right side of heart.

| | | Systolic pressure (mm Hg) | End-systolic volume (mL) | Diastolic pressure (mm Hg) | End-diastolic volume (mL) |
|---|---|---|---|---|---|
| **Left heart** | Left atrium | 4–5 | – | 2–4 | – |
| | Left ventricle | 121 | 50 | 0 | 120–130 |
| | Aorta | 120 | – | 80 | – |
| **Right heart** | Right atrium | 1–2 | – | 0–2 | – |
| | Right ventricle | 25 | 50 | 0 | 120–130 |
| | Pulmonary trunk | 25 | – | 8 | – |

sound and shows a small positive wave in the aortic pulse, called dicrotic notch.

- **Volume:** The Intraventricular volume shows no change during isovolumetric contraction. Once the SLV open, there is rapid and slow ejection of blood during the contraction. It is called as stroke volume (70-90 mL). At the end of systole, some blood still remains in the ventricles called the end systolic volume (ESV = 50 mL). Hence, the fraction of end diastolic volume pumped out in each systole is expressed as ejection fraction (EF). It is calculated as:

$$EF = \frac{EDV - ESV}{EDV} \times 100 = \frac{SV}{EDV} \times 100$$

**Normal EF is between 50–70%**

- When the ventricles begin to relax in the diastole, the SLV and AVV are closed hence there is sudden drop in pressure during the isovolumetric relaxation. The intraventricular pressure drops below the atrial pressure, which passively open the AVV. The blood gushes into the ventricles, during first rapid filling phase, raising the pressure slightly up to the atrial pressure. This phase adds around 75% of blood to the ventricle, which was filled in atria during its diastole. After the atrial and ventricular pressure equalize, the blood flow becomes minimal from atria to ventricles. This is the period of diastasis. Further, the atrial systole pushes the remaining 25% of its blood into the ventricles. And the cycle continues.

## OVERVIEW OF CARDIAC CYCLE

The cardiac cycle begins with atrial contraction, filling the ventricles, followed by ventricular contraction, ejecting blood into the systemic and pulmonary circulations, culminating in a brief period of relaxation before the cycle recommences. The events in cardiac cycle is shown in **Figure 36.3**.

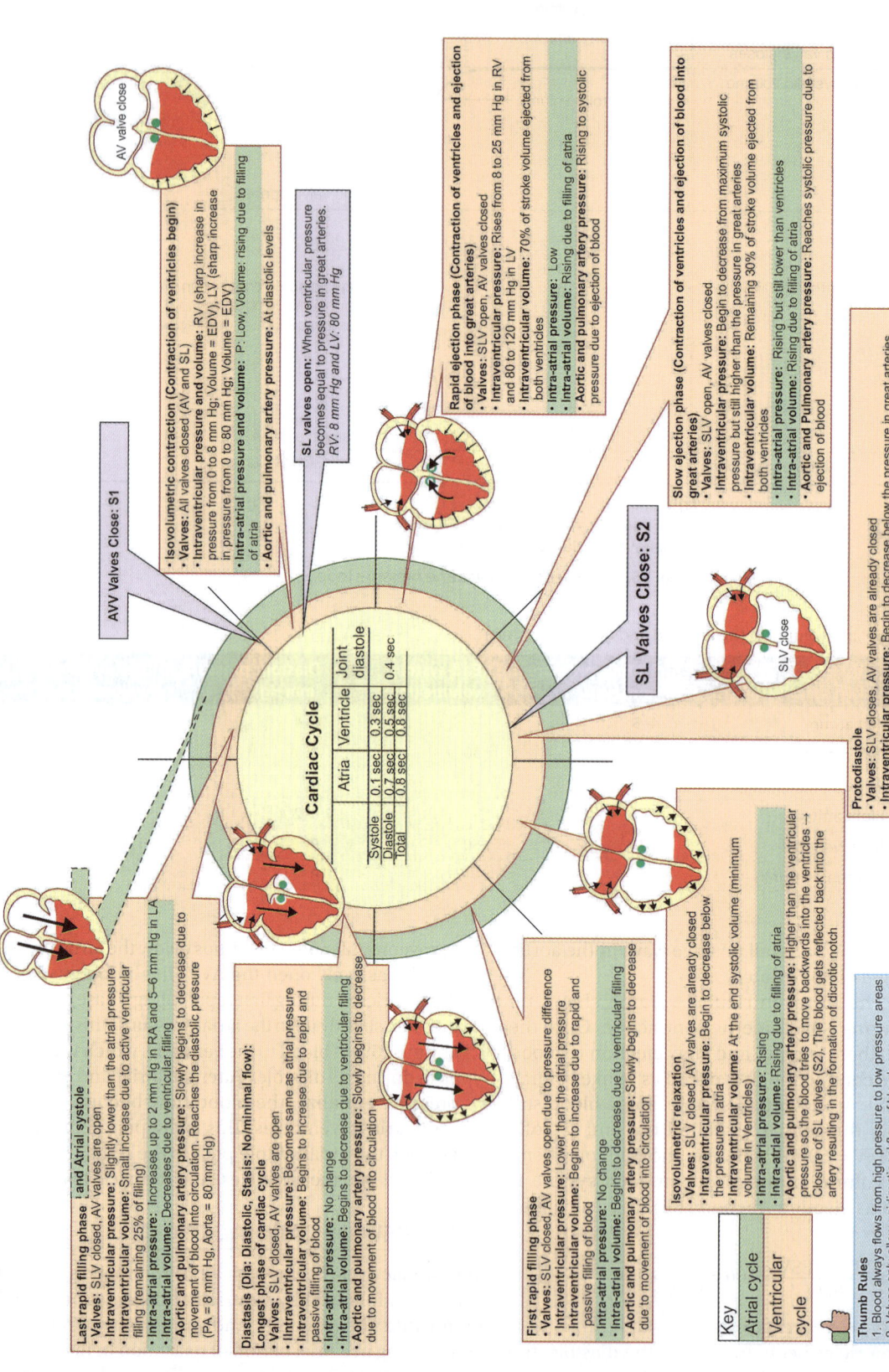

**Fig. 36.3:** Events of cardiac cycle.

## APPLIED PHYSIOLOGY

### Murmurs

Murmurs are abnormal Heart sounds which occur due turbulent flow of blood.

### Causes

- Valvular stenosis
- Valvular incompetence or regurgitation
- Atrial septal defect (ASD), ventricular septal defect (VSD), patent ductus arteriosus (PDA)
- Coarctation of aorta

### Types

Various types of murmurs are Systolic, Diastolic murmur and Continuous murmur. Murmurs according to site of abnormalities are shown in **Table 36.5**.

## Valvular Heart Diseases

Valvular heart diseases disrupt the normal flow of blood through the heart by impairing the function of one or more heart valves. Whether due to stenosis (narrowing) or regurgitation (leakage), these conditions compromise cardiac efficiency, leading to symptoms such as chest pain, shortness of breath, and fatigue, often requiring medical or surgical intervention to manage. **Table 36.6** summarizes the types of valvular heart diseases.

**Table 36.5:** Types of murmur based on site of abnormality.

| Site of abnormality | Type of abnormality | Type of murmur |
|---|---|---|
| Aortic/pulmonary valve (SLV) | Stenosis | Systolic |
| | Insufficiency | Diastolic |
| Mitral/tricuspid valve (AVV) | Stenosis | Diastolic |
| | Insufficiency | Systolic |
| VSD | Congenital hole | Systolic |
| Aorta | Coarctation | Systolic |
| PDA | Patent | Continuous |
| Blood | Anemia | Systolic |

(SLV: semilunar valve, AVV: atrioventricular valve, VSD: Ventricular septal defect)

**Table 36.6:** Effect of valvular diseases of left side of heart on cardiac cycle.

| | Mitral stenosis | Mitral regurgitation | Aortic stenosis | Aortic regurgitation |
|---|---|---|---|---|
| **What's wrong?** | Narrow mitral orifice | Mitral valve does not close properly before systole | Narrow aortic orifice | Aortic valve does not close properly before diastole |
| **So What?** | Impairment of blood flowing from LA to LV. LA has to work more | The blood gets regurgitated back into LA during systole | Ventricle has to exert a lot of effort to pump out blood | 60–70% of ejected blood gets regurgitated into the LV |
| **Ventricular pressure** | Little change or decrease | Normal | Very high | Increased systolic pressure |
| **Arterial pressure** | No change | Slightly decreased | Aortic pressure is not altered | Increased systolic pressure |
| **Left atrial pressure** | Markedly increased | Markedly increased | Normal | Normal |
| **Type of load on muscle** | After load for LA only | Decreased after load | After load | Increased preload due to increased EDV |
| **Murmur** | Diastolic | Systolic | Systolic | Diastolic |
| | Mitral stenosis | Mitral regurgitation | Aortic stenosis | Aortic regurgitation |
| **Effect on heart** | Left atrial hypertrophy | Left atrial hypertrophy | Concentric hypertrophy of ventricle | Eccentric hypertrophy of ventricle |

## SUMMARY

In this chapter, we have learnt that:
- The cardiac cycle is defined as the sequence of events occurring in the heart between two heart beats. The normal cardiac cycle time is 0.8 sec.
- The atria and ventricles undergo contraction (systole) and relaxation (diastole).
- The ventricular cycle has the following phase: The systole (isovolumetric contraction, rapid ejection phase, slow ejection phase) and diastole (isovolumetric relaxation, first rapid filling phase, diastasis and last rapid filling phase).

## LET US SEE, HOW MUCH YOU HAVE LEARNT?

### Review Questions

#### Long/Short Answer Questions

Q1. Define cardiac cycle. Describe the methods to measure cardiac cycle.
Q2. Describe the pressure changes with the help of a diagram, in left atrium, left ventricle and aorta during the cardiac cycle.
Q3. Describe the volume changes in the left ventricle during the cardiac cycle.
Q4. How is electrocardiography correlated with the cardiac cycle?
Q5. How is jugular venous pulse correlated with the cardiac cycle?
Q6. Define stroke volume, end systolic and end diastolic volume.
Q7. Define ejection fraction. What is its physioclinical significance?

#### Explain Why? (Reasoning Questions)

Q1. The atria contract before the ventricles during the cardiac cycle.
Q2. The left ventricular wall is thicker than the right ventricular wall.
Q3. The heart sounds are associated with the closing of heart valves rather than their opening.
Q4. The refractory period of cardiac muscle is longer than that of skeletal muscle.

### Critical Thinking Case-Based Questions

Q1. Ajay, a 65-year-old male, was brought emergency room with complaints of fatigue, shortness of breath, and occasional chest pain. He also noted swelling in his ankles and feet. Upon examination and echocardiography (ECG), Ajay was diagnosed with aortic stenosis.

Based upon the given scenario, answer the following questions:
a. Explain how aortic stenosis affects the phases of the cardiac cycle.
b. What are the key phases of the cardiac cycle?
c. Enumerate the other valvular heart diseases.

### Multiple Choice Questions

Q1. What is the primary function of the cardiac cycle?
   a. To regulate blood pressure
   b. To pump blood throughout the body
   c. To maintain electrolyte balance
   d. To filter waste products from the blood
Q2. During which phase of the cardiac cycle does ventricular contraction occur?
   a. Atrial systole
   b. Ventricular diastole
   c. Ventricular systole
   d. Atrial diastole
Q3. Which valve prevents the backflow of blood from the aorta into the left ventricle?
   a. Pulmonary valve
   b. Aortic valve
   c. Mitral valve
   d. Tricuspid valve
Q4. What initiates the electrical impulse that triggers the cardiac cycle?
   a. SA node            b. AV node
   c. Bundle of His      d. Purkinje fibers
Q5. What is the function of the atrioventricular (AV) node in the cardiac cycle?
   a. Initiates the heartbeat
   b. Conducts electrical impulses to the ventricles
   c. Delays the impulse to allow for atrial contraction
   d. Regulates blood flow between the atria and ventricles
Q6. Which of the following describes diastole in the cardiac cycle?
   a. Relaxation of the heart chambers
   b. Contraction of the heart chambers
   c. Closure of the atrioventricular valves
   d. Opening of the semilunar valves

Q7. In a patient with congestive heart failure, which phase of the cardiac cycle is most affected?
   a. Atrial systole
   b. Ventricular diastole
   c. Ventricular systole
   d. Atrial diastole
Q8. How does hypertension affect the cardiac cycle?
   a. Increases heart rate and contractility
   b. Decreases heart rate and contractility
   c. Increases heart rate but decreases contractility
   d. Decreases heart rate but increases contractility
Q9. In a patient with atrial fibrillation, which phase of the cardiac cycle is disrupted?
   a. Atrial systole
   b. Ventricular diastole
   c. Ventricular systole
   d. Atrial diastole
Q10. In a patient with mitral valve regurgitation, which chamber of the heart experiences increased workload?
   a. Right atrium
   b. Right ventricle
   c. Left atrium
   d. Left ventricle
Q11. How does aging affect the cardiac cycle?
   a. Increases heart rate and contractility
   b. Decreases heart rate and contractility
   c. Increases heart rate but decreases contractility
   d. Decreases heart rate but increases contractility
Q12. A patient presents with symptoms of shortness of breath and edema in the lower extremities. Which phase of the cardiac cycle is likely impaired?
   a. Atrial systole
   b. Ventricular diastole
   c. Ventricular systole
   d. Atrial diastole
Q13. A marathon runner experiences an increase in heart rate and cardiac output during a race. Which phase of the cardiac cycle is predominantly affected?
   a. Atrial systole
   b. Ventricular diastole
   c. Ventricular systole
   d. Atrial diastole
Q14. A patient is diagnosed with aortic valve stenosis. Which phase of the cardiac cycle is directly affected, leading to a decrease in stroke volume?
   a. Atrial systole
   b. Ventricular diastole
   c. Ventricular systole
   d. Atrial diastole
Q15. A hypertensive individual develops left ventricular hypertrophy. Which phase of the cardiac cycle is primarily affected due to increased afterload?
   a. Atrial systole
   b. Ventricular diastole
   c. Ventricular systole
   d. Atrial diastole
Q16. A patient with a history of myocardial infarction undergoes a radionuclide angiography test. The end-diastolic volume (EDV) is found to be 160 mL, and the end-systolic volume (ESV) is 90 mL. What is the ejection fraction of the patient's left ventricle?
   a. 25%
   b. 35%
   c. 45%
   d. 55%

## ANSWERS

1. b  2. c  3. b  4. b  5. b  6. a  7. c  8. a  9. a  10. d  11. b  12. b  13. c  14. c  15. c  16. b

# Basics of Electrocardiography

**CHAPTER 37**

> **COMPETENCY ADDRESSED**
> PY5.5: Describe the physiology of electrocardiogram (ECG), its applications and the cardiac axis.

>  **LEARNING OBJECTIVES**
> **At the end of this chapter, the learner should be able to:**
> - Describe the basic principles of electrocardiography.
> - Describe the spread of cardiac impulse resulting the electrical changes in heart.
> - Describe the physiological basis of various components of ECG.
> - Describe the normal ECG and its physiological significance.

Myocardium is an excitable tissue which responds to electrical changes and results in myocardial contraction. The cardiac impulse generated by the SA node spreads through the entire heart through the conducting system of the heart (discussed in Chapter 5.2). While spreading from the SA node to Purkinje fibers, a dipole is created in the heart, resulting in the *flow of current from areas of depolarization (negatively charged areas) to polarized/resting (positively charged) areas creating a current sink* (**Fig. 37.1**).

These electrical changes vary with the flow of current from one point to another, hence altering the magnitude and direction of dipole created. These changes result in variations in the instantaneous vector of current in terms of direction and magnitude of current and voltage of myocardium (discussed later). There are two main ways to record these changes, either by directly inserting the recording electrodes at various points of the myocardium *(monophasic recording)* or by picking up these electrical changes from the body surface *(electrocardiography)*. The simple explanation that can be given for this procedure is that our body is mainly composed of water and electrolytes, which act as volume conductor and allows these electrical changes to be transmitted to our body surface which can be picked up by simple electrodes. Hence, electrocardiography is defined as *surface recording of electrical changes taking place in heart from beat to beat (i.e., recording of the electrical changes during the cardiac cycle)*.

It is similar to cardiac action potential (**Fig. 37.2**). The differences between ECG with that of cardiac action potential is shown in **Table 37.1**.

The surface recording is done using 2 electrodes, hence they yield a biphasic recording, as shown in **Figure 37.3**.

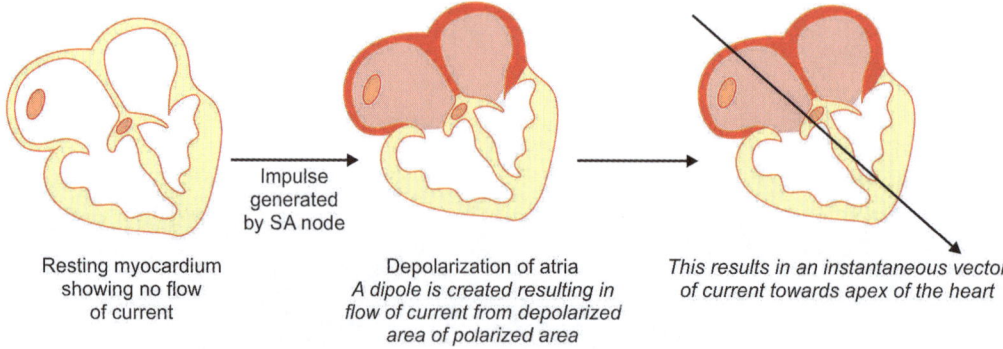

**Fig. 37.1:** Principle of dipole for flow of current in heart.

**Table 37.1:** Features of ECG vs cardiac action potential.

| Features | ECG | Cardiac action potential |
|---|---|---|
| Type of event | Electrical event showing the phases of depolarization and repolarization. | Electrical event showing the phases of depolarization and repolarization. |
| Electrode placement | On the surface of the body | One electrode on the surface of muscle and another inside the cardiac muscle |
| Resting membrane potential | Zero, as both the electrodes have no potential difference at rest | –90 mV, as both the electrodes measure resting potential difference across the cell membrane |
| Type of action potential recorded | Biphasic | Monophasic |
| Magnitude of maximum potential difference | 2–4 mV | 100–110 mV |
| Electrical events captured from | It shows the changes in both the atria and the ventricles | It shows the electrical changes in only one chamber, in which the electrodes are placed |
| Voltage time graph showing both the recordings | 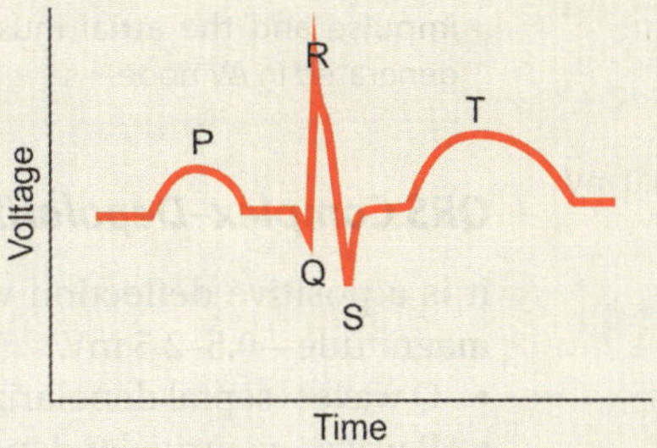 ECG waveform showing P, Q, R, S, T waves on Voltage vs Time axes | 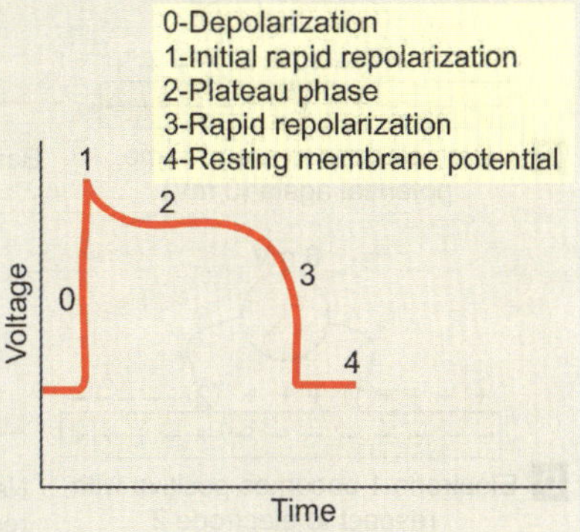 Cardiac action potential curve with phases: 0-Depolarization, 1-Initial rapid repolarization, 2-Plateau phase, 3-Rapid repolarization, 4-Resting membrane potential |
| Correlation between ECG and monophasic AP | 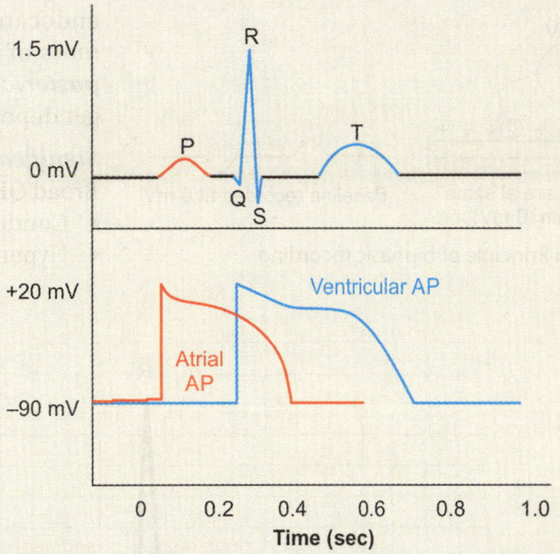 Fig. 37.2: Correlation of ECG and myocardial action potentials (AP). Shows ECG (P, Q, R, S, T) at top with scale 0 mV to 1.5 mV, and below it Atrial AP and Ventricular AP from –90 mV to +20 mV across 0 to 1.0 sec. | |

*Normal ECG:* The record of the electrical activity of heart in terms of voltage-time graph in a normal disease free heart is called as normal ECG.

## COMPONENTS OF NORMAL ECG

- **Waves:** Any deviation above and below the isoelectric line.
- **Intervals:** Intervals between 2 wave including the waves.
- **Segments:** Intervals between 2 waves excluding the waves, i.e., only on isoelectric lines.

### Waves

**Figures 37.4A and B** for physiological basis of waves.

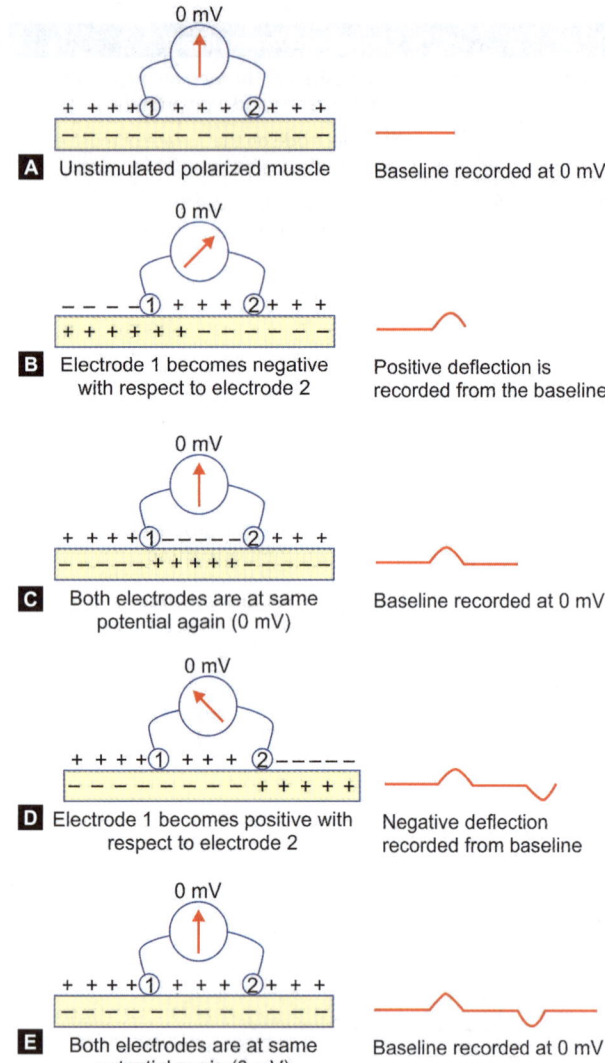

**Fig. 37.3:** Principle of biphasic recording.

## P Wave–Depolarization of Atria

- It is a positive deflection with duration: 0.08–0.1 seconds and magnitude –0.2 mV.
- Depolarization begins in SA node and spreads in all directions.
- It is in the direction of mean cardiac vector, hence positive in all leads.

***Significance of P wave:*** A normal P wave signifies that:
- Impulse is originating in SA node
- Spread of impulse is in usual direction (towards the apex)
- There is no defect in conduction
- Atrial musculature is normal

> **What is the significance of an inverted P wave?**
> An inverted P wave indicates that SA node fails to generate impulse and the atrial muscle is depolarizing by impulse generated in AV node.

## QRS Complex–Depolarization of Ventricles

It is a positive deflection with duration: 0.08–0.12s and magnitude—0.5–2.5 mV.
- Q wave—septal depolarization
- R wave—ventricular depolarization
- S wave—depolarization of basal parts of heart

The first part of the ventricle to become depolarized is ***left endocardial surface of septum***. Followed by endocardial surface of both ventricles. The ventricular mass of left ventricle is more than the right ventricle, ***posterior basal part of left ventricle*** is the last part to get depolarized.

***Significance of QRS complex:***
Broad QRS complexes are seen in:
- Conduction blocks especially bundle branch block
- Hypercalcemia

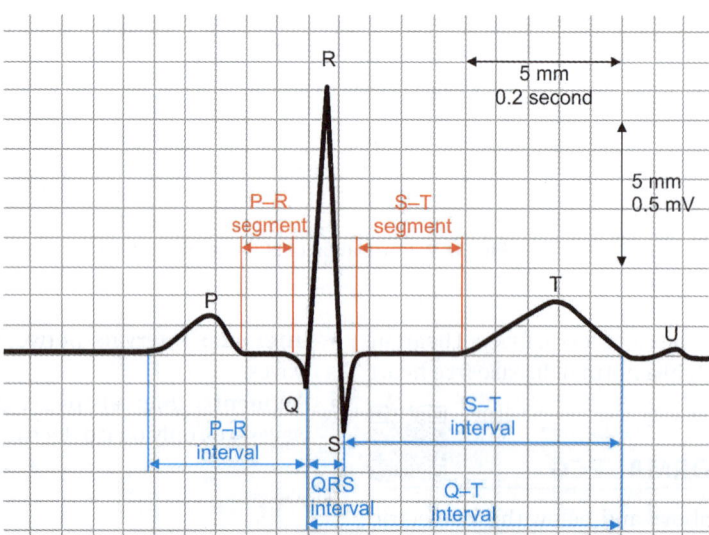

**Fig. 37.4A:** Physiological basis of waves.

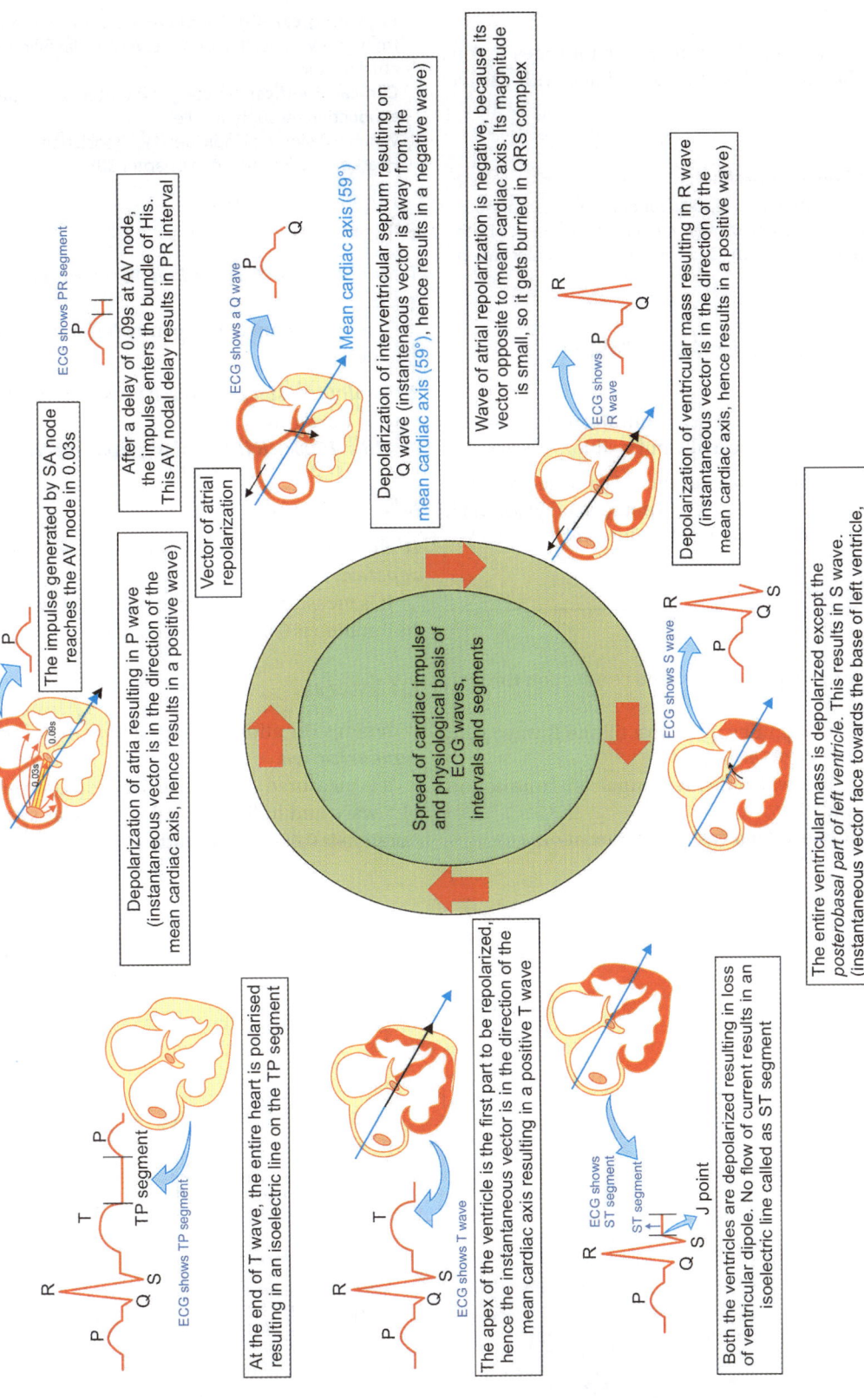

**Fig. 37.4B:** The physiological basis of generation of waves, intervals and segments of ECG.

## T Wave–Repolarization of Ventricles

It is a positive deflection with duration: 0.27 s and magnitude—0.5 mV.

*Significance of T wave:* T wave inversion indicates serious myocardial damage and is often associated with cardiac hypoxia.

> **R wave and T wave are positive**
> During depolarization and repolarization, the instantaneous vectors are in the direction of mean cardiac axis and hence both the waves of depolarization (QRS complex) and repolarization (T wave) are positive.

## U Wave–Slow Repolarization of Papillary Muscles

It is a positive deflection with duration: 0.08 s and magnitude—0.2 mV. It is usually not visible.

*Note:* Wave of atrial repolarization: It is a negative wave, buried in QRS complex. Hence it is not seen on ECG. But it can be seen in cases of prolonged PR interval.

## INTERVALS (FIG. 37.5)

### PR Interval

- Indicates atrial depolarization and conduction through AV node.
- It starts from beginning of P wave till the R wave with duration: 0.12–0.20 seconds.
- Longer PR interval indicates impaired conduction through bundle.
- Variable PR interval indicates AV dissociation.

> **What is the significance of PR interval?**
> **Physiological significance:** Denotes conduction delay through AV node. It allows the ventricular filling at the end of atrial systole.
> **Clinical significance:** Longer PR interval indicates impaired conduction through bundle.
> Variable PR interval indicates AV dissociation.
> Heart blocks (discussed in Chapter 38)

### RR Interval

It denotes the *time taken to complete one cardiac cycle*.

It is the distance between two R waves. Its duration is 0.8 seconds.

*Physiological significance:* It is used to calculate the heart rate by the formula:

*HR = 1500/RR interval at paper speed of 25 mm/s.*

### QRS Duration

It denotes *ventricular depolarization* and *atrial repolarization*.

It is measured as distance between Q wave and S wave. Its duration is 0.08 to 0.10 seconds.

### QT Interval

It denotes duration of *ventricular depolarization* and *repolarization*.

It is measured as distance between Q wave and the end of T wave and indicates total ventricular systolic time. Its duration is 0.40–0.43 seconds.

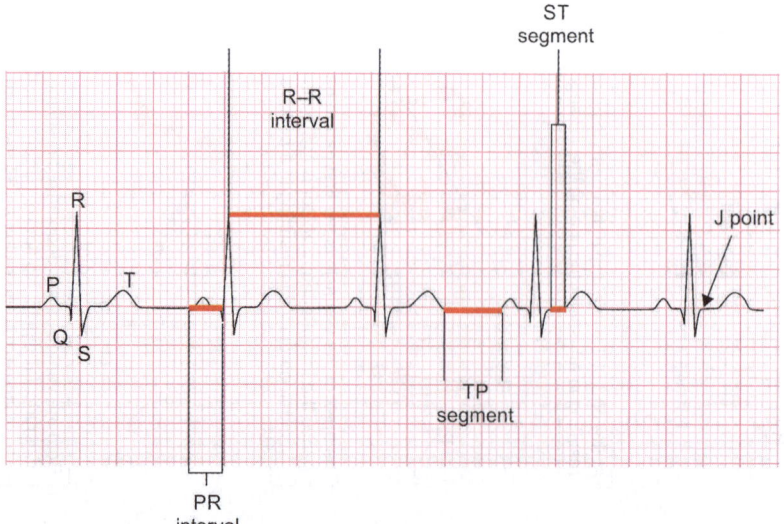

**Fig. 37.5:** The normal ECG trace showing intervals and segments.

*Clinical significance of QTc interval:* QTc interval denotes QT interval corrected for the heart rate. It is measured as the QT interval divided by square root of RR interval:

$$\text{QTc} = \frac{\text{QT interval}}{\sqrt{\text{RR interval}}}$$

A normal QTc interval should be *0.36–0.44 s in males and 0.36–0.46 s in females*. If this QTc interval is more than 0.47 seconds it acts as the predictor of cardiac disease. But a QTc interval of more than 0.5 s predicts increased risk of life-threatening cardiac disease. It also helps in diagnosis of *long QT syndrome*.

## ST Interval

It is measured from end of QRS complex to end of T wave. Its duration is 0.32 seconds.

## TP Interval

It denotes diastolic period of the heart. It is measured from end of T wave and onset of P wave.

*Clinical significance of TP interval:* Variable TP interval indicates AV dissociation.

## SEGMENTS (FIG. 37.5)

### PR Segment

- It denotes time taken by AV node to conduct the impulse.
- It is measured as the isoelectric line between end of P wave and beginning of R wave.
- Its duration is 0.04 to 0.08 seconds.

### ST Segment

It denotes time gap between depolarization and repolarization of the ventricles.

It is measured as isoelectric line at the end of S wave till the beginning of T wave. Its duration is 0.04–0.08 seconds.

*Physiological significance:* The ST segment is the important period during the electrical changes in the ventricle, as no current flows through the ventricles at this time. It marks the period of no electrical activity in depolarized ventricle.

*Clinical significance:* In case of the myocardial injury occurring due to ischemia or infarction, the infarcted muscle does not get depolarized. Hence, this segment shows peculiar changes owing to the dipole so created between the healthy and infarcted myocardium. The current flow in this case is called the *current of injury*. It appears as *elevation and sagging* of this segment indicating myocardial damage or hypoxia respectively.

The point at the beginning of ST segment, when the heart is just completely depolarized and no current flows, is called *J point*. It is the reference point to see or diagnose the changes in ST segment.

### TP Segment

It denotes the polarized or resting state of the heart. In this period, no current flows through the heart and all the chambers are polarized. Its duration is 0.2 s at HR 75/min, which is inversely related to HR.

## RECORDING OF ECG

After we have studied the basics of ECG, let us become familiar with certain terms and basics related to recording and analysis of ECG:
- **Electrocardiography:** It is branch of physiology related to recording and analysis of electrical activity of heart
- **Electrocardiogram:** Recording of the electrical changes in heart during the cardiac cycle
- **Electrocardiograph:** Instrument for making permanent record of small potential variations occurring in different parts of body due to electrical activity of heart.

### ECG Paper (Fig. 37.6)

It is a *heat sensitive/thermal paper* with a graphic pattern, on which the electrocardiograph records the electric fluctuations of heart in terms of voltage and time graph. At the paper speed of 25 mm/s, the small 25 boxes (25 mm) or

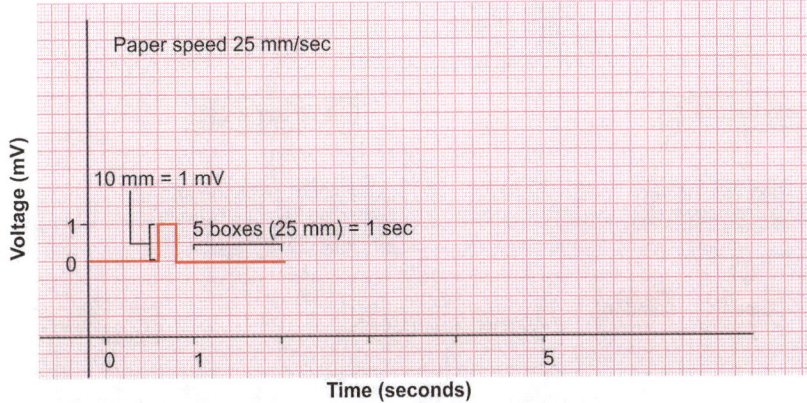

**Fig. 37.6:** The ECG paper showing calibration.

5 big boxes represent one second on the time scale, whereas 10 mm or two large boxes denote 1 mV of potential change.

## ECG Jelly

It is the conducting paste, which contains very fine sand/glass particles, which produce local erythema.

## Electrodes and Leads (Fig. 37.7)

The rectangular flat metallic discs (7.5 × 5 cm) are called *electrodes*, which are placed on the body surface.

In terms of physical lead, it defined as a set of two electrodes connected by a wire. However, the electrical picture of heart recorded between two electrodes on the paper is also called a lead.

*Father of ECG:* **William Einthoven** (1903), discovered the ECG and proposed the Einthoven's laws, which became the basis of recording ECG. He proposed the *Einthoven's triangle* (**Fig. 37.8**) formed by joining 2 acromion processes and the pubic symphysis with heart in the center.

*Einthoven's Law:* It states that "if the ECGs are recorded simultaneously with the three limb leads, the sum of the potentials recorded in leads I and III will equal the potential in lead II".

*Potential of Lead I + Potential of Lead III = Potential of Lead II*

This also implies that, if the electrical potential of any two of the bipolar leads are known at any given instance, the third one can be determined mathematically from first two by simply summing the first two, i.e., mathematical sum of all the leads is zero:

$$LI + LII + LIII = 0$$

## Mean Cardiac Axis

It is the resultant vector of heart which is produced by the sum of instantaneous vectors during the series of electrical changes.

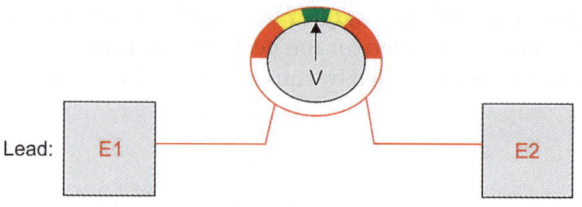

**Fig. 37.7:** Electrodes and leads.

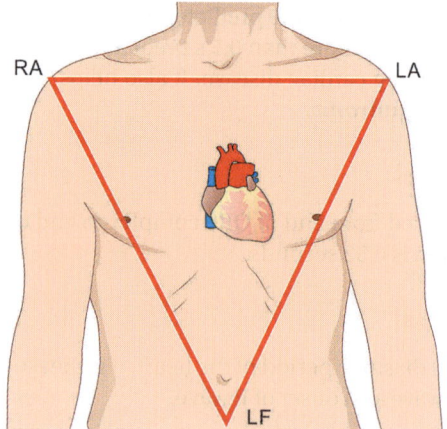

**Fig. 37.8:** Einthoven's triangle.

*Normal Mean QRS vector is 59 degrees.*
Limit of normal cardiac axis is *–30 to +110 degrees*.

*Physiological significance:* If the mean cardiac axis lies to the left of -30°, it is called *left axis deviation*, while to the right of +110° is called *right axis deviation*.

## ECG Leads

Based on the nature of electrodes, the basic 12 ECG leads are classified as (**Flowchart 37.1**):

1. **Bipolar leads:** It is also called as standard limb leads, having 2 active electrodes (positive and negative electrodes):
   - Lead I → between RA and LA (0°)

**Flowchart 37.1:** Types of ECG leads.

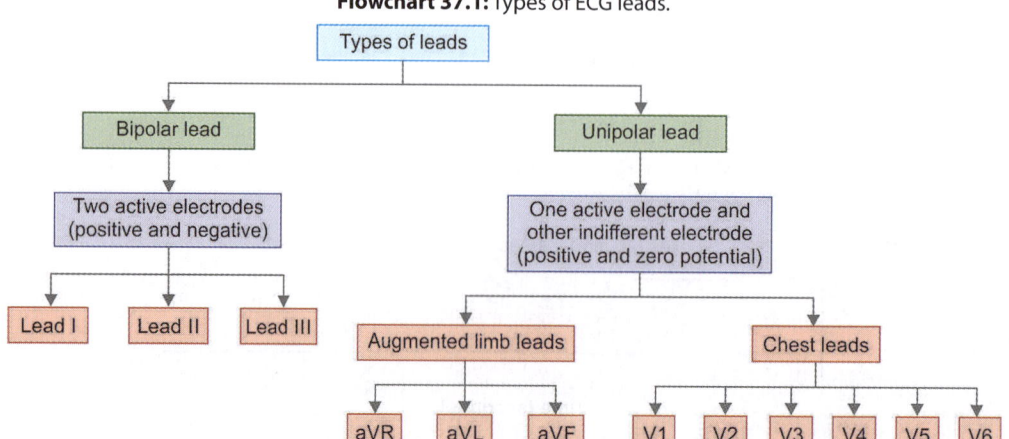

- Lead II → between RA and LF (60°).
  *This lead has the maximum voltage because it is in the direction of mean cardiac axis (59°)*
- Lead III → between LA and LF (120°).

2. **Unipolar leads**: These have 1 active/exploring electrode and another indifferent electrode with zero potential, hence called as unipolar leads. They are of two types:
   i. **Augmented limb leads (Figs. 37.9 and 37.10):** These are called as augmented because the signal is augmented by **50%**:
      **aVR** → The active electrode is at RA and reference/indifferent electrode is average of LA and LF. The *instantaneous vector of aVR is at 210°*, which is opposite to the mean cardiac axis. Hence, this lead is also called the '*inverted lead.*'
      **aVL** → The active electrode at LA and reference/indifferent electrode is average of RA and LF. The *instantaneous vector of aVL is at –30°*

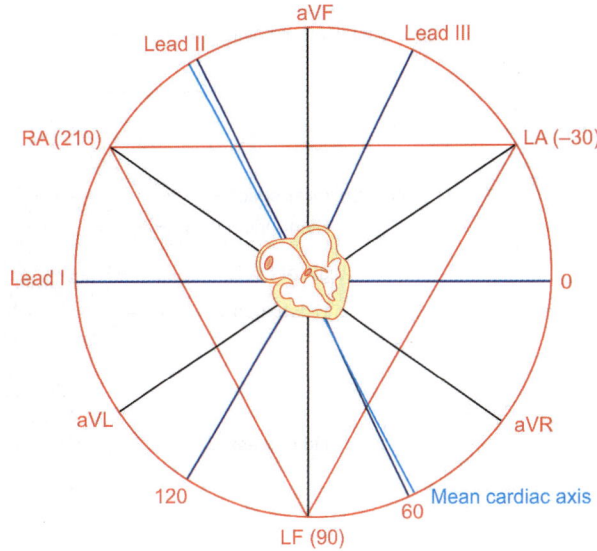

**Fig. 37.10:** Hexagonal arrangement showing directions of limb leads.

**aVF** → The active electrode at LF and reference/indifferent electrode is average of LA and RA. The *instantaneous vector of aVF is at 90°*.

   ii. **Chest Leads (Fig. 37.11):**
      - V1—placed in 4th intercostal space 2.5 cm to right of sternum.
      - V2—placed in 4th intercostal space 2.5 cm to left of sternum.
      - V3—placed between V2 and V4.
      - V4—places in 5th intercostal space in midclavicular line.
      - V5—placed in the 5th intercostal space in anterior axillary line.
      - V6—placed in the 5th intercostal space in posterior axillary line.

      Based on the position of these standard chest electrodes with respect to the heart, they are also called:
      - Right sided chest leads (V1 V2)
      - Inferior chest leads (V3 V4)
      - Left sided chest leads (V5 V6)

## Normal Wave Patterns in All the Standard ECG Leads (Table 37.2)

### Lead I, II and III

- All characteristics are same except for voltage which is maximum in lead II
- P wave: Positive/upward
- Q wave: Absent
- RS wave: Positive R wave
- T wave: Positive

### *Significance of Lead I, II and III*

- For diagnosis of cardiac axis
- For diagnosis of cardiac arrhythmias
- For studying functional abnormality of heart

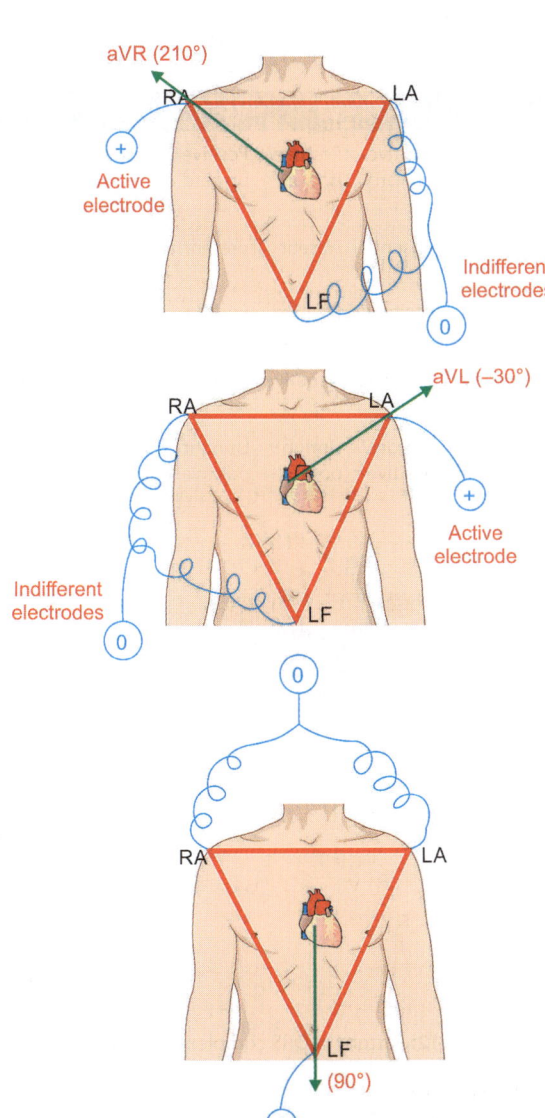

**Fig. 37.9:** The augmented limb leads.

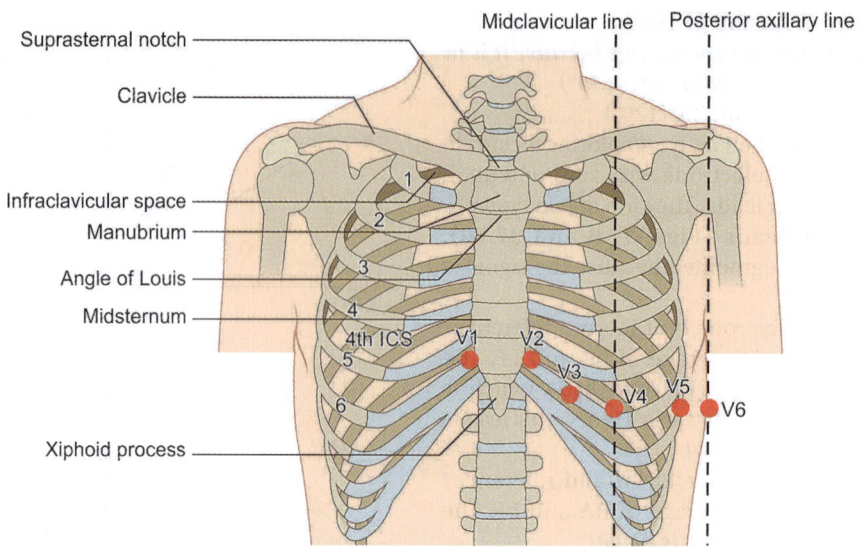

**Fig. 37.11:** Placement of chest leads.

**Table 37.2:** Normal wave patterns in all the standard ECG leads.

| | I | II | III | aVR | aVL | aVF | V1 | V2 | V3 | V4 | V5 | V6 |
|---|---|---|---|---|---|---|---|---|---|---|---|---|
| **P wave** | Positive/upward | Positive/upward | Positive/upward | Negative/Downward | May be upward/Downward | Positive/upward | Positive/upward | Positive/upward | Positive/upward | Positive/upward | Positive/upward | Positive/upward |
| **Q wave** | Absent | Absent | Absent | Absent | Absent | Absent | Absent | Absent | Absent | present | present | present |
| **R wave** | Positive | Positive | Positive | Negative | Biphasic | Positive | Positive r<<S | Positive r<S | Positive R=S | Positive R=S | Positive R>s | Positive R>s |
| **S wave** | Negative | Negative | Negative | Positive | Biphasic | Negative | Negative r<<S | Negative r<S | Negative R=S | Negative R=S | Negative R>s | Negative R>s |
| **T wave** | Upright/positive | Upright/positive | Upright/positive | Inverted | Inverted | Upright/positive | Upright/positive | Upright/positive | Upright/positive | Upright/positive | Upright/positive | Upright/positive |

## Augmented Limb Leads

| Waves | aVR | aVL | aVF |
|---|---|---|---|
| P wave | Inverted | Biphasic | Upright |
| Q wave | Absent | Absent | Absent |
| R wave | Inverted | Positive (Biphasic RS wave) | Positive |
| T wave | Inverted | Inverted | Positive |

*Significance of augmented leads*
- To find out position of heart
- Confirming ventricular damage or hypertrophy

## Chest Leads
- P wave: Positive in all chest leads
- Q wave: Absent in V1, V2 and V3
- RS wave: R increases and S decreases from V1-V6
- T wave: Positive if R>S; negative if R<S *(it is in the direction of QRS complex)*

*Q Wave is Present Only in V4, V5 and V6 (Fig. 37.12)*
- V1: rS pattern
- V2: rS pattern
- V3: RS pattern
- V4: qRs pattern
- V5: qRs pattern
- V6: qRs pattern

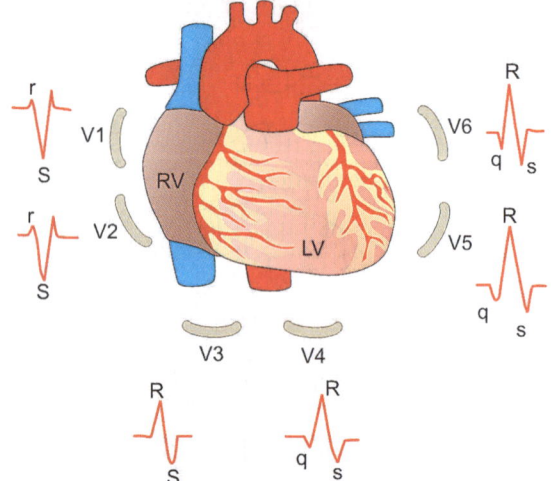

**Fig. 37.12:** Pattern of QRS complex in chest leads.

*Significance of chest leads*
- Localization of recent or old ventricular damage
- Bundle branch block
- Ventricular hypertrophy

## SUMMARY

- In this chapter, we have studied about electrocardiography (ECG), focusing on its basic principles, physiological basis, and clinical significance.
- An Electrocardiogram (ECG) is a graphic representation of the electrical activity of the heart. It comprises several key components:
  a. P Wave: Represents atrial depolarization, the contraction of the atria.
  b. QRS Complex: Depicts ventricular depolarization, the contraction of the ventricles.
  c. T Wave: Reflects ventricular repolarization, the recovery phase of the ventricles.
  d. PR Interval: Indicates the time it takes for the electrical impulse to travel from the atria to the ventricles.
  e. QT Interval: Represents the total time for ventricular depolarization and repolarization.
- A normal Electrocardiogram (ECG) consists of several segments:
  a. PR Segment: The flat line between the end of the P wave and the beginning of the QRS complex, representing the delay at the atrioventricular (AV) node.
  b. ST Segment: The flat, isoelectric line between the end of the QRS complex and the beginning of the T wave, indicating the period when the ventricles are electrically depolarized but not yet repolarized.
  c. TP Segment: The interval between the end of the T wave and the beginning of the next P wave, representing the time when the ventricles are fully repolarized.
- ECG leads are electrodes placed on the body to record the heart's electrical activity. The standard 12-lead ECG includes:
  a. Bipolar Limb Leads (I, II, III): Record electrical activity between two limbs.
  b. Augmented Voltage Leads (aVR, aVL, aVF): Measure electrical activity from a single limb and the augmented (combined) electrical activity of the other two limbs.
  c. Precordial (Chest) Leads (V1-V6): Record electrical activity across the chest, providing a comprehensive view of the heart's horizontal plane.
- Applied aspects of ECG involve utilizing electrocardiography for clinical purposes and patient care. Key applications include:
  a. Diagnosis of Heart Conditions: ECG is crucial for diagnosing various heart conditions such as arrhythmias, myocardial infarction, and conduction abnormalities by analyzing the waveform patterns and intervals.
  b. Monitoring Cardiac Health: ECG monitoring is used in hospitals and ambulatory settings to continuously track and assess a patient's cardiac activity, providing real-time information about rhythm changes and potential issues.
  c. Risk Stratification: ECG findings contribute to assessing the risk of cardiovascular events, aiding healthcare professionals in determining appropriate interventions and treatments.
  d. Exercise Stress Testing: ECG is commonly employed during exercise stress tests to evaluate the heart's response to physical activity, helping diagnose coronary artery disease and assess cardiovascular fitness.
  e. Electrolyte Imbalance Detection: ECG can reveal abnormalities associated with electrolyte imbalances, such as potassium or calcium, which can impact cardiac function.

## LET US SEE, WHAT YOU HAVE LEARNT?

### Review Questions

#### Long/Short Answer Questions

Q1. Define electrocardiogram. Describe the physiological basis of the genesis of ECG waves and intervals.
Q2. Draw a well labeled diagram of normal electrocardiogram.
Q3. Describe the physiological basis of PR interval. Describe the clinical significance of PR interval.
Q4. What is relationship of ECG waves with cardiac action potential?
Q5. Name the inverted lead, why it is called inverted?

#### Explain Why? (Reasoning Questions)

Q1. P wave on an ECG represents atrial depolarization.
Q2. QRS complex on an ECG is larger in amplitude than the P wave.
Q3. PR interval on an ECG is important for assessing atrioventricular (AV) conduction.
Q4. ST segment should be isoelectric (flat) in a normal ECG.

### Critical Thinking Case-Based Questions

Q1. A 25-year-old healthy male, came for a routine physical examination. His physician suggested an electrocardiogram (ECG) as part of the examination due to a family history of heart disease. The ECG showed a normal sinus rhythm with no abnormalities. Depending upon given scenario, answer the following question:

a. Describe the physiological basis of a normal electrocardiogram (ECG) tracing.
b. How does the ECG reflect the different phases of the cardiac cycle?
c. What are the physiological significance of ECG leads?

# Multiple Choice Questions

**Q1.** Vagal stimulation of the heart causes:
  a. Increased heart rate
  b. Increased R-R interval in ECG
  c. Increased force of heart contraction
  d. Increased cardiac output.

**Q2.** Einthoven's triangle, what is the value of Lead III when Lead I = 2 mV and Lead II = 1 mV?
  a. 1    b. 2
  c. 3    d. 4

**Q3.** In a standard electrocardiogram, an augmented limb lead measures the electrical potential difference between:
  a. Two limbs
  b. One limb and two other limbs
  c. One limb and neutral (zero)
  d. Two limbs and two other limbs

**Q4.** QRS complex indicates:
  a. Atrial repolarization
  b. Atrial depolarization
  c. Ventricular repolarization
  d. Ventricular depolarization

**Q5.** The ECG of a 40-year-old male was recorded using standard bipolar limb leads. The sum of voltage of the three standard leads was found to be 5 millivolts. This indicates:
  a. A normal heart
  b. Right ventricular hypertrophy
  c. Left ventricular hypertrophy.
  d. Increased cardiac muscle mass.

**Q6.** A male long-term smoker who is 62-year-old, weighs 110 kg. He had the following ECG recorded at his local hospital. Which of the following is the mean electrical axis calculated from standard Leads I, II and III shown in his ECG?

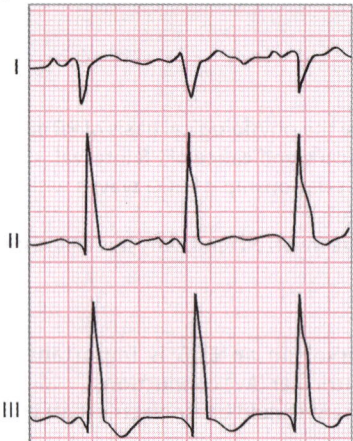

  a. –110°
  b. –20°
  c. +90°
  d. +105°

**Q7.** The phases of the ventricular muscle action potential is given below:

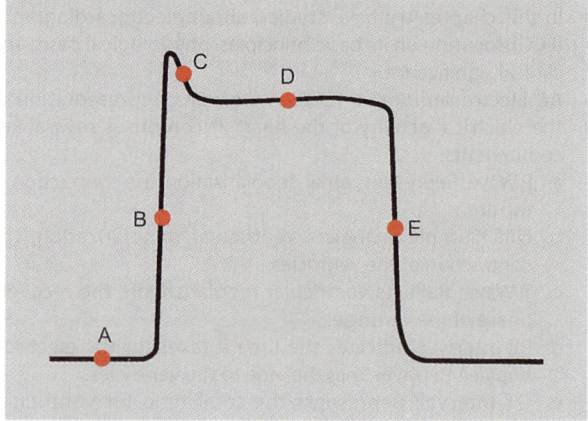

At which point on the above ventricular action potential is membrane potential most dependent on calcium permeability?
  a. Point B
  b. Point C
  c. Point D
  d. Point E

**Q8.** The 58-year-old male is brought to cardiac emergency unit with chest pain. From his symptoms and lab diagnosis, he is diagnosed with inferior wall myocardial infarction. His ECG shows ST segment elevation and T wave inversion. Which phase of cardiac cycle is affected in this patient?
  a. Atrial depolarization and repolarization
  b. Ventricular depolarization and repolarization
  c. Ventricular repolarization
  d. Ventricular depolarization

**Q9.** What is the mean cardiac axis of a patient if the net magnitude of Lead I is +6mV, Lead II is +10 mV and lead III is +5mV. It shows
  a. Right axis deviation
  b. Left axis deviation
  c. Data is insufficient
  d. Normal axis, no deviation

**Q10.** How is the heart rate, calculated in the given ECG strip, recorded at 25 mm/sec?

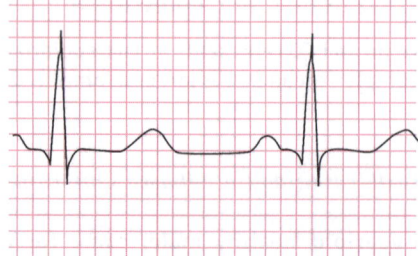

a. 25 × 60/RR interval (in mm)
b. 1500/RR interval (in cm)
c. 25/RR interval (in cm)
d. 150/RR interval (in mm)

Q11. ECG (electrocardiogram) was developed first by:
   a. Wilhelm His
   b. Steward
   c. Hubert Mann
   d. Willem Einthoven

Q12. A normal ECG report must consist of the following information:
   a. Rhythm, cardiac axis
   b. Conduction intervals
   c. Description of the ST segments, QRS complexes, T-waves
   d. All of these

Q13. For the normal heartbeat, depolarization stimulus originates in:
   a. His-bundle areas
   b. Epicardium
   c. Sinoatrial (SA) node
   d. Atrioventricular (AV) node

Q14. P wave indicates:
   a. Depolarization of right ventricle
   b. Depolarization of left ventricle
   c. Depolarization of both atria
   d. Atria to ventricular conduction time

Q15. Ventricular muscle depolarization is indicated by:
   a. PR interval
   b. P wave
   c. U wave
   d. The QRS complex

**ANSWERS**

1. b    2. c    3. c    4. d    5. d    6. d    7. c    8. c    9. d    10. a    11. d    12. d    13. c    14. c    15. d

# Physiological Basis of Abnormalities of Electrocardiogram

**CHAPTER 38**

> **COMPETENCY ADDRESSED**
>
> **PY5.6:** Describe abnormal electrocardiogram (ECG), arrhythmias, heart block and myocardial Infarction.

> **LEARNING OBJECTIVES**
>
> At the end of this chapter, the learner should be able to:
> - Describe the physiological basis of abnormalities of cardiac rhythm, conduction, axis deviation and chamber enlargement on electrocardiogram.
> - Describe the physiological basis of analysis of ECG report.

In the previous chapter, we discussed the wave patterns of normal electrocardiogram (ECG) in all the standard leads. Once we have recorded the ECG, it is analyzed for:

- Heart rate
- Rhythm
- Conduction
- Cardiac axis
- Chamber size
- Changes in wave pattern (as seen in electrolyte disturbances)

## HEART RATE

The heart rate is calculated from the ECG by measuring the RR interval (in mm). At the paper speed of 25 mm/s, the heart rate is calculated by the formula:

$$\text{Paper speed} \times \frac{60}{\text{RR interval (in mm)}} = \frac{1500}{\text{RR interval (in mm)}}$$

## RHYTHM

The normal ECG shows the regular rhythm, i.e., every beat follows the previous beat at the regular interval. The normal sinus rhythm results in a heart rate between 60–100 beats/min. Any alteration in the sinus rhythm is called arrythmia (Fig. 38.1).

The physiological and pathological variations of heart rate are discussed in Chapter 41 in detail.

**Arrhythmias (abnormality of rhythm) (Table 38.1)**

- **Sinus arrhythmia:** It is the variation in sinus rhythm with respiration. It is very clearly observed in children.
    - The heart rate increases with inspiration
    - The heart rate decreases with expiration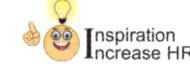
- **Sinus tachycardia:** Increase in heart rate >100 beats/min.
    - *Physiologically*, it occurs during sympathetic stimulation such as anxiety, exercise etc.
    - *Pathologically*, it occurs during **F**ever, **A**nemia and **T**hyrotoxicosis (Tip: **FAT**achy)
- **Sinus bradycardia:** Decrease in heart rate <60 beats/min.
    - *Physiologically it is seen in trained athletes due to increased vagal tone in them.*
    - *Pathologically*, bradycardia is the most important sign of hypothyroidism.

The chain reaction mechanism of current flow is demonstrated by brief exposure of the cardiac muscle to 60 Hz alternating current, as seen in electric shock. It results in spread of impulse in all directions, leaving multiple

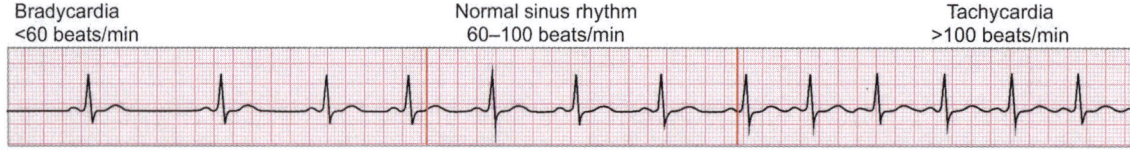

**Fig. 38.1:** Sinus rhythm.

**Table 38.1:** Differences between atrial and ventricular rhythm disorders.

| Disorder | Atrial | Ventricular |
|---|---|---|
| Ectopic | Premature beat, abnormal P wave and normal QRS complex | Abnormal wide QRS complexes with abnormal ST-T change followed by long pause called as compensatory pause<br><br>Ventricular ectopic |
| Tachycardia | Abnormal P waves occurring at higher rate (150–250 beats/min), normal QRS complexes, all P waves not conducted<br><br>Atrial tachycardia | Abnormal wide QRS complexes with abnormal ST-T change without identifiable P waves<br><br>Ventricular tachycardia |
| Flutter | Atrial rate 250–350 beats/min, undulating abnormal P waves (flutter waves), Saw toothed appearance<br><br>Saw tooth appearance<br>Atrial flutter | Large, wide, monophasic, bizarre QRS complexes, P and T waves not identifiable<br>Ghost waves (dire emergency)<br><br>Ventricular flutter |
| Fibrillation | Widely variable RR interval, atrial rate >350/min, irregularly irregular pulse, P waves are totally absent or wide variability (fibrillatory waves), variable degrees of AV block<br><br>Atrial fibrillation | Bizarre QRS complexes, extremely serious and terminal arrhythmia, may end in cardiac arrest<br><br>Ventricular fibrillation |

areas of depolarization and refractory period in the muscle. Some areas repolarize faster than others resulting in islands of refractory muscle. The impulse generated travels through excitable areas and sets in multiple pathways of current flow resulting in fibrillation.

### What will happen, if a patient is exposed to 60 Hz AC current?

Islands of refractory muscle result in irregular spread of cardiac impulse

Chain reaction of current flow sets in resulting in ventricular fibrillation

Physiology of chain reaction set in on brief exposure to 60 Hz alternating current.

### Role of defibrillator in controlling this chain reaction (Fig. 38.2)

The defibrillator is a machine that delivers a high voltage of direct current (1,000 V) to the fibrillating cardiac muscle resulting in the refractory period of the entire ventricular mass. Hence, it helps to restore the rhythm of fibrillating ventricle.

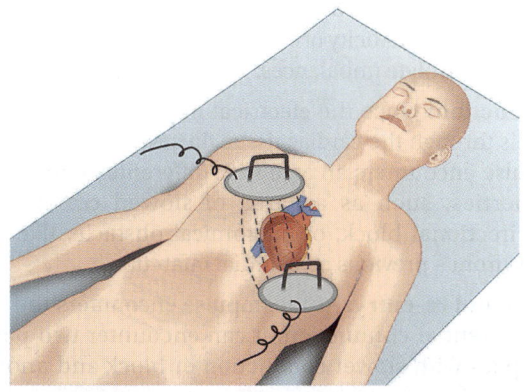

**Fig. 38.2:** Mechanism of action of defibrillator.

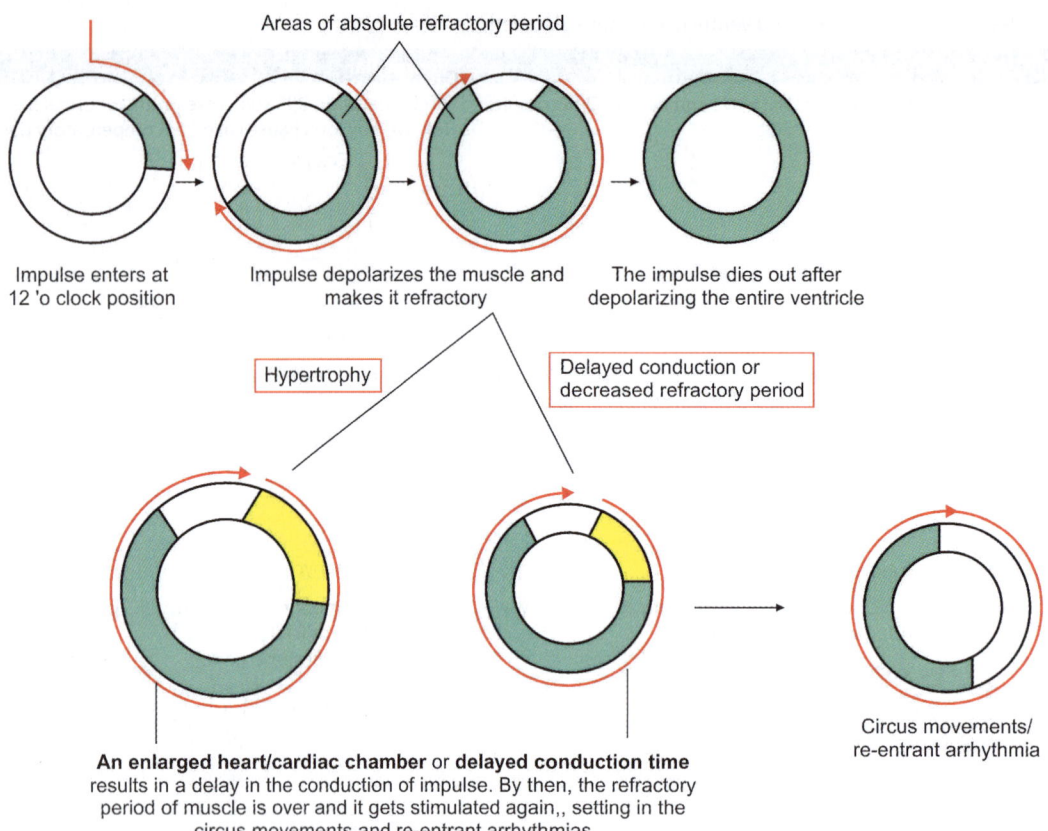

**Fig. 38.3:** Physiology of re-entrant current resulting in circus movements.

## DISORDERS OF RHYTHM

### Physiology of Re-entrant Currents Causing Circus Movements (Fig. 38.3)

They resulting in circus movements are a fundamental aspect of certain cardiac arrhythmias. This phenomenon occurs when an electrical impulse in the heart circulates repeatedly around a re-entry pathway, leading to sustained and often rapid heart rhythms. Let's break down the physiology of re-entrant currents resulting in circus movements:

**Initiation:** The re-entry circuit begins with the initiation of an electrical impulse in the heart. This impulse can be triggered by various factors, such as ectopic beats, abnormal automaticity of cardiac cells, or triggered activity due to electrolyte imbalances.

**Conduction:** Once the electrical impulse is initiated, it travels through the cardiac tissue. In cases of re-entry, the impulse encounters an area with differential conduction properties, such as an area of slowed conduction, unidirectional block, or anatomical obstacle, like scar tissue from a previous myocardial infarction.

**Block and re-entry:** As the impulse encounters the area of differential conduction, it can encounter two paths: one path with slower conduction or block and another with faster conduction. The impulse travels along the faster path and exits the region, while simultaneously, due to refractoriness or anatomical constraints, it cannot proceed through the slower path. Instead, it returns to the region where it originated from, setting up a re-entry circuit.

**Circus movement:** The impulse re-enters the excitable tissue and continues to circulate around the re-entry pathway, perpetuating a circular or spiral movement of electrical activity. This repetitive circuit of electrical activation leads to a sustained, often rapid, and irregular heart rhythm characteristic of certain arrhythmias, such as atrial flutter or ventricular tachycardia.

Circus movements are self-sustaining because the re-entry circuit can perpetuate itself without the need for external stimuli. As long as the conditions necessary for re-entry persist, such as the presence of unidirectional block or slowed conduction, the circus movement can continue indefinitely.

Circus movements can terminate spontaneously if the conditions supporting the re-entry circuit change. For example, alterations in refractoriness, changes in autonomic tone, or interventions like antiarrhythmic medications or electrical cardioversion can disrupt the re-entry circuit and restore normal sinus rhythm.

For the remaining arrhythmias refer to **Table 38.1**

## DISORDERS OF CONDUCTION

The cardiac impulse travels from SA node to AV node through the internodal branches and then passes on to the ventricles through the bundle of His. In normal course, the conduction of the impulse is recorded on the ECG as a P wave is followed by the QRS complex hence we say that the P waves are conducted. If they P waves are not conducted it is referred to as a *heart block* or *conduction block*. Another type of conduction defect which is seen is the presence of the aberrant conducting tissue in between the atria and the ventricles called as *Wolff-Parkinson-White syndrome*. Let's discuss both these conditions one by one.

### Heart Block

Heart block is defined as a defect of conduction of the cardiac impulse where the impulse is not allowed to travel beyond the blockage. The conduction blocks can occur due to the ischemia of the conducting pathways. Depending on the site of blockage they are classified as:
- Atrioventricular blocks
- Bundle branch blocks

#### Atrioventricular Block

This refers to the blockage of impulse from the SA node to the AV node. The AV block can be partial or complete depending on the conduction of the P waves hence they are classified as:
- *Incomplete block some P waves are not conducted*
    - First degree block
    - Second degree block
        - Mobitz type I or Wenckebach phenomenon
        - Mobitz type II
- *Complete block all P waves are not conducted*
    - Third degree block

### FIRST DEGREE HEART BLOCK

It is characterized by a *long PR interval (>0.20 sec)*; impulse is taking a long time to travel from SA node to AV node.

Physiologically, it can be seen in increased vagal tone or athletic training. It is also seen in certain pathological conditions like inferior wall myocardial infarction, myocarditis, hyperkalemia and in patients on beta blockers or other drugs which increase the AV nodal delay. If PR interval becomes >0.30 sec, the P waves get buried in the T waves.

### SECOND DEGREE HEART BLOCK

(Some P waves are **NOT** conducted)
- **Mobitz type I:** There is *progressive lengthening of PR interval till one P wave is not conducted*, i.e., it does

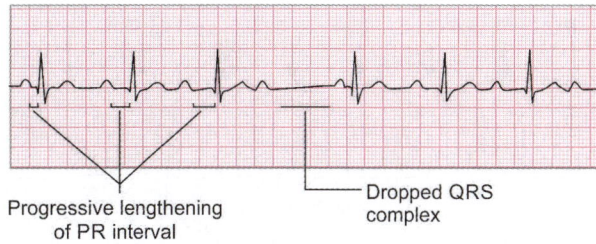

**Fig. 38.4:** Mobitz type I.

not have a QRS complex "dropped beat", also called as *Wenckebach phenomenon* (Fig. 38.4).

It can occur in people:
- With increased vagal tone
- On medications like beta blockers, calcium channel blockers, etc.
- Inferior wall myocardial infarction
- Myocarditis
- After valvular surgeries, damaging the conductive system.

- **Mobitz type II:** In this type of block *some P waves are conducted while others are not, depending upon this categorized as 2:1, 3:1, 4:1 block*. A 2:1 block means that every second P wave is not followed by a QRS complex, similarly a 3:1 block means that every third P wave is not followed by a QRS complex and so on. Hence, we can see continued marching of P waves with variable appearance of QRS complexes. It is usually associated with the bifascicular block (in bundle of His) (Fig. 38.5).

It is seen in patients with:
- Anterior wall myocardial infarction
- Hyperkalemia
- Myocarditis
- Medications such as beta blockers, calcium channel blockers

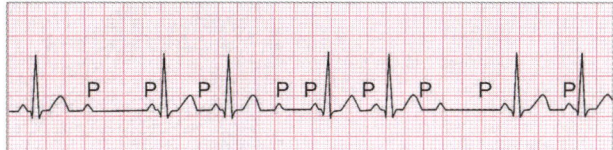

**Fig. 38.5:** Mobitz type II.

### COMPLETE HEART BLOCK

It is the serious form of the heart block where none of the P waves are conducted and there is no fixed PR interval (Fig. 38.6). The ventricles generate their own *idioventricular rhythm (30–40 beats/min)* and there is no coordination between the atrial and ventricular activity. This results in asynchronous activity and fall in the cardiac output. In case, the complete heart block sets up suddenly, thus a patient of *Stokes-Adams syndrome* (sudden onset complete heart block) usually presents with sudden attack of dizziness and fainting (syncope).

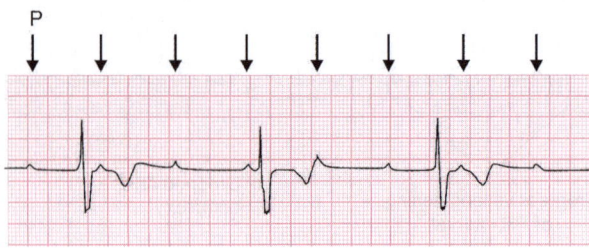

**Fig. 38.6:** Complete heart block.

## SICK SINUS SYNDROME

- Sick sinus syndrome (SSS) is a condition of the sinoatrial node that develops over time such that the SA node is unable to perform its function as the pacemaker of the heart. It most commonly affects the elderly and is often idiopathic.
- **Multiple manifestations on the ECG:** Sinus bradycardia, sinoatrial block, and alternating tachycardia/bradycardia. Thus, it is also known as *tachybrady syndrome*.

---

**Accelerated AV conduction/Pre-excitation syndrome [Wolff-Parkinson-White (WPW) syndrome]**

*A 42-year-old male patient arrived at the emergency department with sudden onset of palpitation and giddiness. He gave a history of similar episodes from the last 12 years. There is no significant history of chronic medication, drugs or substance abuse. His vitals show an increased heart rate with normal blood pressure. The cardiovascular examination was not significant, but his electrocardiogram (ECG) shows narrow QRS complexes with a slurred upstroke (delta wave) PR interval was shortened.*

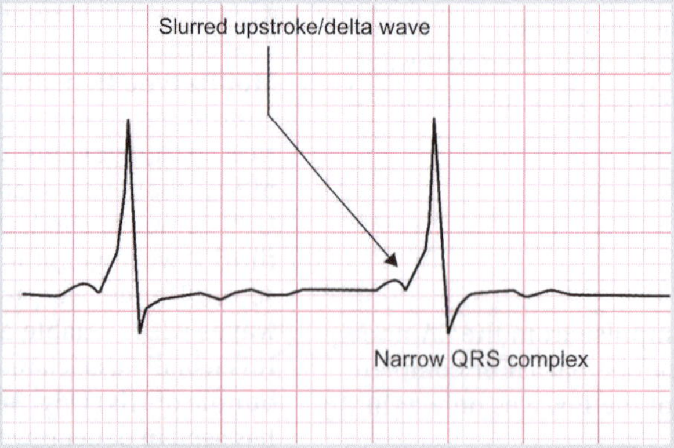

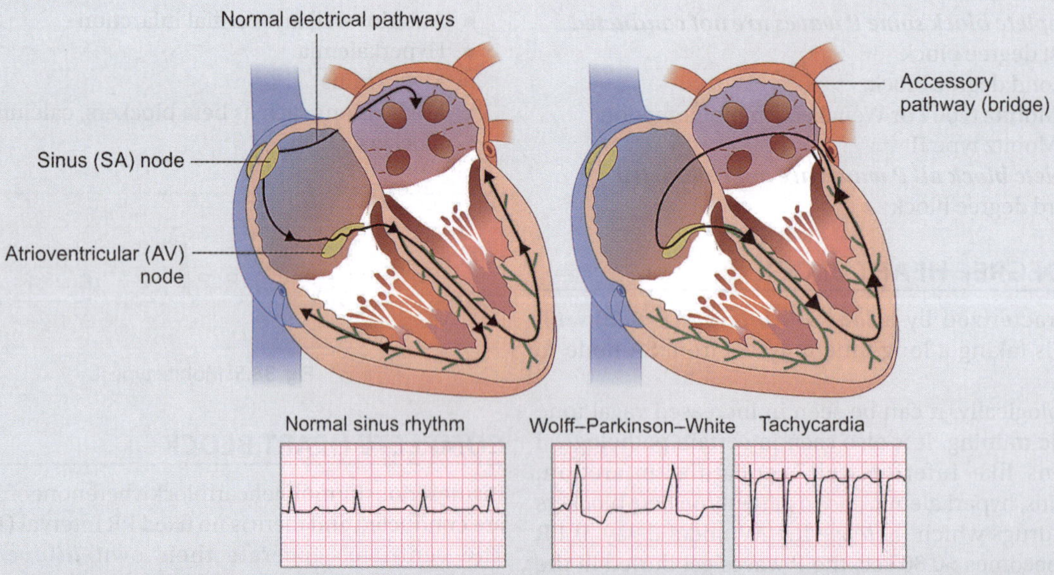

The ECG of this patient is suggestive of pre-excitation syndrome called as WPW syndrome, which occurs due to an additional aberrant nodal tissue connection between atria and ventricles (Bundle of Kent). This conducts more rapidly than AV node and one ventricle is excited early hence resulting in a short PR interval along with a slurred upstroke of QRS complex (delta wave) and narrow QRS complex. There is accompanied by atrial tachycardia resulting in palpitation and syncopal attack. These patients require radio-ablation of the aberrant conductive tissue resulting in pre-excitation.

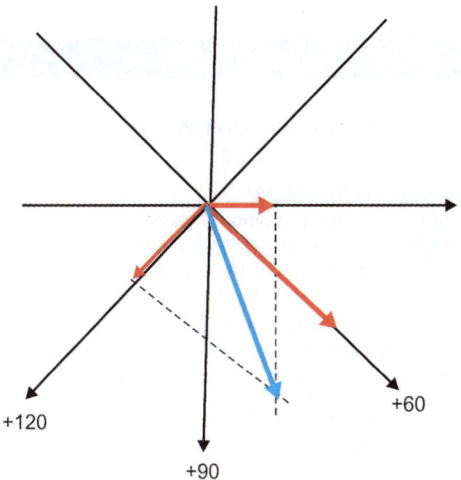

**Fig. 38.7:** Axis deviation.

## AXIS DEVIATION (FIG. 38.7)

- Normal cardiac axis → –30 to +110°
- If axis is lying to left of –30° left axis deviation
- If axis is lying to right of +110° right axis deviation

### Axis Calculation

Lead I: Net magnitude +5 mm
Lead II: Net magnitude +15 mm
Lead III: Net magnitude +10 mm

## CHAMBER ENLARGEMENT

Various cardiological disorders have implications on chamber enlargement. This can be of any side and any chamber depending upon the condition. This can be seen on ECG as shown in **Table 38.2**.

## MYOCARDIAL INFARCTION

Electrocardiogram shows typical findings during myocardial ischemia and infarction These changes occur due to the current of injury resulting from the dipole created between the healthy and injured muscle during the period between complete depolarization and beginning of repolarization of heart, i.e., during the ST segment in the respective chest leads.

- The cardiac ischemia presents as ST **segment depression, T wave inversion.**
- Myocardial injury presents as ST **elevation and upward convexity.**
- However, myocardial infarction (**Fig. 38.8**) is characterized by:
  - **Appearance of Q waves**
  - **ST elevation**
  - **T wave inversion**

## ELECTROLYTE DISTURBANCES IN ECG

Electrolyte disturbances can manifest on an ECG through various abnormalities such as prolonged QT intervals, T-wave changes, and arrhythmias. Recognizing these patterns is crucial in identifying underlying electrolyte imbalances like hyperkalemia or hypokalemia, guiding prompt intervention to restore electrolyte balance and prevent potentially life-threatening cardiac complications (**Table 38.3**).

**Table 38.2:** Electrocardiogram findings in different chamber enlargement conditions.

| | Right side | Left side |
|---|---|---|
| Atrial hypertrophy (P waves in lead II, $V_1$ and $V_2$) | Amplitude of P wave >2.5 mm | Width if P wave >2.5 mm (>0.1s) |
| Ventricular hypertrophy | Tall R waves in leads $V_1$ and $V_2$ Deep S waves in leads $V_5$ and $V_6$ | • Amplitude of R wave in leads $V_5$ and $V_6$ ≥25 mm<br>• Amplitude of S wave in leads $V_1$ and $V_2$ ≥20 mm<br>• Sum of amplitudes of R wave in leads $V_5$ and $V_6$ and S wave in leads $V_1$ and $V_2$ ≥35 mm |

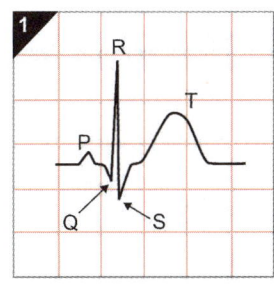
Normal ECG

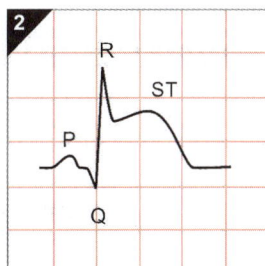

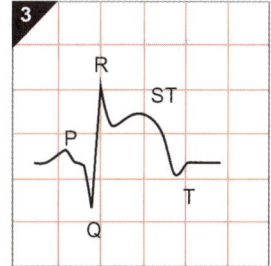
Early myocardial injury showing ST elevation and T wave inversion

**Fig. 38.8:** Electrocardiogram changes in myocardial infarction.

Table 38.3: Electrocardiogram (ECG) changes in electrolyte disturbances.

| Electrolyte | Normal range | ECG changes in decreased level (Hypo) | ECG changes in increased level (Hyper) |
|---|---|---|---|
| Sodium | 135–145 mmol/L | **Hyponatremia**<br>• No effect on rhythm or conduction<br>• Results in low voltage graph | **Hypernatremia**<br>No effect on rhythm or conduction |
| Potassium | 3.5–5.5 mmol/L | **Hypokalemia (Fig. 38.9A)**<br>• Wide T wave, ST depression (T wave inversion can occur in severe cases)<br>• P waves amplitude, duration and PR interval increase<br>• U waves appear in leads $V_2$ and $V_3$<br>• It can result in long QT syndrome (LQTS) | **Hyperkalemia (Fig. 38.9B)**<br>• **Mild** (<6.0 mmol/L): Pointed T waves<br>• **Moderate** (6–7.5 mmol/L): Pointed T waves, wide P wave with decreased amplitude. Conduction blocks can occur.<br>• **Severe** (>7.5 mmol/L): All above changes become more pronounced. Wide QRS complexes, which may fuse with T wave resulting in sine wave pattern. This may result in ventricular fibrillation |
| Calcium | 8.5–10 mg/dL | **Hypocalcemia (Fig. 38.9C)**<br>• Lengthened QT interval<br>• Nodal block | **Hypercalcemia (Fig. 38.9D)**<br>• Shortened QT interval<br>• Lengthened QRS duration<br>• Bradycardia |

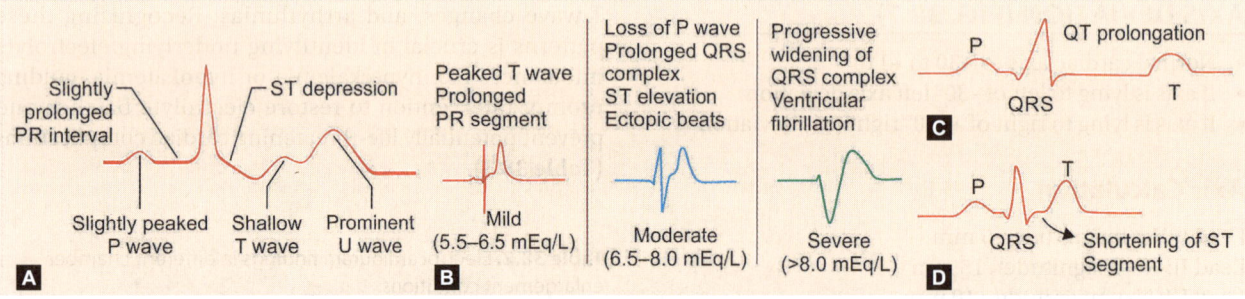

**Figs. 38.9A to D:** ECG changes in (A) Hypokalemia; (B) Hyperkalemia; (C) Hypocalcemia; (D) Hypercalcemia.

## SUMMARY

In this chapter we have further explored the clinical significance of the ECG. We had learnt about the basic analysis of ECG in terms of:
- Calculating the heart rate by measuring the distance between two R waves (R-R interval).
- Analyzing the rhythm of ECG as regular or irregular. The irregularity with respiration is called as the sinus arrythmia, while the normal rhythm produced by SA node, is called as sinus rhythm.

This rhythm can be disturbed in the patients experiencing ectopic beats, flutter and fibrillation.
- The mean cardiac axis is 59 degrees (-30 to +110 degrees). It can be calculated by plotting the net potential of the bipolar limb leads. Hence, it can be used for axis deviation.
- The pattern of waves, segments and intervals are analyzed for various abnormalities.
- The chamber enlargement can also be diagnosed from the ECG.

## LET US SEE, WHAT YOU HAVE LEARNT?

 *Review Questions*

Q1. Define sinus arrhythmia.
Q2. Describe the second degree heart block.
Q3. Describe the mechanism of action of defibrillator in a patient of fibrillation.

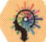 *Critical Thinking Case-Based Questions*

Q1. A 35-year-old man presented in emergency with palpitations. He has been drinking heavily with friends over the weekend. This is his ECG.

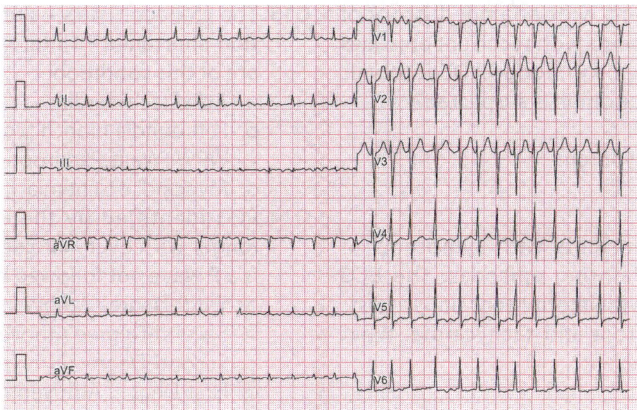

a. What is the diagnosis?
b. Explain the physiological reason behind this condition.
c. What are the investigations and treatment?

Q2. A 45-year-old businessman presented in emergency with a feeling that his heart is racing. He also has some shortness of breath. This is his ECG.

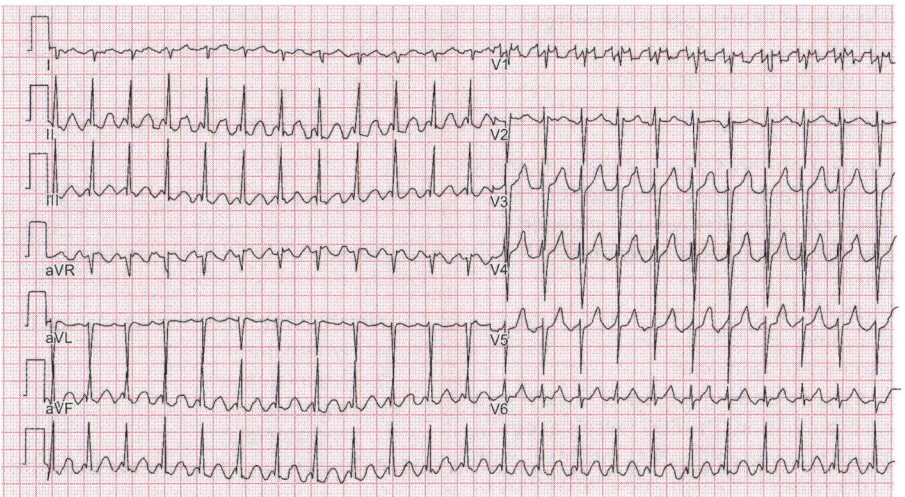

a. What is the diagnosis?
b. Explain the physiological reason behind this condition.
c. What are the investigations and treatment?

## Multiple Choice Questions

Q1. A 55-year-old male patient with a history of hypertension presents to the emergency department with chest pain. The ECG reveals ST-segment elevation in leads II, III, and aVF. What is the most likely diagnosis?
   a. Myocardial infarction involving the inferior wall
   b. Atrial fibrillation
   c. Ventricular tachycardia
   d. Left ventricular hypertrophy

Q2. A 40-year-old female patient presents with palpitations and dizziness. On ECG, irregularly irregular QRS complexes are observed, and no distinct P waves are visible. What arrhythmia is suspected?
   a. Atrial fibrillation
   b. Sinus bradycardia
   c. Ventricular fibrillation
   d. Paroxysmal supraventricular tachycardia (PSVT)

Q3. A 60-year-old male patient complains of shortness of breath and swelling in the legs. The ECG shows evidence of atrial enlargement with a prolonged P wave duration (>120 ms) in lead II. Which condition is most likely present?
   a. Atrial fibrillation      b. Left atrial enlargement
   c. Right atrial enlargement  d. Ventricular hypertrophy

Q4. A 65-year-old female patient with a history of diabetes and hypertension presents with crushing chest pain radiating to the left arm. The ECG shows ST-segment depression and T-wave inversion in leads V1-V4. What is the most likely diagnosis?
   a. Non-ST-segment elevation myocardial infarction (NSTEMI)
   b. Atrial fibrillation
   c. Ventricular tachycardia
   d. Pericarditis

Q5. A 50-year-old male patient with a family history of sudden cardiac death presents with recurrent episodes of syncope. The ECG reveals prolonged QT intervals (>450 ms). What cardiac condition is suspected?
   a. Long QT syndrome
   b. Wolff-Parkinson-White syndrome
   c. Brugada syndrome
   d. Sick sinus syndrome

Q6. A 70-year-old patient presents with symptoms of dizziness, fatigue, and fainting episodes. The ECG shows sinus bradycardia with intermittent sinus arrests and alternating bradycardia and tachycardia. What condition is most likely present?
   a. Sick sinus syndrome
   b. Atrial fibrillation
   c. Ventricular tachycardia
   d. Wolff-Parkinson-White syndrome

Q7. A 60-year-old patient with a history of myocardial infarction presents with syncope. The ECG reveals regular P waves, but not all P waves are followed by QRS complexes. What type of heart block is suspected?
   a. First-degree heart block
   b. Mobitz Type I (Wenckebach) heart block
   c. Mobitz Type II heart block
   d. Third-degree heart block

Q8. A 25-year-old patient presents with palpitations and a history of intermittent rapid heart rates. The ECG shows a shortened PR interval, a delta wave, and widened QRS complexes. What condition is most likely present?
   a. Atrial fibrillation
   b. Ventricular tachycardia
   c. Sick sinus syndrome
   d. Wolff-Parkinson-White syndrome

Q9. A 20-year-old patient undergoes an ECG during a routine physical examination. The ECG reveals a regular rhythm with heart rate variability that increases with inspiration and decreases with expiration. What type of arrhythmia is observed?
   a. Sinus bradycardia
   b. Sinus tachycardia
   c. Sinus arrhythmia
   d. Sinus arrest

Q10. This is the classic ECG change in MI (myocardial infarction).
   a. ST-segment elevation
   b. T-wave inversion
   c. Development of an abnormal Q wave
   d. All of these

Q11. In which of these conditions can widen QRS and Tall-tented T waves be observed?
   a. Hyponatremia
   b. Hyperkalemia
   c. Hyperglycemia
   d. Hyperphosphatemia

Q12. Hypokalemia is the condition of low potassium levels in your blood. Hypokalemia ECG changes are observed by:
   a. ST segment elevation
   b. U wave (a position deflection after the T wave)
   c. Tall peaked T waves
   d. Widening of the QRS complex and increased amplitude

Q13. The characteristics—slurring of the initial QRS deflection, shortened PR interval, and prolonged QRS duration are of this condition:
   a. Atrial tachycardia
   b. Left bundle branch block
   c. WPW (Wolff-Parkinson-White) syndrome
   d. Myocardial ischemia

Q14. ECG identified by the PR interval tends to become longer with every succeeding ECG complex until there is a P wave not followed by a QRS is observed in:
   a. Third-Degree Atrioventricular Block
   b. Second-Degree Atrioventricular Block, Type II
   c. Second-Degree Atrioventricular Block, Type I
   d. First-Degree Atrioventricular Block, Type II

Q15. A 65-year-old male with a history of renal failure presents to the emergency room with weakness and palpitations. On examination, his blood pressure is 160/90 mm Hg, heart rate is 82 bpm, and respiratory rate is 20 breaths/min. An ECG is ordered and reveals tall, peaked T waves.

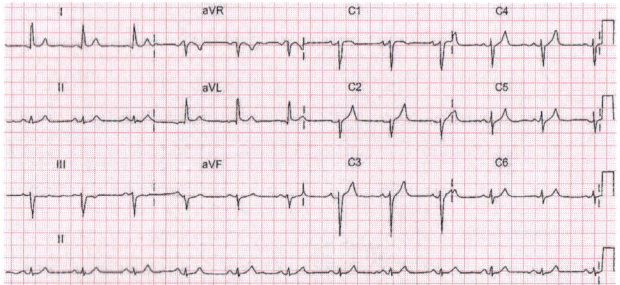

Which of the following is the most likely diagnosis?
   a. Hypernatremia
   b. Hyperkalemia
   c. Hypocalcemia
   d. Hypokalemia

Q16. A 70-year-old male presents to the cardiology clinic for a routine follow-up appointment. He has a history of hypertension, heart failure with reduced ejection fraction, and chronic obstructive pulmonary disease. He reports occasional palpitations but denies any other symptoms. On examination, his heart rate is irregularly irregular at 90 bpm, blood pressure is 140/90 mm Hg, and lung auscultation reveals scattered wheezes. An ECG reveals absence of distinct P waves and irregularly spaced QRS complexes. What is the most likely diagnosis?

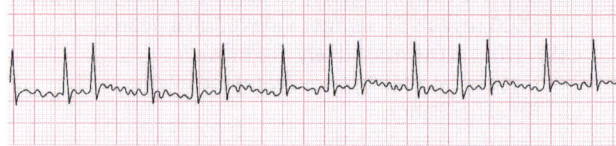

   a. Atrial flutter
   b. Ventricular fibrillation
   c. Atrial fibrillation
   d. Sinus rhythm with frequent premature ventricular contractions

Q17. A 25-year-old female presents to her primary care physician for a routine check-up. She mentions feeling well overall but reports occasional episodes of feeling her heart racing, especially when she takes deep breaths.

She denies any other symptoms. On examination, her heart rate is noted to vary with her breathing cycle, increasing during inspiration and decreasing during expiration. Which of the following conditions is most likely responsible for her symptoms?

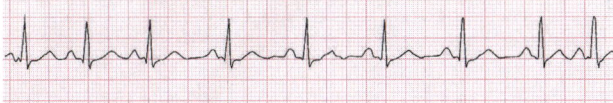

a. Sinus bradycardia
b. Sinus tachycardia
c. Sinus arrhythmia
d. Atrial fibrillation

Q18. A 55-year-old male with a history of myocardial infarction and heart failure presents to the emergency room complaining of sudden onset palpitations and dizziness. He appears diaphoretic and anxious. His blood pressure is 90/60 mm Hg, heart rate is 180 bpm, and respiratory rate is 24 breaths/min. An ECG shows wide QRS complexes with a rate of 180 bpm, lack of discernible P waves, and an irregular rhythm. Which of the following is the most likely diagnosis?

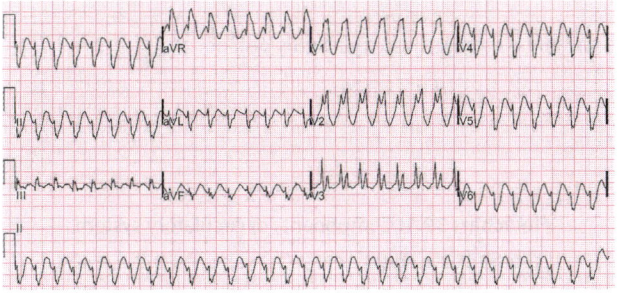

a. Sinus tachycardia
b. Atrial fibrillation
c. Ventricular fibrillation
d. Ventricular tachycardia

Q19. A 45-year-old male with a history of untreated hypertension presents to the emergency room complaining of chest pain and shortness of breath. Suddenly, he becomes unresponsive, and his pulse cannot be palpated. The monitor shows a rapid, chaotic rhythm with no discernible QRS complexes or organized electrical activity. CPR is immediately initiated, and a code blue is called. The team prepares to administer advanced cardiac life support (ACLS) protocols. What is the most likely cardiac rhythm disturbance in this scenario?

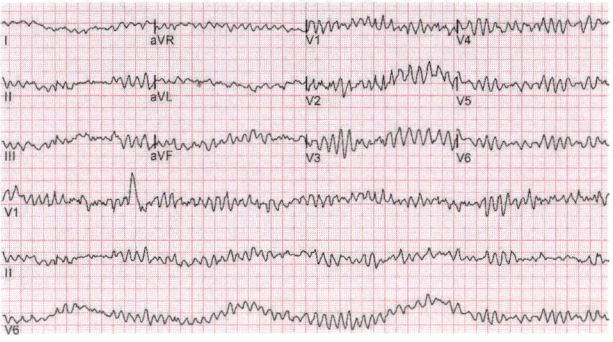

a. Sinus tachycardia
b. Atrial fibrillation
c. Ventricular fibrillation
d. Ventricular tachycardia

Q20. A 60-year-old male collapses suddenly while playing tennis. Bystanders rush to his aid and find him unresponsive with no pulse. CPR is initiated, and an automated external defibrillator (AED) is brought to the scene. The AED pads are placed on the patient's chest, and a shockable rhythm is detected. The AED charges and delivers a shock. Which of the following best describes the mechanism of action of defibrillation in this scenario?

a. Stimulation of the heart to increase cardiac output
b. Restoration of normal sinus rhythm by synchronized pacing
c. Interruption of chaotic electrical activity to allow the heart's natural pacemaker to regain control
d. Induction of temporary asystole to reset the heart's electrical system
e. Prevention of further electrical impulses from reaching the heart

## ANSWERS

1. a  2. a  3. b  4. a  5. a  6. a  7. c  8. d  9. c  10. d  11. b  12. b  13. c  14. c
15. b  16. c  17. c  18. d  19. c  20. c

# Circulation and Hemodynamics

**CHAPTER 39**

### COMPETENCY ADDRESSED
PY5.7: Describe and discuss hemodynamics of circulatory system.

### LEARNING OBJECTIVES
**At the end of this chapter, the learner should be able to:**
- Describe general organization of circulatory system.
- Describe the principles of hemodynamics (interrelation of flow, pressure and resistance) in the circulatory system.
- Describe the factors affecting the blood flow in the circulatory system.
- Describe the regulation of blood flow in the circulatory system.
- Describe the relevant clinical correlations, wherever applicable.

## CIRCULATORY SYSTEM

The circulatory system forms an important part of the cardiovascular system. It comprises of both the major divisions of the circulatory system viz. systemic circulation or greater circulation and pulmonary circulation or lesser circulation. Some of the main functions of circulation are as follows:

**Primary functions:**
- Distribution of nutrients and oxygen to all body cells
- Collection of waste products and $CO_2$ from all body cells to excretory system

**Secondary functions:**
- Thermoregulation
- Distribution of hormones to the target tissues
- Delivery of antibodies, platelets, and leukocytes to aid body defense mechanisms.

The main components of circulator system are aorta, large elastic arteries, small muscular arteries, arterioles, meta-arterioles and through fare channels, capillaries, venules, large veins, inferior and superior vena cava, in a sequence arising from left ventricle and ending in right atrium (**Flowchart 39.1**).

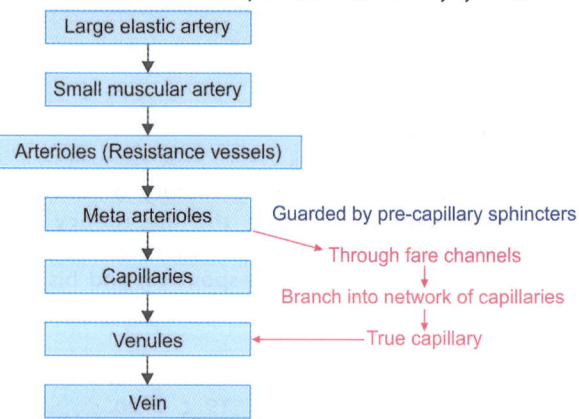

Flowchart 39.1: Components of circulatory system.

The main differences in the major divisions of circulation are shown in **Table 39.1**.

## Windkessel Effect (Fig. 39.3)

This effect is responsible for the continuous flow of blood in blood vessels even during the diastolic phase of cardiac

**Table 39.1:** Differences between artery, arteriole, capillary and veins.

|  | Artery | Arteriole | Capillary | Veins |
|---|---|---|---|---|
| Histology | Strong vascular wall with abundant elastic tissue | Strong vascular wall with less elastic tissue and more smooth muscle | Single-layered, thin-walled having minute pores. Precapillary sphincters are present at the opening of capillaries | Thin walled with smooth muscle, elastic fibers are less, valves are present |

*Contd...*

Contd...

|  | Artery | Arteriole | Capillary | Veins |
|---|---|---|---|---|
| **Pressure (Fig. 39.1)** | *'High pressure system'.* The systolic pressure is 120 mm Hg and diastolic pressure is 80 mm Hg. | *'High pressure system'.* The systolic pressure is 120 mm Hg and diastolic pressure is 80 mm Hg. Mean systemic arterial pressure: 95 mm Hg | *Low pressure.* There is no systolic or diastolic pressure. The flow is continuous with pressure at the arterial end of 35 mm Hg and at venous end of 10 mm Hg. Mean systemic capillary pressure is 17 mm Hg | *'Low pressure system'* The pressure in the veins gradually declines from 10 mm Hg (at venules) to 0 mm Hg (in IVC, when it reaches right atrium) |
|  | *In pulmonary circulation* |  |  |  |
|  | Systolic BP: 25 mm Hg<br>Diastolic BP: 8 mm Hg | Systolic BP: 25 mm Hg<br>Diastolic BP: 8 mm Hg<br>Mean pulmonary arterial pressure: 16 mm Hg | Mean pulmonary capillary pressure: 7 mm Hg |  |
| **Functions** | Transports blood under high pressure. Maintain blood flow during diastole by the elastic recoil *(Windkessel effect)* | Acts as control conduits or STOPCOCKS. Due to abundant smooth muscle and high sympathetic innervation, they act as **resistance vessels** | *'Exchange vessels':* Exchange of gases and nutrients | *'Capacitance vessels':* Acts as a *reservoir* of blood |
| **Lumen diameter** | Aorta—2.5 cm<br>Artery—0.4 cm | 30 µm | 5 µm at arterial end<br>9 µm at venous end | Venules—2 µm<br>Veins—0.5 cm<br>IVC—1.5 cm |
| **Wall thickness** | Aorta—2 mm<br>Artery—1 mm | 20 µm | 1 µm | Venule—2 mm<br>Veins—0.5 mm<br>IVC—1.5 mm |
| **Blood volume** | 13% | 2% | 5% | 64% |
|  | *Heart has 7% and pulmonary circulation has 9% blood* |  |  |  |
| **Cross sectional area** | Aorta—4.5 cm<br>Artery—20 cm | 400 cm | 4,500 cm | 4,000 cm<br>40 cm<br>18 cm |
| **Velocity of flow** | 22.5 m/s | 0.5 m/s | 0.6 m/s | 1.2 m/s |
| **Specific properties** | Windkessel vessel | Resistance vessels | Exchange vessels | Capacitance vessels |
| **Type of blood flow** | Phasic | Phasic but decrease during diastole is less | Continuous | Continuous |
| **Innervation (Fig. 39.2)** | Smooth muscles in the arteries are innervated by sympathetic nerves | High amount of smooth muscles have rich sympathetic innervation | Not innervated as the capillaries don't have the smooth muscles | Slight sympathetic innervation |
| **Effect of sympathetic stimulation** | Arterio-constriction | Arteriolar constriction increases the total peripheral resistance | No effect | Veno-constriction. It leads to the forward propulsion of blood toward the heart |

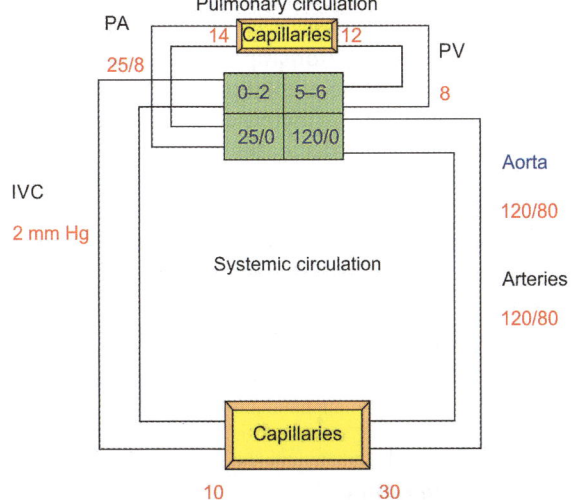

**Fig. 39.1:** Mean pressure (mmHg) in different parts of circulation.
(IVC: inferior vena cava; PA: pulmonary artery; PV: pulmonary vein)

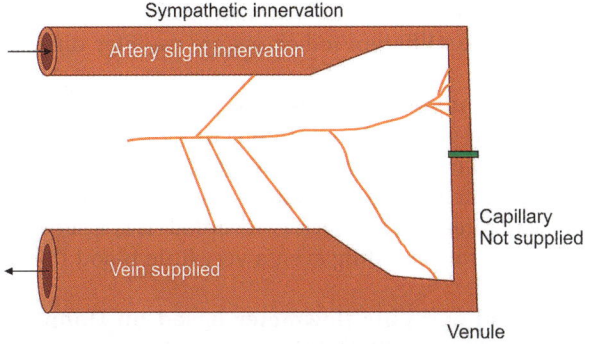

**Fig. 39.2:** Sympathetic innervation of different segments of circulation.

cycle. When the blood enters the aorta during systole, it stretches the walls of elastic arteries. The recoil produced by these arteries during diastole leads to the forward propulsion of blood.

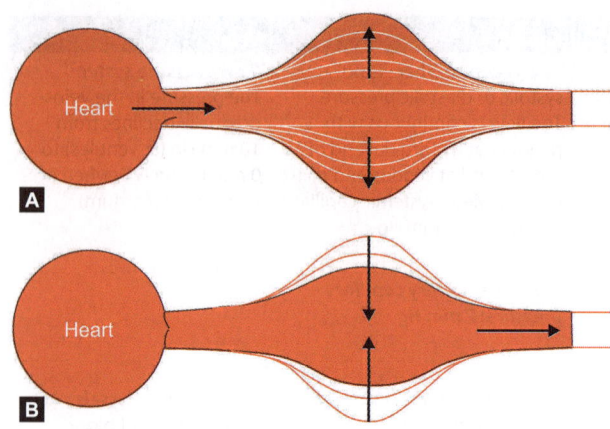

**Figs. 39.3A and B:** Windkessel effect: (A) During ventricular systole; (B) During ventricular diastole.

## HEMODYNAMICS

It refers to the study of various factors affecting blood flow, blood pressure and peripheral resistance in the body. It can be described as:
- **Blood flow and factors affecting it:** Pressure gradient, resistance, viscosity of blood.
- Types of blood flow
- Regulation of blood flow in different situations.

Let's discuss all these factors in detail.

### Blood Flow

Blood flow is defined as the *amount of blood passing from a given point within a specified time*. It is represented as mL/min or L/min. The cardiac output is the sum of the blood flow to all organs of the body.

### Measurement of Blood Flow

- **Fick's principle**: The blood flow to any organ can be measured using the method based on Fick's principle which *measures the consumption of the indicator substance by the organ and its arteriovenous* difference. Different indicators are used for different organs.
- **Electromagnetic flowmeter:** It is based on the principle on generation of electromotive force by a moving wire in magnetic field. When a magnetic field is generated around the blood vessel, carrying blood, it generates e.m.f., which is recorded. It is a sensitive method for recording even a very little blood flow in an organ.
- **Ultrasonographic flowmeter based on Doppler's principle (Fig. 39.4):** It is recorded by an ultrasonic device on which a minute piezo crystal is mounted which emits ultrasonic waves which get reflected from the moving red cells at a lower frequency, which are picked up by the crystal. This is called the Doppler's effect. It is also a sensitive method to record the blood flow in an organ.

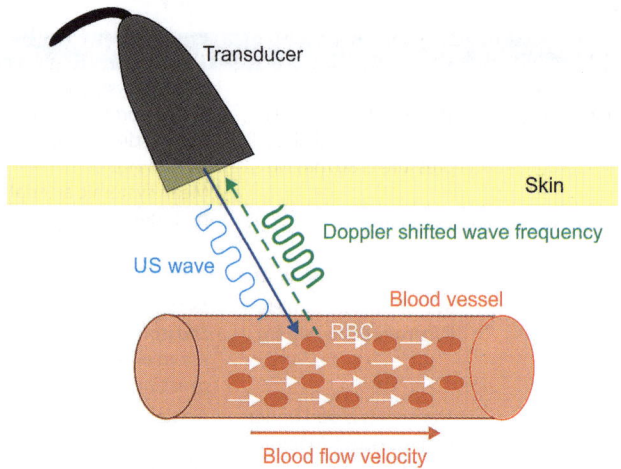

**Fig. 39.4:** Ultrasonographic flowmeter.

- **Para-aminohippuric acid clearance method:** It is the clearance method used to measure renal blood flow. It is discussed in detail in renal blood flow.
- **Plethysmography**

The various principles affecting the blood flow dynamics in circulation are based on the principles of fluid dynamics describing the interrelation of pressure (P), flow (Q) and resistance (R). The various principles/laws are discussed below.

### Hagen Poiseuille's Equation (Fig. 39.5)

Represents the factors affecting blood flow in a long narrow tube.

$$Q = \pi(P_1 - P_2)r^4/8\eta L$$

Q = blood flow
P1 – P2 = effective perfusion pressure
r = radius of blood vessel
L = length in cm
η = viscosity in poise

- **Pressure gradient:**
  - Pressure gradient in the circulation from arterial system to venous system results in constant blood flow in the circulation.
  - **Pressure flow relationship:** Usually the pressure is autoregulated in the circulation. Apart from creating a pressure gradient, an increased pressure distends the elastic vessels and decreases the vascular resistance (due to the stress relaxation property of smooth muscle) while fall in pressure collapses the blood vessels resulting in increased vascular resistance. If the pressure falls below a critical value, the blood

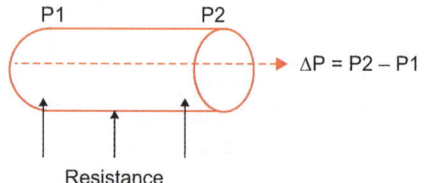

**Fig. 39.5:** Hagen Poiseuille's equation.

vessels become completely collapse, called *critical closing pressure*.

For rigid tube, the critical closing pressure is 0 mm Hg but for blood vessels it is **20 mm Hg for whole blood** and **5–10 mm Hg for plasma**. Under sympathetic stimulation, the critical closing pressure is 60 mm Hg, while during sympathetic inhibition, it is 0 mm Hg.

- **Vascular wall tension:** Transmural pressure gradient causes the stretching of vascular smooth muscle and endothelium resulting in production of shearing stress. It is expressed by the Laplace law, in which wall tension (T) is expressed in terms of pressure gradient (ΔP), radius of blood vessel (r) and thickness of blood vessels (h).

$$T = \Delta P \times \frac{r}{h}$$

Which means larger vessels, withstanding high pressures (elastic arteries) have thicker and reinforced walls while capillaries with lower pressures have delicate walls.

*A 57-year-old male complains of chest pain and visits a cardiologist. After the investigations and angiography, the cardiologist reports that there is 50% occlusion of left anterior descending artery. What do you think would have happened to coronary blood flow in this area?*

a. The coronary blood flow in left anterior descending is reduced by 50%
b. The coronary blood flow in left anterior descending is halved
c. The coronary blood flow in left anterior descending becomes 1/8th
d. The coronary blood flow in left anterior descending becomes 1/16th

*Answer:* d

- **Radius of blood vessel (r):** With the same pressure gradient and viscosity, radius of blood vessels play a very important role in blood flow. **Figure 39.6** shows that reducing the radius to half decreases the blood flow by 16 times, i.e., it varies by 4th power of radius.
- **Viscosity of blood:** The viscosity of blood is about 3 times the viscosity of water. Any clinical condition that alters the viscosity affects the blood flow. In anemia, there is a decrease in viscosity, hence increasing the blood flow, while in polycythemia the viscosity increases which decreases the blood flow.

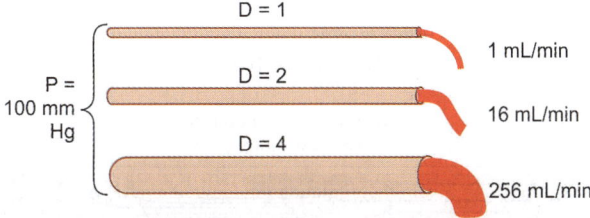

**Fig. 39.6:** The increase in blood flow is 16 times, when ever the radius doubles. It varies by the 4th power of radius.

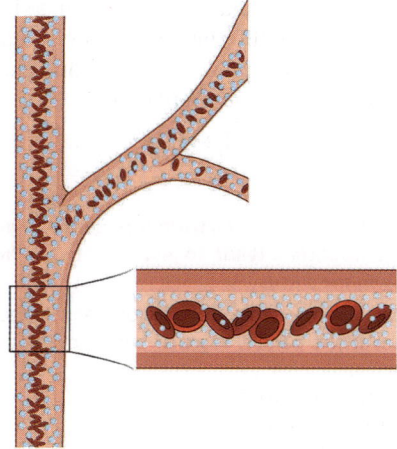

**Fig. 39.7:** Fåhræus-Lindqvist effect.

## Fåhræus-Lindqvist Effect (Plasma Skimming Effect)

This refers to satisfactory blood flow even in small BV due to plasma skimming effect. When the blood enters smaller blood vessels, the cells flowing in the central stream during laminar flow don't enter in same proportions in smaller branches. This maintains the viscosity in smaller branches and maintains the blood flow (**Fig. 39.7**).

## Ohm's Law

It is quite similar to Ohm's law, which states that the flow of current is directly proportional to potential difference and inversely proportional to resistance. Substituting it for fluids, we get the blood flow is directly proportional to the pressure difference and inversely proportional to TPR.

$$Q = \Delta P / R$$

## Resistance

It is defined as impedance to the blood flow.

It is measured as peripheral resistance units (PRU) or dyne sec/cm. From the Hagen Poiseuille's equation and Ohm's law, the resistance can be calculated as:

*Substituting the value of Q in both equations,*

$$\Delta P / R = \pi (P_1 - P_2) r^4 / 8 \eta L$$

$$R = 8 \eta L / \pi r^4$$

Hence, we can see that *resistance is directly proportional to viscosity and varies inversely with the 4th power of the radius.*

The TPR, calculated from the entire systemic circulation is 1 PRU. Strong vasoconstriction of all the blood vessels of our body, results in a peripheral resistance of 4 PRU whereas, mass vasodilation can result in a fall in TPR up to 0.2 PRU.

The pulmonary system has a pulmonary vascular resistance of about 0.14 PRU.

**Vascular resistance is less in parallel vascular circuits:** The extensive branching of the circulation results in much more total resistance than a single blood vessel. Hence, the different regional circulations are arranged in parallel and each tissue contributes to the conductance of systemic circulation.

$$1/R_{total} = 1/R_1 + 1/R_2 + 1/R_3 ....$$

*A 30-year-old man met a road traffic accident and got his left lower limb amputated. What do you think would happen to his hemodynamic status?*

Amputation of limb or removal of a major organ (kidney) results in the removal of a parallel vascular bed from the circulation resulting in:
1. Reduced cardiac output
2. Reduced vascular conductance
3. Reduced blood flow
4. Increased total peripheral resistance

- **Effect of sympathetic discharge:** The blood vessels have only the sympathetic supply and no parasympathetic supply. Hence, they remain in sympathetic vasoconstrictor tone at all times. Increased sympathetic discharge results in vasoconstriction and vice versa **(Fig. 39.8)**.

*A 26-year young female met an road accident and suffered the complete transaction of her spinal cord at the level of T4-T5. On examination, she is found to have severe hypotension. Why is she not able to maintain her blood pressure?*

The transaction of spinal cord in thoracolumbar region damages the sympathetic nerves originating from this area. This leads to loss of sympathetic vasoconstrictor tone and results in massive vasodilation, causing neurogenic shock.

- **Effect of velocity:**

$$Q = V \times A \text{ or } V = Q/A$$

The blood flow to any organ is directly proportional to velocity and area of cross-section. Hence the blood flow will decrease if the velocity of flow is sluggish.

## Types of Blood Flow

Depending upon the number of particles flowing through a certain cross-sectional area, the blood flow is classified as laminar or turbulent. Hence, the type of flow depends on the Reynolds number.

Reynolds number (Re) depends upon velocity of blood flow (v), diameter of blood vessel (d), density of blood (and viscosity of blood). It is represented as the given formula:

$$Re = \frac{v.d.\rho}{\eta}$$

*When Re rises above 2,000, it results in turbulence in smooth straight blood vessels.*

Re can increase due to:
- High blood velocity
- High pulsatility
- Sudden narrowing of blood vessel
- Large vessel diameter

- **Laminar/streamline flow (Fig. 39.9):**
  - Molecules of fluid moves in one direction. Blood flows in layers at steady rate
  - Less energy lost
  - Flow is silent
  - The Reynolds number is <2,000
- **Turbulent flow (Fig. 39.10):**
  - Molecules of fluid move in different directions; colliding with each other
  - Laminar arrangement is lost
  - Greater energy lost
  - Creates a sound
  - The Reynolds number is >2,000

**Physiological significance of turbulence:** The turbulence in the blood vessels is responsible for the Korotkoff's

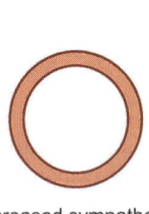

Increased sympathetic discharge resulting in vasoconstriction

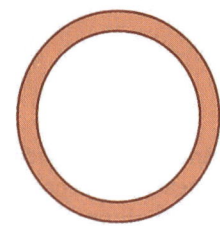

Normal sympathetic vasoconstrictor tone

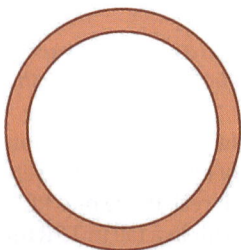

Decreased sympathetic vasoconstrictor tone resulting in vasodilation

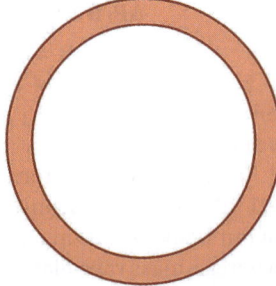

Loss of sympathetic vasoconstrictor tone resulting is massive vasodilation and hypotension

**Fig. 39.8:** Blood vessel diameters showing sympathetic vasoconstrictor tone.

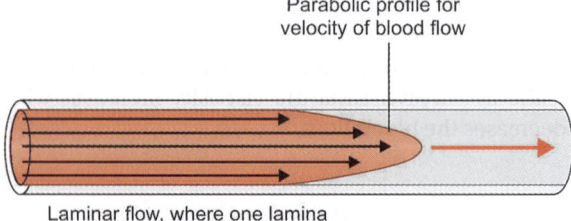

**Fig. 39.9:** Laminar blood flow.

**Fig. 39.10:** Turbulent blood flow.

sounds for measuring blood pressure, audible heart sounds due to the closure of valves.

**Clinical significance:** For diagnosing bruit and murmurs.

## Regulation of Blood Flow

The blood flow to any organ is regulated by various mechanisms. Depending on rapidity of action it is classified as acute control and long-term control.

### Acute Control of Blood Flow

It occurs due to rapid increase or decrease in blood fall to maintain the tissue need of blood. It is primarily affected by rate of metabolism in the tissues. It is explained by two main factors:

- **Oxygen lack:** Due to many factors wherever there is decrease in oxygen availability to tissues, it increases the blood flow to the tissues. Various physiological and clinical conditions like high altitude, pneumonia, carbon monoxide poisoning and cyanide poisoning increase the blood flow.

> **Why there is increased blood flow in cyanide poisoning?**
> The cyanide blocks the mitochondrial enzyme cytochrome P450 and completely blocks the utilization of oxygen by the tissues resulting in extreme and acute hypoxia. Due to oxygen lack in the tissues, there is increased blood flow.

- **Nutrient lack:** Lack of various nutrients like riboflavin, niacin and thiamine also results in high blood flow
- **Accumulation of vasodilator substances:** Various vasodilator substances are released by tissues due to increased metabolism and oxygen lack viz. adenosine, $CO_2$, histamine, $K^+$, and $H^+$. These vasodilator substance and hypoxia leads to opening of precapillary sphincters which opens the capillary circulation to increase the blood flow in the tissues.

Hence, both these theories i.e., oxygen lack theory or better called as *nutrient lack theory* and *vasodilator theory* closely regulates the blood flow in the tissues.

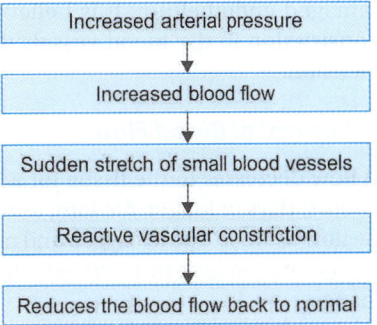

**Flowchart 39.2:** Myogenic theory.

**Active versus reactive hyperemia**
- **Active hyperemia:** Increase in blood flow due to increased tissue metabolism.
- **Reactive hyperemia:** Increase in blood flow in response to transient stoppage of blood.

### Autoregulation of Blood Flow

Acute rise in arterial pressure transiently increases the blood flow but it is reduced back to the normal blood flow within a minute, this mechanism is called autoregulation. It is explained by two mechanisms:

- **Metabolic theory:** The metabolic theory suggests that the blood flow is regulated by the oxygen and nutrient lack along with accumulation of vasodilator substances due to increased metabolism of tissues.
- **Myogenic theory (Flowchart 39.2):** This theory is based on the property of stress relation of smooth muscle.
- **Endothelium derived factors (Fig. 39.11):** Endothelium releases many actors which affect the blood flow. Various factors released are:
  - ***Endothelium derived relaxing factor (EDRF):*** It is very potent vasodilator substance, nitric oxide (NO), which is released by the endothelium in response to shear stress. The half-life of NO is 6 seconds; hence it produces its effect locally on the vascular smooth muscles. The formation of NO and its mechanism of action is shown in the **Figure 39.11**.

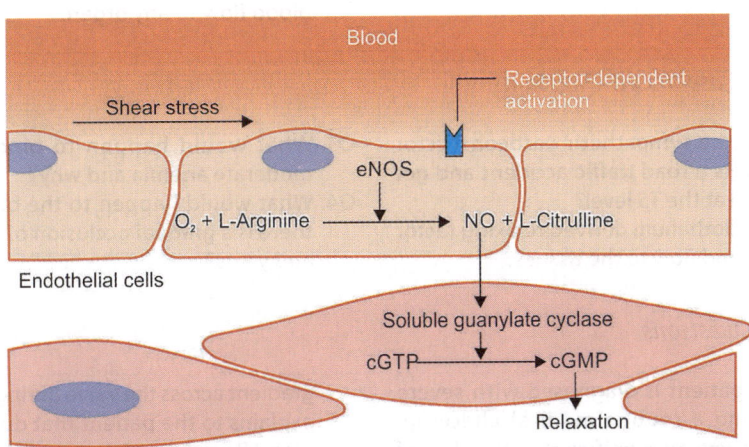

**Fig. 39.11:** Endothelium derived factor.

- **Endothelin:** It is potent vasoconstrictor released by the damaged endothelium. It is believed to cause vasoconstriction in the blood vessels damaged by hypertension.

## Long-term Control of Blood Flow

If the blood flow decreases to the tissue for a long period of time say hours, days or longer, the long term regulation increases the flow of blood due to oxygen and nutrient lack. There is chronic oxygen lack in tissue which induce the following changes:
- Increased vascularity in the tissue
- **Angiogenesis:** Formation of new blood vessels
- Formation of collateral circulation to restore the blood supply to the tissues.

## Hormonal Control

| Vasoconstrictors | Vasodilators |
|---|---|
| Norepinephrine | Bradykinin |
| Epinephrine | Vasopressin |
| Angiotensin II | Histamine |
| Vasopressin | |

## Role of Ions and Other Chemical Factors

- **Increase in intracellular calcium:** Vasoconstriction
- **Increase in $K^+$:** Vasodilation
- **Increase in $Mg^{2+}$:** Powerful vasodilation, $Mg^{2+}$ inhibits smooth muscle contraction
- **Increase in $H^+$:** Arteriolar dilation

### SUMMARY

- In this chapter we have learnt that the circulation follows all the laws of fluid mechanics (Hemodynamics).
- The blood flow to any organ is governed by the pressure gradient, radius of blood vessel and viscosity of blood (Hagen Poiseuille's equation). The increase in the diameter of blood vessel, increases the blood flow by the fourth power of the radius and vice versa.
- Similarly, the resistance offered to the blood flow in the blood vessels is inversely proportional to the fourth power of radius of the blood vessels.
- In smooth blood vessels, the blood flow is silent due to laminar flow but it is converted to the turbulent flow, when the Reynolds number becomes more than 2000.
- The blood flow is regulated to all the tissues by the sympathetic vasoconstrictor tone, hormones like adrenaline dopamine etc. But the most important regulatory mechanism is the 'Autoregulation', which is occurs due to the metabolic demand of the tissues or regulated by the myogenic theory.
- Whenever there is obstruction to blood flow due to atherosclerotic plaques, the vascular angiogenic factors promote angiogenesis to restore the blood flow to the tissue. If there is sudden occlusion of the blood flow to any organ, it causes ischemia and tissue damage.

### LET US SEE, WHAT YOU HAVE LEARNT?

#### Review Questions

Q1. What is Hagen Poiseuille's equation. Describe the factors affecting the blood flow?
Q2. What is peripheral resistance? What are the factors affecting the peripheral resistance?
Q3. How does the peripheral resistance affect the blood flow to the tissues?
Q4. Differentiate between the laminar and the turbulent blood flow.
Q5. Describe the mechanism of autoregulation of blood flow.
Q6. Describe the methods, that can be used to measure the blood flow to any organ.

#### Critical Thinking Case-Based Questions

Q1. What will happen to the sympathetic vasoconstrictor tone, if a patient meets a road traffic accident and get his spinal cord injured at the T5 level?
Q2. What is the role of endothelium derived relaxing factor in maintaining the blood flow to the tissues?
Q3. What would happen to blood flow in a patient of moderate anemia and why?
Q4. What would happen to the blood flow to an organ, if there is a gradual occlusion of the arteries over months and years?

#### Multiple Choice Questions

Q1. A 55-year-old male patient is diagnosed with severe aortic stenosis during a routine medical check-up. His echocardiogram reveals significant narrowing of the aortic valve orifice, leading to increased pressure gradient across the valve during systole. The cardiologist explains to the patient that due to the narrowed valve, blood flow through the aortic valve becomes turbulent. Which of the following parameters is most likely

associated with quantifying the degree of turbulence in the blood flow?
- a. Cardiac output
- b. Stroke volume
- c. Ejection fraction
- d. Reynolds number

Q2. A 60-year-old male patient with a history of hypertension presents to the cardiology clinic with complaints of leg pain during walking. Physical examination reveals diminished peripheral pulses in the lower extremities. An arterial Doppler ultrasound is ordered to assess blood flow in the lower limbs. During the interpretation of the ultrasound findings, the radiologist mentions the importance of considering the Hagen-Poiseuille equation. Which of the following scenarios best illustrates the application of the Hagen-Poiseuille equation in this context?
- a. Assessing the relationship between hematocrit and blood flow rate in the femoral artery
- b. Predicting the change in blood flow velocity in a narrowed segment of the femoral artery due to atherosclerosis
- c. Calculating the resistance to blood flow in the femoral arteries during exercise stress testing
- d. Estimating the velocity of blood flow in the femoral artery based on its diameter and pressure gradient

Q3. Which of the following factors primarily determines vascular resistance in the circulatory system?
- a. Blood viscosity
- b. Heart rate
- c. Cardiac output
- d. Blood pressure

Q4. Which of the following factors contributes to an increase in venous return to the heart?
- a. Decreased sympathetic activity
- b. Increased venous compliance
- c. Constriction of systemic arterioles
- d. Skeletal muscle pump activity

Q5. What is the main determinant of preload in the heart?
- a. Afterload
- b. End-diastolic volume
- c. Stroke volume
- d. Ejection fraction

Q6. What is the primary factor regulating stroke volume (SV) in the heart?
- a. Heart rate
- b. Preload
- c. Afterload
- d. Venous return

Q7. Which of the following represents the Frank-Starling law of the heart?
- a. An increase in ventricular filling results in a decrease in stroke volume
- b. Stroke volume is directly proportional to afterload
- c. The heart pumps more blood when it is filled with a larger volume of blood
- d. Cardiac output is inversely related to heart rate

Q8. Which of the following conditions is associated with decreased peripheral resistance (PR)?
- a. Hypertension
- b. Hemorrhage
- c. Anaphylaxis
- d. Heart failure

Q9. What effect does increased sympathetic nervous system activity have on peripheral resistance (PR)?
- a. Decreases PR
- b. Increases PR
- c. No effect on PR
- d. Increases cardiac output

Q10. Which of the following factors is responsible for the maintenance of blood pressure during diastole?
- a. Elastic recoil of arteries
- b. Contraction of the left ventricle
- c. Sympathetic nervous system activity
- d. Compliance of the veins

Q11. Which of the following is a measure of the force against which the heart must pump to eject blood during systole?
- a. Preload
- b. Afterload
- c. Contractility
- d. Compliance

Q12. What is the primary determinant of diastolic blood pressure (DBP)?
- a. Cardiac output
- b. Mean arterial pressure
- c. Peripheral resistance
- d. Heart rate

Q13. Which of the following conditions is characterized by an elevation in both systolic and diastolic blood pressure?
- a. Hypotension
- b. Hypertension
- c. Orthostatic hypotension
- d. Hypovolemic shock

Q14. Which of the following statements regarding laminar blood flow is correct?
- a. Laminar flow occurs when blood moves in random, chaotic patterns
- b. Laminar flow is characterized by layers of blood moving at different velocities
- c. Laminar flow is typically seen in stenotic arteries
- d. Laminar flow is associated with increased turbulence

Q15. What effect does an increase in blood vessel diameter have on resistance to blood flow?
- a. Increases resistance
- b. Decreases resistance
- c. No effect on resistance
- d. Increases turbulence

Q16. Which of the following factors would lead to increased pulse pressure?
- a. Decreased stroke volume
- b. Increased arterial compliance
- c. Decreased arterial stiffness
- d. Increased heart rate

Q17. What is the term for the resistance to blood flow encountered in the microcirculation, primarily the arterioles?
- a. Systemic vascular resistance (SVR)
- b. Total peripheral resistance (TPR)
- c. Venous return
- d. Capillary resistance

Q18. Which of the following factors contributes to increased venous pressure?
a. Increased sympathetic stimulation
b. Venous vasoconstriction
c. Decreased skeletal muscle activity
d. Increased venous compliance

Q19. Which of the following equations accurately represents the Hagen-Poiseuille equation for laminar flow?
a. Flow = Pressure × Resistance
b. Flow = (Pressure × Radius$^4$)/(Viscosity × Length)
c. Flow = Pressure × Velocity
d. Flow = (Pressure × Length)/(Radius$^4$ × Viscosity)

## ANSWERS

1. d   2. b   3. a   4. d   5. b   6. b   7. c   8. c   9. b   10. a   11. b   12. c   13. b   14. b
15. b   16. d   17. b   18. a   19. b

# Cardiovascular Regulatory Mechanisms

**40**
CHAPTER

### COMPETENCY ADDRESSED
**PY5.8:** Describe and discuss local and systemic cardiovascular regulatory mechanisms.

### LEARNING OBJECTIVES
**At the end of this chapter, the learner should be able to:**
- Describe the various short-term, intermediate-term and long-term regulatory mechanisms.
- Describe the local regulatory mechanisms.

The physiological mechanism by which homeostasis is maintained is called regulation. The cardiovascular regulatory mechanisms are primarily driven by the autonomic nervous system. For a detailed review of autonomic nervous system, you can read Chapter 91. Here we will do a quick review of the role of sympathetic and parasympathetic division of ANS in cardiovascular regulation **(Table 40.1)**.

## HIGHER CENTERS IN BRAIN AND BRAINSTEM FOR CARDIOVASCULAR REGULATION

The **vasomotor center (VMC)** is located bilaterally in the reticular substance of medulla and lower one third of pons. The entire organization of VMC is shown in **Figure 40.1**.

## CLASSIFICATION OF CARDIOVASCULAR REGULATORY MECHANISMS

Various processes in the cardiovascular system, viz. heart rate, arterial pressure, blood flow, etc., are closely regulated at different levels viz the nervous system (both, the higher centers and the autonomic nervous system), hormones and local factors discussed below:

- **Systemic regulation:**
  - *Short-term regulatory mechanisms, which gets activated in seconds to minutes:*
    - Baroreceptor reflex mechanism
    - Chemoreceptor reflex mechanism
    - CNS ischemic response
  - *Intermediate term regulatory mechanisms, which gets activated with minutes to hours:*
    - Renin angiotensin mechanism
    - Stress relaxation of vasculature
    - Capillary fluid shift mechanism
  - *Long-term regulatory mechanisms, which gets activated in hours to days:*
    - Renin angiotensin aldosterone mechanism
- **Local regulation:**
  - Autoregulation of blood flow:
    - Acute regulation
    - Long-term regulation of blood flow
  - Coronary chemoreflex/Bezold Jarish reflex
  - Bainbridge reflex
  - Marey law
  - Cushing's reflex
- **Hormonal regulation**

**Table 40.1:** Role of autonomic nervous system in regulation of cardiovascular mechanisms.

|  | Sympathetic nervous system | Parasympathetic nervous system |
|---|---|---|
| **Heart** | Increases heart rate and contractility | Decreases heart rate. Decreases contractility on a strong stimulation. Keeps the SA node inhibited (vagal tone) |
| **Blood vessels** | Provides sympathetic vasoconstrictor tone to all the blood vessels | No parasympathetic supply to blood vessels |

## SHORT-TERM REGULATORY MECHANISMS

### Baroreceptor Reflex Mechanism ('Baro' Means Pressure)

The baroreceptor reflex mechanism is based on the pressure changes in the large elastic arteries originating

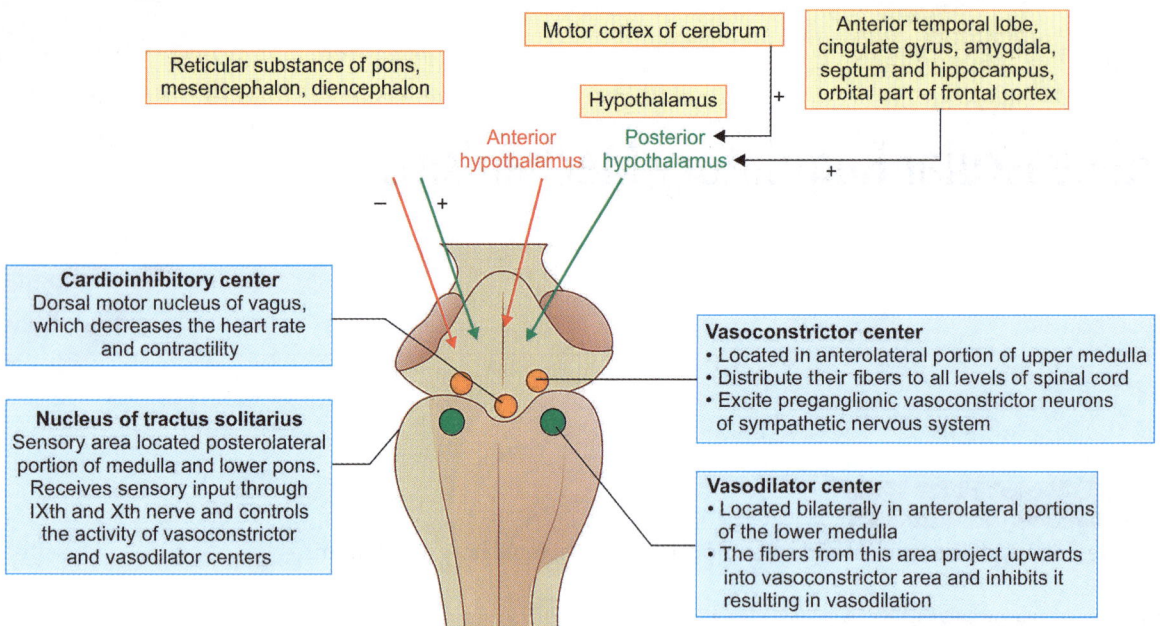

**Fig. 40.1:** Vasomotor center in brainstem and control of vasoconstrictor system.

from the left ventricle, i.e., in the arch of aorta and the carotid sinus located at the root of the internal carotid artery. This reflex buffers the mean arterial pressure changes in the blood and keeps it within the normal range of between *60 to 180 mm Hg*. It gets *activated within 10–15 seconds*, hence quickly restores the blood pressure to the normal limits. Baroreceptor reflex is particularly important in maintaining normal blood pressure with the change of posture and after maximal sympathetic stimulation, as seen in exercise. Since it is a reflex, it has the components of the reflex arc namely:

- **Stimulus:** *Distention of walls of arteries or cardiac chambers due to increased pressures.*
- **Baroreceptors**: Receptors sensitive to *pressure changes in aorta and carotid sinus*. The baroreceptors are the tonic receptors, i.e., they discharge at all the times and send the signals to the vasomotor center. When stimulated by increased pressure, the rate of discharge increases and inhibited by decreased pressure, the firing rate decreases **(Fig. 40.2)**.

*Located in (Fig. 40.3A):*
- Arch of aorta
- Carotid sinus
- Walls of heart at subendocardial position

- **Afferent (Fig. 40.3B):** Glossopharyngeal nerve (IX) from carotid sinus and vagus nerve (X) from arch of aorta. Since these nerves maintain the blood pressure through the baroreceptor reflex mechanism, they are also called *'Buffer nerves'*.
- **Center:** Vasomotor center located in the brain stem
- **Efferent:** Vagus
- **Effector organ:** Blood vessels and heart
- **Effect:**
  - **Increased blood pressure inhibits sympathetic outflow** by inhibiting the vasoconstrictor area and stimulating the dorsal motor nucleus of vagus **(Flowchart 40.1)**. This decreases the sympathetic outflow from vasomotor center and results in vasodilation and decreases heart rate and contractility.
  - However, *decreased blood pressure decreases the stimulation of baroreceptors*, which results in stimulation of vasoconstrictor area and inhibition of vagal nucleus. This increases the sympathetic discharge and increases the sympathetic vasoconstrictor tone and cardiac contractility and heart rate, thus increasing the blood pressure.

It is interesting to see that the baroreceptors are very effective in the acute corrections of blood pressure, but it

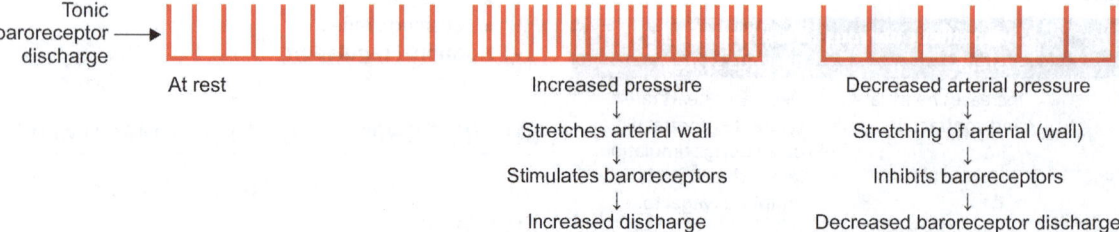

**Fig. 40.2:** Effects of arterial pressure on baroreceptors discharge.

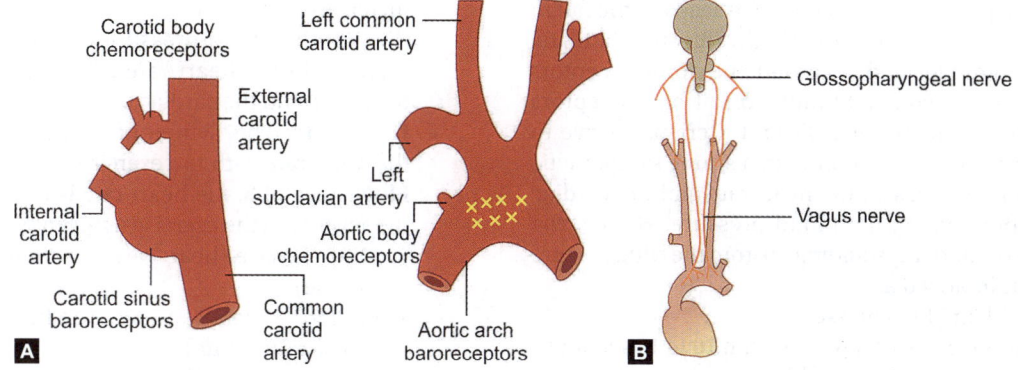

**Figs. 40.3A and B:** (A) Location of baroreceptors and chemoreceptors; (B) Afferent nerve supply.

becomes ineffective in long standing hypertension, called **"Baroreceptor resetting"**.

## Baroreceptor Reflex (Fig. 40.4)

The baroreceptor reflex, a vital regulatory mechanism, swiftly adjusts blood pressure by detecting changes in vessel stretch and signaling adjustments in heart rate and vascular tone. This reflex ensures rapid adaptation to maintain cardiovascular stability, crucial for overall physiological equilibrium.

## Physiological Significance of Baroreceptors

- **Regulation of blood pressure in the change of posture (Flowchart 40.2):** When a person stands up suddenly from the lying posture, the blood from the upper part of the body move towards the feet, resulting in the

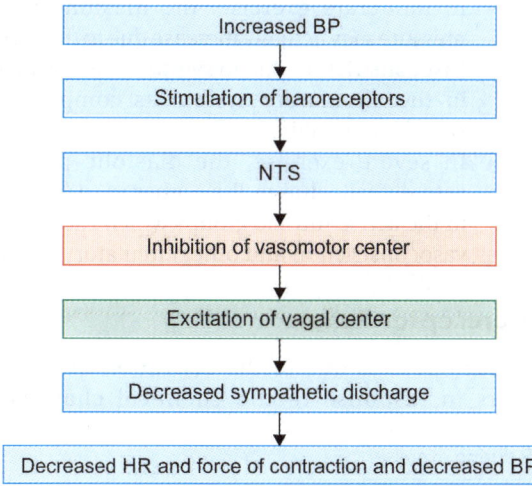

Flowchart 40.1: Effect of increased BP on sympathetic flow.

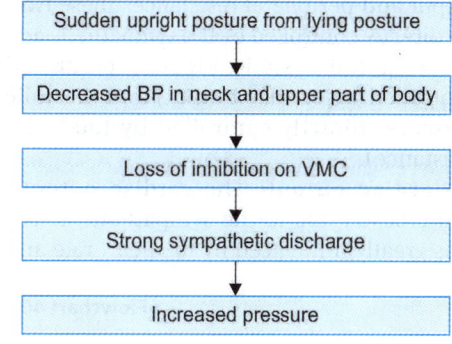

Flowchart 40.2: Regulation of BP with change of posture.

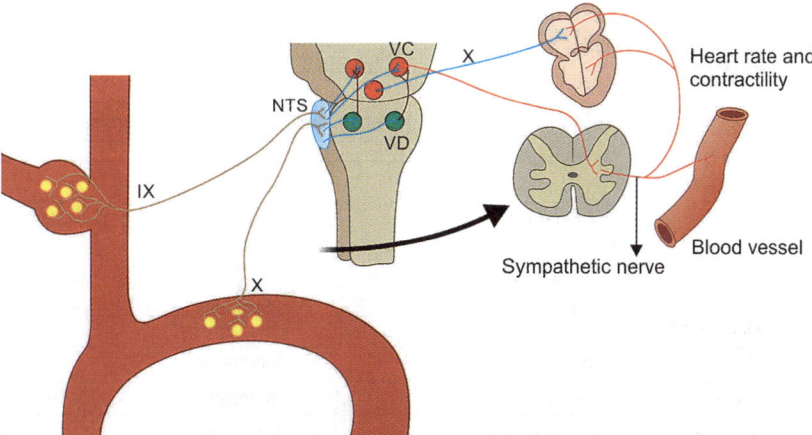

**Fig. 40.4:** Baroreceptor reflux.
(NTS: nucleus of the solitary tract)

peripheral pooling of the blood. This leads to the fall in blood pressure in upper part of body. This stimulates the Baro receptors located in carotid and aortic receptors within 10–15 seconds. Stimulation of baroreceptors sends the signals through IX and X cranial nerve to vasomotor center which initiates a strong sympathetic stimulation, increasing the heart rate and the cardiac output thus raising the blood pressure. Hence, the response of suddenly standing up from the lying posture can be summarized as:

- Initial fall in blood pressure
- Activation of baroreceptors within 10 to 15 seconds
- Increase of heart rate and blood pressure
- This increase settled down over the next two to three minutes.

- **Regulation of blood pressure during exercise (Flowchart 40.3):** When a person begins to exercise, even the thought of exercise increases the heart rate with slight increase in blood pressure due to initial sympathetic activation.
  - During exercise, the increased demand of oxygen by the tissues results in the increased blood flow due to local regulatory mechanisms.
  - The sympathetic activation further adds to the vasodilatation by stimulation of the cholinergic sympathetic fibers; increasing the blood flow to the tissues.
  - The blood pressure is regulated primarily by cardiac output and peripheral resistance. These two factors are directly controlled by the sympathetic activation, affecting the systolic blood pressure (directly controlled by cardiac output) and diastolic blood pressure (directly controlled by total peripheral resistance).
    - **Cardiac output:** The cardiac output is also increased due to the sympathetic activation. It is greatly influenced by the heart rate and hence increases with the severity of the exercise. Hence, the systolic blood pressure increases with the increase in the heart rate as it depends on the heart rate and the cardiac output.
    - **Heart rate:** This sympathetic activity increases the heart rate with the exercise. As we can see in **Flowchart 40.3**, the heart rate is used to classify the severity of the exercise as given below:
      - Mild exercise (heart rate less than 100 beats/minute)
      - Moderate exercise (heart rate between 100 to 125 beats/minute)
      - Severe exercise (heart rate above 125 beats/minute)
    - **Total peripheral resistance:** The diastolic blood pressure depends on the total peripheral resistance of the circulatory system. This further depends on the balance between the net vasodilation and vasoconstriction. We can further discuss that:
      - In the mild exercise, the total peripheral resistance is not affected much and hence the diastolic blood pressure may or may not be increased.
      - In moderate exercise, the diastolic blood pressure may actually increase due to the higher vasoconstriction due to sympathetic activation in the circulatory system as compared to vasodilation in the active muscle groups.
      - In severe exercise, the diastolic pressure actually falls due to the higher vasodilatation in the active muscle groups which exceeds the vasoconstriction and other circulatory beds.

## Chemoreceptor Reflex

This reflex operates due to the activation of chemo-receptors in response to the chemical changes in

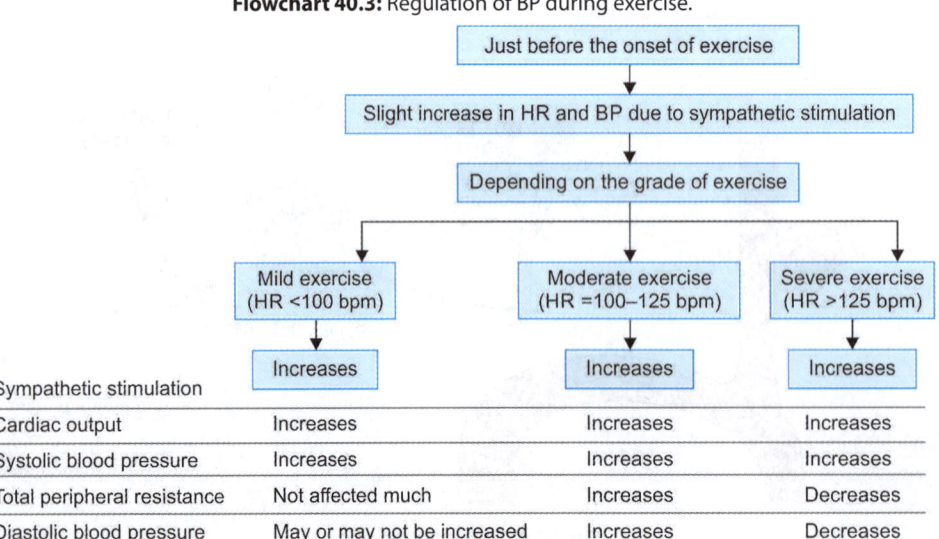

**Flowchart 40.3:** Regulation of BP during exercise.

the blood viz. hypoxia, hypercarbia and acidosis (stimulus). Receptors sensitive to *chemical changes in blood (PO$_2$, PCO$_2$ and pH) are called* **chemoreceptors**. The chemoreceptors are broadly classified as the central chemoreceptors (located in brainstem) and peripheral chemoreceptors, located in arch of aorta (aortic bodies) and carotid sinus (carotid bodies).

The peripheral chemoreceptors have **hypoxia-sensitive glomus cells**, which respond to **decreased oxygen concentration in plasma**. Hence, they are only stimulated by dissolved oxygen (the details about the chemoreceptors are given in the regulation of the respiratory system). *The peripheral chemoreceptors get activated at PO$_2$ levels of 60 mm Hg.* The central chemoreceptors are strongly stimulated by increased PCO$_2$ concentration.

When there is a fall in mean arterial pressure (hypotension) below 60 mm Hg, there is a fall in PO$_2$ levels in the blood resulting in the activation of the chemoreceptor reflex. Hence, this reflex acts as the compensatory mechanism to bring back the falling blood pressure.

The stimulated chemoreceptors send the signals to the nucleus of tractus solitarius which in turn stimulates the vasoconstrictor area and inhibits the vagal nucleus. There is increased sympathetic discharge which increases the blood pressure, heart rate and cardiac contractility.

HYPOXIA stimulates Peripheral Chemoreceptors, HYPERCAPNIA stimulates Central Chemoreceptors.

### CNS Ischemic Response

As the name suggests, whenever there is *severe hypotension*, i.e., the recorded systolic blood pressure is *40 mm Hg or below* there is cerebral ischemia which results in the direct stimulation of the vasomotor center. It is also called as the *last ditch resort* as it is the last attempt of the compensatory mechanisms to raise the blood pressure of an individual. It is accompanied by a rapid and thready pulse rate.

### Cushing's Reflex (Fig. 40.5)

A similar condition is seen when there is *raised intracranial tension* due to a space occupying lesion (hematoma or tumor). There is cerebral ischemia due to the compression of the arteries supplying the brain and thus resulting in the stimulation of vasomotor center. The increased blood pressure stimulates the baroreceptors which leads to reflex bradycardia. *Hence, the patient with raised intracranial tension presents with bradycardia which is called the Cushing reflex.*

### THE LIE DETECTOR POLYGRAPH TEST

During a polygraph examination, a subject is asked a series of questions, including ones related to a recent incident

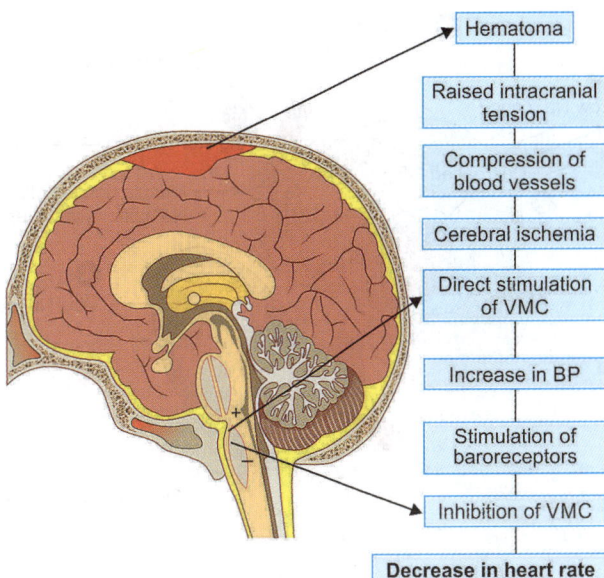

**Fig. 40.5:** Cushing reflex: Raised IC tension presents with bradycardia.

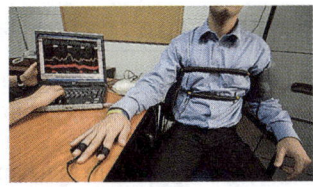

under investigation. As the questions become more probing and personal, the subject's anxiety level rises, and they start to feel increasingly nervous. The subject's palms may become sweaty, and their heart begins to race. The polygraph machine, sensitive to physiological changes, detects a significant increase in heart rate and blood pressure readings.

As the examiner notices the physiological response, they pause and reassure the subject, asking them to remain calm and relaxed. However, the subject's anxiety persists, and they continue to feel the pressure of the interrogation.

Amidst the tense atmosphere, the subject's body responds to the perceived threat by activating the body's stress response system. In the brain, the amygdala signals the hypothalamus to trigger the release of stress hormones, including adrenaline and cortisol. These hormones activate the sympathetic nervous system, leading to increased heart rate and blood pressure.

As the subject's heart pounds and their blood pressure rises, the examiner observes the polygraph machine's readings, noting the significant changes in cardiovascular parameters. The examiner understands that the subject's physiological response reflects their emotional state, potentially indicating heightened stress or anxiety associated with specific questions.

In this scenario, the subject's increased heart rate and blood pressure serve as physiological markers of their emotional arousal, affecting the polygraph test results. The examiner recognizes the role of the central nervous

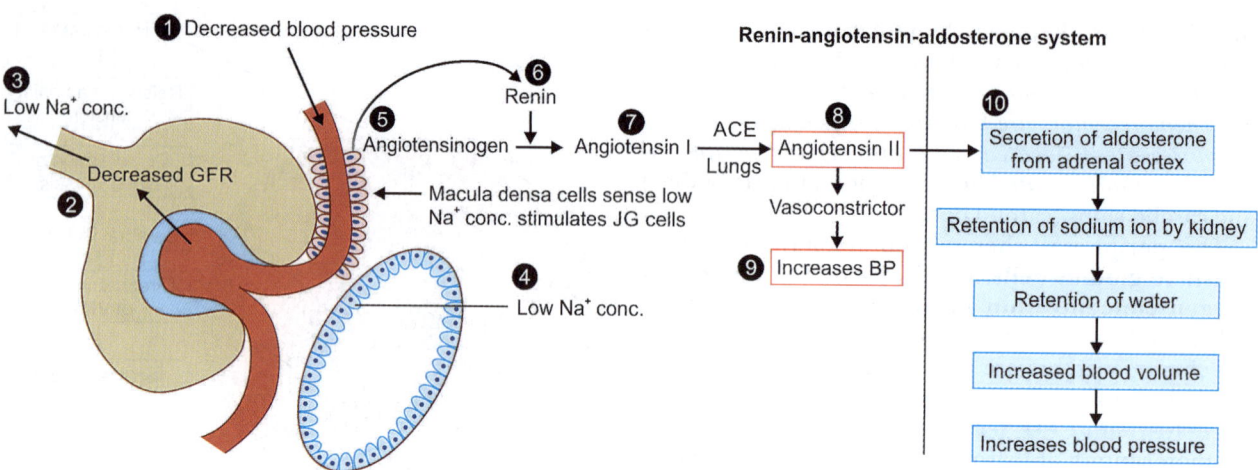

Fig. 40.6: Regulation of BP through RAAS.

system's stress response in modulating cardiovascular function and its implications for interpreting the polygraph examination.

## INTERMEDIATE TERM REGULATION

It takes a few hours to few days to get activated. The various mechanisms which regulate in the intermediate term regulation are:
- Renin-angiotensin mechanism
- Stress relaxation of the vasculature
- Capillary fluid shift mechanism

### Renin-angiotensin Mechanism

This mechanism operates during hypotension when there is decreased renal blood flow which decreases the glomerular filtration rate. There is a decrease in the level of sodium ions in the filtrate which leads to the activation of tubuloglomerular feedback mechanism. There is release of renin from juxtaglomerular cells, which converts the inactive angiotensinogen to active angiotensin I. The angiotensin I is further converted to angiotensin II by angiotensin-converting enzyme (secreted by lungs). The angiotensin II is a potent vasoconstrictor and hence raises the blood pressure **(Fig. 40.6)**.

### Stress Relaxation of the Vasculature

Whenever there is increase in the blood pressure it stretches the smooth muscles of the blood vessels which in turn relax at that pressure due to their inherent property of plasticity. Hence, this reduces the pressure within the vasculature.

### Capillary Fluid Shift Mechanism

According to the Starling forces, which operate in the microvasculature; An increase in blood pressure increases the capillary hydrostatic pressure and hence the net filtration pressure. So, there is movement of fluid from

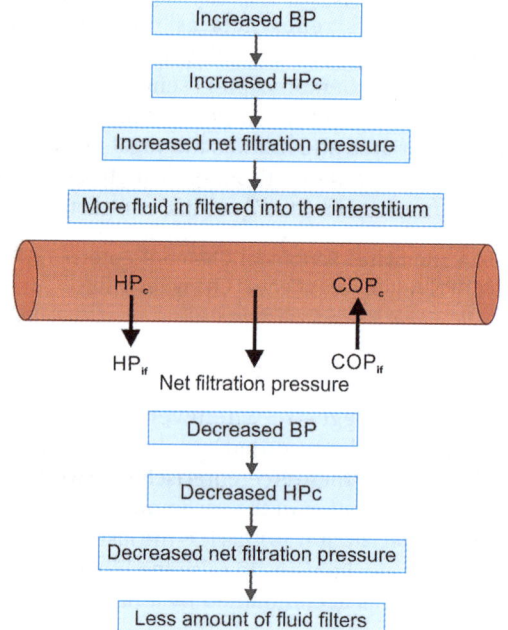

Fig. 40.7: Capillary fluid shift mechanism.

the capillaries into the interstitium, decreasing the blood volume which results in fall in blood pressure **(Fig. 40.7)**.

## LONG-TERM REGULATION

It takes a few days or two months to get activated. It is primarily controlled by the kidneys and the adrenal cortex. Hence, it operates through the renin angiotensin aldosterone mechanism.

The angiotensin-II formed by the renin angiotensin mechanism, during hypotension simulates the adrenal cortex to produce aldosterone which results in increase of the blood volume by retaining sodium and water. Hence, during hypotension the aldosterone levels would increase increasing the blood volume and vice versa.

## Local Regulation

### Autoregulation of the Blood Flow

It means the regulation of the blood flow to the tissues by the tissues. It is discussed in detail in hemodynamics.

### Role of Cardiac Receptors in Cardiovascular Regulation

There are specific stretch receptors located in the atria for various cardiovascular regulatory mechanisms. Based on their location these receptors are classified as:
- **Atrial stretch receptors (discovered by Dr AS Paintel)** located at junction of **right atrium and vena cava**. These are further of two types:
  1. *Type A receptors:* Which get activated during atrial systole
  2. *Type B receptors:* Which get activated during late atrial diastole

  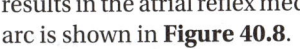
  Dr AS Paintel

  These receptors are **stimulated** by the **stretching of atrial wall** either **due to increased venous return** or **decreased forward movement of blood** due to right ventricular failure. It results in the atrial reflex mediated through vagus, reflex arc is shown in **Figure 40.8**.
  - Afferent: Vagus
  - Center: Medulla oblongata
  - Efferent: Vagosympathetic trunk
  - Response: Increase in heart rate

  It is called as *Bainbridge reflex*. It is a true reflex as it is abolished by vagotomy. The **physiological significance** of this reflex is that it *prevents damming of blood* and results in *forward movement of blood* toward right ventricle. This reflex increases the heart rate only when the initial heart rate is low.

- **Atrial volume receptors:**
  - Located at junction of pulmonary vein and left atrium
  - Stimulus: Stretching of left atrium
  - Afferent: Vagus
  - Response: Inhibition of ADH release and release of ANP resulting in diuresis and decreased blood volume

### Marey's Law

It states that blood pressure is inversely proportional to heart rate.

$$BP \propto \frac{1}{HR}$$

It is not applicable in sleep and exercise.

### Bezold-Jarish Reflex

It is also called as coronary chemoreflex (**Fig. 40.9**).

A similar response is seen, when the injection serotonin, capsaicin, veratridine and phenyl guanine is injected into pulmonary artery, called *pulmonary chemoreflex/ J reflex*.

## Hormonal Regulation

Hormonal regulation controls vascular tone and fluid balance, ensuring optimal perfusion and blood pressure control. This plays important role in cardiovascular homeostasis, harmonizing the body's vital circulatory functions.

### Vasodilator Hormones

- Acetylcholine
- Histamine
- Prostaglandins
- Atrial natriuretic peptide (ANP)
- VIP
- Kinins

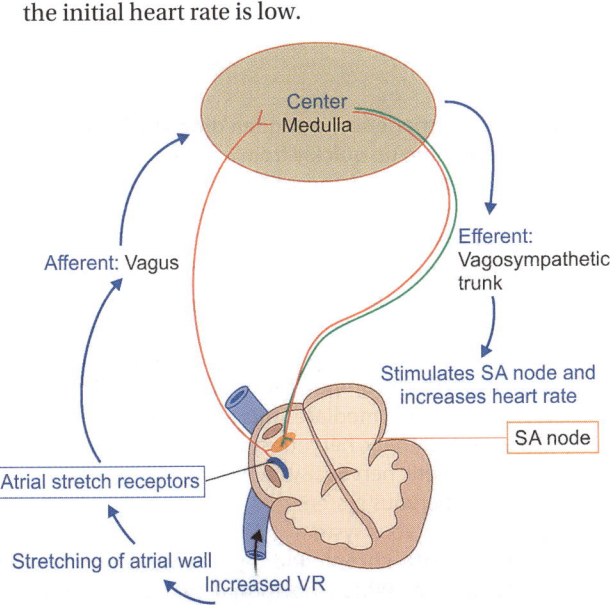

**Fig. 40.8:** Bainbridge reflex mechanism.
Bainbridge reflex: Prevents damming of blood
'Increased blood volume increases the heart rate, if initial heart rate is low'

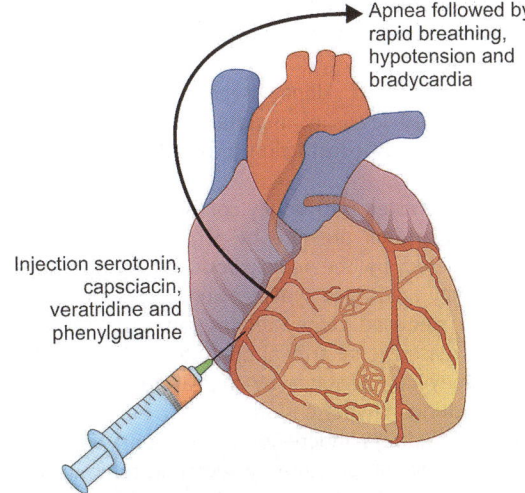

**Fig. 40.9:** Bezold-Jarish reflex.

## Vasoconstrictor Hormones

- Nor epinephrine
- Antidiuretic hormone (ADH)/Vasopressin
- Angiotensin II
- Thyroxine
- 5-HT

## SUMMARY

In this chapter we have learnt that:
- Various mechanisms are involved in the regulation of cardiovascular mechanisms like heart rate, blood pressure, etc. It is mainly classified as:
    - Systemic regulation: It involves the neural control through
        - The baroreceptor reflex mechanism which detects the change in the arterial pressure. It buffers the pressure changes in day-to-day activities.
        - The chemoreceptor reflex mechanism which detects the change in $PO_2$, $PCO_2$ and the $H^+$ concentration. It is primarily active in hypotension.
- CNS ischemic response is seen when the vasomotor center in brain is directly stimulated by the severe hypotension.
    - The local regulation is maintained by the process of:
        - Metabolic demand and waste product accumulation
        - Autoregulation of blood flow
- Various hormones are also involved in the regulatory mechanisms like: Acetylcholine, histamine, catecholamines, etc.

## LET US SEE, WHAT YOU HAVE LEARNT?

### Review Questions

#### Long/Short Answer Questions

Q1. Describe the baroreceptor reflex mechanism and its physiological importance.
Q2. Describe the role of kidneys in regulation of blood pressure.
Q3. Describe the short-term regulatory mechanism and their physiological importance.
Q4. Describe renin angiotensin mechanism and its physiological importance.

#### Explain Why? (Reasoning Questions)

Q1. What happens to blood pressure when a person suddenly stands up from lying position?
Q2. There is increase in the heart rate of an individual, when he gets scared.
Q3. Sympathetic nervous system increases heart rate and contractility during exercise.

### Multiple Choice Questions

Q1. In a patient with stenosis of only one renal artery, hypertension can develop due to compensatory mechanisms involving both kidneys. Which of the following best explains how hypertension arises in this scenario?
   a. The stenosed kidney secretes renin, leading to increased levels of angiotensin II and aldosterone, causing vasoconstriction and salt retention in both kidneys
   b. The non-stenosed kidney compensates for decreased renal arterial pressure by retaining salt and water, triggered by the renin produced by the stenosed kidney, leading to hypertension
   c. The stenosed kidney retains salt and water due to decreased renal arterial pressure, while the opposite kidney compensates by increasing renin secretion, resulting in hypertension
   d. Both kidneys independently respond to decreased renal arterial pressure by secreting renin, leading to increased angiotensin II levels and hypertension

Q2. A patient experiences a sudden drop in blood pressure while standing up quickly from a seated position. Which reflex mechanism is primarily responsible for rapidly adjusting the heart rate and vascular tone to maintain blood pressure?
   a. Baroreceptor reflex        b. Chemoreceptor reflex
   c. Bainbridge reflex          d. Marey's law

Q3. During a stressful situation, a patient's heart rate and blood pressure increase to prepare the body for "fight or flight." Which component of the autonomic nervous system primarily mediates this response?
   a. Parasympathetic nervous system
   b. Sympathetic nervous system
   c. Enteric nervous system
   d. Central nervous system

Q4. A patient with chronic kidney disease presents with hypertension. Which hormonal system is primarily responsible for long-term regulation of blood pressure by modulating fluid and electrolyte balance?
   a. Renin-angiotensin system

b. Aldosterone system
c. Vasopressin system
d. Endothelin system

Q5. A patient with severe dehydration experiences a decrease in blood pressure. Which physiological mechanism primarily responds to low blood volume by releasing antidiuretic hormone (ADH) to promote water reabsorption in the kidneys?
a. Chemoreceptor reflex
b. Bainbridge reflex
c. Baroreceptor reflex
d. Renin-angiotensin system

Q6. A patient with heart failure develops fluid overload, leading to increased preload and elevated blood pressure. Which mechanism of cardiac regulation plays a role in preventing excessive stretching of the cardiac chambers?
a. Bainbridge reflex
b. Frank-Starling mechanism
c. Chemoreceptor reflex
d. CNS ischemic response

Q7. A patient experiences a sudden drop in blood pressure due to hemorrhage. Which reflex mechanism is activated to increase sympathetic outflow and vasoconstriction, thereby restoring blood pressure?
a. Bainbridge reflex
b. Chemoreceptor reflex
c. Baroreceptor reflex
d. Marey's law

Q8. A patient with obstructive sleep apnea exhibits episodes of bradycardia followed by tachycardia upon awakening. Which reflex mechanism is primarily responsible for these heart rate fluctuations during apneic episodes?
a. Bainbridge reflex
b. Chemoreceptor reflex
c. Baroreceptor reflex
d. Marey's law

Q9. A patient with a traumatic brain injury experiences increased intracranial pressure, leading to cerebral ischemia. Which reflex mechanism responds to the decrease in cerebral perfusion pressure by increasing systemic blood pressure?
a. Bainbridge reflex
b. CNS ischemic response
c. Baroreceptor reflex
d. Chemoreceptor reflex

Q10. A patient with heart failure develops pulmonary congestion. Which reflex mechanism is activated to increase heart rate and respiratory rate in response to decreased oxygen levels in the blood?
a. CNS ischemic response
b. Chemoreceptor reflex
c. Bainbridge reflex
d. Baroreceptor reflex

Q11. A patient with hypertension experiences a sudden increase in blood pressure. Which reflex mechanism is activated to decrease sympathetic outflow and promote vasodilation, thereby reducing blood pressure?
a. Baroreceptor reflex
b. Chemoreceptor reflex
c. Bainbridge reflex
d. Marey's law

## ANSWERS

1. b  2. a  3. b  4. a  5. d  6. b  7. c  8. a  9. b  10. a  11. a

# Heart Rate and Regulation

**CHAPTER 41**

> **COMPETENCY ADDRESSED**
> PY5.9: Describe the factors affecting heart rate, regulation of cardiac output and blood pressure.

>  **LEARNING OBJECTIVES**
> **At the end of this chapter, the learner should be able to:**
> - Explain the innervation of the heart and its effect on the cardiac function.
> - Define heart rate.
> - Describe the variations and factors affecting in the heart rate.
> - Explain the reflexes involved in the regulation of heart rate.

## INTRODUCTION

The heart rate is controlled intrinsically by the pacemaker SA node of the heart but the autonomic nervous system modulates the heart rate. Hence, before studying the heart rate, we would quickly try to understand the innervation of heart.

The heart is innervated by both the sympathetic and parasympathetic nervous system through the cardiac plexus (**Fig. 41.1**).

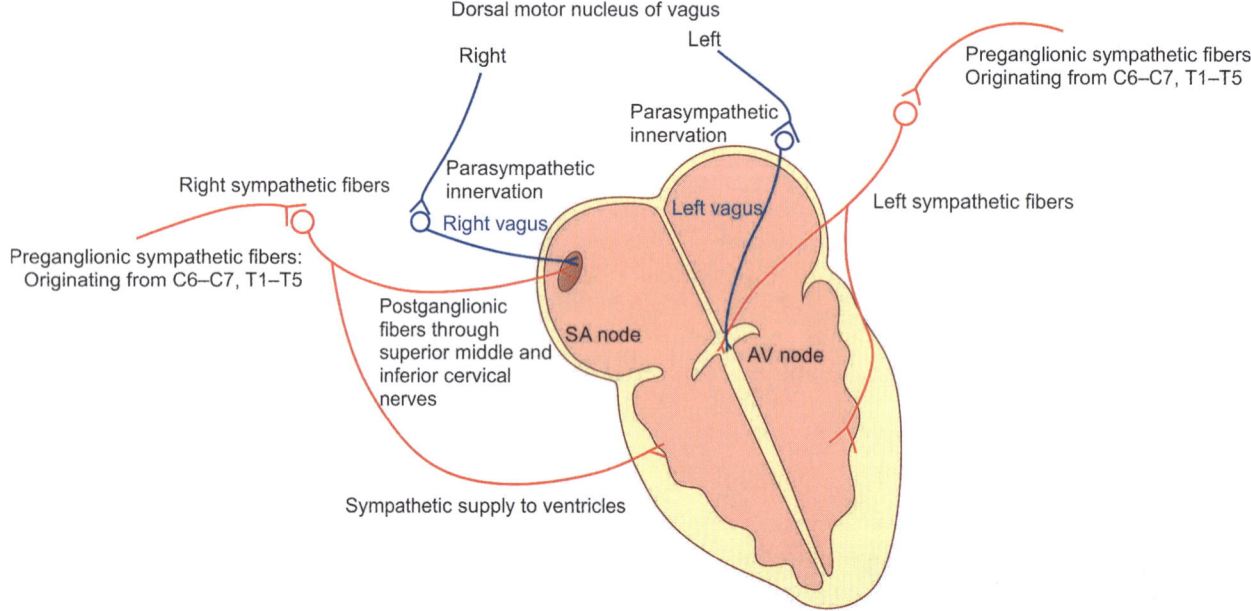

**Fig. 41.1:** Nerve supply of heart.

## Sympathetic Innervation: Thoracolumbar Division (T1–L2)

- *Preganglionic sympathetic fibers* (C6–C7, T1–T5) pass into sympathetic trunk to *superior, middle and inferior cervical ganglia and upper thoracic ganglia*
- *Postganglionic fibers* leave ganglia and pass via superior, middle and inferior cardiac sympathetic nerves and supply to nodal tissues and cardiac muscles
- Sympathetic fibers from *right side innervates SA node and cardiac muscle*
- Sympathetic fibers from *left side innervates AV node and cardiac muscle*

## Parasympathetic Innervation (Right and Left Vagus)

- Distributed to atria, SA node, AV node and AV bundle
- *Right vagus innervates SA node*
- *Left vagus innervates AV node*
- There is **NO** parasympathetic supply to ventricles

## Vagal Tone

It refers to the activity level of the vagus nerve, arising from dorsal motor nucleus of vagus, located in medulla oblongata.

High vagal tone indicates that the parasympathetic nervous system is highly active, leading to a lower heart rate, better regulation of digestion, and overall relaxation. On the other hand, low vagal tone suggests that the parasympathetic nervous system is less active, which may result in a faster heart rate, poor digestion, and increased stress levels. It is increased in athletes; hence, the athletes have resting bradycardia. The old people however have a higher resting heart rate due to lower vagal tone.

What is the physiological significance of higher vagal tone/bradycardia in athletes?

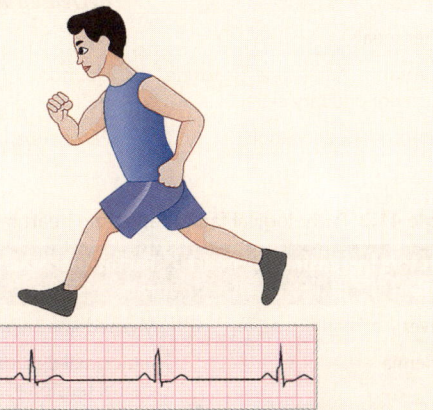

Bradycardia is a common physiological adaptation seen in athletes, particularly those who engage in endurance sports like long-distance running, cycling, or swimming.

- **Improved stroke volume:** Athletes with bradycardia often have a larger stroke volume, which is the amount of blood pumped out of the heart with each beat. A slower heart rate allows the heart more time to fill with blood during diastole, leading to a more efficient ejection of blood during systole.
- **Enhanced cardiac efficiency:** Bradycardia can indicate a well-conditioned heart that is capable of pumping a greater volume of blood with each contraction. This efficiency means the heart doesn't need to work as hard to maintain cardiac output, which is the volume of blood pumped by the heart per minute.
- **Increased aerobic capacity:** Athletes with bradycardia often have a higher aerobic capacity, meaning their bodies can efficiently utilize oxygen during exercise. This is partly due to adaptations in the cardiovascular system, including increased capillarization, improved oxygen delivery to muscles, and enhanced mitochondrial function.
- **Reduced risk of cardiovascular disease:** Studies have shown that individuals with lower resting heart rates, such as athletes with bradycardia, tend to have a reduced risk of developing cardiovascular diseases like hypertension, coronary artery disease, and stroke.

## Effect of Sympathetic Stimulation

- Increased HR → positive chronotropic effect
- Increased conduction → positive dromotropic effect
- Increased excitability → positive bathmotropic effect
- Increased force of contraction → positive inotropic effect

## Effect of Parasympathetic Stimulation

- Decreased HR → negative chronotropic effect
- Decreased conductivity → negative dromotropic effect
- Decreased excitability → negative bathmotropic effect

**Let's learn the meaning of these terms:**

1. **Chronotropic effect:** The term "chronotropic" refers to the heart rate (chronos means time in Greek). Thus, the chronotropic effect involves the modulation of heart rate. Positive chronotropic effects increase heart rate, while negative chronotropic effects decrease it. The primary regulator of chronotropy is the autonomic nervous system, particularly the sympathetic and parasympathetic branches. Sympathetic stimulation, often through the release of adrenaline (epinephrine), increases heart rate by activating beta-adrenergic receptors in the heart's pacemaker cells (sinoatrial node), while parasympathetic stimulation, mediated by the vagus nerve, decreases heart rate by activating muscarinic receptors in the sinoatrial node.

2. **Dromotropic effect:** Dromotropy relates to the conduction velocity of electrical impulses within the heart (dromos means running in Greek). Positive dromotropic effects increase conduction velocity, while negative dromotropic effects decrease it. The main site of dromotropic modulation is the atrioventricular (AV) node. Sympathetic stimulation enhances AV node conduction speed, leading to shorter PR intervals on electrocardiograms (ECGs), while

parasympathetic stimulation slows conduction through the AV node, prolonging PR intervals.

3. **Bathmotropic effect:** Bathmotropy pertains to the excitability or threshold for depolarization of cardiac muscle cells (bathmos means threshold in Greek). Positive bathmotropic effects lower the threshold for depolarization, making cells more excitable, while negative bathmotropic effects raise the threshold, making cells less excitable. The threshold potential is the level of membrane potential that must be reached to trigger an action potential. Factors influencing bathmotropy include ion concentrations (especially calcium and potassium), neurotransmitters, and certain medications.

4. **Inotropic effect:** Inotropy refers to the force of cardiac muscle contraction (inos means fiber or sinew in Greek). Positive inotropic effects increase contractility, leading to stronger contractions and greater ejection of blood from the heart, while negative inotropic effects decrease contractility. Inotropic modulation primarily involves changes in intracellular calcium levels, which affect the interaction between actin and myosin filaments during muscle contraction. Sympathetic stimulation and certain medications (such as digitalis glycosides) exert positive inotropic effects, while factors like acidosis or myocardial depressant drugs induce negative inotropy.

## HEART RATE

The heart rate is defined as the rate at which the heart beats in one minute. *Normal heart rate is between 60 to 100 beats per minute with an average of 75 bpm.*

### Physiological Basis of Generation of Heart Rate

The heart rate is generated by the SA node (the pacemaker of the heart) due to the property of auto-rhythmicity. *The inherent rate of impulse generation by the SA node is at the rate of 100 bpm.* The vagus nerve continuously keeps this rate under check, i.e., up to 75 bpm, called as the vagal tone. Hence, a higher vagal tone would further lower the heart rate, as we have discussed above.

> *What should happen to heart rate in a transplanted heart/all nerve supply to heart is cut/the vagal supply to heart is cut?*
>
> In a transplanted heart or if all the nerve supply to heart is cut, the heart regulates the functioning based on the intrinsic mechanisms and activity of SA node. Hence, the heart will beat at the rate of 100 bpm. There will be no direct effect of sympathetic stimulation on heart. The heart rate is regulated to venous return and stroke volume.
>
> But if only vagus is cut, the vagal tone is abolished. Whereas the sympathetic fibers are intact (presumably), the heart rate will be affected by the sympathetic fibers.

### Variations in Heart Rate

- Normal heart rate ranges between *60 to 100 bpm*
- **Tachycardia** is defined as the increased heart rate *more than 100 bpm*
- **Bradycardia** is defined as the decreased heart rate *less than 60 bpm*

Usually in clinical practice, the pulse rate from a peripheral pulse is used to determine the heart rate. But ideally it should be measured form the cardiac impulse or from the chest with the help of stethoscope.

### Factors Affecting Heart Rate

There are many factors that can affect the hear rate, these are tabulated below for an easy reference.

#### Physiological Factors

These factors occur due to normal physiological processes and are not involved in any disease process **(Table 41.1)**.

#### Pathological Factors

These factors occur due to disease process **(Table 41.2)**.

### Regulation of Heart Rate

(All these reflexes have been discussed in detail in Chapter 40 Cardiovascular Regulatory Mechanisms)
- Baroreceptor reflex
- Chemoreceptor reflex

**Table 41.1:** Physiological factors affecting heart rate

| Factors increasing the heart rate | Factors decreasing the heart rate |
|---|---|
| Excitement, anxiety | Fear, frustration |
| Pregnancy | Trained athletes have resting bradycardia due to increased vagal tone |
| Muscular exercise | Decreases with age<br>At birth: 130–140 bpm;<br>Adults: 60–90 bpm;<br>Old age: 100 bpm (due to decreased vagal tone) |
| After meals | |
| Hormones: Adrenaline, thyroxine, posterior pituitary extract | Hormones: Acetylcholine (ACh) |
| Sympathetic activation | Parasympathetic activation |

**Table 41.2:** Pathological factors affecting heart rate.

| Factors increasing the heart rate | Factors decreasing the heart rate |
|---|---|
| Fever | Myxoedema/hypothyroidism |
| Anemia | Intacranial disorders: Raised intra-cranial tension (Cushing's reflex) |
| Thyrotoxicosis | Heart block |
| Congestive heart failure (CHF), myocardial infarction (MI) | |
| Shock | |

- Other reflexes:
  - Bezold–Jarisch reflex
  - Bainbridge reflex
  - Cushing's reflex
  - Marey's law

> ### SUMMARY
>
> - The heart produces its own impulse through SA node, but is regulated by the autonomic nervous system.
> - The sympathetic nervous system stimulates the cardiac activity as it supplies SA node, AV node and cardiac muscle. Hence, it increases the heart rate and force of contraction.
> - The parasympathetic nervous system, has an inhibitory effect on the heart decreasing the heart rate but it doesn't affect the force of contraction, as there is no parasympathetic supply to ventricles.
> - The normal heart rate in a healthy individual ranges between 60–100 beats per minutes with an average of 75 bpm.
> - It can show variation in various physiological and pathological conditions.
> - Most common cause of resting bradycardia is a trained athlete whose has a high vagal tone.

## LET US SEE, HOW MUCH YOU HAVE LEARNT?

### *Review Questions*

#### Long/Short Answer Questions

Q1. Explain the nerve supply of the heart and its effect on its function.
Q2. What would happen to the heart rate if all the nerve supply to heart is cut?
Q3. What is the physiological significance of resting bradycardia in athletes?
Q4. Define tachycardia. What are the causes of tachycardia?
Q5. Define bradycardia. What are the causes of bradycardia?

#### Explain Why? (Reasoning Questions)

Q1. The heart rate increases during physical exercise.
Q2. The heart rate decreases during deep breathing or meditation.
Q3. Hypoxia (low oxygen levels) can lead to an increased heart rate.

### *Critical Thinking Case-Based Questions*

Q1. Deepak, a 28-year-old athlete, came to the OPD for a routine check-up. During the examination, his resting heart rate was noted to be 45 beats per minute (bpm), which is lower than the average resting heart rate. He reported feeling well, with no symptoms of dizziness, fatigue, or palpitations. He mentioned that he had been training intensively for a marathon and engaged in regular endurance exercises. Depending upon given scenario, answer the following questions:
   a. Explain the physiological mechanisms behind Deepak's lower resting heart rate.
   b. What role does the autonomic nervous system play in regulating heart rate?
   c. Enumerate different variations of heart rate.

### *Multiple Choice Questions*

Q1. What is the primary neurotransmitter released by the parasympathetic nervous system to decrease heart rate?
   a. Norepinephrine
   b. Epinephrine
   c. Acetylcholine
   d. Dopamine

Q2. Which nerve primarily carries parasympathetic innervation to the heart?
   a. Vagus nerve (cranial nerve X)
   b. Glossopharyngeal nerve (cranial nerve IX)
   c. Trigeminal nerve (cranial nerve V)
   d. Hypoglossal nerve (cranial nerve XII)

Q3. What effect does sympathetic stimulation have on heart rate?
   a. Decreases heart rate
   b. Increases heart rate
   c. No effect on heart rate
   d. Irregular heart rate

Q4. A 25-year-old male athlete experiences an increase in heart rate during a sprint race. Which of the following factors is most likely responsible for this increase?
   a. Increased sympathetic activity
   b. Decreased parasympathetic activity
   c. Decreased adrenaline release
   d. Increased vagal tone

Q5. Which of the following statements is true regarding vagal tone?
   a. Vagal tone refers to sympathetic innervation of the heart.
   b. High vagal tone is associated with decreased heart rate variability.
   c. Vagal tone primarily influences heart rate through the release of norepinephrine.
   d. Vagal tone is highest during periods of stress.

Q6. A patient with high blood pressure experiences a sudden increase in heart rate after standing up quickly. Which reflex is most likely responsible for this compensatory response?
   a. Bainbridge reflex
   b. Chemoreceptor reflex
   c. Baroreceptor reflex
   d. Bezold–Jarisch reflex

Q7. What is the primary role of the baroreceptor reflex in regulating heart rate?
   a. Responds to changes in blood pH
   b. Responds to changes in blood pressure
   c. Responds to changes in blood glucose levels
   d. Responds to changes in blood oxygen levels

Q8. A patient undergoing surgery experiences a sudden increase in heart rate due to anxiety. Which neurotransmitter is most likely responsible for this response?
   a. Acetylcholine
   b. Dopamine
   c. Norepinephrine
   d. Serotonin

## ANSWERS

1. c   2. a   3. b   4. a   5. b   6. c   7. b   8. c

# Cardiac Output

**42 CHAPTER**

### COMPETENCY ADDRESSED
**PY5.9:** Describe the factors affecting heart rate, regulation of cardiac output and blood pressure.

### LEARNING OBJECTIVES
At the end of this chapter, the learner should be able to:
- Define cardiac output.
- Describe the various methods to measure the cardiac output.
- Describe the variations observed in cardiac output.
- Describe the regulation of cardiac output.

## DEFINITION

It is defined as the *amount of blood pumped by each ventricle* into the respective great arteries in *one minute*. It is expressed as the product of stroke volume and heart rate.

$$CO = SV \times HR$$
$$= 70 \times 70$$
$$= 4,900 \text{ mL/min or 5 L/min approx.}$$

(Stroke volume is the amount of blood pumped by each ventricle with each beat. It is roughly equal to 70 mL)

The cardiac output is higher in males (5–6 L/min) while it is 10–20% lower in females.

## Cardiac Index (CI)

When cardiac output is expressed in terms of body surface area, it is called as cardiac index [**Cardiac Output/m² of Body Surface Area (BSA)**].

(where, BSA = $W^{0.425}$ (kg) × $H^{0.725}$ (cm) × 0.007184)

The average cardiac index = *3 L/min/m² of BSA*

It increases up to 10 years of age, i.e., up to 4 L/min/m² and declines with age, so that at 80 years, it remains 2.4 L/min/m². This indicates **declining cardiac activity**.

## Stroke Volume Index

Similarly, stroke volume is also expressed as stroke volume index and is represented as stroke volume/m² of BSA, which is **40 mL/m²**.

## MEASUREMENT OF CARDIAC OUTPUT

### Direct Method

#### Adolf's Method Using Fick's Principle

**Fick's principle:** *It states that blood flow to an organ can be calculated from the consumption of indicator substance divided by its arteriovenous difference of indicator substance.*

To calculate the cardiac output, the indicator substance is oxygen consumption by the tissue and measuring the AV difference. It is a very reliable method for calculating cardiac output, as shown in **Figure 42.1**. The arterial sample is

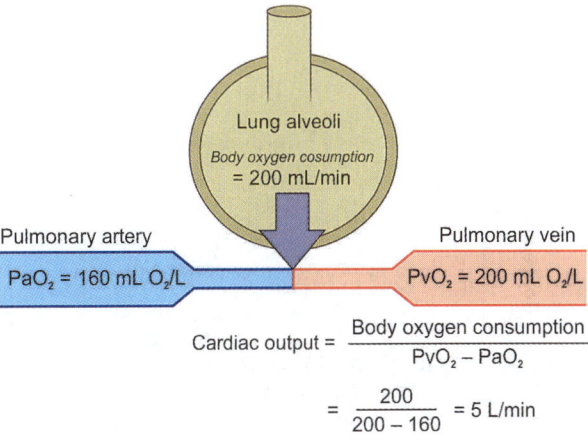

**Fig. 42.1:** Calculation of cardiac output using Fick's principle.

taken from any artery (For $PvO_2$ as it is carrying oxygenated blood) and the venous sample is taken from right ventricle or pulmonary trunk after cardiac catheterization (for $PaO_2$ as it carries deoxygenated blood).

### Indirect Fick's Principle

In patients where Fick's principle does not give reliable results, indirect Fick's principle can be used, which uses $CO_2$ is used instead of $O_2$. This method is used in patients with pulmonary arterial hypertension (PAH).

$$\text{Cardiac output} = \frac{CO_2 \text{ expired/minute} \times 100}{PaCO_2 - PvCO_2}$$

### Indicator Dye Dilution Method

In this invasive method, an indicator dye is injected into a peripheral vein, which gets pumped by the ventricle into the peripheral circulation by the left ventricle. Series of blood samples are then collected from the peripheral artery **(Fig. 42.2)**. The concentration of the indicator dye in the artery is measured and plotted against time in seconds.

As seen in graph **(Fig. 42.3)**, the concentration of dye increases with time, reaches a peak and then declines

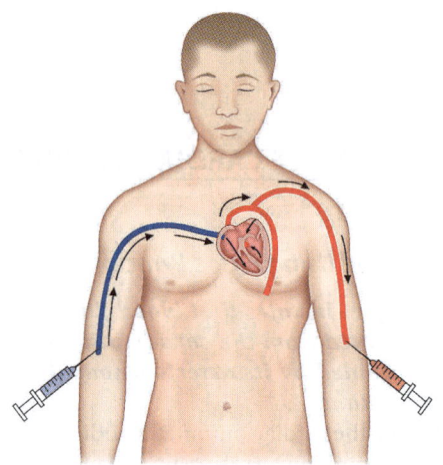

**Fig. 42.2:** Indicator dye dilution method.

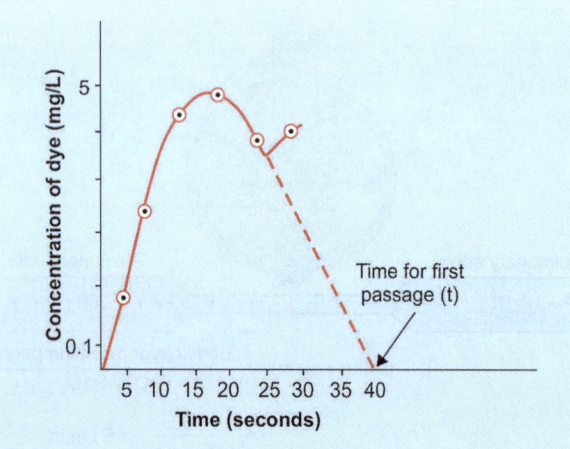

**Fig. 42.3:** Concentration of dye relation with time.

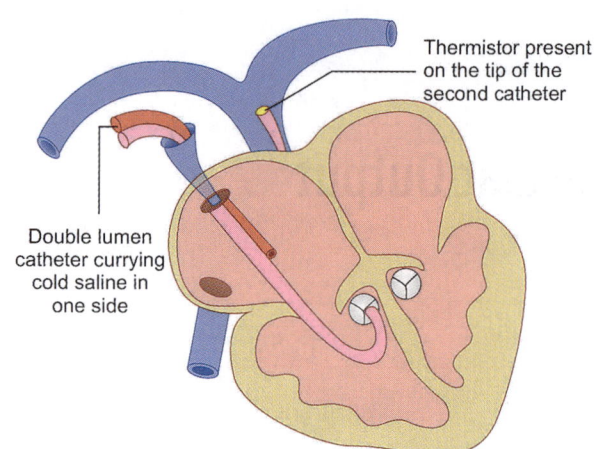

**Fig. 42.4:** Thermodilution method.

gradually, this entire movement of dye in peripheral circulation is called as first pass circulation. During the period of declining concentration (plotted as fall of indicator in arterial blood), the concentration of dye begins to rise again, hence, the second pass begins, i.e., the dye begins to get recirculated again in peripheral circulation. The declining curve on the plot is extended, so that it meets the time axis, which gives us the time duration of first passage of dye (**t**).

From the following parameters, the cardiac out output is calculated using the formula given below:

Q = Quantity of dye injected = 5 mg
C = Mean conc. of dye = 1.5 mg/L
t = Time duration of first passage of dye through the artery = 40 sec

$$\text{Cardiac output} = \frac{Q \times 60}{C \times t}$$

$$= \frac{5 \times 60}{1.5 \times 40} = \mathbf{5 L/min}$$

### Thermodilution Method (Fig. 42.4)

This method is quite similar to the indicator dye dilution method, but the only difference is in the indicator. Cold saline is used instead of dye, through a double lumen catheter, one end in RA and other in pulmonary artery. It carries 2 thermistors, placed in inferior vena cava and pulmonary artery. CO is measured by determining resultant change in the temperature of the blood in pulmonary artery. It is measured with same principle as indicator dilution method.

### Indirect Method

#### Ballistocardiography

- It is based on the principle of recoil, which records the recoil movements of cardiac activity on a highly sensitive table on which the patient is lying. This method is no longer used.
- Roentgenographic method using serial X-rays.

## Other Methods

### Electromagnetic Flowmeter

The flowmeter is placed around the artery through which the blood is flowing. It measures the blood flow through the artery and hence the cardiac output can be measured.

### Doppler Echocardiography

Based on the principle of Doppler sonography, it is the most commonly used method to noninvasively measure the cardiac output.

## FACTORS AFFECTING CARDIAC OUTPUT

- Cardiac output is primarily affected by preload, i.e., the **venous return** and afterload, i.e., **peripheral resistance**.
  - According to Frank Starling law, the cardiac output is directly proportional to the venous return (affecting the initial length of muscle). Hence, an increased venous return into the right atrium from the venous circulation increases the cardiac output.

    **Cardiac output ∞ Venous return**

  - Similarly, Laplace law explains the stress on the ventricular walls due to peripheral resistance. Hence, the cardiac output is inversely proportional to peripheral resistance.

    $$\text{Cardiac output} = \frac{\text{Arterial pressure}}{\text{Peripheral resistance}}$$

  *Hence, all the conditions which either increase the venous return or decrease the peripheral resistance will increase the cardiac output and vice versa.*

- The cardiac output is determined by stroke volume and heart rate as shown below:

    **Cardiac output = Stroke volume × Heart rate**

  Hence, all the factors which increase the stroke volume, i.e., venous return/end diastolic volume, myocardial oxygen demand would increase the cardiac output. Even the factors increasing the heart rate would increase the cardiac output like sympathetic stimulation, drugs, etc.

## VARIATIONS IN CARDIAC OUTPUT

Usually, the cardiac output shows slight variation with various physiological and pathological factors, shown below.

### Physiological Variations

- **Age:** It increases with age up to 10 years, then declines. The decreased cardiac output with increasing age is due to decreased muscle mass.
- **Gender:** It is higher in males as compared to females.
- **Effect of posture:** In the upright standing posture, the cardiac output is more as compared to the recumbent posture.
- **Emotional state:** The cardiac output increases during various psychological states resulting in sympathetic stimulation.
- **Environmental temperature** directly increases the heart rate and hence the cardiac output.
- **Exercise** also increases the cardiac output due to sympathetic stimulation.
- **Pregnancy** is condition of increased demand for nutrients and oxygen, hence, results in hyperdynamic circulation and decreased peripheral resistance. This results in increased cardiac output.
- **High altitude:** Decreased atmospheric oxygen tension results in hypoxic hypoxia in tissues, thus increasing the cardiac output, by decreasing the peripheral resistance.

### Pathological Variations (Table 42.1)

- **Anemia:** As seen in other conditions resulting in tissue hypoxia, anemia also results in decreased oxygen carrying capacity of blood. The other factor is hemodilution occurring in the anemia and decrease in blood viscosity. Hence, it increases the cardiac output. In severe cases of anemia, the patients may even present with systolic murmur.
- **Hemorrhage:** Hemorrhage is blood loss from any cause can that leads to decreased venous return which reduces the cardiac output. As a compensatory mechanism, the sympathetic discharge increases, attempts to increase the heart rate, venous return and cardiac output. But the primary regulating factor is the blood volume and arterial pressure.
- **Hyperthyroidism:** It is the clinical condition where there is excessive production of thyroid hormones. Thyroxine is responsible for regulating the metabolic rate. In thyrotoxicosis, the basal metabolic rate increases resulting in peripheral vasodilation and reduced peripheral resistance. Increased demand of nutrients by the tissues and reduced peripheral resistance increases the cardiac output.

**Table 42.1:** Summary of clinical conditions presenting with abnormal cardiac output.

| Low cardiac output | High cardiac output |
|---|---|
| Myocardial ischemia or hypoxia/decreased coronary perfusion | Beriberi |
| Cardiac tamponade | AV fistula |
| Cardiac metabolic derangements | Hyperthyroidism |
| Hypovolemia | Anemia |
| Acute venous dilation resulting in decreased venous return | Increased metabolic rate of tissues |
| Obstruction of large veins | Decreased total peripheral resistance |
| Decreased muscle mass | |
| Decreased metabolic rate of tissues | |

- **Septicemia:** It increases the cardiac output by decreasing the peripheral resistance due to massive vasodilation.
- **Beriberi:** It is caused due to the deficiency of thiamine. It also increases the cardiac output due to increased nutritional demand of tissues along with decreased peripheral resistance.
- **AV fistula:** An AV fistula shunts the blood from arterial circulation to venous side, hence the tissues become hypoxic and there is decreased peripheral resistance, resulting in increased cardiac output.

## REGULATION OF CARDIAC OUTPUT (FLOWCHART 42.1)

### Factors Affecting Stroke Volume

#### Heterometric Regulation

This is also called intrinsic regulation, i.e., all the factors which are within the cardiac muscle, increasing the stroke volume.

Various factors which are responsible for heterometric regulation are:
- Initial length of cardiac muscle fiber
- Venous return
- Myocardial oxygen demand

Let us discuss all these factors in detail:
- **Initial length of cardiac muscle** depends on the end diastolic volume of the ventricle. Hence, based on Frank Starling's law, which states that the *'within physiological limits, the force of contraction is directly proportional to initial length of muscle fiber or the end diastolic volume.'*
- **Myocardial oxygen demand (MVO$_2$):** It is an important factor which regulates the cardiac output. If the cardiac activity increases, then the MVO$_2$ also increases cardiac output. Myocardial factors play an important role in regulating cardiac output because coronary perfusion also directly depends on the cardiac output.
- **Venous return:** It is amount of blood returning back to the right atrium from the systemic circulation through the inferior and superior vena cava. As discussed earlier, it increases the initial length of muscle fiber and hence increases the cardiac output. The venous return is discussed in detail separately.

#### Homometric Regulation

These factors act on the heart and are present outside the myocardium, hence called extrinsic mechanisms. The various factors acting in this type are:
- Sympathetic stimulation
- Effect of drugs increasing the stroke volume

Let us discuss all these factors in detail:
- **Sympathetic stimulation:** Sympathetic discharge increases during all kinds of physical and emotional stress, thus **increases the force of contraction**, **heart rate** and **venous return** due to venoconstriction.
- **Various drugs/hormones/food items** have **positive inotropic effect** of the heart thus increasing the stroke volume.

### Factors Affecting Heart Rate

We have seen that CO is directly proportional to HR, hence increase in heart rate increases the cardiac output. But this does not go on indefinitely, it shows certain variations as per the heart rate.
- Increase in heart rate up to **180 beats/minute**, results **in increase in CO** because there is shortening of diastasis period in cardiac cycle without comprising filling or emptying of ventricles.

**Flowchart 42.1:** Regulation of cardiac output.

```
                        Regulation of cardiac output
           ┌────────────────────┬──────────────────────┬───────────────────┐
     Factors affecting    Neurohormonal control              Local control
      ┌────────┴────────┐
  Stroke volume      Heart rate
```

**Stroke volume:**

- **Heterometric regulation** (Intrinsic to heart)
  - Initial length of cardiac muscle fiber
  - Oxygen demand
  - Venous return

- **Homometric regulation** (Extrinsic to heart):
  - Sympathetic stimulation
  - Effect of ionotropic drugs
  - Catecholamines → ~ Symp. stimulation
  - Xanthines → + inotropic
  - Glucagon → + inotropic
  - Digitalis → # Na-K ATPase → + inotropic
  - Barbiturates → – inotropic
  - CO$_2$, hypoxia and acidosis → – inotropic

**Heart rate:** All the factors which increase/decrease the HR affect the CO:
- Increase in HR → Inc. CO$_2$, up to 180 bpm, at cost of diastasis
- HR b/w 180–200 bpm → shortening of diastasis, rapid filling and ventricular systole
- HR > 200 bpm → shortening of ventricular → systole → fall in CO

**Neurohormonal control:**
- Control of ANS during emotions, muscular exercise, etc.
- Effect of hormones like catecholamines, thyroxine, glucagon, etc.

**Local control:**
- Tissue oxygen demand
- In peripheral tissues
- Total peripheral resistance CO = 1/ TPR
- Accumulation of metabolic waste products like adenosine and lactic acid

- If heart rate increases **between 180 to 200 beats/minute**, there is shortening of diastasis, rapid filling and ventricular systole. The cardiac may or may not fall in this heart rate range.
- An increase in heart rate **above 200 beats/minute** results in significant shortening of ventricular systole along with filling. This leads to **fall in CO**.

### Neurohormonal Factors

- **Control of ANS** during emotions, muscular exercise, etc. (as mentioned above).
- Effect of **hormones** like catecholamines, thyroxine, glucagon, etc.

These hormones increase the metabolic activity increasing the nutrient demand and increasing the production of metabolites, hence increasing the cardiac output.

### Local Factors

- **Tissue oxygen demand:** The peripheral tissues increase their oxygen demand at the time of increased activity or there is decreased availability of oxygen to the tissues (hypoxia) due to an cause, which results in vasodilation to increase the blood flow to the tissues. This increased blood flow increases the cardiac output.
- **Accumulation of waste products:** Accumulation of lactic acid, adenosine, and other metabolites result in increased cardiac output.
- **Total peripheral resistance:** Decreased total peripheral resistance either due to vasodilation or decreased viscosity of blood results in increased cardiac output.

## CARDIAC FUNCTION CURVES (FIG. 42.5)

This is the graph plotted between right atrial pressure and cardiac output, which shows the efficiency of myocardium, in terms of cardiac output, with respect to above mentioned variables.

As seen in this graph the normal heart can increase the cardiac output up to 13 L/min, without any stimulation, which is 2.5 times the normal cardiac output. However, due to certain factors, the cardiac output can further increase above normal resulting in a hypereffective heart

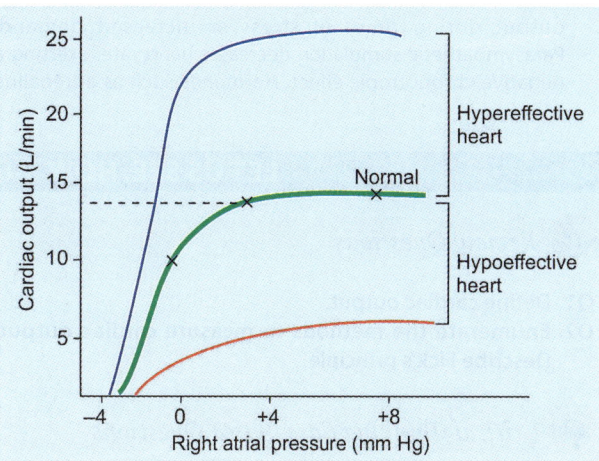

**Fig. 42.5:** Cardiac function curves.

**Table 42.2:** Causes of hypereffective and hypoeffective heart.

| Hypereffective heart | Hypoeffective heart |
|---|---|
| **Nervous stimulation:**<br>• Increased sympathetic stimulation: As seen in stressful conditions or exercise<br>• Parasympathetic inhibition (**Vagal tone**): As seen in athletes<br>Both these factors if work together, can result in maximum increase in cardiac output, as seen in athletes | Increased arterial pressure |
| | Cardiac arryythmias |
| | Coronary artery blockage resulting in decreased myocardial perfusion |
| **Hypertrophy of myocardium:**<br>• Long term training of heart as seen in marathon runners/athletes can result in myocardial hypertrophy resulting in increased cardiac output<br>• Nervous stimulation and cardiac hypertrophy can result in an increased CO up to 40 L/min in athletes | Valvular heart disease |
| | Congenital heart disease |
| | Myocarditis |

and if cardiac output falls below normal, it is referred to as hypoeffective heart. The various causes of both these conditions, are mentioned in **Table 42.2**.

## SUMMARY

- Cardiac output (CO) refers to the volume of blood ejected by the heart per unit of time, typically measured in liters per minute (L/min). It represents the effectiveness of the heart in pumping blood throughout the systemic circulation and is a critical determinant of tissue perfusion and oxygen delivery.
- Several methods are employed to measure cardiac output, including:
  - Fick principle: Calculates cardiac output based on the rate of oxygen consumption and the difference in oxygen content between arterial and venous blood.
  - Thermodilution technique: Utilizes the injection of a cold solution into a central vein and monitoring the resulting temperature changes.
  - Doppler echocardiography: Uses ultrasound to measure blood flow velocity and cross-sectional area to calculate cardiac output.
- Cardiac output can vary in response to physiological and pathological conditions. Factors influencing cardiac output include heart rate, stroke volume, preload, afterload, contractility, and vascular tone. Exercise, stress, blood loss, dehydration, and certain medications can all affect cardiac output.
- Cardiac output is regulated through complex mechanisms involving the autonomic nervous system, hormones, and local factors. The sympathetic nervous system increases heart rate and contractility, thereby enhancing cardiac

output during times of stress or increased demand. Parasympathetic stimulation decreases heart rate, exerting a negative chronotropic effect. Hormones such as adrenaline and noradrenaline, as well as factors like preload and afterload, also play crucial roles in modulating cardiac output.

## LET US SEE, HOW MUCH YOU HAVE LEARNT?

### Review Questions

Q1. Define cardiac output.
Q2. Enumerate the methods to measure cardiac output. Describe Fick's principle.
Q3. What are the variations in cardiac output?
Q4. Describe the regulation of cardiac output.

### Critical Thinking Case-Based Questions

Q1. Why is cardiac output an important parameter to monitor in patients with heart failure?
Q2. Explain how changes in heart rate and stroke volume affect cardiac output.
Q3. Why does cardiac output need to increase during exercise or physical activity?
Q4. Discuss the relationship between cardiac output and tissue perfusion.
Q5. How does the body compensate for a decrease in cardiac output in response to hemorrhage?
Q6. Explain the role of preload, afterload, and contractility in regulating cardiac output.
Q7. Why might a decrease in systemic vascular resistance lead to an increase in cardiac output?
Q8. Discuss how changes in blood volume can impact cardiac output.
Q9. Explain the concept of oxygen delivery and its relationship to cardiac output.
Q10. How does the autonomic nervous system regulate cardiac output in response to stress or changes in activity level?
Q11. Why athletes can increase their cardiac output to 40 L/min as compared to an untrained person who can increase up to 13 L/min.

### Multiple Choice Questions

Q1. Which of the following best describes cardiac output?
   a. The volume of blood ejected by the left atrium per heartbeat
   b. The volume of blood ejected by the ventricles per contraction
   c. The volume of blood ejected by the heart per unit of time
   d. The volume of blood returning to the heart from the systemic circulation

Q2. Which technique involves the insertion of a catheter into the pulmonary artery to directly measure cardiac output?
   a. Doppler echocardiography
   b. Fick principle
   c. Pulmonary artery catheterization
   d. Thermodilution technique

Q3. What factor primarily determines preload, influencing stroke volume and subsequently cardiac output?
   a. Sympathetic nervous system activity
   b. Afterload
   c. Venous return
   d. Contractility

Q4. Which of the following hormones increases heart rate and contractility, thereby enhancing cardiac output during stress?
   a. Insulin
   b. Adrenaline (epinephrine)
   c. Aldosterone
   d. Glucagon

Q5. Scenario: A 60-year-old male presents to the emergency room with chest pain and shortness of breath. Which of the following hemodynamic parameters would be most appropriate to assess his cardiac function?
   a. Blood pressure
   b. Cardiac output
   c. Respiratory rate
   d. Serum electrolytes

Q6. Scenario: During a stress test, a patient's heart rate increases from 70 bpm at rest to 160 bpm during exercise. Which of the following changes in cardiac output is most likely to occur?
   a. Decreased cardiac output
   b. No change in cardiac output
   c. Increased cardiac output
   d. Fluctuating cardiac output

Q7. Scenario: A 55-year-old female with heart failure presents with edema and fatigue. Which of the following factors contributes to her reduced cardiac output?
   a. Decreased afterload
   b. Increased preload
   c. Reduced contractility
   d. Elevated stroke volume

Q8. Scenario: A 40-year-old athlete complains of palpitations and chest discomfort after intense exercise. What hemodynamic response is likely contributing to his symptoms?
   a. Increased preload
   b. Decreased afterload
   c. Elevated cardiac output
   d. Reduced stroke volume

Q9. Which of the following conditions is likely to result in an increase in cardiac output?
   a. Hypovolemia
   b. Systemic hypertension
   c. Pulmonary embolism
   d. Bradycardia

Q10. A patient with severe aortic stenosis is likely to exhibit which of the following adaptations to maintain cardiac output?
   a. Increased preload
   b. Decreased contractility
   c. Elevated afterload
   d. Compensatory tachycardia

Q11. In which of the following situations would the Frank-Starling mechanism play a significant role in regulating cardiac output?
   a. Acute myocardial infarction
   b. Exercise-induced tachycardia
   c. Hypertrophic cardiomyopathy
   d. Systemic vasodilation

Q12. An increase in sympathetic nervous system activity is expected to result in:
   a. Decreased heart rate and contractility
   b. Increased heart rate and contractility
   c. Reduced cardiac output and stroke volume
   d. Elevated afterload and preload

Q13. Which of the following factors primarily determines systemic vascular resistance and influences cardiac output?
   a. Heart rate
   b. Stroke volume
   c. Blood viscosity
   d. Venous return

Q14. A patient with septic shock is likely to exhibit:
   a. Decreased cardiac output and elevated systemic vascular resistance
   b. Increased cardiac output and reduced systemic vascular resistance
   c. Decreased cardiac output and decreased systemic vascular resistance
   d. Increased cardiac output and elevated systemic vascular resistance

Q15. Which of the following conditions would most likely result in an increase in cardiac output?
   a. Decreased preload due to dehydration
   b. Increased afterload due to systemic hypertension
   c. Reduced contractility due to myocardial infarction
   d. Elevated heart rate due to sympathetic stimulation

Q16. An athlete experiences a drop in cardiac output during intense training. What could be a potential explanation for this phenomenon?
   a. Increased venous return
   b. Elevated afterload
   c. Reduced contractility
   d. Enhanced parasympathetic activity

Q17. A patient with chronic obstructive pulmonary disease (COPD) is admitted with exacerbation of symptoms. Which hemodynamic alteration is most likely to occur?
   a. Increased preload due to venous pooling
   b. Decreased afterload due to vasodilation
   c. Reduced cardiac output due to decreased stroke volume
   d. Elevated contractility due to sympathetic activation

Q18. Which of the following interventions is most likely to increase cardiac output in a patient with heart failure?
   a. Administering a beta-blocker to reduce heart rate
   b. Initiating diuretic therapy to decrease preload
   c. Providing inotropic support to enhance contractility
   d. Prescribing an angiotensin-converting enzyme (ACE) inhibitor to reduce afterload

Q19. A patient presents with a myocardial infarction affecting the left ventricle. Which hemodynamic change is expected to compensate for the decreased cardiac output?
   a. Increased preload due to sympathetic stimulation
   b. Decreased afterload due to vasodilation
   c. Elevated heart rate due to baroreceptor reflex
   d. Enhanced contractility due to the Frank-Starling mechanism

Q20. A patient with hypovolemic shock exhibits tachycardia and low blood pressure. What is the primary goal of treatment to restore cardiac output in this scenario?
   a. Administering a beta-blocker to decrease heart rate
   b. Providing intravenous fluids to increase preload
   c. Initiating vasopressor therapy to elevate afterload
   d. Administering a calcium channel blocker to reduce contractility

**ANSWERS**

1. c   2. c   3. c   4. b   5. b   6. c   7. c   8. a   9. c   10. a   11. c   12. b   13. c   14. b
15. d   16. b   17. c   18. c   19. a   20. b

# Venous Return and its Regulation

**CHAPTER 43**

> **COMPETENCY ADDRESSED**
> **PY5.9:** Describe the factors affecting heart rate, regulation of cardiac output and blood pressure.

> **LEARNING OBJECTIVES**
> At the end of this chapter, the learner should be able to:
> - Define venous return.
> - Describe the factors affecting venous return.
> - Describe the role of venous return in regulating cardiac output.
> - Describe the venous function curves.

## INTRODUCTION

It is defined as the amount of blood entering the right atrium per minute from the systemic circulation through superior and inferior vena cava. It is **5–6 L/min**.

Venous return (VR) is an important factor **controlling cardiac output** through changes in diastolic filling of ventricles.

### Right Atrial Pressure (RAP)

Following the principles of fluid dynamics the blood always flows from the areas of high pressure to the low pressure. Hence, in the normal circumstances, the **RAP is less than venous pressure** which results in flow of blood toward RA. If there is an **increase in RAP,** due to any reason, it results in a **decrease in VR.**

> *What will happen to right atrial pressure in a patient of right ventricular failure/pulmonary hypertension?*
>
> In RV failure, the RV fails to effectively pump the blood during systole resulting in reduced stroke volume. Hence, there is an increase in end systolic volume, affecting the filling of the ventricle during diastole. Eventually, there is an increase in RAP, which decreases the VR; which results in peripheral pooling of blood. Hence, a patient with RVF presents with raised JVP, congestive hepatomegaly and edema in dependent parts of body.

### Mean Systemic Filling Pressure (Psf)

It is mean systemic pressure in circulation at any time, hence, it forces systemic blood towards the heart, increasing

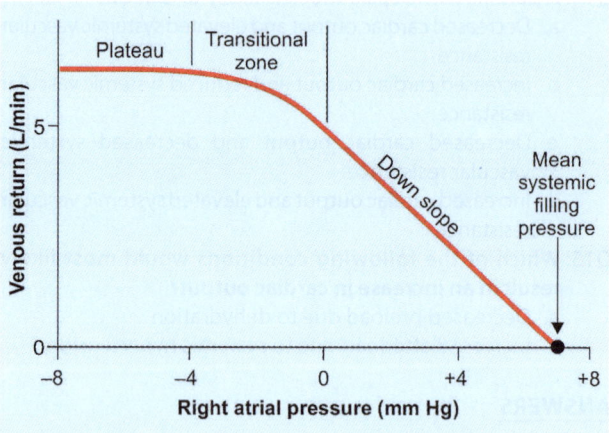

**Fig. 43.1:** Mean systemic filling pressure.

the venous return. It can also be *referred to as a right atrial pressure where the entire circulation comes to a halt*. In a normal individual, the mean systemic filling pressure is *+7 mm Hg* **(Fig. 43.1)**. Hence, from this, we can infer that if the right atrial pressure increases above normal, the venous return remains same for sometime and then it begins to decline till it becomes zero. This point is same as Psf.

### Resistance to Blood Flow between Peripheral Vessels and Heart [Venous Resistance (VR) and Resistance to Venous Return (RVR)]

The *resistance to the blood flowing back toward right atrium, called the resistance to the venous return.* The veins are highly distensible vessels low pressure system, which fail to overcome this resistance. In contrast, the increased arteriolar resistance would increase the arterial pressure to overcome this resistance, and pushes the blood into venous circulation, overcoming some venous resistance. Hence, the resistance to venous return can be expressed as:

$$\text{Venous return} = \frac{Psf - RAP}{\text{Resistance to venous return}}$$

> **Calculate the resistance to VR, if the mean systemic filling pressure is 7 mm Hg, RAP is 0 mm Hg and VR is 5 L/min?**
>
> $$\text{Venous return} = \frac{Psf - RAP}{\text{Resistance to venous return}}$$
> Or
> $$\text{Resistance to venous return} = \frac{Psf - RAP}{\text{Venous return}}$$
> $$\text{Resistance to venous return} = \frac{7 - 0}{5} = 1.4 \text{ mm Hg/L/min}$$
>
> **What will happen to VR, if RVR increases and why?**
>
> An increase in RVR, decreases the VR and vice versa (see figure below). If RVR is doubled, the VR is reduced to half and if RVR is halved, the VR is doubled. But the entire circulation will still come to a halt at RAP of +7 mm Hg, irrespective of RVR.
>
>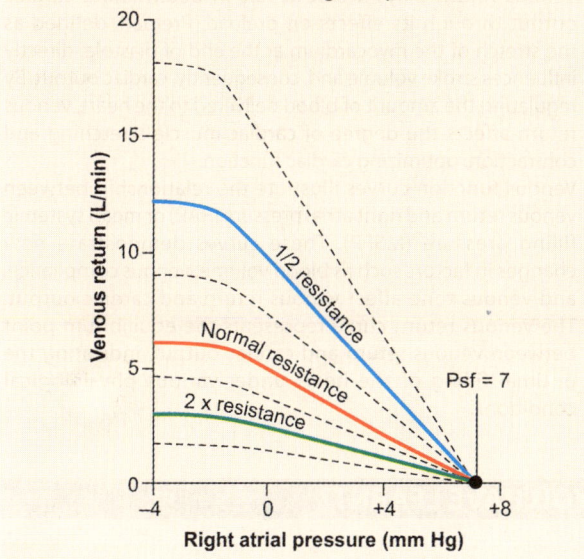

## FACTORS AFFECTING THE VENOUS RETURN

Various factors affecting venous return are summarized below:

| Factors increasing VR | Factors decreasing VR |
|---|---|
| • Sympathetic stimulation<br>• Exercise<br>• Increased vascular tone<br>• Increased blood volume | • Increased TPR<br>• Decreased blood volume |

### Effect of Respiration/Intrathoracic Pressure on Venous Return

Respiration alters intrathoracic pressure, influencing venous return by enhancing venous blood flow during

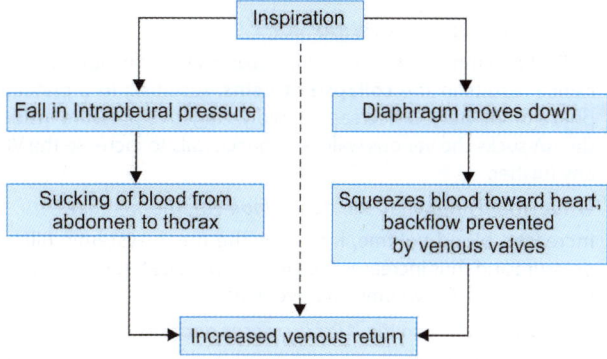

**Flowchart 43.1:** Effects of inspiration on venous return.

inhalation and momentarily impeding it during exhalation, regulating cardiac preload dynamics (**Flowchart 43.1**).

### Effect of Sympathetic Stimulation on VR

The sympathetic stimulation stimulates the entire cardiovascular system.
- It stimulates the heart, increasing the heart rate and force of contraction
- It results in arteriolar constriction, resulting in increased TPR
- The venoconstriction occurring due to sympathetic stimulation results in forward movement of blood toward right atrium, hence, increasing the venous return.

### Relation of RAP, VR and CO

As seen in **Figure 43.2**, RAP directly affects the VR and hence controls the cardiac output. During recordings of various measurements of RAP, the VR and CO shows following changes:
- At RAP = 0; VR = CO = 5 L/min
- At RAP > 0; VR decreases, CO initially increases but then remains same
- At RAP < 0; VR initially increases but then remains same; CO decreases

At rest:
- VR becomes zero at RAP = Psf = 7 mm Hg
- CO becomes zero when RA <0

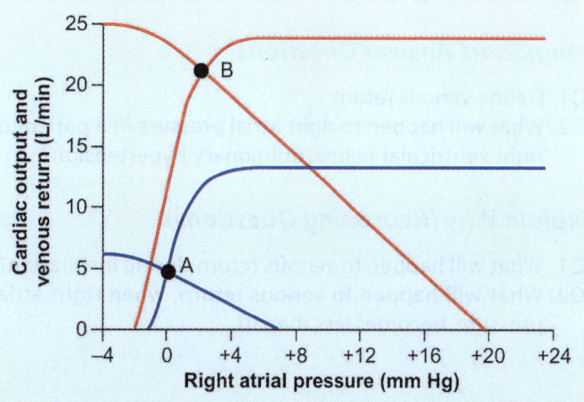

**Fig. 43.2:** Relationship between RAP, VO and cardiac output.

**Why CO falls to zero, with RAP <0?**
At RAP of 0 mm Hg, the pressure becomes subatmospheric and hence results in the **collapse of veins**, resulting in a plateau phase of VR, but CO decreases rapidly. Negative pressure inside the RA sucks the venous walls and hence fails to increase the VR any further.

**What would happen to VR, if the blood volume increases?**
Increased blood volume, increases the mean systemic filling pressure and thus increases the VR. The opposite happens during decrease in blood volume (hypovolemia).

**What will happen to VR, if Psf increases and why?**
Mean systemic filling pressure indicates the tightness with which the blood vessels are filled with blood. In an increased Psf, the VR increases and Venous return curve shifts upward. However, when there is decreased Psf, the venous return curve moves downward.

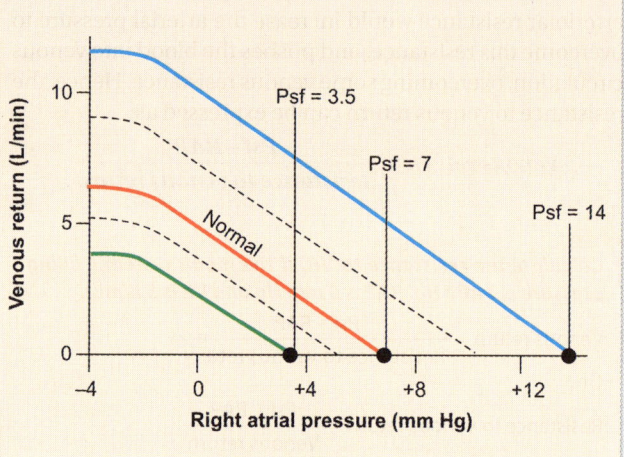

## SUMMARY

- Venous return refers to the volume of blood that returns to the heart from the systemic circulation, primarily through the venous system. It represents the amount of blood delivered to the right atrium, which ultimately determines preload, stroke volume, and cardiac output.
- Several factors influence venous return:
  - Venous tone: Constriction or dilation of venous vessels affects venous capacitance and the ability of veins to store blood.
  - Blood volume: Changes in blood volume, such as dehydration or hemorrhage, directly impact venous return.
  - Skeletal muscle pump: Contractions of skeletal muscles during physical activity compress peripheral veins, aiding in venous return to the heart.
  - Respiratory pump: Changes in intrathoracic pressure during respiration facilitate venous return by enhancing blood flow towards the heart.
  - Venous valves: Prevent backflow of blood, ensuring unidirectional flow towards the heart.
- Sympathetic nervous system activity: Sympathetic stimulation can increase venous tone, reducing venous compliance and enhancing venous return.
- Venous return plays a crucial role in determining cardiac output through its effects on preload. Preload, defined as the stretch of the myocardium at the end of diastole, directly influences stroke volume and, consequently, cardiac output. By regulating the amount of blood delivered to the heart, venous return affects the degree of cardiac muscle stretching and contraction, optimizing cardiac function.
- Venous function curves illustrate the relationship between venous return and right atrial pressure (RAP) or mean systemic filling pressure (MSFP). These curves demonstrate how changes in factors such as blood volume, venous compliance, and venous tone affect venous return and cardiac output. The venous return curve represents the equilibrium point between venous return and cardiac output, indicating the optimal filling of the heart under various physiological conditions.

## LET US SEE, HOW MUCH YOU HAVE LEARNT?

 *Review Questions*

### Long/Short Answer Questions

Q1. Define venous return.
Q2. What will happen to right atrial pressure in a patient of right ventricular failure/pulmonary hypertension?
Q3. Calculate the resistance to VR, if the mean systemic filling pressure is 7 mm Hg, RAP is 0 mm Hg and VR is 5 L/min.

### Explain Why (Reasoning Questions)

Q1. What will happen to venous return during inspiration?
Q2. What will happen to venous return, when right atrial pressure becomes less than 0?
Q3. What will happen to venous return, when right atrial pressure becomes more than 7?
Q4. What will happen to VR, if Psf increases and why?

## Multiple Choice Questions

**Q1.** What is the definition of venous return?
   a. The amount of blood pumped out by the ventricles per minute
   b. The volume of blood returning to the heart from the systemic circulation per minute
   c. The volume of blood returning to the heart from the pulmonary circulation per minute
   d. The pressure exerted by blood in the veins

**Q2.** Which of the following factors affects venous return?
   a. Blood viscosity
   b. Peripheral resistance
   c. Venous compliance
   d. All of the above

**Q3.** What is the role of sympathetic stimulation in venous return?
   a. Decreases venous tone
   b. Increases venous compliance
   c. Increases venous return
   d. Decreases venous pressure

**Q4.** How does skeletal muscle pump contribute to venous return?
   a. By increasing venous resistance
   b. By decreasing venous compliance
   c. By compressing veins during muscle contraction
   d. By decreasing blood viscosity

**Q5.** Which of the following statements about venous return and cardiac output is correct?
   a. Venous return is directly proportional to cardiac output
   b. Cardiac output is inversely proportional to venous return
   c. Venous return is the primary determinant of cardiac output
   d. Cardiac output has no relationship with venous return

**Q6.** What happens to venous return during exercise?
   a. Increases due to increased sympathetic activity
   b. Decreases due to decreased skeletal muscle pump activity
   c. Remains unchanged
   d. Increases due to decreased venous tone

**Q7.** Which of the following curves illustrates the relationship between right atrial pressure and cardiac output?
   a. Frank-Starling curve
   b. Venous return curve
   c. Cardiac function curve
   d. Pressure-volume loop

**Q8.** What does the slope of the venous function curve represent?
   a. Venous pressure
   b. Venous compliance
   c. Venous return
   d. Venous resistance

**Q9.** What does a shift to the right in the venous function curve indicate?
   a. Decreased venous return
   b. Increased venous return
   c. Decreased venous compliance
   d. Increased venous resistance

**Q10.** How does increased blood volume affect the venous function curve?
   a. Shifts it to the left
   b. Shifts it to the right
   c. No effect on the curve
   d. Causes a steeper slope

**Q11.** A patient with chronic venous insufficiency complains of leg pain and swelling, especially after prolonged standing. Which of the following interventions would be most appropriate for improving venous return in this patient?
   a. Encouraging prolonged sitting to reduce gravitational pressure on the legs
   b. Advising regular walking and calf muscle exercises to promote venous blood flow
   c. Prescribing bed rest to minimize leg movement and reduce venous pooling
   d. Suggesting elevation of the legs above heart level to decrease venous pressure

**Q12.** A pregnant woman in her third trimester presents with symptoms of dizziness and fainting spells. Which of the following physiological changes associated with pregnancy is likely contributing to her symptoms?
   a. Decreased blood volume
   b. Increased venous return
   c. Reduced cardiac output
   d. Constriction of peripheral blood vessels

**Q13.** A patient recovering from major surgery is at risk of developing deep vein thrombosis (DVT). Which of the following interventions is most effective for preventing DVT in this patient?
   a. Maintaining prolonged bed rest to reduce movement
   b. Applying warm compresses to the affected limbs
   c. Administering anticoagulant medications as prophylaxis
   d. Encouraging frequent leg elevation above heart level

**Q14.** A marathon runner complains of cramping and fatigue during a long-distance race. Which of the following factors contributes to maintaining venous return and cardiac output during intense exercise?
   a. Decreased sympathetic nervous system activity
   b. Increased venous compliance
   c. Skeletal muscle pump activity
   d. Reduced blood volume

**Q15.** A patient with heart failure experiences worsening dyspnea and edema despite optimal medical therapy. Which of the following interventions directly targets improving venous return in this patient?
   a. Increasing diuretic dosage to reduce fluid overload
   b. Prescribing angiotensin-converting enzyme (ACE) inhibitors to decrease afterload
   c. Recommending regular aerobic exercise to enhance cardiac function
   d. Applying compression stockings to promote venous return

## ANSWERS

1. b  2. d  3. c  4. c  5. c  6. a  7. b  8. c  9. a  10. a  11. b  12. b  13. c  14. c  15. d

# Blood Pressure and its Regulation

**CHAPTER 44**

**COMPETENCY ADDRESSED**

PY5.9: Describe the factors affecting heart rate, regulation of cardiac output and blood pressure.

**LEARNING OBJECTIVES**

At the end of this chapter, the learner should be able to:
- Define the blood pressure.
- Describe the various components of blood pressure.
- Describe the determinants of blood pressure.
- Describe the factors affecting blood pressure.
- Describe the regulation of blood pressure.

Blood pressure is defined as the lateral pressure exerted by the column of blood on the walls of arteries.

**Components of blood pressure (Fig. 44.1)**
- **Systolic blood pressure:** It is the **maximum pressure** in the arteries and is due to ventricular ejection. Hence, it is directly related to cardiac output. Normal range of systolic blood pressure is **100–140 mm Hg**.
- **Diastolic blood pressure:** It is the **minimum pressure** in the arteries. It occurs during ventricular diastole when no blood enters the aorta from the ventricles. The blood flows **due to the Windkessel effect**. It is directly related to total peripheral resistance. Normal diastolic pressure is **60–90 mm Hg**.
- **Pulse pressure:** The **difference between the systolic and diastolic pressure** is called as pulse pressure. Normal pulse pressure is **40 mm Hg**.
- **Mean arterial pressure:** It is the **mean pressure in the arteries**. It is calculated as DBP + ½PP. This pressure is close to DBP. Normal range is **95 mm Hg**.

## DETERMINANTS OF BLOOD PRESSURE

***BP = Cardiac output (CO) × Peripheral resistance (TPR)***

(Peripheral resistance: It is the resistance which blood has to overcome while passing through the periphery. **The main site of resistance is the arterioles).**

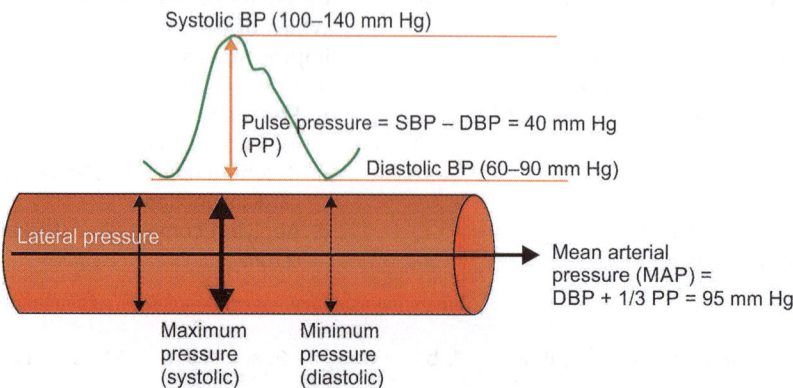

**Fig. 44.1:** Blood pressure and its components.
(SBP: systolic blood pressure; DBP: diastolic blood pressure; PP: pulse pressure)

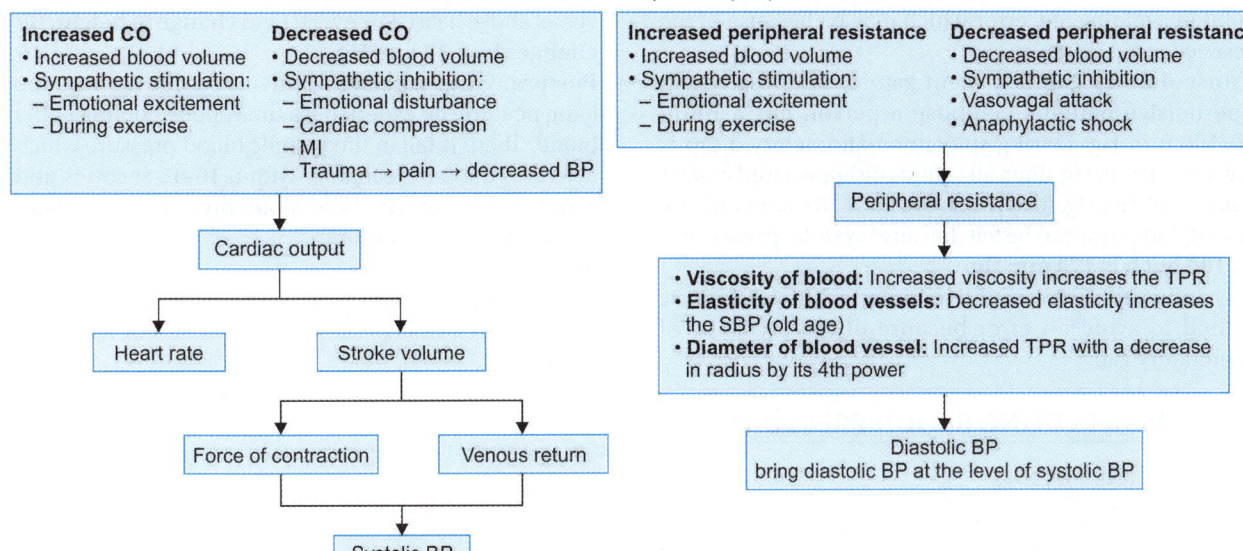

Flowchart 44.1: Effects of cardiac output and peripheral resistance on BP.

We have already learnt that, cardiac output = heart rate × stroke volume. In turn, stroke volume = force of contraction × venous return. Hence, any change in HR, SV, force of contraction or venous return will affect the blood pressure, as seen in **Flowchart 44.1**.

## MEASUREMENT OF BLOOD PRESSURE

Methods:
- Direct method—used in experimental studies
- Indirect method—sphygmomanometery:
  - Palpatory—to find out the systolic blood pressure, before measuring BP by auscultatory method
  - Oscillatory
  - Auscultatory—used in practice

### Sphygmomanometery

The subject lies on his back and the Riva Rocci cuff is tied on the arm. The sphygmomanometer, heart and arm should be in the same level **(Fig. 44.2)**. The cuff is inflated with the help of pump, simultaneously palpating the radial artery. Pressure is increased slightly above the disappearance of radial pulse. The cuff is deflated at the speed of 2–3 mm/sec. *The pressure at which radial pulse becomes palpable is systolic pressure by palpatory method*. Again, the cuff is inflated after deflation, 30 mm above the systolic blood pressure measured by palpatory method and the bell of the stethoscope is placed on brachial artery (in antecubital space). The cuff is slowly deflated. Initially there is no sound but soon a **tap is heard this is systolic BP, continuation of deflation reduces the pressure inside the cuff and the turbulent flow in rachial artery becomes laminar and at that point all sounds disappear this is diastolic BP.** These sounds are called *Korotkoff sounds* **(Fig. 44.3)**.

Recording by palpatory method is very important, though it only gives some idea about systolic BP and

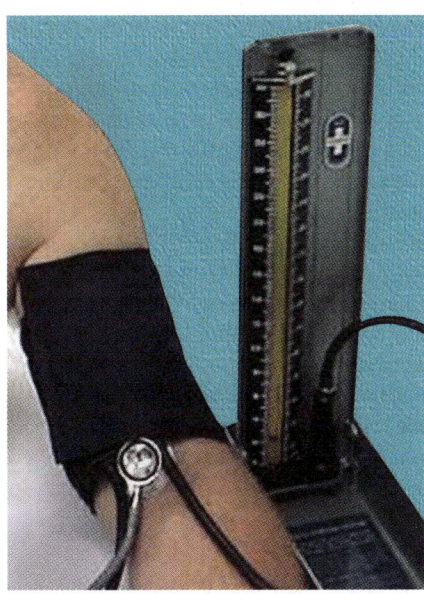

**Fig. 44.2:** Measurement of BP using sphygmomanometer.

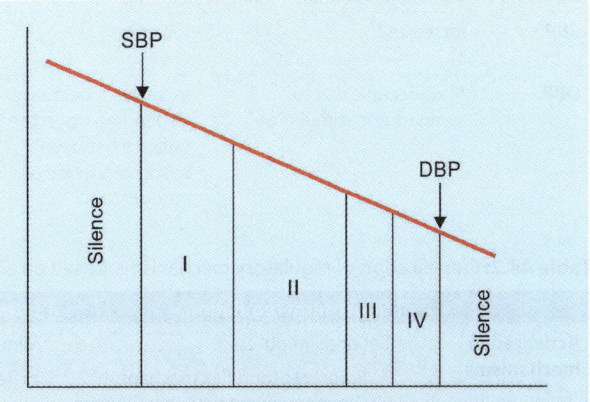

**Fig. 44.3:** Korotkoff's sound between SBP and DBP.

diastolic cannot be measured at all. As this method is useful in avoiding any error which may be because of the presence of auscultatory gap.

**Auscultatory gap** is a silent gap sometimes seen in hypertensive patients. Suppose a person has a BP of 170/100 mm Hg. During sphygmomanometry a tap is heard at 170 mm Hg. Then all sounds disappear and appear again at 130 mm Hg. In between 170 and 130 sounds are not present, but pulse can be felt, because **systolic pressure is not 130 but it is 170 mm Hg.**

Systolic pressure must be recorded first by palpatory method to avoid an error because of the presence of auscultatory gap.

## FACTORS AFFECTING BLOOD PRESSURE

### Physiological Factors

- **Age:** Both systolic and diastolic pressure increase with age.
- **Gender variation:** Before menopause, BP is slightly less in females by 4–6 mm Hg (because of presence of estrogen). No gender difference is seen after menopause.
- **Meals:** Systolic BP increase by 4–6 mm Hg after the meals and lasts for about one hour but diastolic BP shows no change or may decrease as there is fall in peripheral resistance due to vasodilatation in splanchnic vessels.
- **Emotions:** Fear, anxiety cause increase in BP (↑Sympathetic activity).
- **Temperature:** Cold increases the BP because of increase in PR due to cutaneous vasoconstriction [action through hypothalamus whereas heat ↓ BP because of ↓ PR caused by cutaneous vasodilatation (through hypothalamus)].
- **Diurnal variation:** BP is more in the morning due to the increased sympathetic activity.
- **Exercise:** Generally systolic blood pressure increases and diastolic BP varies with the intensity of exercise. Both return to normal within 5 minutes of stoppage of exercise **(Table 44.1)**.
- **Gravity:** It is more in vessels below the heart and less in vessel above heart. **For every 1 cm change in height, BP changes by 0.77 mm Hg.**
- **Posture:** When a person suddenly stands up from the lying posture, he experiences the venous pooling of the blood. There is fall in the systolic blood pressure which activates the baroreceptors within 10–15 seconds and results in the return of the blood pressure to the base line within a few minutes.
- **Sleep:**
  - Early hours of sleep—fall by 15–20 mm Hg
  - In disturbed sleep BP rises as sympathetic activity is more
  - Body built—systolic pressure is more in obese.

## REGULATION OF BLOOD PRESSURE

(Discussed in detail in cardiovascular regulatory mechanisms)

The blood/arterial pressure is an circulatory pressure required for the proper functioning of various body systems and organs. Fall in the arterial pressure severely jeopardize the functioning of other organs. Hence, it is closely regulated by the neural, hormonal and local regulatory mechanisms. Depending on the response time of each of the mechanisms, the regulatory mechanisms are classified as short-term regulation (activated in seconds to minutes), intermediate term (activated in hours to days) and long-term (activated in days to months). The short-term, intermediate and long-term regulation of blood pressure is tabulated in **Table 44.2**.

### Short-term Regulation of Blood Pressure (Table 44.3)

Short-term regulation of blood pressure involves rapid adjustments primarily mediated by the autonomic nervous system, altering heart rate and vascular tone. Baroreceptors

**Table 44.1:** Effects of exercise on BP (also discussed on p. 336).

| | Mild exercise | Moderate exercise | Severe exercise | Reason |
|---|---|---|---|---|
| **Heart rate** | Up to 100 bpm from baseline | 100–125 bpm | >125 bpm | |
| **SBP** | Increases | Increases | Increases | Increase is seen due to increased sympathetic activity |
| **DBP** | May increase due to sympathetic stimulation | Increase or decrease depending upon the balance between vasoconstriction or vasodilation | Decreases | DBP will increase with increased TPR (vasoconstriction due to sympathetic activation) and decrease (vasodilation due to release of metabolic end products and local regulation) due to vasodilatation |

**Table 44.2:** Classification of regulatory mechanisms, based on activation and response time to change in blood pressure.

| | Short-term regulation | Intermediate-term regulation | Long-term regulation |
|---|---|---|---|
| **Activated in mechanisms** | Seconds-minutes | Minutes-hours | days |
| | • Baroreceptor reflex mechanism<br>• Chemoreceptor reflex mechanism<br>• CNS ischemic response | • Renin angiotensin mechanism<br>• Stress relaxation<br>• Capillary fluid shift mechanism | Role of kidney (renin angiotensin mechanism and aldosterone) |

**Table 44.3:** Different responses of short-term, intermediate term an long-term regulation of BP.

| | Short-term regulatory mechanisms | | | Intermediate term regulatory mechanisms | | | Long-term regulatory mechanisms | |
|---|---|---|---|---|---|---|---|---|
| | Baroreceptor reflex | Chemoreceptor reflex | CNS ischemic response 'Last ditch resort' | Renin angiotensin mechanism | Stress relaxation of vasculature | Capillary fluid shift mechanism | Aldosterone | Role of kidney (renin angiotensin aldosterone mechanism) |
| Gets activated within | | Seconds to minutes | | | Minutes to hours | | Days to months | |
| Gets activated when blood pressure | Works between the mean BP range of 60–180 mm Hg. It doesn't get stimulated below 60 mm Hg. (buffers day to day changes in BP) | When mean BP falls below 60 mm Hg (activated in hypotension) | When mean BP falls below 40 mm Hg (activated in severe hypotension and shock) | Decreased blood pressure → Decreases the renal blood flow → Decrease the GFR → Decreases the sodium ion concentration in the filtrate → Release of renin from JG cells through tubuloglomerular feedback mechanism → Renin converts inactive angiotensinogen into Angiotensin I → Which is converted into Angiotensin II by ACE (angiotensin converting enzyme present in lungs). → Angiotensin II is a potent vasoconstrictor and hence increases the BP. Also it increases the secretion of aldosterone which results in retention of sodium and water → Increases the BP (Increased BP will be regulated in the same manner but with opposite effects.) | Increased blood volume → Increased pressure → Relaxation of smooth muscle of blood vessels → Fall in BP | Increased BP → Increased hydrostatic pressure → Increased filtration → Lowers BP | Increased BP → Aldosterone inhibition → Sodium loss in urine (NATRIURESIS); Sodium and water loss brings back the BP to normal | Increased BP → Inhibition of release of angiotensin → Vasodilation → Diuresis |
| Receptor | Baroreceptors-sensitive to pressure changes | Chemoreceptors-sensitive to chemical changes in blood | CNS ischemia | | | | | |
| Location of receptors | Carotid sinus & Arch of Aorta | Carotid and aortic body | Direct stimulation of brain | | | | | |
| Afferents | IXth and Xth cranial nerve | IXth and Xth cranial nerve | | | | | | |
| Center | Vasomotor center | Vasomotor center | Vasomotor center | | | | | |
| Efferent | Xth nerve and sympathetic fibers | Xth nerve and sympathetic fibers | Xth nerve and sympathetic fibers | | | | | |
| Response | Decrease sympathetic discharge, if BP is high whereas it increases sympathetic discharge, if BP is low | Increases the sympathetic discharge | Increases the sympathetic discharge | | | | | |
| Effect | Maintains BP within normal range | Increases BP | Increases BP | | | | | |

in arteries sense changes and trigger reflex adjustments, while hormones like adrenaline and noradrenaline play crucial roles in modulating blood pressure during acute stress or activity.

### Intermediate Control
- **Renin angiotensin mechanism:** Decreased blood pressure → decreases the renal blood flow → decrease the GFR → decreases the sodium ion concentration in the filtrate → Release of renin from JG cells through tubuloglomerular feedback mechanism → Renin converts inactive angiotensinogen into angiotensin I → which is converted into angiotensin II by ACE (angiotensin converting enzyme present in lungs).
Angiotensin II is a potent vasoconstrictor and, hence, increases the BP. Also it increases the secretion of aldosterone which results in retention of sodium and water → increases the BP.
*Increased BP will be regulated in the same manner but with opposite effects.*
- **Stress relaxation of vasculature:** Increased blood volume → increased pressure → relaxation of smooth muscle of blood vessels → fall in BP
- **Capillary fluid shift mechanism:** Increased BP → Increased hydrostatic pressure → Increased filtration → Lowers BP

### Long-term Control
- **Renin angiotensin-aldosterone-system:** Increased BP → Inhibition → Vasodilation → Diuresis
- **Aldosterone mechanism:** Sodium retaining hormone Increased BP → Aldosterone inhibition → Sodium loss in urine (Natriuresis); Sodium and water loss brings back the BP to normal

## APPLIED ASPECTS

### Hypertension

Hypertension involves persistent elevation of blood pressure, often stemming from complex interactions among genetic, lifestyle, and environmental factors. Physiologically, it strains the cardiovascular system, leading to increased risk of heart disease, stroke, and other complications if left uncontrolled. Blood pressure classification and causes are shown in **Table 44.4**.

---

**What would happen if one kidney is removed or one renal artery is constricted?**

**Constricted kidney response:** When the artery to one kidney is constricted, it experiences decreased renal arterial pressure. As a response to this decreased pressure, the kidney secretes renin. Renin is an enzyme that plays a key role in the renin-angiotensin-aldosterone system (RAAS).

Additionally, the constricted kidney retains salt and water. This is a natural physiological response to maintain fluid balance in the body, compensating for the reduced renal arterial pressure.

**Opposite kidney response:** The "normal" kidney, sensing the increased levels of renin circulating in the bloodstream from the constricted kidney, interprets this as a signal of decreased systemic blood pressure.

In response to the increased renin, the opposite kidney also begins to retain salt and water. This response is mediated by the RAAS cascade. Renin triggers the conversion of angiotensinogen to angiotensin I, which is then converted to angiotensin II. Angiotensin II stimulates aldosterone release from the adrenal glands, promoting salt and water retention in the kidneys.

**Resulting effect:** Both kidneys, although for different reasons, become salt and water retainers. The constricted kidney retains salt and water due to decreased renal arterial pressure and the consequent renin secretion. The opposite kidney retains salt and water due to the effects of the renin produced by the ischemic kidney.

Consequently, hypertension develops as the body retains more fluid, leading to an increase in blood volume and pressure.

**Clinical implications:** This mechanism mirrors the process observed in two-kidney Goldblatt hypertension, where hypertension occurs due to stenosis of a single renal artery, such as in cases of atherosclerosis. Even though the patient has two kidneys, the stenosis of one renal artery triggers a cascade of events that lead to hypertension through mechanisms involving both kidneys.

**What would happen if one kidney is removed and other renal artery is constricted?**

This leads to the development of hypertension known as one-kidney Goldblatt hypertension, which occurs when one kidney is removed, and a constrictor is placed on the renal artery of the remaining kidney.

---

**Table 44.4:** Blood pressure classification of hypertension and causes.

| Blood pressure classification | Systolic (mm Hg) | Diastolic (mm Hg) |
|---|---|---|
| Normal | <120 | <80 |
| Prehypertension | 120–139 | 80–89 |
| Stage 1 hypertension | 140–159 | 90–99 |
| Stage 2 hypertension | ≥160 | ≥100 |
| Isolated systolic hypertension | ≥140 | <90 |
| **Causes** | **Primary** | **Secondary** |
|  | Essential hypertension | - *Renal:* Parenchymal disease<br>- *Renovascular:* Arteriosclerotic, fibromuscular dysplasia<br>- *Adrenal:* Primary aldosteronism, Cushing's syndrome<br>- Coarctation of aorta<br>- Pre-eclampsia/Eclampsia<br>- *Thyroid:* Hypothyroidism, hyperthyroidism |

**Immediate effect:** The placement of the constrictor on the renal artery immediately reduces pressure in the renal artery beyond the constriction. This leads to poor blood flow through the kidney.

**Early rise in arterial pressure:** Due to decreased blood flow, the kidney responds by secreting large quantities of renin into the bloodstream. Renin initiates the renin-angiotensin-aldosterone system (RAAS) cascade. Renin leads to the production of angiotensin II and aldosterone, both of which cause vasoconstriction and retention of salt and water in the body. The increased angiotensin II levels lead to an acute rise in arterial pressure.

**Second rise in arterial pressure:** The constricted kidney retains salt and water due to the effects of angiotensin II and aldosterone.

Over time (5–7 days), the body fluid volume increases due to salt and water retention, leading to a sustained rise in arterial pressure.

**Normalization of renal arterial pressure:** As arterial pressure increases, the renal arterial pressure beyond the constriction returns almost to normal levels.

Renin secretion decreases gradually over 5–7 days as renal arterial pressure rises back to normal, and the kidney is no longer ischemic.

**Clinical implications:** This mechanism mirrors the process observed in patients with stenosis of the renal artery of a single remaining kidney, such as after kidney transplantation, or in conditions with functional or pathological increases in resistance of the renal arterioles (e.g., due to atherosclerosis or excessive vasoconstrictor levels).

The sustained rise in arterial pressure is determined by the degree of constriction of the renal artery and the need to maintain normal urine output.

## Hypotension

- Resting blood pressure below 90/60 mm Hg.
- Causes:

| Causes of hypotension |
|---|
| • Dehydration |
| • Orthostatic hypotension (sudden drop in blood pressure while standing up or sitting down) |

## SUMMARY

- The blood pressure/arterial pressure is the lateral pressure exerted by the column of blood on the walls of the blood vessels.
- The maximum pressure in the blood vessels is the systolic pressure, while the minimum pressure is called the diastolic pressure. The difference in systolic and diastolic pressure is called the pulse pressure. The fourth and most important component of pressure is mean arterial pressure (DBP + 1/3 PP).
- All the regulatory mechanisms respond to the mean arterial pressure.
- The regulatory mechanism are classified on the basis of response time to change in arterial pressure.
- Short-term regulation: Baroreceptor reflex mechanism, chemoreceptor

## LET US SEE, HOW MUCH YOU HAVE LEARNT?

### Review Questions

**Q1.** Define blood pressure. What are the components of the blood pressure? Describe the factors affecting blood pressure.

**Q2.** What are the determinants of blood pressure? Describe their role in determining the blood pressure. (Hint: BP= CO x TPR)

**Q3.** What will happen to the blood pressure of a patient whose one kidney is removed?

### Critical Thinking Case-Based Questions

**Q1.** A 32-year-old primigravida at 20 weeks of gestation presented to obstetrics OPD for her routine ANC visit. She complaints of severe headache, vision changes and dizziness. On examination, her blood pressure was 150/90 mm Hg.
  a. What is the most likely diagnosis?
  b. Explain the physiological reason behind this condition.
  c. Describe the regulation of the blood pressure.

**Q2.** A 13-year-old male patient was brought by his parents to casualty with complaints of sudden collapsing episodes. His parents gave history of sickness since one week. Physical examination revealed sunken eyes and dry mucous membrane. Vitals: BP—88/60 mm Hg, $SPO_2$—99% @RA, HR—98/min.
  a. What is the most likely diagnosis?
  b. Explain the physiological reason behind this condition.
  c. What are the investigations and treatment?

**Q3.** A 63-year-old female patient presented to medicine OPD with complaints of headache, blurring of vision and palpitation. She has a history of hyperthyroidism since past 8 years for which she was on medication. On physical examination, fourth heart sound was noted. ECG revealed left ventricular hypertrophy.

a. What is the most likely diagnosis?
b. Explain the physiological reason behind this condition.
c. What are the investigations and treatment?

## Multiple Choice Questions

**Q1. Match the following:**

| Regulation of blood pressure | Mechanism |
|---|---|
| A. Short-term regulation | 1. Renin angiotensin mech and aldosterone |
| B. Intermediate term regulation | 2. Baroreceptor reflex mechanism, chemoreceptor reflex mechanism, CNS ischemic response |
| C. Long-term regulation | 3. Renin angiotensin mechanism, stress relaxation, capillary fluid shift mechanism |

a. A-2; B-3; C-1
b. A-1; B-2, C-3
c. A-3; B-2; C-1
d. A-1; B-3; C-2

**Q2. Mean pressure in the arteries is calculated as:**
a. SBP + ⅓PP
b. DBP + PP/2
c. DBP + ⅓PP
d. SBP + PP/2

**Q3. Blood is determined by:**
a. Cardiac output × peripheral resistance
b. Heart rate × stroke volume
c. Force of contraction × venous return
d. Cardiac output × pulse rate

**Q4. What will be the effect of moderate exercise on diastolic blood pressure?**
a. Decreases
b. Increase due to sympathetic stimulation
c. Increase or decrease depending upon the balance between vasoconstriction or vasodilation
d. Remains unchanged

**Q5. What is the SI unit of measuring blood pressure?**
a. mm Hg
b. Torr
c. Barr
d. kPa

**Q6. Which of the following statement is true about chemoreceptor complex?**
a. Sensitive to pressure changes
b. Receptors are located at carotid and aortic body
c. Decreases the sympathetic discharge
d. Activated in severe hypotension and shock

**Q7. Korotkoff's sound is produced because of:**
a. Arterial turbulence
b. Closure of AV valve
c. Vibration of ventricular wall
d. Closure of mitral and tricuspid valve

**Q8. Match the following:**

| Classification of blood pressure | Blood pressure | |
|---|---|---|
| | Systolic | Diastolic |
| A. Prehypertension | 1. ≥140 | <90 |
| B. Stage I hypertension | 2. ≥160 | ≥100 |
| C. Stage II hypertension | 3. 120–139 | 80–89 |
| D. Isolated systolic hypertension | 4. 140–159 | 90–99 |

a. A-1, B-2, C-3, D-4
b. A-2, B-3, C-4, D-1
c. A-3, B-4, C-1, D-2
d. A-4, B-1, C-2, D-3

### ANSWERS

1. a  2. c  3. a  4. c  5. d  6. b  7. a  8. c

# Coronary Circulation

**CHAPTER 45**

### COMPETENCY ADDRESSED

**PY5.10:** Describe and discuss regional circulation including microcirculation, lymphatic circulation, coronary, cerebral, capillary, skin, fetal, pulmonary, and splanchnic circulation.

### LEARNING OBJECTIVES

At the end of this chapter, the learner should be able to:
- Describe the functional anatomy of coronary circulation.
- Describe the methods to measure the coronary blood flow.
- Describe the peculiarities of the coronary circulation.
- Describe the factors affecting the coronary blood flow.
- Describe the regulation of coronary blood flow.

The blood flow to the myocardium, by the coronary arteries is called as the coronary circulation. There are two main coronaries originating from the root of aorta, viz. right and left coronary arteries (RCA and LCA). The left coronary artery further divides into 2 main branches left anterior descending (LAD) and left circumflex artery (LCX). The functional anatomy and the areas supplied by these are shown in **Figure 45.1**.

## CORONARY BLOOD FLOW

The blood flowing through the coronaries is around *4–5% of the cardiac output*, amounting to about *225 mL/min*. It is the only source of blood supply to the myocardium. Hence, it is very important to study the myocardial perfusion. The coronary blood flow can be measured by many methods, given below:

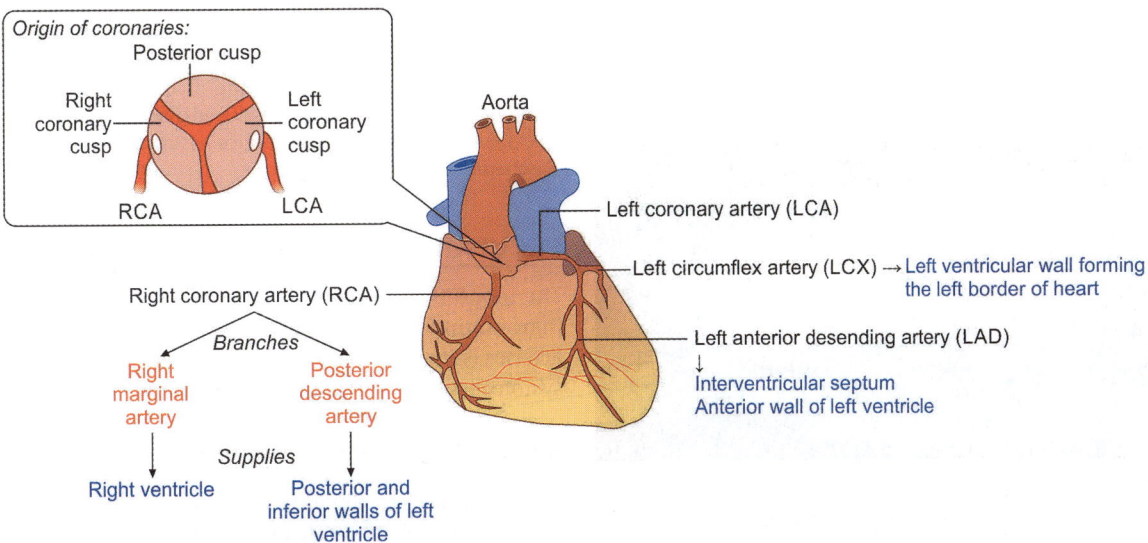

**Fig. 45.1:** Coronary circulation and blood supply of heart.

## Measurement of Coronary Blood Flow

### Kety's Method

It is based on Fick's principle, but the *indicator substance used is nitrous oxide ($N_2O$)*. The patient is asked to inhale $N_2O$, and the total body consumption of the gas is noted. The arteriovenous difference of the $N_2O$ is measured by taking the sample from the root of aorta and coronary sinus, indicating the consumption of gas by the heart. The coronary blood flow is measured by the formula:

$$CBF = \frac{QN_2O}{\text{Arteriovenous difference of } N_2O}$$

### Radionucleotide Study

It is used to study the regional blood flow in heart, using the radionucleotides.
- **Thallium ($^{201}$Tl):** The areas of ischemia show low $^{201}$Tl uptake **(Fig. 45.2)**.
- **Technetium -99 m:** It is selectively taken up by infarcted area, hence, the hot spots indicate the reduced blood supply.
- **$^{133}$Xe wash out method** combined with angiography is used to outline the distribution of blood in the myocardium.

### Coronary Angiography (Fig. 45.3)

A catheter is inserted into the coronary arteries, through femoral/radial artery, through which the contrast medium is injected into the coronary circulation. The angiogram is obtained which is used to study the flow of blood and blockade in the coronary arteries, if any.

## BLOOD FLOW IN THE CORONARIES

The blood flow in the coronary arteries is phasic and depends on the **pressure gradient** created **between aorta and ventricular pressure** during ventricular systole and diastole. It is also affected by the intramuscular pressure built in the muscle during systole. Let us try to visualize, how the blood vessels are arranged in the myocardium **(Fig. 45.4)**. In the thickness of the cardiac muscle, the coronary

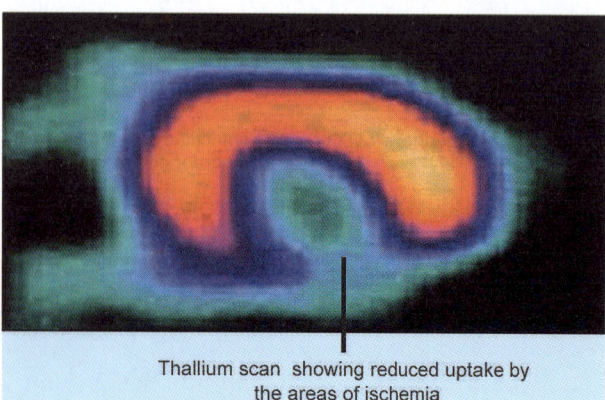

Thallium scan showing reduced uptake by the areas of ischemia

**Fig. 45.2:** Thallium radionucleotide scan.

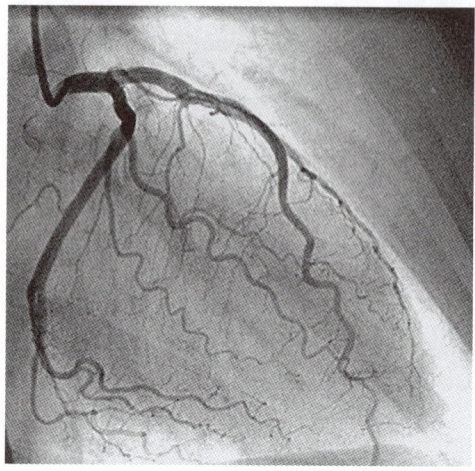

**Fig. 45.3:** Coronary angiogram.

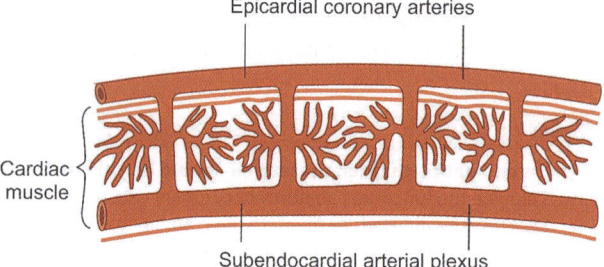

**Fig. 45.4:** Blood supply of cardiac muscle.

arteries are arranged in a specific pattern having epicardial arteries and subendocardial plexus which are connected through small intramuscular arteries. Whenever the pressure in the muscle (intramuscular pressure) increases during systole the subendocardial plexus gets compressed, compromising the blood flow to the subendocardial area of cardiac muscle.

> **Why the subendocardial infarcts are more common?**
> The subendocardial muscle has higher oxygen consumption and blood intramuscular arteries along with subendocardial plexus gets squeezed during systole reducing the blood supply to subendocardial regions of the myocardium. During the coronary artery occlusion, the reduced blood supply is sufficient to salvage the muscle and hence results in subendocardial ischemia and infarcts.

## PECULARITIES OF CORONARY BLOOD FLOW

The blood flow in the coronary arteries is **Phasic**, rather than continuous **(Fig. 45.5)**. The blood flow in the coronary arteries is maximum during diastole and minimum during systole, especially in left coronary artery.

### Reason for Phasic Blood Flow

- High pressure develops in the myocardium during systole, which **squeezes and obliterates** the subendocardial and epicardial branches of coronary

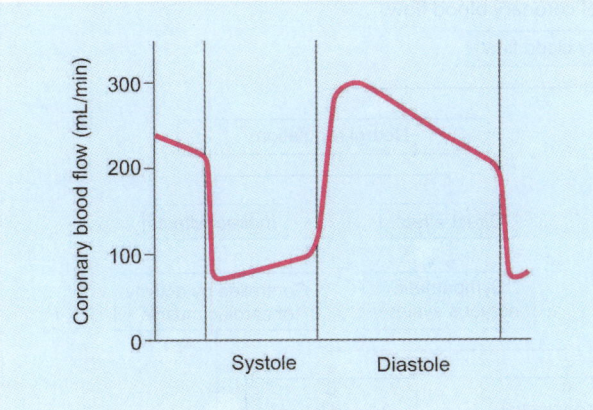

**Fig. 45.5:** Phasic blood flow of coronary arteries.

arteries and hence raises the pressure inside the coronaries too.
- The blood fills up in the arch of aorta during ventricular systole. Aorta being a Windkessel vessel accommodates a large quantity of blood during systole.
- At the beginning of diastole, the pressure inside the myocardium and the coronaries drops and the blood accumulated in aorta, flows into the coronaries.
- Depending upon pressure gradient between aorta and the ventricles, the filling of LCA and RCA is shown in **Figures 45.6A and B**, which determine the filling of coronaries during systole and diastole.

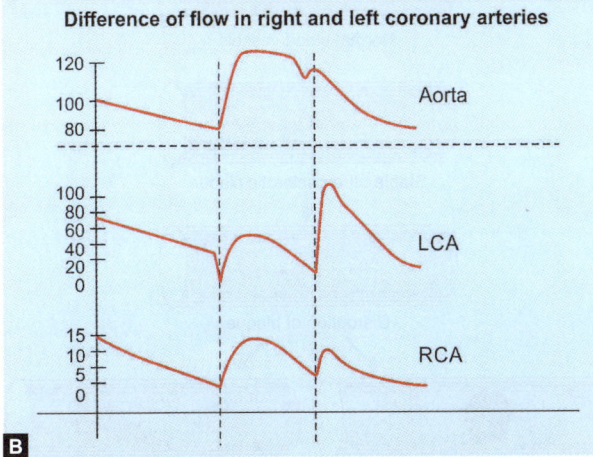

**Figs. 45.6A and B:** (A) Pressure in systole and diastole; (B) difference of flow in right and left coronary arteries.

## FACTORS AFFECTING CORONARY CIRCULATION

- **Mean aortic pressure:** The increased mean aortic pressure directly increases the pressure gradient between the aorta and ventricles, increasing the filling of coronaries and hence, increases the coronary blood flow.
- **Cardiac output:** Increased CO, increases mean aortic pressure and hence CBF, as discussed above.
- **Metabolic factors:** Accumulation of metabolic waste products increases the coronary blood flow by increasing the metabolic demand of the myocardium. The myocardial oxygen demand ($MVO_2$) is an important determinant of the coronary blood flow.
- **Effect of ions:** Ions which increase the heart rate and contractility results in accumulation of metabolites, hence increasing the coronary blood flow.
- **Adenine nucleotides:** It is a metabolic waste product, hence increases the myocardial blood flow.
- **Autonomic nerves:** Sympathetic stimulation affects the myocardial perfusion. Usually, the sympathetic vasoconstrictor tone results in vasoconstriction but the coronaries show vasodilation and increased blood flow. It has been proposed that it occurs due to indirect effect of sympathetic stimulation by increasing the heart rate, contractility and increasing the $MVO_2$.
- **Heart rate:** Increased heart rate increases the myocardial oxygen demand and hence increases the myocardial blood flow.
- **Hormones:** The thyroid hormones, catecholamines result in increased myocardial oxygen demand by increasing the metabolism or through cardiostimulatory effect, increases the myocardial blood flow.
- **Temperature:** It is the property of cardiac muscles, that heart rate increases by 10 beats with each degree rise in the temperature. Hence, high temperature increases the myocardial blood flow.
- **Anemia:** It decreases the delivery of oxygen to the tissues, resulting in increased heart rate and contractility, for which the heart has to work more, this results in increased myocardial oxygen demand and increases the myocardial blood flow.

## REGULATION OF CORONARY BLOOD FLOW (FLOWCHART 45.1)

The regulation of blood flow in coronary arteries is by following mechanisms:
- **Autoregulation:** Coronary blood flow adjusts to meet the heart's oxygen demands by dilating or constricting coronary arterioles in response to changes in perfusion pressure.
- **Metabolic regulation:** Metabolic byproducts like adenosine and potassium ions promote coronary vasodilation, ensuring adequate blood flow during increased myocardial metabolism.

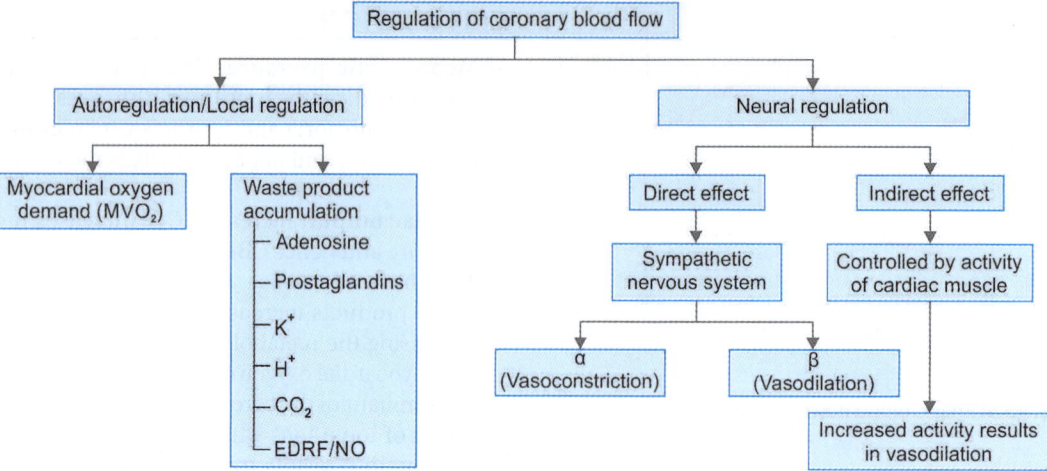

Flowchart 45.1: Regulation of coronary blood flow.

(EDRF: endothelial derived relaxation factor)

- **Neural regulation:** Sympathetic stimulation enhances coronary vasodilation via β-adrenergic receptors, while parasympathetic activity has a minor influence, primarily through indirect mechanisms.

## CORONARY ARTERY DISEASE (CAD) OR ISCHAEMIC HEART DISEASE (IHD)

Ischemia is defined as the imbalance between demand and supply of blood or decreased perfusion of the tissue. The ischemia can present in a patient in various ways, depending on its severity. It is broadly clubbed under the *Myocardial ischemic syndrome*, which includes:

- **Angina pectoris:** It refers to compromised myocardial perfusion and is an early sign of myocardial ischemia. Angina can present with varied severity ranging from pain during exertion (in early stages) to angina at rest (in severely compromised perfusion). It presents as referred pain in the left arm, neck or jaw (the pain of angina is felt in the left arm due to the common dermatomal origin).
- **Myocardial infarction:** The complete occlusion of the coronary artery or its branch supplying the myocardium results in a myocardial injury called as infarction.
- **Chronic ischemic heart disease (IHD):** When a patient is suffering from chronic or long term myocardial ischemia, due to varied degree of coronary occlusion, the condition is referred to as ischemic heart disease. A patient of IHD can present with angina, breathlessness and congestive cardiac failure. The pathogenesis of IHD can be explained by the coronary artery occlusion by the atherosclerotic plaque and thrombus formation (explained below). When the myocardium is subjected to chronic ischemia, the collateral circulation begins to form in the myocardium as a long term regulation of the blood flow. The IHD can present with any of the following symptoms:
    - *Angina:* When there is >75% stenosis of coronary artery
    - *Unstable angina:* Occurring during the plaque rupture
    - *Myocardial infarction:* Plaque rupture with complete occlusion sudden death severe multivessel disease

## Acute Coronary Artery Occlusion (ACAO)

It is the syndrome of ischemia leading to disruption of function and myocardial damage. It is commonly called as heart attack.

### Etiopathogenesis (Fig. 45.7)

The most common cause of IHD is **atherosclerosis** (deposition of cholesterol in the arterial walls resulting in occlusion of lumen of the coronary arteries and decrease in coronary blood flow).

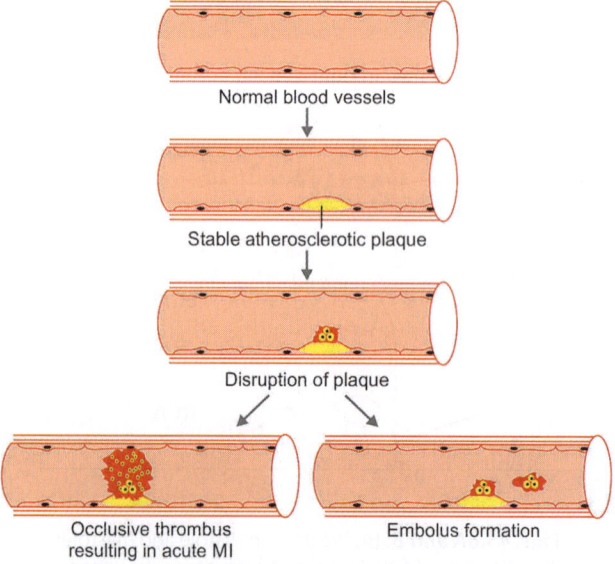

**Fig. 45.7:** Pathogenesis of thrombus/embolus formation.

## Pathogenesis of Ischemic Heart Disease

The **most common artery** affected by the atherosclerosis is *left anterior descending artery* followed by the right coronary artery and then the left circumflex artery (**LAD > RCA > LCX**). The *commonest site of development of atherosclerotic plaques is near the origin of the coronary arteries*. It is important to understand that high grade slowly developing plaques open up **collateral circulation** due to the long-term regulation of the blood flow.

## Various Risk Factors Associated with CAD

- **Males and postmenopausal women:** The premenopausal women are protected from atherosclerosis by the estrogen hormone. Estrogen induces the LDL receptors in the liver and enhances the metabolism of LDL receptors. However, the males and post-menopausal women are at equal risk of atherosclerosis and myocardial ischemia. Recently, the incidence of ischemic heart disease has been on the rise even in premenopausal women.
- **Atherosclerosis:** It is single most important risk factor which result in IHD, pathogenesis is explained above.
- **Hyper lipoproteinemia:** Increase in the levels of LDL, VLDL cholesterol, triglycerides and decreased the HDL:LDL ratio are potential risk factors for the development of atherosclerosis.
- **Cigarette smoking:** It is a serious risk factor as it affects the myocardium in many ways:
    - The nicotine in cigarette smoke results in increased heart rate and vasoconstriction. This further results in worsening of hypertension and myocardial workload.
    - It adds to the alteration of lipid profile by increasing the LDL levels and decreasing the HDL cholesterol.
    - It stimulates the increase in fibrinogen levels resulting in platelet aggregation, triggering the thrombus formation.
    - The carbon monoxide present in the smoke displaces oxygen from hemoglobin and decreases oxygen delivery to tissues.
- **Hypertension:** Long standing hypertension results in an increase in the afterload, which increases the workload of the left ventricle. This results in the ventricular hypertrophy and failure. Overtime, the $MVO_2$ increases and the myocardial blood flow is not sufficient for adequate perfusion of muscle, hence, resulting in IHD.
- **Diabetes mellitus:** It is an independent risk factor for the development of IHD. Lack of insulin results in the metabolic derangements resulting in hyperlipoproteinemia, predisposing to atherosclerosis and IHD. The patients with diabetes mellitus often suffer from 'silent MI', i.e., myocardial infarction without pain.
- **Genetic predisposition:** There is a strong genetic predisposition for the IHD, probably due to the increased incidence of other risk factors, lifestyle diseases, etc.

### Myocardial Infarction

The ACAO, results in cessation of blood flow beyond the occlusion and result in the myocardial cell death and shows changes as described in **Flowchart 45.2**.

> Oxygen requirement of *myocardial cells at rest is 8 mL/100 g/min while it is 1.3 mL/100 g/min to remain alive,* i.e., the minimum requirement.
> The central portion of infarct does not receive any blood supply, hence, it undergoes necrosis and become non-functional. Later it is replaced by fibrous tissue or scar.

### Clinical presentation

- Pain:
    - Deep, visceral, radiating to arm, abdomen, back, lower jaw and neck
- Other features:
    - Weakness
    - Sweating

**Flowchart 45.2:** Changes in myocardial cells following artery occlusion.

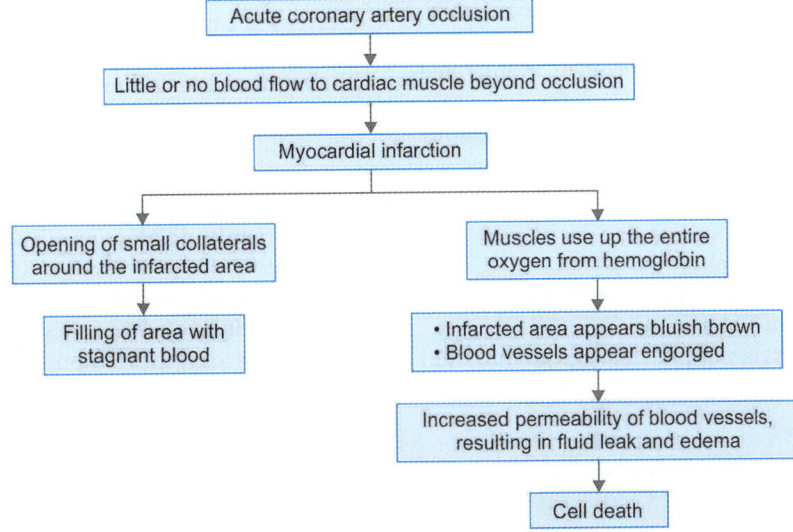

- Nausea, vomiting
- Anxiety
- Sense of impending doom

*Physical findings*
- Patient is appears pale, anxious, restless, sweating with cold extremities
- Complains of substernal chest pain, usually keeps the fist over chest. The aim is explained as deep, boring, and constricting or squeezing in nature
- Heart rate and blood pressure are normal within first hour
- There is decreased carotid pulse volume
- Decreased systolic BP

*Laboratory diagnosis*
- ECG:
  - ST wave elevation and T wave inversion due to current of injury (discussed in the chapter on ECG)
  - Q waves are usually absent in all leads except V4–V6. Abnormal Q waves appear after 24 hours after the injury. The presence of Q waves indicates a scarred or injured myocardium.
  - Changes in the:
    - Lateral leads (I, aVL, V5-V6) indicate the blockage in LCX or diagonal LAD
    - Anterior leads V1-V4 indicate blockage in LAD artery
    - Inferior leads: II, III, aVF indicate the blockage in RCA and or LCX
- **Serum cardiac markers:**
  - ***CPK-MB:*** (Creatine phosphokinase—muscle and brain) indicates cardiac muscle injury, as this enzyme is specific for myocardium. It is raised within 3-6 hours and peak levels are seen between 6-30 hours.
  - ***Cardiac specific troponin-T:*** Begin to rise after 2 hours and remain elevated for 1-2 weeks.
- **Cardiac imaging:** 2D echocardiography shows the cardiac wall motion and ejection fraction.
- **Radionucleotide study:**
  - To study the regional blood flow in heart
  - Thallium ($^{201}$Tl) is used shows areas of ischemia show low Tl uptake
  - Technetium –99 m is selectively taken up by infarcted area
  - $^{133}$Xe wash out method combined with angiography to outline the distribution of blood

*Management*
- $O_2$ inhalation
- Inj. Morphine to control pain
- Thrombolysis with inj. Streptokinase within 6 hours
- Low molecular weight heparin
- Low dose aspirin (acts as antiplatelet aggregation drug)

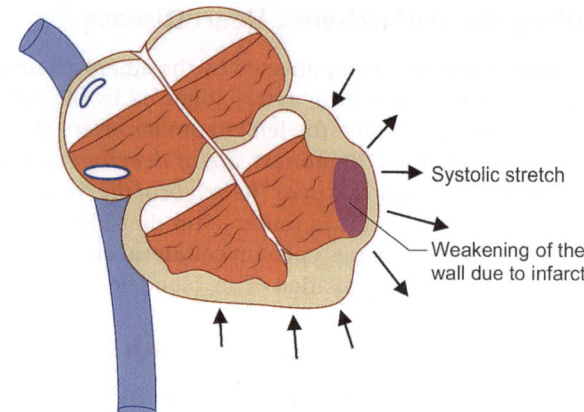

**Fig. 45.8:** Systolic stretch.

- **Operative treatment:**
  - Percutaneous transluminal coronary angioplasty with stenting
  - Coronary artery by-pass grafting (CABG)

*Complications*
- **Arrythmias:** The *most common complication* is arrythmia, which are most commonly seen during 3 dangerous periods post MI:
  - During first 10 minutes of infarction
  - One to few hours after MI
  - 3 days to several weeks after MI

  The physiological basis of fibrillation can be described as:
  - Acute coronary occlusion rapidly depletes the intracellular potassium and increases its concentration in extracellular fluid, which is a potential trigger for the development of arrhythmias.
  - The injured myocardium results in a current of injury and elicits abnormal impulses resulting in fibrillation.
  - The powerful sympathetic stimulation increases the irritability of cardiac muscle predisposing to fibrillation.
  - Weak cardiac muscle results in ventricular dilation and predispose to development of circus movement.
- Decreased cardiac output due to **systolic stretch** and cardiac shock **(Fig. 45.8)**.

  The injured myocardium loses its contractility; hence, it gets stretched instead of contraction during systole. This reduces the cardiac output and results in cardiogenic shock.
- **Damming of blood in venous system:** The low cardiac output results in decreased urinary output, which increases the blood volume. There is pooling of the blood in the veins resulting in pulmonary edema.
- **Rupture of infarcted area:** It is very serious complication which leads to cardiac tamponade and sudden death.

## SUMMARY

- Coronary circulation is the network of blood vessels that supply oxygenated blood to the heart muscle (myocardium). It plays a crucial role in maintaining cardiac function by ensuring adequate oxygen and nutrient delivery to the myocardial cells.
- Coronary circulation originates from the coronary arteries, which arise from the aortic sinuses (right and left coronary arteries).
- The major coronary arteries include the left main coronary artery, left anterior descending artery, left circumflex artery, and right coronary artery.
- Coronary arteries branch into smaller arterioles and capillaries that penetrate the myocardium, facilitating nutrient and gas exchange at the cellular level.
- Venous blood from the myocardium is drained primarily by the coronary sinus, which empties into the right atrium.
- Coronary blood flow is regulated by various factors, including metabolic demands, autonomic nervous system activity, and local factors such as nitric oxide.
- Techniques for measuring coronary blood flow include Doppler flowmetry, and positron emission tomography (PET).
- Coronary flow reserve, defined as the ratio of maximal coronary blood flow to resting flow, provides insights into the functional status of coronary circulation.
- Coronary blood flow exhibits autoregulation, ensuring adequate perfusion despite changes in systemic blood pressure.
- Blood flow is highest during diastole when the myocardium relaxes, allowing for optimal perfusion of coronary arteries.
- Endothelial dysfunction, characterized by reduced nitric oxide bioavailability, contributes to coronary artery disease by impairing vasodilation and promoting atherosclerosis.
- CAD encompasses various pathologies, including atherosclerosis, coronary artery spasm, and microvascular dysfunction.
- Atherosclerosis involves the buildup of plaque within coronary arteries, leading to luminal narrowing and reduced blood flow to the myocardium.
- Clinical manifestations of CAD include angina pectoris (stable and unstable), myocardial infarction, and heart failure.
- Diagnostic modalities for CAD include electrocardiography (ECG), stress testing, coronary angiography, and non-invasive imaging techniques (e.g., CT angiography, MRI).

## LET US SEE, HOW MUCH YOU HAVE LEARNT?

### Review Questions

#### Long/Short Answer Questions

Q1. Describe the peculiarities of coronary blood flow.
Q2. Discuss methods of measurements of coronary blood flow.
Q3. Describe the ECG changes in myocardial ischemia, infarction and necrosis.
Q4. What are the factors affecting coronary blood flow?
Q5. Write a long note on pathophysiology of coronary artery diseases.

#### Explain Why? (Reasoning Questions)

Q1. Collateral circulation can develop in individuals with chronic coronary artery disease.
Q2. The maximum blood flow in left coronary artery is occurs during the diastole, while in right coronary artery it occurs during systole.
Q3. The subendocardial region is more vulnerable to ischemic injury.
Q4. The premenopausal women are protected against atherosclerosis.
Q5. Coronary arteries are more susceptible to atherosclerosis compared to other arteries in the body.

### Critical Thinking Case-Based Questions

Q1. A 61-year-old man with **Type II diabetes mellitus** presents to the emergency room you are working at complaining of "**heaviness**" in his chest. He says the discomfort began as a pressure pain sensation in the middle of his chest shortly after starting some minor physical activity. He is **sweaty** and **complains of nausea**. He says the pain subsided somewhat when he sat down, but has persisted as a heaviness. He revealed on detailed history that he is a **smokes 2 packs of cigarettes every day** and takes **has 2–3 alcohol drinks daily**.

Physical examination reveals that he is **obese**, holding his fist over his sternum in apparent mild-moderate discomfort.
*Vitals signs are:* HR—110/min; BP—146/100 mm Hg; RR—22/min; Temp—98.6°F; $SpO_2$—93% on room air. JVP is within normal limits but shows a rapid carotid pulse. His peripheral pulses are decreased, and his capillary refill is delayed. His abdominal and respiratory examinations are unremarkable.
*ECG shows:* **Q waves in V1–V4** with **elevation of ST segment** due to acute MI.

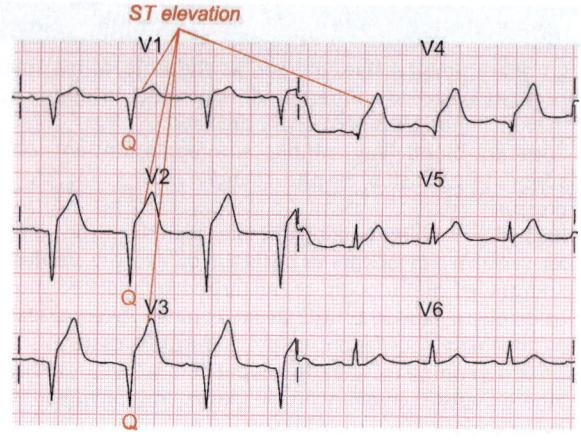

a. What is the most likely diagnosis in this patient?
b. What are the risk factors associated in this patient to support your answer?
c. How does cigarette smoking affect his condition?
d. What is the pathogenesis of this condition?
e. What laboratory tests would help you to confirm his diagnosis?
f. What would you expect to find in his ECG?

## Multiple Choice Questions

**Q1.** Which vessel supplies oxygenated blood directly to the myocardium?
 a. Pulmonary artery
 b. Coronary artery
 c. Aorta
 d. Superior vena cava

**Q2.** Which layer of the heart receives blood supply from the coronary arteries?
 a. Epicardium
 b. Myocardium
 c. Endocardium
 d. Pericardium

**Q3.** Which of the following substances is predominantly responsible for regulating coronary blood flow?
 a. Nitric oxide
 b. Epinephrine
 c. Angiotensin II
 d. Insulin

**Q4.** What is the primary determinant of coronary blood flow during diastole?
 a. Myocardial oxygen demand
 b. Coronary artery diameter
 c. Heart rate
 d. Systemic blood pressure

**Q5.** During exercise, which of the following occurs in coronary circulation?
 a. Coronary blood flow decreases due to increased sympathetic activity.
 b. Coronary vessels dilate to meet increased oxygen demand.
 c. Coronary resistance increases due to parasympathetic stimulation.
 d. Coronary blood flow remains constant regardless of metabolic demand.

**Q6.** A patient with hypertension complains of chest pain. Which phenomenon contributes to the pain?
 a. Decreased myocardial oxygen demand
 b. Increased afterload on the heart
 c. Coronary vasodilation
 d. Elevated levels of HDL cholesterol

**Q7.** Which condition results from an imbalance between myocardial oxygen supply and demand?
 a. Coronary artery disease
 b. Atherosclerosis
 c. Myocardial infarction
 d. Bradycardia

**Q8.** In a patient with coronary artery disease, which diagnostic test measures the functional significance of stenotic lesions?
 a. Coronary angiography
 b. Coronary artery calcium scoring
 c. Coronary flow reserve measurement
 d. Stress echocardiography

**Q9.** What effect does sympathetic stimulation have on coronary circulation during fight or flight response?
 a. Decreases coronary blood flow by constricting vessels
 b. Increases coronary blood flow by dilating vessels
 c. Reduces myocardial oxygen demand
 d. None of the above

**Q10.** Which medication is commonly prescribed to dilate coronary arteries and improve blood flow?
 a. Beta-blockers
 b. Calcium channel blockers
 c. Angiotensin-converting enzyme (ACE) inhibitors
 d. Nitrates

**Q11.** How does endothelial dysfunction contribute to coronary artery disease?
 a. By increasing vasodilation
 b. By reducing nitric oxide production
 c. By enhancing coronary blood flow
 d. By decreasing platelet aggregation

**Q12.** What role do collateral vessels play in coronary circulation?
 a. They shunt blood away from the heart during exercise.
 b. They provide an alternative route for blood flow in case of coronary artery blockage.
 c. They regulate coronary resistance.
 d. They carry deoxygenated blood back to the heart.

**Q13.** Which coronary artery is most commonly affected in a condition known as the "widow-maker" heart attack?
 a. Left anterior descending artery
 b. Right coronary artery
 c. Left circumflex artery
 d. Posterior descending artery

**Q14.** What is the term for the phenomenon where coronary blood flow is maximized during diastole?
 a. Coronary autoregulation
 b. Ventricular contractility
 c. Coronary steal syndrome
 d. Myocardial perfusion reserve

**Q15.** A patient presents with chest pain relieved by rest. Which term best describes this clinical condition?
  a. Unstable angina
  b. Stable angina
  c. Variant (Prinzmetal's) angina
  d. Acute myocardial infarction

**Q16.** During an angioplasty procedure, a stent is placed to widen a narrowed coronary artery. What effect does this have on coronary blood flow?
  a. Decreases resistance and increases blood flow
  b. Increases resistance and decreases blood flow
  c. No significant effect on blood flow
  d. Causes vasospasm and reduces blood flow

**Q17.** How does exercise training contribute to improved coronary circulation?
  a. By reducing myocardial oxygen demand
  b. By increasing collateral vessel formation
  c. By decreasing coronary artery diameter
  d. By decreasing coronary blood flow

**Q18.** Which physiological factor primarily determines coronary perfusion pressure?
  a. Heart rate
  b. Left ventricular end-diastolic pressure
  c. Aortic pressure
  d. Pulmonary artery pressure

**Q19.** What is the role of adenosine in coronary circulation?
  a. Causes vasoconstriction in coronary arteries
  b. Acts as a vasodilator during ischemia
  c. Inhibits platelet aggregation
  d. Stimulates sympathetic nervous activity

## ANSWERS

**1.** b  **2.** b  **3.** a  **4.** b  **5.** b  **6.** b  **7.** c  **8.** c  **9.** b  **10.** d  **11.** b  **12.** b  **13.** a  **14.** a
**15.** b  **16.** a  **17.** b  **18.** c  **19.** b

# Blood Flow in Systemic Circulation: Arterial, Capillary, Venous and Lymphatic Circulation

## CHAPTER 46

### COMPETENCY ADDRESSED
**PY5.10:** Describe and discuss regional circulation including microcirculation, lymphatic circulation, coronary, cerebral, capillary, skin, fetal, pulmonary, and splanchnic circulation.

### LEARNING OBJECTIVES
**At the end of this chapter, the learner should be able to:**
- Describe the characteristics of blood flow in the various segments of systemic circulation.
- Describe the factors affecting flow in each of the segments.
- Describe the related applied physiology.

## COMPONENTS OF SYSTEMIC CIRCULATION

The various components of the circulation are arteries, microvasculature and veins. The differences in each one of these have been discussed in detail in the chapter of hemodynamics. However, to understand the blood flow in these segments it is important that we discuss two very important properties of the vasculature, namely **vascular distensibility and compliance**.

Both arteries and veins have the property of distensibility, which allows the arteries to accommodate the pulsatile output of the ventricle and convert this pulsatile flow into a smooth continuous flow in the capillaries. **The veins are the most distensible of all the vessels in the circulation,** being **eight times** more distensible than the arteries. It is interesting to note that the pulmonary veins have similar distensibility as systemic veins, but pulmonary arteries are six times more distensible, as they work under six times less pressure, as compared to systemic arteries.

Considering the **vascular compliance or vascular capacitance**, it is expressed as total quantity of blood that can be stored in each portion of circulation for each mm Hg. Vascular compliance is defined as *'Increase in volume per unit increase in pressure'.* It is also expressed as distensibility × volume.

*The compliance of a systemic vein is about 24 times that of the corresponding artery because it is 8 times more distensible and has 3 times more volume than it.*

From these above two properties, we have understood that volume and pressure play a very important role in

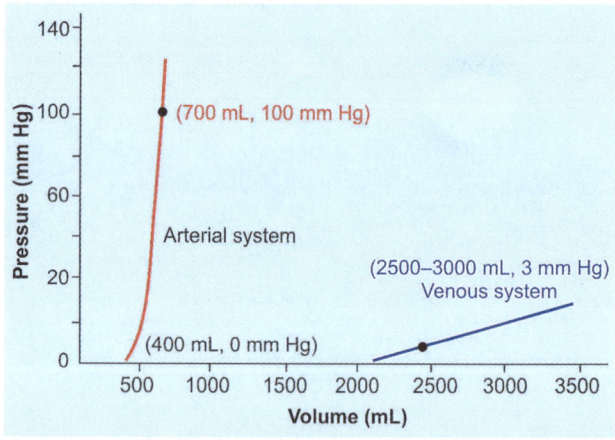

**Fig. 46.1:** Pressure volume curve for arterial and venous system.

circulation. The relationship between volume and pressure can be expressed in terms of the volume pressure curve of the arterial and the venous circulation **(Fig. 46.1)**.

*What would happen to circulatory function, if we transfuse around half a liter of blood into the veins of a healthy patient?*

The circulatory function would show no change. This could be explained by the high distensibility and compliance of veins, due to which they can accommodate a very large amount of blood to actually show a measurable increase in venous pressure. Hence, according to the volume pressure relationship of veins, a large increase of blood volume in veins is required to show an increase of pressure from 3 to 5 mm Hg.

The **delayed compliance** of the blood vessels is also an important property of the vasculature, in which a sudden increase in volume initially reflects a sharp increase in the intravascular pressure due to the elastic distension of the vessel but later shows a drop in pressure due to stress relaxation of the vascular smooth muscle (which is the inherent property of the smooth muscle).

Let us now discuss the characteristics of each segment of the circulation with special emphasis on its physiological functions.

## ARTERIAL CIRCULATION (FROM HEART TO CAPILLARIES)

As discussed previously, in the chapter of hemodynamics, depending on structural details in terms of arterial wall, amount of elastic fibers and smooth muscle, the arteries are classified as:
- Aorta
- Large elastic arteries
- Arterioles

The thick and elastic walls of the aorta, accommodates the large amount of blood entering it at the time of ventricular systole The elastic fibers present in the aorta, distend it and recoils during the diastolic phase resulting the forward propulsion of blood into the large arteries. *A wave of receptive relaxation of arterial wall precedes the blood flow, which is recognized as arterial pressure pulse (commonly called pulse).*

The arterial pressure pulse recorded at the root of aorta shows the following characteristics as shown in **Figure 46.2**.

The peak pressure corresponds to the systolic pressure (120 mm Hg) and the minimum pressure corresponds to the diastolic pressure (80 mm Hg). The difference in systolic and diastolic pressure is pulse pressure. There are two main factors, which affect the pulse pressure:
1. **Stroke volume output:** Directly increases the amount of blood that can be accommodated in the arteries.
2. **Compliance (total distensibility) of arterial tree:** Inversely proportional to rise in systolic pressure. Hence, lower compliance would result in a higher systolic pressure.

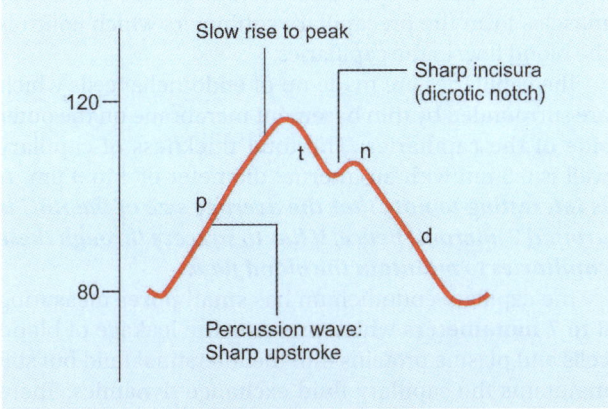

**Fig. 46.2:** Characteristic of arterial pulse.

***Why does the systolic pressure increase in old age?***
In old age, the arterial walls get stiffened due to arteriosclerosis and become noncompliant. Hence, the systolic blood pressure increases in old age.

Hence, any change in the above two factors can affect the pulse pressure.

### Abnormalities of Pulse Contours

There are various abnormalities in pulse pattern due to various disease conditions. They are described in **Table 46.1**.

### Transmission of Pressure Pulse to Peripheral Arteries

The velocity of transmission is faster in less compliant arteries; hence, it is 3–5 m/s in aorta, 7–10 m/s in large arteries and 15–35 m/s in smaller arteries. The mechanism of transmission is shown in **Flowchart 46.1**. These pulses become progressively damped in smaller arteries, arterioles and capillaries. It occurs due to resistance to the movement of blood in these vessels and decreased compliance in peripheral vessels. Hence, *the degree of dampness is directly proportional to the product of resistance and compliance.*

## MICROCIRCULATION AND CAPILLARY CIRCULATION

The fine vascular channels linking the arterial segment with the venous segment is called as **microcirculation**. It is composed of capillaries and venules having a single cell thick lumen. These capillaries are responsible for adequate perfusion of all the tissues. However, the blood flow in these capillaries is determined by two main factors:
1. **Active metabolism** in the tissue, resulting in increased nutrient demand and accumulation of waste products.
2. **Precapillary sphincters** which control the flow at rest and during high demand. These sphincters are sensitive to the oxygen concentration in the blood. A drop in oxygen concentration results in relaxation of sphincteric smooth muscles and opens capillary network.

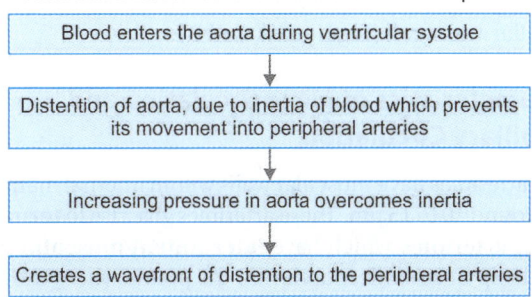

**Flowchart 46.1:** Mechanism of transmission of pulse.

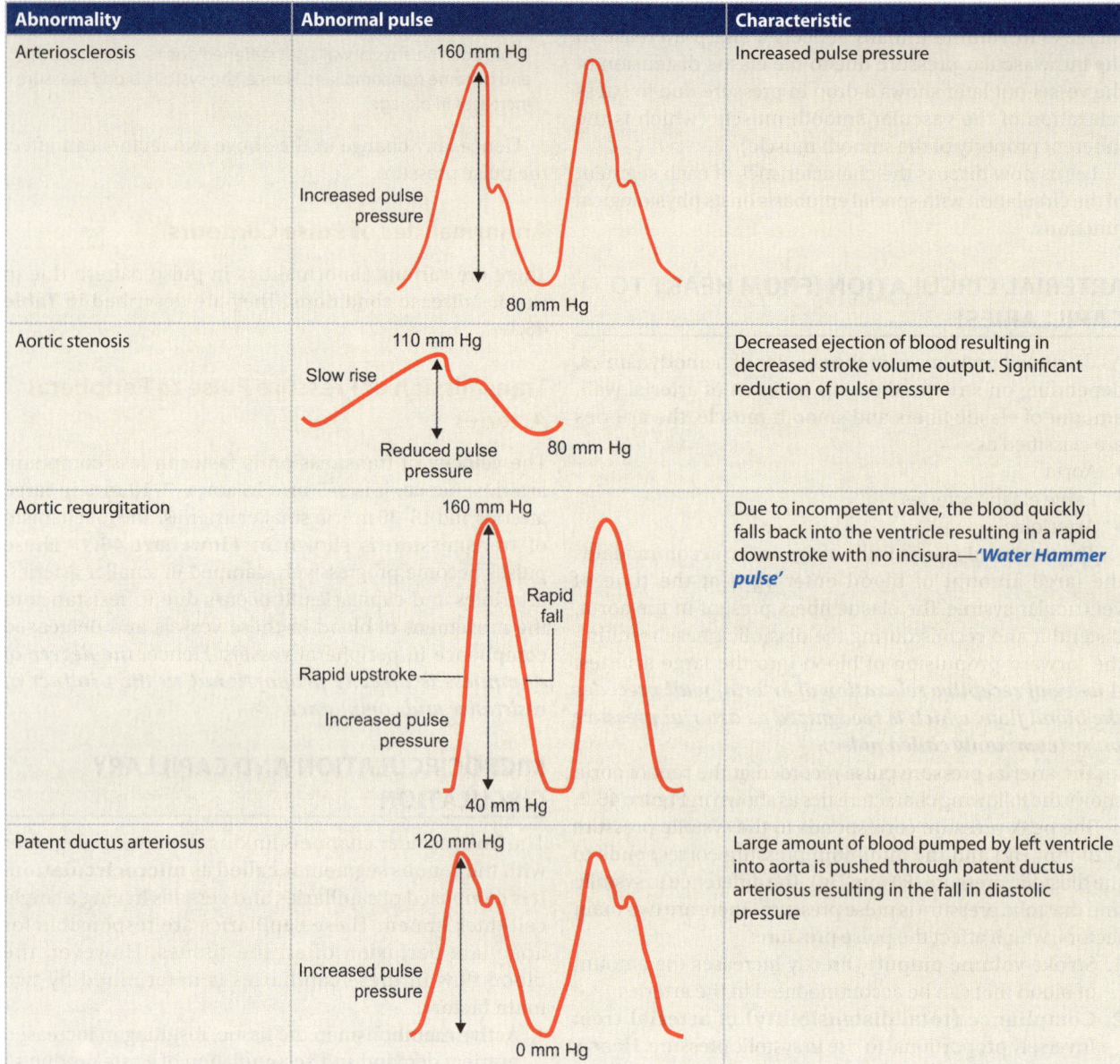

Table 46.1: Abnormal pulses and their characteristics.

| Abnormality | Abnormal pulse | Characteristic |
| --- | --- | --- |
| Arteriosclerosis | 160 mm Hg / 80 mm Hg — Increased pulse pressure | Increased pulse pressure |
| Aortic stenosis | 110 mm Hg / 80 mm Hg — Slow rise, Reduced pulse pressure | Decreased ejection of blood resulting in decreased stroke volume output. Significant reduction of pulse pressure |
| Aortic regurgitation | 160 mm Hg / 40 mm Hg — Rapid upstroke, Rapid fall, Increased pulse pressure | Due to incompetent valve, the blood quickly falls back into the ventricle resulting in a rapid downstroke with no incisura—**'Water Hammer pulse'** |
| Patent ductus arteriosus | 120 mm Hg / 0 mm Hg — Increased pulse pressure | Large amount of blood pumped by left ventricle into aorta is pushed through patent ductus arteriosus resulting in the fall in diastolic pressure |

In the resting state, these precapillary sphincters remain closed which directs the blood into venules by using **throughfare channels**, intermittently opening up the capillaries. However, at the times of increased tissue oxygen demand, these oxygen sensitive precapillary sphincters relax which allows the blood flow though the capillary network **(Figs. 46.3A and B)**.

## Characteristics of Microcirculation and Capillary Circulation

The arterioles have muscular walls within internal diameter of around 10 to 15 μm. These arterioles give rise to **terminal meta arterioles** which have **intermittent muscular coat** made up of smooth muscles. At the points where the true capillaries originate from these meta arterioles, the smooth muscles form the precapillary sphincters which controls the blood flow in the capillaries.

The capillaries are made up of endothelial cells which are surrounded by thin basement membrane on the outer side of the capillaries. The total thickness of capillary wall is 0.5 μm with an internal diameter of 4 to 9 μm. *It is interesting to note that the average size of the RBC is around 7 microns; hence, it has to squeeze through these capillaries to maintain the blood flow.*

The capillary endothelium has **small pores** measuring **6 to 7 nanometers** which prevents the leakage of blood cells and plasma proteins into the interstitial fluid but still maintains the capillary fluid exchange dynamics. There are some **special type of pores** in the capillaries of certain

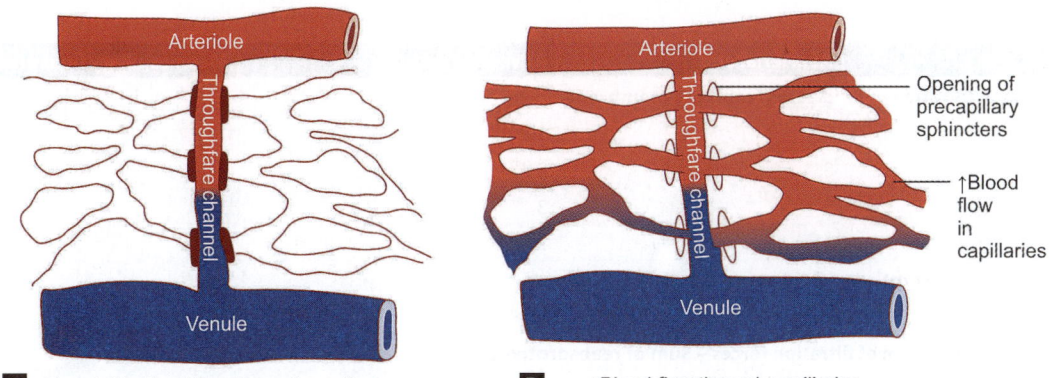

**Figs. 46.3A and B:** Blood flow through capillaries. (A) At rest; (B) Increased oxygen demand.

organs like brain has tight junctions between the capillary endothelial cells, which forms the blood brain barrier and allows the movement of very small molecules such as water, oxygen and carbon dioxide. Liver has clefts which allows the easy passage of plasma its dissolved substances and the plasma proteins in liver. The fenestrations present in the glomerular capillaries of kidney allows the movement of tremendous amount of small molecular and ionic substances but prevents the movement of plasma proteins and cells.

**Vasomotion:** The blood flow in the capillaries is intermittent, i.e., it is turned on and off every few seconds or minutes. This *intermittent blood flow* is called as vasomotion, which means the intermittent contraction of meta-arterioles and precapillary sphincters.

## Functions of Capillaries

The main function of the capillaries is exchange of water nutrients and other substances between the blood and the interstitial fluid in various tissue beds. Hence, the capillaries are also called the *exchange vessels*. The various factors which effect the exchange of these substances are mentioned below:

1. **Lipid solubility:** The lipid soluble substances like oxygen, carbon dioxide easily diffuse through the cell membrane of the capillary endothelial cells. However, the nonlipid soluble substances like water, various ions (sodium, chloride), glucose are not freely permeable and depend on their molecular size and pore size of the endothelium.
2. **Molecular size of the substance:** The average pore size of the capillaries is around 6 to 7 nanometers which allows the passage of water molecules through it. Hence, the permeability of various substances depends on their molecular size, thus determining their permeability.
The permeability of NaCl is closer to water followed by urea. The least permeable substance is albumin, which is the smallest plasma protein. Hence, the plasma proteins remain in the vascular compartment and do not enter the interstitial fluid.
3. **Concentration gradient of the substance:** The rate of capillary exchange is directly proportional to the concentration gradient of the substance across the capillary membrane.

## Capillary Fluid Dynamics

As the main purpose of the capillaries is fluid exchange, it is governed by Starling forces viz.

a. **Hydrostatic pressure of capillaries (Pc) and interstitial fluid (Pif):** It is primarily due to the fluid pressure in that compartment. In the capillaries, it is affected by the blood pressure.
Pc varies from the arterial to the venous end and also with the change in the blood pressure. The average Pc at the arterial end in 30 mm Hg and at venous end is 10 mm Hg. The Pc is however 28.3 mm Hg. Pif is subatmospheric, averaging about –3 mm Hg due to the negative pressure created due to pumping by the lymphatic system.
b. **Colloid osmotic pressure of capillaries (πc) and interstitial fluid (πif):** It occurs by the virtue of plasma proteins (exerting 19 mm Hg of colloid osmotic pressure in plasma) and the Donnan effect, due to osmotically active ions like $Na^+$, $K^+$ and other captions (contributing another 9 mm Hg of pressure). Hence, the resultant πc is 28 mm Hg.
The interstitial colloid osmotic pressure is however less than the plasma, averaging to about 8 mm Hg.

## Starlings' Equilibrium of Fluid Dynamics

Starling's equilibrium governs the intricate interplay of hydrostatic and oncotic pressures within systemic circulation, facilitating the precise regulation of vascular fluid dynamics crucial for nutrient exchange and metabolic waste clearance throughout the body's vasculature **(Table 46.2)**.

## Capillary Filtration Coefficient (Kf)

As seen above in table, the mean filtration pressure is 0.3 mm Hg which causes the filtration in the entire body at

Table 46.2: Fluid dynamics.

| | At arterial end | At venous end | Mean capillary fluid pressures |
|---|---|---|---|
| **Forces resulting in filtration of fluid across capillary membrane** | | | |
| Pc | 30 | 10 | 17.3 |
| πif | 8 | 8 | 8 |
| Negative Pif | 3 | 3 | 3 |
| Resultant filtration force | 41 | 21 | 28.3 |
| **Forces resulting in reabsorption of fluid across capillary membrane** | | | |
| πc | 28 | 28 | 28 |
| **Net filtration pressure = Sum of filtration forces – Sum of reabsorptive forces** | | | |
| | 13 mm Hg | –7 mm Hg | 0.3 mm Hg |
| | Filtration | Reabsorption | Filtration |

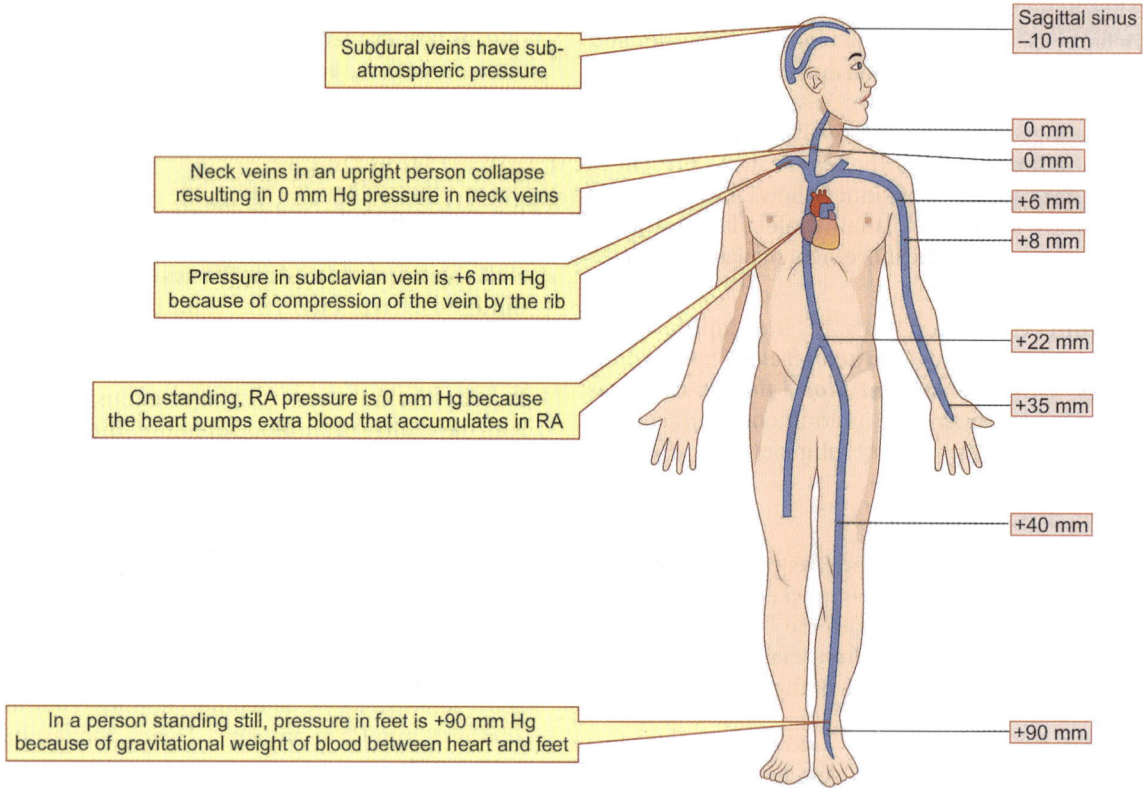

Fig. 46.4: Venous pressure throughout the body in standing position.

the rate of 2 mL/min. Hence, we can deduce that the net filtration rate across all the capillaries is **6.67 mL/min/mm Hg**.

Due to the differences in the capillaries in different tissues, the filtration coefficient can vary in different organs.

## VENOUS CIRCULATION (FROM CAPILLARIES TO HEART)

The veins provide an important segment of circulation performing a vital function of storage of blood and providing extra blood at times of need. The peripheral veins serve another important function of *venous pump* which helps in regulating the venous return and hence the cardiac output.

### Venous Pressures (Fig. 46.4)

The venus circulation has very low pressure but still the blood flow is maintained from the veins into the right atrium by the pressure gradient. Since the right atrium receives the venous blood from this systemic circulation it is also called the *central venous pressure (CVP)*. In normal healthy individuals, the **right atrial pressure** (at the level of the **tricuspid valve**) is **0 mm Hg**, i.e., it is equivalent to the atmospheric pressure.

Right **atrial pressure (RAP)** can **increase** in certain abnormal conditions like **serious heart failure** and a **massive increase** in the **blood volume** (as seen in massive transfusion). However, the right atrial pressure can become **less** than the atmospheric pressure that is up to **– 5 mm Hg**, when the heart is **pumping vigorously**.

### Role of Venous Valves

The veins in the legs have valves, which direct the blood flow toward heart. This peripheral pumping system is called *venous pump* or *muscle pump*. It keeps the venous pressure under control at +20 mm Hg, when a person is walking, as compared to +90 mm Hg when standing still, due to gravitational pull.

The veins of the lower limbs have venous valves which provide unidirectional flow of blood toward the heart. In people with raised intra-abdominal pressure or having long standing hours; tend to raise the venous pressure resulting in incompetence of these valves. They usually present with pedal edema and tortuous veins of the lower limbs called varicose veins.

*What would happen to venous pressure in lower limbs in a patient with raised intra-abdominal pressure above +20 mm Hg (pregnancy, ascites or abdominal tumor)?*

The blood from the legs (pressure in femoral vein is +20 mm Hg) would not be able to flow toward abdominal veins (normal pressure +6 mm Hg raised to +20 mm Hg or more) due to loss of pressure gradient. Hence, it leads to venous stasis and edema. Long standing venous stasis result in incompetent venous valves and leads to the enlargement and increased tortuosity of veins called varicose veins.

*Why the cranium is opened in the sitting posture, during the neurosurgery?*

The subatmospheric pressure (–10 mm Hg) in dural sinuses can lead to suction of air, if sagittal sinus is opened during the surgery, sucking the air into the venous system which may result in air embolism and death. In sitting posture, the risk of air embolism becomes less.

*What is the mean arterial pressure in feet, in an upright person, if mean arterial pressure at the level of heart is 100 mm Hg?*

a. 100 mm Hg  b. 120 mm Hg
c. 160 mm Hg  d. 190 mm Hg

Ans: 100 mm Hg

### Functions of Venous Circulation

- The venous circulation is responsible for maintaining the venous return to the right atrium and hence regulates the cardiac output.
- Since the veins have a high distensibility and capacitance; they act as the reservoir of blood and stores around 62% of the blood in the circulation.
- The sympathetic stimulation results and venoconstriction and increases the venous return hence affecting the cardiac output.
- The right atrial pressure is also called as the central venous pressure which acts as an indicator of ability of the heart to pump out the blood out of right atrium and the ventricle into lungs, i.e., right ventricular function.

## LYMPHATIC CIRCULATION

They lymphatic circulation represents an accessory route of lymphatic vessels, which drains the excessive fluid from interstitial spaces along with the large molecules and proteins into the main circulation. Like any other circulation it is also composed of lymphatic capillaries and lymphatic ducts which drain into the blood vessels. The lymphatics from the right and the left side of the body drain into right lymphatic duct and thoracic duct respectively (**Fig. 46.5**).

All the organs and the tissues of our body have special lymph channels that drain excess fluid from interstitial spaces into the blood *except skin, central nervous system, endomysium of muscle and bones* which has a few interstitial prelymphatics instead of well-developed lymphatic system.

The lymphatic capillaries are formed from endothelial cells which are held by anchoring filaments to the

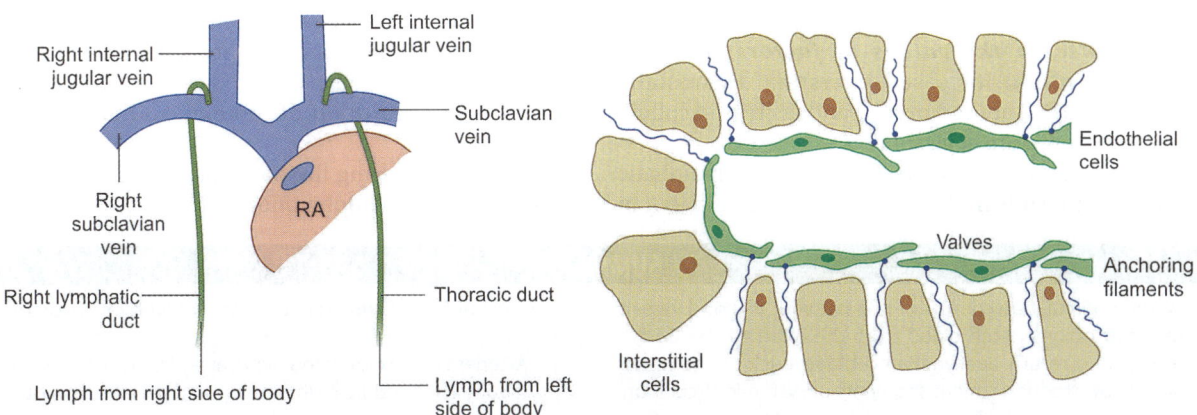

**Fig. 46.5:** Lymphatic circulation.

surrounding connective tissue. The edge of endothelial cell overlaps the adjacent cell in such a way that the overlapping edge is free and forms a minute valve, which helps in forward movement of lymph.

### Formation of Lymph

The initial lymph is formed in the interstitial space, which contains water and the large molecules such as proteins, etc. This lymph is formed in the terminal lymphatic capillaries, from where it flows toward the collecting lymphatics (**Fig. 46.6**). The average rate of *lymph flow in the thoracic duct is around 100 mL/hr*, along with 20 mL/hr from the other lymphatic channels; hence, there is **120 mL/hr** of lymphatic flow rate in the entire body amounting to **2–3 L/day**. The **protein content** of the lymph is same as the interstitial fluid that is **2 g/dL**. However, the lymph formed in **liver** has higher protein content of **6 g/dL** because liver is the site of synthesis of plasma proteins. Even the lymph from the **intestines** also has a higher protein content of **3 to 4 g/dL**, because the proteins are absorbed from intestine. The lymph also carries the larger fat droplets from the intestine and is the major route for absorption of fats through lacteals, which drain into lymphatic vessels. It is interesting to note that the fat concentration in thoracic duct may be as high as 1 to 2% after a fatty meal. The other larger substances like bacteria can also enter the lymphatic circulation through the endothelial cells. These bacteria are removed from the circulation, when the lymph passes through the lymph nodes.

### Factors Affecting the Lymphatic Flow

- **Interstitial fluid pressure:** Usually the interstitial fluid pressure is subatmospheric, i.e., less than 0, resulting in the baseline lymphatic flow. If there is an increase in the interstitial fluid pressure to 0 mm Hg, the lymphatic flow increases by 20 folds. Hence, all the factors which increase the interstitial fluid pressure like:
    - *Increase in values of the factors favoring filtration:* **Capillary hydrostatic pressure (Pc)** and **colloid osmotic pressure** of the interstitial fluid **(πif)**. An increased **permeability of capillaries** also plays an important role in increasing the interstitial fluid pressure
    - *Decrease in the values of factors favoring reabsorption:* Increased interstitial hydrostatic pressure **(Pif)** above 0 mm Hg and decreased colloid osmotic pressure of plasma **(πc)**.
- **Lymphatic pump:** When the fluid enters the lymphatic channels it results in the stretching of the segment in

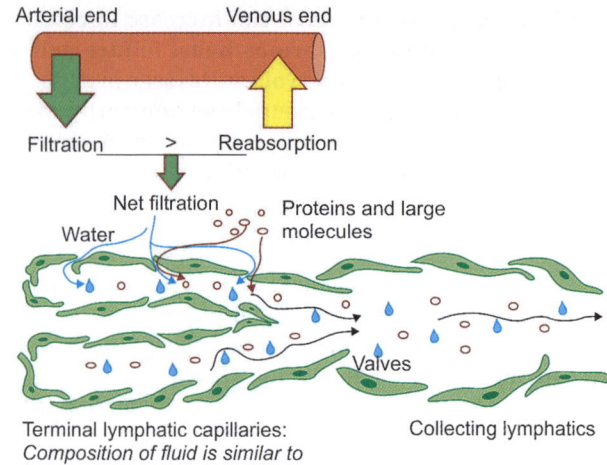

**Fig. 46.6:** Lymphatic capillaries and collection of lymph.

which the fluid is entering. This stretching results in the reflex contraction of the lymphatic channel, pushing the lymph forward into the next section. This property is called the lymphatic pump. It can generate pressure up to 50 to 100 mm Hg. This lymphatic pump plays an important role in draining excessive fluid from the interstitial spaces and maintains the interstitial fluid balance. In lungs, it is responsible for keeping the alveoli in the dry state.
- **Role of external compression on lymphatic circulation:** The external intermittent compresses of the lymphatic vessels due to the contraction of surrounding skeletal muscles or the pulsations of the adjacent arteries add to the lymphatic pump, which further increases the lymphatic flow from 10 to 30 folds.

### Functions of the Lymphatic Circulation

- It maintains the interstitial fluid volume and pressure.
- It maintains the colloid osmotic pressure of the interstitial fluid by removing the excessive proteins and returning them back to the blood.
- It returns the proteins to the circulation, which were lost from the capillaries into the interstitium. If the lymphatics fail to return this protein back into circulation, the person will die in 24 hours.
- The negative interstitial fluid pressure holds the body tissues together.
- It helps in absorption of proteins and fats from the intestine.
- It helps in removing the bacteria from the circulation with the help of lymph nodes.

---

### SUMMARY

- Systemic circulation consists of the network of blood vessels that carry oxygenated blood from the heart to the body's tissues and return deoxygenated blood back to the heart. Blood flow through various segments of systemic circulation, including arterial, capillary, venous, and lymphatic circulation, exhibits distinct characteristics influenced by physiological factors.
    - Arteries carry oxygenated blood away from the heart to the tissues. They endure high pressure and pulsatile flow due to ventricular contraction during systole.

- Elasticity of arterial walls allows for accommodation of blood volume during systole and maintenance of pressure during diastole.
- Arterial resistance, determined by vessel diameter and vascular tone, regulates blood flow distribution to different tissues.
- Factors affecting blood flow in arteries:
  - Vascular tone: Constriction and dilation of arterial smooth muscle influence blood flow resistance.
  - Blood viscosity: Increased viscosity reduces flow, while decreased viscosity enhances flow.
  - Arterial compliance: Reduced compliance affects pressure wave propagation and arterial stiffness.
- Capillaries are thin-walled vessels where exchange of gases, nutrients, and waste products occurs between blood and tissues.
- They are low pressure and continuous flow. They have extensive network provides large surface area for exchange.
- Precapillary sphincters regulate blood flow into capillary beds based on tissue metabolic demands.
- Factors affecting flow:
  - Metabolic activity: Increased metabolic demand leads to vasodilation and enhanced blood flow.
  - Capillary density: Higher capillary density in metabolically active tissues facilitates nutrient exchange.
  - Autoregulation: Local factors such as oxygen tension, pH, and carbon dioxide regulate capillary blood flow.
- Veins return deoxygenated blood from the tissues to the heart. They have low pressure and continuous flow with minimal pulsatility.
- Veins contain valves to prevent backflow and aid in venous return. Capacitance vessels capable of storing large volumes of blood.
- Factors affecting flow:
  - Skeletal muscle pump: Contraction of skeletal muscles compresses veins, promoting venous return.
  - Respiratory pump: Changes in thoracic pressure during breathing assist venous return to the heart.
  - Venous tone: Sympathetic stimulation regulates venous tone and affects venous capacitance.
- Lymphatic vessels collect excess interstitial fluid and return it to the bloodstream. They are also low-pressure system driven by intrinsic contractions of lymphatic vessels and external factors such as muscle movement. Lymph nodes filter lymph and play a role in immune response.
- Factors affecting flow:
  - Muscle activity: Contractions of skeletal muscles and smooth muscles in lymphatic vessels propel lymph flow.
  - Pressure differentials: Interstitial fluid pressure gradients facilitate lymphatic drainage.
  - Lymphatic vessel integrity: Damage or obstruction to lymphatic vessels impairs lymph flow.

## LET US SEE, HOW MUCH YOU HAVE LEARNT?

 *Review Questions*

### Long/Short Answer Questions

Q1. Describe the role of Starling forces in maintaining capillary fluid dynamics.

Q2. What are the functions of venous circulation?

Q3. What are the functions of lymphatic circulation?

### Explain Why? (Reasoning Questions)

Q1. What would happen to circulatory function, if we transfuse around half a litre of blood into the veins of a healthy patient?

Q2. What would happen to venous pressure in lower limbs in a patient with raised intra-abdominal pressure above +20 mm Hg (pregnancy, ascites or abdominal tumor)?

Q3. Why the cranium is opened in the sitting posture, during the neurosurgery?

Q4. What will happen, if the venous valves become incompetent?

Q5. What will happen, if the lymphatics are blocked?

### Multiple Choice Questions

Q1. What type of blood vessels carry oxygenated blood away from the heart?
   a. Veins
   b. Capillaries
   c. Arteries
   d. Venules

Q2. Which segment of systemic circulation is characterized by low pressure and continuous flow?
   a. Arterial circulation
   b. Venous circulation
   c. Capillary circulation
   d. Lymphatic circulation

Q3. During exercise, which factor contributes to increased blood flow in skeletal muscles?
   a. Constriction of arterioles
   b. Vasodilation of capillaries
   c. Decreased cardiac output
   d. Increased resistance in veins

Q4. A patient presents with swollen ankles and feet after prolonged standing. Which mechanism is likely impaired?
   a. Skeletal muscle pump
   b. Respiratory pump
   c. Venous tone regulation
   d. Lymphatic vessel integrity

Q5. How does increased sympathetic stimulation affect venous return to the heart?
   a. Enhances venous tone and decreases venous return
   b. Promotes vasodilation and increases venous return
   c. Constricts arterioles and decreases venous return
   d. Augments skeletal muscle pump activity and increases venous return

**Q6.** What role do precapillary sphincters play in regulating blood flow in capillary beds?
   a. They prevent backflow of blood into arterioles.
   b. They regulate blood flow based on tissue metabolic demands.
   c. They control blood pressure within capillaries.
   d. They facilitate exchange of gases between blood and tissues.

**Q7.** In which segment of systemic circulation does the majority of nutrient exchange occur between blood and tissues?
   a. Arterial circulation
   b. Capillary circulation
   c. Venous circulation
   d. Lymphatic circulation

**Q8.** What physiological mechanism ensures continuous flow of blood in veins despite low pressure?
   a. Presence of one-way valves
   b. Elasticity of vein walls
   c. Constriction of venous smooth muscle
   d. Arterial-venous pressure gradient

**Q9.** How does increased metabolic activity in a tissue affect blood flow in the corresponding capillary bed?
   a. Decreases blood flow due to vasoconstriction
   b. Increases blood flow due to vasodilation
   c. No significant effect on blood flow
   d. Causes blood to bypass the capillary bed

**Q10.** What is the primary function of lymphatic vessels in systemic circulation?
   a. Transporting oxygenated blood to tissues
   b. Collecting excess interstitial fluid and returning it to the bloodstream
   c. Filtering blood and removing toxins
   d. Regulating blood pressure in capillaries

**Q11.** During a long-haul flight, a passenger experiences swelling in the lower limbs. Which physiological mechanism is primarily responsible for this condition?
   a. Skeletal muscle pump dysfunction
   b. Venous vasoconstriction
   c. Reduced capillary density
   d. Arterial vasodilation

**Q12.** A marathon runner collapses at the finish line due to dehydration and extreme fatigue. Which factor contributes to decreased venous return in this scenario?
   a. Increased sympathetic stimulation
   b. Reduced blood viscosity
   c. Enhanced skeletal muscle pump activity
   d. Insufficient fluid intake

**Q13.** A patient with congestive heart failure presents with edema in the legs and abdominal distension. What mechanism exacerbates fluid accumulation in this condition?
   a. Increased lymphatic drainage
   b. Elevated arterial blood pressure
   c. Impaired venous return
   d. Enhanced capillary filtration

**Q14.** Following a severe injury, a patient experiences hypovolemic shock characterized by decreased blood pressure and tachycardia. Which compensatory mechanism aims to maintain tissue perfusion in this situation?
   a. Arterial vasoconstriction
   b. Skeletal muscle pump activation
   c. Capillary dilation
   d. Lymphatic vessel contraction

**Q15.** A person spends several hours sitting without moving, leading to numbness and tingling in the lower extremities. Which mechanism contributes to this sensation?
   a. Increased capillary permeability
   b. Reduced arterial pressure
   c. Impaired lymphatic drainage
   d. Venous stasis

**Q16.** A pregnant woman complains of swollen ankles and feet. Which physiological change during pregnancy contributes to venous insufficiency?
   a. Increased lymphatic drainage
   b. Enhanced venous tone
   c. Elevated cardiac output
   d. Compression of pelvic lymphatic vessels

**Q17.** A person experiences a sudden drop in blood pressure upon standing up from a lying position, leading to dizziness. Which mechanism fails to compensate for the change in posture?
   a. Activation of the skeletal muscle pump
   b. Constriction of arterioles
   c. Venous valve incompetence
   d. Rapid increase in heart rate

**Q18.** After a prolonged period of physical inactivity, a person notices swelling in the legs and ankles. What factor contributes to impaired venous return in this situation?
   a. Increased sympathetic stimulation
   b. Enhanced skeletal muscle pump activity
   c. Arterial vasodilation
   d. Venous valve dysfunction

### ANSWERS
1. c  2. b  3. b  4. a  5. d  6. b  7. b  8. a  9. b  10. b  11. a  12. d  13. c  14. a  15. d  16. d  17. a  18. d

# Physiological Basis of Cardiovascular Diseases

**CHAPTER 47**

**COMPETENCY ADDRESSED**

PY5.11: Describe the pathophysiology of shock, syncope and heart failure.

**LEARNING OBJECTIVES**

At the end of this chapter, the learner should be able to:
- Describe the physiological basis of clinical presentation of various cardiovascular diseases, viz., shock, syncope and heart failure.
- Describe the physiological basis of management of various cardiovascular diseases, viz., shock, syncope and heart failure.

## SHOCK

### Definition

It is defined as decreased perfusion of vital organs resulting in inadequate supply of nutrients and inadequate removal of the waste products from the tissues.

*What is the difference in hypoxia, shock and anemia, where all three of them result in decreased oxygenation of tissues?*

Hypoxia is a broad term that is defined as **decreased availability** of oxygen to tissues. It could be due to any reason, resulting either due to decreased oxygen-carrying capacity (as seen in anemia; or anemic hypoxia) or due to decreased perfusion (as seen in shock, or stagnant hypoxia).

### Etiopathogenesis

Depending on the etiology, the shock can be classified as:
- **Pump failure/heart failure:** It is also called *cardiogenic shock*. In this type of shock, the inadequate pumping of the ventricle results in decreased cardiac output and hence resulting in inadequate perfusion, resulting in shock.
- **Decreased venous return:** The decreased venous return due to any of the following causes, may result in decreased cardiac output resulting in decreased perfusion and shock.
  - ***Decreased blood volume (hypovolemic shock):*** The most common cause of the hypovolemia is hemorrhage, however, the other causes resulting in plasma loss occurring due to severe dehydration, burns, intestinal obstruction, etc. which could lead to shock.
  - ***Distributive shock:*** In this type of shock, there is no loss of blood but redistribution of plasma volume into the other fluid compartments. It is seen in:
    - Anaphylactic shock
    - Septic shock
    - Neurogenic shock
  - ***Obstructive shock:*** In this type of shock, there is obstruction to the flow of blood, hence resulting in decreased cardiac output.

Different types of shocks and their features are described in **Table 47.1**.

*Why a person with intestinal obstruction goes into shock?*

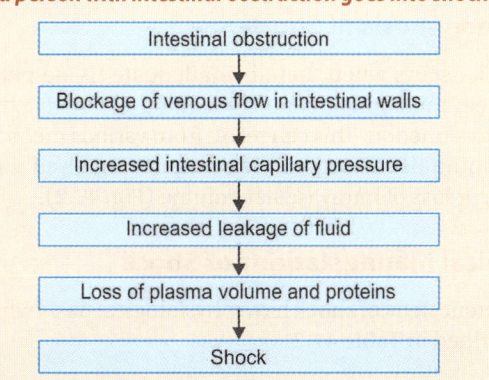

**Table 47.1:** Features of different types of shock.

| | Hypovolemic shock | Distributive shock | Cardiogenic shock | Obstructive shock |
|---|---|---|---|---|
| Causes | Loss of blood volume | Blood is distributed into other compartments | Failure of the heart to pump adequate blood for perfusion | Obstruction to blood flow |
| Examples | • **Hemorrhage (most common)**<br>  ▪ Trauma<br>  ▪ Surgery<br>  ▪ Internal bleeding<br>• **Loss of plasma volume**<br>  ▪ Burns<br>  ▪ Intestinal obstruction<br>• **Loss of body fluids**<br>  ▪ Severe vomiting<br>  ▪ Severe diarrhea<br>• **Increased water loss from kidneys**<br>  ▪ Diuretics<br>  ▪ Diabetes insipidus | • **Anaphylactic shock**<br>  ▪ Severe allergic reaction<br>  ▪ Mediated by antigen antibody reaction, primarily due to release of histamine from mast cells<br>  ▪ Massive vasodilation, increased capillary permeability, reduction in venous return<br>• **Neurogenic shock**<br>  ▪ Deep general anesthesia, spinal anesthesia, brain damage resulting in vasomotor failure and transaction of spinal cord in thoracolumbar segments<br>  ▪ Massive vasodilation due to loss of sympathetic vasoconstrictor tone<br>  ▪ Reduces mean systemic filling pressure, resulting in venous pooling of blood<br>• **Septic shock**<br>  ▪ Most common cause of shock<br>  ▪ Occurs due to widespread infection by gram-positive bacteria followed by release of endotoxin by gram-negative bacteria<br>  ▪ There is high-grade fever, marked vasodilation, high cardiac output, sludging of blood, formation of microthrombi leading to disseminated intravascular coagulation | **Pump failure**<br>• Heart failure<br>• Results from severe depression of cardiac performance<br>• Shock occurs when >40% of ventricular muscle is damaged | **Obscured filling or emptying of heart**<br>Compression of great veins, pulmonary artery, aorta and myocardium<br>• Pulmonary embolism: prevents emptying of RV<br>• Pericardial tamponade: prevents filling during diastole<br>• Tension pneumothorax: displaces IVC, decreases VR |

## Stages of Shock

Shock progresses through various stages—starting with the initial compensatory phase where the body activates mechanisms to maintain blood pressure and perfusion. As shock worsens, the compensatory mechanisms become overwhelmed, leading to the progressive stage characterized by tissue hypoperfusion and metabolic acidosis. Finally, if untreated, shock enters the irreversible stage marked by widespread cellular damage and organ failure **(Fig. 47.1)**.

## Pathogenesis of Shock

Shock occurs when there is inadequate tissue perfusion to meet metabolic demands, leading to cellular hypoxia and dysfunction. This can result from various mechanisms including decreased cardiac output, impaired vascular tone, or loss of intravascular volume **(Fig. 47.2)**.

## Clinical Manifestations of Shock

Different signs of shock have physiological basis which are described in **Table 47.2**.

## Physiological Basis of Management of Shock

- **Replacement therapy:**
  - Blood and plasma transfusion: The best therapy is whole blood transfusion, but in patients with only plasma loss, plasma is the replacement of choice.
  - Plasma substitutes (dextran) are made of large molecules of polysaccharide polymer of glucose. It is used as a substitute for plasma transfusion.
- **Drugs:**
  - **Sympathomimetic drugs:** These drugs are particularly useful in the treatment of anaphylactic shock and neurogenic shock.
  - **Antibiotics:** These are particularly useful in septic shock.
  - **Glucocorticoids:** These drugs increase myocardial strength in later stages of shock, stabilize the lysosomal membrane and prevent the cellular injury. They also aid in glucose metabolism.
- **Oxygen therapy:** It is usually considered in the first line of treatment but it is not as effective as it appears because the problem is inadequate perfusion, not the availability of oxygen.

| | Stage I<br>Compensatory shock | Stage II<br>Progressive shock | Stage III<br>Irreversible shock |
|---|---|---|---|
| Pathogenesis | Body responds to hypotension and compensatory mechanisms come into play<br>• Baroreceptor reflex mechanism<br>• Chemoreceptor reflex mechanism<br>• CNS ischemic response<br>• Renin angiotensin system is activated<br>• Reverse stress relaxation<br>• Capillary fluid shift into the blood vessels<br>• Release of ADH by posterior pituitary<br>• Water and salt conservation by kidney<br>• Increased thirst and appetite | Decreased tissue perfusion<br><br>*If compensatory mechanism fails* → | • Microcirculatory failure<br>• Cellular death<br>• Depletion of ATP<br><br>*If shock is not treated efficiently* → |
| Outcome | Body tries to restore BP by sympathetic stimulation | • BP falls<br>• Systemic effects of shock present | Death is imminent |
| | • Adrenal hormones<br>  – Stimulation of sympathetic system<br>  – Mineralocorticoids: Retention of sodium<br>  – Glucocorticoids: Increases blood glucose level<br>• Increased thirst<br>• Increased salt intake<br>**Late compensatory mechanisms**<br>• Increased plasma protein synthesis<br>• Red cell mass restoration | • Compensatory mechanisms fail to restore BP<br>• Cardiac depression: Decreased arterial pressure, decreased coronary blood flow resulting in weakening of myocardium. This further decreases the cardiac output<br>• Vasomotor failure: Initial cerebral ischemia results in strong stimulation of vasomotor center but a continued cerebral ischemia of 10–15 minutes and arterial pressure falls below 30 mm Hg, it results in depression of vasomotor center<br>• Increased capillary permeability: Capillary hypoxia increases the capillary permeability resulting in transudation of fluids and further decreasing the cardiac output<br>• Release of endotoxins by ischemic tissues: Various toxic mediators like histamine, serotonin are released during shock. Release of endotoxins from the gram-negative bacteria increases the cellular metabolism especially of myocardium. All these factors depresses the cardiac efficiency and further decreas the cardiac output<br>• Cellular deterioration:<br>  – Depletion of ATP due to exhaustion and inability of cell to form new ATP<br>  – Decreased activity of Na+ K+ ATPase pump, resulting in accumulation of sodium and chloride inside the cells. This results in osmotic swelling of cells<br>  – Depression of mitochondrial activity<br>  – Lysosomal lysis and increased enzymatic activity (hydrolases) resulting in tissue injury<br>  – Depression of cellular metabolism and hormonal secretion | • Body becomes refractory to all treatments<br>• Multiple organ failure<br>• Severe cellular deterioration<br>• Severe depletion of energy<br>• Death is imminent |
| Homeostatic mechanisms | It is regulated by strong negative feedback mechanism | It is primarily regulated by the positive feedback mechanism, because of which the vicious cycle is set up leading to irreversible shock. The active intervention in this stage breaks this cycle and increases the chances of recovery from shock | The positive feedback cycle further progresses and leads to the irreversible shock, which is resistant to all the treatments. The patient in this stage of shock cannot be saved because of the microemboli formed during this stage. The acidosis due to accumulation of carbonic acid and lactic acid results in formation of micro emboli which affects various vital organs resulting in multiple organ failure |

**Fig. 47.1:** Stages of shock physiology and their effects.

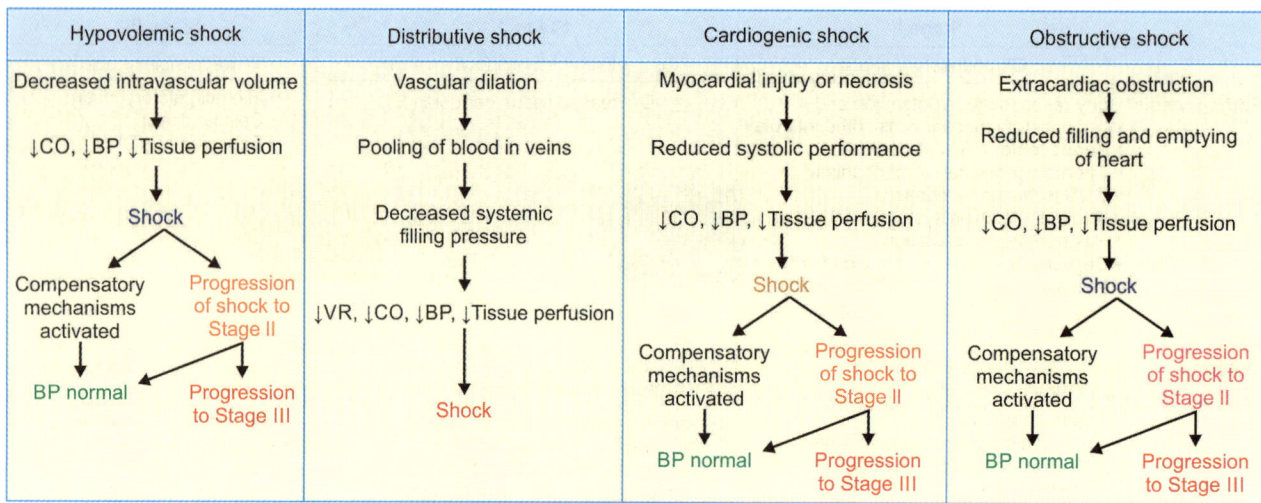

**Fig. 47.2:** Pathogenesis of different types of shock.

Table 47.2: Physiological basis of clinical manifestations of shock.

| Clinical manifestation | Physiological basis |
|---|---|
| Hypotension | It is the main presentation of shock. Decreased systemic blood pressure leads to inadequate perfusion, hence resulting in shock |
| Rapid and thready pulse | Hypotension results in activation of compensatory mechanisms, which results in sympathetic activation, increasing the heart rate. Hence, Marey's law (HR $\propto$ 1/BP) is not applicable here |
| Rapid and shallow breathing | The accumulation of $CO_2$, and hypoxia results in the stimulation of chemoreceptor areas and the stimulation of respiration |
| Cold clammy skin except in distributive shock | Sympathetic stimulation results in cutaneous vasoconstriction and activates the sweat glands resulting in sweaty cold extremities. Hence, resulting in cold shock. Distributive shock occurs due to massive vasodilation, the extremities remain warm, hence called warm shock |
| Thirst | Hypotension stimulates the osmoreceptors and hence activates the thirst mechanism, in order to maintain blood volume |
| Decreased urine output | Hypotension decreases the renal blood flow, which decreases the GFR and blood flows through the vasa recta resulting in the formation of concentrated urine. ADH also increases the water reabsorption from the kidneys, decreasing urine output |
| Hypothermia | Hypotension and sympathetic activation cause hypothermia |
| Nausea and vomiting | Hypotension stimulates the chemoreceptor trigger zone resulting in nausea and vomiting |
| Metabolic acidosis | Hypotension and hypoxia results in increased anaerobic glycolysis resulting in the production of excessive lactic acid. The excessive carbon dioxide in tissues also reacts with water to produce carbonic acid |
| Cyanosis | Decreased perfusion of peripheral tissues presents with bluish discoloration of the extremities and acral parts, resulting in cyanosis |

- **Posture:** In case of hemorrhagic and neurogenic shock, the head of the patient should be placed 12 inches lower than the feet, promoting the venous return. It is the first essential step in most of the patients of shock.

## Complications of Shock

- **Cardiac complications:** Cardiac arrest, ventricular fibrillation
- **Neural complications:** It has been observed that 5–8 minutes of cerebral hypoxia results in brain damage and if the circulatory arrest continues for more than 10–15 minutes, there is permanent brain damage. However, it has been observed that if intravascular clotting is prevented by effective thrombolysis immediately, the brain can withstand the hypoxia for up to 30 minutes.

## CARDIAC FAILURE

It is defined as failure of the heart to pump enough blood to meet the demands of the body.

### Causes

- Intrinsic pump failure—weakening of ventricular muscle
- Increased work load on heart—increased afterload and preload

- Restricted filling of cardiac chambers—cardiac tamponade, constrictive pericarditis.

## Classification of Cardiac Failure

Cardiac failure is commonly classified into systolic and diastolic dysfunction. Systolic dysfunction involves impaired contractility, while diastolic dysfunction relates to impaired relaxation and filling of the ventricles (**Table 47.3**).

For the case based learning, refer author's Early Clinical Exposure in Clinical Physiology.

## Pathophysiology of Cardiac Failure

See **Figure 47.3**.

**Table 47.3:** Classification of cardiac failure.

| | Depending upon ventricular involvement | |
|---|---|---|
| **Single ventricular involvement** | **Right ventricular failure** | **Left ventricular failure** |
| | Inability of RV to pump the blood into pulmonary artery (cor pulmonale) | Inability of LV to pump the blood into aorta |
| Signs | Raised JVP, liver congestion and pedal edema | Pulmonary edema, pulmonary crepitations present, dyspnea, orthopnea, decreased LV output, ischemic acute tubular necrosis (ATN), hypoxic encephalopathy, muscular weakness and fatigue |
| Biventricular failure (congestive heart failure) | Signs of both LVF and RVF are present | |
| | **Based on phase of cardiac cycle** | |
| | Systolic failure | Diastolic failure |
| | Decreased stroke volume due to weak ventricular contraction | Increased myocardial stiffness leads to decreased ventricular filling |
| | **Based on cardiac output** | |
| | Low output failure | High output failure |
| | Occurs due to decreased venous return<br>• Myocardial infarction<br>• Cardiogenic shock<br>• Cardiomyopathies | Occurs due to increased venous return<br>• Thyrotoxicosis<br>• AV fistula<br>• Beriberi |

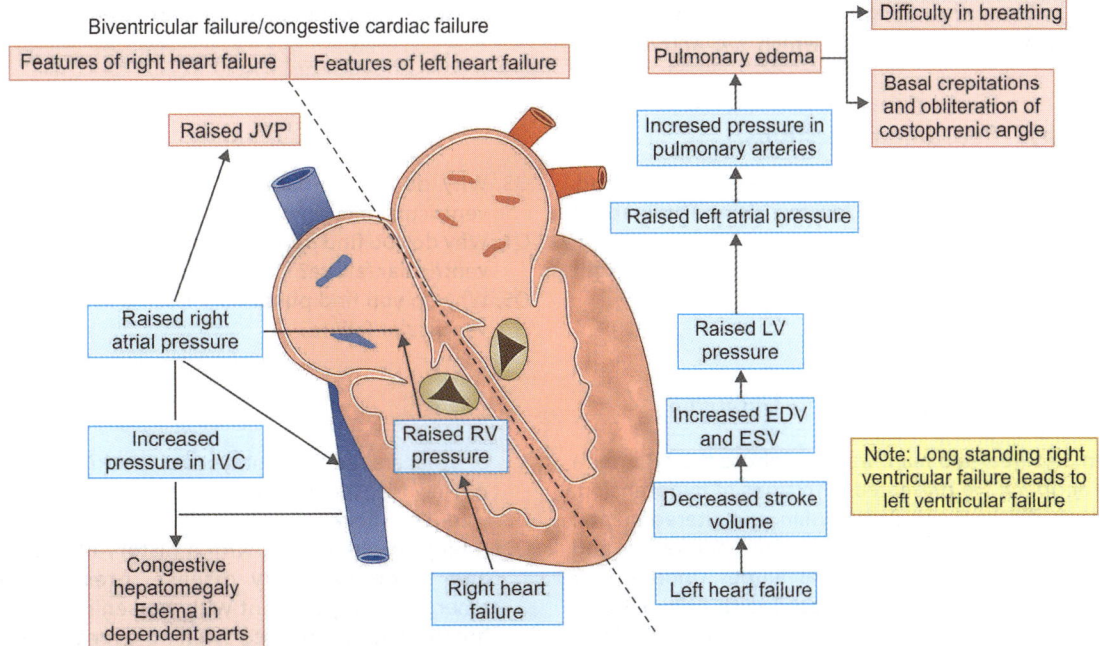

**Fig. 47.3:** Pathophysiology of congestive cardiac failure.

## SUMMARY

Cardiovascular diseases, including shock and heart failure, are characterized by impaired cardiovascular function, leading to inadequate tissue perfusion and systemic symptoms.

- Shock:
  - Shock is a life-threatening condition characterized by systemic hypoperfusion and inadequate oxygen delivery to tissues.
  - Types of shock include hypovolemic, cardiogenic, distributive (septic, anaphylactic, neurogenic), and obstructive shock.
  - Clinically, it presents with hypotension, tachycardia, cold, clammy skin, altered mental status.
  - Physiologically, it is explained as Inadequate cardiac output leads to decreased tissue perfusion. Compensatory mechanisms include sympathetic activation, vasoconstriction, and redistribution of blood flow to vital organs.
  - It is managed by fluid resuscitation to restore intravascular volume, vasopressor therapy to improve vascular tone and blood pressure and treatment of underlying cause (e.g., hemorrhage, myocardial infarction, sepsis).
- Heart failure:
  - Heart failure is a chronic condition characterized by the heart's inability to pump blood effectively, leading to inadequate tissue perfusion.
  - Types of heart failure include systolic heart failure (reduced ejection fraction) and diastolic heart failure (preserved ejection fraction).
  - Clinical presentation of heart failure includes dyspnea, fatigue, peripheral edema, orthopnea.
  - Physiological basis of these symptoms could be explained as impaired contractility of the myocardium leads to reduced cardiac output, activation of compensatory mechanisms such as the renin-angiotensin-aldosterone system and sympathetic nervous system, ventricular remodeling and neurohormonal activation contribute to disease progression.
- Management:
  - Pharmacological therapy including diuretics, ACE inhibitors, beta-blockers, and aldosterone antagonists to reduce symptoms and improve outcomes.
  - Lifestyle modifications such as sodium restriction, fluid restriction, and regular exercise.
  - Device therapy (e.g., implantable cardioverter-defibrillator, cardiac resynchronization therapy) and surgical interventions (e.g., coronary artery bypass grafting, heart transplant) in advanced cases.

## LET US SEE, HOW MUCH YOU HAVE LEARNT?

### Review Questions

#### Long/Short Answer Questions

Q1. Define shock. Describe the stages of shock.
Q2. What is compensated shock? Describe the various compensatory mechanisms which are activated in shock?
Q3. Define cardiac failure. How would you differentiate between the right and left heart failure?

#### Explain Why? (Reasoning Questions)

Q1. What will happen, if a person allergic to sea food, inadvertently consumes a lobster? (Hint: Think about anaphylactic shock)
Q2. Why do you find hepatomegaly in a patient of right ventricular failure?
Q3. Why do you find raised JVP in a patient of right ventricular failure?
Q4. Why do you find dependent edema in a patient of right ventricular failure?
Q5. Why do you find pulmonary edema in a patient of left ventricular failure?

### Critical Thinking Case-Based Questions

Q1. Ram a 45-year-old man, was brought to the ER after a car accident. He presented with signs of hypotension, tachycardia, cool and clammy skin, and altered mental status. His medical history was unremarkable, and there were no apparent external injuries. Upon further evaluation, David was diagnosed with hemorrhagic shock due to internal bleeding from a ruptured spleen. Depending upon the given scenario, answer the following questions:
  a. Explain the physiological mechanisms underlying hemorrhagic shock.
  b. What are the different types of shock?
  c. How do the compensatory mechanisms activated during shock?

Q2. A 65-year-old woman with a history of hypertension and coronary artery disease, presented to the emergency department with worsening shortness of breath, fatigue, and leg swelling over the past week. She reported difficulty breathing when lying flat and waking up at night gasping for air. On examination, crackles were heard in her lung bases, and her jugular venous pressure was elevated. An echocardiogram

revealed reduced left ventricular ejection fraction and signs of pulmonary congestion. Depending upon given scenario, answer the following questions:
a. What is the probable diagnosis?
b. Explain the pathophysiological mechanisms underlying this patient's condition.
c. How do the compensatory mechanisms contribute to patient's symptoms and clinical findings?

## Multiple Choice Questions

Q1. What is the primary characteristic of shock?
a. Hypertension
b. Hyperglycemia
c. Systemic hypoperfusion
d. Bradycardia

Q2. Which type of shock results from an acute loss of intravascular volume?
a. Cardiogenic shock
b. Distributive shock
c. Hypovolemic shock
d. Obstructive shock

Q3. What is the hallmark symptom of heart failure?
a. Peripheral edema
b. Tachypnea
c. Bradycardia
d. Hypernatremia

Q4. Which type of heart failure is characterized by reduced ejection fraction?
a. Systolic heart failure
b. Diastolic heart failure
c. Acute heart failure
d. Chronic heart failure

Q5. A patient presents with hypotension, tachycardia, and cool, clammy skin following a severe allergic reaction. What type of shock is most likely occurring?
a. Septic shock
b. Anaphylactic shock
c. Neurogenic shock
d. Cardiogenic shock

Q6. A patient involved in a motor vehicle accident exhibits signs of shock, and imaging reveals pericardial tamponade. Which type of shock is evident in this case?
a. Cardiogenic shock
b. Obstructive shock
c. Distributive shock
d. Hypovolemic shock

Q7. A patient with a history of hypertension presents with dyspnea on exertion and bilateral lower extremity edema. What is the likely diagnosis?
a. Systolic heart failure
b. Diastolic heart failure
c. Septic shock
d. Neurogenic shock

Q8. A patient with heart failure exhibits signs of fluid overload despite adherence to medication. Which pharmacological intervention is most appropriate?
a. Aldosterone antagonists
b. Loop diuretics
c. Beta-blockers
d. ACE inhibitors

Q9. How do vasopressor medications such as norepinephrine benefit patients in shock?
a. By increasing venous return to the heart
b. By improving myocardial contractility
c. By constricting blood vessels and raising blood pressure
d. By enhancing capillary permeability

Q10. What is the primary mechanism by which ACE inhibitors improve outcomes in heart failure?
a. By increasing sympathetic nervous system activity
b. By reducing preload on the heart
c. By enhancing ventricular remodeling
d. By promoting vasoconstriction

Q11. How does chronic kidney disease contribute to the development of heart failure?
a. By decreasing fluid retention and reducing cardiac output
b. By increasing sympathetic activity and impairing ventricular function
c. By causing electrolyte imbalances and promoting arrhythmias
d. By inducing volume overload and exacerbating myocardial stress

Q12. Which diagnostic test is most useful in assessing left ventricular function in heart failure patients?
a. Echocardiography
b. Electrocardiography
c. Cardiac catheterization
d. Coronary angiography

Q13. How does the loss of sympathetic tone lead to hypotension in neurogenic shock?
a. By causing vasodilation and reducing systemic vascular resistance
b. By increasing myocardial contractility and cardiac output
c. By stimulating the release of vasopressin and angiotensin II
d. By promoting vasoconstriction and elevating blood pressure

Q14. What is the primary characteristic of cardiac failure?
a. Increased myocardial contractility
b. Impaired cardiac pump function
c. Elevated stroke volume
d. Enhanced diastolic filling

Q15. Which type of cardiac dysfunction is characterized by reduced ejection fraction?
a. Systolic dysfunction
b. Diastolic dysfunction
c. Ischemic dysfunction
d. Valvular dysfunction

Q16. What is the main consequence of neurohormonal activation in cardiac failure?
a. Vasodilation
b. Fluid excretion
c. Ventricular remodeling
d. Bradycardia

Q17. Which compensatory mechanism is activated in response to reduced cardiac output in cardiac failure?
   a. Parasympathetic nervous system inhibition
   b. Renin-angiotensin-aldosterone system activation
   c. Decreased sympathetic activity
   d. Vasodilation of systemic arteries

Q18. What effect does sympathetic nervous system activation have on the heart in cardiac failure?
   a. Decreases heart rate and contractility
   b. Increases heart rate and contractility
   c. Promotes vasodilation
   d. Reduces systemic vascular resistance

Q19. How does ventricular remodeling contribute to the progression of cardiac failure?
   a. It improves myocardial contractility
   b. It reduces systemic vascular resistance
   c. It leads to chamber dilation and myocardial hypertrophy
   d. It decreases preload and afterload

Q20. Which factor is associated with the development of diastolic dysfunction in cardiac failure?
   a. Increased left ventricular end-diastolic volume
   b. Reduced left ventricular wall thickness
   c. Impaired relaxation of the myocardium
   d. Elevated ejection fraction

Q21. How does myocardial ischemia contribute to systolic dysfunction in cardiac failure?
   a. By increasing myocardial contractility
   b. By reducing preload on the heart
   c. By impairing oxygen delivery to myocardial tissue
   d. By decreasing afterload on the heart

## ANSWERS

1. c    2. c    3. a    4. a    5. b    6. b    7. a    8. b    9. c    10. b    11. d    12. a    13. a    14. b
15. a    16. c    17. b    18. b    19. c    20. c    21. c

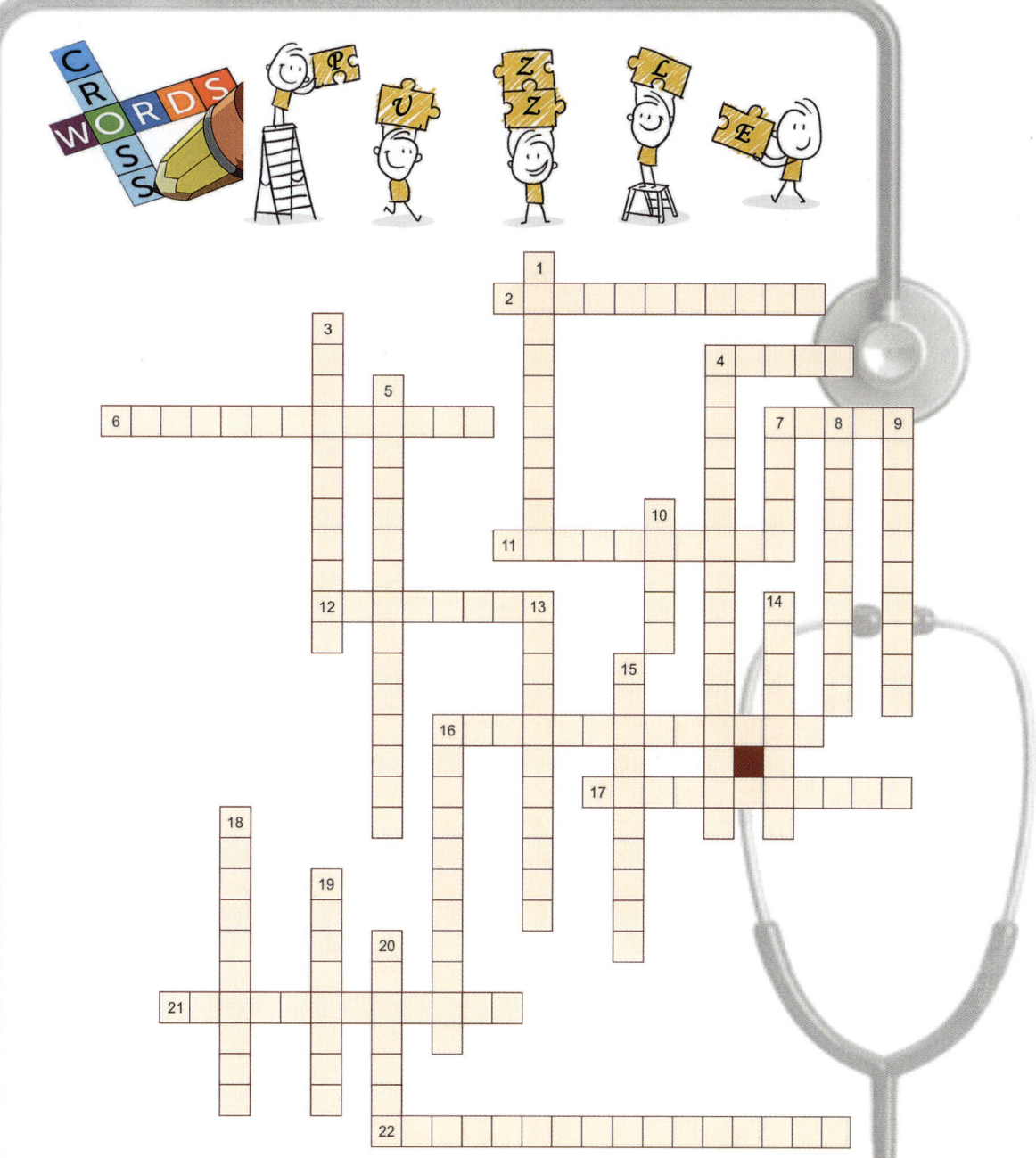

### Across

2. Outermost covering of the heart
4. Nerve that decreases heart rate when stimulated
6. Amount of blood pumped by each ventricle into the respective great arteries in one minute
7. Depolarization of atria resulting in positive deflection on ECG
11. Impedance to the blood flow
12. Condition caused by reduced blood flow in coronary arteries
16. Receptors sensitive to pressure changes in aorta and carotid sinus
17. Hormone that raises blood pressure by vasoconstriction
21. Chronic disease characterized by high blood pressure
22. Most used non-invasive method for the study of cardiac cycle

### Down

1. Most common cause of hypovolemic shock
3. Condition in which ECG shows peak T waves and wide P waves
4. Effect of high intracellular calcium on blood flow
5. Disease caused by plaque buildup in arteries
7. A wave of receptive relaxation of arterial wall precedes the blood flow
8. Rapid, irregular heart beats detectable on ECG
9. Potent vasoconstrictor released by the damaged endothelium
10. Thin-walled chambers located at the top of the heart
13. Study of flow of blood and blockage in the coronary arteries
14. Pattern of T wave in ECG in aVR and aVL leads
15. Used in radionucleotide study and selectively taken up by infarcted area
16. Most important sign of hypothyroidism related to heart rhythm
18. Leg vein valves that causes blood flow towards heart
19. Atrial and ventricular relaxation during cardiac cycle
20. Sudden attack of dizziness and fainting

# SECTION 6

# RESPIRATORY PHYSIOLOGY

## Section Outline

**Chapter 48:** Functional Anatomy of Respiratory System
**Chapter 49:** Mechanics of Pulmonary Ventilation (Chest Movements, Pressure Changes, Alveolar Surface Tension, Compliance, Airway Resistance)
**Chapter 50:** Pulmonary Ventilation (Diffusion of Gases Across Respiratory Membrane)
**Chapter 51:** Pulmonary Function Tests
**Chapter 52:** Pulmonary Circulation
**Chapter 53:** Transport of Respiratory Gases (Oxygen and Carbon Dioxide)
**Chapter 54:** Regulation of Respiration
**Chapter 55:** Respiration in Special Conditions (In Different Barometric Pressures)
**Chapter 56:** Physiological Basis of Respiratory Disorders

# Functional Anatomy of Respiratory System

**48 CHAPTER**

**COMPETENCY ADDRESSED**
PY6.1: Describe the functional anatomy of the respiratory system.

**LEARNING OBJECTIVES**

At the end of this chapter, the learner should be able to:
- Describe the different phases of respiration and describe their importance.
- Enlist the parts of the respiratory tract and describe their importance.
- Explain the division of airways into conducting and respiratory zones.
- Enlist and analyze functions of the respiratory system.

## INTRODUCTION

The term "respiration" has its roots in the Latin word "Respirae," which means "to breathe." The respiratory system possesses a distinct structure that facilitates its primary function, transporting gases in and out of the body. This chapter describes the fundamental anatomy and cellular physiology that contribute to the respiratory system and its distinguishing characteristics. Moreover, the chapter explores how the anatomical features contribute to the basic mechanics of breathing, highlighting non-respiratory physiology in the pulmonary system.

**Respiration comprises of two processes:**
1. The external respiration
2. The internal respiration

## The Internal Respiration or Tissue Respiration

Refer to utilization of $O_2$ and production of $CO_2$ by the tissue and gaseous exchange the cells and their fluid medium.

## The External Respiration

Includes supply of $O_2$ to the tissues from the environment and excretion of $CO_2$ released by the tissues into the atmosphere.

The process of external respiration involves three major events:
1. **Pulmonary ventilation** refers to the exchange of gases between the environment and lungs, which involves the mechanics of respiration.
2. **Pulmonary diffusion**, also known as gaseous exchange, is the transfer of gases from the alveoli to the blood through the respiratory membrane. To understand the process of pulmonary diffusion, it is essential to grasp the facts about pulmonary circulation, as well as the properties of gases and the laws governing diffusion of gases.
3. **Transport of gases**, or the carriage of blood gases from the blood to the body cells and back, also occurs, and exchange of blood gases (oxygen and carbon dioxide) happens at the tissue level.

**Respiratory adjustments in health and disease** are essential to life, and to comprehend these, knowledge about the **regulation of respiration** is crucial.

## FUNCTIONAL ANATOMY OF THE RESPIRATORY TRACT

The respiratory tract is the anatomical structure responsible for the movement of air in and out of the body. It is divided into two portions:
1. The upper respiratory tract, which includes the nostrils, nasopharynx, oropharynx, and larynx.

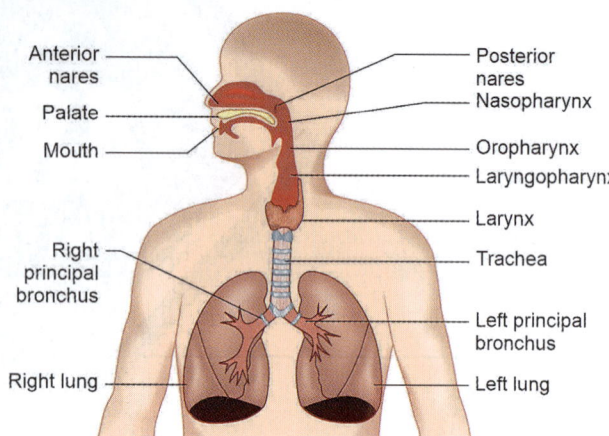

Fig. 48.1: Respiratory system and passages.

2. The lower respiratory tract, which includes the trachea, bronchi, lungs, and alveoli.

When we breathe in, the air enters the respiratory tract through either the nostrils or the mouth, and passes through the upper respiratory tract before moving on to the lower respiratory tract **(Fig. 48.1)**.

## Respiratory Passages

**Nasal cavities** warm and humidify the air due to the blood vessels in the mucosa. Nostril hairs and mucus trap, clean, and filter particulate content. They create 50% of respiratory system airflow resistance, which may increase during upper respiratory tract infections.

## *Applied Physiology*

- Nasal breathing is better than mouth breathing. Congestion can cause mouth breathing, which can lead to dry mouth and gum infections.
- Cold air can trigger bronchospasms in asthmatics if it enters the lower respiratory tract. Air goes through the lower respiratory tract to reach the alveoli for gas exchange.

**Paranasal sinuses** are air-filled spaces around the nasal passage. They include maxillary, sphenoid, ethmoid, and frontal sinuses. They offer voice resonance, lighten the skull, and protect the brain from facial trauma.

**The pharynx** is divided into three parts:
1. **The nasopharynx** is located behind the nose and connects to the eustachian tubes and posterior nares. Infections of the nasopharynx are common.
2. **The oropharynx** is behind the mouth and the laryngopharynx extends from the hyoid bone to the esophagus.
3. **The laryngopharynx** is located behind the opening of the larynx.

**The larynx** consists of the epiglottis, arytenoids, and vocal cords. During swallowing, the epiglottis and arytenoids cover the vocal cords to prevent food from entering the respiratory tract.

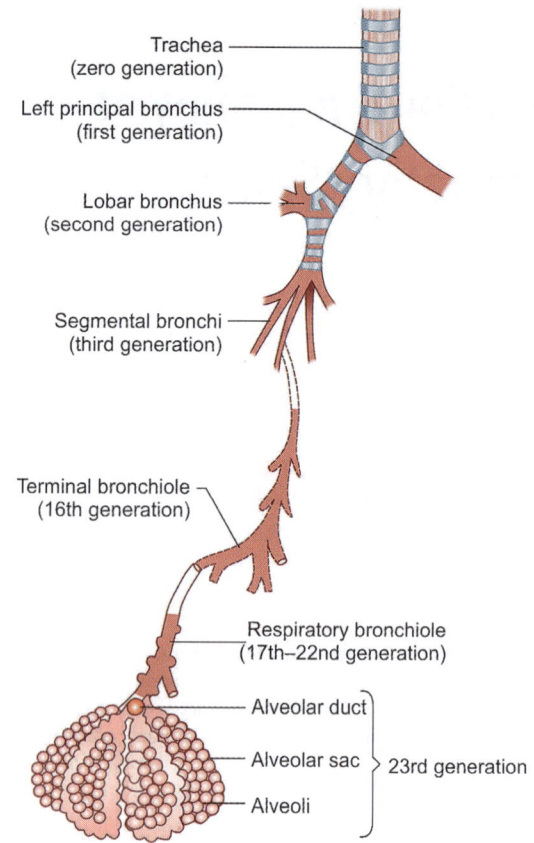

Fig. 48.2: The tracheobronchial tree.

**The trachea** is supported by 16–20 C-shaped cartilaginous rings, which prevent it from collapsing and allow for head movement.

## Tracheobronchial Tree

Air passages divide 23 times, creating the tracheobronchial tree. This increases the airway's cross-sectional area and reduces airflow velocity in small airways **(Fig. 48.2)**.

The tracheobronchial tree divides *23 times* between the trachea and alveoli, increasing the total cross-sectional area of the airway from **2.5 to 11,800 cm²** in the alveoli. This results in a significant decrease in airflow velocity in the small airways. The 23 generations of divisions in the tracheobronchial tree have been numbered as follows:

- The trachea is the starting point, designated as the zero generation.
- The principal bronchi, the right and left major divisions of the trachea, are the first generation.
- The lobar bronchi are the second generation and are formed by the division of principal bronchi.
- Segmental bronchi from the third generation.
- **Terminal bronchioles** is the *16th generation* of division and no exchange of gases is possible in this tube. These are medium sized bronchioles having the maximum amount of smooth muscle. They are hence the *seat of airway resistance*.
- **Respiratory bronchioles** is the name given to the *17th to 22nd generation* of divisions. These are labeled as

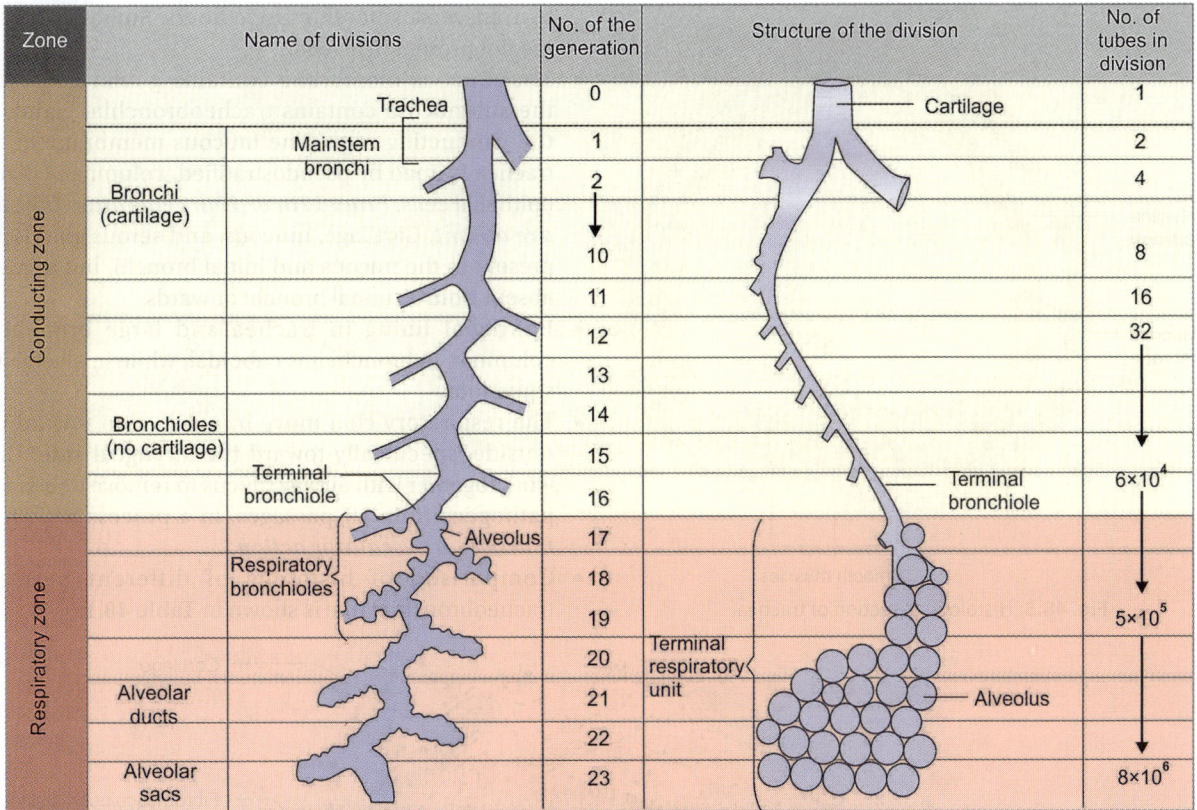

**Fig. 48.3:** Conducting and respiratory airways zones.

respiratory bronchioles because some exchanges of gases are possible in this tube.
Alveolar ducts and the alveoli or the alveolar sacs are part of the **23rd-generation** division. It is here most of the $O_2$ and $CO_2$ exchange occurs. The alveoli are the structural and functional units of the respiratory system. There are around 300 million alveoli in an adult human.

**The tracheobronchial tree** can be divided into two zones from a function point of view: *the conducting and respiratory zones* (Fig. 48.3).

1. **The conducting zone** is composed of the first 16 generations of air passages, which include the trachea to terminal bronchioles. This zone only transports gases and there are no gas exchanges taking place here. Hence, the area from the nose to the terminal bronchioles is referred to as the dead space. The dead space has a total capacity of approximately 150 mL.
2. **The respiratory zone** is formed by the 17th to 23rd generations of air passages, which include the respiratory bronchioles to alveoli. In this zone, gas exchange occurs and it has a volume of around 4L.
    - **Alveoli** are the functional units of gas exchange in our lungs. Each alveolus has an average diameter of about 0.2 mm. Adults have around 300 million of them in both lungs with a total surface area of 50–100 m², roughly the size of a tennis court. That makes them *one of the largest biological membranes* in the human body.

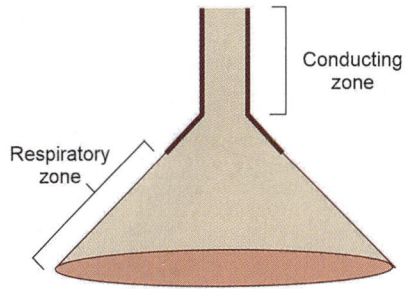

**Fig. 48.4:** Inverted funnel view of tracheobronchial tree.

The conducting zone has a narrow mean diameter, causing high-velocity air movement. Conversely, the larger mean diameter of the respiratory zone slows down the air movement. Visualize the tracheobronchial tree as an inverted funnel. *The total cross-sectional area of the conducting zone is small (about 2.5 cm²), whereas the total cross-sectional area of the respiratory zone is about 12,000 cm²* (Fig. 48.4).

## Histology

Trachea and bronchi are made up of (from inside to outside) a mucous membrane, submucosa, smooth muscles, cartilage and fibers (**Figs. 48.5 and 48.6**).
- The trachea has 16–20 C-shaped cartilaginous rings. Ends of cartilaginous rings of trachea are approximated

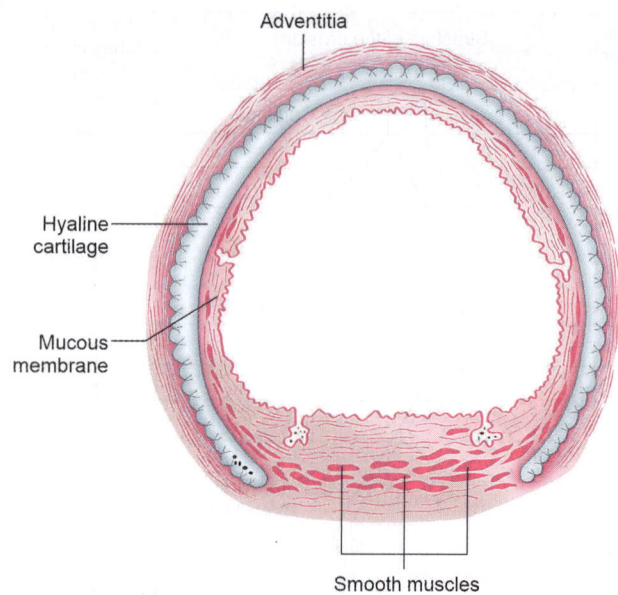

**Fig. 48.5:** Histological section of trachea.

by transverse smooth muscle fibers. Smooth muscles are not present in alveoli.

- The mucous membrane contains goblet cells, and the submucosa contains tracheobronchial glands in the conducting zone. The mucous membrane of the trachea is lined by pseudostratified, columnar, ciliated epithelial cells. *From 17th or 18th generation the cilia are absent*. Cartilage, mucous, and serous glands are present in the trachea and initial bronchi, but they are absent from terminal bronchi onwards.
- Epithelial lining in trachea and large bronchi is columnar, in bronchi it is cuboidal, while in alveoli it is squamous.
- The respiratory cilia move in a direction toward the outside, specifically toward the laryngeal side. Cilia work together with airway mucus to remove debris and pathogens from air passages, in a process known as *mucociliary escalator action*.
- Comparison of histology of different parts of tracheobronchial tree is shown in **Table 48.1**.

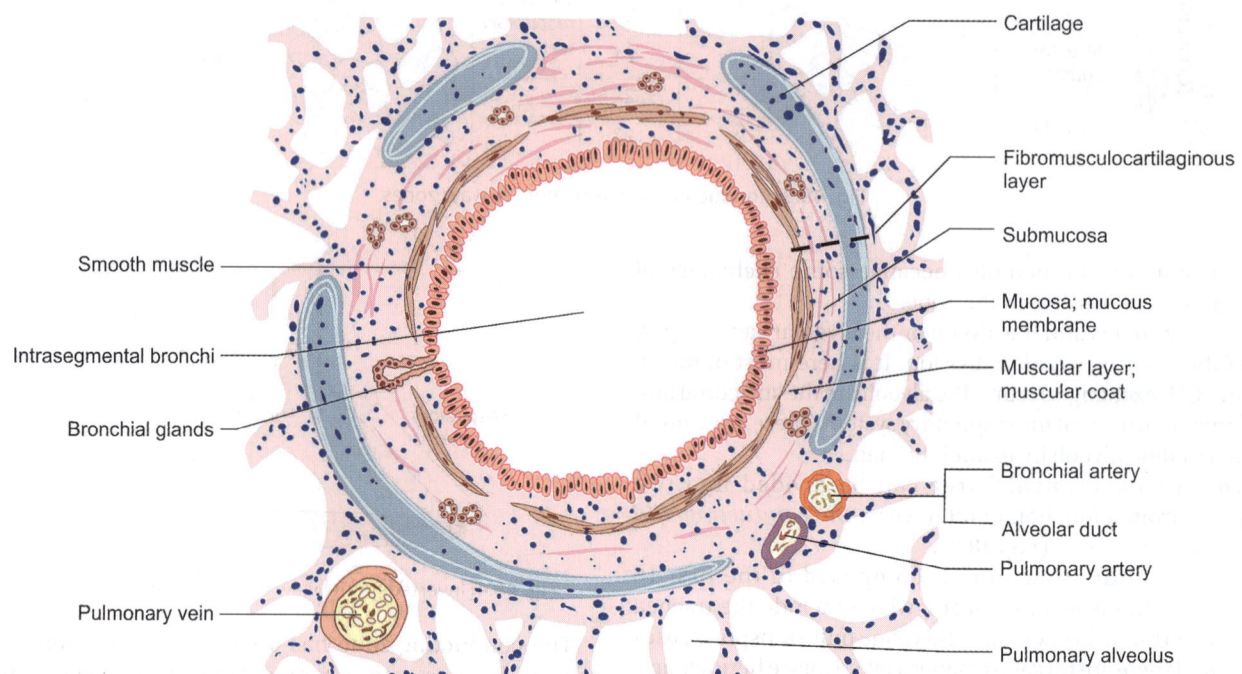

**Fig. 48.6:** Histological section of bronchi.

**Table 48.1:** Histological characteristics of tracheobronchial tree.

|  | Cartilage | Epithelium | Cilia | Glands mucous and serous | Blood supply |
|---|---|---|---|---|---|
| **Trachea** | Present 16–20 C-shaped rings | Columnar | Present | Present | Bronchial arteries |
| **Bronchi** | Present | Columnar | Present | Present | Bronchial arteries |
| **Terminal bronchioles** | Absent | Cuboidal | Present | Absent | Bronchial arteries |
| **Respiratory bronchioles** | Absent | Cuboidal | Present | Absent | Pulmonary arteries |
| **Alveoli** | Absent | Simple squamous | Absent | Absent | Pulmonary arteries |

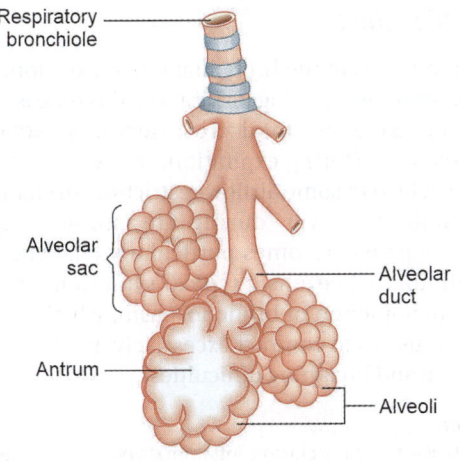

Fig. 48.7: Respiratory unit.

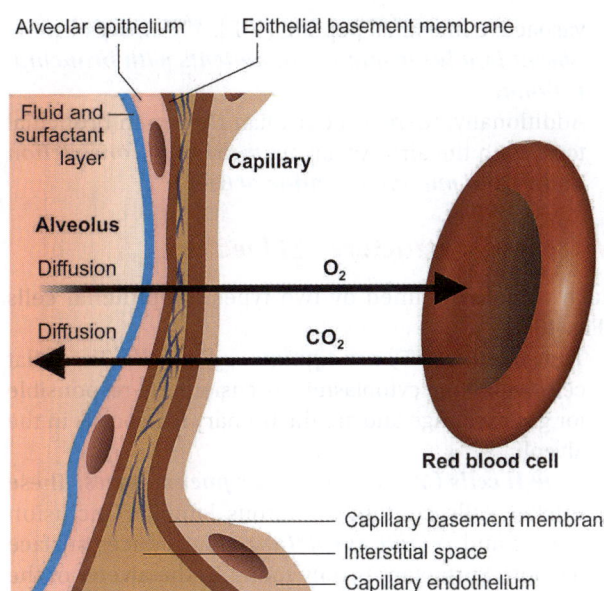

Fig. 48.8: Alveolar respiratory membrane.

Cigarette smoking destroys cilia and thus facilitates the development of chronic bronchitis and chronic obstructive pulmonary disease (COPD).

## Respiratory Unit

It is the terminal portion of the respiratory tract (**Fig. 48.7**). The respiratory unit begins with *respiratory bronchioles*. Each respiratory bronchiole is divided into *alveolar ducts*. These ducts lead to an enlarged structure called the *alveolar sac*, which contains a space called the *antrum*. The wall of the alveolar sack contains the *alveoli*. Few alveoli are also present in the wall of the alveolar duct. Each alveolus is a small pouch, approximately 0.2–0.5 mm in diameter, lined with epithelial cells.

## Respiratory Membrane

It is the name given to the tissues that separate the capillary blood from the alveolar air. The respiratory membrane is composed of various layers that facilitate the exchange of oxygen and carbon dioxide between the lungs and blood capillaries (**Fig. 48.8**).
- A layer of fluid that lines the alveolus and reduces surface tension
- The alveolar epithelium
- An epithelial basement membrane
- A thin interstitial space
- A capillary basement membrane
- The capillary endothelial membrane

Despite having multiple layers, the *respiratory membrane is quite thin, ranging from 0.2 to 0.6 µm* in thickness, except in areas with cell nuclei. The total surface area of the respiratory membrane is about 70 square meters. The total quantity of *blood in the pulmonary capillaries at any given instant is 70–140 mL*.

The average diameter of the pulmonary capillaries is only about 5 µm, which means that red blood cells must squeeze through them. The red blood cell membrane usually touches the capillary wall, which allows for efficient diffusion of oxygen and carbon dioxide between the alveolus and red blood cells.

## Blood Supply

The lungs receive a dual blood supply through two systems:
1. *The pulmonary arterial system*, and
2. *The bronchial arterial system*.

The conducting airway is supplied by the bronchial circulation through the bronchial artery and drained by the pulmonary veins.

In the respiratory zone, deoxygenated (venous) blood comes through the pulmonary arteries to the lungs. The blood is then oxygenated in the lungs and returned to the left atrium via pulmonary veins.

## Nerve Supply

The lungs are innervated by autonomic nerves that have different effects on bronchial tone.
- The parasympathetic fibers, pass through the *vagus nerve*, when stimulated, cause *bronchoconstriction and increased bronchial secretion* through muscarinic receptors.
- The *sympathetic nerves*, when stimulated cause *bronchodilation* and *decreased bronchial secretion* through adrenergic receptors, predominantly $\beta_2$ receptors.
- Afferent fibers from the lungs also pass through the vagus nerves.
- Noncholinergic nonadrenergic nerves, when stimulated produce bronchodilation due to the release of mediator

vasoactive intestinal peptide (VIP). *VIP is deficient or absent in a large number of patients with bronchial asthma.*
- Additionally, there is a circadian rhythm in bronchial tone, with the airways having *maximum constriction at 6 AM and maximal dilation at 6 PM.*

## Microscopic Structure of Alveolus

Each alveolus is lined by two types of epithelial cells **(Fig. 48.9)**.
- *Type I cells (95%) are squamous flat cells.* These flat cells with large cytoplasmic extensions are responsible for gas exchange and are the primary living cells in the alveoli.
- *Type II cells (5%) are granular pneumocytes.* These thicker cells contain numerous lamellar inclusion bodies and *secrete surfactant*, that reduces surface tension. Surfactant is only found in the alveoli of the lungs.
*Communication between 2 alveoli occurs through the pores of Kohn.* This allows air to flow from one alveolus to another.
- *Pulmonary alveolar macrophages (PAM)* or dust cells are active phagocytic cells. They are the last defense and janitors of the respiratory epithelium. The black staining seen in the lungs of smokers results from macrophages cleaning and sequestering particles that make their way inside.
- Lymphocytes
- Plasma cells that form and secrete immunoglobulins.
- *Clara cells*, act as stem cells, and detoxify noxious substances.
- *Amine precursor uptake and decarboxylation (APUD) cells* store and secrete biologically active peptides such as VIP and substance P. Mast cells contain heparin, lipids, histamine, and proteases involved in allergic reactions.

## Bronchial Tone

Smooth muscles of the bronchial tree have a tone known as *bronchial tone*. During inspiration, this tone is reduced, thus increasing the total cross-sectional area of the bronchial tree. During expiration, the tone is increased, which can lead to some airflow restriction, even in healthy individuals. However, during an asthma attack, the expiratory phase becomes particularly challenging, and an expiratory wheeze is a typical symptom. This is due to the phenomenon of bronchospasm, which causes the smooth muscles to contract excessively, leading to airway narrowing and breathing difficulties.

---

**Asthma**

Bronchial asthma is a chronic inflammatory disease that affects the airways, causing bronchospasm and variable airway obstruction, especially during exhalation. The condition is diagnosed based on the patient's clinical history, physical examination, and pulmonary function tests.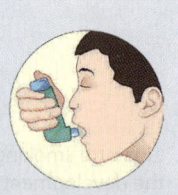

The cause of bronchospasm is inflammation of the bronchial mucosa, which makes the bronchial muscles hypersensitive to stimuli. In the case of allergic asthma, allergens are the primary cause of inflammation. When allergens enter the bronchial tubes, they trigger the degranulation of mast cells in the alveoli. These mast cells release various mediators such as leukotrienes and prostaglandins, which cause the bronchial muscles to constrict.

**Treatment of asthma:** (i) Bronchodilators like salbutamol ($\beta_2$ agonist). (ii) Inhalation of anti-inflammatory agents (glucocorticosteroids). (iii) Anti-leukotriene agents (e.g., montelukast)

---

## Pleura

**The pleura** is a layer that covers the lungs. It consists of two layers: the parietal pleura and the visceral pleura. **The parietal pleura** is the outer layer of the pleural sac and

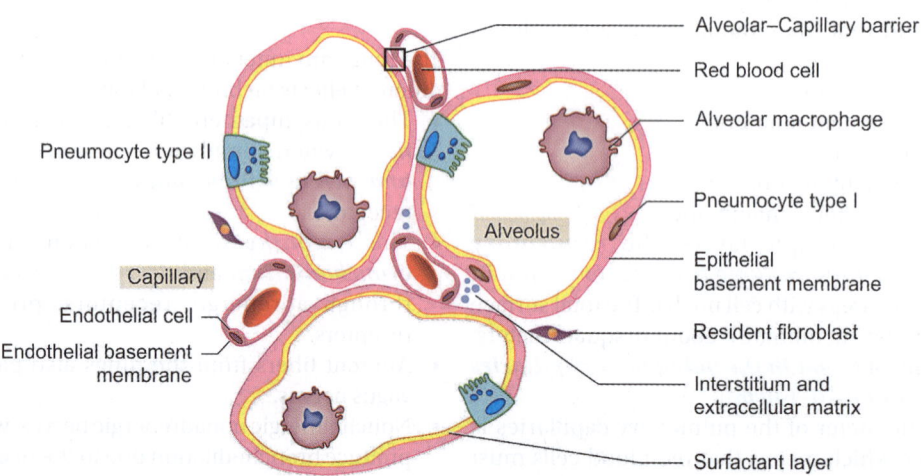

**Fig. 48.9:** Structure of alveolar tissues.

contains blood vessels. **The visceral pleura**, on the other hand, lies directly on the lung. Normally, about 2–10 mL of this fluid is present in the pleural cavity. The viscous pleural fluid acts as a lubricant allowing the lungs to slide against the chest wall, but it is difficult to separate the pleura due to the adhesive nature of the fluid. Therefore, pleural fluid facilitates the change in size and shape of the lungs during respiration and protects them from external damage.

> Take 2 unused slides from the hematology laboratory. Place them together. Try to slide them against each other, and then try to pull them apart. What happens?
> Now add 1 or 2 drops of water on one slide. Place two slides together again. Try to slide them against each other. Now try to pull them apart. What happens?
> This simple model will help you to understand the functioning of the pleura and pleural fluid.

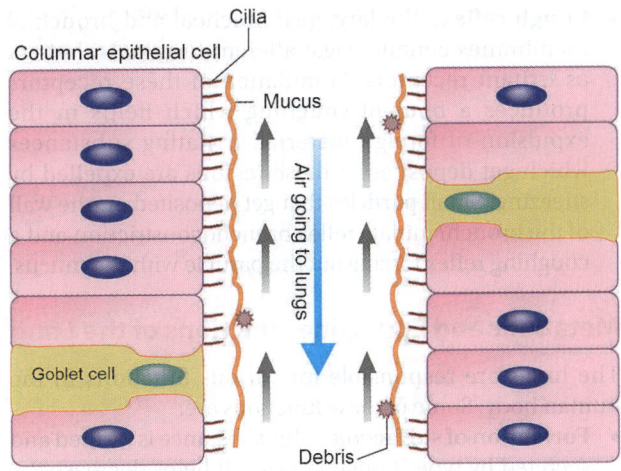

**Fig. 48.10:** Defense mechanism of epithelial lining of respiratory system.

## NONRESPIRATORY FUNCTIONS OF THE RESPIRATORY SYSTEM

The primary function of the respiratory system is the exchange of gases between the atmosphere and blood. Just as the respiratory system has developed unique systems to bring in and transport oxygen and simultaneously transport and expel carbon dioxide, it has also developed many other unique functions, which include:
- Lung defense systems
- Metabolic and endocrine functions of the lung
- Functions of pulmonary circulation
- Miscellaneous

### Lung Defense Systems

The respiratory tract is continuously exposed to various foreign substances such as dust, pollen, toxic gases, and chemicals, as well as microorganisms like bacteria and viruses. These substances are processed and disposed of by the specialized mucosal immune system, phagocytosis, and mucociliary clearance.
- **Particles of different sizes** tend to settle in different regions of the respiratory system. Larger particles, with a diameter of over 10 μm, are strained out by hairs of nostrils or are trapped in the oropharynx and larynx through impaction. Particles with a diameter of 2–10 μm are typically acted upon by ciliary escalator action or deposited in the tracheobronchial region. The smallest particles, with a diameter of 0.5–2 μm, are deposited in the alveoli and small conducting airways due to gravitational sedimentation and acted upon by PAMS.
- **The ciliary escalator action** is a defense mechanism that protects against airborne infections and particulate matter **(Fig. 48.10)**. These particles are trapped in the mucosal layer of the respiratory passages and are moved upwards toward the pharynx by the rhythmic upward beating action of the cilia. However, cigarette smoking can interfere with the ciliary functions, which explains why smokers are more susceptible to infections compared to nonsmokers.
- **Pulmonary alveolar macrophages**, also known as PAMS, play a vital role in the body's defense mechanism. They are responsible for phagocytosing foreign substances, processing inhaled antigens for the immunological attack, secreting substances like cytokines that attract polymorphonuclear cells (PMNs) to the lungs, and stimulating granulocytes and monocyte formation in the bone marrow.

> *Kartagener syndrome* is a rare genetic disorder characterized by a triad of symptoms:
> - Situs inversus (organs in mirror-image reversal),
> - Chronic sinusitis, and
> - Bronchiectasis (damaged airways).
>
> It is caused by defective cilia, leading to impaired mucociliary clearance. Patients may also exhibit infertility due to impaired sperm motility in males.

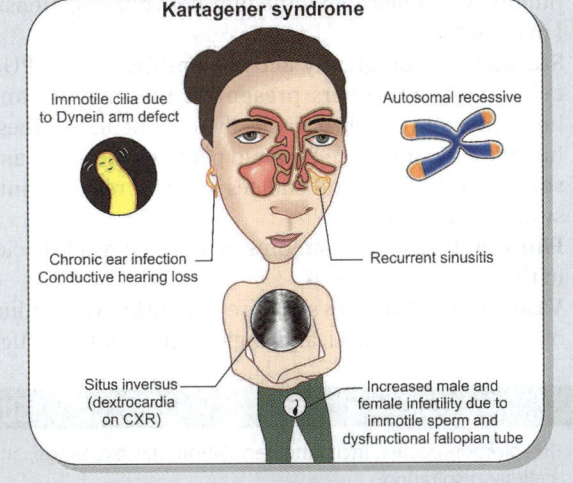

- IgA is secreted in the bronchial secretion protects against respiratory infections and maintains the integrity of the mucosal lining.
- PGE2 protects pulmonary epithelial cells.

- **Cough reflex:** The laryngeal, tracheal and bronchial membranes contain vagal afferent terminals that act as irritant receptors. Stimulation of these receptors produces a bout of coughing which helps in the expulsion of foreign material. Irritating substances which get deposited in these regions are expelled by sneezing. Small particles that get deposited on the wall of the bronchi initiate reflex bronchoconstriction and a coughing reflex forcing out the particle with the mucus.

## Metabolic and Endocrine Functions of the Lung

The lungs are responsible for various functions in the human body. Some of these functions are:

- **Formation of surfactant**—this substance is formed and secreted by type II pneumocytes. It helps decrease the surface tension and aids in increasing compliance while decreasing the work done for breathing.
- **Protein synthesis**—the lungs create proteins that help in the maintenance of the structural framework.
- **Hormone synthesis**—locally active hormones like prostaglandins (PGs), thromboxane (Tx), and leukotrienes (LTs), are synthesized and secreted by the lungs. These hormones are also degraded locally, so their functions are confined to the lung alone. Most of them are proinflammatory.
- **Mast cells**—the lungs contain mast cells that may degranulate in sensitive people to release mediators' histamine, heparin, serotonin, and others responsible for asthmatic attacks. Dendritic cells capture, process and present the antigen to T-lymphocytes. Natural killer (NK) cells are large granular cells considered as 3rd type of lymphocytes. Its granules contain hydrolytic enzymes which destroy micro-organisms. They also destroy malignant cells.
- **Conversion of angiotensin I to angiotensin II**—angiotensin converting enzyme (ACE), present in pulmonary capillary endothelium, converts angiotensin I to angiotensin II.
- **Storage of biologically active peptides**—the APUD cells and nerve fibers present in the alveoli store hormones and certain biologically active peptides. These include VIP, substance P, opioid peptides, CCK-PZ, and somatostatin. These substances are later released into systemic circulation.
- **Fibrinolytic mechanism** present in the lungs lyse clot in the pulmonary vessels.
- **Vasoactive substances** such as epinephrine, dopamine, oxytocin, gastrin, ADH, and angiotensin II pass through the lungs without being metabolized. However, the lungs partially remove prostaglandins, bradykinin, adenosine, serotonin, acetylcholine and norepinephrine from blood.

## Functions of Pulmonary Circulation

- **Reservoir for left ventricle:** The right ventricle pumps the entire cardiac output into the pulmonary circulation. The pulmonary circulation has a high compliance and can accommodate about 0.5 L of blood. When the left ventricle output momentarily exceeds systemic venous return, the blood stored in the pulmonary circulation helps to maintain the left ventricular output for a few strokes.
- Pulmonary circulation acts as a **filter**.
- Pulmonary vasculature captures and removes micro emboli such as blood clots, fats, or air bubbles, preventing them from entering systemic circulation and causing tissue damage. However, larger emboli can damage lung tissue.
- **Removal of fluid from alveoli:** Pulmonary hydrostatic pressure is low, therefore, the fluid entering the alveoli is absorbed by the capillaries. This prevents the transudation of fluid from capillaries to the alveoli.
- **Absorption of drugs:** Certain drugs that pass through the alveolar-capillary membrane by diffusion can be administered through inhalation. This includes anesthetic gases, aerosols, and bronchodilators.

## Miscellaneous

The lungs perform various other vital functions in the body which include:

- **Maintenance of water balance:** Expiration leads to evaporation of water from the lungs which helps in maintaining the body's water balance.
- **Regulation of body temperature:** Expiration leads to loss of heat from the body which helps in regulating body temperature.
- **Regulation of acid-base balance:** By controlling carbon dioxide output from the body, the lungs control plasma bicarbonate concentration which helps in regulating the acid-base balance.
- **Speech:** The larynx, along with other structures, forms the sound box which is essential for speech.
- **Olfaction:** Olfactory receptors present in the upper part of the nostrils are responsible for olfactory sensation which helps in detecting various smells.

## SUMMARY

- Respiration occurs, including ventilation, gas exchange, and cellular respiration.
- From the nasal cavity and pharynx to the bronchi and alveoli, each component serves a unique purpose in the process of respiration, such as filtering air, humidifying it, and facilitating gas exchange with the bloodstream.
- The conducting zone encompasses the passages through which air is transported into the lungs, while the respiratory zone comprises the structures where gas exchange occurs.
- Understanding this division is essential for comprehending how air flows through the respiratory system and how oxygen is delivered to tissues.

- Lastly, the functions of the respiratory system are enumerated. Beyond mere gas exchange, the respiratory system plays diverse roles, including maintaining acid-base balance, regulating blood pressure, and assisting in vocalization. Through a detailed analysis, we gain insight into the multifaceted nature of respiratory function and its integral role in sustaining life. Overall, this chapter provides a comprehensive overview of the respiratory system, equipping readers with a thorough understanding of its anatomy, physiological processes, and functional significance.

## LET US SEE, HOW MUCH YOU HAVE LEARNT?

### Review Questions

#### Long/Short Answer Questions

Q1. Explain the tracheobronchial tree as a branching structure of several generations.
Q2. Explain the division of airways into conducting and respiratory zones.
Q3. Write a short note on the respiratory/pulmonary capillary membrane.
Q4. Enlist and describe the nonrespiratory functions of the lung.

#### Explain Why? (Reasoning Questions)

Q1. The alveoli are structured to maximize gas exchange in the lungs.
Q2. The pleural cavity is essential for normal lung expansion during breathing.

### Multiple Choice Questions

Q1. Pulmonary surfactant is secreted by:
   a. Type-I pneumocytes    b. Type-II pneumocytes
   c. Clara cells           d. Bronchial epithelial cell
Q2. In cigarette smoking, surfactant is:
   a. Increased
   b. Decreased
   c. Increased followed by decrease
   d. Unaltered
Q3. Sympathetic stimulation on the bronchus causes:
   a. Bronchial constrictions
   b. Increased secretion of glands in bronchi
   c. No effect
   d. Bronchial dilatation
Q4. True about "dead space" in tracheobronchial tree is:
   a. Increases in coughing
   b. Humidifies air
   c. Increases with adrenaline
   d. In all respiratory diseases the anatomical dead space coincides with the physiological dead space.
Q5. A 55-year-old factory worker, who has worked in the insulation industry for over 25 years, develops progressive shortness of breath and persistent dry cough. A chest X-ray is consistent with an alveolus from asbestos inhalation. Which of the following is the major route for the removal of small particles from the alveoli?
   a. Bulk flow             b. Diffusion
   c. Expectoration         d. Phagocytosis
   e. Ciliary transport
Q6. The largest airways in the lungs where gaseous exchange takes place are:
   a. Respiratory bronchioles  b. Segmental bronchioles
   c. Terminal bronchioles     d. Alveolar sacs
Q7. Which conversion occurs in due to the presence of certain enzyme in lungs
   a. Angiotensinogen to angiotensin-I
   b. Prorenin to renin
   c. Angiotensin-I to angiotensin-II
   d. Angiotensin II to angiotensin-III
Q8. Bronchoconstriction is produced in response to:
   a. Parasympathetic discharge
   b. Sympathetic discharge
   c. Exposure to cold air
   d. Exposure to dust
   Please choose the best response:
   i. Option b, c, d are correct
   ii. Option 'a' is correct
   iii. Option 'b' is correct
   iv. Option a, c, d are correct
Q9. The lowest airway resistance is offered by:
   a. Small airways         b. Trachea
   c. Large airways         d. Medium airways
Q10. Vasoactive substances that pass through the lungs without getting metabolized is:
   a. Norepinephrine        b. Acetylcholine
   c. Epinephrine           d. Serotonin
Q11. All are functions of paranasal sinuses, *except*:
   a. Voice resonance.
   b. Lighten the skull
   c. Olfaction
   d. Protect the brain from trauma

### ANSWERS

1. b    2. b    3. d    4. b    5. d    6. a    7. c    8. d    9. a    10. c    11. c

# Mechanics of Pulmonary Ventilation
## (Chest Movements, Pressure Changes, Alveolar Surface Tension, Compliance, Airway Resistance)

**CHAPTER 49**

### COMPETENCY ADDRESSED
**PY6.2:** Describe the mechanics of normal respiration, pressure changes during ventilation, lung volume and capacities, alveolar surface tension, compliance, airway resistance, ventilation, V/P ratio, diffusion capacity of lungs.

### LEARNING OBJECTIVES
**At the end of this chapter, the learner should be able to:**
- Explain the mechanics of normal respiration, including the role of respiratory muscles and diaphragm in ventilation.
- Describe the pressure changes that occur during ventilation, particularly during inspiration and expiration.
- Describe the role of alveolar surface tension in maintaining lung stability and preventing collapse.
- Describe the concept of compliance in the context of lung physiology and its relationship to lung elasticity.
- Explain the factors affecting airway resistance and its impact on ventilation.

As discussed in the previous chapter, we have learned that the main function of the respiration is to provide $O_2$ to the tissues and remove $CO_2$ from there. Hence, the respiratory system is involved is involved in breathing, diffusion of gases across the respiratory membrane and the transport of these gases to the tissues and back. Hence, it becomes clear that breathing and respiration are two different terms.

## MECHANICS OF RESPIRATION

Breathing refers to the inspiration and expiration of air, into and out of lungs respectively whereas respiration means the breathing along with utilization of oxygen and release of $CO_2$ by the tissues (internal respiration).

The **inspiration**, is defined as breathing in of air from atmosphere into lungs. It is shorter and lasts for 1 second (**Fig. 49.1**). It is an active process and requires the expansion of chest for the air to enter into the lungs, brought about by the contraction of intercostal muscles and the diaphragm (mentioned below).

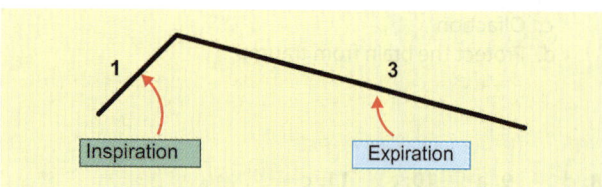

**Fig. 49.1:** Inspiration and expiration duration.

While the expiration is defined as breathing out of air from lungs into atmosphere. This phase is longer and lasts for 3 seconds. It is a passive process as it is initiated by the elastic recoil of the lungs and the chest wall.

## Modes of Respiration

During inspiration the air enter inside the lungs, along with the pressure gradient created inside the lungs. This pressure gradient is created by the descent of diaphragm and contraction of intercostal muscles. These result in the movement of thoracic wall and the abdomen. However, one of these (thorax or abdomen) shows a predominance. Hence, the mode of respiration is classified as:
- *Thoracoabdominal*, where the main component is thoracic. It is seen in females and children.
- *Abdomino-thoracic*, where the main component is abdominal. It is seen in males.

## Diameters of Chest

In an upright person, three diameters can be identified in the chest/thorax **(Fig. 49.2)**.
1. **Transverse diameter:** The distance across the chest from one side to the other, usually taken at the level of the nipples. It represents the widest part of the chest from left to right.
2. **Vertical diameter:** This measurement refers to the distance from the top to the bottom of the chest. It is

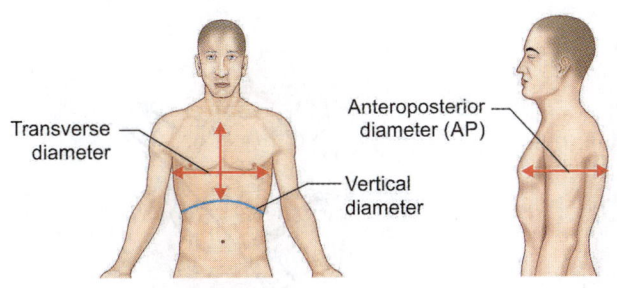

**Fig. 49.2:** Various diameters of chest.

taken along the midline of the body, from the top of the sternum or clavicles down to the lowest ribs or the bottom of the rib cage. The vertical diameter provides an indication of the height or length of the chest.
3. **Anteroposterior diameter:** This measurement refers to the distance from the front (anterior) to the back (posterior) of the chest. It is typically taken at the level of the thorax, from the sternum (breastbone) to the spine. The anteroposterior diameter gives an indication of the depth of the chest cavity.

## MUSCLES OF RESPIRATION

The mechanism of breathing requires expansion of lungs and chest wall for inspiration and retraction of chest wall for expiration. The combination of lungs and chest wall make a mechanical device for which the muscles of respiration provide force. Inspiratory and expiratory muscles are tabulated in **Table 49.1**.

### Diaphragm

- It is the *principal muscle* for quiet breathing.
- Contraction of **central tendinous portion** of diaphragm results in **increased vertical** diameter.
- Contraction of **peripheral part of diaphragm** results in **upward and outward movement** of **ribs**. This increases **anteroposterior and transverse** diameter of the thorax.
- Vertical descent during quiet breathing = 1.5 cm, which accommodates 500–700 mL of air in the lungs, this descent is 7.0 cm during forceful inspiration.
- *'Diaphragmatic descent leads to expansion of lower parts of lungs'.*

**Table 49.1:** Muscles of respiration.

| Sl. No. | Inspiratory muscles | Expiratory muscles |
|---|---|---|
| 1. | Diaphragm | Abdominal muscles |
| 2. | External intercostals | Internal intercostals |
| 3. | Sternocleidomastoids | Serratus posterior inferior |
| 4. | Scapular elevators | Transverse thoracis |
| 5. | Serratus anterior | Subcostalis |
| 6. | Scaleni | |
| 7. | Erector muscles of spine | |

### External Intercostal Muscles

- They elevate the ribs during inspiration.
- Along with diaphragm maintains adequate ventilation at rest.
- Prevents the bulging of intercostal spaces during inspiration.

> **REMEMBER**
> Diaphragm and External intercostal muscles are the main muscles of inspiration, rest all are the accessory muscles of respiration and they work during forceful inspiration or labored breathing.

### Internal Intercostal Muscles

- Prevents the retraction of intercostal space during expiration.
- Helps in expiration during forceful expiration.

## MECHANISM OF INSPIRATION

The inspiration allows the air to enter in the thorax by increasing the negative pressure inside the thorax. Hence, this fall in intrathoracic pressure is brought by 2 mechanisms: by increasing the intrathoracic volume and decreasing the intrathoracic pressure.

### By Increasing the Intrathoracic Volume

You must be quite familiar with *Boyle's law*, which states that '*at constant temperature, the pressure of a gas is inversely proportional to its volume. So, if you decrease the volume of a gas while keeping the temperature constant, the pressure of the gas will increase, and vice versa*'.

Hence, if we increase the intrathoracic volume, the pressure inside the thorax will fall. The intrathoracic volume is increased by increasing the thoracic diameters by the movements of the ribs and the descent of the diaphragm.

The diaphragm contracts, increasing the vertical diameter of the chest. External intercostal muscles elevate the ribs, increasing the AP and transverse diameter through two distinct movements: the pump handle movement and the bucket handle movement.

#### Pump Handle Movement

- Occurs in 2nd–6th ribs.
- At rest, the ribs slope downwards and forwards. During inspiration, they swing upwards to assume more horizontal position from their joints with spine. This raises the sternum upwards, increasing the AP diameter of the chest **(Fig. 49.3)**.

#### Bucket Handle Movement

- Occurs in 7th–10th ribs.
- Increases transverse diameter.
- It is effective to a lesser degree.

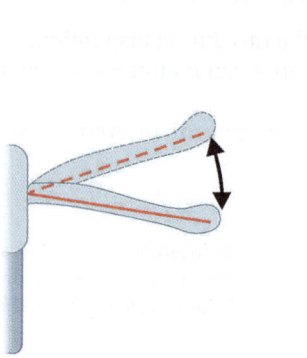
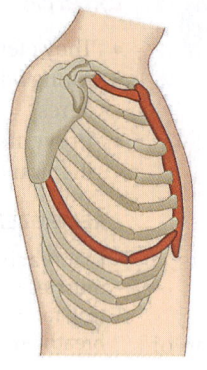
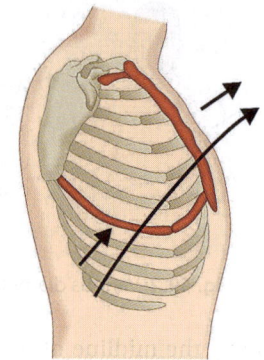

**Fig. 49.3:** Pump handle movement.

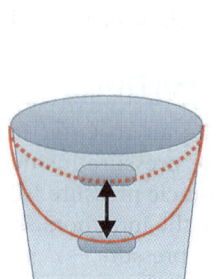
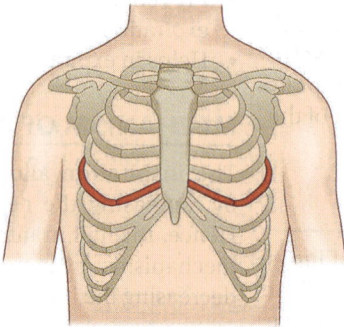
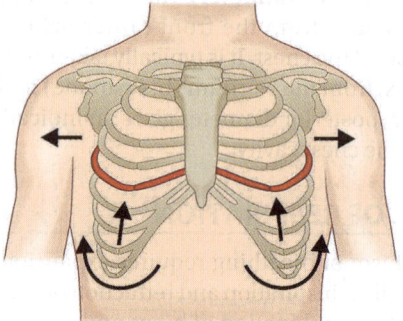

**Fig. 49.4:** Bucket handle movement.

- These ribs swing upwards and outwards increasing the transverse diameter of the chest **(Fig. 49.4)**.

### By Decreasing the Intrathoracic Pressure

The air flow in any hollow and elastic bag (say a balloon) can occur in two ways; either by blowing air into it (positive pressure filling; **Fig. 49.5**) of by creating a negative pressure outside the balloon (negative pressure filling; **Fig. 49.6**).

Our lungs are filled by the negative pressure filling, i.e., fall in the alveolar pressure results in the movement of air into the lungs.

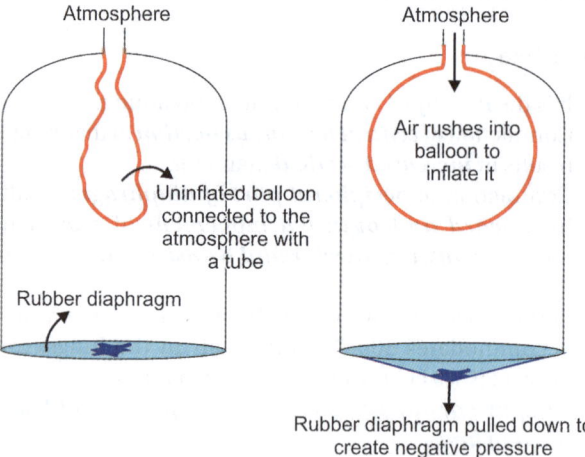

**Fig. 49.6:** Negative pressure filling.

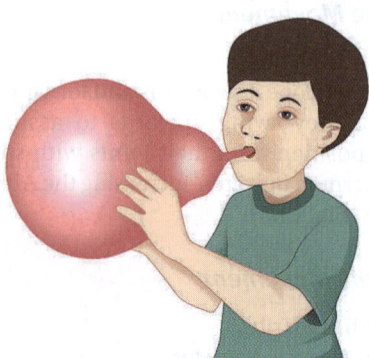

**Fig. 49.5:** Positive pressure filling.

Well, do you know that the net pressure (transpulmonary pressure) affecting the intrathoracic pressure is an interplay of two different types of pressures, namely:
1. Intrapulmonary pressure/alveolar pressure
2. Intrapleural pressure

The transpulmonary pressure (TPP) is calculated mathematically by subtracting intrapleural pressure (IPP) from alveolar pressure (AP).

$$TPP = AP - IPP$$

## MECHANISM OF EXPIRATION

Muscles of expiration are required only during forceful expiration. Internal intercostal muscles and anterior abdominal muscles pull the ribs downwards and increase the intraabdominal pressure and push the diaphragm upwards.

Hence, from the above discussion, we have learned that the mechanism of breathing is mainly influenced by the pressure gradients in the chest and the muscles of respiration (inspiration) influencing the diameters of the chest. Let's learn about these pressure gradients in detail.

## PRESSURE GRADIENTS

The various pressure gradients responsible for the normal breathing are:
a. Alveolar pressure/intrapulmonary pressure
b. Intrapleural pressure
c. Transpulmonary pressure
d. Intrathoracic pressure

### Alveolar Pressure (AP, $P_{alv}$)

- It is also called as *intrapulmonary pressure*.
- It is the pressure which is present inside the alveoli.
- It varies from *–1 to 0 to +1 cm of water* from inspiration to expiration.
- It means that during inspiration it is –1 cm of water less than the atmospheric pressure and it pulls 500 mL (equal to tidal volume) of air inside to lungs. At the end of inspiration, it becomes zero, i.e., it becomes equal to the atmospheric pressure and hence the inflow of air stops. During expiration it is +1, i.e., it becomes more than the atmospheric pressure and hence the expiration, exhaling 500 mL of air.

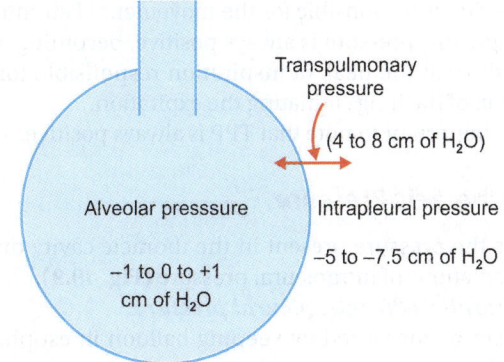

**Fig. 49.7:** Relation between alveolar and intrapleural pressure.

### Intrapleural Pressure (IP, $P_{ip}$)

*'Keeps the lungs in expanded state'*
- *Pressure between the visceral and the parietal pleura.*
- Always subatmospheric (i.e., negative).
- It varies from *–5.0 to –7.5 cm of water at base of the lungs*, which means it is –5 cm of water at the beginning of inspiration which decreases further to –7.5 cm during inspiration at the base. It is as low as –10 cm of water at the apex **(Fig. 49.7)**.

### Transpulmonary Pressure (TPP)

- It is the pressure across the alveolar membrane.
- It is the difference between alveolar pressure and the intrapleural pressure **(Fig. 49.8)**.
- TPP = AP – PP
- At the beginning of inspiration: –1 – (–5) = +4 cm water
  At the peak of inspiration: +1 – (–7.5) = +8.5 cm of water

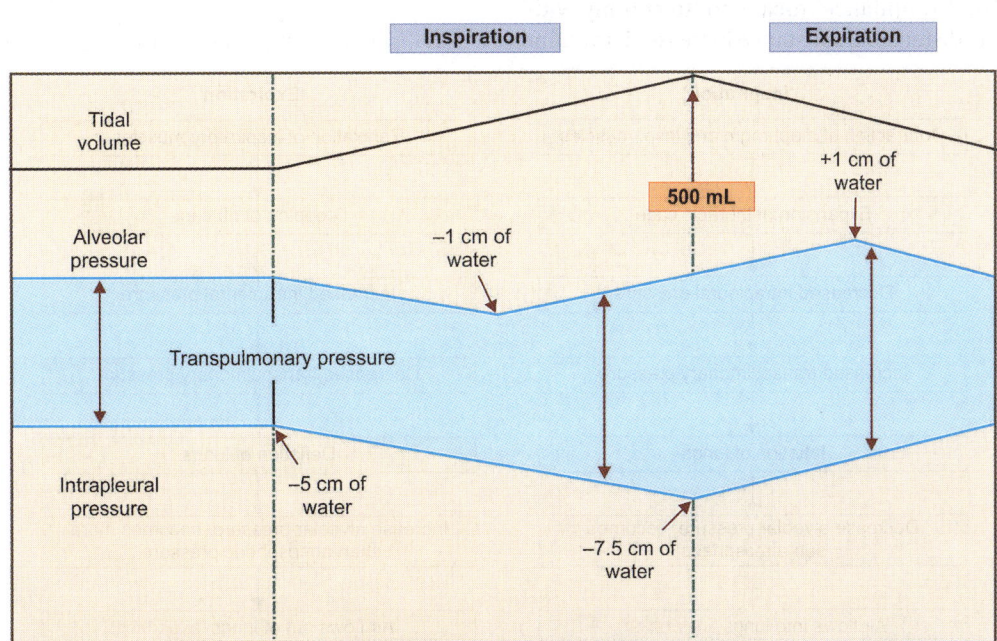

**Fig. 49.8:** Transpulmonary pressure.

- The TPP is responsible for the movement of air into the lungs. This pressure is always positive, becoming more positive at the peak of inspiration responsible for the recoil of the lungs initiating the expiration.
- It is important to note that TPP is always positive.

### Intrathoracic Pressure

- It is the pressure present in the thoracic cavity due to fluctuations of intrapleural pressure (**Fig. 49.9**).
- *It parallels the intrapleural pressure.*
- It can be measured by keeping balloon in esophagus and measuring intra esophageal pressure.
- It acts as a *'Respiratory pump'* which builds up a pressure gradient and helps in sucking blood from abdomen into thorax during inspiration.
- It is important during exercise to increase the cardiac output.

> **SUMMARY OF INSPIRATION (FIG. 49.10)**
> 1. Diaphragm contracts → Increases vertical diameter
> 2. External intercostal muscles contract → Increases AP and transverse diameter
> 3. Fall in intrapleural pressure (Alveolar pressure) to sub atmospheric levels
> 4. All these lead to airflow into lungs → "INSPIRATION"

## LUNG COMPLIANCE

### Definition

Compliance is defined as *the change in the volume per unit change in the pressure.*

$$C = \Delta V/\Delta P$$

It means that capacity of lungs to distend with increasing pressure OR it is a measure of distensibility of lungs. In simple English, 'compliance' means to 'to comply with' that means, the distensible substance increases its volume in response to the pressure applied to distend it, i.e., the substance is complying to pressure gradient.

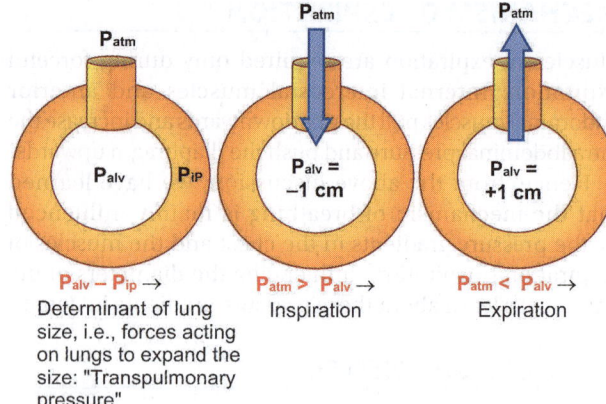

**Fig. 49.9:** Inter-relationship of various pressures.
($P_{alv}$: alveolar pressure, $P_{atm}$: atmospheric pressure, $P_{ip}$: intrapleural pressure)

In order to understand compliance, let's do a practical with two different balloons. Take a balloon made of soft good quality rubber (let's call it balloon 1) and the other one which is made of a low quality hard rubber (balloon 2). When we try to inflate these balloons, balloon 1 gets easily inflated as compared to balloon 2. Now what do you think, which out of two ballons, has a high a compliance?

Definitely its balloon 1, where small increase in pressure, increases the volume more efficiently.

The normal value of compliance of:
- *Lungs alone is measured to be 220 mL/cm of water.*
- *Thorax alone is measured to be 200 mL/cm of water.*
- *Lungs and thorax together are measured to be 110 mL/cm of water.*

Therefore, total compliance

$$= \frac{1}{\text{Lung compliance}} + \frac{1}{\text{Thoracic compliance}}$$

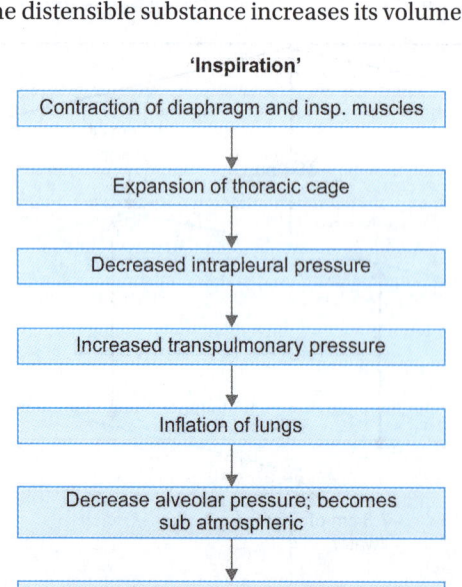
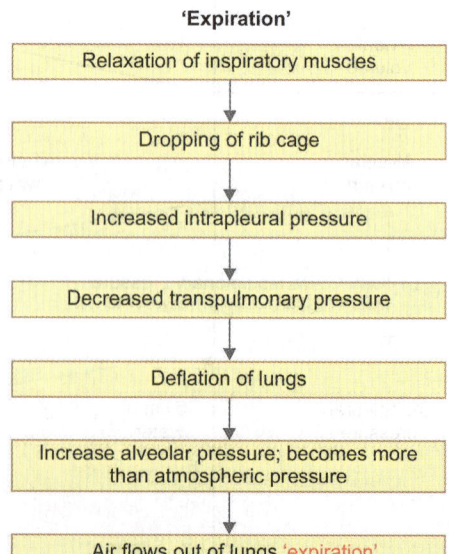

**Fig. 49.10:** Process of inspiration and expiration.

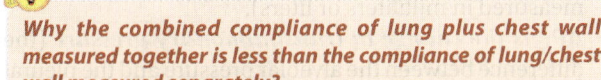

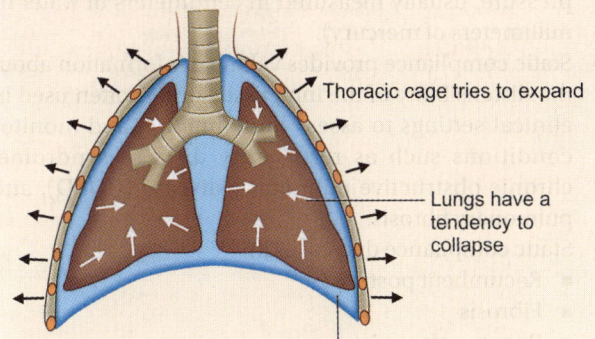

The expansion of chest wall and collapse of lungs tends to exert an opposite pressure on both the layers of pleura, which result in the:
- Negative intrapleural pressure
- Decrease in the combined lung and chest wall compliance, as compared to when measured separately

## Specific Compliance

When the compliance is expressed as a fraction of functional residual capacity, it is called specific compliance, i.e.,

$$\text{Specific compliance} = \frac{\text{Compliance}}{\text{Functional residual capacity (FRC)}}$$

**Controversies:**
The compliance is measured in healthy adults but there are certain controversies, that arise due to certain.
- In cases where the patient has only one normally functional lung, the compliance will be ½ of the normal compliance.
- It is different in children.

**Uses:**
- Removes the controversies of compliance
- It is not affected by age

## Compliance Loop/Hysteresis

The compliance of the lung thorax system is plotted on the pressure volume graph, in which the lung volumes of the subject are plotted against different values of intrapleural pressure, to understand the variations in the compliance at the lower and higher lung volumes and also during the different phases of respiration (inspiration and expiration). It is called compliance loop/P-V loop (Pressure-volume loop)/Hysteresis loop. To study this graph, let's study each parameter on by one.

### Effect of Lung Volume on Compliance

As we see in the **Figure 49.11** showing the compliance loop, we find that:
- The compliance is *lowest at very low volumes* (during the lag phase of the graph). Such a condition is seen

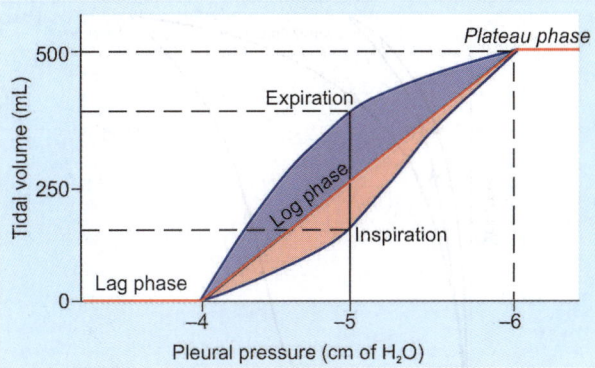

**Fig. 49.11:** Compliance loop.

in *newborn babies at the time of their first breath* into this world or in patients of *total lung collapse (atelectasis)*.
- On the other hand, the *patients of emphysema have a high compliance* which can be due to the following reasons:
  - *Loss of elastic recoil:* Emphysema is characterized by the destruction of the alveolar walls, leading to a reduction in the surface area available for gas exchange and a loss of elastic recoil in the lung tissue. As a result, the lungs become more distensible and compliant, meaning they can expand more easily with changes in pressure.
  - *Decreased lung tissue resistance:* The destruction of alveolar walls in emphysema also leads to a reduction in lung tissue resistance. This means that the lungs encounter less resistance to expansion during inhalation, contributing to increased compliance.
  - *Air trapping:* In emphysema, air can become trapped in the lungs due to the collapse of small airways during exhalation. This trapped air increases lung volume, further enhancing lung compliance.
  - *Loss of supportive structures:* Emphysema can cause destruction of the supporting structures of the lungs, including the elastin fibers in the alveolar walls. This loss of support allows the lungs to expand more easily, contributing to increased compliance.

### Effect of Phase of Respiration on Compliance (Hysteresis)

Compliance curve *of inspiration lags behind the expiration phase*, forming the loop called the Hysteresis Loop. Hysteresis refers to the phenomenon where the pressure-volume relationship of the lungs during inspiration differs from that during expiration. This difference occurs because of the presence of surfactant in the alveoli.

During inspiration, surfactant molecules at the air-liquid interface reduce surface tension, allowing the alveoli to expand more easily at lower pressures. However, during *expiration, some surfactant molecules remain adsorbed to the alveolar surface, maintaining a lower surface*

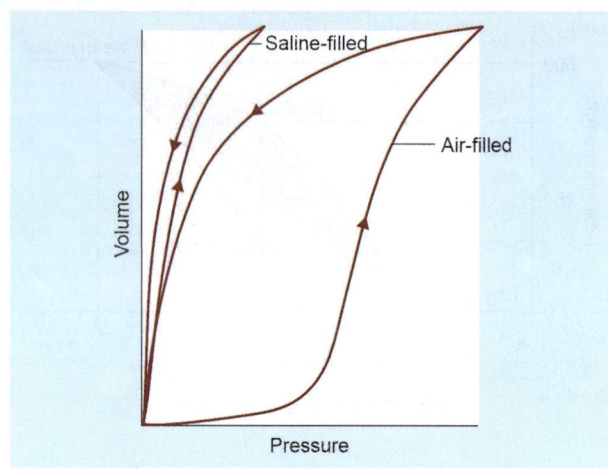

**Fig. 49.12:** Saline-filled lungs vs Air-filled lungs.

*tension and preventing the alveoli from collapsing completely at higher pressures.*

This hysteresis loop represents the energy required to inflate and deflate the lungs and ensures the stability of the alveoli throughout the breathing cycle. It's an important concept in respiratory physiology and plays a role in maintaining lung function and preventing alveolar collapse.

Hence, the loop is formed due to the viscous resistance (resistance to the movement offered by surfactant and air). If the viscous resistance is absent then the loop is not formed, the P-V relationship is linear.

### Saline Filled Lungs Vs Air Filled Lungs (Fig. 49.12)

In experimental settings, when a lung is filled with saline, it essentially eliminates the surface tension forces that occur at the air-liquid interface within the alveoli. This reduction in surface tension allows the lung to expand more readily with changes in pressure, resulting in higher compliance compared to when it is filled with air.

Saline-filled lungs exhibit a phenomenon known as *"zero surface tension compliance."* This means that the lung's compliance is primarily determined by the elastic properties of the lung tissue rather than the surface tension forces that contribute to hysteresis in air-filled lungs.

### Static Compliance

- When the adequate time is given for the lung volumes to stabilize in response to the distending pressure. Static compliance refers to the ability of the lungs to stretch and expand in response to a given change in pressure when the lungs are not in motion, i.e., when airflow has ceased, and the system is in a static state. It is a measure of the elasticity of the lung tissue and is calculated by dividing the change in lung volume by the change in transpulmonary pressure.
- Mathematically, static compliance ($C_{st}$) can be expressed as:

$$C_{st} = \Delta V / \Delta P_{tp}$$

- Where: **$\Delta V$ is the change in lung volume** (usually measured in milliliters or liters).
- *$\Delta P_{tp}$ is the change in transpulmonary pressure* (the difference between the alveolar pressure and the pleural pressure, usually measured in centimeters of water or millimeters of mercury).
- Static compliance provides valuable information about the distensibility of the lung tissue and is often used in clinical settings to assess lung function and monitor conditions such as respiratory distress syndrome, chronic obstructive pulmonary disease (COPD), and pulmonary fibrosis.
- Static compliance decreases in:
  - Recumbent posture
  - Fibrosis
  - Pneumonia

### Dynamic Compliance

Dynamic compliance refers to the ability of the lungs to stretch and expand during breathing cycles, specifically during the movement of air in and out of the lungs (i.e., during inspiration and expiration). Unlike static compliance, which measures lung elasticity when the lungs are not in motion, dynamic compliance takes into account the resistance to airflow within the airways during breathing.

Mathematically, dynamic compliance ($C_{dyn}$) is calculated by dividing the change in lung volume by the change in airway pressure (the difference between the pressure at the airway opening and the pressure inside the alveoli), and it is often expressed in milliliters per centimeter of water (mL/cmH$_2$O):

$$C_{dyn} = \Delta V / \Delta P_{aw}$$

Where: *$\Delta V$ is the change in lung volume* (usually measured in milliliters or liters); *$\Delta P_{aw}$ is the change in airway pressure*. Dynamic compliance accounts for the resistance encountered by the air as it flows through the airways during breathing. Factors such as airway resistance, compliance of the lung tissue, and the properties of the chest wall influence dynamic compliance. It is an important parameter in assessing lung function, particularly in conditions such as asthma, chronic bronchitis, and other obstructive lung diseases, where airway resistance may be increased.

### Factors Affecting Compliance

Compliance is affected by the factors which are:
- Present in the lungs.
- Present in the chest wall.

### Factors Present in the Lungs

- **Elasticity of lung tissue:**
  - *Elastic fibers of the lungs:* These fibers provide structural support and recoil properties to the lung

tissue, influencing its ability to stretch and recoil during breathing.
- **Surface tension:** Surface tension at the air-liquid interface within the alveoli can affect lung compliance. Surfactant molecules reduce surface tension, preventing alveolar collapse and enhancing compliance.
- **Interdependence of the alveoli:** All the neighboring alveoli pull the collapsing alveolus and prevent collapse (Newton's third law) at the end-expiratory volume. This phenomenon, known as interdependence, helps maintain alveolar stability and prevents lung collapse, especially during exhalation.
- **Volume of lung at which compliance is measured:** Compliance is influenced by the volume of the lung at which it is measured. Generally, compliance is higher when the lung volume is lower and decreases as lung volume increases for the tidal volume.
- **Degree of congestion in pulmonary capillaries:** Increased congestion in pulmonary capillaries, as seen in conditions such as pulmonary edema or pulmonary hypertension, mechanically opposes the expansion of the lungs, decreasing lung compliance.

### Factors Present in the Chest Wall

- **Chest wall deformities:** The compliance of the chest wall, including the ribs and muscles, affects overall lung compliance. Stiffness or reduced compliance of the chest wall can limit lung expansion.
  **There is barrel chest in emphysema:** Due to decreased elastic recoil of lungs in emphysema, the wall remains expanded even during expiration leading to poor ventilation and dyspnea.
- **Airway resistance:** Resistance to airflow within the airways can affect lung compliance, particularly during dynamic breathing cycles. Increased airway resistance, as seen in conditions such as asthma or chronic obstructive pulmonary disease (COPD), can reduce lung compliance.

## SURFACE TENSION

Surface tension is a property of the surface of a liquid that causes it to behave like a stretched elastic membrane. It is the result of the cohesive forces between the molecules in the liquid. Essentially, molecules at the surface of a liquid experience an inward force due to the unbalanced attractions between them and the neighboring molecules, as there are no molecules above them to balance out these forces. This creates a sort of "skin" or tension at the surface of the liquid.

Considering this concept of surface tension of fluids, let's see what happens in alveoli. The inner side of alveolus has a thin (monomolecular) layer of fluid. These molecules attract each other through Vander Walls forces. These molecules cling to each other and resist separation;

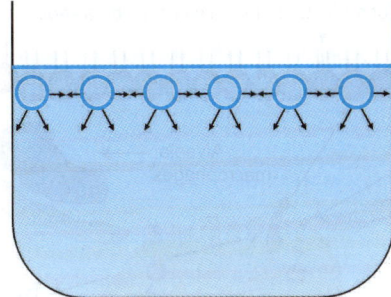

**Fig. 49.13:** Surface tension.

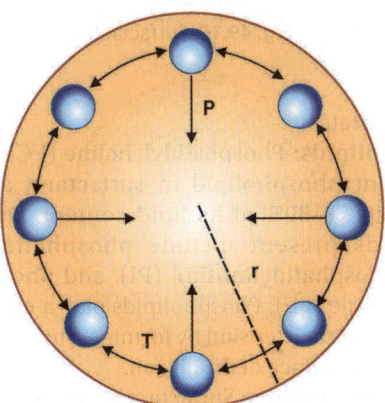

**Fig. 49.14:** Surface tension and resultant force.

the force generated by these molecules is called *surface tension (T)* **(Fig. 49.13)**.

The direction of this resultant force *(P, transmural pressure)* is such that, if this force is sufficiently strong, it can lead to *collapse of the alveoli* **(Fig. 49.14)**.

According to Laplace Law: $P = \dfrac{2T}{r}$

Where, T is the surface tension
P is the transmural pressure (sum of all forces trying to decrease the radius of the sphere)
R is the radius of the sphere/alveoli

> **REMEMBER**
> An increase in surface tension or decrease in the radius, increases the collapsing tendency of the alveoli.

## SURFACTANT

A fluid lines the alveoli which lowers the surface tension and prevents the collapse of the alveoli. It is secreted by *Type II pneumocyte cells* **(Fig. 49.15)**.

This fluid is a lipid surface tension lowering agent which is a mixture of:
1. ***Dipalmitoylphosphatidylcholine (DPCC)***
2. ***Phosphatidylglycerol***
3. Other phospholipids
4. Neutral lipids

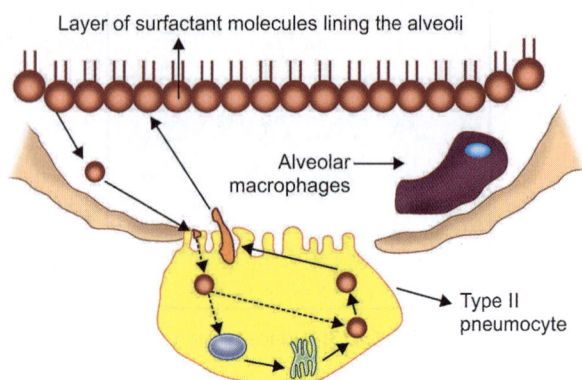

**Fig. 49.15:** Surfactant.

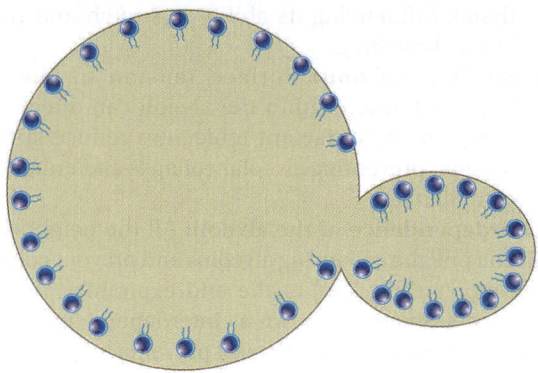

**Fig. 49.16:** Mechanism of action of surfactant.

5. Proteins
6. Carbohydrates

- **Phospholipids:** Phosphatidylcholine (PC) is the predominant phospholipid in surfactant, accounting for about 70–80% of its lipid content. Other phospholipids present include phosphatidylglycerol (PG), phosphatidylinositol (PI), and phosphatidylethanolamine (PE). Phospholipids play a crucial role in reducing surface tension by forming a monolayer at the air-liquid interface of the alveoli.
- **Surfactant proteins:** Surfactant proteins are classified into two main groups: hydrophobic proteins (SP-B and SP-C) and hydrophilic proteins (SP-A and SP-D).
  - *SP-B and SP-C:* These hydrophobic proteins are involved in stabilizing the lipid layer and reducing surface tension.
  - *SP-A and SP-D:* These hydrophilic proteins have roles in immune defense, regulating surfactant metabolism, and modulating inflammation.
- **Neutral lipids:** Surfactant also contains neutral lipids, such as cholesterol, which contribute to the overall structure and function of surfactant.

## Mechanism of Action of Surfactant

The primary function of surfactant is to reduce the surface tension at the air-liquid interface within the alveoli. As air enters the alveoli during inspiration, the surface tension at the air-liquid interface tends to cause the alveoli to collapse. Surfactant molecules, particularly phospholipids like phosphatidylcholine, are hydrophobic on one end and hydrophilic on the other. When surfactant is secreted onto the alveolar surface, the hydrophobic tails of the phospholipids embed themselves into the air-facing surface, while the hydrophilic heads orient themselves toward the liquid, disrupting the cohesive forces between water molecules. This reduces surface tension, making it easier for the alveoli to expand during inspiration and preventing collapse during expiration (**Figs. 49.16** and **49.17**).

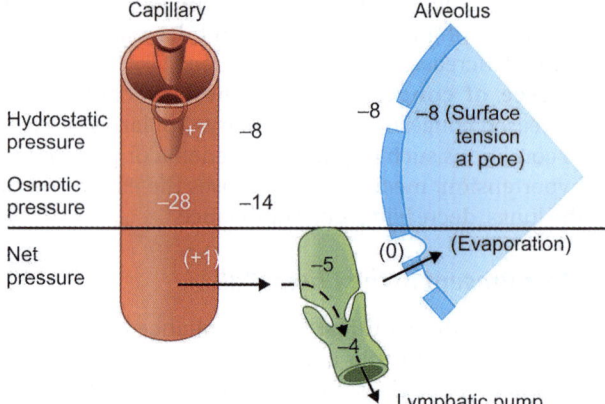

**Fig. 49.17:** Pressure causing fluid movement.

## Functions of Surfactant (Fig. 49.18)

- It prevents collapse of alveoli.
- Helps to prevent pulmonary edema:
  - If surfactant is absent, there is unopposed surface tension producing a force of 20 mm Hg, resulting in transudation of fluid from blood into alveoli.

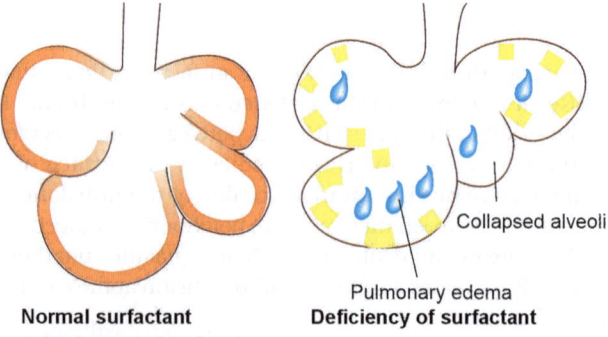

**Normal surfactant**
1. Reduces surface tension
2. Prevents the collapse of alveoli
3. Keeps the alveoli dry

**Fig. 49.18:** Effects of deficiency of surfactant.

**CASE BASED SELF-DIRECTED LEARNING MODULE**

**Infant Respiratory Distress Syndrome (IRDS):**

- **Case scenario:** You are a neonatologist, working in a busy neonatal intensive care unit (NICU). A 32-year-old woman, G2P1, has just given birth to a male infant at 30 weeks gestation via emergency cesarean section due to fetal distress. The infant, weighing 1,400 grams, is admitted to the NICU for further management.
- **Presenting complaint:** Upon admission to the NICU, the infant exhibits signs of respiratory distress shortly after birth. The infant is tachypneic, with a respiratory rate of 70 breaths per minute, nasal flaring, and grunting. The infant appears cyanotic around the lips.
- **Initial assessment:**
  - Vital signs: Heart rate 160 bpm, respiratory rate 70 bpm, oxygen saturation 86% on room air.
  - Apgar scores: 5 at 1 minute, 7 at 5 minutes.
  - Physical examination: Decreased breath sounds bilaterally, intercostal retractions, and grunting.
  - Lab tests: Arterial blood gas (ABG) shows pH 7.25, $PaO_2$ 45 mm Hg, $PaCO_2$ 60 mm Hg, $HCO_3^-$ 24 mEq/L, and base excess -3 mmol/L.

*(Hints for Case Discussion for Self-directed Learning)*

- **Risk factors assessment:** Discuss maternal and neonatal risk factors for RDS, including prematurity, maternal diabetes, and fetal distress.
- **Clinical assessment Interpretation:** Interpret the clinical signs and symptoms observed in the infant, correlating them with the diagnosis of RDS.
- **Diagnostic evaluation:** Review the diagnostic workup for RDS, including chest X-ray findings consistent with diffuse bilateral atelectasis and ground-glass opacities.
- **Differential diagnosis:** Consider other causes of neonatal respiratory distress, such as transient tachypnea of the newborn (TTN) and meconium aspiration syndrome (MAS).

**Pathophysiology review:**

- **Alveolar surfactant deficiency:** Explore the pathophysiological mechanisms underlying RDS, focusing on surfactant deficiency and lung immaturity in premature infants.
- **Surfactant production:** Explain that surfactant is a complex mixture of phospholipids and proteins produced by type II alveolar cells. It reduces surface tension at the air-liquid interface, preventing alveolar collapse.
- **Lung immaturity:** Describe how premature infants may have insufficient surfactant production due to immature type II cells and reduced alveolar surface area, leading to increased surface tension and alveolar collapse during expiration.
- **Consequences of surfactant deficiency:** Discuss the impact of surfactant deficiency on lung compliance, gas exchange, and respiratory function.
- **Atelectasis:** Explain that surfactant deficiency results in increased alveolar surface tension, causing collapse of alveoli, decreased lung compliance, and impaired gas exchange.
- **Ventilation-perfusion mismatch:** Describe how atelectasis leads to ventilation-perfusion mismatch, resulting in hypoxemia and respiratory acidosis.
- **Inflammatory response:** Discuss the inflammatory response triggered by surfactant deficiency, leading to further lung injury and inflammation.

**Treatment:**

- **Supportive care:** Implement supportive care measures, including thermal regulation, oxygen supplementation, and fluid management.
- **Respiratory support:** Initiate noninvasive respiratory support with nasal continuous positive airway pressure (NCPAP) and prepare for potential intubation and mechanical ventilation.
- **Surfactant replacement therapy:** Discuss the indications for surfactant replacement therapy and the timing of administration.
- **Exogenous surfactant:** Explain the administration of exogenous surfactant via endotracheal tube to improve lung compliance and prevent alveolar collapse.
- **Complications management:** Address potential complications of RDS, such as pneumothorax and pulmonary hemorrhage, and their management strategies.

**Prevention and prognosis:**

- **Preventative strategies:** Review strategies for preventing RDS, such as antenatal corticosteroid administration and maternal magnesium sulphate for neuroprotection.
- **Prognosis:** Discuss the prognosis of RDS, including potential long-term respiratory sequelae and developmental outcomes.

## INFANT RESPIRATORY DISTRESS SYNDROME

Infant respiratory distress syndrome (IRDS), also known as respiratory distress syndrome (RDS) of the newborn or neonatal respiratory distress syndrome, is a common respiratory disorder affecting premature infants characterized by surfactant deficiency and resulting in respiratory distress shortly after birth.

### Physiological Basis

Surfactant is a complex mixture of lipids and proteins produced by type II alveolar cells in the lungs. Its primary function is to reduce surface tension at the air-liquid interface within the alveoli, preventing alveolar collapse during expiration and promoting lung compliance.

### Pathophysiology (Fig. 49.19)

Premature infants have immature lungs with inadequate surfactant production. Surfactant deficiency leads to increased surface tension, causing alveolar collapse, decreased lung compliance, and ventilation-perfusion mismatch. This results in impaired gas exchange, hypoxemia, and respiratory distress.

### Clinical Features

Infants with IRDS typically present shortly after birth with signs of respiratory distress, including:
- Tachypnea
- Nasal flaring
- Intercostal retractions
- Grunting
- Cyanosis

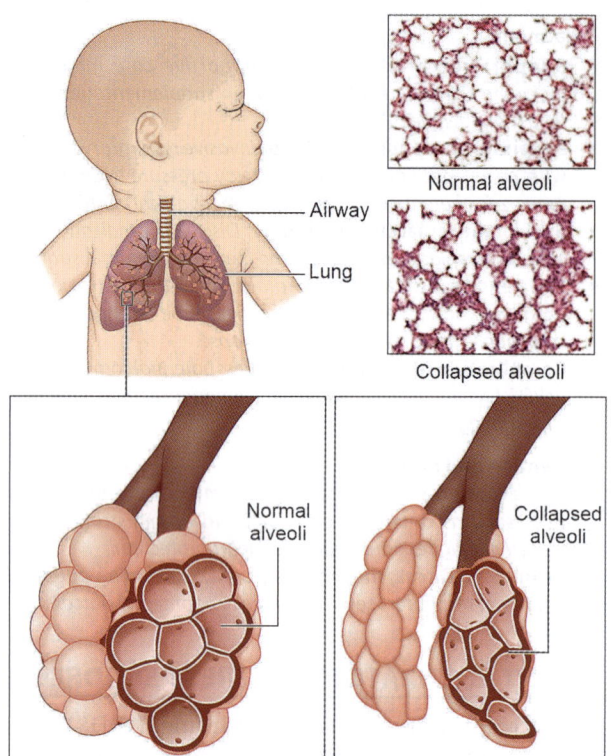

**Fig. 49.19:** Pathophysiology of IRDS.

## Diagnosis and Management

- **Diagnostic evaluation for IRDS includes:**
  - Clinical assessment of respiratory distress signs and symptoms
  - Chest X-ray findings consistent with diffuse bilateral atelectasis and ground-glass opacities
  - Arterial blood gas analysis showing hypoxemia, hypercapnia, and respiratory acidosis
- **Management:**
  - Supportive care measures, including thermal regulation, oxygen supplementation, and fluid management
  - Respiratory support with noninvasive methods such as nasal continuous positive airway pressure (NCPAP)
  - Surfactant replacement therapy via endotracheal tube for severe cases
- **Complications:** Pneumothorax and pulmonary hemorrhage
- **Prevention:** Injection betamethasone to mother near term or in preterm labor can accelerates the surfactant formation in lungs.

## ADULT RESPIRATORY DISTRESS SYNDROME

When the deficiency of surfactant occurs in adults, it is called the adult respiratory distress syndrome (ARDS).

It can occur in chronic cigarette smokers, which leads to decrease in the surfactant. Even prolonged inhalation of 100% oxygen also decreases the surfactant. Various other factors can cause the same like infections, embolism, sepsis, etc.

## AIRWAY RESISTANCE

It is defined as the resistance offered by the airways to the airflow due to diameter and the patency of the bronchi.

In healthy individuals, maximum airway resistance is seen in *medium sized airways (seat of airway resistance)*, because they have maximum amount of smooth muscle in them. Further, the large airways are too wide to offer resistance and small airways are too numerous with overall large cross-sectional area.

### Factors Determining Airway Resistance

- **Radius of airways:**
  - $R = 8\eta l/\pi r^4$
  - According to this formula, the resistance 'R' is inversely proportional to the fourth power of the radius, which means that the resistance will increase with the decreased radius and vice versa. The smaller bronchioles will thus have larger resistance as compared to the larger bronchi. Also, the resistance increases during the expiratory phase due to decreased radius of the airways as compared to the inspiratory phase.
- **Flow of air (turbulence and velocity of flow):**
  - The turbulence and the velocity of airflow directly increases the airway resistance. More the turbulence, more is the velocity.
  - Flow is laminar through straight portions. Laminar flow poses less resistance to the airflow.
  - Turbulent through branching points. The laminar flow becomes turbulent at the branching points and hence increased airway resistance.
  - Turbulence increases at higher flow rates, hence R also increases at higher flow rates.
- **Bronchial musculature:**
  - Sympathetic nervous system causes bronchodilation and decreases airway resistance.
  - Parasympathetic nervous system causes bronchoconstriction and increases the airway resistance.
- **Lung volume:** Expansion of lungs results in stretching of airways which decreases airway resistance.
- **Breathing:** Airway resistance is lower during inspiration and is more during expiration due to compression of the smaller airways by the increased intrathoracic pressure **(Fig. 49.20)**. This decreases the lumen of the bronchioles. It results in prolongation of the expiratory phase to 3 times of the inspiratory phase.

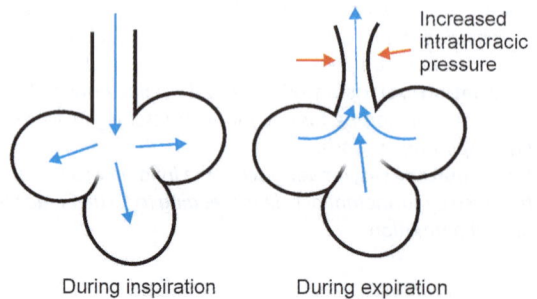

**Fig. 49.20:** Intrathoracic pressure.

- **Dust and smoke:** Airway resistance increases in polluted environment.

> **Emphysema:** It is a type of chronic obstructive pulmonary disease (COPD) characterized by irreversible damage to the alveoli, leading to airway obstruction and impaired gas exchange. Inhalation of irritants such as cigarette smoke triggers inflammation and destruction of alveolar walls, resulting in enlarged air spaces and reduced lung elasticity.
>
> **Asthma:** It involves chronic inflammation of the airways, leading to bronchial hyperresponsiveness and airflow obstruction. Triggered by allergens or irritants, inflammation causes airway constriction, mucus production, and edema. Smooth muscle contraction further narrows airways. Treatment focuses on anti-inflammatory medications and bronchodilators to alleviate symptoms and prevent exacerbations.

## WORK OF BREATHIING

The work of breathing refers to the amount of effort required by the respiratory muscles to overcome the resistance of the respiratory system and move air into and out of the lungs during breathing.

*Work done = force × distance*
- Force is analogous to change in pressure.
- Distance is analogous to change in volume.
- W = change in pressure × change in volume.

> **Closing volume**
> It is the lung volume at which the finest bronchioles are virtually closed; no air flow occurs despite the best effort

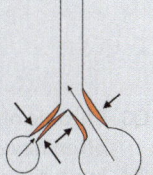

## Components of Work of Breathing

### Elastic Work

- Elastic work refers to the energy expended by the respiratory muscles to overcome the elastic recoil of the lungs and chest wall during breathing.
- The lungs and chest wall have elastic properties that allow them to stretch during inspiration and recoil passively during expiration. However, to expand the lungs during inspiration, the respiratory muscles must overcome this elastic recoil force. Similarly, during expiration, energy is required to counteract the tendency of the lungs and chest wall to recoil inward.
- Elastic work is calculated as the product of the force required to overcome the elastic recoil and the distance moved during breathing.
- *Elastic Work = Force × Distance.*

### Work Done to Overcome Viscous Resistance

- This component of work refers to the energy expended to overcome the resistance encountered by airflow due to viscosity within the airways.
- Viscous resistance occurs as air flows through the airways, particularly at higher velocities during inspiration. This resistance is related to the frictional forces between the air and the airway walls.
- Work done to overcome viscous resistance is maximum at the middle of inspiration when the velocity of air flow is highest.
- Work done to overcome viscous resistance is calculated as the integral of the product of air flow velocity and the pressure drop across the airways over the duration of inspiration.

### Work Done to Overcome Tissue Resistance (WTR)

- This component represents the energy expended by the respiratory muscles to overcome resistance encountered by lung tissues during breathing.
- Lung tissues have inherent resistance to deformation, requiring energy expenditure by the respiratory muscles to stretch and recoil the lung parenchyma during ventilation.
- While smaller compared to other components, work done to overcome tissue resistance contributes to the overall work of breathing.
- Work done to overcome tissue resistance is not typically quantified separately but is considered as part of the overall work of breathing.

### Work Done to Overcome Airway Resistance (WAR)

- This component represents the energy expended to overcome the resistance encountered by airflow through the airways.
- Airway resistance arises due to the frictional forces between the air and the airway walls as air flows through the conducting airways.
- Airway resistance is a significant component of the work of breathing, particularly in conditions where the airways are narrowed or obstructed, such as asthma or chronic obstructive pulmonary disease (COPD).
- Work done to overcome airway resistance is calculated as the product of the pressure drop across the airways and the volume of air moved during breathing.

## Energy Cost of Breathing (Fig. 49.21)

- During quiet breathing, there is less than 5% of total oxygen consumption.
- Increases enormously during exercise or lung disease.

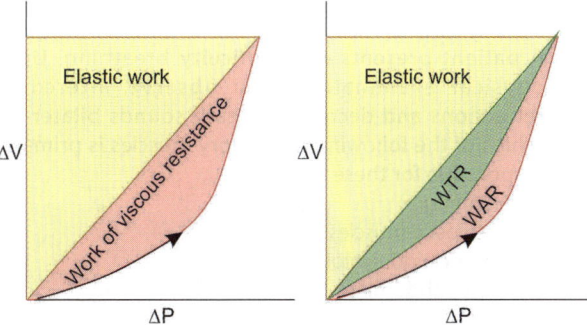

**Fig. 49.21:** Energy cost of breathing.

## SUMMARY

- The respiration involves breathing (inspiration and expiration), transport of gases and utilization of these gases at the tissue level.
- Inspiration is an active process occurring due to the contraction of the diaphragm and intercostal muscles, which increases the thoracic diameters dropping the intrathoracic pressure and the filling of the lungs with air. Whereas the expiration is a passive process occurring due to the recoil of the lungs.
- The alveoli are lined with fluid, which is responsible for the development of surface tension inside the alveoli. This surface tension increases the collapsing tendency of alveoli and renders them vulnerable to pulmonary edema, decreased pulmonary ventilation and increased work of breathing.
- However, the surfactant secreted by the type II pneumocytes secrete the surfactant which reduces the surfactant and protects the lungs from all above problems.
- We had also learned about the compliance of the lungs, which refers to the change in volume per unit change in pressure. We had learned about the conditions that affect compliance.
- The airway resistance is primarily dependent on the radius of bronchus, patency of bronchus, velocity of airflow and the intrathoracic pressure.

## LET US SEE, HOW MUCH YOU HAVE LEARNT?

### Review Questions

#### Long/Short Answer Questions

Q1. Describe the process of inspiration in terms of thoracic diameters and pressure gradients.
Q2. Explain why the expiratory phase is longer than the inspiratory phase?
Q3. Define compliance. Enumerate/describe the factors affecting compliance.
Q4. What is specific compliance? What is its significance?
Q5. What is the difference between static and dynamic compliance?
Q6. Define surface tension. What is the physiological basis of development of surface tension?
Q7. Define surfactant. What is the composition of surfactant? What are the functions of surfactant?
Q8. What will happen if there is deficiency of surfactant in a patient?
Q9. What are the various factors affecting the airway resistance?

#### Explain Why? (Reasoning Questions)

Q1. Surfactant is crucial for normal lung function, particularly in newborns.
Q2. The diaphragm is the primary muscle involved in quiet breathing.
Q3. Chronic obstructive pulmonary disease (COPD) patient often have an increased work of breathing.
Q4. Lung compliance is higher during expiration compared to inspiration.

### Critical Thinking Case-Based Questions

Q1. Mahira, a 28-week preterm infant, was admitted to the NICU shortly after birth with severe respiratory distress. She was exhibiting rapid breathing, grunting, and cyanosis. A chest X-ray revealed diffuse ground-glass opacities, and her arterial blood gases indicated hypoxemia and respiratory acidosis. The attending neonatologist suspected neonatal respiratory distress syndrome (NRDS) due to surfactant deficiency. Based upon the given scenario, answer the following questions:
  a. Explain the role of surfactant in the lungs.
  b. Discuss how its deficiency leads to the clinical presentation observed in this case.
  c. Why are preterm infants particularly at risk for developing neonatal respiratory distress syndrome?

### Multiple Choice Questions

Q1. A patient presents with difficulty breathing. Upon physical examination, you observe intercostal retractions and decreased breath sounds bilaterally. Which of the following respiratory muscles is primarily responsible for these findings?
  a. Diaphragm
  b. Intercostal muscles
  c. Sternocleidomastoid
  d. Rectus abdominis

Q2. A 35-year-old male is admitted to the emergency department with acute respiratory distress. Chest X-ray reveals diffuse bilateral opacities. Which of the following best explains the role of alveolar surface tension in this patient's condition?
  a. Increased surface tension leads to lung collapse.
  b. Decreased surface tension facilitates lung expansion.
  c. Surface tension has no effect on lung stability.
  d. Surface tension enhances gas exchange in the alveoli.

Q3. During a physical exam, a physician hears wheezing upon auscultation of a patient's chest. Which of the following conditions is most likely to cause increased airway resistance?
   a. Pulmonary fibrosis
   b. Chronic obstructive pulmonary disease (COPD)
   c. Pulmonary embolism
   d. Normal lung function

Q4. A 28-year-old female presents with shortness of breath and a history of asthma. Which of the following factors primarily contributes to airway resistance in this patient?
   a. Increased lung compliance
   b. Narrowing of bronchioles
   c. Decreased alveolar surface tension
   d. Strengthening of respiratory muscles

Q5. A patient is experiencing difficulty exhaling air during expiration. Which of the following conditions is most likely causing increased resistance during expiration?
   a. Asthma      b. Pneumonia
   c. Pulmonary fibrosis      d. Pulmonary embolism

Q6. A premature infant is born at 28 weeks gestation and requires mechanical ventilation. Which of the following factors contributes to increased work of breathing in this infant?
   a. Increased lung compliance
   b. Surfactant deficiency
   c. Decreased airway resistance
   d. Elevated tidal volume

Q7. Which of the following statements accurately describes the mechanics of normal respiration?
   a. Inspiration is an active process requiring contraction of the diaphragm.
   b. Inspiration involves relaxation of the diaphragm and external intercostal muscles.
   c. During normal breathing, intrapleural pressure is higher than atmospheric pressure.
   d. During expiration, the thoracic cavity expands, leading to lung expansion.

Q8. Which of the following pressure changes occurs during inspiration?
   a. Intrapulmonary pressure decreases below atmospheric pressure.
   b. Intrapleural pressure becomes more positive.
   c. Alveolar pressure exceeds atmospheric pressure.
   d. Extrapulmonary pressure decreases.

Q9. Alveolar surface tension primarily affects which of the following lung properties?
   a. Compliance      b. Elasticity
   c. Airway resistance      d. Ventilation

Q10. Compliance of the lungs refers to:
   a. The ability of the lungs to stretch and expand.
   b. The resistance encountered by airflow through the airways.
   c. The frictional forces between the air and the airway walls.
   d. The force required to overcome elastic recoil during expiration.

Q11. Which of the following factors affects airway resistance?
   a. Lung compliance
   b. Alveolar surface tension
   c. Diameter of the airways
   d. Lung elasticity

Q12. A patient with asthma experiences bronchoconstriction, leading to:
   a. Decreased airway resistance
   b. Increased lung compliance
   c. Increased work of breathing
   d. Improved gas exchange

Q13. Chronic obstructive pulmonary disease (COPD) is characterized by:
   a. Increased alveolar surface tension
   b. Decreased airway resistance
   c. Decreased alveolar surface tension
   d. Increased airway resistance

Q14. In patients with pulmonary fibrosis, increased lung stiffness results in:
   a. Decreased airway resistance
   b. Increased lung compliance
   c. Decreased work of breathing
   d. Increased work of breathing

Q15. Which of the following conditions is most likely to cause decreased lung compliance?
   a. Pulmonary embolism
   b. Pulmonary edema
   c. Emphysema
   d. Acute respiratory distress syndrome (ARDS)

Q16. A patient with emphysema has destruction of lung tissue, resulting in:
   a. Decreased airway resistance
   b. Increased lung compliance
   c. Decreased work of breathing
   d. Increased alveolar surface tension

Q17. During normal expiration, which of the following pressure changes occurs?
   a. Intrapleural pressure becomes more negative.
   b. Intrapulmonary pressure exceeds atmospheric pressure
   c. Alveolar pressure decreases.
   d. Extrapulmonary pressure increases.

Q18. Which of the following conditions is most likely to result in increased work of breathing?
   a. Increased lung compliance
   b. Decreased airway resistance
   c. Strengthening of respiratory muscles
   d. Surfactant deficiency

## ANSWERS
1. b    2. a    3. b    4. b    5. a    6. b    7. a    8. a    9. d    10. a    11. c    12. c    13. d    14. d
15. d    16. b    17. c    18. d

# Pulmonary Ventilation
## (Diffusion of Gases Across Respiratory Membrane)

**CHAPTER 50**

### COMPETENCY ADDRESSED
**PY6.2:** Describe the mechanics of normal respiration, pressure changes during ventilation, lung volume and capacities, alveolar surface tension, compliance, airway resistance, ventilation, V/P ratio, diffusion capacity of lungs.

### LEARNING OBJECTIVES
**At the end of this chapter, the learner should be able to:**
- Describe the layers of the respiratory membrane.
- Define the process of diffusion across the respiratory membrane.
- Explain the factors affecting diffusion.
- Analyze the process of diffusion in a patient with damage to the respiratory membrane.
- Describe the process of evaluation of diffusion capacity of the respiratory membrane.
- Describe the ventilation-perfusion ratio. Apply this knowledge to assess the shunt and dead space air.

As discussed earlier, the main function of the respiratory system is to provide the oxygen to the tissues and remove the carbon dioxide, produced by the tissues. This involves the exchange of respiratory gases ($O_2$ and $CO_2$) at the alveolar level and at the tissue level. At both these places, the respiratory gases diffuse though the biological membranes.

**At the lungs:** The gaseous exchange takes place through the respiratory membrane, which is made up of 6 layers, as discussed in Chapter 48. But for a quick reference, they are enumerated below:
1. Layer of fluid lining the alveolus
2. Alveolar epithelium
3. Epithelial basement membrane
4. Interstitial space between alveolar epithelium and capillary membrane
5. Capillary basement membrane
6. Capillary endothelial membrane

*The average thickness of the respiratory membrane is 0.6 μm with total surface area of 70 m². The average diameter of pulmonary artery is 5 μ and the total quantity of blood in lungs at any instance is around 60–140 mL.*

**At the tissue level:** The gaseous exchange takes place through the tissue cell membrane having the following layers:
1. Cell membrane
2. Epithelial basement membrane
3. Interstitial space between cellular epithelium and capillary membrane
4. Capillary basement membrane
5. Capillary endothelial membrane

The respiratory gases are lipid soluble, hence, can easily move across these membranes but, their movement depends on the diffusion coefficient of the gas.

## DIFFUSION OF GASES ($O_2$ AND $CO_2$)

It is defined as the movement of the particles from its higher concentration to its lower concentration. Since we are going to talk about the movement of the gases we can rephrase it as, 'movement of a gas from its higher partial pressure to its lower partial pressure,' i.e., along its pressure gradient.

### Factors Affecting the Rate of Diffusion

1. **Pressure difference of gas:** The pressure gradient across the biological membranes is responsible for the movement of gases across it.
   - At lungs/alveoli **(Fig. 50.1)**:
     - The $PO_2$ of alveoli is 100 mm Hg while $PO_2$ of pulmonary capillary blood is 40 mm Hg. Hence, the $O_2$ moves from the alveoli to the capillary.
     - The $PCO_2$ of alveoli is 40 mm Hg while $PCO_2$ of pulmonary capillary blood is 40 mm Hg. Hence, the $CO_2$ moves from the capillary to the alveoli.

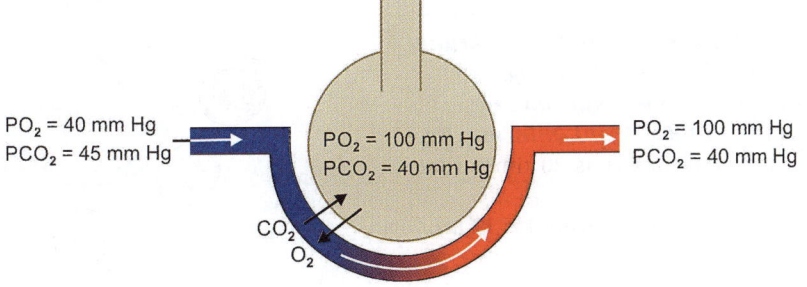

**Fig. 50.1:** Pressure differences of gases at the level of alveoli.

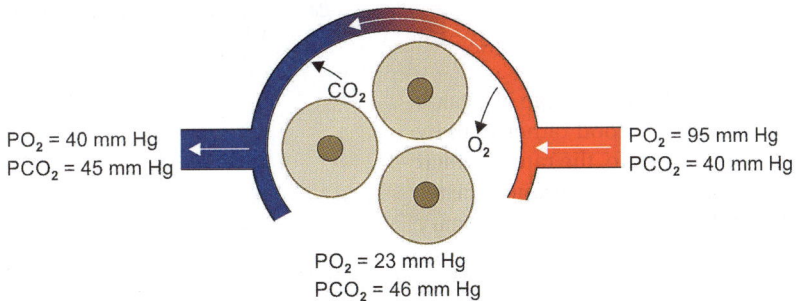

**Fig. 50.2:** Pressure differences of gases at the level of tissues.

- At tissues **(Fig. 50.2)**:
    - The $PO_2$ of tissues is 23 mm Hg while $PO_2$ of capillary blood is 95 mm Hg. Hence, the $O_2$ moves from the capillary to the tissues.
    - The $PCO_2$ of tissues is 46 mm Hg while $PCO_2$ of capillary blood is 40 mm Hg. Hence, the $CO_2$ moves from the tissue to the capillaries.
2. **Diffusion coefficient of gas:** It is defined as the ease with which the lipid soluble molecule can diffuse through a biological semipermeable membrane. It depends of the solubility of the gas and its molecular weight. It is expressed as:

$$\frac{Solubility}{\sqrt{Molecular\ weight}}$$

- The diffusion coefficient of $O_2$ is 1.0
    - $CO_2 \to 20.3$
    This means *carbon dioxide is 20.3 times more diffusible than the oxygen*.
3. **Area of cross-section:** The greater area of cross-section increases the rate of rate of diffusion and vice versa. Hence, the bronchial tree ends in alveolar membrane and pulmonary arteries split to form capillary network, greatly increasing the surface area for the optimum rate of diffusion.
4. **Thickness of respiratory membrane:** The thickness of respiratory membrane adversely affects the rate of diffusion. Thicker respiratory membrane, as seen in fibrosis of basement membrane or interstitial lung diseases, have decreased rate of diffusion. Diffusion of gases through tissues is almost equal to the diffusion of gases in water.

Factors affecting diffusion **(Fig. 50.3)**:
- Pressure difference of gas
- Diffusion coefficient of gas →
    - S/√ MW (solubility/square root of molecular weight)
    - $O_2 \to 1.0$
    - $CO_2 \to 20.3$
- Area of cross-section
- Thickness of respiratory membrane

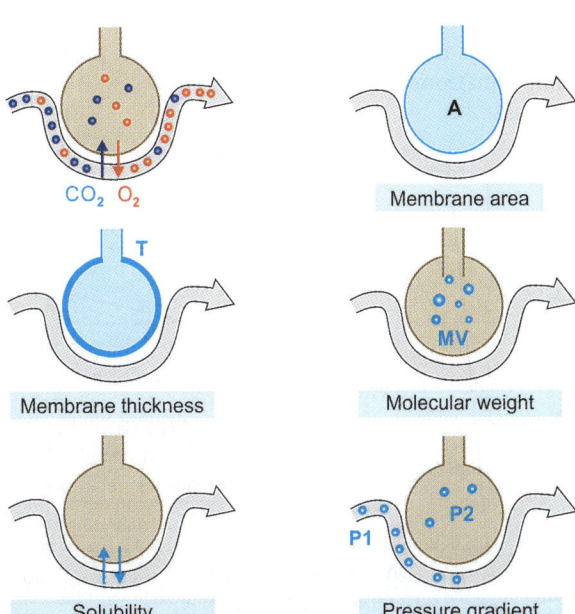

**Fig. 50.3:** Factors affecting diffusion rate.

## DIFFUSION CAPACITY

It is defined *amount of gas diffusing across the membrane in 1 minute with pressure difference of 1 mm Hg*.
- Diffusion capacity of *$O_2$ is 21-25 mL/min/mm Hg*
- Diffusion capacity of *$CO_2$ is 400-450 mL/min/mm Hg*, because diffusion coefficient of $CO_2$ is 20 times that of $O_2$)
- Diffusion capacity of CO (carbon monoxide) is *17 mL/min/mm Hg*

### Limitations of Gaseous Exchange in Diffusion (Fig. 50.4)

#### Flow Limited

This limitation occurs when the rate of exchange of a gas is primarily determined by the flow of blood rather than by the process of diffusion. In this scenario, the rate at which the gas can diffuse across the alveolar membrane is faster than the rate at which blood flows through the pulmonary capillaries. An example is nitrous oxide ($N_2O$). It diffuses very quickly (in 0.1 seconds) across the alveolar membrane but the flow of blood through the pulmonary capillary takes longer (0.75 seconds). Therefore, the rate of exchange is limited by the flow of blood.

#### Diffusion Limited (Fig. 50.5)

This limitation occurs when the rate of exchange of a gas is primarily determined by the ability of the gas to diffuse across the alveolar membrane. In this case, the gas is taken up by the blood (usually by binding to hemoglobin) at such a high rate that the partial pressure of the gas in the capillary remains low, and equilibrium is not reached. An example is CO. It binds to hemoglobin with such high affinity that even though it can diffuse rapidly across the alveolar membrane, the partial pressure of CO in the capillary remains low because it is rapidly bound by hemoglobin, preventing equilibrium from being reached.

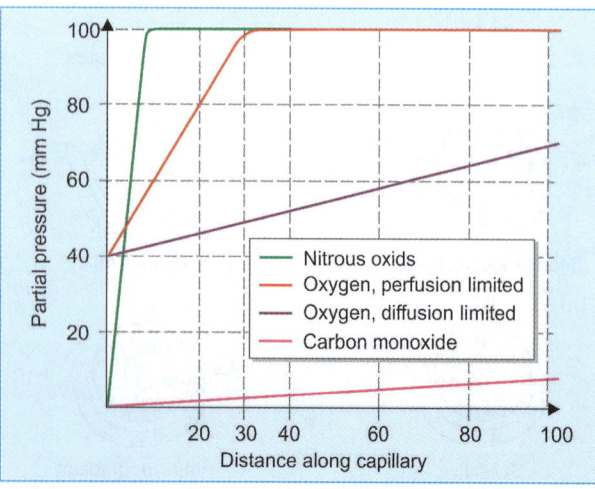

**Fig. 50.4:** Diffusion of various gases in capillaries.

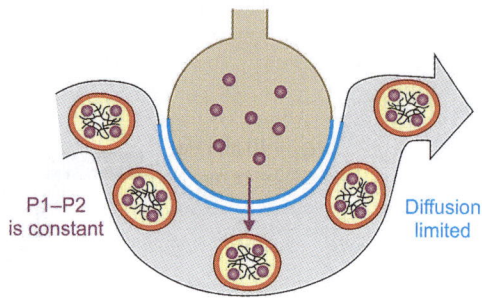

Inspired carbon monoxide rapidly enters red blood cells and binds to hemoglobin, creating a constant maximal partial pressure of carbon monoxide in the plasma. Therefore, carbon monoxide absorption is diffusion limited and depends on diffusion characteristics of the alveolar-capillary membranes, and not on the amount of pulmonary blood flow

**Fig. 50.5:** Diffusion limited.

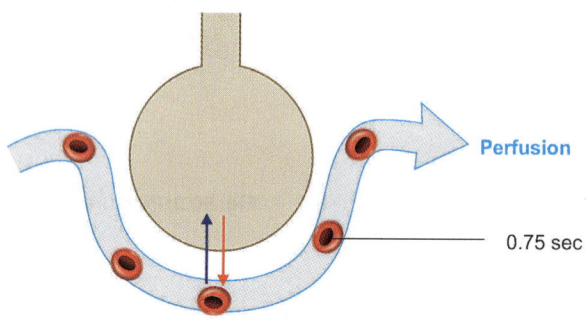

**Fig. 50.6:** Perfusion determining the diffusion capacity.

#### Perfusion Limited (Fig. 50.6)

This limitation occurs when the rate of exchange of a gas is primarily determined by the blood flow and the capacity of blood to pick up the gas, rather than by the diffusion across the alveolar membrane.

In this case, the gas is taken up by the blood and reaches equilibrium with the capillary blood quickly. An example is oxygen ($O_2$). It diffuses rapidly across the alveolar membrane and is taken up by hemoglobin, reaching equilibrium with the capillary blood in a short time (0.35 seconds). Therefore, the rate of exchange is primarily limited by the rate of blood flow and the capacity of blood to pick up oxygen.

### Measurement of Diffusing Capacity Using DLCO (Diffusing Capacity of the Lung for Carbon Monoxide)

DLCO is a *measure of the lung's ability to transfer gases from inspired air to the red blood cells in the pulmonary capillaries*. It specifically measures the diffusion capacity of the lung for CO, as CO has a high affinity for hemoglobin and diffuses readily across the alveolar-capillary membrane.

#### Indications

DLCO testing is commonly used to assess various lung diseases, including:
- Chronic obstructive pulmonary disease (COPD)

- Interstitial lung diseases (ILDs)
- Pulmonary vascular diseases
- Pulmonary hypertension
- Evaluation of pulmonary function before lung surgery or transplantation

## Method

DLCO is typically measured using a technique called *the single-breath CO uptake test*. The patient breathes in a small quantity of CO mixed with a test gas, usually helium or methane, for a short period of time (usually 10 seconds). Then, the patient exhales the gas mixture, and the concentration of CO in the exhaled breath is measured. By comparing the concentration of CO inhaled with that exhaled, the DLCO can be calculated.

DLCO is calculated using the formula:

$$DLCO = \frac{(C1-C2) \times VA}{PCO}$$

*Where:*

$C1$ = Concentration of CO in the inhaled gas sample (in mL/min/mm Hg)
$C2$ = Concentration of CO in the exhaled gas sample (in mL/min/mm Hg)
$VA$ = Alveolar volume or lung volume (in liters)
$PCO$ = Pressure of CO in the alveolar gas (in mm Hg)

The DLCO value may need to be adjusted or corrected for factors such as hemoglobin concentration, age, sex, and altitude. These adjustments ensure that the DLCO measurement is standardized and comparable across different individuals and conditions.

## Interpretations

- **Reduced DLCO:** A decreased DLCO suggests impaired gas exchange in the lungs, which can be indicative of various lung diseases. It may signify conditions such as emphysema, pulmonary fibrosis, pulmonary hypertension, or other disorders affecting the alveolar-capillary membrane.
- **Normal DLCO:** A normal DLCO indicates that gas exchange in the lungs is within the expected range. However, it's essential to consider other clinical findings and tests when interpreting DLCO results.
- **Increased DLCO:** An increased DLCO is less common but may occur in certain conditions such as polycythemia, left-to-right cardiac shunts, or during exercise.

## Normal Values Measured

**Normal value of DLCO is 17 mL/min/mm Hg.** From this, we can deduce the diffusion capacity of oxygen, $DLO_2 = 1.23 \times DLCO = 21–25\ mL/min/mm\ Hg$ and carbon dioxide as $DLCO_2 = 20 \times DLO_2 = 400–450\ mL/min/mm\ Hg$.

## INSPIRED, ALVEOLAR AND EXPIRED AIR

- **Inspired air:** It is the air which is inspired inside the lungs and its composition is same as the atmospheric air.
- **Alveolar air:** It is the air present in the alveoli is called as the alveolar air **(Fig. 50.7)**. *Last 350 mL of expired air during quite breathing* is composed of the alveolar air. Alveolar air is slowly renewed by the atmospheric air. Each breath replaces only 1/7th of total alveolar air. Even 16 breaths are not enough to renew the entire alveolar air.
- **Expired air:** It is the air which is expired out of the lungs and the respiratory passages. First 150 mL of expired air comes from the conducting passages, where no gaseous exchange takes place, hence its composition is similar to the expired air. While last 350 mL of expired air is from the respiratory zone, where the gaseous exchange takes place.

Composition of these airs are shown in **Table 50.1**

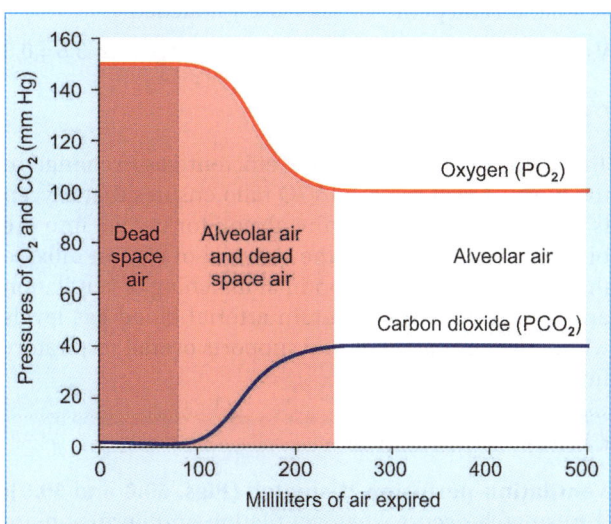

**Fig. 50.7:** $PO_2$ and $PCO_2$ of dead space and alveolar air.

**Table 50.1:** Composition of different air in lungs.

|  | Inspired air | Alveolar air | Expired air |
|---|---|---|---|
| $PO_2$ (mm Hg) | 158 | 100 | 116 |
| $PCO_2$ (mm Hg) | 0.3 | 40 | 32 |
| $PH_2O$ (mm Hg) | 3.7 | 47 | 47 |
| $PN_2$ (mm Hg) | 596 | 573 | 565 |

**Pressures in Arteries and Veins**

|  | Arteries | Veins |
|---|---|---|
| $PO_2$ (mm Hg) | 95 | 40 |
| $PCO_2$ (mm Hg) | 40 | 45 |
| $PH_2O$ (mm Hg) | 47 | 47 |
| $PN_2$ (mm Hg) | 573 | 573 |

# VENTILATION-PERFUSION RATIO ($V_A/Q$)

- $V_A \rightarrow$ alveolar ventilation
- $Q \rightarrow$ perfusion
- $VA/Q = 4.2/5.5 = 0.8$
- If VA is zero (no ventilation)
  - $0/Q =$ zero (base of lungs)
- If Q is zero (no perfusion)
  - $VA/0 =$ infinity (perfusion of lungs)

The ventilation-perfusion ratio (V/Q ratio) is a physiological parameter that describes the matching of ventilation (V) and perfusion (Q) in the lungs. It represents the ratio of the amount of air reaching the alveoli (ventilation) to the amount of blood flow through the pulmonary capillaries (perfusion) in a given time.

## Normal Values

Under normal conditions, the V/Q ratio is relatively balanced throughout the lungs. The average V/Q ratio in healthy individuals is approximately 0.8, indicating that ventilation and perfusion are closely matched

V = 4.2 L/min, Q = 5.5 L/min, therefore, V/Q = 4.2/5.5 = 0.8

## Physiological Significance

The V/Q ratio is essential for efficient gas exchange in the lungs. A well-matched V/Q ratio ensures that oxygen is effectively delivered to the alveoli for uptake into the blood while allowing for the removal of carbon dioxide through exhalation. This optimal matching of ventilation and perfusion helps maintain arterial blood gas levels within the normal range and supports overall respiratory function.

## Clinical Significance

**Ventilation-perfusion Mismatch (Figs. 50.8 and 50.9):** A mismatch occurs when ventilation and perfusion are not well-matched. This can lead to areas of the lung where ventilation exceeds perfusion (high V/Q ratio, termed dead space) or areas where perfusion exceeds ventilation (low V/Q ratio, termed shunt). Conditions such as pulmonary embolism, pneumonia, COPD, and pulmonary hypertension can disrupt the normal V/Q ratio.

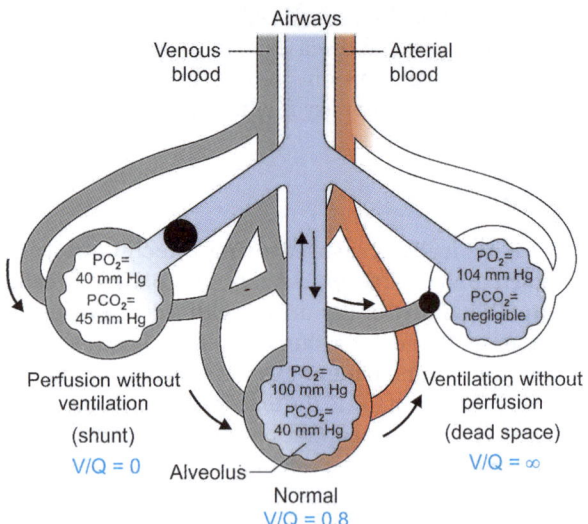

Fig. 50.9: Possible causes of ventilation-perfusion disturbances.

**A: Normal ventilation and perfusion**
- V/Q → 0.8
- Alveolar air composition is normal, i.e., $PO_2 = 100$ mm Hg, $PCO_2 = 40$ mm Hg

**B: Complete airway blockage (VA is zero)**
- No ventilation, i.e., V = 0
- V/Q → 0/Q = 0
- Alveolar air composition is similar to composition of venous blood, i.e., $PO_2 = 40$ mm Hg, $PCO_2 = 45$ mm of Hg
- It occurs in clinical conditions such as foreign body impaction or obstruction of airflow by mucus during severe asthmatic exacerbation. It creates a shunt where the blood doesn't get oxygenated due to ventilatory block.

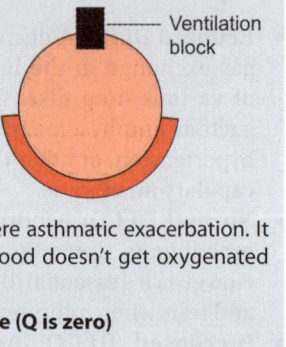

**C: Complete perfusion blockage (Q is zero)**
- No perfusion
- V/Q → V/0 = ∞
- Alveolar air composition is similar to inspired air, i.e., $PO_2 = 104$ mm Hg, $PCO_2 =$ negligible
- It occurs in clinical conditions which blocks the pulmonary blood vessels like pulmonary embolism. It creates a dead space air where the alveolar air is not able to oxygenate the blood.

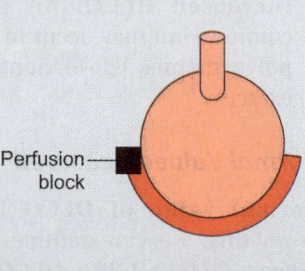

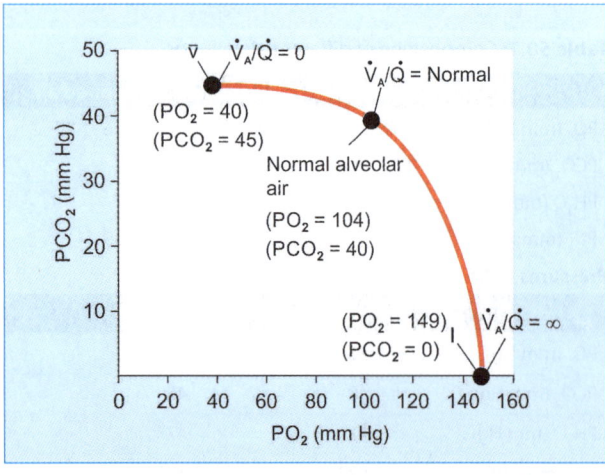

Fig. 50.8: Values of ventilation-perfusion ratio.

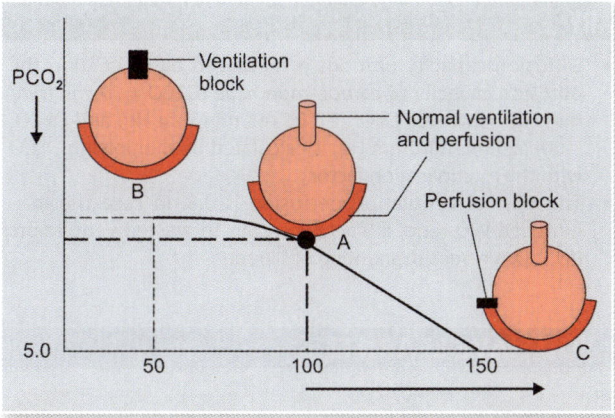

> **REMEMBER**
> - The apices of the lungs are well ventilated but poorly perfused, hence causing the V/Q mismatch, decreasing the ratio, leading to predilection for tubercle bacilli to grow.
> - The bases of the lungs are well perfused but poorly ventilated, hence causing the V/Q mismatch, decreasing the ratio, can cause basal edema in hypertension.

## PHYSIOLOGICAL SHUNT

A physiological shunt refers to a condition in which blood flows through the pulmonary circulation without undergoing oxygenation due to a mismatch between ventilation and perfusion **(Fig. 50.10)**. It occurs due to two reasons:

1. **Blood flowing through bronchial circulation:** The bronchial arteries (carrying 2% of cardiac output) supply oxygenated blood to the lung tissue itself but some of this blood mixes with deoxygenated blood returning to the heart via the pulmonary veins. This mixes the deoxygenated blood from bronchial circulation with the oxygenated blood in pulmonary circulation, contributing to a small degree of physiological shunting.

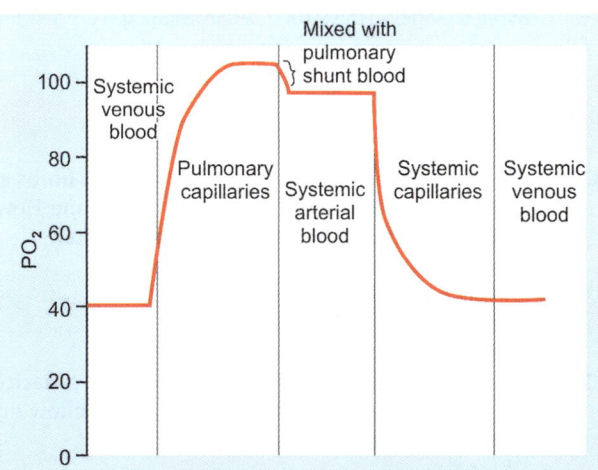

**Fig. 50.10:** Graph showing physiological shunt.

2. **Anatomical variations in pulmonary vasculature:** There may be anatomical variations or differences in the distribution of pulmonary blood flow. The apex of the lung has more ventilation and less perfusion where as the base of lungs have more perfusions and compared to ventilation creating V/Q mismatch.

## DEAD SPACE AIR

It refers to the portion of each breath that does not participate in gaseous exchange with the pulmonary capillaries. It represents the volume of air that fills the conducting airways (trachea, bronchi, and bronchioles) and does not reach the alveoli, where gas exchange occurs.

### Types

1. **Anatomical dead space:**
   - Anatomical dead space is the volume of the conducting airways where gas exchange does not occur. This includes the air in the trachea, bronchi, bronchioles, and terminal bronchioles.
   - It is relatively constant and does not vary significantly during normal breathing.
2. **Physiological dead space:**
   - Physiological dead space includes both anatomical dead space and any additional volume of alveoli that are poorly perfused or ventilated.
   - It can vary depending on factors such as lung pathology, lung volume, and distribution of ventilation and perfusion.
   - Physiological dead space contributes to *wasted ventilation* as it does not participate in gas exchange but still requires energy for ventilation.

### Physiological Significance

- Dead space air plays a role in maintaining lung function by conducting air to and from the alveoli for gas exchange.
- Anatomical dead space helps humidify, warm, and filter the inspired air before it reaches the alveoli.
- Physiological dead space can increase in conditions such as pulmonary embolism, lung injury, or diseases affecting lung compliance, leading to inefficient gas exchange and hypoxemia.

### Clinical Significance

- Measurement of dead space can provide valuable information about lung function and gas exchange efficiency.
- Monitoring changes in dead space can help diagnose and manage respiratory conditions such as pulmonary embolism, acute respiratory distress syndrome (ARDS), COPD, and asthma.
- Elevated dead space can indicate impaired ventilation-perfusion matching, lung pathology, or the need for adjustments in mechanical ventilation strategies.

## SUMMARY

- The respiratory membrane is made up of 6 layers across which the respiratory gases have to diffuse.
- The diffusion of these gases depends on the diffusion coefficient, which depends on solubility of gas and its molecular weight. Other factors affecting diffusion are area of cross-section, thickness of membrane and pressure gradient of gases.
- Diffusion capacity of lungs is measured by estimating the diffusion capacity of carbon monoxide (DLCO = 17 mL/min/mm Hg). However, $DLO_2$ (21–25 mL/min/mm Hg) and $DLCO_2$ (400–425 mL/min/mm Hg) is calculated by multiplying DLCO with the multiplication factor.
- The normal ventilation perfusion is 0.8. In case the mismatched V/Q ratio, if V > Q, it results in wasted ventilation. If V < Q, it results in shunting of blood.

## LET US SEE, HOW MUCH YOU HAVE LEARNT?

### Review Questions

#### Long/Short Answer Questions

Q1. Describe the layers of the respiratory membrane with diagram.
Q2. What is diffusion? Enumerate the factors affecting diffusion. How can the diffusion capacity of lungs be measured?
Q3. What will happen to diffusion in a patient of pulmonary fibrosis?
Q4. Define dead space air. What is the physiological significance of dead space air?
Q5. Define physiological shunt. What is the significance of physiological shunt?
Q6. Explain the factors limiting the diffusion across the respiratory membrane.

#### Explain Why? (Reasoning Questions)

Q1. The arterial $PO_2$ in alveoli is 100 mm Hg but remains 95 mm Hg when it reaches left atrium.
Q2. The carbon dioxide diffuses more easily across the cell membranes as compared to oxygen.
Q3. The thickness of the respiratory membrane affects the rate of gas diffusion.
Q4. Pulmonary edema can impair gas exchange across the respiratory membrane.

### Critical Thinking Case-Based Questions

Q1. Radha, a 60-year-old woman, presented to OPD with progressive shortness of breath, particularly during exertion. She had a long history of smoking and was recently diagnosed with chronic obstructive pulmonary disease (COPD). On physical examination, she had a prolonged expiratory phase and diminished breath sounds. Pulmonary function tests revealed reduced diffusing capacity for carbon monoxide (DLCO). A high-resolution CT scan of the chest showed areas of emphysema and interstitial fibrosis. Based on this clinical scenario, answer the following questions:
   a. Explain the physiological mechanisms affecting the diffusion of gases across the respiratory membranes in this case.
   b. How does the structure of the respiratory membrane facilitate the diffusion of gases?
   c. What changes in this structure can impair gas exchange?

### Multiple Choice Questions

Q1. Which process describes the movement of gases across the respiratory membrane?
   a. Filtration
   b. Osmosis
   c. Diffusion
   d. Active transport
Q2. Which of the following factors affects the rate of diffusion across the respiratory membrane?
   a. Partial pressure gradient
   b. Thickness of the membrane
   c. Surface area available for diffusion
   d. All of the above
Q3. A patient has been diagnosed with pulmonary fibrosis, leading to thickening of the respiratory membrane. How would this affect diffusion across the membrane?
   a. Diffusion would increase
   b. Diffusion would be unaffected
   c. Diffusion would decrease
   d. Diffusion would stop
Q4. A patient presents with a decreased diffusion capacity of the respiratory membrane. Which of the following tests would be used to evaluate this?
   a. Chest X-ray
   b. Spirometry

c. Arterial blood gas analysis
d. Diffusion capacity testing

Q5. A patient with chronic obstructive pulmonary disease (COPD) experiences an imbalance in ventilation-perfusion ratio. What would be the expected effect on dead space air?
a. Increase in dead space air
b. Decrease in dead space air
c. No change in dead space air
d. Dead space air becomes fully functional

Q6. A patient is diagnosed with a pulmonary embolism, leading to a mismatch in ventilation and perfusion. Which condition is likely to result from this mismatch?
a. Shunt
b. Wasted ventilation
c. No effect on dead space air
d. V/Q ratio = 0

Q7. How would an increase in the surface area of the respiratory membrane affect diffusion?
a. Diffusion would increase
b. Diffusion would decrease
c. Diffusion would be unaffected
d. Diffusion would stop

Q8. Explain how changes in altitude affect diffusion across the respiratory membrane.
a. Decreased oxygen levels result in increased diffusion
b. Increased pressure at higher altitudes decreases diffusion
c. Increased altitude leads to decreased diffusion due to decreased oxygen levels
d. Diffusion remains unaffected by changes in altitude

Q9. Describe the steps involved in evaluating the diffusion capacity of the respiratory membrane.
a. Spirometry and bronchoscopy
b. Arterial blood gas analysis and pulmonary function tests
c. Measurement of carbon monoxide uptake and lung volume
d. Chest X-ray and computed tomography (CT) scan

Q10. How does exercise affect the ventilation-perfusion ratio?
a. It decreases ventilation and increases perfusion
b. It increases ventilation and decreases perfusion
c. It increases both ventilation and perfusion proportionally
d. It decreases both ventilation and perfusion proportionally

Q11. In the graph, given below, showing the rate of alveolar ventilation in which the half of alveolar is renewed in 17 seconds. Choose one correct response, from the graph.

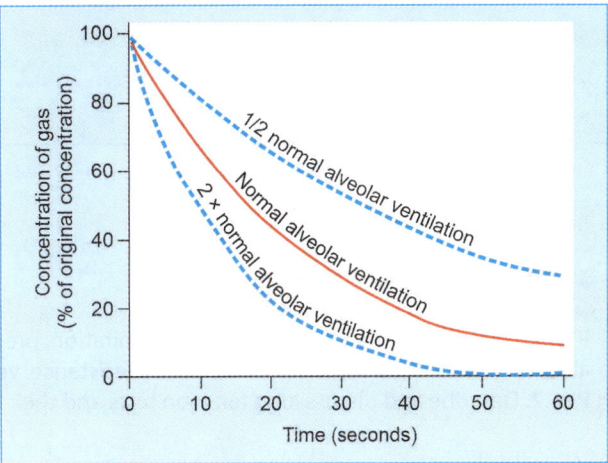

a. If alveolar ventilation is one-half normal, one half the gas is removed in 50 seconds
b. If alveolar ventilation is doubled, one half the gas is removed in 8 seconds
c. If alveolar ventilation is one-half normal, one half the gas is removed in 60 seconds
d. If alveolar ventilation is doubled, one half the gas is removed in 12 seconds

12. If the mean $O_2$ pressure difference across the respiratory membrane during normal, quiet breathing is about 11 mm Hg. What is the net diffusing capacity of oxygen through the respiratory membrane?
a. 17 mL/min
b. 21 mL/min
c. 230 mL/min
d. 400 mL/min
[Hint $DLO_2$ is 21 mL/min/mm Hg, if pressure gradient is 11 mm Hg, the $DLO_2 = 21 \times 11 = 230$ mL/min)

## ANSWERS

1. c   2. d   3. c   4. d   5. a   6. b   7. a   8. c   9. c   10. c   11. b   12. c

# Pulmonary Function Tests

**CHAPTER 51**

> **COMPETENCY ADDRESSED**
>
> **PY6.2:** Describe the mechanics of normal respiration, pressure changes during ventilation, lung volume and capacities, alveolar surface tension, compliance, airway resistance, ventilation, V/P ratio, diffusion capacity of lungs.
> **PY6.7:** Describe and discuss lung function tests and their clinical significance.

> **LEARNING OBJECTIVES**
>
> At the end of this chapter, the learner should be able to:
> - Define the pulmonary function tests.
> - Enumerate all the tests for the assessment of the pulmonary functions.
> - Describe the spirometric and nonspirometric lung volumes and capacities in terms of definition, measurement and functions.
> - Describe the dynamic lung volumes and capacities.

The tests conducted for the assessment of the functional status of the respiratory system are called as the *Pulmonary function tests*.

The various pulmonary function tests are enumerated in **Box 51.1**. As per the learning objectives of a first year MBBS students, we will discuss, the spirometry in detail.

## SPIROMETRY

It is defined as the assessment of lung volumes and capacities using the **Simple Spirometer (Fig. 51.1).** Now a days, the computerized spirometry is more popular and convenient to use than the simple spirometry.

### Lung Volumes (TV, IRV, ERV and RV)

Volume of air breathed in or out by a subject, in different phases of respiration, e.g., *tidal volume, inspiratory reserve*

> **Box 51.1:**
>
> **Pulmonary function tests.**
>
> - Spirometry
> - Diffusion capacity of lung with carbon monoxide (DLCO)
> - 6-minute walk test (6-MWT)
> - Fractional exhalation of NO (FeNO)
> - Body plethysmography
> - Cardiopulmonary exercise testing (CPET)
> - Bronchoprovocation test (Methacholine challenge test)
> - Forced oscillometry (FOT)

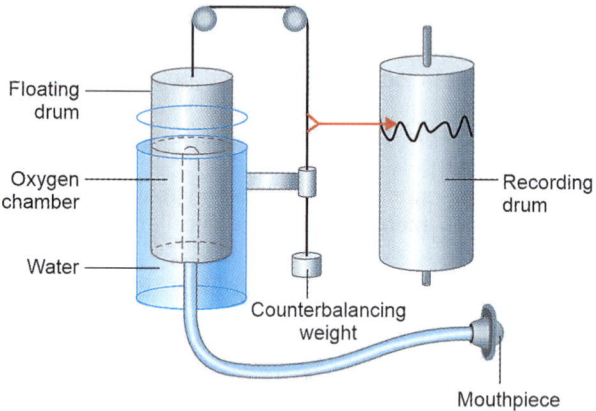

**Fig. 51.1:** A simple spirometer.

*volume and expiratory reserve volume.* These volumes can be measured by spirometer and hence are called as the *spirometric lung volumes*.

The volumes which cannot be measured by spirometer are called *the nonspirometric lung volume*, e.g., *residual volume*.

### Lung Capacities ( IC, EC, VC, FRC and TLC)

When two or more lung volume are taken together, they are called Lung capacities, e.g., *inspiratory capacity, expiratory capacity and vital capacity.*

Nonspirometric capacities are *functional residual capacity (FRC) and the total Lung capacity (TLC).*

## STATIC LUNG VOLUMES AND CAPACITIES VS. DYNAMIC LUNG VOLUMES AND CAPACITIES

- **Static lung volumes and capacities:** When the time factor is not considered or in other words, when enough time is given before the assessment, so that the volumes are stabilized. For example, TV, IRV, ERV, VC, etc.
  *In the static LV and capacities, the rate of change of volume per unit time is not considered. It is the net change in the volume which is measured.*
- **Dynamic lung volumes and capacities:** When the time factor is considered/the lung volumes are measure, as they change with time. For example, Timed forced expiratory volume ($FEV_1$, $FEV_2$, MVV, etc.). *In dynamic lung volumes and capacities, the rate of change of lung volumes per unit time is measured*, e.g., $FEV_1$ measures the forced expiratory volume in the first second of the expiration. Hence, when the volumes are timed, they are called dynamic LV and C.

## Static Lung Volumes

### Tidal Volume

It is the amount air breathed in and out in a single breath. Technically, it is the amount of air which is inspired normally at the end of normal relaxed expiration and vice versa. It is about 500 mL or 0.5 L/breath.

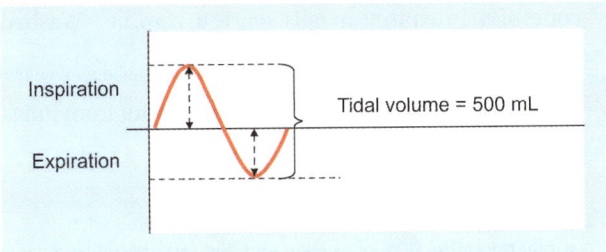

### Inspiratory Reserve Volume (IRV)

It is the maximum amount of air that can be inspired *at the end of normal tidal inspiration* with the maximum inspiratory effort. It is about 2,500 mL.

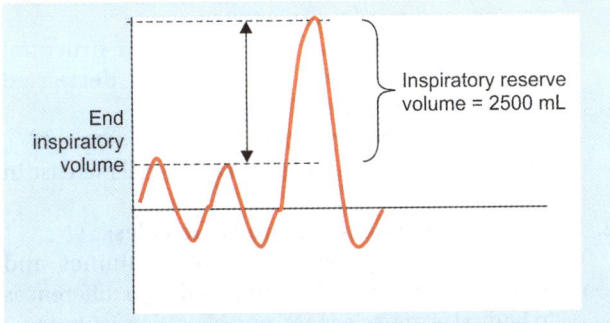

### Expiratory Reserve Volume (ERV)

It is the maximum amount of air that can be expired out at the end of normal tidal expiration with maximum expiratory effort. It is about 1,000 mL.

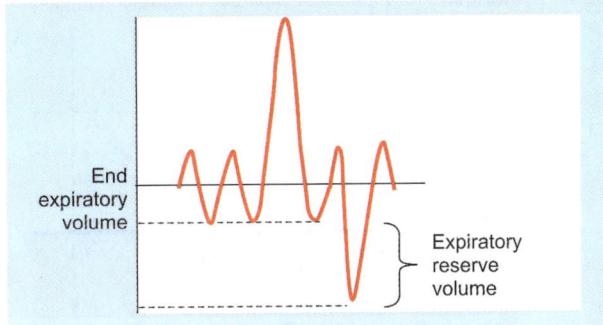

## Static Lung Capacities (Fig. 51.2)

### Inspiratory Capacity (IC)

It is the maximum amount of air that can be inspired at the end of normal tidal expiration with maximum inspiratory effort. It is sum of TV and IRV (500 mL + 2,500 mL) = 3,000 mL or 3 L.

### Expiratory Capacity (EC)

It is the maximum amount of air that can be expired at the end of normal tidal inspiration with maximum expiratory effort. It is sum of TV and ERV (500 mL + 1,000 mL) = 1,500 mL or 1.5 L.

### Vital Capacity (VC)

It is the maximum amount of air that can be expired at the end of maximum inspiration with maximum inspiratory and expiratory effort. It is sum of TV, IRV and ERV (500 mL + 3,000 + 1,000 mL) = 4,500 mL or 4.5 L.

## Nonspirometric Static Lung Volumes and Capacities (Fig. 51.2)

### Residual Volume (RV)

It is the amount of air present in the lungs at the end of maximal expiration, and this air cannot be expelled out from the lungs even with maximal expiratory effort. It is 1,200 mL or 1.2 L.

### Total Lung Capacity

It is the total volume of the air present in the lungs at the end of inspiratory reserve volume:

$$\begin{aligned}\text{TLC} &= \text{IRV} + \text{TV} + \text{ERV} + \text{RV} \\ &\quad OR \\ &= \text{VC} + \text{RV} \\ &\quad OR \\ &= \text{IC} + \text{EC} + \text{RV}\end{aligned}$$

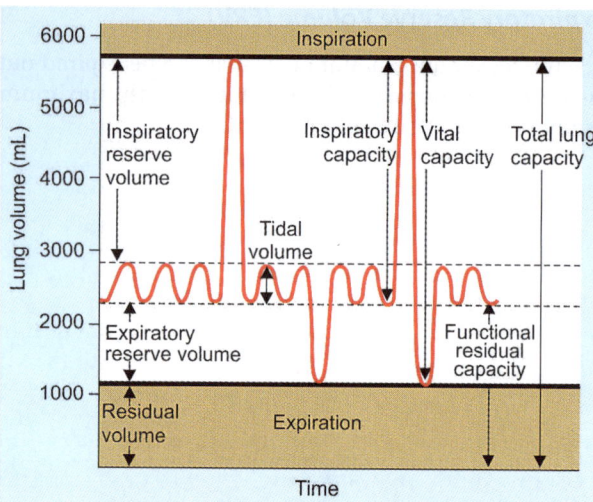

**Fig. 51.2:** Static lung volumes and capacities.

## Functional Residual Capacity (FRC)

It is the amount of air present in the lungs after normal tidal expiration.

FRC = ERV + RV = 1,000 + 1,200 = 2,200 mL or 2.2 L

### Measurement of FRC

- **Closed circuit method:** Helium dilution method
- **Open circuit method:** Nitrogen wash out method
- Whole body plethysmography

### Closed Circuit Method: Helium Dilution Method (Fig. 51.3)

**Principle:** It is based on the principle of closed circuit method (called so because the air is inspired from and expired into the bag).

**Procedure:** The subject is given to re breathe a known volume of gas mixture containing 80% $O_2$ and 20% helium. The helium concentration stabilizes in 5 minutes, i.e., diluted in bag and enters lungs. The fall in He concentration at equilibrium indicates extent of dilution, which is proportional to FRC:

$$V_1 C_1 = V_2 C_2$$

- $V_1$ = Total volume of the bag
- $V_2$ = Total volume of the bag and lungs after equilibrium

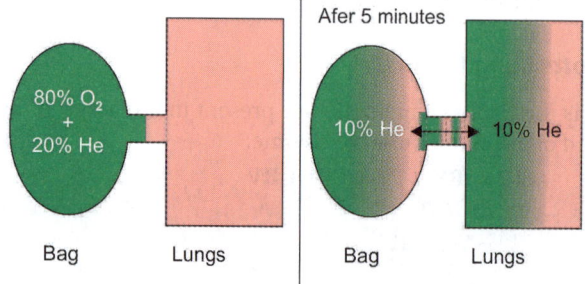

**Fig. 51.3:** Helium dilution method.

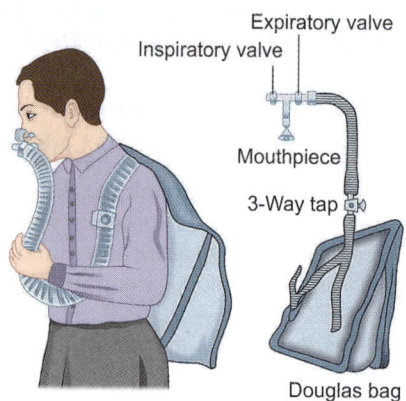

**Fig. 51.4:** Nitrogen washout method.

- $C_1$ = Initial conc. of gas
- $C_2$ = Final conc. of gas

$$V_2 = V_1 C_1 / C_2$$

Hence, FRC = $V_2 - V_1$

> **Solve it yourself:**
> A subject rebreathes in 2L reservoir containing 20% He and 80% oxygen. After equilibrium the conc. of He falls to 10%. Find out the FRC of the subject.

### Nitrogen Washout Method (Fig. 51.4)

It is based on the open circuit method:

- **Procedure:** The subject breathes in 100% oxygen and breathes out into a large Douglas bag
- As breathing continues, the conc. of $N_2$ falls in lungs till conc. of $N_2$ in expired air falls nearly to zero, i.e., 'Washed Out'
- $Q = C \times V$
    - Q = Total amount of nitrogen washed out from lungs
    - C = Conc. of nitrogen
    - V = Volume of expired air collected

> **Solve it yourself:**
> A subject breathes 40 L of oxygen and expired gas mixture has a nitrogen conc. of 5%. Total volume of expired gas mixture is 40 L. The amount of nitrogen in lungs is 80%.

### Variations in FRC

1. **It increases with age:**
    - As individuals age, there is a natural loss of lung elasticity and chest wall compliance.
    - Weakening of respiratory muscles and structural changes in the lungs contribute to decreased efficiency in exhalation.
    - These factors result in a higher residual volume (RV), which is part of FRC, leading to an overall increase in FRC with age.
2. **It is more in males as compared to females:**
    - Males typically have larger lung volumes and dimensions compared to females due to differences in body size, muscle mass, and chest configuration.

- This difference in lung size and morphology results in a higher FRC in males compared to females.
3. **FRC is more in taller individuals:**
   - Taller individuals tend to have larger lung volumes and greater chest wall compliance.
   - The increased lung size and better expansion capacity lead to a higher residual volume (RV) and, consequently, a higher FRC in taller individuals.
4. **Effect of posture on FRC:**
   - When standing, the chest wall is more expanded, and the diaphragm is in a lower position compared to when lying down.
   - This standing position allows for better lung expansion and increased residual volume (RV), leading to a higher FRC compared to lying down.
5. **Effect of weight on FRC:**
   - Obesity can lead to reduced chest wall compliance and increased airway resistance.
   - Fat deposits around the chest and abdomen can compress the lungs, limiting their expansion capacity.
   - These factors result in a decrease in residual volume (RV) and, consequently, a decrease in FRC in obese individuals.
6. **Effect of pregnancy on FRC:**
   - During pregnancy, hormonal changes lead to increased chest circumference and upward displacement of the diaphragm due to the growing uterus.
   - This reduces the space available for lung expansion and decreases chest wall compliance.
   - As a result, there is a decrease in residual volume (RV) and, consequently, a decrease in FRC during pregnancy.
7. **In anesthetized person:** An anesthetized person has less Functional Residual Capacity (FRC) due to anesthesia-induced effects such as depressed respiratory drive, muscle relaxation, loss of conscious control over breathing, and the supine position during surgery, all of which contribute to incomplete lung emptying and reduced FRC. The FRC reduced by 400 mL.

### Significance of FRC

- Maintains constant levels of $PO_2$ and $PCO_2$ in blood
- Fall in $PCO_2$ would have taken away the respiratory drive
- Dilutes the toxic effects of the gases
- Keeps the lungs expanded state at the end of expiration, prevents them from collapsing

## Dynamic Lung Volumes (Fig. 51.5)

When the lung volumes are expressed as a function of time, i.e., expressed as 'per unit time':
- $FEV_1$, $FEV_2$, $FEV_3$
- FVC
- $FEV_1$/FVC
- FEFR
- MVV
- RMV

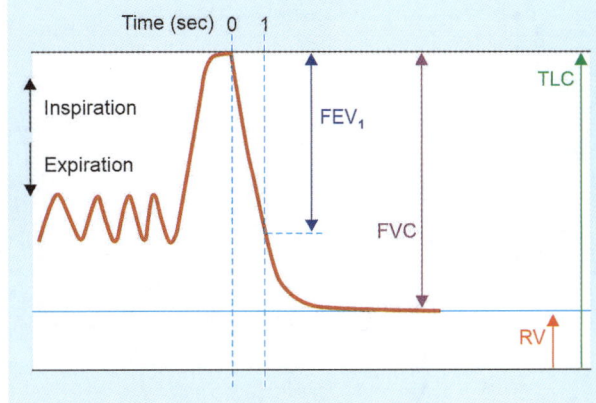

**Fig. 51.5:** Dynamic lung volumes.

### Forced Expiratory Volume (FEV)

It is also called as timed vital capacity. It is the volume of air expired forcefully in a specified time interval.

**$FEV_1$:** The maximum amount of air which a subject breathes out in first second of forceful expiration. It is 83% of the total forceful expiration. $FEV_2$ = 94%, $FEV_3$ = 97%.

### FEV/FVC

- It is a more meaningful ratio than only $FEV_1$
- It is important for diagnosis of obstructive lung disease
- $FEV_1$/FVC = 83%, $FEV_2$/FVC = 94% and $FEV_3$/FVC = 97%
- A decrease in $FEV_1$/FVC <70% indicates obstructive lung disease **(Fig. 51.6)**.

### Significance of FEV

- Diagnosis of obstructive lung diseases
- Differentiation of obstructive and restrictive lung diseases

### Forced Expiratory Time

- Time taken for completing the respiration forcefully
- 4 seconds

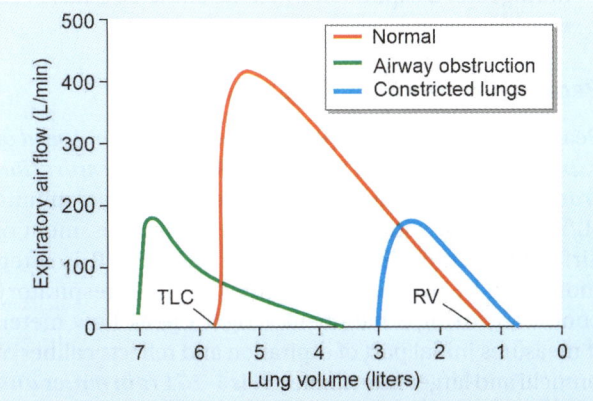

**Fig. 51.6:** Normal and abnormal lung volumes.

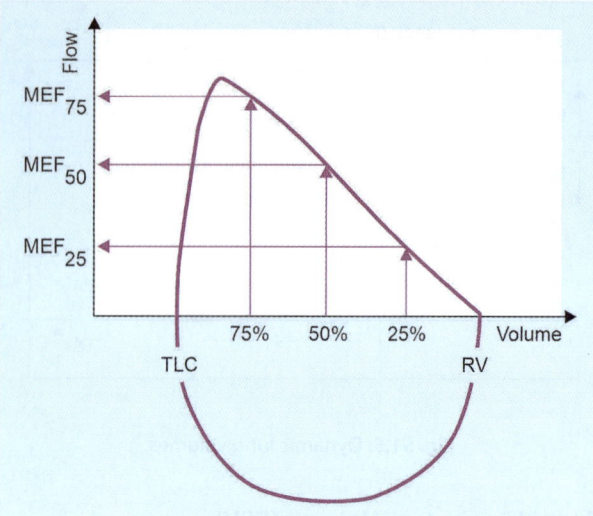

**Fig. 51.7:** Expiratory phases.

- >4 seconds indicates airway obstruction
- >6 seconds indicates airway obstruction

### Expiratory Flow Rates

Expiratory flow rates refer to the rate at which air is expelled from the lungs during expiration.

Expiratory phase is divided into 4 quarters **(Fig. 51.7)**:
1. **MEFR 25%:** This refers to the Maximal Expiratory Flow Rate at 25% of the Forced Vital Capacity (FVC). It indicates the rate of airflow during forced expiration when approximately 25% of the FVC has been exhaled.
2. **MEFR 50%:** This indicates the Maximal Expiratory Flow Rate at 50% of the Forced Vital Capacity (FVC). It represents the rate of airflow during forced expiration when approximately 50% of the FVC has been exhaled.
3. **MEFR 75%:** This refers to the Maximal Expiratory Flow Rate at 75% of the Forced Vital Capacity (FVC). It signifies the rate of airflow during forced expiration when approximately 75% of the FVC has been exhaled.
4. **MEFR 100%:** This denotes the Maximal Expiratory Flow Rate at 100% of the Forced Vital Capacity (FVC). It represents the maximum rate of airflow achieved during forced expiration when the entire FVC has been exhaled.

### Peak Expiratory Flow Rate

Peak expiratory flow rate (PEFR) is the *maximum speed of expiration achieved during a forced maximal expiration from full lung inflation*. It is measured in liters per minute (L/min) and provides a simple and quick assessment of airflow limitation in the larger airways. PEFR is often monitored by patients with asthma or other respiratory conditions using a handheld Wright's peak flow meter. It measures initial part of expiration and reflects caliber of bronchi and larger bronchioles. *It is 5–15 L/s in males and 2.5–10 L/s in females.*

### Maximal Mid-expiatory Flow Rate

Maximal mid-expiratory flow rate (MMEFR) is a *measure of airflow during the middle portion of forced expiration*. It is also known as forced mid-expiratory flow (FMEF).

**FEF 25–75%:** MMEF is typically calculated as the average flow rate over the middle half of the forced vital capacity (FVC) curve, usually between 25% and 75% of the FVC. This parameter provides information about the function of small and medium-sized airways in the lungs.

## PULMONARY VENTILATION

It is defined as the amount air inspired or expired over a period of 1 minute at rest. It is also called as *respiratory minute volume (RMV)/minute ventilation*.

RMV = Tidal volume × Respiratory rate
- Normal RR = 12–16/min, TV = 500 mL
- Hence, RMV = 6 L/min

### Alveolar Ventilation

It is the amount of air entering the alveoli and taking part in the respiratory gas exchange. Here, we calculate the rate by multiplying it with the alveolar ventilation.

Alveolar ventilation = Tidal volume – Dead space air
= 500 – 150
= 350 mL

Hence, alveolar ventilation = 350 × RR

> **Solve it yourself:**
> Calculate the respiratory minute volume and alveolar ventilation of the patient with tidal volume of 400 mL with a respiratory rate of 16 breaths per minute. Consider the patient has a normal dead space air volume.
>
> **Answer:** RMV = 6.4 L/min, AV = 4 L/min

### Maximum Voluntary Ventilation (MVV)/ Maximum Breathing Capacity (MBC)

Maximum voluntary ventilation (MVV) is a measure of *the maximum amount of air a person can breathe in and out of their lungs in one minute* during hyperventilation/ vigorous exercise. It's often used as an indicator of overall respiratory function. During this, the MVV, the respiratory rate can increase to 30–40 breaths/min. Hence, the MVV, can be as high as 125 ± 25 L/min in healthy individuals.

### Breathing Reserve

- The breathing reserve refers to the difference between the maximum amount of air a person can breathe in and out during forced breathing [Maximum Voluntary Ventilation (MVV)] and their normal breathing rate at rest.
- In other words, it represents the additional capacity of the respiratory system that can be recruited during times of increased demand, such as during exercise or

in response to respiratory challenges. The breathing reserve is typically expressed in liters per minute (L/min) and is calculated by subtracting the resting minute ventilation (the volume of air breathed in one minute at rest) from the MVV.
- *BR = MVV – RMV*
- The breathing reserve serves as a measure of the capacity of the respiratory system to respond to increased oxygen demand or to compensate for decreased lung function. It can be an important indicator of overall respiratory health and fitness.

### Dyspneic Index

In this context, it seems to represent the proportion of the breathing reserve in relation to the individual's maximum ventilatory capacity (MVV). The breathing reserve is the difference between the maximum ventilation that an individual can achieve (MVV) and their resting ventilation. By expressing the breathing reserve as a function of MVV, you can assess how much of the total ventilatory capacity is being utilized during a specific activity or condition, which may be relevant in evaluating respiratory function.

Mathematically, it might be expressed as follows:

$$Dyspneic\ index = \frac{Breathing\ reserve}{MVV} \times 100$$

This index could provide insights into respiratory efficiency, especially in situations where individuals may experience dyspnea (breathlessness) due to limitations in their breathing reserve compared to their maximum ventilatory capacity.

## OTHER METHODS FOR ASSESSMENT OF PFT

### DLCO, or Diffusing Capacity of the Lung for Carbon Monoxide

It measures the lung's ability to transfer gas from inhaled air to the bloodstream. It's a crucial test in diagnosing and monitoring lung diseases like COPD and interstitial lung disease. DLCO provides insights into gas exchange efficiency. We have discussed DLCO in detail, in chapter 50.

### The 6-minute Walk Test (6MWT)

It is a simple, widely used assessment of functional exercise capacity. It measures the distance an individual can walk in 6 minutes on a flat, hard surface. Used in various clinical settings, especially for cardiopulmonary diseases, it provides valuable information about exercise tolerance, functional status, and prognosis. The test is easy to administer, requiring minimal equipment and supervision. Results can help guide treatment decisions, monitor disease progression, and assess response to interventions.

### Fractional Exhalation of Nitric Oxide (FeNO)

Fractional exhaled nitric oxide (FeNO) is a noninvasive biomarker for airway inflammation, particularly in asthma. It measures the concentration of nitric oxide in exhaled breath, reflecting eosinophilic airway inflammation. FeNO testing aids in diagnosis of asthma, monitoring, and management, guiding treatment decisions such as adjusting corticosteroid therapy. This quick and easy-to-perform test *helps assess airway inflammation levels and monitor response to anti-inflammatory medications*.

### Body Plethysmography

It is a pulmonary function test that measures lung volumes and airway resistance. It involves a person sitting inside a sealed chamber while breathing through a mouthpiece. By monitoring pressure changes inside the chamber during breathing maneuvers, the test calculates lung volumes, including total lung capacity, residual volume, and functional residual capacity. Additionally, it assesses airway resistance, aiding in the diagnosis and management of respiratory conditions such as COPD, asthma, and restrictive lung diseases. Body plethysmography provides valuable insights into lung mechanics, helping clinicians understand pulmonary function and tailor treatment plans for optimal respiratory health.

### Cardiopulmonary Exercise Testing (CPET)

This assesses the integrated function of the heart, lungs, and muscles during exercise. It measures various parameters such as oxygen consumption, carbon dioxide production, heart rate, and ventilatory response to exercise. CPET provides valuable insights into cardiorespiratory fitness, exercise capacity, and the presence of underlying cardiopulmonary diseases. Used in clinical and research settings, CPET aids in diagnosing conditions like heart failure, COPD, and pulmonary hypertension, guiding treatment decisions and exercise prescription. By evaluating exercise tolerance and physiological responses, CPET helps optimize patient care, rehabilitation programs, and enhances understanding of cardiopulmonary physiology.

### Bronchoprovocation Testing

It is a diagnostic procedure used to assess airway hyper-responsiveness, a hallmark of conditions like asthma. During the test, a bronchoconstrictor agent like methacholine or histamine is inhaled in gradually increasing concentrations. Lung function, typically measured through spirometry, is monitored before and after each dose to detect changes indicative of airway narrowing. Bronchoprovocation tests help confirm a diagnosis of asthma, assess its severity, and guide treatment decisions. While generally safe, they require careful monitoring for potential bronchoconstriction and may not be suitable for individuals with certain pre-existing conditions.

Overall, bronchoprovocation testing plays a crucial role in asthma management and research.

## Forced Oscillation Technique (FOT)

This is a noninvasive pulmonary function test used to assess respiratory mechanics. It measures the impedance of the respiratory system by applying small-amplitude pressure oscillations during tidal breathing. By analyzing the response of the respiratory system to these oscillations, FOT provides valuable information about airway resistance, compliance, and reactance. FOT is particularly useful in assessing lung function in individuals who may have difficulty performing traditional spirometry maneuvers, such as young children or patients with severe respiratory conditions. It aids in diagnosing and monitoring diseases like asthma, COPD, and cystic fibrosis, contributing to personalized treatment strategies.

### SUMMARY

- PFTs are diagnostic procedures that assess the function of the lungs and airways. They measure various parameters such as lung volumes, capacities, airflow rates, and gas exchange efficiency.
- PFTs are crucial for diagnosing respiratory conditions, monitoring disease progression, and evaluating treatment effectiveness.
- PFTs encompass a range of tests, including spirometry, lung volume measurements, diffusion capacity testing, bronchoprovocation tests, and cardiopulmonary exercise testing.
- Spirometric volumes include tidal volume, inspiratory reserve volume, expiratory reserve volume, and residual volume.
- Nonspirometric volumes and capacities, such as total lung capacity, functional residual capacity, and vital capacity, are measured using techniques like body plethysmography and gas dilution.
- Dynamic lung volumes and capacities reflect airflow rates and respiratory mechanics during breathing maneuvers.
- These include forced vital capacity (FVC), forced expiratory volume in one second ($FEV_1$), peak expiratory flow rate (PEFR), and maximal voluntary ventilation (MVV).
- Dynamic lung volumes and capacities are essential for evaluating airway patency, assessing ventilatory reserve, and predicting exercise tolerance.

### LET US SEE, HOW MUCH YOU HAVE LEARNT?

### Review Questions

#### Long/Short Answer Questions

Q1. Enumerate various lung volumes and capacities. Describe the static lung volumes and capacities with a help of well labeled spirogram.

Q2. What are dynamic lung volumes? What is the physiological significance of $FEV_1$/FVC in a healthy subject? How can it help in the diagnosis of obstructive lung disease?

Q3. Define forced expiratory volume. What is its physiological significance?

Q4. What is functional residual capacity? How can it be measured? What is the physiological significance of FRC?

#### Explain Why? (Reasoning Questions)

Q1. A reduced forced vital capacity (FVC) can indicate restrictive lung disease.

Q2. The ratio of forced expiratory volume in 1 second ($FEV_1$) to forced vital capacity (FVC) is a critical parameter in differentiating between obstructive and restrictive lung diseases.

Q3. A peak flow meter is used to monitor asthma control in patients.

#### Multiple Choice Questions

Q1. What are pulmonary function tests (PFTs)?
 a. Tests to measure heart function
 b. Diagnostic procedures to assess lung function
 c. Tests to evaluate liver function
 d. Imaging studies for bone density

Q2. Which of the following is NOT a type of pulmonary function test?
 a. Spirometry
 b. Electrocardiography
 c. Lung volume measurements
 d. Diffusion capacity testing

Q3. What is the main purpose of spirometry?
 a. To measure gas exchange efficiency
 b. To assess lung volumes and capacities
 c. To evaluate airway resistance
 d. To monitor heart function

Q4. Which of the following is a spirometric lung volume/capacity?
 a. Total lung capacity (TLC)
 b. Functional residual capacity (FRC)
 c. Residual volume (RV)
 d. Vital capacity (VC)

Q5. A 45-year-old smoker presents with shortness of breath. Which pulmonary function test would be most appropriate for assessing airflow limitation?
   a. Spirometry
   b. Diffusion capacity testing
   c. Bronchoprovocation test
   d. Cardiopulmonary exercise testing

Q6. A patient with suspected asthma complains of episodic wheezing and chest tightness. Which test would help confirm the diagnosis?
   a. Bronchoprovocation test
   b. Cardiopulmonary exercise testing
   c. Spirometry
   d. Lung volume measurements

Q7. A 60-year-old patient with COPD experiences difficulty exhaling completely. Which lung volume is most likely to be increased in this patient?
   a. Inspiratory reserve volume (IRV)
   b. Expiratory reserve volume (ERV)
   c. Tidal volume (TV)
   d. Residual volume (RV)

Q8. A 35-year-old athlete presents with exercise intolerance. Which dynamic lung volume would be most relevant to assess exercise capacity?
   a. Forced vital capacity (FVC)
   b. Forced expiratory volume in one second ($FEV_1$)
   c. Peak expiratory flow rate (PEFR)
   d. Maximal voluntary ventilation (MVV)

Q9. How does spirometry measure lung volumes and capacities?
   a. By assessing gas exchange efficiency
   b. By analyzing airflow rates during forced breathing maneuvers
   c. By measuring diffusion capacity
   d. By monitoring heart function

Q10. In which condition would you expect to see a decreased forced expiratory volume in one second ($FEV_1$)?
   a. Chronic obstructive pulmonary disease (COPD)
   b. Pulmonary fibrosis
   c. Asthma
   d. Pneumonia

Q11. What is the significance of total lung capacity (TLC) in pulmonary function testing?
   a. It reflects the maximum volume of air the lungs can hold
   b. It measures the efficiency of gas exchange
   c. It assesses airway resistance
   d. It evaluates lung compliance

Q12. How does body plethysmography measure lung volumes?
   a. By analyzing gas exchange efficiency
   b. By assessing airflow rates during forced breathing maneuvers
   c. By measuring changes in pressure within a sealed chamber
   d. By monitoring heart function

Q13. Which pulmonary function test is most appropriate for evaluating gas exchange efficiency?
   a. Spirometry
   b. Diffusion capacity testing
   c. Lung volume measurements
   d. Bronchoprovocation test

Q14. A patient with suspected restrictive lung disease would likely have which characteristic spirometric finding?
   a. Decreased forced vital capacity (FVC)
   b. Decreased forced expiratory volume in one second ($FEV_1$)
   c. Decreased residual volume (RV)
   d. Decreased peak expiratory flow rate (PEFR)

Q15. What is the primary purpose of measuring bronchial hyperresponsiveness in pulmonary function testing?
   a. To evaluate gas exchange efficiency
   b. To assess lung volumes and capacities
   c. To confirm the diagnosis of asthma
   d. To monitor heart function

Q16. Which lung volume represents the maximum amount of air the lungs can hold after a maximum inhalation?
   a. Inspiratory reserve volume (IRV)
   b. Expiratory reserve volume (ERV)
   c. Total lung capacity (TLC)
   d. Functional residual capacity (FRC)

Q17. In which condition would you expect to see an increased total lung capacity (TLC)?
   a. Asthma
   b. Chronic obstructive pulmonary disease (COPD)
   c. Pulmonary fibrosis
   d. Pneumonia

Q18. What is the primary function of measuring dynamic lung volumes and capacities?
   a. To assess gas exchange efficiency
   b. To evaluate lung compliance
   c. To monitor airway resistance
   d. To assess airflow rates during breathing maneuvers

Q19. A patient with chronic bronchitis presents with chronic cough and sputum production. Which pulmonary function test would be most useful in assessing airway obstruction?
   a. Spirometry
   b. Diffusion capacity testing
   c. Lung volume measurements
   d. Cardiopulmonary exercise testing

Q20. Which of the following conditions is characterized by decreased diffusion capacity?
   a. Asthma            b. Pulmonary embolism
   c. Pulmonary fibrosis  d. Pleural effusion

**ANSWERS**

1. b  2. b  3. b  4. d  5. a  6. a  7. d  8. d  9. b  10. a  11. a  12. c  13. b  14. a
15. c  16. c  17. c  18. d  19. a  20. c

# Pulmonary Circulation

**CHAPTER 52**

> **COMPETENCY ADDRESSED**
>
> **PY5.10:** Describe and discuss regional circulation including microcirculation, lymphatic circulation, coronary, cerebral, capillary, skin, fetal, pulmonary and splanchnic circulation.

> **LEARNING OBJECTIVES**
>
> At the end of this chapter, the learner should be able to:
> - Describe the physiological anatomy of the pulmonary circulation.
> - Describe the blood volume, blood flow and pressures in the pulmonary circulation.
> - Describe the zones of the pulmonary circulations and their physio-clinical significance.
> - Describe the capillary fluid dynamics in the pulmonary circulation.
> - Describe the physiological basis, pathophysiology, clinical features and management of pulmonary edema and pleural effusion.

## PHYSIOLOGICAL ANATOMY OF PULMONARY CIRCULATION (FIG. 52.1)

Our body has the two major circulatory systems, connected in series, the pulmonary circulation and the systemic circulation. The pulmonary circulation makes the low-pressure system, originating from the right ventricle through the pulmonary trunk, carrying the deoxygenated blood to the lungs. The lungs also receive the oxygenated blood from the bronchial arteries, arising from the descending aorta. The bronchial arteries supply the bronchi and the connective tissue septa. Hence, the lungs have a dual blood supply; the major supply from pulmonary arteries and minor supply (2% of cardiac output) from bronchial arteries.

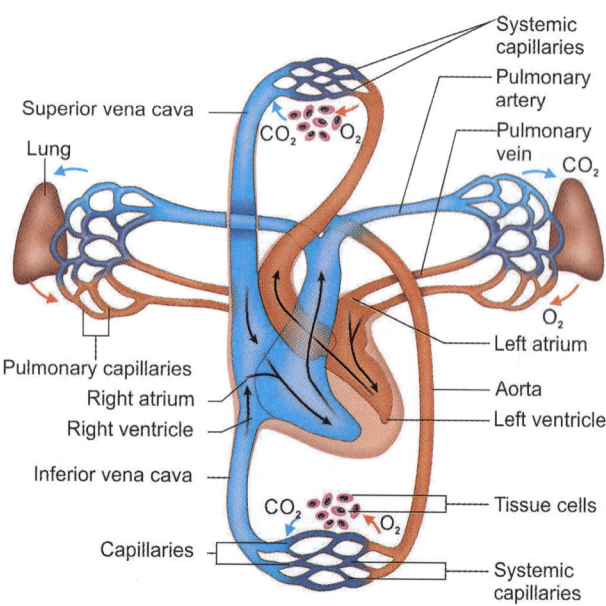

**Fig. 52.1:** Pulmonary circulation.

### Pulmonary Vessels (Fig. 52.2)

The pulmonary artery originates from the pulmonary trunk, after it bifurcates into the right and left main branches. It further divides into pulmonary arteries, arterioles, and capillaries. The pulmonary vessels have thin walls and large diameters exhibiting higher compliance (7 mL/mm Hg). The pulmonary circulation accommodates the stroke volume of the right ventricle. The pulmonary capillaries form a network of capillaries surrounding the alveoli. There are four short pulmonary veins which drain the oxygenated blood into the left atrium.

### Bronchial Circulation

In addition to pulmonary circulation, the bronchial vessels form a distinct circulatory system supporting the lung tissues.

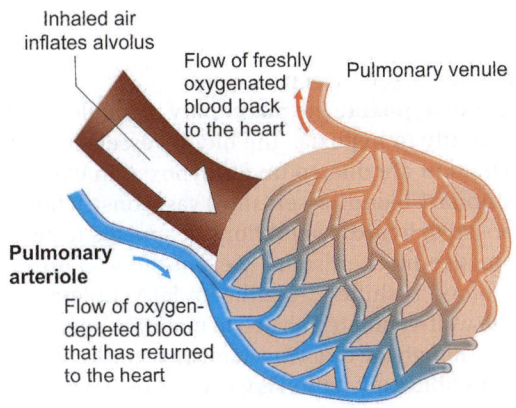

**Fig. 52.2:** Pulmonary vessels.

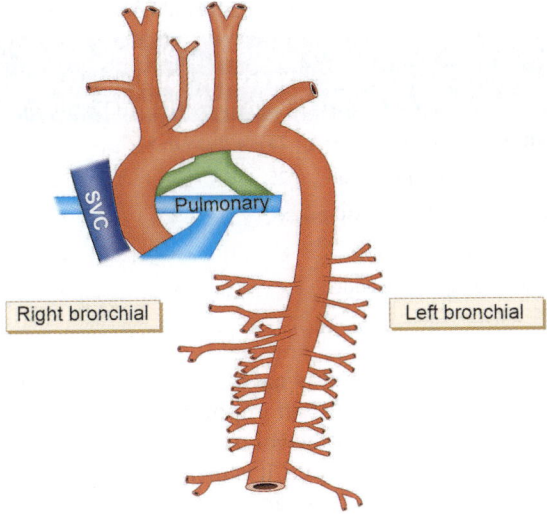

**Fig. 52.3:** Bronchial arteries originating from descending thoracic aorta.

Bronchial arteries originate from the descending thoracic aorta **(Fig. 52.3)** supplying oxygenated blood to the supporting tissues of lungs, including connective tissue and bronchi.

There are no separate bronchial veins; the deoxygenated blood drains into the pulmonary veins and then to the left atrium. Together, the venous drainage is known as bronchopulmonary anastomosis along with the drainage into mediastinal veins **(Fig. 52.4)**. It is worth mentioning here that the deoxygenated blood of bronchial circulation mixes with the oxygenated blood of pulmonary veins, returning to the left atrium of heart. Hence the blood volume of the left atrium is slightly higher than the volume of the right atrium.

## Lymphatic Circulation

The lymphatic system plays a crucial role in maintaining pulmonary health by facilitating fluid drainage and immune function. Lymphatics extend from lung tissues to the hilum and drain into the right thoracic lymphatic duct. Lymphatic circulation aids in removing particulate matter and plasma proteins, thus preventing lung edema.

## Pressures in Pulmonary Circulation

The pressure in the pulmonary circulation is much lower compared to the systemic circulation. It is primarily a reflection of left atrial pressure. Before discussing the various other details, let's go through the basic pressures in pulmonary circulation **(Table 52.1)**.

### Pulmonary Capillary Wedge Pressure (PCWP)

It is a measure of the pressure within the small blood vessels (capillaries) in the pulmonary circulation. Specifically, it reflects the pressure in the left atrium at the end of diastole when the mitral valve is closed.

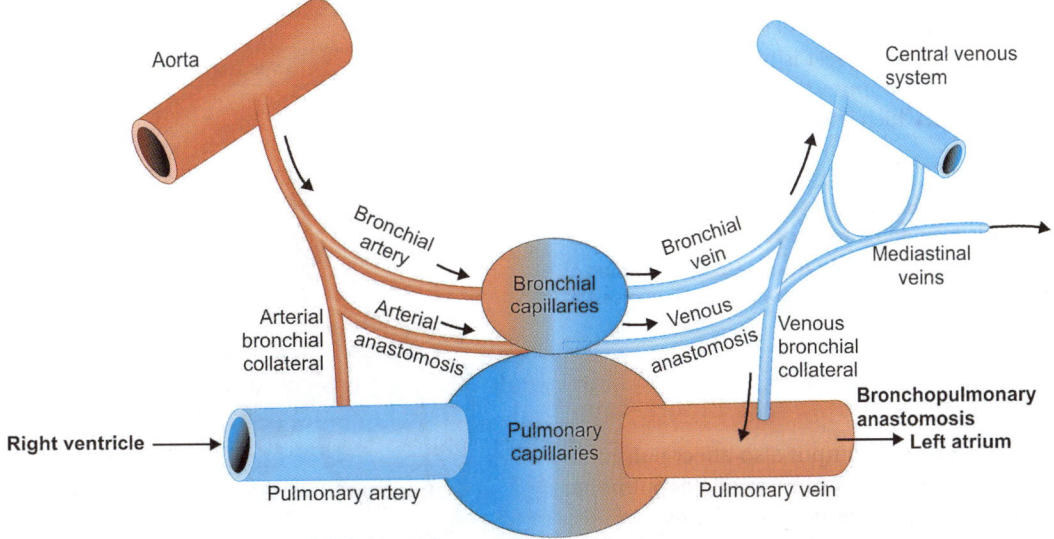

**Fig. 52.4:** Bronchopulmonary anastomosis.

**Table 52.1:** Pressures of different areas of pulmonary circulation.

| | Systolic pressure (mm Hg) | Diastolic pressure (mm Hg) | Mean pressure (mm Hg) |
|---|---|---|---|
| Right ventricle pressure | 25 | 0–1 | - |
| Pulmonary artery pressure | 25 | 8 | 15 |
| Pulmonary capillary pressure | x | x | 7 |
| Left atrial pressure | x | x | 2 |
| Pulmonary capillary wedge pressure | x | x | 5 |

PCWP is often used as an *indirect estimate of left atrial pressure*, which is an important *indicator of left ventricular preload* or the volume of blood entering the left ventricle during diastole. It is measured by inserting a catheter into a small pulmonary artery and then advancing it until it wedges into a small pulmonary blood vessel. This allows the catheter to directly measure the pressure within the pulmonary capillaries, providing valuable information about the filling pressure of the left side of the heart. *The normal PCWP is measured as 5 mm Hg, which is 2–3 mm Hg greater than the left atrial pressure.*

Clinically, PCWP measurement is frequently used in the management of patients with heart failure, pulmonary hypertension, and other cardiopulmonary conditions to assess left ventricular function, guide fluid management, and monitor response to therapy.
- A high PCWP may indicate fluid overload, left heart failure, pulmonary hypertension.
- A low PCWP may suggest hypovolemia, reduced left ventricular filling.

## BLOOD VOLUME AND FLOW IN PULMONARY CIRCULATION

The volume and flow dynamics of blood within the pulmonary circulation are crucial for understanding its function.

Approximately 450 mL, constituting around 9% of the total cardiac output. Out of this 450 mL, 70 mL is present in pulmonary capillaries, the rest is present in pulmonary arteries and veins. In one minute, the pulmonary blood flow ranges from 5–6 L/min which is equivalent to cardiac output.

> **Q: What will happen to pulmonary blood volume, in a patient of mitral regurgitation/mitral stenosis?**
> The pulmonary blood volume increases due to the damming of blood in the lungs, increasing the pulmonary capillary pressure and resulting in pulmonary edema.

### Factors Affecting the Pulmonary Blood Flow

All factors affecting cardiac output also affect pulmonary blood flow, as right ventricular output regulates pulmonary blood flow. These factors are enumerated below:
1. Stroke volume of right ventricle
2. Heart rate
3. Venous return
4. Exercise
5. Increased tissue oxygen demand
6. **Effect of hypoxia:** The pulmonary blood flow behaves differently to hypoxia. The blood vessels in systemic circulation are dilated under hypoxia. In contrast the pulmonary blood vessels show vasoconstriction when exposed to hypoxic conditions. It appears to act as the protective mechanism to prevent the V/Q mismatch. The blood is shifted from the under-ventilated alveoli to the well-ventilated alveoli to maintain adequate V/Q ratio. Though the exact mechanism of this is not known, the possible explanation is given in the **Flowchart 52.1**.

## Role of Hydrostatic Pressure Gradients

The lowermost part of the lungs is 30 cm below the uppermost part, having a pressure of 23 mm Hg **(Fig. 52.5)**. Out of this 23 mm Hg, 15 mm Hg is above and 8 mm Hg is below the level of heart. This pressure difference creates three different zones of perfusion in the lungs depending on the perfusion pressure of capillaries (which distends the capillaries) and the alveolar air pressure (which compresses the capillaries from the outside) **(Fig. 52.6)**.

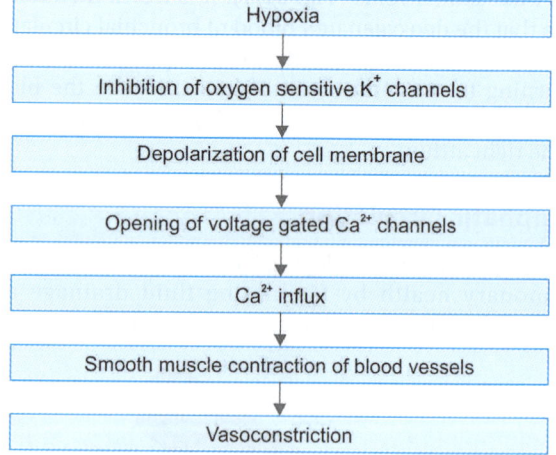

**Flowchart 52.1:** Mechanism of effect of hypoxia.

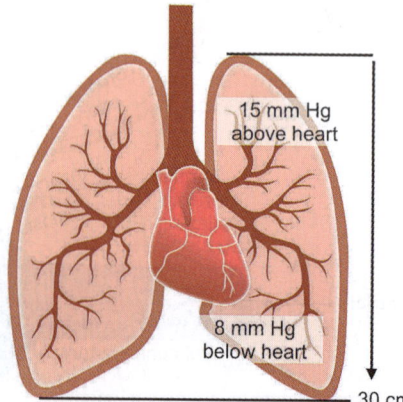

**Fig. 52.5:** Pressure differences in parts of lungs.

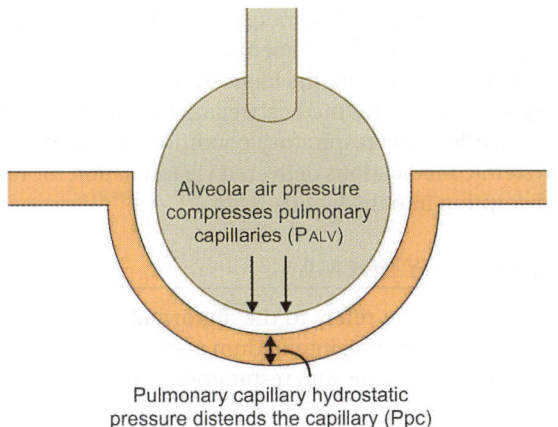

**Fig. 52.6:** Effects of alveolar air pressure and hydrostatic pressure on capillaries.

**Zone 1: No blood flow during any phase of cardiac cycle.** The alveolar air pressure ($P_{ALV}$) remains higher than the capillary hydrostatic pressure (Ppc) through all the phases of cardiac cycle. Hence, even during the systolic phase, there is no blood flow. This zone does not occur in healthy individuals. But it can be seen if Ppc becomes low as seen in patients with hypotension, severe hemorrhage. Even the patients with a high $P_{ALV}$ due to positive pressure ventilation (for a patient on artificial ventilation on positive pressure, PEEP mode).

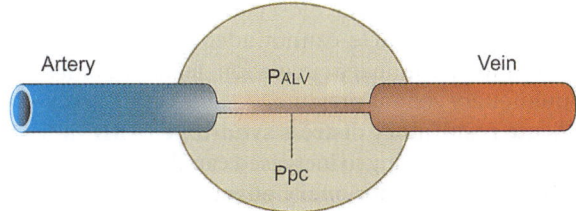

**Zone 2: Intermittent blood flow** during peaks of pulmonary arterial pressure due to systole of right ventricle, but there is no flow in diastolic phase. This zone is seen in the apices of the lungs, about 10 cm above mid-level of heart to the top of lungs. Blood flow will occur during the phases where Ppc is more than $P_{ALV}$.

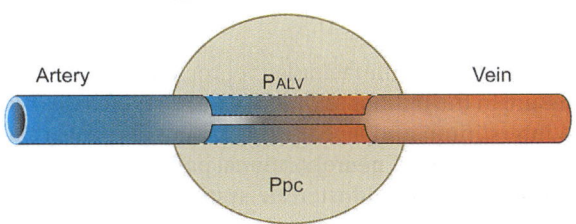

**Zone 3: Continuous blood flow during all phases of cardiac cycle.** It is seen in the lower regions of the lungs, where the Ppc is always more than $P_{ALV}$, i.e., from 10 cm above mid-level of heart to the base of heart. When a patient is lying down, the entire lung is converted into zone 3. That is why patients with left ventricular failure develop breathlessness on lying down (orthopnea).

During exercise, there is an increase in blood flow to all parts of lungs, converting the entire lung into zone 3.

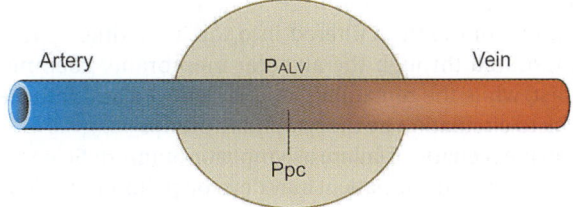

### Role of Pulmonary Circulation with Increased Left Atrial Pressure in Left Sided Heart Failure

In left heart failure, the left atrial pressure increases from 1 to 5 mm Hg to 40–50 mm Hg. If the left atrial pressure becomes more than 7–8 mm Hg, the increase in pulmonary arterial pressure causes pulmonary edema.

### Capillary Exchange and Fluid Dynamics (Fig. 52.7)

Like any other capillaries, the fluid dynamics follow the Starling Forces of the fluid dynamics. From the **Figure 52.7**, we can deduce that the mean net filtration pressure of +1 mm Hg is generated by the mathematical sum of the starling forces. Furthermore, the surface tension at the

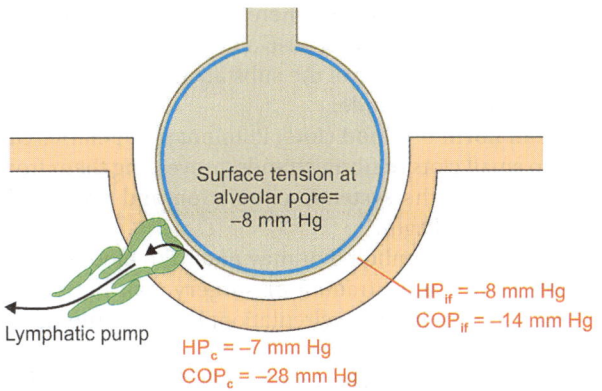

| | mm Hg |
|---|---|
| *Forces tending to cause movement of fluid outward from the capillaries and into the pulmonary Interstitium:* | |
| Capillary pressure | 7 |
| Interstitial fluid colloid osmotic pressure | 14 |
| Negative interstitial fluid pressure | 8 |
| Total outward force | 29 |
| *Forces tending to cause absorption of fluid into the capillaries:* | |
| Plasma colloid osmotic pressure | 28 |
| Total inward force | 28 |
| Total outward force | +29 |
| Total inward force | −28 |
| Mean filtration pressure | +1 |

The mean filtration pressure of +1 mm Hg leads to increased fluid in the interstitial fluid, which is pumped back into the circulation by the lymphatics

**Fig. 52.7:** Capillary exchange and fluid dynamics.

alveolar pore is present, creating a pressure gradient of –8 mm Hg, which increases further with the deficiency of surfactant.

Some of the fluid filtered into the interstitial space is evaporated through the alveolar membrane, keeping it moist, while the remaining fluid is removed and returned back to circulation by the lymphatic pump.

In the scenario of failure of lymphatic pump/deficiency of surface tension, the patient may develop pulmonary edema.

## FUNCTIONS OF PULMONARY CIRCULATION

### Reservoir for the Left Ventricle

Pulmonary circulation serves as a reservoir for the left ventricle by accommodating a portion of the blood pumped by the right ventricle during systole. This reservoir function helps regulate blood volume and maintain optimal cardiac output. During diastole, when the left ventricle relaxes, blood from the pulmonary circulation flows back into the left atrium and ventricle, ensuring a continuous blood supply to the systemic circulation.

### It Acts as a Filter

Pulmonary circulation acts as a filter by trapping and removing various substances that may be present in the bloodstream. This filtration process occurs primarily in the pulmonary capillaries, where the thin walls allow for the exchange of gases while also allowing certain particles to be filtered out. Some of the substances that pulmonary circulation filters include:

- **Small fibrin or blood clots:** Pulmonary capillaries can trap small clots or fibrin strands, preventing them from traveling to the systemic circulation and potentially causing blockages.
- **Fat cells:** Fat emboli that may enter the bloodstream, particularly after trauma or surgery, can be filtered out by the pulmonary circulation, reducing the risk of embolic events.
- **Detached cancer cells:** Cancer cells that have detached from primary tumors and entered the bloodstream can be captured by pulmonary capillaries, preventing their dissemination to other organs and potentially reducing the risk of metastasis. They are removed by the Pulmonary alveolar macrophages (PAM cells).
- **Gas bubbles:** In conditions such as decompression sickness or iatrogenic air embolism, gas bubbles may enter the bloodstream. The pulmonary circulation helps to filter out these gas bubbles, preventing them from causing harm to other organs.

### Fluid Exchange and Drug Absorption

- Pulmonary circulation facilitates fluid exchange between the bloodstream and the surrounding lung tissue. This exchange is important for maintaining the balance of fluids within the lungs, preventing conditions such as pulmonary edema.
- Additionally, the thin membrane of the pulmonary capillaries allows for efficient absorption of drugs and other substances into the bloodstream. This property is exploited in various medical treatments, such as inhaled medications for respiratory conditions like asthma or systemic medications delivered via inhalation for rapid absorption into the bloodstream.

## PULMONARY EDEMA

Pulmonary edema refers to the abnormal accumulation of fluid within the lung interstitium and alveoli, leading to impaired gas exchange and respiratory distress.

### Physiological Basis

Pulmonary edema disrupts the delicate balance between fluid filtration and reabsorption in the lungs. Under normal circumstances, the pulmonary capillaries maintain a low hydrostatic pressure that prevents excessive fluid leakage into the interstitium. However, conditions such as increased capillary permeability, elevated pulmonary venous pressure, or decreased lymphatic drainage can disrupt this balance, resulting in fluid accumulation.

### Causes

- **Left heart failure:** The most common cause, where the failing left ventricle cannot adequately pump blood out of the pulmonary circulation, leading to increased pulmonary venous pressure.
- **Acute respiratory distress syndrome (ARDS):** Severe lung injury leading to increased capillary permeability.
- **High-altitude pulmonary edema (HAPE):** Occurs at high altitudes due to hypoxic pulmonary vasoconstriction and increased capillary pressure.
- **Fluid overload:** Excessive intravenous fluid administration or renal failure leading to volume overload.
- **Infection:** Pneumonia or other lung infections can cause inflammation and increased capillary permeability.

### Pathogenesis

In left heart failure, the failing left ventricle leads to increased pressure in the pulmonary veins, causing fluid to leak into the interstitium and alveoli. This process is exacerbated by the activation of neurohormonal pathways, such as the renin-angiotensin-aldosterone system, which promotes sodium and water retention. As fluid accumulates, it impairs gas exchange and leads to respiratory distress.

### Clinical Features

- **Dyspnea:** Initially on exertion, progressing to orthopnea and paroxysmal nocturnal dyspnea.
- Tachypnea and respiratory distress.
- Pink, frothy sputum due to blood-tinged pulmonary edema fluid.

- Crackles or rales on auscultation of the lungs.
- Hypoxemia and cyanosis.
- Anxiety and restlessness.

> **CASE SCENARIO: LEFT HEART FAILURE WITH PULMONARY EDEMA**
>
> Mr Kamlesh, a 65-year-old male with a history of hypertension and coronary artery disease, presents to the emergency department with severe shortness of breath and coughing up pink, frothy sputum. He reports worsening dyspnea over the past few days, especially when lying flat.
>
> On examination, Mr Kamlesh appears anxious and tachypneic. Auscultation reveals bilateral crackles in the lung bases. His oxygen saturation is 88% on room air. An electrocardiogram shows evidence of left ventricular hypertrophy and strain pattern.
>
> Based on the clinical presentation and history, Mr Kamlesh is diagnosed with acute pulmonary edema secondary to left heart failure exacerbation.
>
> Treatment involves oxygen supplementation, diuretics to reduce fluid overload, and medications to improve left ventricular function, such as angiotensin-converting enzyme inhibitors or beta-blockers.

## Management

- Oxygen therapy is used to improve oxygenation.
- Diuretics are used to reduce fluid overload and pulmonary congestion.
- Vasodilators (e.g., nitroglycerin) to reduce preload and afterload on the heart.
- Positive pressure ventilation in severe cases to improve oxygenation and reduce respiratory distress.
- Treating the underlying cause, such as optimizing heart failure management.
- Monitoring fluid balance and electrolytes closely to prevent dehydration or electrolyte imbalances.

## PLEURAL EFFUSION

Pleural effusion refers to the accumulation of excess fluid in the pleural space, the thin fluid-filled space between the layers of the pleura (the membranes surrounding the lungs) **(Fig. 52.8)**. This accumulation of fluid can impair lung function and lead to respiratory symptoms.

## Physiological Basis

Under normal conditions, there is a small amount of fluid present in the pleural space, which helps lubricate the surfaces of the pleura and facilitates smooth lung expansion during breathing. However, when there is an imbalance between fluid production and absorption or when there is increased leakage of fluid into the pleural space, pleural effusion can occur.

## Causes

- **Congestive heart failure:** Elevated pressure in the blood vessels surrounding the lungs can lead to leakage of fluid into the pleural space.
- **Pneumonia or lung infections:** Inflammatory processes in the lungs can lead to increased production of pleural fluid.
- **Malignancy:** Cancer cells can spread to the pleura and stimulate fluid production or block lymphatic drainage, leading to pleural effusion.
- **Pulmonary embolism:** Blood clots in the pulmonary blood vessels can cause inflammation and leakage of fluid into the pleural space.
- **Liver disease:** Conditions such as cirrhosis can lead to increased pressure in the veins surrounding the lungs, resulting in pleural effusion.

## Pathogenesis

The pathogenesis of pleural effusion involves the disruption of the normal balance between fluid production and absorption in the pleural space. This imbalance can occur due to increased hydrostatic pressure, decreased oncotic pressure, increased permeability of the pleural membranes, or impaired lymphatic drainage. As a result, fluid accumulates in the pleural space, compressing the lung and causing respiratory symptoms.

## Clinical Features

- **Dyspnea:** Shortness of breath, especially with exertion.
- **Pleuritic chest pain:** Sharp chest pain worsened by deep breathing or coughing.
- **Decreased breath sounds:** On auscultation of the lungs, there may be decreased or absent breath sounds over the affected area.
- **Dullness to percussion:** Percussion of the chest may reveal a dull sound over the area of pleural effusion.
- **Decreased tactile fremitus:** Palpation of the chest may reveal decreased or absent tactile fremitus over the affected area.
- **Pleural friction rub:** In some cases, a pleural friction rub may be heard on auscultation, indicating inflammation of the pleural membranes.

> **CASE SCENARIO: CONGESTIVE HEART FAILURE WITH PLEURAL EFFUSION**
>
> Mr Gupta, a 70-year-old male with a history of hypertension and coronary artery disease, presents to the clinic with progressive shortness of breath and pleuritic chest pain. He reports increased swelling in her legs and weight gain over the past month.

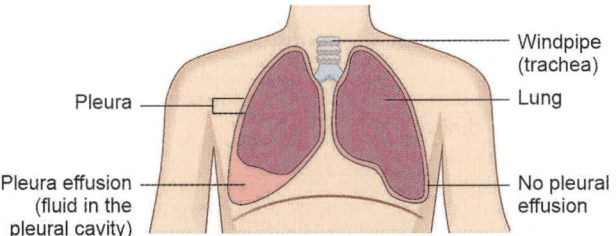

**Fig. 52.8:** Pleural effusion.

On examination, Mr Gupta appears tachypneic and in respiratory distress. Chest auscultation reveals decreased breath sounds and dullness to percussion over the right lower lung field. An ultrasound or chest X-ray confirms the presence of a moderate-sized pleural effusion on the right side.

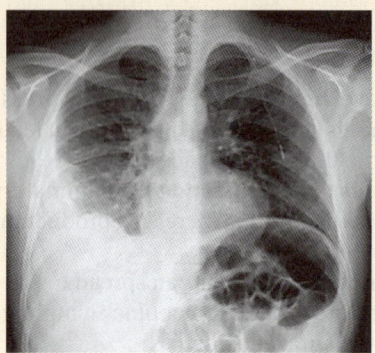

Based on the clinical presentation and history, Mr Gupta is diagnosed with pleural effusion secondary to congestive heart failure exacerbation. Treatment involves addressing the underlying heart failure with diuretics to reduce fluid overload and medications to improve cardiac function. Thoracentesis may be performed to drain the pleural fluid and relieve respiratory symptoms.

## Management

1. Treating the underlying cause, such as heart failure, pneumonia, or malignancy.
2. **Thoracentesis:** Draining excess pleural fluid using a needle inserted into the pleural space.
3. **Pleurodesis:** Inducing adhesion between the layers of the pleura to prevent recurrence of pleural effusion.
4. **Chest tube insertion:** In severe cases or when thoracentesis is not feasible, a chest tube may be inserted to drain the pleural fluid continuously **(Fig. 52.9)**.
5. **Symptomatic relief:** Analgesics may be prescribed to alleviate pleuritic chest pain, and supplemental oxygen may be provided to improve oxygenation.

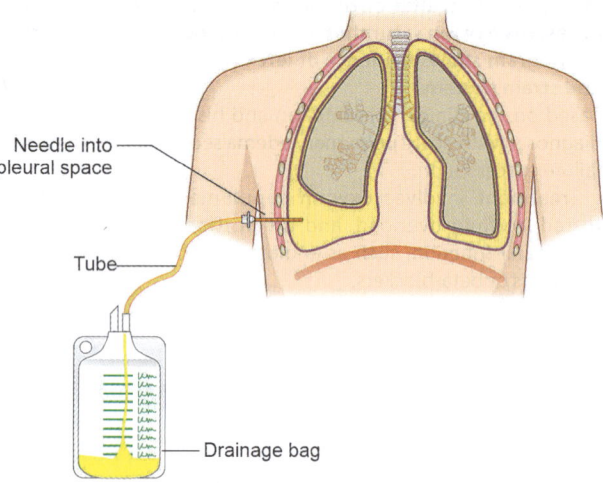

**Fig. 52.9:** Chest tube insertion for drainage of fluid.

## SUMMARY

This chapter provides a comprehensive overview of the physiological anatomy, hemodynamics, and clinical aspects of pulmonary circulation, focusing on pulmonary edema and pleural effusion.

In this chapter we have learnt that:
- Lungs have a dual blood supply from pulmonary artery and bronchial arteries.
- The bronchial veins form the bronchopulmonary anastomosis and drain deoxygenated blood into the oxygenated blood carried by the pulmonary veins.
- The total blood flow though lungs is equal to cardiac output and around 450 mL of blood is present in the lungs at any given time.
- Depending on the blood flow during different phases of cardiac cycle, the lungs are divided into three zones. Zone 1 doesn't exist in healthy individuals. Upper part of lungs form zone 2 whereas lower part forms the zone 3.
- Accumulation of fluid in the lungs due to various causes, most common being left heart failure, results in pulmonary edema.
- However the accumulation of fluid in the pleural space is called pleural effusion.

## LET US SEE, HOW MUCH YOU HAVE LEARNT?

 *Review Questions*

### Long/Short Answer Questions

Q1. Describe the peculiarities of pulmonary circulation.
Q2. Why does the pulmonary capillaries undergo vasoconstriction in hypoxia?
Q3. What will happen to lungs, in a patient of left heart failure?
Q4. What is pulmonary capillary wedge pressure? What is its physio-clinical significance?

### Explain Why? (Reasoning Questions)

Q1. The pulmonary arteries have thinner walls compared to systemic arteries.
Q2. Pulmonary vascular resistance decreases in response to increased oxygen levels in the alveoli.

Q3. Blood flow through the pulmonary circulation increases during exercise.

Q4. Pulmonary embolism can lead to increased pulmonary vascular resistance.

## Critical Thinking Case-Based Questions

Q1. A 55-year-old man, presented with complaints of worsening shortness of breath, especially with exertion, and occasional chest pain. He had a history of hypertension and type 2 diabetes. On examination, his blood pressure was elevated, and auscultation revealed bilateral crackles in the lung bases. An echocardiogram shows signs of right ventricular hypertrophy, and a pulmonary artery catheterization indicated elevated pulmonary artery pressure. Based on the given scenario, answer the following questions:
   a. What is the probable diagnosis?
   b. Explain the physiological mechanisms underlying the pulmonary circulation in this case.
   c. What are the consequences of elevated pulmonary artery pressure on right ventricular function and pulmonary circulation?

## Multiple Choice Questions

Q1. Mr Patel, a 55-year-old male, presents to the emergency department with severe dyspnea and frothy pink sputum. His medical history includes hypertension and coronary artery disease. Based on the provided scenario, what is the most likely cause of his symptoms?
   a. Pulmonary embolism
   b. Left heart failure
   c. Pneumonia
   d. Chronic obstructive pulmonary disease (COPD)

Q2. In a patient with left heart failure, which of the following changes is most likely to occur in the pressures within the pulmonary circulation?
   a. Decrease in pulmonary artery pressure
   b. Increase in mean pulmonary capillary pressure
   c. Decrease in left atrial pressure
   d. Increase in right ventricular pressure

Q3. A patient with congestive heart failure presents with orthopnea and bilateral crackles on lung auscultation. Which of the following findings is most consistent with pulmonary edema?
   a. Decreased oxygen saturation
   b. Absent tactile fremitus
   c. Hyperresonance to percussion
   d. Wheezing on auscultation

Q4. What effect would a decrease in left ventricular preload have on pulmonary capillary wedge pressure (PCWP) in a patient with heart failure?
   a. Increase in PCWP
   b. Decrease in PCWP
   c. No change in PCWP
   d. Increase in PCWP followed by a decrease

Q5. A patient with a history of cirrhosis presents with progressive dyspnea and dullness to percussion over the right lung base. What is the most likely cause of these findings?
   a. Pulmonary embolism     b. Right-sided heart failure
   c. Pleural effusion             d. Pneumothorax

Q6. How does hypoxia affect pulmonary vascular resistance and blood flow distribution in the lungs?
   a. Increases pulmonary vascular resistance and shifts blood flow to poorly ventilated areas
   b. Decreases pulmonary vascular resistance and shifts blood flow to well-ventilated areas
   c. Increases pulmonary vascular resistance and shifts blood flow to well-ventilated areas
   d. Decreases pulmonary vascular resistance and shifts blood flow to poorly ventilated areas

Q7. A patient with acute respiratory distress syndrome (ARDS) presents with severe hypoxemia and diffuse bilateral infiltrates on chest X-ray. Which of the following mechanisms is most likely contributing to the development of pulmonary edema in this patient?
   a. Increased pulmonary capillary permeability
   b. Left ventricular failure
   c. Pulmonary artery vasoconstriction
   d. Lymphatic obstruction

Q8. How does thoracentesis help in the management of pleural effusion?
   a. By increasing pleural pressure
   b. By removing excess pleural fluid and relieving respiratory symptoms
   c. By promoting pleural adhesion and preventing fluid accumulation
   d. By decreasing pleural compliance

Q9. A patient presents with sudden onset dyspnea and pleuritic chest pain. Imaging reveals a wedge-shaped infiltrate in the lung parenchyma. What is the most likely diagnosis?
   a. Pulmonary edema        b. Pneumothorax
   c. Pulmonary embolism    d. Pleural effusion

Q10. How does the hydrostatic pressure gradient between the pulmonary capillaries and interstitium contribute to fluid movement in pulmonary circulation?
   a. It promotes fluid reabsorption into the capillaries
   b. It promotes fluid filtration into the interstitium
   c. It has no effect on fluid movement
   d. It regulates fluid distribution within the alveoli

**ANSWERS**

1. b    2. b    3. a    4. a    5. c    6. a    7. a    8. b    9. c    10. b

# Transport of Respiratory Gases
## (Oxygen and Carbon Dioxide)

**CHAPTER 53**

> **COMPETENCY ADDRESSED**
> PY6.3: Describe and discuss the transport of respiratory gases: Oxygen and carbon dioxide.

> **LEARNING OBJECTIVES**
> **At the end of this chapter, the learner should be able to:**
> - Describe the transport of oxygen from lungs to the tissues in combined and dissolved form.
> - Explain the mechanism of formation of oxygenated hemoglobin.
> - Describe the relationship between oxygen hemoglobin binding through the oxygen-hemoglobin dissociation curve under normal circumstance and special circumstances.
> - Draw a labeled diagram of the $O_2$-hemoglobin dissociation curve.
> - Explain the mechanism of oxygen delivery to the tissue and various factors affecting it.
> - Define Bohr's effect and describe the factors responsible for it.
> - Explain the mechanism of transport of carbon dioxide in blood, in combined and dissolved form.
> - Explain the delivery of the carbon dioxide in the lungs and the $CO_2$ dissociation curves.
> - Define Haldane effect and its physio-clinical significance.

## TRANSPORT OF OXYGEN

As we have discussed in detail about the diffusion of respiratory gases across the respiratory membrane in chapter 50, let's do a brief recap of the same. At the respiratory membrane, where the alveolar and capillary walls meet, gases move across the membranes, with oxygen entering the bloodstream and carbon dioxide diffuses into blood stream. The actual exchange of gases occurs due to simple diffusion, allowing gases to flow from a higher partial pressure to lower pressures. This allows for $O_2$ to cross the alveoli and re-oxygenate the blood in the pulmonary vasculature, while $CO_2$ leaves the bloodstream and enters the alveoli where it is expired.

As studied earlier, the partial pressure of oxygen varies in different samples of air (inspired, alveolar and expired air) and in blood. Let us have a quick look at oxygen content (mL/dL) in them **(Table 53.1)**.

From the **Table 53.1**, we deduce that 100 mL of blood, extracts 5 mL of oxygen from the lungs and an equal amount of (5 mL) is delivered to the tissues.
**Oxygen enters the pulmonary capillaries in two forms:**
- **Dissolved form (3%; 0.3 mL/dL in arterial blood and 0.12 mL/dL in venous blood):**
  It delivers 0.17 mL of $O_2$ to tissues

**Table 53.1:** The partial pressures and composition of oxygen in the body.

| | $PO_2$ (mm Hg) | $O_2$ content (mL/dL of blood) |
|---|---|---|
| Inspired air | 158 | 21 |
| Expired air | 116 | 16 |
| Alveolar air | 100–104 | 13–14 |
| Arterial blood | 97–100 | 19 |
| Venous blood | 40 | 14 |

(Alveolar air to Arterial blood: 5 mL; Arterial blood to Venous blood: 5 mL)

The oxygen gets dissolved in the plasma, which is in accordance with **Henry's law**. Henry's law states that, the concentration of gas in a liquid; to which it is not chemically combined; is directly proportional to the solubility and partial pressure of that gas.

Content of dissolved $O_2$ in blood = Partial pressure of $O_2$ in arterial blood ($PaO_2$) × Solubility co-efficient ($\alpha$).

$PO_2$ of arterial blood = 100 mm Hg; $\alpha$ = 0.003 mL $O_2$ (100 mL plasma/mm Hg)

Content of dissolved $O_2$ in blood = 100 mm Hg ($PO_2$) × 0.0031 mL/mm Hg/dL ($\alpha$) = **0.31 mL/dL of blood**.

- Also, as per Henry's law, if the partial pressure of $O_2$ increases, as in the person breathing hyperbaric oxygen or 100% oxygen, the amount of dissolved oxygen would increase.

*Calculate the concentration of dissolved oxygen in person breathing at high altitude with $PO_2$ = 60 mm Hg*

Dissolved $O_2$ = $PaO_2$ × α
= 60 × 0.003
= 0.18 mL/dL

- **Combined form (97%; 19.5 mL/dL in arterial blood and 15.1 mL/dL in venous blood) Delivers 5 mL of $O_2$ to tissues.**
  In combined form, the oxygen is transported in the blood bound to the hemoglobin, an iron containing protein packed in the RBCs. Each molecule of Hb can bind 4 molecules of $O_2$. Further, *1 g/dL of Hb carries 1.34 mL of $O_2$*. This quantity is called the oxygen-binding capacity of blood. Note that oxygen carrying capacity of blood is proportional to the hematocrit of the blood.

*Calculate the oxygen carrying capacity of 100 mL of blood of a person with Hb level of 15 g/dL*

1 g/dL of Hb can carry 1.34 mL of $O_2$ in combined form
Therefore, 15 g/dL of Hb, carries 15 × 1.34 = 20.1 mL/dL

## OXYGENATION OF HEMOGLOBIN

The hemoglobin molecule has porphyrin ring have a $Fe^{2+}$ ion, which binds 4 molecules of $O_2$ to form oxy Hb (oxygenated). The oxygen combines loosely and reversibly to Hb molecule. It is an effective system for the transport of $O_2$ from lungs to the tissues. The process of oxygenation reaction takes place in 0.01 seconds.

*Remember its oxygenation and not oxidation:* Oxygenation means reversible addition of $O_2$ to the Hb molecule whereas oxidation refers to loss of electron from the $Fe^{2+}$ to form $Fe^{3+}$, forming meth Hb.

Depending on its affinity and oxygen binding, the hemoglobin exists in two interconvertible forms, taut (T) form and the relaxed or (R form) **(Fig. 53.1)**.

- **T Form (Taut form):**
  - Deoxygenated Hb, exists in T form
  - It has low affinity for $O_2$
  - Stabilized by salt bridges and 2,3 bisphosphoglycerate (2,3 BPG)
- **R Form (Relaxed form):**
  - When the first molecule of oxygen combines with the Hb, it converts the T form into R form, exposing more $O_2$ binding sites. Due to breakage of salt bridges.
  - There is 500-fold in increase in oxygen affinity, resulting in the steep phase of $O_2$-Hb dissociation curve.
  - As $O_2$ binds, 2,3-BPG and $CO_2$ are expelled out.

*Saturation of hemoglobin:* It is defined as the percentage of Hb that is combined with $O_2$.
- **At 100 mm Hg of $PO_2$** = Hb is 97.5% saturated with $O_2$ (Arterial blood)

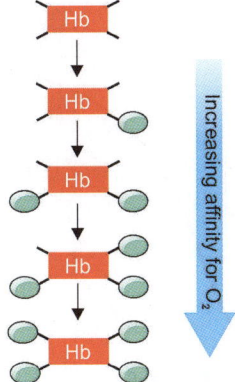

**Fig. 53.1:** Affinity of oxygen in T and R form.

- At 90 mm Hg of $PO_2$ = Hb is 96.5% saturated with $O_2$
- At 80 mm Hg of $PO_2$ = Hb is 94.5% saturated with $O_2$
- At 70 mm Hg of $PO_2$ = Hb is 92.7% saturated with $O_2$
- At 60 mm Hg of $PO_2$ = Hb is 89% saturated with $O_2$
- **At 40 mm Hg of $PO_2$** = Hb is 75% saturated with $O_2$ (Venous blood)
- % age saturation of Hb with $O_2$

$$= \frac{O_2 \text{ content of blood}/100 \text{ mL} \times 100}{O_2 \text{ carrying capacity of blood}}$$

*Saturation of Hb with Oxygen*
Arterial blood → 97% saturated
Venous blood → 75% saturated

## OXYGEN HEMOGLOBIN DISSOCIATION CURVE

It is a graphical representation of the relationship between the partial pressure of oxygen ($PO_2$) in the blood and the saturation of hemoglobin with oxygen. *It is S shaped/sigmoid curve* **(Fig. 53.2)**.

At low partial pressures of oxygen (such as in tissues), hemoglobin has a lower affinity for oxygen, meaning it releases oxygen more readily to the tissues. As the partial pressure of oxygen increases (such as in the lungs), affinity of hemoglobin for oxygen increases, allowing it to bind more readily. It has two phases, steep phase and plateau phase.

### Steep Phase

It is seen between the $PO_2$ of 10–60 mm Hg. The hemoglobin has very high affinity to bind with oxygen. The loading of hemoglobin (binding of oxygen with Hb) occurs in lungs. *It is equally important to understand that the affinity decreases as rapidly, when the $PO_2$ decreases from 60 to 10 mm Hg.* In a healthy individual, it is seen in tissues where $PO_2$ decreases in tissues, resulting in unloading of oxygen.

**Physio-clinical significance:** If a person ascends to the high altitude, where $PO_2$ below 60 mm Hg, the oxygen

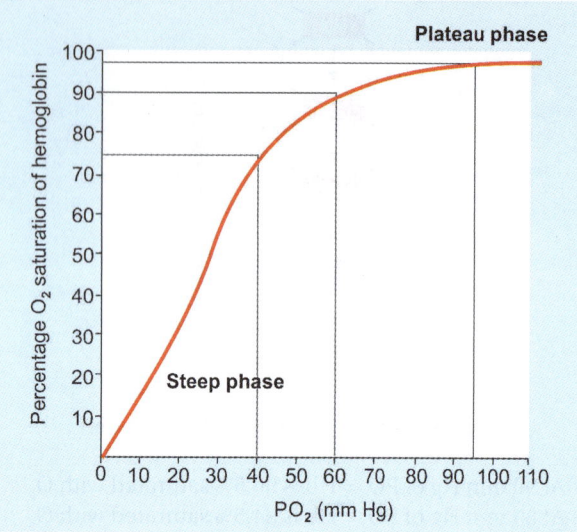

**Fig. 53.2:** Oxygen Hb dissociation curve (*At 40 mm Hg, Hb is 75% saturated; at 60 mm Hg it is 89% saturated and at 95 mm Hg, it is 97% saturated*).

dissociation will be very rapid. Hence, the person may require oxygen cylinders to maintain oxygen saturation.

## Plateau Phase

The oxygen dissociation curve plateaus at *above 60 mm Hg and flattens at 70 mm Hg, meaning that an increase in $PO_2$ above 60 mm Hg only results in a small increase in oxygen binding.*

**Physiological significance of plateau phase:**
- The plateau phase is seen between the $PO_2$ level of 60 to 100 mm Hg. This provides a safety factor for the percentage saturation of Hb with $O_2$. *This applies that the saturation doesn't fall below 90% even if the $PO_2$ falls to 60 mm Hg.*
- When the partial pressure of oxygen in the alveoli fluctuates widely, the saturation of hemoglobin with oxygen remains relatively constant. This means that even with variations in the concentration of oxygen in the lungs, the blood is still efficiently loaded with oxygen.

  At sea level, where the atmospheric pressure is relatively high, breathing 100% oxygen or hyperventilating doesn't significantly increase the oxygen content in the blood for healthy individuals. This is because under normal conditions, hemoglobin is already almost fully saturated with oxygen when the partial pressure of oxygen in the alveoli is around 100 mm Hg. However, in individuals with lung diseases or at high altitudes where the partial pressure of oxygen in the alveoli is lower than normal, hyperventilating or breathing pure oxygen can indeed increase the saturation of hemoglobin with oxygen. This is because these individuals may initially have more deoxygenated hemoglobin in their blood, so providing more oxygen allows them to reach higher levels of hemoglobin saturation.

## SHIFT OF $O_2$-Hb DISSOCIATION CURVE

The $O_2$-Hb dissociation curve, discussed above, is shown in the ideal conditions. It can be shifted to the right when the Hb needs to deliver the oxygen (as seen in tissue) or it can be shifted to left, when the Hb needs to bind with $O_2$. Let's what are all the factors, which result in shifting of the curve to right or left.

### Shift to Right

A right shift indicates a decrease in hemoglobin's affinity for $O_2$, causing release of $O_2$ to the tissues. This leads to a lower level of oxygen saturation of hemoglobin at every level of $PO_2$, compared to the normal curve. Consequently, more offloading of $O_2$ occurs (**Fig. 53.3**).

> **Factors shifting the curve to right:**
> 1. Decreased $PO_2$
> 2. Increased $PCO_2$
> 3. Increased temperature
> 4. Increased $H^+$
> 5. Increased 2,3, BPG

Factors resulting in right shift are:
- **Decreased $PO_2$:** Due to rapid consumption of $O_2$ by the metabolically active tissues.
- **Increased $PCO_2$:** Due to the accumulation of $CO_2$ resulting from rapid metabolism in the tissues.
- **Increased $H^+$ concentration:** Due to accumulation of lactic acid and other acids by the metabolically active tissues.
- **Increased body temperature:** In the metabolically active tissues.
- **Increased 2,3 BPG:** An increase in the concentration of 2,3-BPG decreases the affinity of Hb for $O_2$ and shifts the normal $O_2$-Hb dissociation curve to the right. *The causes of increased levels of 2,3-BPG are thyroid hormone,*

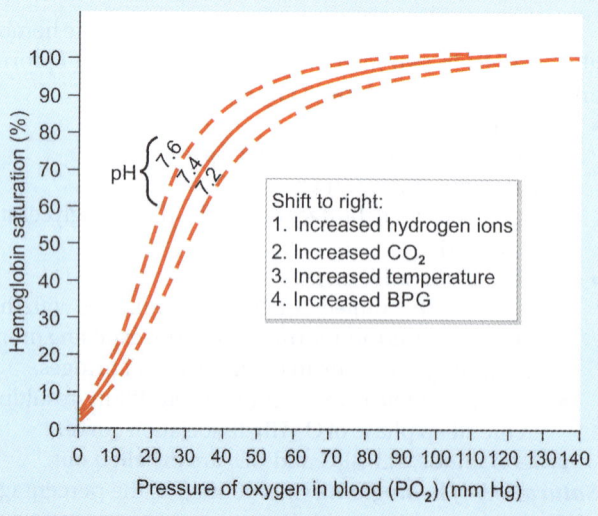

**Fig. 53.3:** Graph showing shift to right decreasing hemoglobin affinity.

growth hormone, androgen, anemia, exposure to chronic hypoxia at high altitudes, and certain pulmonary diseases. However, acidosis decreases the level of 2,3-BPG.

*In stored blood (blood bank blood), 2,3-BPG also falls, and the ability to release oxygen in the tissues is reduced. Hence, transfusion of stored blood is less effective for hypoxic patients.*

While the right shift has its advantage at the level of tissues, it is of disadvantage at the lung level.

### Bohr's Effect
The Bohr effect refers to the phenomenon where the affinity of hemoglobin for oxygen decreases as the partial pressure of carbon dioxide ($PCO_2$) or the acidity (pH) of the blood increases. It was first described by Danish physiologist Christian Bohr in 1904.

**Factors:**
1. **Carbon dioxide ($PCO_2$):** An increase in carbon dioxide levels in the blood leads to a decrease in pH due to the formation of carbonic acid. This decrease in pH causes hemoglobin to release oxygen more readily.
2. **pH:** As pH decreases, the affinity of hemoglobin for oxygen decreases, facilitating oxygen release to the tissues.
3. **Temperature:** Higher temperatures also promote the release of oxygen from hemoglobin, though the Bohr effect primarily operates through changes in $PCO_2$ and pH.

**Physiological significance:** The Bohr effect plays a crucial role in the transport and delivery of oxygen to tissues. When tissues are metabolically active and produce carbon dioxide and acidic byproducts, such as during exercise, the Bohr effect helps ensure that oxygen is released from hemoglobin where it's needed most. This mechanism ensures efficient oxygen delivery to tissues with increased metabolic demands.

**Clinical significance:**
1. **Exercise physiology:** During physical activity, muscles generate carbon dioxide and lactic acid, leading to localized increases in $PCO_2$ and acidity. The Bohr effect facilitates oxygen release from hemoglobin in active tissues, optimizing oxygen delivery for energy production.
2. **Respiratory diseases:** In conditions such as chronic obstructive pulmonary disease (COPD) or emphysema, where there's impaired gas exchange and increased $PCO_2$ levels, the Bohr effect helps compensate by promoting oxygen release from hemoglobin despite lower levels of oxygen in the blood.
3. **Acid-base disorders:** Disorders affecting blood pH, such as metabolic acidosis or alkalosis, can influence the Bohr effect. For example, in conditions like diabetic ketoacidosis, where there's increased acidity, the Bohr effect assists in oxygen unloading to tissues despite potential hypoxemia.

## Shift to Left

A shift to the left of the $O_2$-Hb dissociation curve means that hemoglobin has an increased affinity for $O_2$. This results in a higher oxygen saturation level of hemoglobin at every $PO_2$ level, compared to a normal curve.

**Factors shifting the curve to left:**
1. Increased $PO_2$
2. Decreased $PCO_2$
3. Decreased temperature
4. Decreased $H^+$
5. Decreased 2,3, BPG

Various factors responsible for shifting the curve to left are:
1. **Increased $PO_2$ and decreased $PCO_2$:** The high concentration of oxygen and low $PCO_2$ favours loading of Hb with $O_2$ in lungs.
2. **Decreased $H^+$ concentration:** The decreased metabolic activity, with reduced production of $H^+$, shifts the curve to left.
3. **Decreased body temperature**
4. **Decreased 2,3 BPG**

There are some special conditions, where the curve lies to the left of $O_2$-Hb dissociation curve, which hampers the binding of oxygen to Hb and increased its own binding to $O_2$ like the fetal Hb, carboxy Hb and myoglobin. The physiological basis of these are mentioned below:

- **Fetal hemoglobin:** The structure, fetal hemoglobin (HbF) consists of two α-subunits and two γ-subunits ($\alpha_2\gamma_2$). This structural difference decreases the affinity of HbF for 2,3-BPG.

  The 2,3 DPG normally decreases the affinity of hemoglobin for oxygen, in the absence of 2,3-DPG binding the oxyhemoglobin dissociation curve of HbF is left-shifted. Hemoglobin F (HbF) demonstrates a greater affinity for oxygen compared to hemoglobin A (HbA). Consequently, even when exposed to relatively low partial pressure of oxygen ($PO_2$) values in the maternal blood within the placenta, fetal blood exhibits significantly higher oxygen affinity. This characteristic proves advantageous in utero, enabling the fetus to extract oxygen more efficiently from the maternal circulation. *The p50 value of HbF is recorded at 19 mm Hg.*

  *The oxy-Hb dissociation curve in also sigmoid but to the left of HbA* (Fig. 53.4)

- **Myoglobin:** Myoglobin is a type of red protein that contains heme. It is responsible for carrying and storing oxygen in muscle cells. Although its structure is similar to that of hemoglobin, myoglobin is capable of binding only one molecule of oxygen per mole. This binding causes the oxygen-hemoglobin dissociation curve to shift to the left, creating a *rectangular hyperbola* and losing its sigmoid shape **(Fig. 53.5)**.

  This feature helps muscle cells to efficiently pick up oxygen from the blood, particularly when blood flow is disrupted during sustained muscle contraction.

  Myoglobin is more abundant in regularly exercising muscles, especially those trained in isometric exercise (such as leg and heart muscles). Since it can take up oxygen at low pressure more readily, the rate of association of myoglobin with oxygen is very fast. Unlike hemoglobin, myoglobin *doesn't exhibit Bohr's effect*.

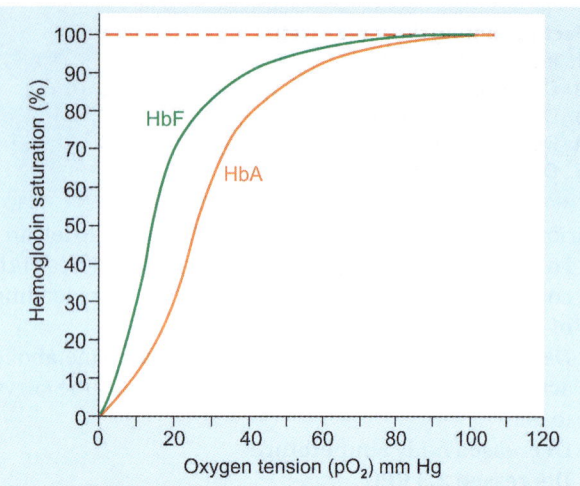

**Fig. 53.4:** Oxygen Hb dissociation curve of HbA and HbF.

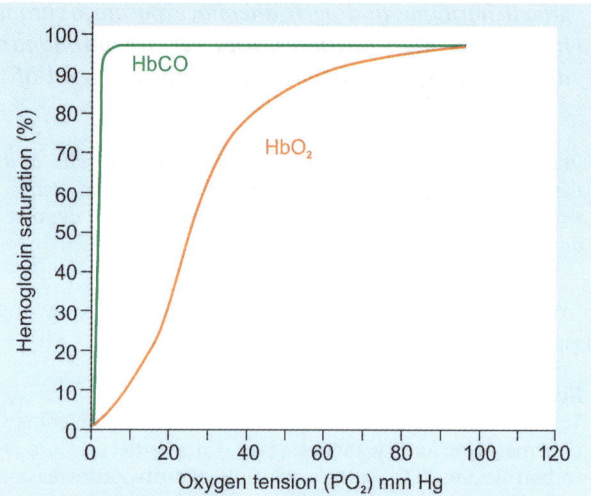

**Fig. 53.6:** $HbO_2$ and HbCO saturation curves.

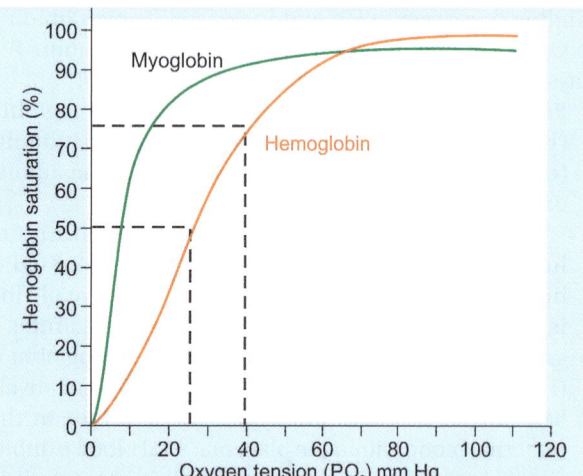

**Fig. 53.5:** Oxygen dissociation curve of myoglobin vs hemoglobin.

At a partial pressure of oxygen *($PO_2$) of 40 mm Hg, myoglobin is 95% saturated*, while hemoglobin is only 75% saturated. Even at $PO_2$ of 5 mm Hg, myoglobin is saturated by slightly <60%. Therefore, it acts as a temporary oxygen storage in the muscles.

- **Carbon monoxide:** The affinity of carbon monoxide for hemoglobin is 240 times that of oxygen, which interferes with oxygen transport by competing for the same binding sites on hemoglobin. When CO binds to hemoglobin, it forms carboxyhemoglobin (HbCO). The binding of one CO molecule to hemoglobin increases the affinity of the other binding spots for oxygen, leading to a left shift in the dissociation curve. This shift prevents oxygen unloading from hemoglobin (keeping hemoglobin in the tense state) in peripheral tissue and therefore the oxygen concentration of the tissue is much lower than normal.

Despite a greater proportion of saturated hemoglobin molecules, total $O_2$ content is decreased because of the high affinity of CO for hemoglobin. This may lead to severe tissue hypoxia. In healthy individuals CO occupies 1–2% of Hb binding sites. Chronic smokers, traffic personnel, and those in crowded traffic areas have increased CO concentration in plasma, occupying about 10% of Hb-binding sites. The concentration of dissolved oxygen remains normal, hence it does not stimulate the respiratory center even when there is severe hypoxia **(Fig. 53.6)**.

**$P_{50}$:** $P_{50}$ is the level of $PO_2$ at *which 50% of hemoglobin is saturated with oxygen*. It assesses binding affinity of hemoglobin for oxygen. In healthy adults at sea level, normal $P_{50}$ is at a $PO_2$ of 27 mm Hg. High $P_{50}$ means there is less affinity of Hb for oxygen and a right-shift in the oxygen-hemoglobin equilibrium curve. Conversely, low $P_{50}$ signifies a left-shift curve and more Hb affinity for oxygen.

## OXYGEN RELEASE IN TISSUES AT REST (FIG. 53.7)

During rest, the amount of oxygen that is delivered to the body cells is known as oxygen delivery.

Oxygen delivery = Arterial oxygen content × Cardiac output.

If the arterial blood contains 100 mL of oxygen at a $PO_2$ of approximately 100 mm Hg, then with a cardiac output of about 5 L/min, the normal oxygen delivery to the body is

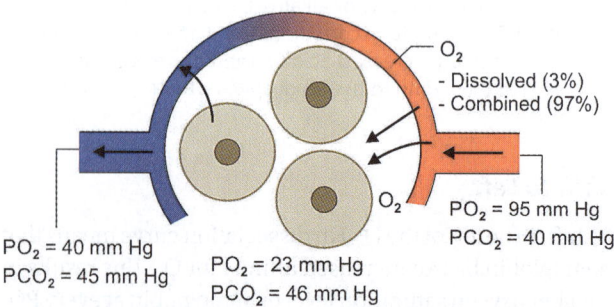

**Fig. 53.7:** Oxygen release in tissues at rest.

about 1 L/min. However, when the arterial oxygen content or cardiac output decreases, the oxygen delivery to tissues also decreases.

## OXYGEN CONSUMPTION

When the arterial blood reaches the tissues with a $PO_2$ of around 40 mm Hg, approximately *5 mL of oxygen diffuses from the tissue capillaries to the interstitial fluid* per minute due to the pressure gradient. The cardiac output at rest is 5 L/min, hence $5/100 \times 5000 = 250$ mL of $O_2$/min is transported from blood to the tissues, called the oxygen consumption for the whole body at rest.

## CO-EFFICIENT OF UTILIZATION OF $O_2$

The utilization coefficient refers to the percentage of oxygen consumed out of oxygen delivered to the tissue. During exercise, oxygen release is increased.

Co-efficient of utilization
$$= \frac{\text{Oxygen consumption/min}}{\text{Oxygen delivered per minute}} \times 100$$

The oxygen content of arterial blood that feeds the tissue = 19 mL/min

The oxygen content of venous blood that drains the tissue = 14 mL/min

The tissues are extracting 19 mL/min – 14 mL/min = 5 mL of $O_2$/100 mL of blood flow.

The co-efficient of $O_2$ utilization ($O_2$ extraction/100 mL of oxygen flow) is:

$$\frac{19 - 14}{19} \times 100 = 26\%$$

Coefficient of utilization of $O_2$ varies from tissue to tissue. In coronary it is quite high, about 60%, but there is no scope for improvement. In skeletal muscles at rest, it is quite low but can rise sharply during exercise to reach around 90%.

## VEHICLES FOR THE TRANSPORT OF OXYGEN: A COMPARISON OF PLASMA, HEMOGLOBIN AND WHOLE BLOOD

The oxygen dissociation curves of plasma, hemoglobin solution and whole blood and the amount of oxygen that can be loaded and unloaded by different transport vehicles reveal that the *whole blood is an ideal vehicle for the transport of $O_2$*, to load itself in lungs with $O_2$ and to release $O_2$ in tissues as per requirement **(Fig. 53.8)**.

> *At maximum hemoglobin saturation, the whole blood can release:*
> - 5 mL of $O_2$ at rest when tissue $PO_2$ is about 40 mm Hg
> - 13 mL of $O_2$ during moderate exercise when tissue $PO_2$ is about 25 mm Hg, and
> - 15–16 mL of $O_2$ during severe exercise, when tissue $PO_2$ is about 15 mm Hg.

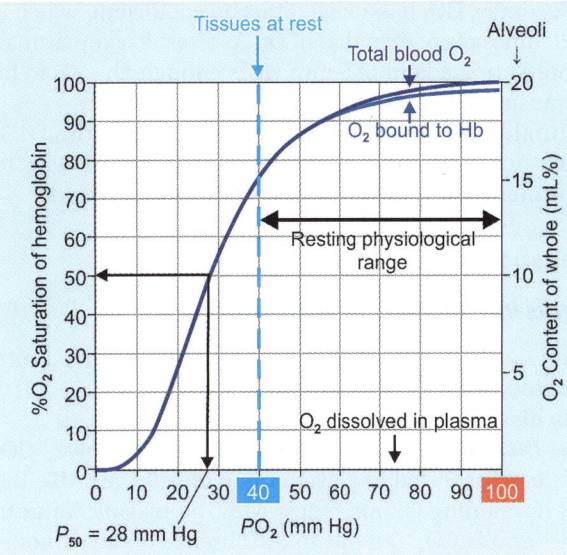

**Fig. 53.8:** Graph showing oxygen saturation of Hb in tissues and alveoli.

**Measurement of Oxygen Saturation of Hb Pulse Oximetry**
A pulse oximeter is a noninvasive device used to measure oxygen saturation and pulse rate. It's essential in clinical settings for monitoring respiratory and cardiac conditions, guiding oxygen therapy, and detecting hypoxemia early. Portable versions allow home monitoring for patients with chronic respiratory illnesses, aiding in timely intervention and improved patient management.

## TRANSPORT OF CARBON DIOXIDE

Carbon dioxide ($CO_2$) is mainly produced during the aerobic cellular metabolism of glucose and the conversion of carbohydrates to fat. After being produced, $CO_2$ is transported in the venous blood to the lungs and then exhaled in the expired air.

When our body tissues are active, they produce $CO_2$ as a metabolic byproduct; which enters our blood. This is due to three reasons:

1. Firstly, there is a difference in $PCO_2$ between the arterial blood and the tissues. Arterial blood has a $PCO_2$ of 40 mm Hg while the tissues have a $PCO_2$ of 46 mm Hg **(Fig. 53.9)**.

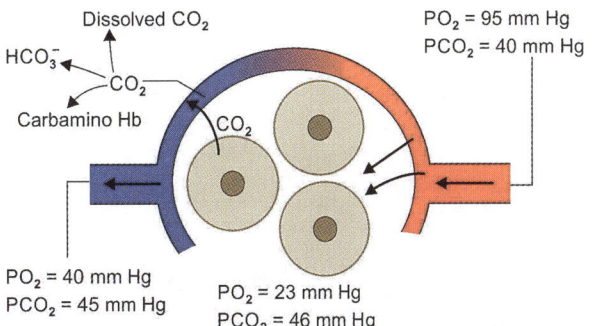

**Fig. 53.9:** Transport of $CO_2$ from tissues to plasma.

2. Secondly, $CO_2$ has a high diffusion coefficient, which is 20 times more than that of $O_2$. As a result, even a small pressure gradient of 6 mm Hg is enough for $CO_2$ to be transported.
3. Finally, a decrease in $O_2$ content causes the "$CO_2$ dissociation" curve to shift to the left, which leads to further loading of $CO_2$ from the tissues to the blood.

## Transport of $CO_2$ in Blood

### Forms in Which $CO_2$ is Transported

Like $O_2$, $CO_2$ is transported in blood in dissolved and combined form.
- **In dissolved form:**
  - ***Dissolved $CO_2$ (7%, 0.3 mL/dL):*** The dissolved $CO_2$ is transported in plasma up to only 0.1 mL/dL. The remaining 0.2 mL reacts with the plasma water to form $H_2CO_3$. But due to the absence of the carbonic anhydrase, this reaction is extremely slow.
  - ***$HCO_3^-$ in plasma (70%):*** Most of the bicarbonate present in the plasma, is transported out of the RBCs in exchange with chloride (chloride shift). Some amount of bicarbonate in also present in the RBC, which also gets subsequently exchanged with chloride.
- **In combined form:**
  - ***Carbamino hemoglobin (23%, 0.6 mL/dL):*** The $CO_2$ combines with the Hb to form the carbamino-Hb.

## Chloride Shift (Fig. 53.10)

The chloride shift, also known as the Hamburger phenomenon, refers to the exchange of chloride ions ($Cl^-$) and bicarbonate ions ($HCO_3^-$) by **anion exchanger 1 (AE1)**, between red blood cells and plasma in response to changes in carbon dioxide ($CO_2$) levels. It occurs in the tissues and lungs as part of the bicarbonate buffer system, helping to maintain acid-base balance.

### Physiological Significance

During gas exchange in the tissues, carbon dioxide is produced as a byproduct of cellular metabolism. This $CO_2$ diffuses into RBCs, where it combines with water to form carbonic acid ($H_2CO_3$), which then dissociates into bicarbonate ions ($HCO_3^-$) and hydrogen ions ($H^+$). To maintain electrochemical neutrality, chloride ions ($Cl^-$) move from plasma into the RBCs, in exchange of the bicarbonate ions by the anion exchanger. The chloride shift is a rapid process and is essentially complete within 1 second. As a result of this chloride shift:
- The $Cl^-$ content of the red cells in venous blood is significantly greater than that in arterial blood (increased hematocrit). A small amount of fluid in the arterial blood returns via the lymphatics rather than the veins, the hematocrit of venous blood is usually 3% greater than that of arterial blood.
- For each $CO_2$ molecule added to a red cell, there is an increase of one osmotically active particle in the cell—$HCO_3^-$ or $Cl^-$; hence the red cells take up water and increase in size in the venous blood.
- In the lungs, the $Cl^-$ moves back out of the cells and they shrink.
- The pH also drops from 7.4 to 7.36 after entry of carbon dioxide into the blood, hence *the venous blood is more acidic than the arterial blood*.

### Clinical Significance

- **pH regulation:** The chloride shift helps regulate pH by facilitating the transport of carbon dioxide as bicarbonate ions, which helps buffer changes in blood pH caused by metabolic or respiratory disturbances.
- **Respiratory disorders:** Dysfunctions in the chloride shift mechanism can contribute to acid-base imbalances seen in respiratory disorders such as chronic obstructive pulmonary disease (COPD) or emphysema.
- **Diagnostic tool:** Monitoring chloride levels in conjunction with bicarbonate and carbon dioxide levels can aid in diagnosing acid-base disorders and assessing respiratory function.
- **Therapeutic targets:** Understanding the chloride shift is essential for developing treatments aimed at correcting acid-base disturbances, such as administering bicarbonate therapy in cases of metabolic acidosis.

## CARBON DIOXIDE DISSOCIATION CURVES

There are two separate $CO_2$ dissociation curves—one for oxygenated and second for deoxygenated blood **(Fig. 53.11)**.

Carbon dioxide dissociation curves depict the relationship between the partial pressure of carbon dioxide ($PCO_2$) and the amount of carbon dioxide ($CO_2$) carried in the blood, typically as dissolved $CO_2$ or as bicarbonate ions ($HCO_3^-$) formed via the carbonic acid-bicarbonate buffer system.

### Physiological Basis

- **Carbonic acid-bicarbonate buffer system:** The majority of $CO_2$ in the blood is transported in the

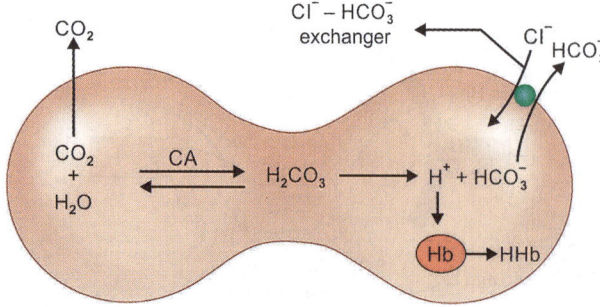

**Fig. 53.10:** Chloride shift.

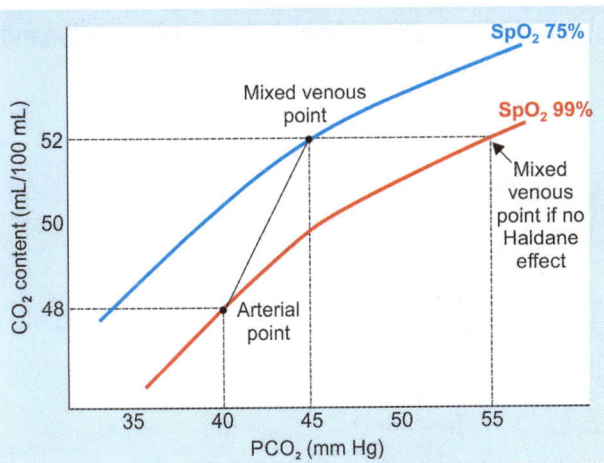

**Fig. 53.11:** $CO_2$-dissociation curves—for oxygenated blood (red curve) and deoxygenated blood (blue curve).

form of bicarbonate ions through the carbonic acid-bicarbonate buffer system. Carbon dioxide produced in tissues diffuses into red blood cells, where it combines with water to form carbonic acid in the presence of carbonic anhydrase enzyme. Carbonic acid rapidly dissociates into bicarbonate ions ($HCO_3^-$) and hydrogen ions ($H^+$). Bicarbonate ions are then transported out of the RBCs into plasma in exchange for chloride ions ($Cl^-$) through the chloride shift, while carbon dioxide diffuses into the plasma.

**Haldane effect:** The Haldane effect is a phenomenon first described by John Scot Haldane, the where the oxygenation of hemoglobin affects its ability to bind and releases carbon dioxide. *Deoxygenated hemoglobin has a higher affinity for $CO_2$ and $H^+$ ions,* facilitating the binding of $CO_2$ and $H^+$ ions to hemoglobin in the tissues. Conversely, when hemoglobin is oxygenated in the lungs, its affinity for $CO_2$ decreases, leading to the release of $CO_2$.

*Haldane effect causes increased unloading of $CO_2$ upon oxygenation of blood.* As blood passes through the lungs an influx of $O_2$ causes a right shift of the carbon dioxide dissociation curve while the partial pressure of carbon dioxide drops from 45 mm Hg to 40 mm Hg. This serves to release greater amount of $CO_2$ into the alveolar spaces.

Hence, venous blood carries more carbon dioxide than the arterial blood.

2. **Direct dissolution:** A small fraction of $CO_2$ (around 5–10%) is transported in the blood directly dissolved in plasma, without undergoing conversion to bicarbonate ions. This dissolved $CO_2$ is directly proportional to the $PCO_2$ in the blood.

## Clinical Significance

The clinical significance of carbon dioxide dissociation curves lies in their utility for diagnosing and managing various respiratory and metabolic disorders, as well as assessing acid-base balance in clinical settings:

- **Respiratory disorders:** Carbon dioxide dissociation curves help clinicians evaluate respiratory function and diagnose respiratory disorders such as chronic obstructive pulmonary disease (COPD), asthma, and respiratory acidosis. Changes in the shape or position of the curve can indicate abnormalities in $CO_2$ transport and elimination.
- **Metabolic disorders:** Disorders affecting the carbonic acid-bicarbonate buffer system, such as metabolic acidosis or alkalosis, can be assessed using carbon dioxide dissociation curves. Changes in bicarbonate levels and their relationship with $PCO_2$ provide valuable insights into metabolic abnormalities.
- **Ventilation management:** In critical care settings, carbon dioxide dissociation curves assist in managing mechanical ventilation and optimizing ventilator settings. Monitoring changes in $PCO_2$ and bicarbonate levels helps ensure adequate ventilation and oxygenation.
- **Acid-base balance:** Carbon dioxide dissociation curves are essential for assessing acid-base balance and diagnosing acid-base disorders such as respiratory acidosis, respiratory alkalosis, metabolic acidosis, and metabolic alkalosis. Clinicians use these curves to interpret blood gas analysis results and guide appropriate treatment.
- **Monitoring therapy:** Monitoring changes in carbon dioxide dissociation curves over time can help assess the effectiveness of respiratory therapy, such as oxygen therapy, mechanical ventilation, or treatments targeting acid-base imbalances. It allows clinicians to adjust treatment plans and optimize patient care accordingly.

## SUMMARY

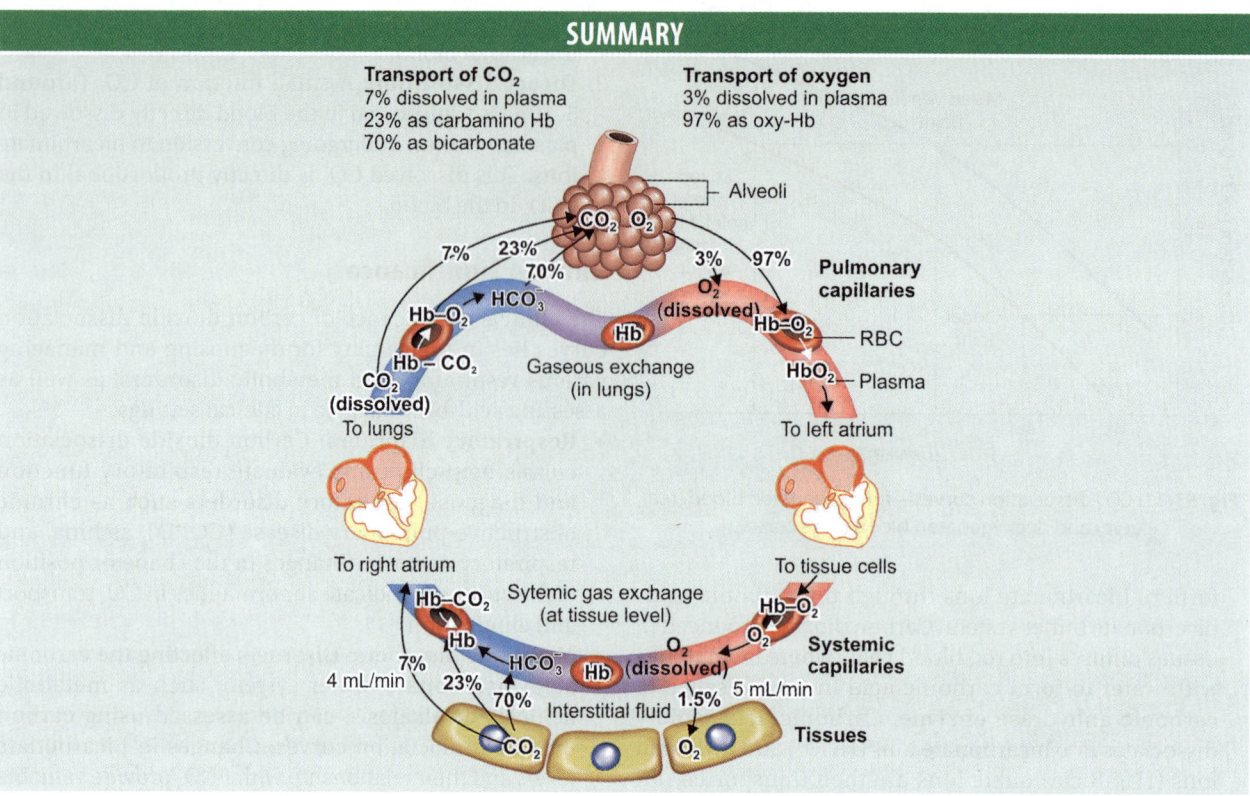

## LET US SEE, HOW MUCH YOU HAVE LEARNT?

 *Review Questions*

### Long/Short Answer Questions

Q1. Describe the mechanism of transport of oxygen from the lungs to the tissues.
Q2. Draw a well labeled self-explanatory diagram of oxygen Hb dissociation curve.
Q3. What is the physiological significance of steep phase and plateau phase of oxygen Hb dissociation curve?
Q4. What is P50? What is its physiological significance?
Q5. Calculate the amount of dissolved and combined oxygen of the blood of a patient of severe anemia, with Hb level of 6 g/dL.
Q6. What is Bohr's effect? What is its physiological significance?
Q7. How is carbon dioxide carried in the blood from tissues to lungs?
Q8. Define chloride shift. What is its physio-clinical significance?
Q9. What is Haldane effect? What is its physio-clinical significance?
Q10. Describe the carbon dioxide dissociation curves for arterial and venous blood.
Q11. What is the $CO_2$ content of the blood at $PCO_2$ of 45 mm Hg? Describe with the help of a diagram.

### Explain Why? (Reasoning Questions)

Q1. The stored blood cannot be given to the patients of hypoxia.
Q2. There is higher hemotocrit of venous blood.
Q3. The venous blood is more acidic than arterial blood.
Q4. Hemoglobin saturation with oxygen is higher in the lungs compared to the tissues.
Q5. Carbon dioxide is transported in the blood in multiple forms, including dissolved $CO_2$, bicarbonate ions, and carbaminohemoglobin.
Q6. The oxyhemoglobin dissociation curve shifts to the right during exercise.
Q7. Carbon monoxide poisoning can lead to tissue hypoxia despite normal arterial oxygen levels.

# Multiple Choice Questions

**Q1.** Most of the $CO_2$ transported in the blood is:
a. Dissolved in plasma
b. In carbamino compounds formed from plasma proteins
c. In carbamino compounds formed from hemoglobin.
d. In $HCO_3$

**Q2.** Which of the following has the greatest effect on the ability of blood to transport oxygen?
a. Capacity of the blood to dissolve oxygen
b. Amount of hemoglobin in the blood
c. pH of plasma
d. Temperature of the blood

**Q3.** Which of the following is true of the system?

$$CO_2 + H_2O \overset{1}{\rightleftharpoons} H_2CO_3 \overset{2}{\rightleftharpoons} H^+ + HCO_3^-$$

a. Reaction 2 is catalyzed by carbonic anhydrase
b. Because of reaction 2, the pH of blood declines during hyperventilation
c. Reaction 1 occurs in the red blood cell
d. Reaction 1 occurs primarily in plasma

**Q4.** What is the main form of oxygen transport in the blood?
a. Oxygenated hemoglobin
b. Dissolved oxygen
c. Oxygen-bound plasma proteins
d. Oxygenated RBCs

**Q5.** In which form does most of the carbon dioxide transport in the blood?
a. Dissolved $CO_2$
b. Bicarbonate ions
c. Carbaminohemoglobin
d. Carbonic acid

**Q6.** Which factor primarily affects the oxygen-hemoglobin dissociation curve?
a. Temperature
b. pH
c. Partial pressure of oxygen
d. Partial pressure of carbon dioxide

**Q7.** What is the Bohr effect primarily associated with?
a. Oxygen transport in the lungs
b. Oxygen release to tissues
c. Carbon dioxide transport in the blood
d. Hemoglobin synthesis

**Q8.** A patient with chronic obstructive pulmonary disease (COPD) presents with decreased oxygen saturation. Which factor is primarily responsible for this?
a. Increased carbon dioxide levels
b. Decreased pH
c. Reduced lung compliance
d. Elevated levels of 2,3-BPG

**Q9.** A patient with diabetic ketoacidosis (DKA) is admitted to the emergency room with altered mental status. Which acid-base disorder is most likely present in this patient?
a. Respiratory acidosis
b. Respiratory alkalosis
c. Metabolic acidosis
d. Metabolic alkalosis

**Q10.** During exercise, which factor contributes to increased oxygen delivery to tissues?
a. Decreased pH
b. Increased temperature
c. Elevated levels of 2,3-BPG
d. All of the above

**Q11.** A pregnant woman undergoes labor and experiences hyperventilation. How does this affect oxygen delivery to the fetus?
a. Increases oxygen delivery due to the Bohr effect
b. Decreases oxygen delivery due to decreased $CO_2$ levels
c. Increases oxygen delivery due to increased Haldane effect
d. Decreases oxygen delivery due to increased 2,3-BPG levels

**Q12.** In which scenario would you expect a leftward shift of the oxygen-hemoglobin dissociation curve?
a. Hyperventilation
b. Exercise
c. High altitude
d. Decreased pH

**Q13.** A patient with severe anemia presents with decreased oxygen saturation. Which compensatory mechanism is activated in response to this?
a. Increased respiratory rate
b. Increased oxygen affinity of hemoglobin
c. Decreased cardiac output
d. Increased 2,3-BPG levels

**Q14.** A patient with chronic obstructive pulmonary disease (COPD) presents with increased carbon dioxide levels in the blood. Which compensatory mechanism is activated in response to this condition?
a. Increased respiratory rate
b. Decreased bicarbonate reabsorption in the kidneys
c. Enhanced oxygen affinity of hemoglobin
d. Decreased 2,3-BPG levels

**Q15.** During a mountain climbing expedition, climbers experience decreased oxygen saturation due to reduced partial pressure of oxygen at high altitudes. Which physiological adaptation occurs to compensate for this hypoxia?
a. Leftward shift of the oxygen-hemoglobin dissociation curve
b. Increased respiratory rate
c. Decreased ventilation-perfusion matching
d. Elevated levels of carbon monoxide in the blood

**Q16.** A patient with severe anemia undergoes blood transfusion. Which immediate effect is expected on the oxygen-hemoglobin dissociation curve following the transfusion?
a. Rightward shift of the curve
b. Leftward shift of the curve
c. Decreased affinity of hemoglobin for oxygen
d. No change in the curve position

**Q17.** In a patient with metabolic alkalosis, which alteration in the oxygen-hemoglobin dissociation curve is most likely to occur?
  a. Leftward shift of the curve
  b. Rightward shift of the curve
  c. Increased oxygen affinity of hemoglobin
  d. Decreased oxygen delivery to tissues

**Q18.** During severe exercise, which factor primarily contributes to increased oxygen delivery to the tissues?
  a. Decreased temperature
  b. Increased pH
  c. Decreased carbon dioxide levels
  d. Elevated levels of 2,3-BPG

**Q19.** A patient with diabetic ketoacidosis (DKA) presents with deep, rapid breathing. How does this hyperventilation affect the oxygen-hemoglobin dissociation curve?
  a. Rightward shift of the curve
  b. Leftward shift of the curve
  c. Decreased oxygen affinity of hemoglobin
  d. Increased oxygen delivery to tissues

**Q20.** In a patient with chronic hypoxemia, which compensatory mechanism enhances oxygen delivery to tissues?
  a. Increased production of carbon monoxide
  b. Decreased 2,3-BPG levels
  c. Leftward shift of the oxygen-hemoglobin dissociation curve
  d. Enhanced erythropoietin production

**Q21.** A patient with severe pneumonia experiences respiratory acidosis. How does this acidosis affect the dissociation curve of oxygen from hemoglobin?
  a. Rightward shift of the curve
  b. Leftward shift of the curve
  c. Decreased oxygen saturation of hemoglobin
  d. Increased oxygen affinity of hemoglobin

## ANSWERS

| 1. d | 2. b | 3. c | 4. a | 5. b | 6. c | 7. b | 8. a | 9. c | 10. d | 11. b | 12. a | 13. d | 14. a |
| 15. a | 16. a | 17. a | 18. d | 19. b | 20. c | 21. a | | | | | | | |

# Regulation of Respiration

## CHAPTER 54

### LEARNING OBJECTIVES

**At the end of this chapter, the learner should be able to:**
- Enumerate the different levels of regulatory controls of respiration.
- Explain the nervous regulation of respiration in terms of respiratory centers, respiratory reflexes.
- Describe the respiratory changes, in case of damage to the different levels of respiratory center.
- Describe the mechanism of stimulation of the central and peripheral chemoreceptors.
- Describe the role of local receptors and reflexes in the regulation of respiration.

The regulation of respiration refers to the regulate the rate and depth of respiration, which is needed to maintain the normal arterial level of the respiratory gases (oxygen and carbon dioxide), along with maintenance of the normal arterial pH. It is interesting to note that the respiration is both under the voluntary as well as in the involuntary nervous control. To know more about the regulation, lets first learn the different levels of controls of respiration. The **Flowchart 54.1** demonstrates the nervous, chemical and nonchemical regulation.

Flowchart 54.1: Schematic representation of regulation of respiration.

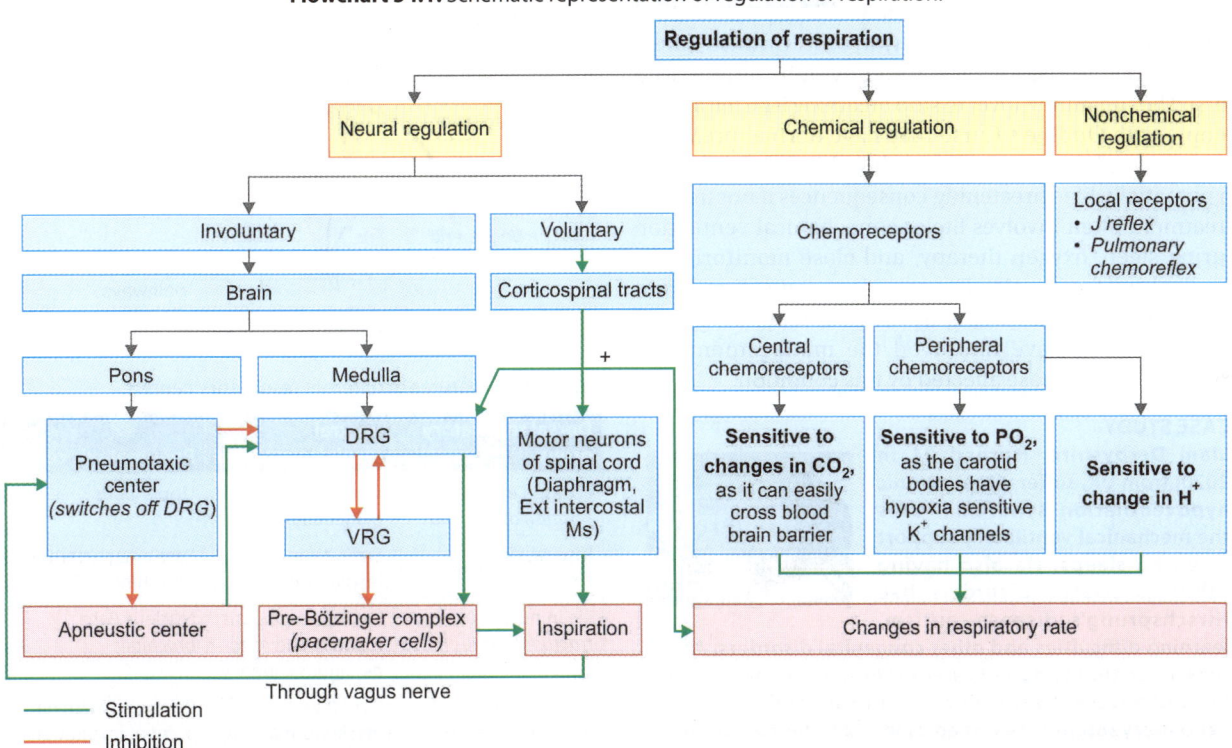

## NERVOUS REGULATION

Respiratory system is controlled by automatic involuntary system as well as voluntary cortico-spinal tracts.

- **Nervous regulation**
  - *Respiratory centers:*
    - Dorsal respiratory group
    - Ventral respiratory group
    - Pneumotaxic center
    - Apneustic center
- **Chemical regulation**
  - $PO_2$, $PCO_2$, pH
- **Nonchemical regulation**
  - *Local receptors (J receptors):*
    - J-reflex
    - Pulmonary chemoreflex

### Voluntary Control

The respiration is under the voluntary control of the cerebral cortex. It sends signals through corticospinal tract to the muscle of respiration. Hence, we can voluntarily alter the rate and depth of our respiration.

Imagine a scenario where autonomic control of respiration is lost while the voluntary control is retained. It is seen in one of the rare genetic neurological disorder, due to a *mutation in the PHOX2B gene*, which plays a crucial role in the development of the autonomic nervous system, including the part that controls breathing. It is called the *chronic hypoventilation syndrome/Ondine curse*.

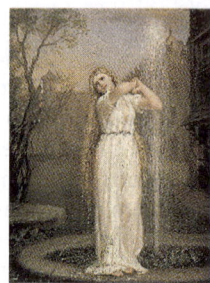

It's named after the mythical water nymph Ondine, who cursed her unfaithful lover to stop breathing if he fell asleep. People with Ondine's Curse may have normal breathing when awake but struggle to breathe while asleep, leading to potentially life-threatening consequences if not treated. Treatment often involves lifelong mechanical ventilation during sleep, oxygen therapy, and close monitoring by medical professionals. Though it presents significant challenges, advancements in medical technology and understanding have improved the management and quality of life for those affected by this condition.

**CASE STUDY**
Liam Derbyshire, (turned 21 in 2020) from UK, suffers from chronic hypoventilation syndrome, uses the mechanical ventilatory support when he sleeps. He also having other associated disorders like Hirschsprung's disease, autism, learning difficulties and other congenital disorders. At the time of birth, his parents were told that he may not live beyond 6 weeks, but with constant care and mechanical ventilatory support, he turned 21 in 2020. This condition has not more than 1500 patients world-wide.

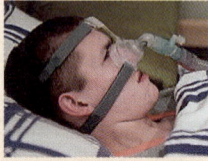

### Involuntary Control

The involuntary autonomic control of the respiration, makes the respiration automatic, and is controlled by a complex multitier system of respiratory centers located in pons and medulla.

### Respiratory Centers

The respiratory centers **(Fig. 54.1)** in the brainstem play a crucial role in generating and regulating the inspiratory ramp during natural breathing **(Table 54.1)**.

- **Pons:**
  - Pneumotaxic center
  - Apneustic center (at pontomedullary junction)
- **Medulla oblongata:**
  - Dorsal respiratory group (DRG) of neurons—inspiratory center
  - Ventral respiratory group (VRG) of neurons—inspiration and expiration
  - Pre-Bötzinger Complex (pre-BÖTC)

### Inspiratory Ramp Signal

The inspiratory ramp refers to the gradual increase in airflow or volume of air in lungs during inspiration followed by

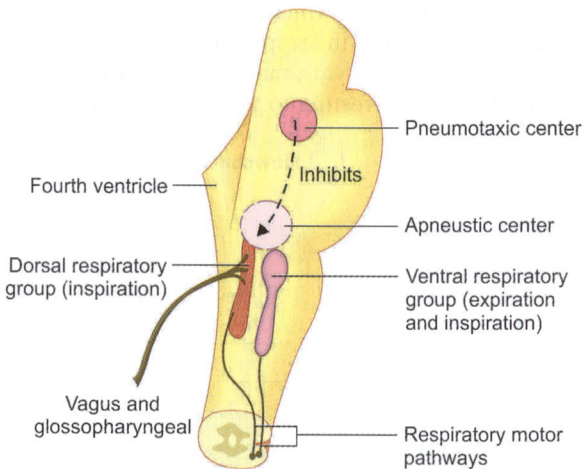

**Fig. 54.1:** Respiration control centers in brain.

**Table 54.1:** Features of different respiratory centers.

| Dorsal respiratory group | Ventral respiratory group | Pneumotaxic center |
|---|---|---|
| Located in *dorsal position of medulla* | *Ventro lateral* part of *medulla* | Upper *pons* |
| Inspiration | Expiration/Inspiration | Rate and pattern of breathing |
| Lie in nucleus of *tractus solitarius (NTS)* | Nucleus *Ambiguus* rostrally and *retro-ambiguus* caudally | Nucleus *Para brachialis* |
| Most *fundamental role* in respiratory control | *Overdrive mechanism* during exercise | Controls *switch off point* of inspiration |

the passive expiration due to recoil. It is again followed by another cycle of inspiration and expiration after a brief pause. This increase in airflow during inspiration is controlled by a switch off point, controlling the tidal volume during inspiration and rate of respiration. Hence, understanding the inspiratory ramp is important to understand the nervous regulation of respiration.

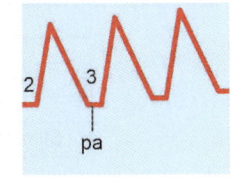

## Dorsal Respiratory Group (DRG)

It is a group of inspiratory neurons (I-neurons), located in nucleus of tractus solitarius. *These neurons discharge during inspiration.* The DRG responds to the receptors present in the lungs, carotid sinus, carotid bodies and the local receptors in lungs. The DRG then stimulates the phrenic nerve to stimulate the diaphragm and external intercostal muscles, initiating contraction and causing inspiration. The DRG neurons are involved in the gradual increase in neural drive to respiratory muscles, contributing to the inspiratory ramp.

- **Receptors:**
  - Peripheral chemoreceptors
  - Baro receptors
  - Receptors in lungs
- **Afferents:** Through vagus and glossopharangeal nerve
- **Center:** DRG
- **Efferents:** Via phrenic nerve to diaphragm

The DRG primarily regulates the basic rhythm of breathing, including the timing and duration of inspiration and expiration.

## Ventral Respiratory Group (VRG)

It is a group of neurons having both E-neurons and I-neurons, located in the nucleus ambiguus and retro-ambiguus on ventrolateral part of medulla. It does not participate in the quiet respiration but is active in the overdrive mechanism during exercise.

The VRG coordinates the activity of accessory respiratory muscles, which may be recruited during increased respiratory effort. It also contributes to the modulation of respiratory rhythm and pattern, potentially influencing the shape of the inspiratory ramp.

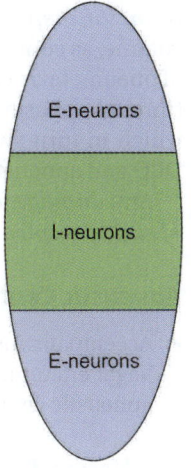

## The Pre-Bötzinger Complex (Pre-BÖTC)

It is a crucial part of the respiratory rhythm generator located in the medulla oblongata. It is thought to be the primary site for generating the rhythm of breathing, specifically controlling the inspiratory phase. It is also called as the pacemaker for regulating inspiratory ramp signal.

This complex consists of a network of interconnected neurons that fire rhythmically, generating the basic pattern of breathing. It receives the inputs from DRG and other sensory receptors and adjusts the respiratory rhythm accordingly.

## Pneumotaxic Center (Fig. 54.2)

It is the pontine respiratory center containing E and I neurons. It fine tunes the inspiratory signals of the

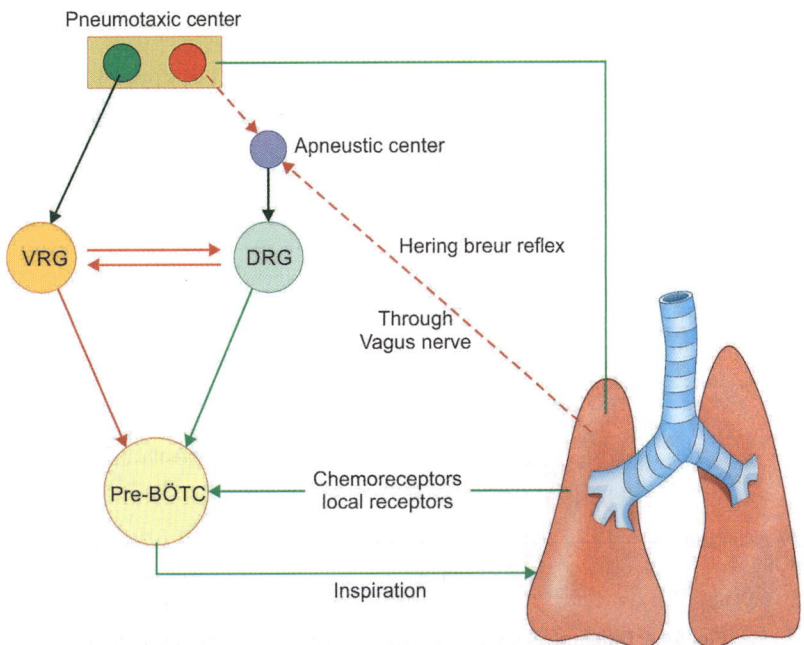

**Fig. 54.2:** Control of respiration by pneumotaxic center.

medullary respiratory centers. It *'Controls switch off point of inspiratory ramp,'* hence controls the tidal volume, as controls filling phase of lung cycle. Stimulation of pneumotaxic center by the pulmonary stretch receptors (through vagus nerve) stimulates the pneumotaxic center, which in turn switches off the inspiration by inhibiting DRG and apneustic center.

Any *damage* to pneumotaxic center results *in slowing of rate of respiration and increased tidal volume.*

## Apneustic Center

- Accentuates inspiration by stimulating inspiratory center.
- Vagal efferents from stretch receptors in lungs inhibits apneustic center once lung expansion >800 mL.

## The Hering-Breuer Reflex

It is a protective reflex, named after its discoverers Karl Ewald Hering and Josef Breuer, involved in the regulation of breathing, particularly in controlling the depth and frequency of breathing. It primarily acts to prevent overinflation of the lungs during inspiration **(Fig. 54.3)**.

The reflex is initiated by stretch receptors, also known as pulmonary stretch receptors or slowly adapting pulmonary stretch receptors (SARs), which are located in the smooth muscle of the airways and lung parenchyma. These receptors are sensitive to changes in lung volume and are activated when the lungs are inflated beyond a certain threshold. When lung inflation occurs, such as during deep inspiration, the SARs are stretched, leading to the initiation of the Hering-Breuer reflex. *Activation of these stretch receptors sends inhibitory signals via the vagus nerve (cranial nerve X) to the medulla oblongata, specifically to the inspiratory neurons in the apneustic center, pre-Bötzinger complex and the dorsal respiratory group.*

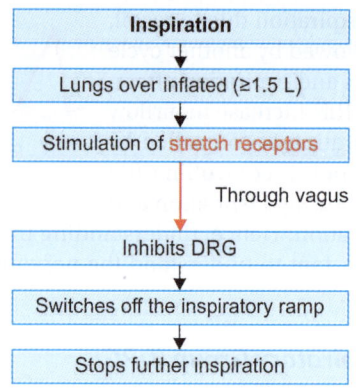

**Fig. 54.3:** Hering-Breuer inflation reflex.

As a result, the Hering-Breuer reflex causes the termination of inspiration, preventing further lung inflation and promoting the onset of expiration. *This reflex helps regulate tidal volume*—the volume of air breathed in and out during normal breathing—and ensures that the lungs are not excessively inflated, which could lead to damage or compromise gas exchange efficiency.

The Hering-Breuer reflex is most active in newborns and young infants, playing a role in regulating breathing patterns during different phases of development. However, it continues to function throughout life, contributing to the maintenance of respiratory homeostasis in response to changes in lung volume and respiratory demands.

## Effect of Lesion/Damage to Brainstem/Respiratory Centers

Damage to brainstem or respiratory centers can affect can lead to various effects on respiration (**Fig. 54.4** and **Table 54.2**)

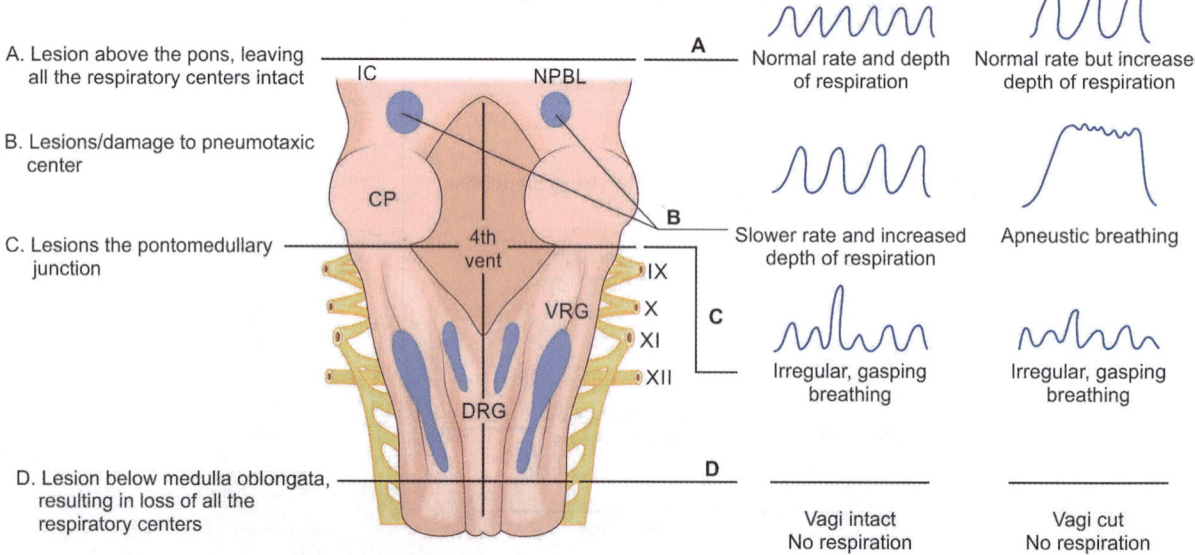

**Fig. 54.4:** Different levels of lesions of brainstem affecting respiration.

Table 54.2: Features of lesions due to damage to brainstem and respiratory center (Fig. 54.4).

| | Level of lesion | Response with vagus intact | Response with vagotomy | Discussion |
|---|---|---|---|---|
| A | Above the pons. All the neural groups regulating the respiration are preserved | Normal respiratory rate and depth | Normal rate of respiration but depth increases | Since all the respiratory centers are intact, the rate of respiration is not affected. However, vagotomy abolishes the feedback from stretch receptors, increasing the tidal volume |
| B | Damage to pneumotaxic center | Slow rate of respiration with increased tidal volume | *Apneustic breathing* | The pneumotaxic center switches off the inspiratory ramp signal. In case of damage to the pneumotaxic center, the switch off doesn't happen, increasing the tidal volume and hence slowing the respiratory rate. But the vagotomy abolishes the local stretch reflex, causing prolonged inspiration called *apneusis* |
| C | Lesions at the upper border of medulla/at pontomedullary junction | Periodic breathing: Irregular rate of breathing with decreased tidal volume with some deep breaths (gasps) in between | Periodic breathing: Irregular rate of breathing with decreased tidal volume with some deep breaths (gasps) in between | Damage to the respiratory centers in this area can lead to decreased respiratory drive, resulting in hypoventilation or respiratory depression. This condition can manifest as *shallow breathing*, decreased tidal volume, and a reduction in the rate of breathing<br>*Cheyne-Stokes respiration* is characterized by periods of progressively deeper and faster breathing followed by periods of shallow or absent breathing, while ataxic breathing is marked by unpredictable and irregular breathing patterns |
| D | At the lower border of medulla | No respiration | No respiration | |

## CHEMICAL REGULATION

### (Effect of $PO_2$, $PCO_2$, $H^+$ variations)

The chemical changes occurring in the blood with reference to the respiratory gases ($PO_2$, $PCO_2$) and the $H^+$ affect the rate and depth of respiration. These chemical changes are sensed by the specialized receptors called the chemoreceptors (Fig. 54.5).

The chemoreceptors are broadly classified as the central and peripheral chemoreceptors.

## Central Chemoreceptors (Fig. 54.6)

It refers to the direct chemical control of respiratory center activity by $CO_2$ and $H^+$ ions in the chemosenstive are of respiratory center beneath the ventral surface of medulla. Also called as medullary receptors.

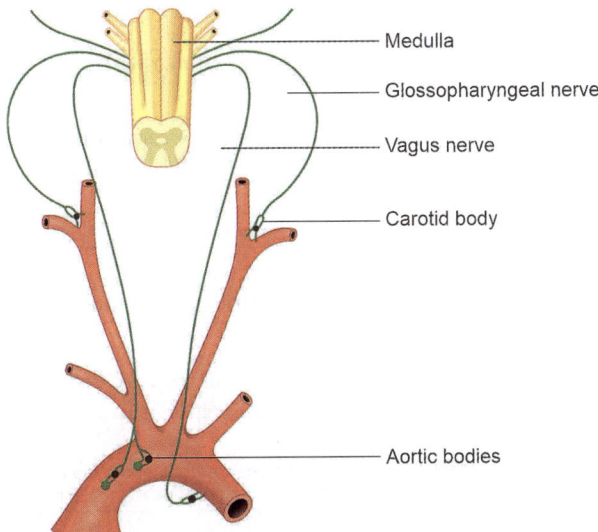

Fig. 54.5: Chemoreceptors in aortic bodies.

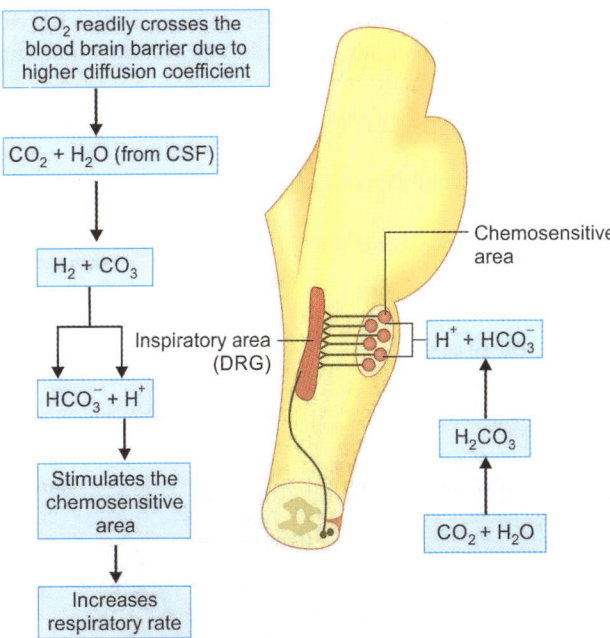

Fig. 54.6: Central chemoreceptors.

An additional neuronal area, a *chemosensitive area* is located bilaterally lying only 0.2 mm beneath the ventral surface of medulla which is highly sensitive to changes in either blood $PCO_2$ or $H^+$ concentration.

The $CO_2$ is highly lipid soluble gas having a quite high diffusion coefficient, easily crosses the blood brain barrier. It then combines with the water present in the CSF to form carbonic acid ($H_2CO_3$). It readily dissociates to form $H^+$, which stimulates the chemosensitive zone. It leads to the *increase in rate and depth of respiration, hence, controlling minute to minute respiration*. It is responsible for 80–85% of the respiratory drive (peripheral chemoreceptors are responsible for 15–20% of respiratory drive). *This makes $CO_2$ the most powerful and the primary regulatory factor for the chemical regulation of respiration.*

## Peripheral Chemoreceptors

These receptors are the special chemical receptors located in several areas outside the brain. They are important for detecting changes in $O_2$ in blood, although they also respond to a lesser extent to change in $CO_2$ and $H^+$ ion concentrations.

For regulation of respiratory system, the chemoreceptors are divided into two groups:
1. **Carotid bodies:** Located in either side near the Bifurcation of common carotid artery
2. **Aortic bodies:** Located near the arch of aorta

These chemoreceptors have two types of cells (**Fig. 54.7**):
1. **Type 1 (Glomus cells):** These cells have dense-core granules containing catecholamines and probably dopamine, acetylcholine and ATP. Dopamine containing unmyelinated nerve endings are closely applied to these cells. When exposed to hypoxia, these type 1 cells release catecholamines stimulates $D_2$ receptors on the nerve endings. Most recently, the studies have shown that the ATP is also the neurotransmitter.
2. **Type 2 cells (Glial cells)** and are closely applied to around 6–8 Type 1 glomus cells.

Nerve fibers (outside the capsule of each body): Afferents from the carotid body join the sinus nerve to form glossopharyngeal nerve and ultimately ascends to medulla; while those from aortic body join aortic nerve forming vagus nerve which ascend to medulla.

The blood flow to the carotid bodies is extremely high, i.e., 20 times the weight of body themselves each minute 2,000 mL/100 g/min. It is the highest amount of blood flow to any organ. The chemo receptors are always exposed to arterial blood, and NOT the venous blood, the arterial $PO_2$ values, i.e., in dissolved form. *That is why the peripheral chemoreceptors are not stimulated in anemia and carbon monoxide poisoning.*

$CO_2$ and $H^+$ ion concentration also stimulate chemoreceptors, in this way, indirectly raising the respiratory activity.

Even the *drugs as cyanide, nicotine and lobeline stimulate the peripheral chemoreceptors.*

### Effect of Stimulation of Peripheral Chemoreceptors

Stimulation of peripheral chemoreceptors result in the increase in respiratory rate and depth.

Since the anemia and carbon monoxide poisoning, does not stimulate peripheral chemoreceptors, the rate and depth of respiration remains unchanged.

### Chemoreceptor Reflex

- **Stimulus:** Chemical changes in blood ($PO_2$, $PCO_2$, pH)
- **Receptors:** Glomus cells in chemoreceptors, sensitive to hypoxia (dissolved oxygen)
- **Location and afferent:** Aortic bodies *(Afferent: Xth nerve)*
  Carotid bodies *(Afferent: IXth nerve)*

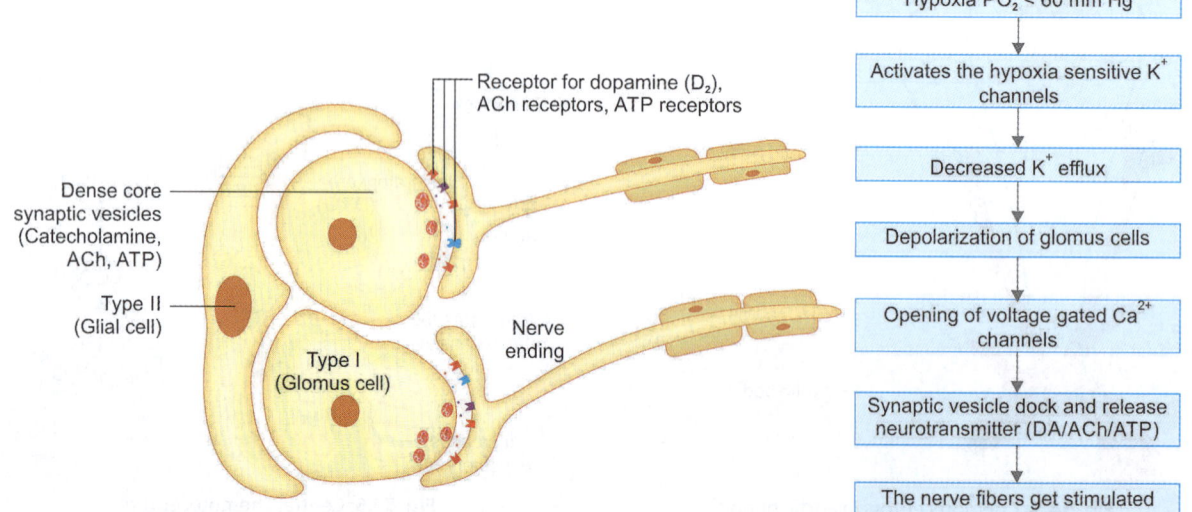

**Fig. 54.7:** Mechanism of glomus and glial cells regulating respiration.

- **Efferent:** Vagus *(Xth nerve)*
- **Center:** Chemo sensitive area in medulla oblongata
- **Response:** Change in rate of respiration through DRG

> **CAROTID BODIES**
> - Blood flow → 2,000 mL/100 g of tissue/min (highest blood flow)
>   - Brain → 54 mL/100 g of tissue/min
>   - Kidney → 420 mL/100 g of tissue/min
> - Senses the dissolved oxygen concentration (sensitive to hypoxia)
> - Maximum sensitivity to hypoxia à 30–60 mm Hg
>
> *Stimulated in:*
> - Arterial $PO_2$ is low
> - Vascular stasis
> - Amount of $O_2$ delivered to receptor/unit time is low
>
> *Not stimulated in:*
> - Anemia
> - CO poisoning

## Carbon Dioxide Narcosis

It is also known as hypercapnic narcosis or $CO_2$ narcosis. It is a condition characterized by an excessive *accumulation of carbon dioxide in the blood*, leading to neurological symptoms and impairment.

Carbon dioxide is a waste product of metabolism that is normally expelled from the body through breathing. However, if ventilation is inadequate or if there is an increased production of $CO_2$, such as in conditions like hypoventilation or respiratory failure, $CO_2$ levels can rise in the blood, resulting in hypercapnia. It occurs when alveolar $PCO_2$ becomes equal to the inspired $PCO_2$. *When the inspired $PCO_2$ becomes more than 7%, it is difficult to eliminate the $CO_2$ from the blood resulting in the retention of $CO_2$ and hence the $CO_2$ narcosis.*

The effects of carbon dioxide narcosis primarily stem from its impact on the central nervous system. $CO_2$ is a potent respiratory stimulant, and elevated levels can lead to vasodilation in the brain, resulting in increased cerebral blood flow. This increased blood flow, in turn, can cause symptoms such as:
- Mental confusion
- Drowsiness or lethargy
- Headaches
- Tremors or muscle twitching
- Flushing of the skin
- Increased heart rate and blood pressure
- In severe cases, carbon dioxide narcosis can progress to respiratory depression, coma, and even death if left untreated.

> **$CO_2$ Narcosis**
> - Accumulation of $CO_2$ in blood
> - Occurs when alveolar $PCO_2$ = inspired air $PCO_2$
> - Inspired $PCO_2$ > 7%
> - Elimination becomes difficult
> - Headache
> - Confusion
> - Eventually coma

Treatment of carbon dioxide narcosis involves addressing the underlying cause of hypercapnia, such as improving ventilation through *supplemental oxygen therapy, mechanical ventilation, or treating the underlying respiratory condition*. In acute cases, interventions may also include respiratory stimulants or medications to enhance respiratory drive. Prompt recognition and management of carbon dioxide narcosis are crucial to prevent further neurological deterioration and complications.

## NONCHEMICAL REGULATION

The local receptors present in lungs and airways are responsible for the non-nervous, nonchemical regulation of the respiration. Based on the location, these receptors are located in the:
- **Receptors in airway epithelium:**
  - Respond to lung hyper inflation
  - Cough, broncho constriction, mucus secretion
- **Receptors in airway smooth muscle cells:**
  - Respond to lung inflation
  - Broncho dilation, Hering-Breuer reflex
- **Receptors lying close to blood vessels (J receptors) (Fig. 54.8)**
  - *J receptors: juxta capillary receptors*
  - Discovered by Dr Autar Singh Paintal
  - Stimulated by Lung hyperinflation and pulmonary edema

## J Reflex

The J reflex, also known as the J-receptor reflex or pulmonary C-fiber reflex, is a respiratory reflex mediated by sensory nerve endings called J-receptors. These receptors are found in the walls of the pulmonary capillaries and are sensitive to changes in pulmonary interstitial fluid pressure.

The J reflex is primarily *activated by pulmonary congestion or edema*, which increases interstitial fluid pressure in the lungs. When the J-receptors are stimulated by this increased pressure, they send sensory signals to the brainstem respiratory centers, including the medulla

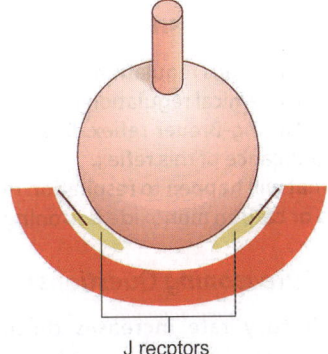

**Fig. 54.8:** Location of J receptors.

oblongata. Activation of the J reflex results in several respiratory responses, including:
- **Bronchoconstriction:** The reflex causes the smooth muscles of the bronchioles in the lungs to constrict, leading to narrowing of the airways. This helps redistribute blood flow away from congested or edematous areas of the lungs, improving ventilation-perfusion matching.
- **Rapid, shallow breathing:** The J reflex can stimulate an increase in the rate and shallowness of breathing, known as tachypnea and shallow breathing. This response aids in reducing pulmonary congestion by increasing the removal of carbon dioxide and maintaining oxygenation.
- **Coughing:** Activation of the J reflex can trigger coughing, which helps clear excessive fluid or mucus from the airways, further aiding in improving ventilation.

*The J reflex plays a protective role in maintaining respiratory function in response to pulmonary congestion or edema.* However, excessive or chronic activation of this reflex can contribute to respiratory symptoms seen in conditions such as heart failure, pulmonary edema, and acute respiratory distress syndrome (ARDS). Therefore, modulation of the J reflex is a potential target for therapeutic interventions aimed at improving respiratory function in these conditions.
- **Stimulus:** Hyperinflation or pulmonary congestion
- **Receptors:** Occurs due to stimulation of J receptors
- **Afferent:** Vagus
- **Center:** DRG
- **Efferent:** Vagus
- **Effect:** Decreased ventilation, rapid shallow breathing, coughing

### Pulmonary Chemoreflex

The intravenous or intracardiac administration of chemicals such as capsaicin results in reflex response characterized by *apnea followed by rapid breathing, bradycardia, and hypotension*. It is also seen in coronaries called as Bezold-Jarish reflex/coronary chemoreflex.

## BREATH HOLDING

### (Voluntary inhibition of respiration)

Breath holding, or voluntary apnea, involves conscious suppression of breathing. When breath holding begins, oxygen levels decrease and carbon dioxide levels increase in the bloodstream, triggering the respiratory centers in the brainstem. Initially, there's a strong urge to breathe due to rising $CO_2$ levels. Overtime, as oxygen levels continue to decline, peripheral chemoreceptors may also contribute to the sensation. Eventually, breath holding leads to involuntary respiratory contractions known as the *"break point,"* prompting the individual to resume breathing. Here, the $PO_2$ *is 60 mm Hg and* $PCO_2$ *is 50 mm Hg*.

---

### SUMMARY

- The regulation of respiration occurs at many levels and is classified as:
    - Nervous regulation: It is controlled by many levels:
        - Cerebral cortex, for voluntary control of respiration
        - Pons (pneumotaxic center and the apneustic center) finetunes the activity of main respiratory centers located in the medulla.
        - Medulla oblongata has the dorsal and ventral respiratory groups of neurons. The DRG exerts its effect through the pacemaker neurons (Pre-BÖTC)
- Chemical regulation is brought about by the central and peripheral chemoreceptors. The central chemoreceptors primarily respond to the $CO_2$ levels and a little bit to the $H^+$. However, the peripheral chemoreceptors respond mainly to hypoxia and a little bit to $H^+$.
- Nonchemical regulation: The regulation is due to the local receptors present in lungs and airways.

---

### LET US SEE, HOW MUCH YOU HAVE LEARNT?

 *Review Questions*

### Long/Short Answer Questions

Q1. Describe the nervous regulation of respiration.
Q2. Describe the chemical regulation of respiration.
Q3. Define the Hering-Breuer reflex. Describe the physiological significance of this reflex.
Q4. Explain what will happen to respiration rate in a patient of anemia or carbon monoxide poisoning.

Q5. Describe the J reflex.
Q6. Explain the mechanism of activation of glomus cells.
Q7. Explain the mechanism of activation of central chemoreceptors with $CO_2$.

### Explain Why? (Reasoning Questions)

Q1. The respiratory rate increases during metabolic acidosis.
Q2. Hyperventilation can lead to respiratory alkalosis.

Q3. Central chemoreceptors are more sensitive to changes in arterial carbon dioxide levels compared to changes in arterial oxygen levels.

Q4. The Hering-Breuer reflex prevents overinflation of the lungs during inspiration.
Q5. Respiratory centers in the brainstem are sensitive to changes in hydrogen ion concentration rather than changes in oxygen concentration.
Q6. Breath-holding can lead to an increase in carbon dioxide levels and a decrease in oxygen levels in the blood.
Q7. What will happen to respiratory rate in CO poisoning?

### Critical Thinking Case-Based Questions

Q1. Teresa, a 35-year-old woman, presented to the ER with complaints of dizziness, confusion, and rapid breathing. She had a history of anxiety disorder and panic attacks but denied any recent episodes. On examination, her respiratory rate was elevated, and she appeared restless. Arterial blood gas analysis reveals respiratory alkalosis with hypoxemia. Based upon the scenario, answer the following questions:

a. Explain the physiological mechanisms involved in the regulation of respiration in this condition.
b. What factors influence respiratory rate and depth?
c. What are the potential causes of respiratory alkalosis, and how might hypoxemia exacerbate respiratory symptoms such as rapid breathing and dizziness in a patient like Teresa?

### Multiple Choice Questions

Q1. Which level of regulatory control involves conscious effort to alter breathing patterns?
   a. Voluntary control
   b. Autonomic control
   c. Chemical control
   d. Mechanical control

Q2. Which level of regulatory control involves feedback mechanisms responding to changes in blood gases?
   a. Voluntary control
   b. Autonomic control
   c. Chemical control
   d. Mechanical control

Q3. Which of the following are primary respiratory centers in the brainstem?
   a. Cerebral cortex
   b. Medulla oblongata
   c. Pons
   d. Hypothalamus

Q4. Which respiratory center is responsible for setting the basic rhythm of breathing?
   a. Dorsal respiratory group (DRG)
   b. Ventral respiratory group (VRG)
   c. Pontine respiratory centers
   d. Pre-Bötzinger complex

Q5. Which of the following reflexes responds to changes in blood pH?
   a. Hering-Breuer reflex
   b. Bezold-Jarisch reflex
   c. Central chemoreceptor reflex
   d. Peripheral chemoreceptor reflex

Q6. Damage to which respiratory center is likely to result in complete cessation of breathing?
   a. Dorsal respiratory group (DRG)
   b. Ventral respiratory group (VRG)
   c. Pontine respiratory centers
   d. Pre-Bötzinger complex

Q7. Damage to which level of the respiratory control center is likely to affect voluntary control of breathing?
   a. Medulla oblongata
   b. Pons
   c. Cerebral cortex
   d. Hypothalamus

Q8. Central chemoreceptors are primarily sensitive to changes in which blood gas?
   a. Oxygen ($O_2$)
   b. Carbon dioxide ($CO_2$)
   c. Hydrogen ions ($H^+$)
   d. Nitrogen ($N_2$)

Q9. Peripheral chemoreceptors are primarily sensitive to changes in which blood gas?
   a. Oxygen ($O_2$)
   b. Carbon dioxide ($CO_2$)
   c. Hydrogen ions ($H^+$)
   d. Nitrogen ($N_2$)

Q10. Which of the following directly stimulate the central chemoreceptors?
   a. Changes in blood $CO_2$ levels
   b. Changes in blood $O_2$ levels
   c. Changes in blood pH
   d. Changes in blood pressure

Q11. Which of the following local receptors are involved in the Hering-Breuer reflex?
   a. Pulmonary stretch receptors
   b. Pulmonary irritant receptors
   c. J-receptors
   d. Central chemoreceptors

Q12. Local reflexes such as the Hering-Breuer reflex are involved in regulating:
   a. Tidal volume
   b. Respiratory rate
   c. Oxygen diffusion
   d. Carbon dioxide transport

Q13. Which of the following local reflexes helps prevent overinflation of the lungs during inspiration?
   a. Hering-Breuer reflex
   b. Bezold-Jarisch reflex
   c. J-receptor reflex
   d. Central chemoreceptor reflex

Q14. A patient presents with damage to the medulla oblongata due to a traumatic brain injury. What respiratory changes would you expect to observe?
   a. Decreased tidal volume and irregular breathing patterns
   b. Increased respiratory rate and depth
   c. Complete cessation of breathing
   d. No change in breathing patterns

Q15. A patient experiences prolonged exposure to high altitude. Which receptors are primarily responsible for detecting changes in oxygen levels in this situation?
   a. Central chemoreceptors
   b. Peripheral chemoreceptors
   c. Pulmonary stretch receptors
   d. J-receptors

Q16. A patient with severe pneumonia develops hyperventilation. Which reflex is most likely responsible for this respiratory response?
   a. Hering-Breuer reflex
   b. Central chemoreceptor reflex
   c. Bezold-Jarisch reflex
   d. Peripheral chemoreceptor reflex

Q17. A patient with chronic obstructive pulmonary disease (COPD) presents with hypercapnia. Which chemoreceptors are primarily responsible for detecting this increase in $CO_2$ levels?
   a. Central chemoreceptors
   b. Peripheral chemoreceptors
   c. J-receptors
   d. Pulmonary stretch receptors

Q18. A patient undergoes surgery under general anesthesia. Which respiratory reflex is most likely suppressed during anesthesia, leading to a risk of hypoventilation?
   a. Hering-Breuer reflex
   b. Bezold-Jarisch reflex
   c. Central chemoreceptor reflex
   d. Peripheral chemoreceptor reflex

Q19. A patient with severe heart failure experiences a sudden decrease in ventricular volume. Which reflex is most likely triggered, leading to bradycardia and hypotension?
   a. Hering-Breuer reflex
   b. Bezold-Jarisch reflex
   c. Central chemoreceptor reflex
   d. Peripheral chemoreceptor reflex

Q20. A patient with chronic respiratory alkalosis presents with compensatory hypoventilation. Which chemoreceptors are primarily responsible for detecting changes in blood pH?
   a. Central chemoreceptors
   b. Peripheral chemoreceptors
   c. Pulmonary stretch receptors
   d. J-receptors

Q21. A patient with acute respiratory distress syndrome (ARDS) experiences dyspnea and increased respiratory rate. Which local reflex is most likely contributing to this respiratory response?
   a. Hering-Breuer reflex
   b. Bezold-Jarisch reflex
   c. J-receptor reflex
   d. Central chemoreceptor reflex

## ANSWERS

| 1. a | 2. c | 3. b | 4. a | 5. c | 6. a | 7. c | 8. b | 9. a | 10. a | 11. a | 12. a | 13. a | 14. a |
| 15. a | 16. a | 17. a | 18. a | 19. b | 20. b | 21. c | | | | | | | |

# Respiration in Special Conditions
## (In Different Barometric Pressures)

**55**
**CHAPTER**

> **COMPETENCIES ADDRESSED**
> **PY6.4:** Describe and discuss the physiology of high altitude and deep-sea diving.
> **PY6.5:** Describe and discuss the principles of artificial respiration, oxygen therapy, acclimatization and decompression sickness.

>  **LEARNING OBJECTIVES**
> At the end of this chapter, the learner should be able to:
> - Explain the change in atmospheric pressure and composition (especially oxygen) at different levels of altitude below and above the sea level.
> - Describe the physiological effects of acute change in the barometric pressure on various body systems.
> - Describe the effect of gravity on the respiratory system.
> - Describe the related applied physiology in various professionals exposed to these special environments like mountaineers, astronauts and deep-sea divers.

We had been studying from our school days that the earth's atmosphere changes with altitude. Most of us live on the earth at the sea level, where the atmospheric pressure is 760 mm Hg. This means, we all living under the pressure of 1 atmosphere (760 mm Hg). There are two ways, we can study the variation of this altitude:
1. Ascending upwards with altitude, like climbing a mountain, flying in an aircraft or even flying in a rocket into the space.
2. Another view is descending below the sea level, into the ocean.

**Figure 55.1** shows us that the $PO_2$ decreases significantly with increase in the altitude.

**Note that:**
- At sea level, atmospheric pressure in 760 mm Hg and $PO_2$ is 21% of 760 mm Hg, i.e., 159 mm Hg.
- On ascending upwards, till 10,000 feet, the atmospheric pressure reduces to 523 mm Hg, further reducing the $PO_2$ to 110 mm Hg.
- While at 50,000 feet, the pressure drops to 87 mm Hg, and $PO_2$ further decreases to 18 mm Hg.

From these values we conclude that as we ascend high up, the $PO_2$ decreases and causes the various changes in body due to acute effects of hypoxia.

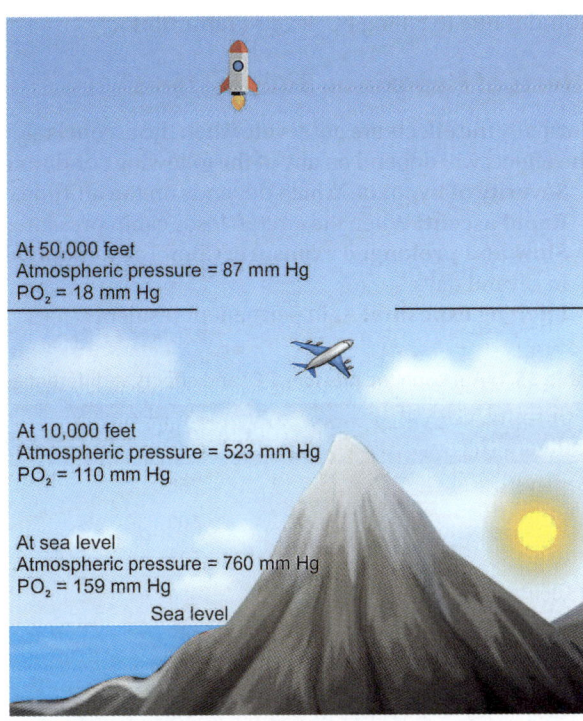

**Fig. 55.1:** $PO_2$ levels decrease with increase in altitude.

However, going deep into the sea the barometric pressure increases considerably with almost 1 atmosphere increase with 33 feet below the sea level. Hence, the person at the bottom of 33 feet will experience 2 atmosphere pressure and it increases with further descent. At 300 feet below the sea level, he will experience the pressure of 10 atmospheres. It is equally important to understand here, that as the atmospheric pressure increase, below the sea level, the gases dissolved in the blood tend to get compressed and reduce in volume, which can result in:

- Reduction in the volume of air in the lungs. Under very high pressures, it can even lead to collapse of the lung.
- The gases form the tiny bubbles and get dissolved in the the tissues (much like the compressed gas in a bottle of Cola).
- Hence when a person ascends up quickly these gases rapidly dissolve in blood, forming tiny bubbles, as would happen, when you suddenly open a bottle of cola.

From these facts we conclude, that as we descend below sea level, the atmospheric pressure increases and causes the gases to dissolve in blood and tissues. On rapid decompression, these gases form bubbles causing the decompression sickness. After this introduction, lets now focus on the high altitude physiology and its effects on respiratory system in the section below.

## HIGH ALTITUDE PHYSIOLOGY

As we have discussed above, the $PO_2$ decreases with the altitude; lets understand the effect of hypoxia at different altitudes due to falling $PO_2$ levels **(Table 55.1)**.

### Effects of Hypoxia on Body Systems

Normally the effects are not severe when the ascent is slow. The effects will depend on any of the following conditions:
- **Severity of hypoxia:** Which depends on the altitude.
- **Rapid ascent:** When the aircraft loses cabin pressure.
- **Slow and prolonged exposure:** Climbing a mountain in several days.
- **Lifelong exposure:** As in permanent residents.

**What will happen if a person ascends up in an unpressurised airplane?**

If a person ascends up in an unpressurized aircraft, he experiences "ceiling effect", which can be explained as under:
- When an aviator breathes air (which contains approximately 21% oxygen), the arterial oxygen saturation decreases as altitude increases due to the reduced atmospheric pressure.
- An unacclimatized person can typically remain conscious until their arterial oxygen saturation falls to around 50%.
- For short exposure times, the ceiling (maximum altitude) for an aviator in an unpressurized airplane when breathing air is approximately 23,000 feet.

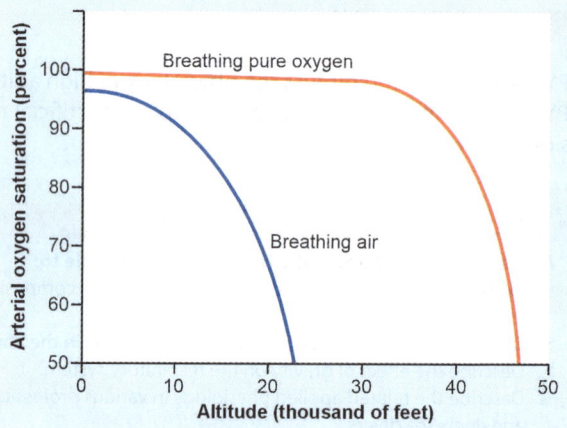

- On the other hand, when an aviator breathes pure oxygen (100% oxygen), the arterial oxygen saturation remains higher at higher altitudes.
- At an altitude of 47,000 feet, an aviator breathing pure oxygen still maintains an arterial saturation of about 50%.
- Therefore, the ceiling for an aviator in an unpressurized airplane when breathing pure oxygen is approximately 47,000 feet.

(It is important to note that these altitudes assume that the equipment supplying the oxygen operates perfectly. If the oxygen supply fails or malfunctions, the aviator's ability to remain conscious would be compromised, regardless of whether they are breathing air or pure oxygen.)

**Table 55.1:** Atmospheric pressure, $PO_2$ and effects at different altitudes.

| Altitude in feet | Atmospheric pressure (mm Hg) | $PO_2$ in air (mm Hg) | Effect |
|---|---|---|---|
| Sea level | 760 | 158 | Normal |
| 5000 | 600 | 132 | No hypoxia |
| 10,000 | 523 | 110 | Hypoxic symptoms appear |
| 15,000 | 400 | 90 | Severe hypoxic effects develop |
| 20,000 | 349 | 73 | Severe hypoxic effects, consciousness may be lost |
| 25,000 | 250 | 62 | Pure $O_2$ breathing essential |
| 30,000 (29,028 is height of Mount Everest) | 226 | 47 | |

*At 63,000 feet (19,200 m), the barometric pressure is 47 mm Hg. At this pressure, the body fluids boil at body temperature. This is an academic speculation, as any individual exposed to such low pressure will die of hypoxia before the bubbles of oxygen "Boiling of blood" could cause death.*

These hypoxic effects can be classified as:
- **Severe hypoxic effects** (It occurs, when altitude is more than 20,000 feet): The effects are mainly on seen on CNS:
  - Causing the development of *cerebral ischemia and cerebral edema*.
  - Within 10-15 minutes the subject may become unconscious.
  - This is similar to rapid arrest of circulation; instant death may ensue due to cerebral ischemia and cerebral edema within 4-5 minutes.
- **Moderate hypoxia** (It is slow onset of hypoxia <15,000 feet):
  - *Nervous system:* Most of the symptoms are seen in nervous system and are similar to alcoholic intoxication. Patient may be depressed or elated, lose control of self, become more talkative, quarrelsome, ill-tempered, or rude. There may be loss of coordination and easy fatiguability, impaired power of judgement, loss of memory and euphoria. Visual and auditory acuity decreases dure to cerebral ischemia.
  - *Respiratory system:* Hypoxia stimulates respiratory centers through peripheral chemoreceptors.
    - *Rate and depth of respiration increases.*
    - Alkalosis may result due to loss of $CO_2$.
    - Pulmonary vasoconstriction results in *pulmonary edema* and *dyspnea*. In some people periodic breathing may develop.
  - *Cardiovascular system:* There is increased sympathetic activity leading to tachycardia and increased myocardial contractility develop. There is increase in blood pressure and cardiac output. There will be increase in cerebral and coronary blood flow and a decrease in cutaneous and splanchnic blood flow. After sometime there is reduction in cardiac output and BP, but tachycardia persists.
  - *Digestive system:* Loss of appetite (anorexia, nausea, vomiting and diarrhea).
  - *Kidney:* Excretion of alkaline urine. Hypoxia stimulates production of erythropoietin.
  - *Blood:* The blood counts increase, resulting in increase in RBC, WBC, platelets. This is due to shift of storage pool to circulation pool.

**Chronic Effects of Hypoxia**
- Increase RBC counts
- Increase hematocrit
- Increase pulmonary arterial pressure
- Increase right ventricular size
- Decreased peripheral arterial pressure
- Chronic heart failure (CHF) followed by death

## Acclimatization to High Altitude

Acclimatization is the ability of the body to adjust to an altered environment. Acclimatization refers to a series of integrated adaptations that take place at high altitudes,

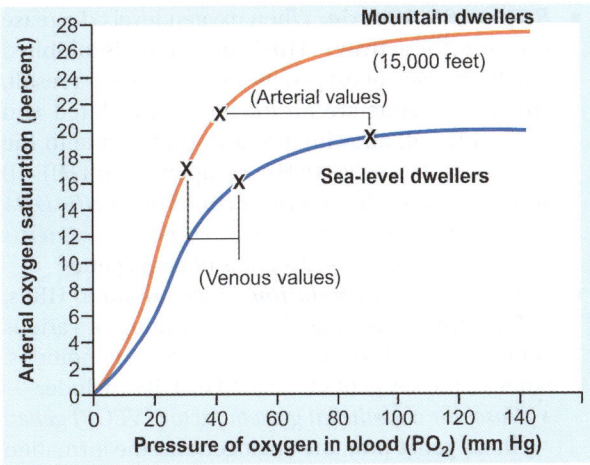

**Fig. 55.2:** Natural acclimatization of human living at mountains.

that tend to restore the $PO_2$ within the tissue to normal sea level values despite lowered $PO_2$ of the atmosphere (**Fig. 55.2**). The adaptive changes appear within 8 hours and may take several days. *The maximum height up to which adaptation occurs is 18,000 feet,* beyond this level, the subject needs $O_2$ inhalation for survival. The following mechanisms are responsible for acclimatization.

### Compensatory Changes

1. *Increase in pulmonary ventilation—earliest response.* Hypoxia *stimulates chemoreceptors* which result in generation of chemoreflex, leading to hyperventilation and decreased $CO_2$. The $CO_2$ washout results in respiratory *alkalosis* (hypocalcemic tetany may occur along with it due to alkalosis). This inhibits hyperventilation and excess bicarbonate is excreted by kidneys (kidneys compensate by decreasing hydrogen secretion and increasing bicarbonate excretion). Respiratory centers become much more responsive to peripheral chemoreceptors stimulus caused by hypoxia after kidneys compensate for alkalosis.
2. *Erythropoietin is increased* which increases the RBC. This is probably the best-known physiological response to chronic hypoxia and a hallmark of high-altitude acclimatization. Hypoxia induces expression of glycoprotein hormone erythropoietin, which mediates increased RBC production. *Erythropoietin level peak after about 24–48 hours of hypoxia.*
3. *Hypoxia-inducible factors (HIFs)* play a crucial role in the body's response to decreased oxygen levels, ensuring that cells can adapt to low oxygen environments:
   - *HIF structure and activation:* HIFs are DNA-binding transcription factors composed of two subunits: *HIF-1α and HIF-1β*. Under normal oxygen conditions, HIF-1α subunits are constantly being hydroxylated by specific HIF hydroxylases, marking them for degradation via the proteasome pathway. This process keeps HIF levels low in oxygen-rich environments.

- ***Response to hypoxia:*** When oxygen levels decrease (hypoxia, the activity of HIF hydroxylases is inhibited due to the lack of oxygen as a substrate. As a result, HIF-1α subunits are no longer hydroxylated and are stabilized, allowing them to translocate to the nucleus and form active HIF complexes with HIF-1β subunits. *These HIF complexes bind to specific DNA sequences known as hypoxia response elements (HREs)* in the promoter regions of target genes.
- ***Gene expression regulation:*** Once bound to HREs, HIF complexes activate the transcription of various genes that facilitate adaptation to hypoxic conditions. Some of the key genes regulated by HIFs include:
  - *Vascular endothelial growth factor (VEGF) genes:* These genes promote angiogenesis, the formation of new blood vessels, which helps improve oxygen delivery to tissues.
  - *Erythropoietin (EPO) genes:* EPO stimulates the production of red blood cells (erythropoiesis), increasing the oxygen-carrying capacity of the blood.
  - *Mitochondrial genes:* HIFs regulate genes involved in mitochondrial biogenesis and function, optimizing energy utilization and metabolism under low oxygen conditions.
  - *Glycolytic enzyme genes:* HIFs enhance the expression of glycolytic enzymes, promoting anaerobic metabolism as an alternative energy source when oxygen availability is limited.
  - *Nitric oxide (NO) genes:* HIFs increase the availability of nitric oxide, a vasodilator, which helps dilate blood vessels in the lungs (pulmonary vasodilation), improving blood flow and oxygen exchange.

  **Master switch for hypoxia response:** HIFs serve as a "master switch" that mediates the body's response to hypoxia by regulating the expression of genes involved in oxygen delivery, energy metabolism, and vascular function. This adaptive mechanism helps cells and tissues survive and function optimally under low oxygen conditions.

4. *Peripheral circulatory system changes:* There is an increase in tissue capillaries, which increases the cardiac output to 30%, as an individual ascends to high altitude as hematocrit increases, the cardiac output decreases towards normal in few weeks. There is an increase in the number of capillaries in nonpulmonary tissues (angiogenesis). Combined effect of hypoxia and excess workload lead to pulmonary hypertension causing increased capillary density in the right ventricular muscle.
5. *Increase in diffusion of gases and diffusion capacity*—due to increase in pulmonary capillary blood volume, increase in lung air volume, increase in pulmonary arterial blood pressure, increased hemoglobin, alveolar volume and membrane diffusion. Reduction in alveolar-capillary barrier resistance is possibly mediated by an increase of sympathetic tone and can develop in 3 weeks.
6. *Cellular acclimatization*—increase in the number of mitochondria, which are the site of oxidation reactions, and increase in myoglobin that facilitates the movement of oxygen in the tissues. There is also an increase in tissue content of cytochrome oxidase. This all leads to an increase in $O_2$ utilization.

## High Altitude Illness

Individuals who ascend from sea level to high altitude (unacclimatized) can experience a sudden decrease in arterial oxygen and rapid onset of signs and symptoms of hypoxia with altered functions of CNS. These same symptoms are seen in people on airplanes when there is a sudden loss of cabin pressure.
- Acute mountain sickness:
  - High altitude cerebral edema (HACE)
  - High altitude pulmonary edema (HAPE)
- Chronic mountain sickness (Monge's disease)

---

**Title: Surviving High Altitude: A First-Time Expedition to K2**

**Learning Objectives:**
a. Understand the symptoms and risks associated with high altitude sickness.
b. Learn how to recognize and respond to hypoxia and pulmonary edema.
c. Acquire knowledge about preventive measures and treatments for altitude-related illnesses.
d. Develop strategies for effective communication and teamwork in challenging environments.

**Case Scenario:**

Meet Sam, an adventurous mountaineer embarking on his first expedition to conquer the mighty K2 peak, the second highest mountain in the world. With a passion for adventure and a thirst for exploration, Sam has meticulously prepared for this journey, equipped with essential gear and guided by experienced sherpas.

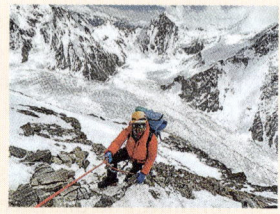

As Sam and his team ascend towards the summit, the air becomes thinner, and the oxygen levels drop drastically. Despite Sam's physical fitness and determination, his body begins to struggle with the altitude. He starts experiencing symptoms of hypoxia, such as dizziness, shortness of breath, and confusion. Ignoring these signs, Sam pushes forward, eager to reach the peak.

However, as Sam climbs higher, his condition worsens. He begins to develop pulmonary edema, marked by a persistent cough, frothy sputum, and extreme fatigue. Recognizing the seriousness of Sam's condition, his sherpa intervenes immediately. With quick thinking and expertise, the sherpa diagnoses Sam's altitude sickness and makes the crucial decision to descend to lower altitudes.

Back at the base camp, Sam receives prompt medical attention and is administered supplemental oxygen to alleviate his symptoms. As he recuperates, Sam reflects on the importance of recognizing the warning signs of altitude sickness and the significance of teamwork and communication in such perilous situations.

*Explore on these points:*
- Symptoms of high altitude sickness: What are the various symptoms of altitude sickness, including hypoxia and pulmonary edema. Emphasize the importance of recognizing these signs early on to prevent further complications.
- Risk factors: Explore the factors that contribute to altitude-related illnesses, such as rapid ascent, dehydration, and individual susceptibility. Encourage participants to assess their own risk factors before embarking on high-altitude expeditions.
- Response and treatment: Analyze the sherpa's response to Sam's condition and discuss the appropriate actions taken to ensure his safety. Highlight the significance of timely intervention and the administration of supplemental oxygen in managing altitude sickness.
- Preventive measures: Outline strategies for preventing altitude-related illnesses, including gradual acclimatization, adequate hydration, and proper nutrition. Encourage participants to incorporate these measures into their expedition plans to mitigate risks.
- Teamwork and communication: Emphasize the importance of effective communication and teamwork in mountain expeditions. Describe how Sam's sherpa effectively communicated and collaborated with the team to ensure Sam's safety during a crisis.

*Conclusion:*
Through Sam's experience on his first expedition to K2, participants gain valuable insights into the challenges and risks associated with high-altitude mountaineering. By understanding the symptoms, risks, and preventive measures for altitude sickness, participants are better equipped to navigate such environments safely and responsibly. Additionally, the scenario underscores the critical role of teamwork and communication in ensuring the well-being of all expedition members, highlighting the importance of collective responsibility in extreme outdoor pursuits.

## Acute Mountain Sickness

At non-extreme altitudes (5000 m), 10–85% of individuals who ascend rapidly may develop acute mountain sickness (AMS). They may lose consciousness and die if they if not given $O_2$ or descend to a low altitude. This syndrome develops 8–24 hours after arrival at altitude and may last 4–8 days. It is characterized by nonspecific symptoms like loss of appetite, nausea, vomiting, disturbed sleep, fatigue, dizziness, and confusion. High-altitude illnesses encompass the pulmonary and cerebral syndromes that occur in nonacclimatized individuals shortly after rapid ascent to high altitude **(Table 55.2)**.

**Table 55.2:** Features of different high altitude sickness.

|  | High altitude cerebral edema (HACE) | High altitude pulmonary edema (HAPE) | Chronic mountain sickness/Monge's disease |
|---|---|---|---|
|  | An extreme form of AMS | Noncardiogenic form of pulmonary edema | Loss of high altitude tolerance after prolonged exposure |
| Manifestation | • Altitude >10,000 feet<br>• Rare but fatal. Seen in individuals who ascend quickly to high altitudes | • Altitudes >8,000 feet<br>• Fatal. Seen in those of quickly ascend and engage in heavy work. Most common cause of altitude illness-related mortality<br>• Also seen in acclimatized individuals who spend 2 weeks or more at sea level. And then re ascend | • Altitude >1,200 feet<br>• Develops in individuals that reside at high altitude (natives of Andes mountains, Tibetan highlanders) |
| Clinical features | Headache, irritability, insomnia, breathlessness, nausea, vomiting. Encephalopathic features-ataxia and/or decreased consciousness | • Headache, irritability, insomnia, breathlessness, nausea, vomiting<br>• Cough, dyspnea, and/or decreased exercise tolerance<br>• Associated with marked pulmonary hypertension, but left arterial pressures are normal | • Fatigue, shortness of breath, aches and pains, and a blue color to the lips and skin (cyanosis)<br>• Pulmonary hypertension, cor-pulmonale<br>• Cough may be the first sign |
| Pathophysiology | • Cerebral edema<br>• Low $PO_2$ causes arteriolar dilatation, increase in capillary pressure, increased transudation of fluids into brain tissue, decreased urine volume | The edema fluid is of a high-permeability type, with a high content of protein and blood cells. It occurs as not all pulmonary arteries have enough smooth muscles to constrict in response to hypoxia. Rise in pulmonary arterial pressure causes a capillary pressure increase that disrupt their walls | • Excess erythrocytosis (due to body's compensatory response to high altitude)<br>• Elevated pulmonary arterial pressure (due to hypoxic vascular constriction)<br>• Greatly enlarged right side of the heart<br>• Peripheral arterial pressure begins to fall<br>• Congestive heart failure ensues<br>• Death follows |
| Treatment | Rest, descent to lower altitude, $O_2$ supplementation, $Ca_2$= channel blocker<br>• Nifedipine, dexamethasone (corticosteroid) | Rest, descent to lower altitude, $O_2$ supplementation, $Ca_2$= channel blocker<br>• Nifedipine, dexamethasone (corticosteroid) | Venesection, acetazolamide (carbonic anhydrase inhibitor)<br>• Dexamethasone |

> **Q: Explain why the cerebral edema develops in high altitude sickness?**
> The local vasodilation occurring in the cerebral blood vessels causing the increased capillary hydrostatic pressure and hence the cerebral edema. It causes the mental symptoms like confusion and disorientation
>
> **Q: Explain why the pulmonary edema develops in high altitude sickness?**
> The pulmonary capillaries have a peculiar property of causing vasoconstriction in hypoxia. Hence, the blood gets shifted to the better oxygenated areas of lungs. The increased blood flow in these areas causes increased capillary hydrostatic pressure resulting in an increased net filtration pressure and hence the development of pulmonary edema.

## SPACE PHYSIOLOGY

*(Effect of acceleratory forces on the body in aviation and space physiology)*

Because of rapid changes in velocity and direction of motion in airplanes and spacecrafts, several types of acceleratory forces effect the body during flight:
- At beginning of flight the astronaut experiences simple linear acceleration.
- At end of flight there is deceleration
- Everytime vehicle turns there is centrifugal acceleration.

### Measurement of Acceleratory Force—"G" (Fig. 55.3)

When an aviator is sitting in his seat, the force with which he is pressing against the seat results from the pull of gravity and is equal to his weight and is said to be +1G because it is equal to the pull of gravity.

If the force with which he presses against the seat becomes five times his normal weight during pull-out from a dive, the force acting on the seat is +5G.

If the airplane goes through an outside loop so that the person is held down by his seat belt, negative G is applied to his body: if the force with which he is held down by his belt is equal to the weight of his body, the negative force is –1G.

### Effect of Centrifugal Acceleratory Force on the Body—Positive G (Fig. 55.3)

- **Effect on circulatory system:** The most important effect is on circulatory system as blood is mobile and can be translocated. When an aviator is subjected to positive G, the *blood is translocated to lower part of the body*. Thus, if the centrifugal acceleratory force is +5G, and the person is in immobilized standing position, the pressure in the veins of the feet becomes greatly increased (450 mm Hg). In sitting pressure becomes nearly 300 mm Hg. *If more blood is pooled in lower parts of the body, there will be a decrease in venous return and therefore cardiac output will decrease.*

  The secondary recovery may be caused by baroreceptor reflex. Acceleration greater than 4 to 6 G, *causes "blackout" of vision* within a few seconds and *unconsciousness* shortly thereafter, and ultimately death ensues, if this acceleration continues unabated.

- **Effects on vertebrae:** Extremely high acceleration forces if continued even for a fraction of a second, may lead to *fracture of vertebrae*. The degree of positive

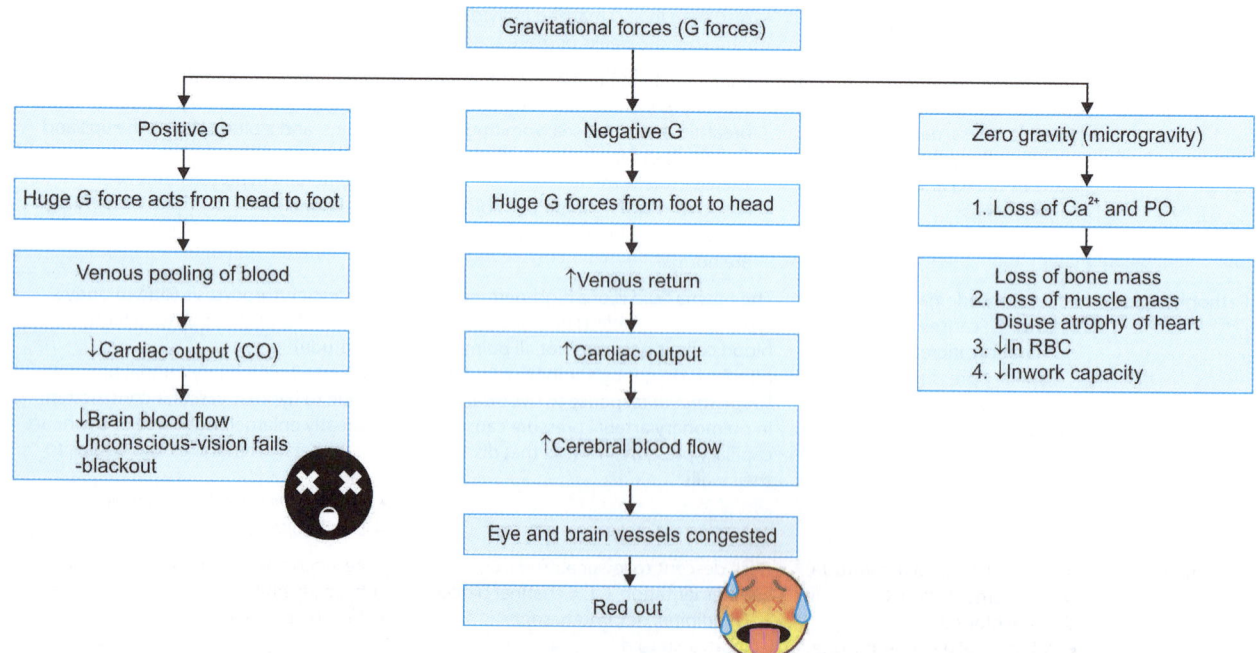

**Fig. 55.3:** Effects of G forces on human body.

acceleration, that a normal individual can withstand in a sitting position before vertebral fracture occurs is 20G.

### The Effects of Negative G (Fig. 55.3)

The effects of negative G are more damaging on the body permanently, then the effects of positive G.

An aviator can usually go through outside loops up to negative acceleratory forces of -4 to -5G without causing permanent harm, although causing intense hyperemia of the head. Occasionally psychotic disturbances lasting for 15 to 20 minutes occur as a result of brain oedema. Sometimes negative G forces can be so great (-20G), that centrifugation of the head is extreme, cerebral BP reaches 300 to 400 mm Hg, causing small vessels on the surface of the head and the brain to rupture. However, the vessels inside the cranium show less tendency to rupture because of the following reason:

- The CSF is centrifuges towards the head, and the blood is centrifuged towards the cranial vessels, and the greatly increased pressure of the CSF act as a 'cushioning buffer' on the outside the brain to prevent intracerebral vascular rupture.
- As the eyes are not protected by the cranium, intense hyperemia occurs in them during strong negative G. As a result, the eyes temporarily become blinded with *"red-out"*.
- Body can be protected against centrifugal acceleratory forces by—tightening abdominal muscles and leaning forward which prevents pooling of blood in lower parts of the body. "Anti-G suits' also compress abdomen and legs.

### Effects of Linear Acceleratory Forces on the Body (Fig. 55.3)

**Acceleratory forces in space travel:** Spacecraft does not make rapid turns, therefore acceleratory forces are of much less significance during space travel. Blast-off acceleration and landing deceleration are both linear accelerations, one positive and other negative. The standing body may not be able to tolerate the blast-off acceleration, but in a semi reclining position, transverse to the axis of acceleration, the amount of acceleration can be withstood with ease. That is how, we see the reason of reclining seats used by astronauts.

Problems also occur when the spacecraft re-enters the atmosphere during deceleration. Deceleration is proportional to square root of velocity. A person traveling at a greater speed will require greater distance for deceleration. Deceleration may be accomplished much more slowly at higher velocities, than is necessary at lower velocities.

## Artificial Climate in Closed Spacecrafts

An artificial atmosphere and climate must be produced in a spacecraft. $O_2$ concentration should be high enough and $CO_2$ concentration low, to prevent suffocation. In modern space shuttles gases equal to those in normal air are used, with total pressure equal to 760 mm Hg. The presence of nitrogen diminishes likelihood of fire and explosion. It also protects development of local patches of lung atelectasis that often occur when breathing pure oxygen, because oxygen is absorbed rapidly when small bronchi are temporarily blocked by mucous plugs. For space travel lasting several months, it is impractical to carry adequate oxygen. So, recycling of oxygen over and over again by electrolysis of water to release oxygen. Other biological methods like algae with its large store of chlorophyll to release oxygen from carbon dioxide by process of photosynthesis.

## Weightlessness in Space

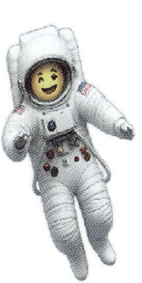

Near zero G force–microgravity. The cause of this is not failure of gravity to pull on the body, because gravity from any nearby heavenly body is still active. However, gravity acts on the spacecraft and the individual at the same time, so that both are pulled at the same time, so that both are pulled at exactly the same acceleratory forces and in the same direction. For this reason, the person is simply not attracted toward any specific wall of the spacecraft.

### Physiological Problems of Weightlessness

- Motion sickness during first few days of travel.
- Translocation of fluids within the body because of failure of gravity to cause normal hydrostatic pressure.
- Diminished physical activity because no strength of muscle contraction is required to oppose the force of gravity.

### The Observed Effects of Staying in Space

- Decreased blood volume
- Decreased red cell mass
- Decrease in muscle strength and work capacity
- Decrease in maximum cardiac output
- Loss of calcium and phosphate from bones, as well as loss of bone mass.

Most of these same effects also occur in people who lie in bed for an extended period of time. For this reason, exercise programs are carried out by astronauts during a prolonged space mission.

### Cardiovascular, Muscle, and Bone De-conditioning during Prolonged Exposure to Weightlessness

The deconditioning occurs despite rigorous exercise during flight. During prolonged stay in space, the astronauts may loose 1.0% of their bone mass every month. Substantial atrophy of cardiac and skeletal muscle also occurs during prolonged stay in microgravity environment. Cardiovascular deconditioning leads to decreased work capacity, reduced blood volume, diminished baroreceptor reflex, and reduced orthostatic tolerance. On returning back to earth, this greatly limits their capacity to stand erect and perform normal daily activities. Astronauts are susceptible to bone fractures, for 4–6 months on return back to normal gravity conditions. They may require several weeks to regain back cardiovascular, muscle and bone health.

## DEEP-SEA DIVING

Deep-sea diving is a challenging and specialized activity that involves exploring the underwater world at depths beyond what is accessible through regular recreational diving. The physiology of deep-sea diving is complex and involves various physiological adaptations and considerations to ensure the safety and well-being of divers.

The relationship between pressure and sea depth is a result of the increasing weight of the water column above a certain point. As you descend deeper into the ocean, the pressure exerted by the water increases **(Table 55.3)**.

In general, the pressure in a fluid, such as water, increases with depth due to the weight of the fluid above. This relationship is described by **Pascal's law**, which states *that the pressure at any point in a fluid is equal in all directions and increases with depth.*

In the case of seawater, the pressure increases by approximately one atmosphere (equivalent to the pressure at sea level) for every 33 feet (10.1 meters) of depth. This means that at a depth of 33 feet, a person would experience a total pressure of 2 atmospheres, with one atmosphere caused by the weight of the air above the water and the other atmosphere caused by the weight of the water itself. At 66 feet, the pressure would be 3 atmospheres, and so on.

The effect of increasing pressure with depth has important implications for diving physiology. It can cause compression of gases, such as air, to smaller volumes. This is described by **Boyle's law**, which states *that the volume of a gas is inversely proportional to the pressure applied to it, assuming the temperature remains constant.* As the pressure increases, the volume of a given quantity of gas decreases.

For example, if a bell jar at sea level contains 1 liter of air, at a depth of 33 feet (2 atmospheres of pressure), the volume of the air would be compressed to half a liter. At a depth of 233 feet (8 atmospheres of pressure), the volume would be compressed to one-eighth of a liter.

## Nitrogen Narcosis and Decompression Sickness at High Pressure

*(Caisson disease, diver's paralysis or dysbarism, bends)*

To study the case related to Caissons disease, refer to the author's early clinical exposure in clinical physiology.

Caisson's disease, also known as decompression sickness or "the bends," is a condition that occurs when nitrogen bubbles form in the bloodstream and tissues due to a rapid decrease in pressure, typically experienced by divers ascending too quickly or workers in pressurized environments like caissons (watertight chambers used in underwater construction).

### *Pathophysiology*

During dives or work in pressurized environments, nitrogen (being most abundant gas) dissolves into body tissues due to increased pressure. As pressure decreases during ascent or decompression, nitrogen can come out of solution and form bubbles in the bloodstream and tissues. These bubbles can obstruct blood flow, cause tissue damage, and trigger inflammatory responses, leading to various symptoms. These symptoms occur due to various reasons, discussed below:

- **Pressure effects:** As divers descend into the deep sea, they encounter increased pressure due to the weight of the water above them. This pressure affects the body in several ways. The most significant impact is on the respiratory and circulatory systems. Breathing compressed gas at depth helps counteract the pressure and prevents the lungs from collapsing. However, it also exposes divers to increased nitrogen levels, which can lead to decompression sickness if ascent is too rapid.
- **Nitrogen narcosis:** About four-fifths of the air is nitrogen. At sea-level pressure, the nitrogen has no significant effect on bodily function, but at high pressures, it can cause varying degrees of narcosis. At greater depths, divers may experience a condition known as nitrogen narcosis or *'the bends' or "rapture of the deep."* Under high-pressure conditions, nitrogen gas can have an anesthetic effect on the nervous system, resulting in impaired judgment, confusion, and a feeling of euphoria. It is similar to being intoxicated and can impair a diver's ability to make critical decisions.

- Increased barometric pressure
- $PIO_2$ and $PIN_2$ will be increased
- Blood plasma holds more nitrogen than at normal barometric pressure
- Can lead to nitrogen narcosis
- Mental confusion, incoherence of speech, etc.
- Motor functions remain normal
- Sudden decompression (rapid ascent)

**Table 55.3:** Sea depth and pressure/volume changes.

| Sea depth | Pressure | Volume |
|---|---|---|
| 33 feet (10 m) | 2 atm *(1 atmosphere of pressure caused by the weight of the air above the water and the second atmosphere caused by the weight of the water)* | ½ liter (Boyles law – Pα 1/V) |
| 66 feet (20 m) | 3 atm | 1/3rd liter |
| 233 feet | 8 atm | 1/8th liter |

## Clinical Symptoms

The symptoms of nitrogen narcosis can resemble alcohol intoxication or general confusion. Common signs include:
- Impaired judgment
- Euphoria
- Dizziness
- Slowed mental processing
- Loss of coordination
- Sometimes hallucinations. It can affect a diver's ability to make rational decisions and execute critical tasks underwater.

**Depth-related:** Nitrogen narcosis generally becomes noticeable at depths below 100 feet (30 meters) but can vary between individuals. The severity of the narcosis increases with increasing depth.

**Decompression sickness (DCS):** When divers spend time at depth, nitrogen dissolves into their tissues. If ascent is too rapid, the nitrogen forms bubbles that can cause decompression sickness, also known as "the bends." DCS can lead to joint and muscle pain (the bends), dizziness, shortness of breath (chokes—due to massive microbubbles in lung capillaries), pulmonary edema, fatigue, and in severe cases, it can be life-threatening. To prevent DCS, divers must ascend slowly, making decompression stops at specified depths to allow the excess nitrogen to safely dissipate from their bodies.

## Prevention and Management

- To prevent nitrogen narcosis, divers often use a dive table or dive computer that provides safe depth and time limits.
- Another approach is to use a gas mixture with lower nitrogen content, such as nitrox or trimix (mixture of oxygen, nitrogen, helium or argon).
    - Using scuba equipment **(Fig. 55.4)**: An open circuit demand type scuba, commonly known as scuba diving equipment, is a *self-contained underwater breathing apparatus* that allows a diver to breathe while submerged. In an open circuit system, the diver inhales from a tank containing compressed air or a breathing gas mixture, and then exhales the used air or gas into the surrounding water. Open circuit demand type scuba systems are the most common type of scuba diving equipment used by recreational divers. They allow for longer dives as the exhaled air is released into the water, and fresh air is supplied from the tank. However, open circuit systems are less efficient than closed circuit rebreathers in terms of gas consumption, making them better suited for shorter dives or dives with easy access to a refill station.
    - **Saturation diving** is a technique used in deep-sea diving where divers work at great depths, typically between 250 feet and nearly 1000 feet. In this type of diving, divers live in a large compression tank for extended periods, often days or weeks, at a pressure level close to the working pressure. This process saturates the diver's tissues and fluids with the gases they will be exposed to during the dive, preventing the occurrence of decompression bubbles when they return to the tank after working.

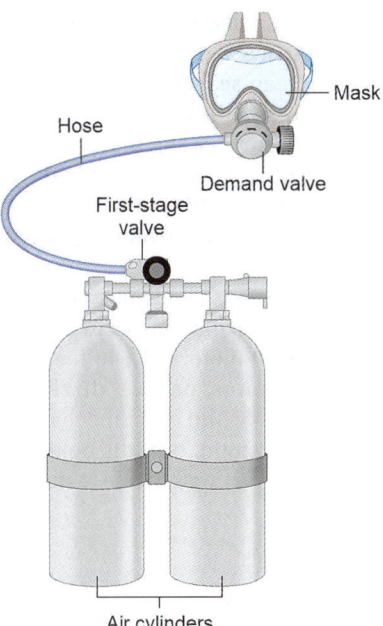

**Fig. 55.4:** Scuba equipment.

To facilitate saturation diving and minimize the risks associated with deep dives, a gas mixture of helium and oxygen is used instead of the traditional nitrogen-oxygen mixture. In addition to using helium, it is also important to reduce the concentration of oxygen ($O_2$) in the gas mixture during very deep dives. High partial pressures of oxygen can lead to oxygen toxicity, which can cause seizures and other severe health issues. By reducing the oxygen concentration in the gas mixture, the risk of oxygen toxicity is minimized.

- In case symptoms of nitrogen narcosis appear during a dive, ascending to a shallower depth usually alleviates the condition. However, severe cases may require immediate ascent to avoid further complications.

## Other Effects

1. **Oxygen toxicity:** While oxygen is essential for sustaining life, it can become toxic at high partial pressures, particularly during prolonged exposures at great depths. Hyperoxic exposure can cause central nervous system toxicity, resulting in symptoms like seizures, dizziness, and nausea. *The toxicity is caused due to conversion of molecular oxygen into active oxygen (oxygen free radicals).* These radicals oxidize polyunsaturated fatty acids and also oxidize cellular enzymes. Nervous tissues are especially susceptible because of their high lipid content, lethal effects therefore are mostly related to

brain dysfunction. Divers must monitor their oxygen exposure limits to avoid oxygen toxicity.
2. **Hypothermia:** Deep-sea diving often takes place in cold water, which increases the risk of hypothermia. The body loses heat much faster in water than in air, and extended exposure can lead to a drop in core body temperature. Proper insulation, wetsuits or drysuits, and thermal protection are crucial to prevent hypothermia during deep-sea dives.
3. **High-pressure nervous syndrome (HPNS):** HPNS is a neurological condition that can occur at extreme depths, typically below 500 meters (1,640 feet). It can cause symptoms like tremors, nausea, dizziness, and even loss of consciousness. The exact mechanisms of HPNS are not fully understood, but it is believed to involve changes in the nervous system due to the high-pressure environment.

### Treatment

Treatment for decompression sickness typically involves administering:
1. 100% oxygen to the affected individual and arranging for them to receive specialized medical care as soon as possible. The primary goal is to reduce the size of the gas bubbles and promote their elimination from the body. This is typically achieved by administering oxygen therapy.
2. Recompression chambers placing the individual in a recompression chamber. The chamber simulates a high-pressure environment, allowing the excess nitrogen to be gradually eliminated from the body.
3. Prevention is crucial in managing decompression sickness. Divers are trained to follow safe diving practices, including proper ascent rates, dive profiles, and decompression stops.
4. Dive tables and dive computers are used to calculate and track the ascent to minimize the risk of developing decompression sickness.

### Hyperbaric Oxygen Therapy (HBOT)

It is a medical treatment that involves the administration of 100% oxygen at higher than normal atmospheric pressure. The increased pressure allows for a greater amount of oxygen to dissolve in the bloodstream, which can have therapeutic effects in certain clinical conditions. One of the main mechanisms of action of HBOT is based on the increased delivery of oxygen to tissues. By breathing pure oxygen under pressure, the oxygen dissolved in the plasma can reach areas of the body with compromised blood flow, leading to improved oxygenation and enhanced healing processes.

HBOT has been found to be beneficial in various medical conditions.
1. **Gas gangrene:** Gas gangrene is a severe and potentially life-threatening infection caused by certain bacteria, such as clostridium species. These bacteria thrive in anaerobic (oxygen-deprived) environments. Hyperbaric oxygenation creates an oxygen-rich environment that inhibits the growth of these bacteria, stopping the infection and promoting healing.
2. **Decompression sickness:** Decompression sickness, also known as "the bends," can occur when a person ascends too quickly after scuba diving or being exposed to high-pressure environments. It is caused by the formation of nitrogen bubbles in the bloodstream. HBOT helps to reduce the size of these bubbles and accelerates their elimination, relieving symptoms and preventing further complications.
3. **Arterial gas embolism:** Arterial gas embolism occurs when gas bubbles enter the arterial circulation, usually due to trauma or medical procedures. HBOT can help dissolve the gas bubbles and restore blood flow to affected tissues, preventing tissue damage and improving outcomes.
4. **Carbon monoxide poisoning:** Carbon monoxide (CO) is a toxic gas that binds to hemoglobin, reducing its ability to transport oxygen. HBOT increases the elimination of CO from the body and facilitates the replacement of carboxyhemoglobin with oxygenated hemoglobin, promoting recovery from CO poisoning.
5. **Osteomyelitis:** Osteomyelitis is a bone infection often caused by bacteria. HBOT can enhance the effectiveness of antibiotics by improving oxygen delivery to infected bone tissues, supporting the body's immune response, and aiding in tissue repair.
6. **Myocardial infarction:** Hyperbaric oxygen therapy has been explored as an adjunctive treatment for myocardial infarction (heart attack). It aims to improve oxygen supply to the damaged heart tissue, reduce inflammation, and promote healing.

### Side Effects of HBOT

1. Ear barotrauma
2. Temporary vision changes
3. Oxygen toxicity

---

### SUMMARY

- The $PO_2$ changes with the barometric pressure. While ascending up, the air thins out, reducing the $PO_2$ and causing the clinical features due to hypoxia.
- If a person ascend too rapidly he shows the signs of acute hypoxia affecting various body systems. However, a person staying at ahigh altitude for a long time shows chronic effects of hypoxia like increased blood counts etc. Hence the persons at high altitudes, get acclimatized by certain physiological changes.
- HIFs play a central role in coordinating the cellular and physiological responses to hypoxia, ensuring the body's ability to adapt and maintain homeostasis in oxygen-deficient environments.
- The space physiology is also quite intriguing, where we had learnt about the concept of effect of positive and negative G

force on the body. We learnt that the astronauts experience these G forces along with rapid acceleration, deceleration and centrifugal forces. The artificial climate in the space ships is required for them to survive for many months in space.
- The similar effects are seen when a person ascends rapidly from the deep sea to the surface. The journey to the ocean bed compresses the respiratory and other gases and dissolves them into the tissues, especially the nitrogen. On the way back to sea surface, these gases get decompressed and get dissolved back in blood. A rapid ascent results in the formation of tiny bubbles chocking the microcirculation. While a slower ascent will gradually dissolve these gases.

## LET US SEE, HOW MUCH YOU HAVE LEARNT?

### Review Questions

#### Long/Short Answer Questions

Q1. What will happen if the pilot ascends up to 30,000 feet rapidly in an unpressurised aircraft while breathing from a cylinder containing air?
Q2. Why the mountain expeditions are planned to be conducted slowly over two to three months?
Q3. Why the person at high altitude more vulnerable to get the pulmonary edema?
Q4. What is caissons disease? Describe the pathophysiology of caisson's disease.
Q5. What are the indications hyperbaric oxygen therapy (HBOT)?
Q6. What would happen if a person is exposed to high concentration of oxygen for a prolonged period?

#### Explain Why? (Reasoning Questions)

Q1. Nitrogen narcosis occurs during deep-sea diving at significant depths.
Q2. Decompression sickness (the bends) can occur during deep-sea diving if ascent is too rapid.
Q3. Altitude sickness occurs when ascending to high altitudes.
Q4. Hypoxia is a concern for individuals in high-altitude environments such as Mount Everest.
Q5. Space motion sickness occurs in astronauts during space missions.

### Critical Thinking Case-Based Questions

Q1. You are a medical officer assigned to a military base stationed at the Siachen Glacier, one of the highest and coldest battlefields on earth. Soldiers are rotated in and out every 6 months due to the extreme conditions. Recently, a new batch of soldiers has arrived after spending the past 6 months stationed at the glacier. As their medical officer, you conduct routine health assessments on the returning soldiers.

During your assessments, you notice significant changes in the soldiers compared to when they arrived 6 months ago. They appear physically and mentally fatigued, with a noticeable decrease in their overall energy levels and morale. Many of them report experiencing difficulty sleeping, constant headaches, and increased irritability. Physical examinations reveal signs of frostbite on their extremities, despite proper cold weather gear usage.

As you delve deeper into their medical histories, you uncover a pattern of respiratory issues, ranging from mild coughs to more severe cases of bronchitis and pneumonia. Some soldiers also mention struggling with memory lapses and difficulty concentrating, which is affecting their ability to carry out their duties effectively.

Upon further inquiry, you learn that the soldiers faced several challenges during their deployment, including extreme cold temperatures, treacherous terrain, and limited access to medical facilities. They recount instances of intense combat, frequent avalanches, and the emotional toll of being separated from their families for extended periods.

Based on the above case study, answer the following questions:
a. What physiological changes would have occurred in these soldiers?
b. Why do you think, these soldiers are experiencing irritability, memory lapses and difficulty in concentrating?

### Multiple Choice Questions

Q1. Which of the following physiological adaptations occurs in response to high altitude exposure?
  a. Increased production of red blood cells
  b. Decreased heart rate
  c. Constriction of blood vessels
  d. Reduced breathing rate

Q2. During deep-sea diving, which gas can cause narcosis when breathed at high pressures?
a. Nitrogen
b. Oxygen
c. Carbon dioxide
d. Helium

Q3. What is the primary goal of artificial respiration?
a. To provide oxygen to the lungs
b. To stimulate the respiratory centers in the brain
c. To prevent aspiration of fluids into the lungs
d. To regulate the body's pH balance

Q4. Which of the following is a potential complication of prolonged oxygen therapy?
a. Hypoxemia
b. Hypocapnia
c. Oxygen toxicity
d. Respiratory alkalosis

Q5. Which of the following is a symptom of decompression sickness?
a. Bradycardia
b. Hypothermia
c. Joint pain
d. Hypertension

Q6. Which of the following devices is commonly used to deliver oxygen therapy?
a. Venturi mask
b. Nebulizer
c. Ambu bag
d. Stethoscope

Q7. What is the primary mechanism of oxygen toxicity during deep-sea diving?
a. Increased blood pressure
b. Formation of reactive oxygen species
c. Excessive carbon dioxide levels
d. Hypoxemia

**ANSWERS**

1. a  2. a  3. a  4. c  5. c  6. a  7. b

# Physiological Basis of Respiratory Disorders

## CHAPTER 56

**COMPETENCY ADDRESSED**

PY6.6: Describe and discuss the pathophysiology of dyspnea, hypoxia, cyanosis, asphyxia; drowning, periodic breathing.

**LEARNING OBJECTIVES**

At the end of this chapter, the learner should be able to:
- Define hypoxia. Classify it and describe the etiopathogenesis of hypoxia.
- Describe various clinical conditions related to respiratory system.

## HYPOXIA

**Definition**: Hypoxia is defined as the decreased availability of oxygen at the level of tissues.

### Classification of Hypoxia

Depending on the cause, hypoxia is classified as:
- Hypoxic hypoxia
- Anemic hypoxia
- Stagnant hypoxia
- Histotoxic hypoxia

### Hypoxic Hypoxia

Hypoxic hypoxia occurs when there's a deficiency of oxygen in the bloodstream, leading to inadequate oxygen delivery to the tissues and cells throughout the body. This can happen due to various factors that impair the uptake or transport of oxygen or reduce the partial pressure of oxygen in the inspired air.
- **High altitude:** At high altitudes, the concentration of oxygen in the air decreases, leading to hypoxic conditions. This is known as altitude hypoxia. As you ascend to higher altitudes, the atmospheric pressure decreases, causing a reduction in the partial pressure of oxygen in the inspired air. People who ascend rapidly to high altitudes without acclimatization may experience symptoms of hypoxia.
- **Respiratory disorders:** Conditions such as chronic obstructive pulmonary disease (COPD), pneumonia, asthma, and respiratory infections can impair the ability of the lungs to take in oxygen or expel carbon dioxide efficiently. This leads to decreased oxygen exchange in the lungs and subsequent hypoxia.

### Physiological Basis

The hypoxic conditions result in decreased oxygen levels in blood and RBC. The oxygen delivery to tissues is reduced, resulting in normal to high arteriovenous difference in $O_2$ (**Fig. 56.1**).

The oxygen-Hb dissociation curve shifts to right in hypoxic hypoxia, due to low $PO_2$.

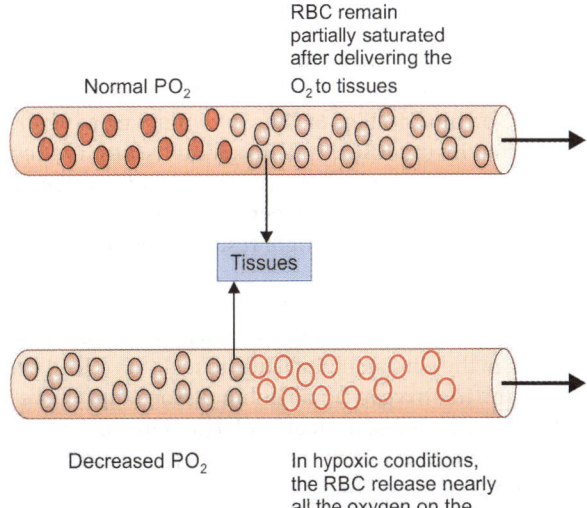

**Fig. 56.1:** Effect of hypoxic on blood and tissues.

**Effect of hypoxic hypoxia on respiratory system:** The decreased $PO_2$ (dissolved form) <60 mm Hg, results in activation of peripheral chemoreceptors and hence stimulates the respiratory center and increases the rate and depth of respiration.

### Management

- If atmospheric $PO_2$ is reduced, then it can be managed by the inhalation of $O_2$. Administering oxygen through nasal cannula, face mask, or other delivery methods can increase the oxygen levels in the blood and alleviate symptoms.
- In various lung diseases, related to diffusion or perfusion disorders, nothing much can be done but to institute the $O_2$ therapy in advance cases. However, mild to moderate cased of lung disorders use bronchodilators, and acclimatize for chronic hypoxia.
- **Lifestyle modifications:** The patient should be advised to quit smoking or avoid going to high altitudes.
- **Treat the underlying cause:** If hypoxic hypoxia is caused by an underlying medical condition, such as lung disease, heart failure, or anemia, treating the underlying condition is essential. This may involve medications, lifestyle changes, or other interventions tailored to the specific condition.

## Anemic Hypoxia

It is defined as the decreased oxygen carrying capacity of the blood. The concentration of dissolved oxygen is normal but the combined oxygen with hemoglobin decreases. It is seen in the following conditions:
- Decreased RBC count
- Low hemoglobin content
- Abnormal hemoglobin present instead of adult hemoglobin/hemoglobinopathies (HbF, thalassemia)
- Carbon monoxide poisoning.

### Physiological Basis

The oxygen carrier (Hb) is either deficient or unable to bind with the oxygen, hence decreasing the oxygen carrying capacity of blood **(Fig. 56.2)**. So, whatever oxygen is transported by the RBCs, is delivered to tissues, reducing the oxygen saturation of the venous blood. Hence, the arteriovenous difference of oxygen is increased. The oxygen hemoglobin curve shifts to right resulting in the increased oxygen delivery in the tissue.

It is interesting to note that the patients of thalassemia are not able to synthesize normal adult hemoglobin, hence resulting in the persistence of fetal hemoglobin (HbF) even after birth. The oxygen hemoglobin dissociation curve of fetal Hb is to the left of normal adult Hb. Depending on the concentration of the HbF, the tissue hypoxia further gets worsened.

**Effect of anemic hypoxia on respiratory system:** Since the dissolved $PO_2$ seldom goes below <60 mm Hg, there is

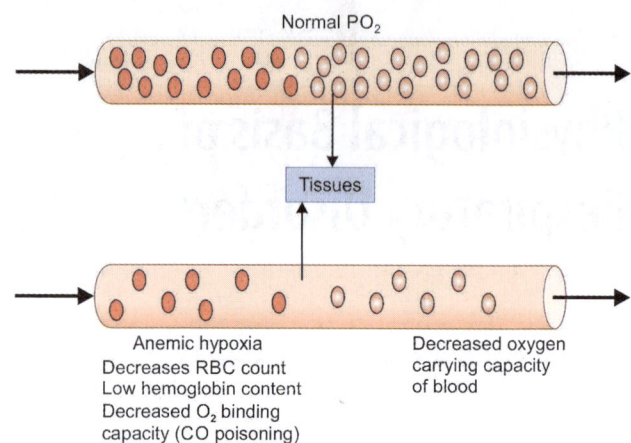

**Fig. 56.2:** Anemic hypoxia.

no activation of peripheral chemoreceptors and hence the respiratory center are not stimulated in the mild to moderate anemia. Moderate anemia presents with breathlessness on exertion (due to respiratory stimulation) while severe anemia can cause respiratory stimulation even at rest.

### Management

- **Treat the underlying cause:** Supplement iron therapy for iron deficiency anemia. Similarly other nutritional deficiencies can be treated by supplementation.
- Repeated blood transfusions are required by the patients of hemolytic anemia, suffering from the hemoglobinopathies.
- The hyperbaric oxygen therapy for the patients of the carbon monoxide poisoning.

## Stagnant Hypoxia

It is defined as the decreased oxygen delivery to the tissues due to decrease in the blood flow (reduced tissue perfusion) due to the following reasons:
- Circulatory shock and hypotension
- Cardiac failure
- Vasoconstriction, reducing the blood flow to the tissues.
- **Thromboembolic events:** Blood clots that travel through the bloodstream (emboli) can obstruct blood vessels, leading to stagnant hypoxia in affected tissues. This can occur in conditions such as pulmonary embolism (clot in the lungs) or systemic embolism affecting other organs.
- **High-altitude pulmonary edema (HAPE):** HAPE is a potentially life-threatening condition that can occur at high altitudes due to a combination of reduced oxygen availability and increased pulmonary artery pressure. It can lead to impaired blood flow to tissues and stagnant hypoxia.
- **Respiratory conditions:** Severe respiratory failure or lung diseases that impair gas exchange can lead to secondary cardiovascular effects, including decreased cardiac output and stagnant hypoxia. Conditions such as acute respiratory distress syndrome (ARDS) or severe

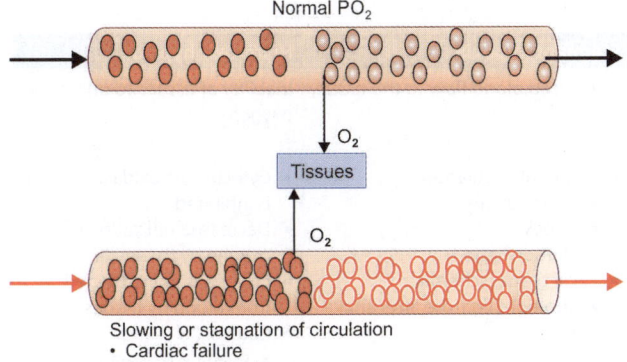

**Fig. 56.3:** Stagnant hypoxia.

chronic obstructive pulmonary disease (COPD) can contribute to stagnant hypoxia.

### Physiological Basis

Slowing of the circulation due to any cause can result in the decreased renewal of the fresh RBCs/blood bringing in more oxygen to the tissues **(Fig. 56.3)**. This results in complete extraction of the oxygen from the blood. The arteriovenous difference is maximum in this type of hypoxia. The oxygen hemoglobin curve shifts to right at the tissues.

### Management

- Treatment of underlying cause
- Oxygen therapy

## Histotoxic Hypoxia

It is also called as the cytotoxic hypoxia. The inability of the tissues to extract/utilize the oxygen due to the *blockage of mitochondrial enzymes like cytP450/cytochrome oxidase* as seen in cyanide poisoning/due to action of diphtheria toxin. The oxygen carrying capacity of blood, blood flow is normal. Since, the tissues are not able to utilize the oxygen, there is practically no arteriovenous difference of oxygen **(Fig. 56.4)**. The normal levels of dissolved oxygen in blood does not stimulate the respiratory centers.

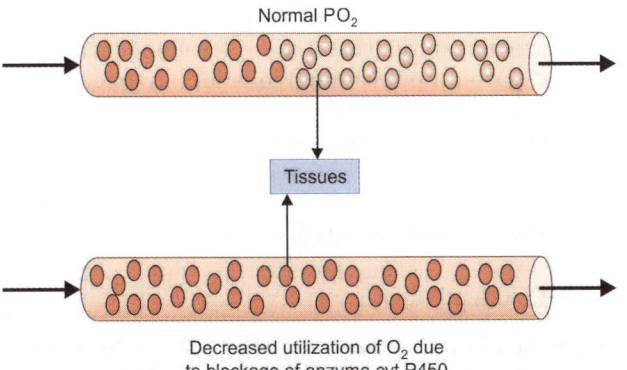

**Fig. 56.4:** Cytotoxic hypoxia.

### Management

- Identify and remove the toxins
- Provide supporting care by maintaining hydration, electrolyte balance etc.
- **Oxygen therapy:** While the primary issue in histotoxic hypoxia is not lack of oxygen in the blood, supplemental oxygen may still be beneficial in supporting cellular function and reducing tissue damage. Administering oxygen through nasal cannula, face mask, or other methods can help alleviate symptoms and improve tissue oxygenation.
- **Antioxidant therapy:** Antioxidants such as vitamin C, vitamin E, and glutathione may help protect cells from oxidative damage associated with histotoxic hypoxia.
- **Support cellular metabolism:** Supporting cellular metabolism is essential in managing histotoxic hypoxia.
  In cases of cyanide poisoning, administering hydroxocobalamin can help convert cyanide into a less toxic form, allowing cellular respiration to continue.
- **Hyperbaric oxygen therapy (HBOT):** In some cases, hyperbaric oxygen therapy may be considered as a treatment for histotoxic hypoxia. HBOT involves breathing 100% oxygen in a pressurized chamber, which can increase the oxygen content in the blood and improve tissue oxygenation. This approach may help overcome cellular dysfunction caused by toxins or metabolic inhibitors.
- **Monitoring and supportive measures:** Continuous monitoring of vital signs, including oxygen saturation, blood pressure, and organ function, is important in managing histotoxic hypoxia. Depending on the severity of the condition and associated symptoms, supportive measures such as intravenous fluids, vasopressors, or mechanical ventilation may be necessary to stabilize the patient and prevent further complications.

**Table 56.1** discusses the features and differences between various types of hypoxia.

## DYSPNEA

Dyspnea, commonly known as shortness of breath or breathlessness, is a distressing sensation of difficult or uncomfortable breathing. It is a subjective experience that varies in intensity and can be caused by a wide range of factors.

### Causes

- **Respiratory conditions:** Chronic obstructive pulmonary disease (COPD), asthma, pneumonia, pulmonary embolism, interstitial lung disease, and respiratory infections are common respiratory causes of dyspnea.
- **Cardiovascular conditions:** Heart failure, myocardial infarction, arrhythmias, and valvular heart disease can lead to dyspnea due to impaired cardiac function.
- **Anemia:** Reduced oxygen-carrying capacity of the blood due to anemia can result in dyspnea.

Table 56.1: Differences between different types of hypoxia.

| Types | Hypoxic hypoxia | Anemic hypoxia | Stagnant hypoxia | Histotoxic hypoxia |
|---|---|---|---|---|
| Definition | Decreased oxygen availability | Decreased oxygen carrying capacity of blood | Decreased blood flow to the tissue | Inability of tissues to utilize the oxygen |
| Causes | • Decreased atmospheric $PO_2$<br>  ▪ High altitude<br>• Lung diseases<br>  ▪ Diffusion diseases<br>  ▪ Decreased ventilation perfusion ratio | • Anemia<br>• CO poisoning—formation of carboxy Hb (Heavy cigarette smokers, professional drivers) | • Stagnant circulation<br>  ▪ Heart failure<br>  ▪ Shock<br>  ▪ Hemorrhage<br>• Local tissue ischemia<br>  ▪ Too tight ligature after snake bite | • Cytochrome oxidase system is inhibited<br>• Decreased utilization of oxygen by tissues<br>• Oxygen is not extracted from blood by tissues<br>• Causes:<br>  ▪ Cyanide poisoning<br>  ▪ Diphtheria toxin |
| Oxygen carrying capacity | Decreased | Decreased | Normal | Normal |
| Dissolved oxygen level $PO_2$ | Decreased | Normal | Normal | Normal |
| Combined $O_2$ | Decreased | Decreased | Normal | Normal |
| AV difference | Normal/Increased | Normal/Increased | High | Nil |

**Anoxia:** Total decrease in the level of oxygen, an extreme form of hypoxia or "low oxygen."

- **Obesity:** Excess weight can lead to mechanical restriction of lung expansion, causing dyspnea.
- **Psychological factors:** Anxiety, panic disorders, and stress can contribute to the sensation of dyspnea.
- **Others:** Environmental factors (e.g., high altitude), neuromuscular disorders, metabolic conditions, and certain medications can also cause dyspnea.

## Physiological Basis

- Dyspnea arises from a complex interplay of sensory, motor, and emotional factors. Physiologically, it involves increased respiratory effort, activation of respiratory muscles, and alterations in respiratory rate and tidal volume.
- Sensory receptors in the airways, lungs, chest wall, and peripheral chemoreceptors monitor changes in oxygen and carbon dioxide levels, pH, and mechanical stretch, triggering the sensation of dyspnea.
- Emotional and cognitive factors, such as anxiety and fear, further amplify the perception of breathlessness.

## Management

- **Treat underlying cause:** Identify and address the underlying condition contributing to dyspnea, whether it is a respiratory, cardiovascular, or other medical issue.
- **Oxygen therapy:** Supplemental oxygen may be beneficial, especially in cases of hypoxemia, to improve oxygen delivery to tissues and alleviate dyspnea.
- **Bronchodilators and anti-inflammatory medications:** In respiratory conditions such as asthma and COPD, bronchodilators and anti-inflammatory medications can help relieve airway constriction and inflammation, reducing dyspnea.
- **Diuretics and vasodilators:** In heart failure and other cardiovascular conditions, medications such as diuretics and vasodilators may be prescribed to reduce fluid overload and improve cardiac function, thereby alleviating dyspnea.
- **Pulmonary rehabilitation:** Exercise training, breathing exercises, and education programs can improve respiratory muscle strength, endurance, and overall functional capacity, leading to reduced dyspnea.
- **Psychological support:** Addressing anxiety, stress, and panic disorders through counseling, relaxation techniques, and cognitive-behavioral therapy can help manage dyspnea associated with psychological factors.
- **Positioning and breathing techniques:** Encourage patients to adopt positions that optimize lung mechanics (e.g., sitting upright) and teach breathing techniques (e.g., pursed-lip breathing) to reduce dyspnea during activities of daily living.
- **Symptom management:** Palliative care approaches, including opioid medications and nonpharmacological interventions, may be necessary for managing dyspnea in advanced or end-stage diseases.

## ASPHYXIA

Asphyxia refers to a condition characterized by insufficient supply of oxygen to the body's tissues, leading to cellular hypoxia and potentially life-threatening consequences. It can result from various causes and requires prompt

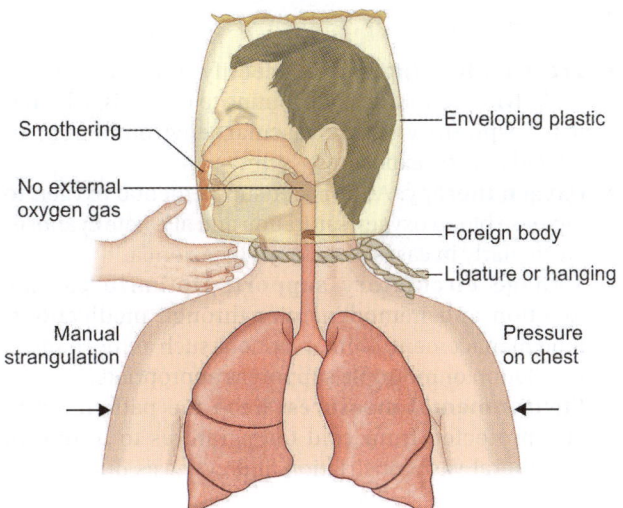

**Fig. 56.5:** Different causes of asphyxia.

intervention to restore adequate oxygenation and prevent complications. In common language, it is also called choking.

## Causes (Fig. 56.5)

- **Airway obstruction:** Blockage of the airway by foreign objects, such as food, vomit, or a swollen tongue, can prevent the entry of air into the lungs, leading to asphyxia.
- **Respiratory failure:** Conditions that impair the respiratory system's ability to exchange oxygen and carbon dioxide, including asthma, chronic obstructive pulmonary disease (COPD), pneumonia, and respiratory muscle weakness, can result in asphyxia.
- **Drowning and suffocation:** Submersion in water or other fluids, or entrapment in confined spaces without access to air, can cause asphyxia due to inability to breathe.
- **Toxic inhalants:** Inhalation of toxic gases (e.g., carbon monoxide, hydrogen sulfide) or exposure to environments with low oxygen concentration can lead to asphyxia.
- **Strangulation:** Compression of the neck, such as in cases of hanging, ligature strangulation, or manual strangulation, can obstruct blood flow to the brain and airway, causing asphyxia.
- **Neonatal asphyxia:** In newborns, birth complications, umbilical cord compression, or meconium aspiration syndrome can lead to inadequate oxygenation and neonatal asphyxia.

## Physiological Basis

Asphyxia disrupts the body's ability to deliver oxygen to tissues and remove carbon dioxide, leading to cellular hypoxia and acidosis. Initially, the body responds to hypoxia by increasing respiratory rate and depth in an attempt to improve oxygenation. However, if the underlying cause persists or worsens, compensatory mechanisms become overwhelmed, resulting in respiratory and metabolic acidosis, decreased cardiac output, and ultimately, organ dysfunction and failure. Hypoxia-induced cellular damage can occur rapidly, particularly in vital organs such as the brain and heart, leading to irreversible injury and death if oxygenation is not restored promptly.

## Management

- **Airway management:** Ensure a patent airway by clearing any obstructions and providing appropriate interventions, such as suctioning, positioning, or advanced airway maneuvers (e.g., intubation).
- **Oxygen therapy:** Administer supplemental oxygen via mask, nasal cannula, or bag-valve-mask ventilation to improve oxygenation and tissue perfusion.
- **Ventilation support:** Provide mechanical ventilation if necessary to support respiratory function and maintain adequate oxygenation and ventilation.
- **Cardiopulmonary resuscitation (CPR):** Initiate CPR, including chest compressions and rescue breathing, in cases of cardiac arrest to restore circulation and oxygenation.
- **Treat underlying cause:** Identify and address the underlying cause of asphyxia, whether it is respiratory, cardiovascular, or related to trauma, and implement appropriate interventions.
- **Neonatal resuscitation:** Follow neonatal resuscitation protocols, including drying, stimulation, and assisted ventilation, in newborns with signs of neonatal asphyxia.
- **Toxicology management:** Administer antidotes or provide supportive care for toxic inhalant exposures, such as carbon monoxide poisoning, to enhance oxygen delivery and remove toxins from the body.

## Prevention

Educate individuals on safety measures to prevent asphyxia-related accidents, such as water safety practices, safe sleep environments for infants, and awareness of environmental hazards.

## CYANOSIS

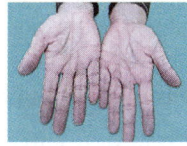

Cyanosis manifests as a bluish or purplish tint to the skin, particularly in areas with high blood flow, such as the lips, tongue, nail beds, and fingertips. It occurs when blood oxygen saturation falls below 85–90%, leading to an increased proportion of deoxygenated hemoglobin, which has a bluish hue.

> **Cyanosis**
> - Bluish or violet discoloration of skin or mucous membrane
> - Reduced hemoglobin >5 g%

- Types:
  - Central cyanosis: Due to heart or lung disease
  - Peripheral cyanosis: Severe vasoconstriction
- **Not Seen in**
  - Severe anemia Hb < 5 g%
  - CO poisoning—cherry red color
  - Histotoxic hypoxia as blood gas content is normal

## Causes

### Central Cyanosis

Cyanosis originating from the central circulation (e.g., lips, tongue) suggests systemic hypoxemia and is commonly associated with respiratory or cardiovascular conditions.

- **Respiratory conditions:** Cyanosis commonly occurs in respiratory conditions that impair oxygen exchange, such as pneumonia, chronic obstructive pulmonary disease (COPD), asthma, pulmonary embolism, and respiratory distress syndrome (RDS).
- **Cardiovascular conditions:** Cyanosis can result from congenital heart defects (e.g., tetralogy of Fallot), heart failure, myocardial infarction, severe valvular disease, or circulatory shock, leading to decreased oxygen delivery to tissues.

### Peripheral Cyanosis

Cyanosis limited to the extremities may be caused by peripheral vasoconstriction due to cold exposure or circulatory disturbances (e.g., Raynaud's phenomenon), rather than systemic hypoxemia.

- **Cold exposure:** Prolonged exposure to cold temperatures can cause peripheral vasoconstriction and cyanosis of the extremities.
- **High altitude:** Cyanosis may occur at high altitudes due to decreased oxygen availability in the atmosphere (hypobaric hypoxia).
- **Methemoglobinemia:** Elevated levels of methemoglobin, a form of hemoglobin that cannot bind oxygen effectively, can lead to cyanosis. This can result from exposure to certain medications, chemicals, or genetic conditions. It occurs when the reduced Hb level becomes more than 5 gm%. Hence it is not seen in severe anemia, where the total Hb level is below 5 g/dL.

## Physiological Basis

Cyanosis occurs when the concentration of deoxygenated hemoglobin exceeds 5 g%, resulting in a visible bluish tint to the skin. Hemoglobin normally appears red when oxygenated and bluish-purple when deoxygenated. The bluish color of deoxygenated hemoglobin becomes more apparent as blood oxygen saturation decreases, reflecting inadequate oxygenation of tissues.

## Management

- **Treat underlying cause:** Identify and address the underlying condition contributing to cyanosis, whether it is respiratory, cardiovascular, environmental, or related to toxic exposures.
- **Oxygen therapy:** Administer supplemental oxygen to increase blood oxygen saturation and alleviate cyanosis, particularly in cases of systemic hypoxemia.
- **Manage circulatory support:** Optimize cardiac function and hemodynamics through medications, fluid management, or interventions such as mechanical ventilation or inotropic support as appropriate.
- **Environmental measures:** Keep the patient warm and protected from cold temperatures to minimize peripheral vasoconstriction and cyanosis due to cold exposure.
- **Address methemoglobinemia:** Administer methylene blue or other antidotes to reduce methemoglobin levels in cases of methemoglobinemia-induced cyanosis.

# PERIODIC BREATHING

Periodic breathing is a breathing pattern marked by regular fluctuations in respiratory rate and depth, with alternating periods of breathing and temporary pauses in breathing (apnea). These cycles typically last for seconds to minutes and can be observed during wakefulness or sleep.

## Causes

- **High altitude:** Periodic breathing commonly occurs at high altitudes due to changes in the body's response to hypoxia (hypobaric hypoxia).
- **Heart failure:** Heart failure can lead to periodic breathing due to alterations in chemoreceptor sensitivity and cardiac function.
- **Central nervous system disorders:** Neurological conditions affecting the respiratory centers in the brainstem, such as brainstem stroke or congenital central hypoventilation syndrome (CCHS), can result in periodic breathing.
- **Drug-induced respiratory depression:** Certain medications, such as opioids, sedatives, or benzodiazepines, can depress the respiratory drive and predispose to periodic breathing.
- **Cheyne-Stokes respiration (CSR):** A specific type of periodic breathing characterized by progressively deeper and faster breathing followed by a gradual decrease and cessation of breathing (apnea). CSR is commonly associated with heart failure, stroke, and central nervous system disorders.

## Physiological Basis

The physiological basis of periodic breathing involves complex interactions between respiratory drive, chemoreceptor sensitivity, and feedback mechanisms. During periods of hypoxia, such as at high altitudes or in conditions like heart failure, chemoreceptors sense changes in arterial oxygen and carbon dioxide levels. This leads to increased ventilatory drive and hyperpnea. As oxygen levels rise and carbon dioxide levels decrease, the respiratory drive diminishes, resulting in apnea. This cyclic pattern repeats as oxygen and carbon dioxide levels fluctuate, causing periodic breathing.

### Types (Fig. 56.6)

- **High-altitude periodic breathing:** Occurs at high altitudes due to hypoxia-induced changes in respiratory control.
- **Cheyne-stokes respiration (CSR) (Fig. 56.7):** Characterized by crescendo-decrescendo patterns of breathing with alternating periods of hyperpnea and apnea, commonly seen in heart failure and neurological disorders.
- **Central periodic breathing/biots breathing:** Results from dysfunction of the central respiratory centers in the brainstem, leading to irregular breathing patterns with periods of apnea.
- **Drug-induced periodic breathing:** Caused by medications that suppress respiratory drive, such as opioids or sedatives.

### Management

- **Treat underlying cause:** Identify and address the underlying condition contributing to periodic breathing, whether it is related to high altitude, heart failure, neurological disorders, or medication side effects.
- **Oxygen therapy:** Oxygen therapy may help stabilize breathing patterns and alleviate hypoxia-related respiratory drive.
- **Medication adjustment:** Review and adjust medications that may depress respiratory drive, such as opioids or sedatives, under medical supervision.
- **Positive airway pressure (PAP) therapy:** Continuous positive airway pressure (CPAP) or bilevel positive airway pressure (BiPAP) may be used to stabilize breathing patterns and improve oxygenation, particularly in cases of CSR or obstructive sleep apnea.
- **Cardiovascular management:** Optimize heart failure management and cardiac function to reduce the risk of CSR and periodic breathing associated with cardiac conditions.

### Apneusis (Fig. 56.8)

- Abnormal pattern of breathing characterized by deep, gasping inspiration with a pause at full inspiration followed by brief, insufficient expiration.

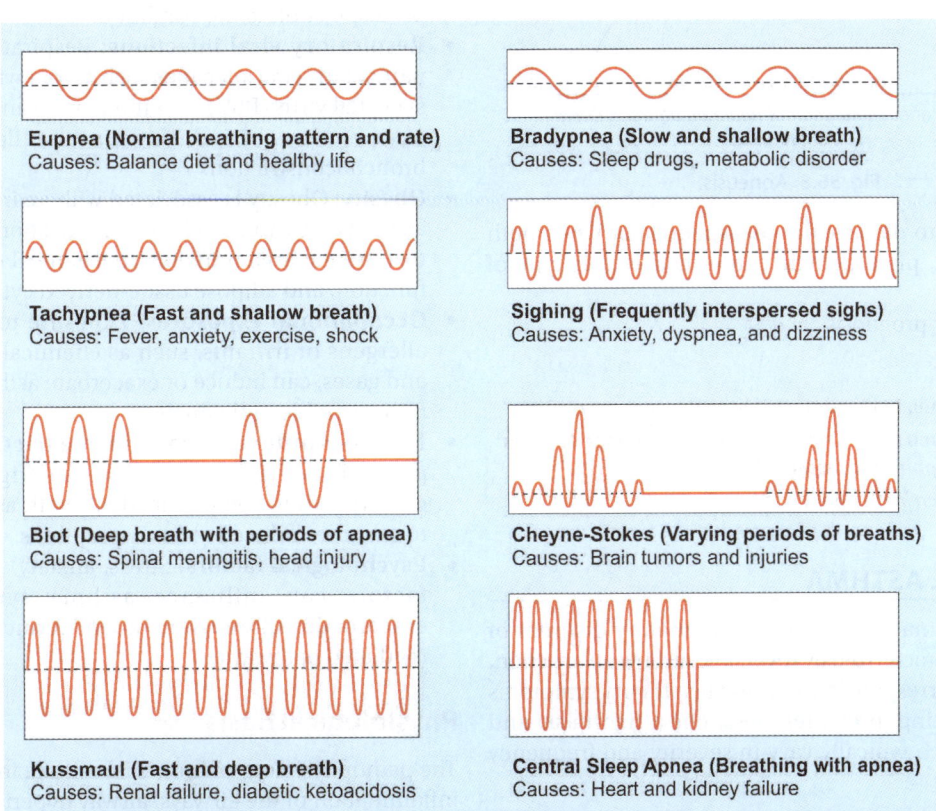

**Fig. 56.6:** Different types of periodic breathing patterns—normal and abnormal.

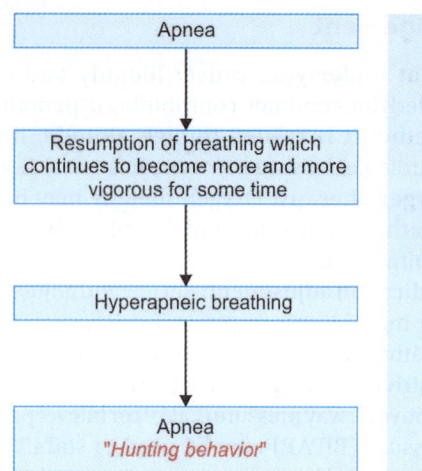
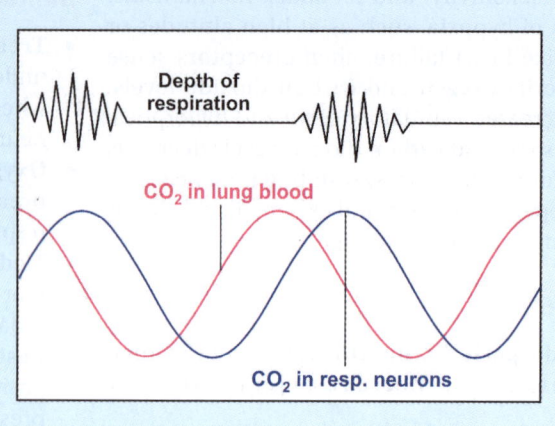

**Fig. 56.7:** Cheyne-Stokes respiration.

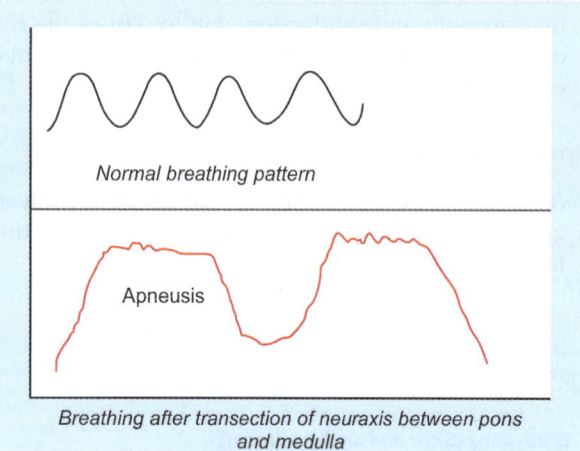

**Fig. 56.8:** Apneusis.

- Occurs due to damage to pons/medulla or when both vagi are cut, pneumotaxic center causes this type of respiration.
- Carries poor prognosis.

*What will happen to respiration if both the vagi are cut?*
*What will happen to respiration if there is a damage to brain stem between pons and medulla?*
Answers are given in the Chapter 54.

## BRONCHIAL ASTHMA

Bronchial asthma is a chronic inflammatory disorder of the airways characterized by reversible airflow obstruction, bronchial hyperresponsiveness, and respiratory symptoms such as wheezing, breathlessness, chest tightness, and coughing, which typically vary in severity and frequency over time.

### Causes

- **Allergic sensitization:** Exposure to allergens such as pollen, dust mites, animal dander, mold, and certain foods can trigger an allergic response in susceptible individuals, leading to airway inflammation and asthma symptoms.
- **Environmental factors:** Exposure to tobacco smoke, air pollution, occupational chemicals, respiratory infections, cold air, and weather changes can exacerbate asthma symptoms and trigger asthma attacks.
- **Genetic predisposition:** Family history of asthma or atopic diseases (e.g., allergic rhinitis, eczema) increases the risk of developing asthma, suggesting a genetic predisposition to the condition.
- **Respiratory viral infections:** Respiratory infections, particularly viral infections such as rhinovirus, respiratory syncytial virus (RSV), and influenza, can trigger asthma exacerbations by inducing airway inflammation and bronchoconstriction.
- **Obesity:** Obesity is associated with an increased risk of asthma and asthma-related complications, possibly due to systemic inflammation, mechanical effects on lung function, and adipose tissue-derived cytokines.
- **Occupational exposures:** Exposure to occupational allergens or irritants, such as chemicals, dust, fumes, and gases, can induce or exacerbate asthma symptoms in susceptible individuals.
- **Exercise-induced bronchoconstriction:** Vigorous physical activity or exercise can trigger bronchoconstriction in some individuals with asthma, leading to exercise-induced asthma symptoms.
- **Psychological factors:** Stress, anxiety, and emotional factors can influence asthma symptoms and exacerbations through neuroendocrine and immune-mediated pathways.

### Physiological Basis

The pathophysiology of bronchial asthma involves chronic inflammation of the airways, airway hyperresponsiveness, and reversible airflow obstruction. Exposure to triggers such as allergens, pollutants, or respiratory infections activates inflammatory cells (e.g., mast cells, eosinophils, T lymphocytes) in the airway mucosa, leading to release of inflammatory mediators (e.g., histamine, leukotrienes, cytokines) and recruitment of inflammatory cells to the airways. This inflammatory response causes airway edema, mucus production, smooth muscle contraction (bronchoconstriction), and structural changes in the airway wall, resulting in airflow limitation and asthma symptoms.

## Management

- **Medical treatment:**
  - Long-term control medications, including inhaled corticosteroids, long-acting beta-agonists, leukotriene modifiers, and mast cell stabilizers, are used to reduce airway inflammation, prevent asthma symptoms, and maintain asthma control.
  - Short-acting bronchodilators (e.g., albuterol) provide rapid relief of acute asthma symptoms and bronchoconstriction during asthma attacks or exacerbations.
- **Avoid the allergen:** Identify and minimize exposure to allergens or triggers that worsen asthma symptoms, such as dust mites, pollen, pet dander, mold, and tobacco smoke.
- **Patient education:** Educate patients about asthma triggers, symptoms, medication adherence, proper inhaler technique, asthma action plans, and when to seek medical attention for worsening symptoms or exacerbations.
- **Immunotherapy:** Consider allergen immunotherapy (allergy shots) for patients with allergic asthma who have persistent symptoms despite optimal medical management, to desensitize the immune system and reduce sensitivity to specific allergens.

## CHRONIC OBSTRUCTIVE PULMONARY DISEASE

Chronic obstructive pulmonary disease (COPD) is a chronic inflammatory lung disease characterized by airflow limitation that is not fully reversible. The airflow limitation is usually progressive and associated with an abnormal inflammatory response of the lungs to harmful particles or gases, most commonly from cigarette smoke.

## Causes

- **Tobacco smoke:** Cigarette smoking is the primary cause of COPD, accounting for the majority of cases. Chronic exposure to tobacco smoke irritates and damages the airways and alveoli, leading to inflammation, mucus production, and destruction of lung tissue.
- **Environmental exposures:** Occupational exposure to dust, fumes, chemicals, and indoor and outdoor air pollution can contribute to the development and progression of COPD, particularly in susceptible individuals.
- **Genetic factors:** Genetic predisposition, including alpha-1 antitrypsin deficiency, a rare genetic disorder, can increase the risk of developing COPD, especially in nonsmokers or individuals with a family history of the disease.
- **Respiratory infections:** Recurrent respiratory infections, particularly during childhood, can predispose to the development of COPD later in life, potentially exacerbating underlying lung inflammation and damage.
- **Aging:** Aging is associated with physiological changes in the respiratory system, including decreased lung elasticity and function, which can contribute to the development of COPD in older adults.

## Physiological Basis

The pathophysiology of COPD involves chronic inflammation, mucus hypersecretion, and structural changes in the airways and lung parenchyma. Prolonged exposure to irritants, such as tobacco smoke or occupational pollutants, activates inflammatory cells (e.g., neutrophils, macrophages) in the airway mucosa, leading to release of inflammatory mediators (e.g., cytokines, proteases) and recruitment of inflammatory cells to the lungs. This chronic inflammation results in airway remodeling, mucus hypersecretion, and narrowing of the airways (bronchoconstriction), leading to airflow limitation and respiratory symptoms.

## Management

- **Smoking cessation:** The most important intervention in managing COPD is smoking cessation, which can slow disease progression, reduce symptoms, and improve quality of life.
- **Medications:** Bronchodilators (e.g., beta-agonists, anticholinergics) and inhaled corticosteroids are the mainstay of pharmacological treatment for COPD, helping to relieve symptoms, improve lung function, and reduce exacerbations.
- **Pulmonary rehabilitation:** Comprehensive pulmonary rehabilitation programs incorporating exercise training, education, nutritional support, and psychosocial interventions can improve exercise tolerance, reduce dyspnea, and enhance quality of life in individuals with COPD.
- **Oxygen therapy:** Long-term oxygen therapy (LTOT) is indicated for patients with severe COPD and chronic hypoxemia to improve survival, reduce complications, and alleviate symptoms.
- **Management of exacerbations:** Prompt recognition and treatment of COPD exacerbations with bronchodilators, corticosteroids, antibiotics (if indicated), and oxygen therapy can help minimize disease progression and improve outcomes.
- **Lifestyle modifications:** Encourage regular physical activity, healthy diet, weight management, and avoidance of environmental triggers (e.g., air pollution, respiratory irritants) to optimize overall health and reduce exacerbation risk.

## RESPIRATORY FAILURE

Respiratory failure is defined as the inability of the respiratory system to maintain adequate oxygenation (hypoxemia) and/or ventilation (hypercapnia) to meet the body's metabolic demands. It is typically characterized by low arterial oxygen partial pressure ($PO_2$) and/or high arterial carbon dioxide partial pressure ($PCO_2$) on arterial blood gas analysis.

### Causes

- **Airway obstruction:** Conditions such as asthma, COPD, bronchiolitis, and foreign body aspiration can obstruct airflow and impair ventilation.
- **Lung parenchymal disease:** Pneumonia, acute respiratory distress syndrome (ARDS), pulmonary edema, pulmonary fibrosis, and lung contusion can impair gas exchange by reducing lung compliance or increasing intrapulmonary shunting.
- **Neuromuscular disorders:** Conditions affecting the respiratory muscles (e.g., Guillain-Barré syndrome, myasthenia gravis, amyotrophic lateral sclerosis) or the central nervous system (e.g., stroke, spinal cord injury) can impair ventilatory function.
- **Chest wall disorders:** Thoracic trauma, kyphoscoliosis, obesity, and neuromuscular conditions affecting chest wall mechanics can restrict lung expansion and impair ventilation.
- **Drug overdose:** Opioids, sedatives, and other central nervous system depressants can suppress respiratory drive and lead to respiratory depression and failure.
- **Cardiogenic pulmonary edema:** Severe heart failure can lead to fluid accumulation in the lungs, impairing gas exchange and causing hypoxemia.
- **High altitude:** Hypobaric hypoxia at high altitudes can lead to hypoxemic respiratory failure due to reduced oxygen availability.
- **Environmental exposures:** Inhalation of toxic gases (e.g., carbon monoxide, hydrogen sulfide) or smoke inhalation can impair oxygenation and lead to respiratory failure.

### Physiological Basis

Respiratory failure results from imbalances in the physiological processes of gas exchange, ventilation, and perfusion. In hypoxemic respiratory failure, there is inadequate oxygenation of arterial blood, typically due to ventilation-perfusion (V/Q) mismatch, shunting, or diffusion impairment. Hypercapnic respiratory failure, on the other hand, is characterized by elevated arterial carbon dioxide levels, indicating inadequate alveolar ventilation relative to metabolic carbon dioxide production. These imbalances disrupt acid-base homeostasis, leading to respiratory acidosis, which can further exacerbate respiratory failure and impair cellular function.

### Types

- **Hypoxemic respiratory failure:** Characterized by low arterial oxygen levels ($PaO_2$ < 60 mm Hg) despite normal or low arterial carbon dioxide levels. It is commonly seen in conditions causing V/Q mismatch, shunting, or diffusion impairment.
- **Hypercapnic respiratory failure:** Characterized by elevated arterial carbon dioxide levels ($PaCO_2$ >45 mm Hg) due to inadequate alveolar ventilation. It is often associated with conditions causing hypoventilation, such as neuromuscular disorders or central respiratory depression.
- **Combined respiratory failure:** Occurs when both hypoxemia and hypercapnia are present, indicating severe impairment of gas exchange and ventilation.

It is also classified as Type I and II respiratory failure **(Fig. 56.9)**

### Management

- **Oxygen therapy:** Administer supplemental oxygen to correct hypoxemia and improve tissue oxygenation, while monitoring oxygen saturation and avoiding hyperoxia.
- **Mechanical ventilation:** Provide invasive or noninvasive mechanical ventilation to support respiratory function, optimize oxygenation and ventilation, and relieve respiratory distress.
- **Treatment of underlying cause:** Identify and address the underlying condition contributing to respiratory failure, such as infection, pulmonary edema, or neuromuscular weakness, through appropriate medical management.

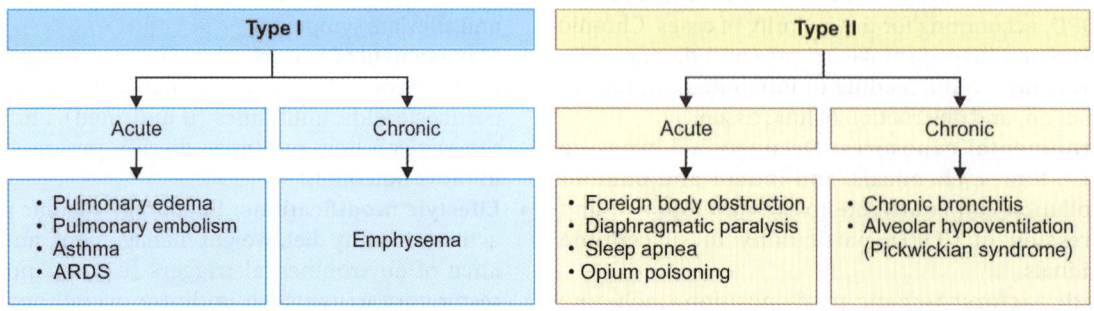

**Fig. 56.9:** Classification of respiratory failure.

- **Airway management:** Ensure a patent airway and adequate ventilation, perform suctioning if necessary, and consider interventions such as bronchodilators or airway adjuncts to optimize respiratory function.
- **Respiratory supportive measures:** Position the patient to maximize lung mechanics, administer bronchodilators or mucolytics as indicated, and provide chest physiotherapy to facilitate airway clearance.
- **Monitoring:** Continuously monitor vital signs, arterial blood gases, pulse oximetry, and clinical status to assess response to treatment and adjust management as necessary.
- **Critical care support:** Transfer patients with severe respiratory failure to an intensive care unit for close monitoring, advanced respiratory support, and multi-disciplinary management of complications.

## SUMMARY

In this chapter we have learnt about various applied aspects of respiratory disorders.

- **Hypoxia:** The decreased availability of oxygen to the tissues is called hypoxia. Based on etiology it is classified as hypoxic hypoxia, anemic hypoxia, stagnant hypoxia and histotoxic hypoxia.
- **Anoxia:** It is severe hypoxia or no availability of oxygen to the tissues.
- **Dyspnea** is a multifactorial symptom with diverse underlying causes and physiological mechanisms. Effective management requires a comprehensive approach tailored to the individual patient, addressing both the underlying condition and the associated distressing sensation of breathlessness.
- **Asphyxia** is a life-threatening condition characterized by oxygen deprivation, which requires prompt recognition and intervention to restore adequate oxygenation and prevent organ damage or death. Effective management involves addressing the underlying cause, supporting respiratory and cardiovascular function, and providing appropriate interventions tailored to the individual patient's needs.
- **Cyanosis** is a clinical sign indicating inadequate oxygenation of tissues, often associated with respiratory, cardiovascular, or environmental conditions. Prompt identification of the underlying cause and appropriate management are essential to address the underlying pathology and improve oxygen delivery to tissues, thereby alleviating cyanosis and preventing complications.
- **Periodic breathing** is a respiratory pattern characterized by alternating cycles of hyperpnea and apnea, which can occur in various clinical contexts. Management involves identifying and addressing the underlying cause, optimizing oxygenation, and considering interventions to stabilize breathing patterns and improve patient outcomes.
- **Bronchial asthma** is a chronic inflammatory respiratory condition characterized by reversible airway obstruction, bronchial hyperresponsiveness, and recurrent episodes of respiratory symptoms. Management involves identifying and avoiding asthma triggers, using appropriate medications for long-term control and acute symptom relief, providing patient education and self-management strategies, and monitoring asthma control to prevent exacerbations and improve quality of life.
- **COPD** is a chronic respiratory condition characterized by airflow limitation, typically caused by exposure to tobacco smoke and other environmental factors. Management involves smoking cessation, pharmacological therapy, pulmonary rehabilitation, oxygen therapy, vaccinations, and lifestyle modifications to reduce symptoms, improve lung function, and prevent exacerbations. Early diagnosis and comprehensive management are essential to slow disease progression and improve outcomes in individuals with COPD.
- **Respiratory failure** is a critical condition characterized by inadequate gas exchange leading to hypoxemia, hypercapnia, and respiratory acidosis. Management involves addressing the underlying cause, providing respiratory support, optimizing oxygenation and ventilation, and monitoring closely to prevent further deterioration and improve patient outcomes.

## LET US SEE, HOW MUCH YOU HAVE LEARNT?

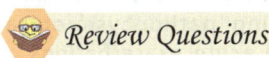

*Review Questions*

### Long/Short Answer Questions

Q1. Define hypoxia. Classify the hypoxia on the basis of etiology. Describe the pathophysiology of each type of hypoxia.

Q2. What will happen, if HbF persists after birth?

Q3. What will happen to respiration if both the vagi are cut?

Q4. What will happen to respiration if there is a damage to brain stem between pons and medulla?

Q5. What will happen to respiration of a person with cardiac failure?

Q6. What will happen to respiration of a patient admitted to the emergency with acidosis?

Q7. What will happen to the respiratory rate of a patient with mild to moderate anemia?

Q8. What will happen to the respiratory rate of a patient with mild to moderate CO poisoning?

Q9. What will happen to the respiratory rate of a patient with visiting a hill station at an altitude of 5,000 feet above sea level?

Q10. What changes occur in the people living in Leh for years together?

## Explain Why? (Reasoning Questions)

Q1. Cyanosis is observed in individuals with low oxygen levels in the blood.
Q2. Bronchial asthma is characterized by bronchoconstriction, mucus production, and airway inflammation.
Q3. Hypoxia occurs in conditions such as high-altitude exposure, respiratory diseases, and cardiovascular disorders.
Q4. Prolonged breath-holding or apneusis can lead to hypoxia and respiratory distress.
Q5. Supplemental oxygen therapy is a common treatment approach for hypoxia in various clinical settings.

## Multiple Choice Questions

Q1. Which of the following conditions is characterized by a bluish discoloration of the skin and mucous membranes due to inadequate oxygenation?
   a. Dyspnea
   b. Hypoxia
   c. Cyanosis
   d. Asphyxia

Q2. Which of the following physiological mechanisms is primarily responsible for the development of hypoxia at high altitudes?
   a. Increased oxygen delivery to tissues
   b. Decreased atmospheric pressure
   c. Enhanced oxygen-binding capacity of hemoglobin
   d. Stimulation of respiratory centers in the brainstem

Q3. A patient presents to the emergency department with sudden onset of shortness of breath, chest tightness, and wheezing. Which of the following conditions is most likely responsible for these symptoms?
   a. Cyanosis
   b. Asthma
   c. Hypoxia
   d. Asphyxia

Q4. A patient with a history of heart failure presents with Cheyne-Stokes respiration. What underlying mechanism contributes to this breathing pattern?
   a. Increased respiratory drive
   b. Delayed response of central chemoreceptors
   c. Fluctuations in blood pressure
   d. Dysfunction of respiratory centers in the brainstem

Q5. Which of the following conditions is characterized by a deficiency in oxygen supply to tissues and organs?
   a. Dyspnea
   b. Hypoxia
   c. Cyanosis
   d. Asphyxia

Q6. How does cyanosis differ from hypoxia in terms of clinical presentation?
   a. Cyanosis is a subjective sensation, while hypoxia is a visible discoloration of the skin.
   b. Cyanosis indicates deoxygenation of hemoglobin, while hypoxia refers to inadequate oxygenation of tissues.
   c. Cyanosis is reversible, while hypoxia is irreversible.
   d. Cyanosis is characterized by increased respiratory rate, while hypoxia leads to decreased respiratory rate.

Q7. A patient with chronic obstructive pulmonary disease (COPD) presents with worsening dyspnea, productive cough, and wheezing. What underlying pathophysiological mechanisms contribute to these symptoms?
   a. Airway inflammation and mucus hypersecretion
   b. Destruction of alveolar walls and loss of lung elasticity
   c. Hypertrophy of respiratory muscles
   d. Decreased respiratory drive

Q8. A newborn infant presents with cyanosis shortly after birth. What condition should be considered as a potential cause of neonatal cyanosis?
   a. Drowning
   b. Asthma
   c. Meconium aspiration syndrome
   d. COPD

Q9. What is the term for the abnormal respiratory pattern characterized by recurrent cycles of breathing alternating between periods of hyperpnea and apnea?
   a. Dyspnea
   b. Hypoxia
   c. Cyanosis
   d. Periodic breathing

Q10. A mountaineer experiences difficulty breathing and fatigue while climbing to high altitudes. What physiological adaptation occurs in response to hypoxic hypoxia at high altitudes?
   a. Increased oxygen delivery to tissues
   b. Decreased respiratory rate and depth
   c. Enhanced production of red blood cells
   d. Expansion of lung volume

Q11. A patient with asthma reports increased wheezing and shortness of breath after exposure to cold air. What type of asthma exacerbation is this likely to be?
   a. Allergic asthma exacerbation
   b. Exercise-induced asthma exacerbation
   c. Cold air-induced asthma exacerbation
   d. Nonallergic asthma exacerbation

Q12. A patient with COPD presents with acute worsening of dyspnea, increased sputum production, and chest tightness. What underlying pathophysiological mechanism contributes to acute exacerbations of COPD?
   a. Airway inflammation and bronchoconstriction
   b. Destruction of alveolar walls and loss of lung elasticity
   c. Decreased respiratory drive
   d. Hypertrophy of respiratory muscles

Q13. A swimmer experiences sudden submersion in water and subsequent loss of consciousness. What is the most likely cause of death in this scenario?
   a. Drowning
   b. Asthma exacerbation
   c. COPD exacerbation
   d. Hypoxia

### ANSWERS

1. c   2. b   3. b   4. d   5. b   6. b   7. a   8. c   9. d   10. c   11. c   12. a   13. a

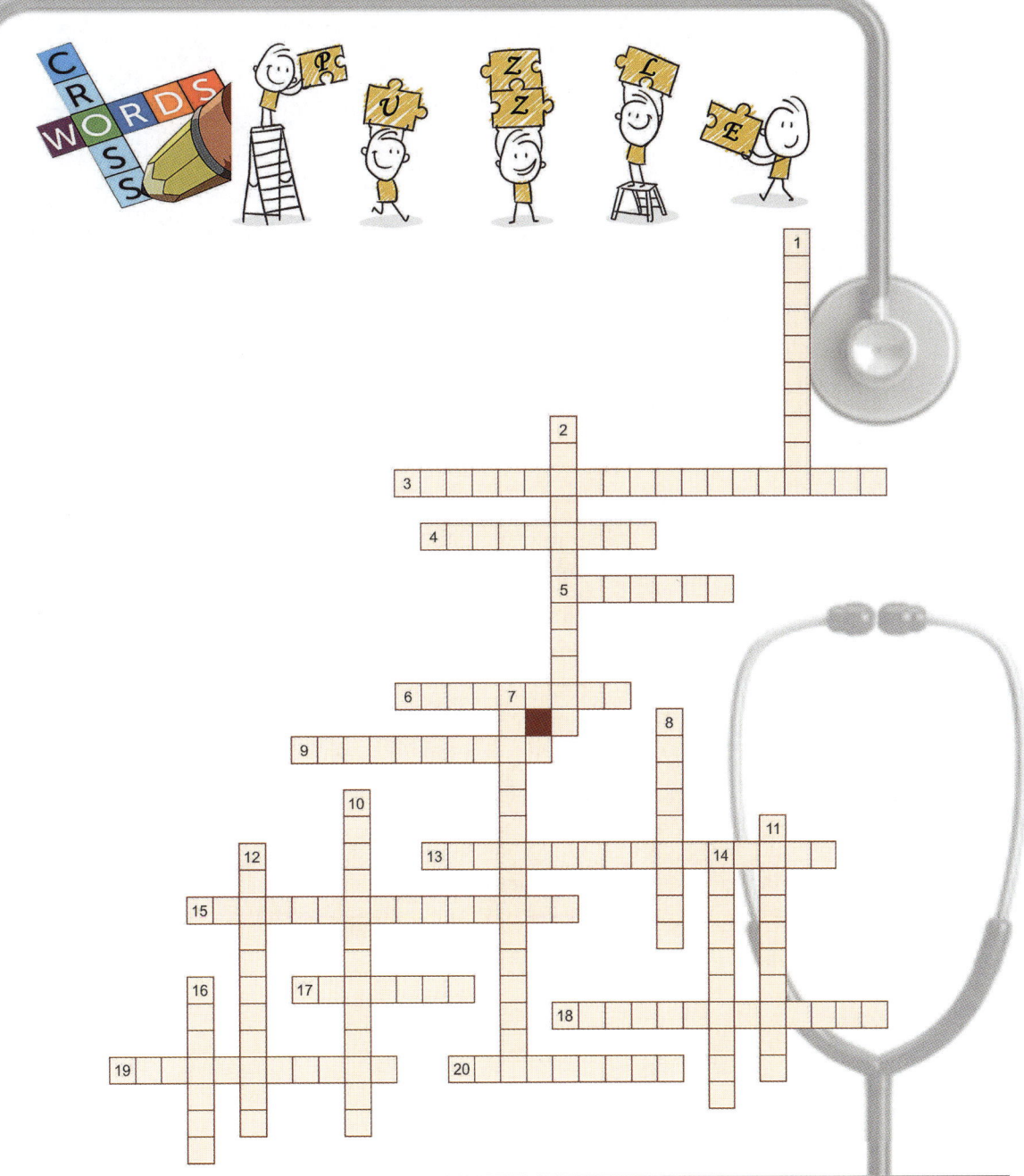

### Across

3. Predominant phospholipid in surfactant
4. Condition in which there is barrel shaped chest
5. The functional units of gas exchange in our lungs
6. Process of loss of electron from the Fe2+ to form Fe3+, forming meth Hb
9. The change in the volume per unit change in the pressure
13. Additional capacity of lungs that can be recruited during times of increased demand
15. The accumulation of excess fluid in the pleural space
17. Decreased availability of oxygen at the level of tissues
18. Draining excess pleural fluid using a needle inserted into the pleural space
19. These nerves causes bronchodilation and decreased bronchial secretions
20. Center at pontomedullary junction which accentuated inspiration

### Down

1. β₂ agonist bronchodilator
2. The volume of air that fills the conducting airways
7. Physiological adaptation to low oxygen levels at high altitudes
8. It is the principal muscle for quiet breathing
10. The maximum amount of air that can be expired at the end of maximum inspiration with maximum inspiratory and expiratory effort
11. Condition characterized by inflammation and narrowing of the airways
12. These cells have lamellar inclusion bodies and secrete surfactant
14. Device used to measure lung volumes and capacities
16. Shortness of breath, especially with exertion

# SECTION 7

# RENAL PHYSIOLOGY

## Section Outline

**Chapter 57:** Functional Anatomy of Kidney
**Chapter 58:** Juxtaglomerular Apparatus and Renin-angiotensin Aldosterone System
**Chapter 59:** Formation of Urine (Glomerular Filtration, Tubular Reabsorption and Secretion, Concentration of Urine)
**Chapter 60:** Renal Function Tests (Including Plasma Clearance)
**Chapter 61:** Physiological Basis of Diuretics and Renal Disorders
**Chapter 62:** Urinary Bladder and its Applied Physiology

# Functional Anatomy of Kidney

**CHAPTER 57**

**COMPETENCY ADDRESSED**

PY7.1: Describe structure and function of kidney.

**LEARNING OBJECTIVES**

**At the end of this chapter, the learner should be able to:**
- Describe the physiological anatomy of kidney and urinary tract.
- Describe the histological and functional anatomy of nephron.
- Differentiate between the cortical and juxtamedullary nephrons
- Describe the excretory and nonexcretory functions of kidney.
- Describe the anatomical characteristics of the renal circulation.
- Describe the renal blood flow, its measurement and regulation.
- Describe the physiological basis for the disparity and consequences of difference in the renal blood flow in various regions of kidney.

## INTRODUCTION

The excretion means the elimination of the waste products from the body. The organs which perform this function are called excretory organs. The main excretory organs of our body which eliminates the nitrogenous waste product are the kidneys or the urinary tract. The other important organs which perform the excretory function in addition to their main functions are skin and lungs. in this chapter we are going to focus on the kidneys as the important excretory organ of our body.

The urinary tract comprises of **(Fig. 57.1)**:
- **Kidneys:** Which will form the main function of filtrating the plasma and formation of urine.

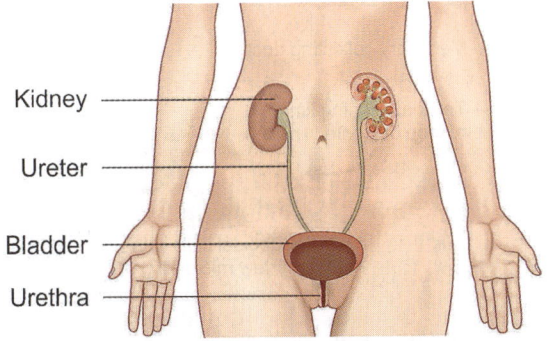

**Fig. 57.1:** Excretory system of human body.

- **Ureters:** These are the thin muscular tubes connecting kidneys to the urinary bladder. They carry the urine formed in the kidney to the urinary bladder.
- **Urinary bladder:** It is a hollow bladder which receives the urine. It collects the urine and stores it until it is voided. It has smooth muscles and it's lined by the transitional epithelium.
- **Urethra:** It is a tubular structure arising from the urinary bladder, opening outside through the urethral opening. It helps in voiding of urine.

## KIDNEY

Each of us have two kidneys situated on the posterior wall of the abdomen, outside the peritoneal cavity. An adult kidney weighs around 150 grams and is of the size of the clenched fist. Structurally it has an indented surface called hilum, on its medial side through which, various important structures (like renal vessels, nerves, ureter) enter and exit the kidney **(Fig. 57.2)**.

It is surrounded by a fibrous capsule which protects the delicate internal structures of kidney. Histologically, it is divided into outer renal cortex and inner renal medulla. The medulla is divided into 8-10 conical structures called renal pyramids, the space between the pyramids is called Columns of Bertini. These inverted pyramids originate at the corticomedullary junctions and end at the apical

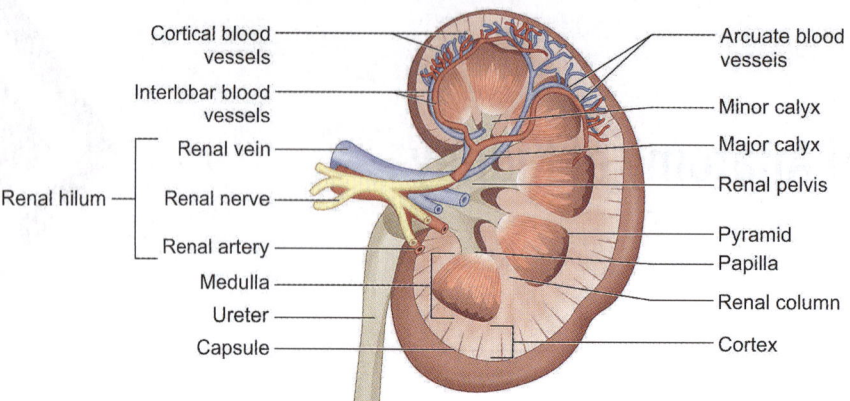

**Fig. 57.2:** Structure of kidney.

papilla, which opens into minor calyces. These minor calyces coalesce to form major calyces, which in turn open into renal pelvis. From there arises the ureter which leaves the kidney through the hilum and enters the urinary bladder. The walls of the calyces, renal pelvis and ureter have smooth muscles, which pushes the urine towards the urinary bladder.

## NEPHRON

The *structural and functional unit* of the kidney is a tubular structure called nephron. Each kidney has around 8 lakhs to one million nephrons. These nephrons cannot regenerate, hence if they are damaged due to ageing, renal injury or disease, their number would decrease compromising the renal function.

> *If the number of nephrons decreases with age, why the renal functions remain unaffected?*
>
> The surviving nephrons undergo adaptive changes, i.e., there is hypertrophy of various structures in the nephrons which decreases the vascular resistance and increases the tubular reabsorption. These adaptive changes permit the person to excrete normal amounts of water, nitrogenous waste products and solutes, even when the kidney mass is reduced to 20–25% of the normal.

### Structure of the Nephron (Fig. 57.3)

A nephron is a tubular structure, which has the following parts:

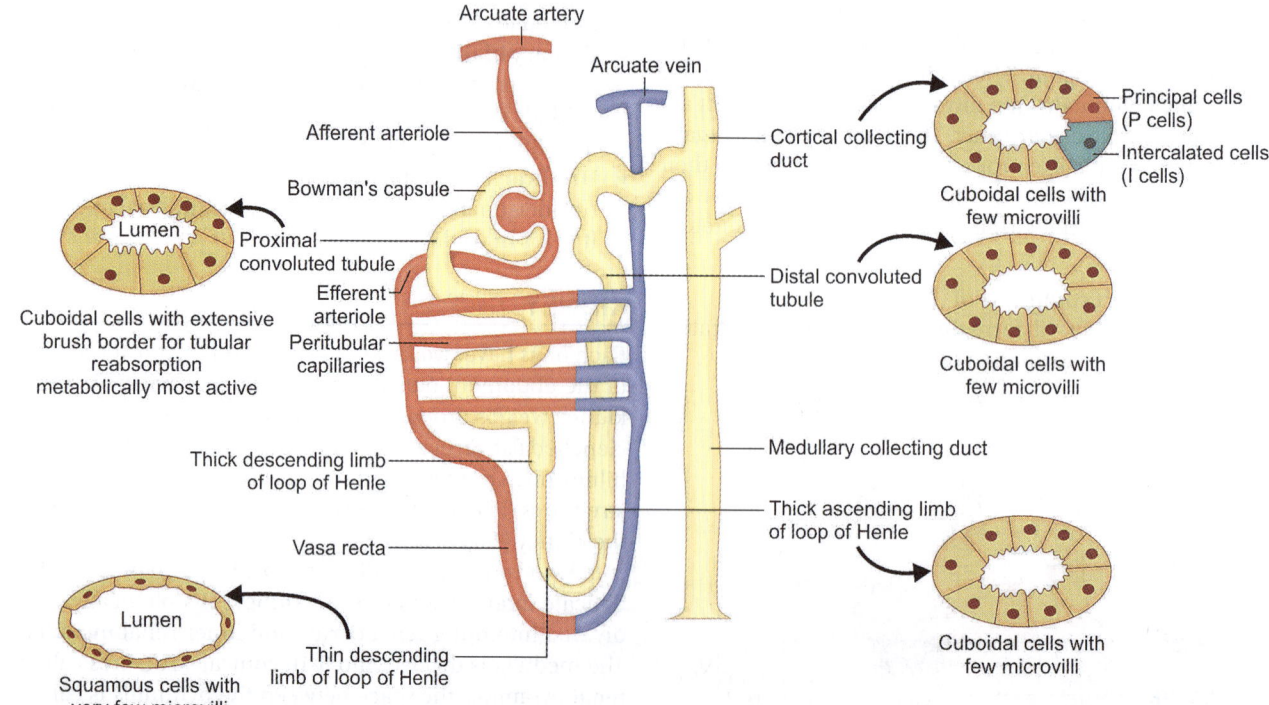

**Fig. 57.3:** Detailed structure of nephron.

> **Parts of nephron in:**
> - **Cortex:**
>   - Glomerulus
>   - Bowman's capsule
>   - Proximal convoluted tubule (PCT)
>   - Distal convoluted tubule (DCT)
>   - Cortical collecting duct (CCD)
> - **Medulla:**
>   - Loop of Henle (LOH)
>   - Medullary collecting duct (CCD)

## Bowman's Capsule and Glomerulus (Fig. 57.4)

It is a double layer structure which is invaginated by the tuft of capillaries, called glomerulus. It is lined by these squamous cells. The Bowman's capsule and glomerulus together form the filtration barrier which results in the ultra filtration of plasma.

*The filtration barrier/glomerular capillary membrane:* The filtration barrier is made-up of three layers **(Fig. 57.5)**.

1. **Capillary endothelium:** There are small openings in the capillary endothelium called *fenestrae*. The endothelial cell proteins have abundant fixed negative charges that do not allow the passage of negatively charged plasma proteins from plasma into the Bowman's capsule.
2. **Basement membrane (Fig. 57.5):** It surrounds the endothelium and consists of *meshwork of collagen and proteoglycan fibrillae*. These strong negative electrical charges of the proteoglycans in this layer does not allow the proteins to filter into the Bowman's capsule.
3. **Layer of epithelial cells (podocytes):** The final, outermost layer is formed of the epithelial cells, podocytes, which means the cell with the foot processes. There are *large slit pores* between the podocytes. These cells also have negative charges on their surface and hence also prevent the passage of the plasma proteins into the Bowman's capsule.

## Proximal Convoluted Tubule

It is highly convoluted portion of the nephron. It plays a very important role in the formation of urine as majority of obligatory tubular reabsorption and secretion takes place in this segment. It is lined by the cuboidal epithelium with extensive brush border and abundant cellular organelles. These cells are metabolically most active. The major activities carried out in PCT are:

- Reabsorption of sodium along with glucose, amino acids, phosphate, other ions like calcium, magnesium, bicarbonate are absorbed with water.
- Secretion of $H^+$, bile acids, bile salts, uric acid and creatinine.
- Bicarbonate buffer to regulate urinary pH.

## Loop of Henle

It is a U-pin bend tubular structure It has three parts **(Fig. 57.6)**:
1. Thin descending limb
2. Thin ascending limb
3. Thick ascending limb

The main function of loop of Henle is the concentration of urine through the counter current mechanism. It creates the hyperosmolar gradient in the medullary interstitium.

## Distal Convoluted Tubule

The next segment of the nephron is also convoluted hence called DCT. It is divided into two subparts:
1. **Early DCT:** It participates in the reabsorption of $Na^+$ and $Cl^-$ through Na-Cl cotransporter.

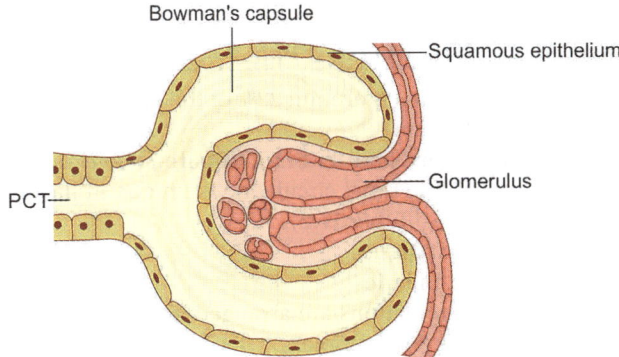

**Fig. 57.4:** Structure of Bowman's capsule and relation to glomerulus.

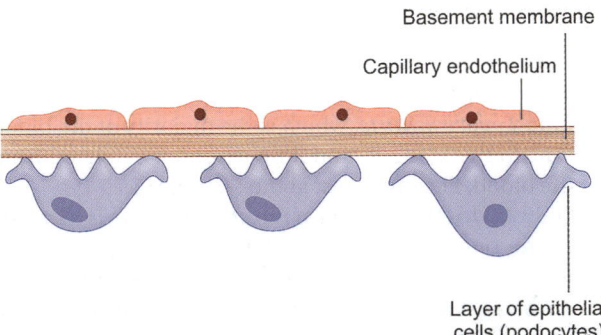

**Fig. 57.5:** Basement membrane showing arrangement of podocytes.

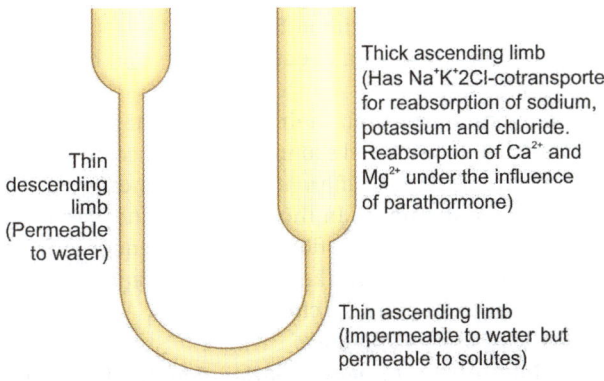

**Fig. 57.6:** Loop of Henle.

2. **Late DCT:** The late DCT apart from the Na-Cl cotransporter also has two specific cells principal cells (P-cells) and intercalated cells (I-cells). These cells are also present in the cortical collecting duct. They have three important functions:
   1. Regulation of Na$^+$ concentration in body.
   2. Regulation of water homeostasis in body due to Na$^+$ levels.
   3. Regulation of pH by the I-cells.

### Collecting Duct

It collects the urine from the nephrons and pours into the minor calyces. The collecting ducts have two subparts:
1. **Cortical collecting duct (CCD):** Similar to the late DCT, the CCD also has the P cells and the I cell and serves a similar function.
   - *P-cells:* They regulate the Na$^+$ concentration in extracellular fluid by regulating the activity of Na$^+$K$^+$ ATPase pump under the influence of aldosterone. It leads to the retention of Na$^+$ and loss of K$^+$ in urine.
   - *I-cells:* They regulate the H$^+$ concentration by H$^+$ ATPase pump.
2. **Medullary collecting duct (MCD):** This segment is responsible for the
   - Facultative reabsorption of water by regulating the water reabsorption under the influence of antidiuretic hormone (ADH) secreted by the posterior pituitary.
   - Reabsorption of urea to create the hyperosmolarity of the medullary interstitium.

### Types of Nephrons

Depending the structural and functional differences, the nephrons are of two types **(Table 57.1)**:
1. Cortical nephrons
2. Juxtamedullary nephrons

## FUNCTIONS OF KIDNEYS

Kidney performs many homeostatic functions like:
- **Excretory function:**
  - Excretion of the nitrogenous waste products like blood urea, S. creatinine, S. uric acid
  - Excretion of foreign chemicals, drugs and hormone metabolites.

  The kidneys carry out their most important tasks by filtering the plasma and eliminating different compounds from the filtrate at different rates, depending on the body's requirements. In the end, the kidneys remove waste products from the filtrate (and subsequently from the blood) by excreting them in the urine and restoring essential products to the circulation.
- **Non-excretory Functions:**
  - *Regulation of water homeostasis:* It occurs through obligatory reabsorption of water at PCT and facultative reabsorption under the influence of ADH at MCD.
  - *Regulation of electrolyte balance:* Various electrolytes like Na$^+$, K$^+$, Mg$^{2+}$, Ca$^{2+}$, HCO$_3^-$ etc., are handled and their balance maintained in ECF.
  - *Regulation of body fluid osmolality:* It regulates the fluid osmolality by handling the water and electrolyte concentrations of body.
  - *Regulation of arterial pressure:* It plays a very important role in maintaining arterial pressure through renin angiotensin mechanism.
  - *Regulation of acid-base balance/pH regulation:* It efficiently regulates the pH of blood through the bicarbonate, phosphate and ammonia buffer systems.
- **Endocrine function:**
  - Secretion of erythropoietin for regulating the erythropoiesis
  - Activation of vitamin D3 (1,25 dihydroxy cholecalciferol)
- **Gluconeogenesis:** Formation of glucose from the other molecules like proteins and fats during the need.

> **Why a patient with chronic renal failure presents with:**
> 1. Anemia
> 2. Vitamin D deficiency
> 3. Acidosis
> 4. Hyperparathyroidism
> 5. Weak bones

## RENAL BLOOD FLOW (FIGS. 57.7A AND B)

The renal blood flow is around 22% of the cardiac output that is 1100 mL/min.

The renal artery and its branches are shown in the diagram below. The renal circulation is unique in having two capillary beds **(Table 57.2)**:
1. Glomerular capillaries
2. Peritubular capillaries

Both these circulations are arranged in series and are separated by efferent arteriole.

Depending on the body homeostatic demands, the glomerular filtration, tubular reabsorption can be adjusted.

### Regional Blood Flow and Oxygen Consumption (Fig. 57.8)

- *The renal cortex receives 5 mL/g of kidney tissue of blood every minute*, which is the majority of the blood flow to the kidneys, and little oxygen is removed from the blood, leaving PO$_2$ at about 50 mm Hg.
- Only *1% to 2% of the total renal blood flow is directed to the renal medulla*, which has relatively low blood flow needs. Blood flow to the medulla is approximately *2.5 mL/g/min in the outer medulla and 0.6 mL/g/min in the inner medulla*. However, metabolic work is being done, particularly to reabsorb Na$^+$ in the thick ascending limb of Henle, so relatively large amounts of

**Table 57.1:** Differences between cortical and juxtamedullary nephrons.

| | Cortical nephrons | Juxtamedullary nephrons |
|---|---|---|
| Location | These nephrons mostly lie in renal cortex | These nephrons start in renal cortex and extend deep into medulla |
| Number | 85% of nephrons | 15% of nephrons |
| Length | Short | Long |
| Bowman's capsule | Small, located in outer renal cortex | Large, located near corticomedullary junction |
| Peritubular capillary network | Extensively present | Present |
| Diameter of efferent arteriole | Large | Small |
| Vasa recta | Absent | Present |
| Loop of Henle | Short | Long |
| Tip of LOH | In outer renal medulla | In inner renal medulla |
| Function | Filtration and reabsorption | Concentration of urine |

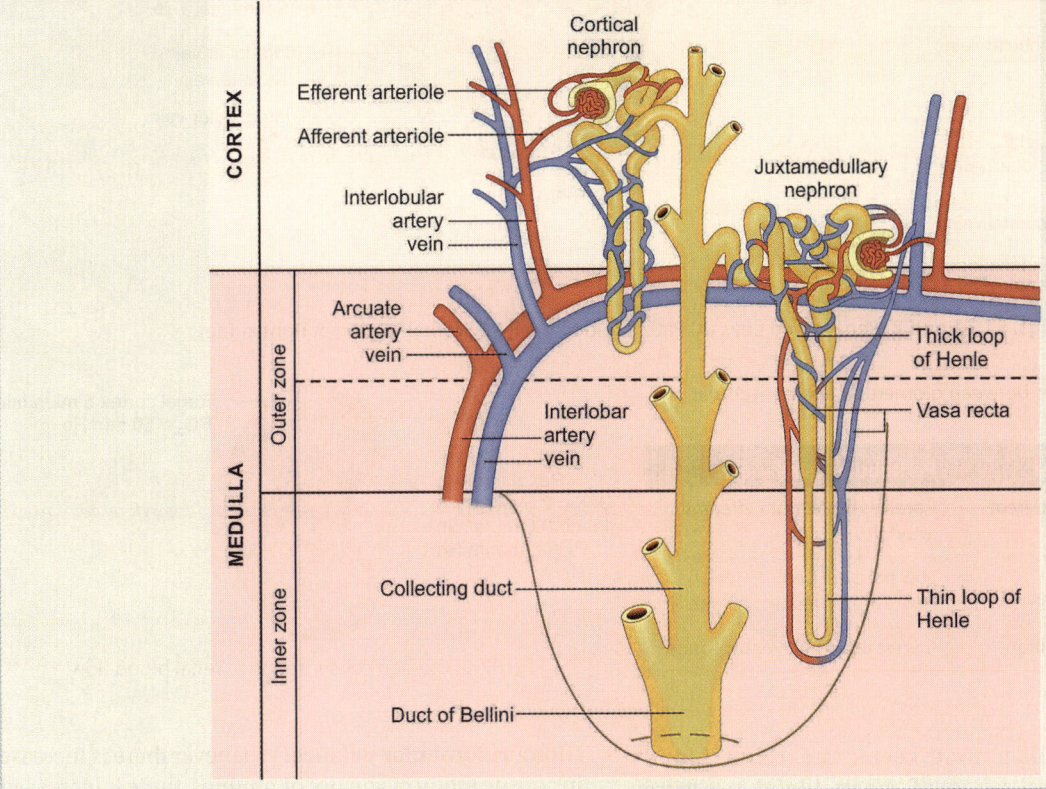

$O_2$ are extracted from the blood in the medulla. The $PO_2$ in renal medulla is roughly 15 mm Hg.

**What would happen, if blood flow through renal medulla increases?**

The low blood flow in renal medulla helps in maintaining the hyperosmolar gradient of medulla, which would get diluted, if the blood flow through medulla is increased.

- The only blood supply to renal medulla is through the vasa recta, which carries a little blood flow to renal medulla. *So, if there is decreased blood flow to renal medulla, it can result in medullary hypoxia.*

**Why is renal medulla more susceptible to hypoxic damage?**
- High metabolic demand due to active reabsorption of Na⁺ in the thick ascending limb of Henle.
- Large amount of oxygen is extracted from the blood in the medulla.
- Less blood flow to the medulla.
- Sluggish blood flow.

## Regulation of Renal Blood Flow

The renal blood flow is very tightly regulated by the following mechanisms:

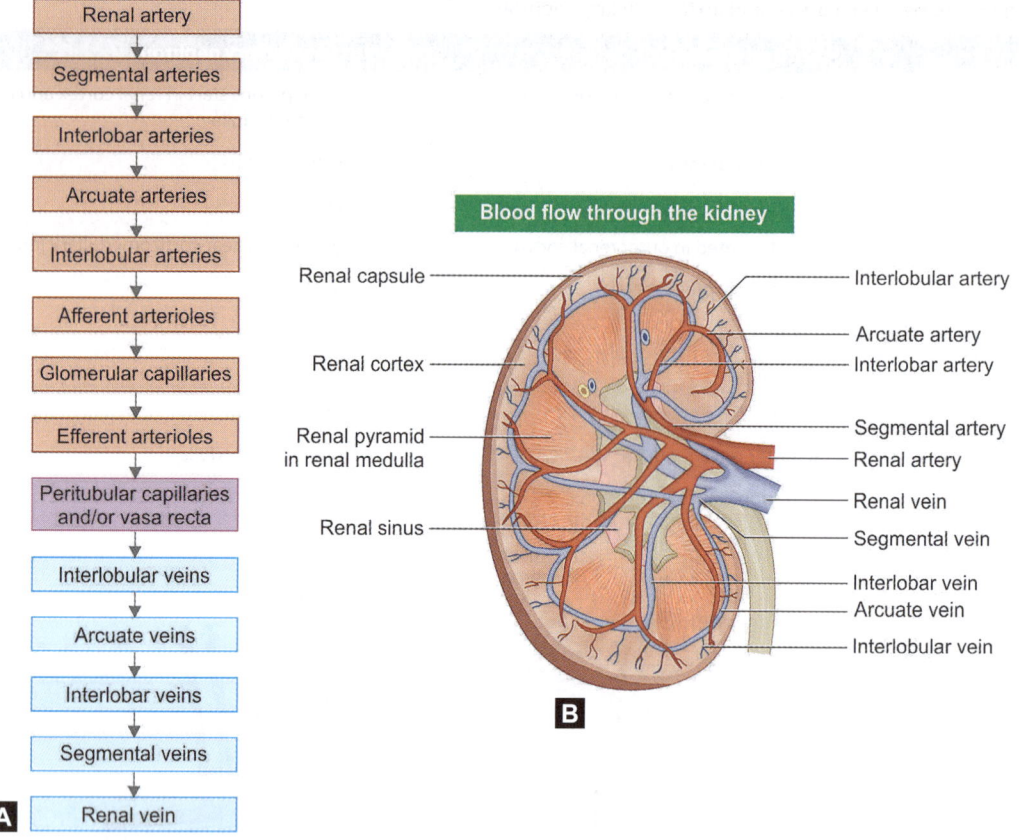

**Figs. 57.7A and B:** Renal blood flow. (A) Path of blood flow; (B) Frontal section of right kidney.

**Table 57.2:** Differences between glomerular and peritubular capillaries.

| Glomerular capillaries | Peritubular capillaries |
| --- | --- |
| Receives blood from afferent arterioles | Receives blood from efferent arterioles |
| High pressure bed Hydrostatic pressure: 60 mm Hg | Low pressure bed Hydrostatic pressure: 13 mm Hg |
| Causes rapid fluid filtration | Causes rapid fluid reabsorption |

**Fig. 57.8:** Oxygen consumption in renal blood flow.

## Autoregulation

It is the mechanism that keeps the renal blood flow constant over range of mean blood pressure (80–200 mm Hg). At 80 mm Hg, smooth muscle cells in arterioles are completely relaxed and renal blood flow is optimal.

### Mechanism for Autoregulation

- **Myogenic mechanism:** Smooth muscle cells in arterioles automatically contract when stretched by high blood pressure (related to increased blood flow).
- **Tubuloglomerular mechanism:** The macula densa cells release adenosine, which increases resistance in the afferent arteriole in response to increased RBF, GFR, and subsequently enhanced salt chloride transport to the distal convoluted tubules.
- **Glomerulotubular balance:** Whenever there is increase in consumption of glucose or proteins, there is increased renal blood flow (**Flowchart 57.1**).

## Hormonal Regulation

Hormones causes either vasoconstriction or vasodilatation which are tabulated in **Table 57.3**.

## Stimulation of Renal Nerves

The proximal and distal tubules and the thick ascending limb of the loop of Henle are richly innervated. Strong stimulation of the sympathetic noradrenergic nerves via $\alpha_1$-adrenergic receptors causes a marked decrease in renal blood flow.

**Flowchart 57.1:** Effect of glucose and protein intake on renal blood flow.

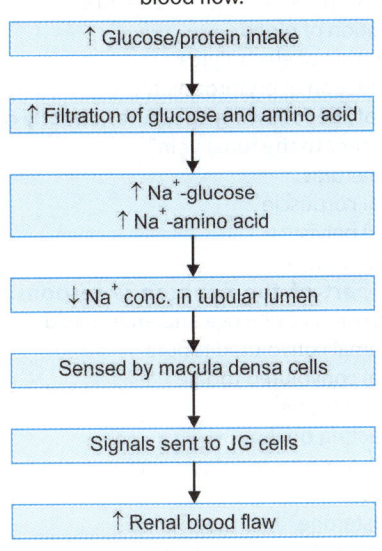

**Table 57.3:** Hormonal regulation of renal blood flow.

| Hormones vasoconstriction/ increasing arteriolar resistance (decrease renal blood flow) | Hormones vasodilatation/ decreasing arteriolar resistance (increase renal blood flow) |
|---|---|
| • Adrenaline<br>• Angiotensin II | • Atrial natriuretic peptide (ANP)<br>• Prostaglandin<br>• Dopamine |

## Measurement of Renal Blood Flow

The renal blood flow is measured with the help of various methods:
- Para amino hippuric acid (PAH) clearance method based on the principle of Plasma clearance (discussed with plasma clearance chapter 60)
- Electromagnetic flowmeter
- Color Doppler ultrasonography

## SUMMARY

In this chapter, we have discussed that
- There are two kidney present retroperitonially in the abdomen. Their main functions apart from excretion of nitrogenous waste products is to synthesize hormones (erythropoietin and vitamin D3), maintain fluid and electrolyte balance, maintain pH of body, etc.
- There are two types of nephrons, the cortical and juxtamedullary nephrons, which have different functions like filtration and reabsorption and concentration of urine, respectively.
- Kidneys receive around 1,100–1,200 mL of blood in a minute which is mostly distributed in renal cortex and the medulla receives very little blood flow. This helps in maintaining the hyperosmolar gradient of the renal medulla but also makes the kidney susceptible to ischemic injuries.

## LET US SEE, HOW MUCH YOU HAVE LEARNT?

 *Review Questions*

### Long/Short Answer Questions

**Q1.** Draw a well labeled diagram of a nephron. Enumerate its parts and discuss each of them.

**Q2.** Differentiate between cortical and juxtamedullary nephrons.

**Q3.** How is the renal blood flow regulated?

### Explain Why? (Reasoning Questions)

**Q1.** The renal function remains normal in old age, despite of decrease in number of nephrons.

**Q2.** The proteins are not filtered across the glomerular filtration barrier.

**Q3.** There is increase in renal blood flow in a person consuming high glucose meal.

 *Multiple Choice Questions*

**Q1.** Which of the following accurately describes the physiological anatomy of the kidney?
   a. It consists of two lobes separated by the renal hilum.
   b. It is made up of nephrons and collecting ducts.
   c. Its main function is the production of insulin.
   d. It primarily serves as a storage organ for urine.

**Q2.** What is the primary function of the nephron?
   a. Filtration of blood
   b. Production of urine
   c. Regulation of blood sugar levels
   d. Absorption of oxygen

**Q3.** Cortical nephrons are characterized by:
  a. A longer loop of Henle
  b. Location mainly in the outer cortex of the kidney
  c. Greater involvement in the production of concentrated urine
  d. More abundant in the medullary region

**Q4.** Which of the following is an excretory function of the kidney?
  a. Regulation of blood pressure
  b. Secretion of hormones
  c. Removal of waste products from the blood
  d. Production of red blood cells

**Q5.** What are the anatomical characteristics of the renal circulation?
  a. It is a low-pressure system
  b. The renal artery branches into interlobar arteries
  c. Veins carry oxygenated blood away from the kidney
  d. The renal vein exits the kidney through the renal cortex

**Q6.** Renal blood flow is primarily regulated by:
  a. Sympathetic nervous system
  b. Parasympathetic nervous system
  c. Hormonal signals from the pancreas
  d. Skeletal muscle contractions

**Q7.** Which of the following accurately describes renal blood flow measurement?
  a. It is typically measured using an electrocardiogram (ECG).
  b. Renal blood flow can be assessed by angiography.
  c. Doppler ultrasound can be used to measure renal blood flow.
  d. Renal blood flow is directly proportional to heart rate.

**Q8.** The physiological basis for the disparity in renal blood flow in various kidney regions is primarily due to:
  a. Differences in oxygen demand
  b. Variances in sympathetic innervation
  c. Concentration gradients of solutes
  d. Hormonal fluctuations

**Q9.** Juxtamedullary nephrons are characterized by:
  a. Shorter loops of Henle
  b. Location mainly in the outer cortex of the kidney
  c. Lesser involvement in the production of concentrated urine
  d. Greater abundance in the medullary region

**Q10.** Which of the following is NOT a non-excretory function of the kidney?
  a. Regulation of blood pressure
  b. Removal of nitrogenous wastes
  c. Regulation of blood pH
  d. Production of erythropoietin

**Q11.** The glomerulus is responsible for:
  a. Filtration of blood
  b. Secretion of hormones
  c. Reabsorption of water
  d. Production of urine

**Q12.** The collecting duct is responsible for:
  a. Reabsorption of water and solutes
  b. Filtration of blood
  c. Secretion of electrolytes
  d. Production of erythropoietin

**Q13.** Which of the following structures directly connects the renal artery to the renal vein?
  a. Glomerulus
  b. Renal corpuscle
  c. Renal pelvis
  d. Renal sinus

**Q14.** Which part of the nephron is responsible for the reabsorption of glucose and amino acids?
  a. Proximal convoluted tubule
  b. Distal convoluted tubule
  c. Loop of Henle
  d. Collecting duct

**Q15.** Which hormone regulates water reabsorption in the kidneys?
  a. Aldosterone
  b. Antidiuretic hormone (ADH)
  c. Renin
  d. Angiotensin II

**Q16.** Which of the following statements is true regarding the renal medulla?
  a. It is mainly responsible for the filtration of blood.
  b. It contains the majority of the nephrons in the kidney.
  c. It has a high concentration of solutes due to the countercurrent mechanism.
  d. It is primarily involved in the secretion of hormones.

**Q17.** Which of the following is NOT a function of the renal pelvis?
  a. Storage of urine
  b. Transportation of urine from the kidneys to the bladder
  c. Filtration of blood
  d. Collection of urine from the calyces

**Q18.** Which of the following substances is primarily excreted through the kidneys?
  a. Oxygen
  b. Glucose
  c. Carbon dioxide
  d. Urea

**Q19.** What is the function of the juxtaglomerular apparatus?
  a. Regulation of blood pressure
  b. Secretion of erythropoietin
  c. Production of urine
  d. Filtration of blood

**Q20.** Which of the following is NOT a component of the renal corpuscle?
  a. Glomerulus
  b. Bowman's capsule
  c. Proximal convoluted tubule
  d. Podocytes

## ANSWERS

1. b  2. a  3. b  4. c  5. b  6. a  7. c  8. a  9. d  10. b  11. a  12. a  13. c  14. a
15. b  16. c  17. c  18. d  19. a  20. c

# Juxtaglomerular Apparatus and Renin-angiotensin Aldosterone System

**CHAPTER 58**

### COMPETENCY ADDRESSED
PY7.2: Describe the structure and functions of juxtaglomerular apparatus and role of renin-angiotensin system.

### LEARNING OBJECTIVES
At the end of this chapter, the learner should be able to:
- Describe the juxtaglomerular apparatus using a well labeled self-explanatory diagram/flowchart.
- Describe the functions of juxtaglomerular apparatus.
- Apply the concept of JG apparatus on physiological basis of management of renal blood flow, GFR and arterial pressure.

## JUXTAGLOMERULAR APPARATUS

The Juxtaglomerular apparatus (JGA) is the specialized anatomical unit situated near the glomerulus of each nephron. It is located in a specialized region of a nephron, where in the afferent arteriole and the distal convoluted tubule (DCT) come in direct contact with each other **(Fig. 58.1)**.

## Components

The juxtaglomerular complex consist of:
- **Juxtaglomerular cells (JG cells):** They are modified epithelioid cells of tunica media in afferent arterioles as they approach the glomeruli. These cells store renin, a protein hormone, released from JG cells as a result

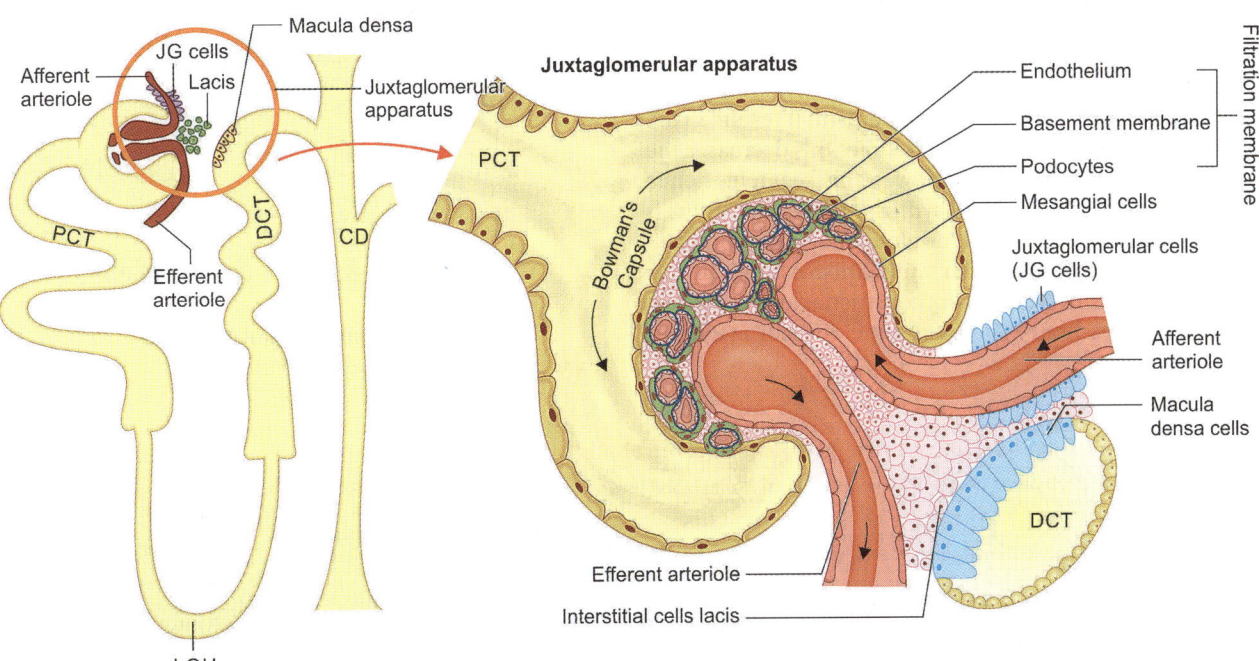

**Fig. 58.1:** Structure of juxtaglomerular apparatus (JGA).
(CD: collecting duct; DCT: distal convoluted tubule; LOH: loop of Henle; PCT: proximal convoluted tubule)

of signals received from macula densa in response to low sodium concentration in tubular filtrate due to low arterial pressure, decreased GFR, increased sympathetic nervous system activity.

- **Macula densa cells:** They are specialized group of columnar cells situated in the distal convoluted tubular, where the afferent and efferent arterioles converge. These cells detect a change in sodium chloride in the tubular filtrate in the distal convoluted tubule and then sends a signals to JG cells through the interstitial cells of lacis.
- **Extraglomerular mesangial cells/lacis cells/agranular cells:** These cells, which are modified interstitial cells located in the triangular region between the afferent and efferent arterioles on sides and macula densa at the base. They transmit signals from macula densa cells to JG cells.

## Physiological Functions of JG Cells

- **Autoregulation of renal blood flow and GFR:** The JG apparatus provide an efficient mechanism for autoregulation of GFR and RBF during changes in arterial pressure by secreting renin and activating the renin angiotensin mechanism.

The renin angiotensin mechanism:

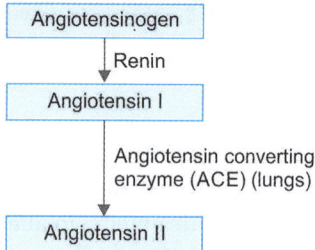

All the physiological actions of renin angiotensin mechanism are because of its end product angiotensin II, which is a potent vasoconstrictor. However, this renin angiotensin mechanism operates through two different mechanisms:

1. **The afferent arteriolar mechanism:** It results in the dilatation of the afferent arteriole. This decreases the resistance to the blood flow in this segment, hence increasing the capillary hydrostatic pressure. There is a resultant increase in the glomerular filtration rate.
2. **The efferent arteriolar mechanism:** Through this mechanism, there occurs constriction of the efferent arterioles hence increasing the efferent arteriolar resistance.

Both these mechanisms result in the increased glomerular hydrostatic pressure and hence the GFR.

Since then, the decreased sodium concentration due to decreased GFR was sensed by distal tubular cells and the feedback sent to JG cells to secrete renin, this mechanism is also called as the *tubuloglomerular feedback mechanism* (**Fig. 58.2**). It serves as an important feedback system for the regulation of GFR and RBF.

Another important mechanism regulating the GFR and RBF is *glomerulotubular balance*. In this mechanism, the glomerulus regulates the filtration rate depending on the reabsorptive capacity of proximal convoluted tubular.

> **Why there is increase in RBF in a person consuming high glucose meal/high protein meal?**
>
> The glucose and the amino acids are reabsorbed back into the body in the proximal convoluted tubular. If the person consumes a meal with high glucose/protein content, there is more reabsorption of sodium due to sodium linked glucose/amino acid transport on the apical membrane of PCT cells.
>
> Decreased sodium concentration results in increased GFR through tubuloglomerular feedback mechanism.
>
> This is an example of glomerulotubular balance. Because the decreased concentration of sodium in the filtrate is due to increased tubular absorption.

- Secretion of erythropoietin by JG cells in response to hypoxia. Kidney secrete 90% of the erythropoietin hormone

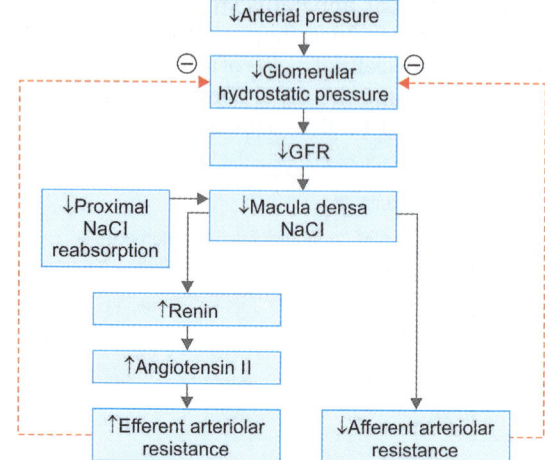

**Fig. 58.2:** Tubuloglomerular feedback.
(GFR: glomerular filtration rate)

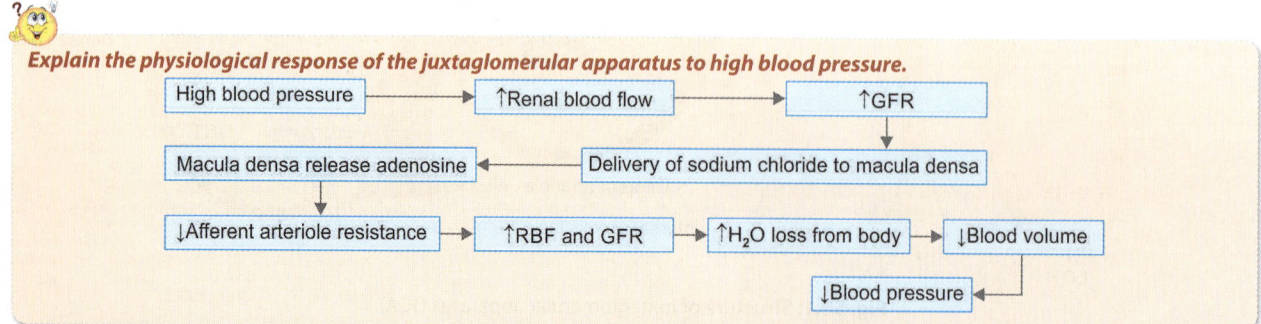

*Explain the physiological response of the juxtaglomerular apparatus to high blood pressure.*

*Explain the physiological response of the juxtaglomerular apparatus to low blood pressure.*

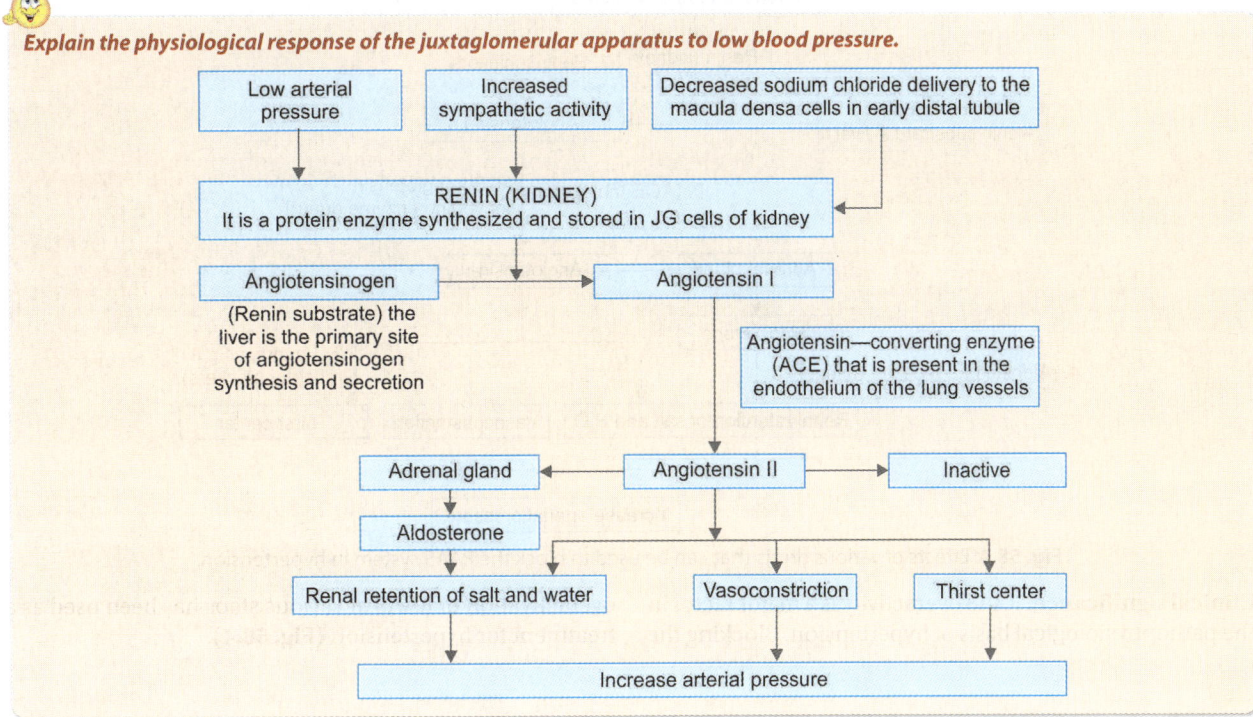

## RENIN-ANGIOTENSIN ALDOSTERONE SYSTEM (RAAS)

The renin-angiotensin-aldosterone system (RAAS) plays a crucial role in controlling systemic vascular resistance, blood volume, and electrolyte balance. By controlling vascular tone and maintaining salt and water homeostasis, it is a critical modulator of cardiac, vascular, and renal physiology.

## Components

- Renin
- Angiotensin II
- Aldosterone

**Physiological function:** One of the most important functions of the renin-angiotensin system is allowing a person to consume very small or very high amounts of salt without significantly altering extracellular fluid volume or arterial pressure **(Fig. 58.3)**.

*Explain the physiological basis for how angiotensin II causes an increase in renal salt and water retention.*

- **Direct renal effect:** Constriction of efferent arterioles thereby diminishing blood flow through kidney and this decreases pressure in the peritubular capillaries, which increases reabsorption of fluid from the tubules.
- It stimulates the release of aldosterone by the adrenal gland and that increases sodium reabsorption by the renal tubules.

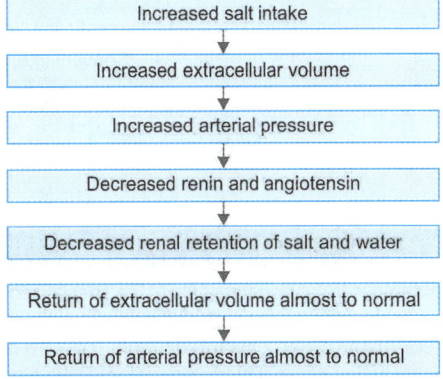

**Fig. 58.3:** A series of processes takes place when salt consumption is increased; nevertheless, a feedback reduction in renin-angiotensin system activity causes the arterial pressure to virtually return to normal.

It is the body's most effective system for allowing a wide range of salt consumption with just little changes in arterial pressure. When the RA system is working properly, a 100-fold increase in salt intake often results in a pressure increase of no more than 4 to 6 mm Hg. On the other hand, when the system is suppressed, the same increase in salt consumption may result in a pressure increase of at least 40 mm Hg.

*Explain the physiological causes of hypertension in cases where renin is secreted in high amounts.*

By releasing angiotensin II that causes
- By vasoconstricting the arterioles
- By causing the kidney to retain salt and water

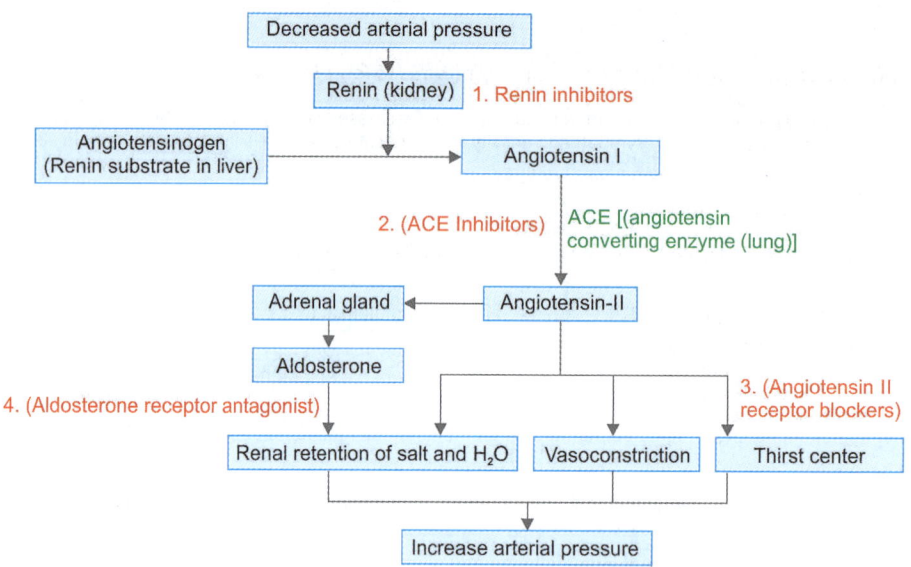

Fig. 58.4: Effects of various drugs that can be used to block the RAAS system in hypertension.

**Clinical significance:** RAAS overactivity is a major factor in the pathophysiological basis of hypertension. Blocking the overactivation of RAAS at various steps has been used as a treatment for hypertension **(Fig. 58.4)**.

*Describe the physiological reasons for coughing when renin-angiotensin system blockers are used as hypertension medications.*

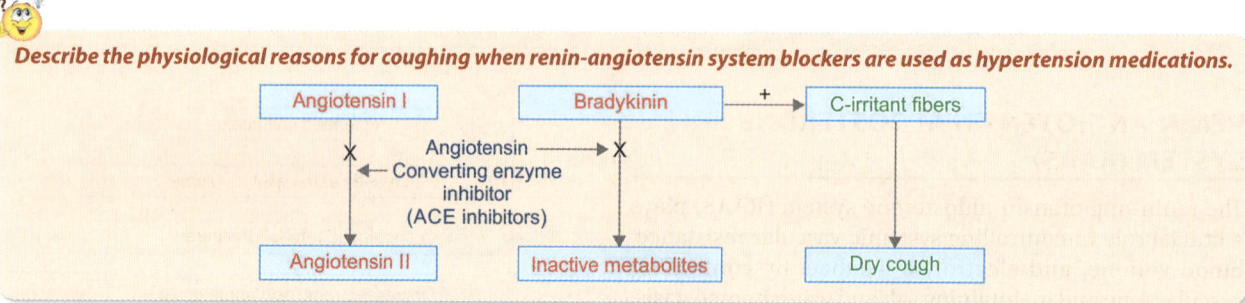

## SUMMARY

- The juxtaglomerular apparatus (JGA) is a specialized structure located in the kidney where the afferent arteriole comes into contact with the distal convoluted tubule. It plays a crucial role in the regulation of renal blood flow, glomerular filtration rate (GFR), and arterial pressure.
- The JGA consists of three main components: the macula densa, granular cells (juxtaglomerular cells), and extraglomerular mesangial cells. These components work together to sense changes in blood pressure and electrolyte concentrations, and to regulate the release of renin, a hormone involved in blood pressure regulation.
- The macula densa cells are specialized cells in the wall of the distal convoluted tubule that monitor the concentration of sodium chloride in the tubular fluid. When there is a decrease in sodium chloride concentration, indicating low blood pressure or low GFR, the macula densa cells signal to the adjacent granular cells.
- The granular cells are modified smooth muscle cells of the afferent arteriole. In response to signals from the macula densa, they release renin into the bloodstream. Renin acts on angiotensinogen to produce angiotensin I, which is then converted to angiotensin II by angiotensin-converting enzyme (ACE).
- Angiotensin II has several effects on the body, including vasoconstriction of the efferent arteriole, stimulation of aldosterone release from the adrenal glands, and stimulation of thirst. These actions collectively help to increase blood pressure, increase renal blood flow, and restore GFR to normal levels.

## LET US SEE, HOW MUCH YOU HAVE LEARNT?

*Review Questions*

### Long/Short Answer Questions

Q1. Describe the juxtaglomerular apparatus using a well labeled self-explanatory diagram/flowchart.
Q2. Describe the functions of juxtaglomerular apparatus.
Q3. Describe the renin angiotensin mechanism.
Q4. Describe the tubuloglomerular apparatus.

## Explain Why? (Reasoning Questions)

Q1. The activation of the renin-angiotensin-aldosterone system (RAAS) leads to an increase in blood pressure.
Q2. Juxtaglomerular cells, located in the walls of the afferent arteriole, are essential for the regulation of blood pressure.
Q3. The macula densa cells, found in the distal convoluted tubule, are critical for sensing sodium chloride concentration in the tubular fluid.
Q4. The inhibition of the RAAS with medications such as ACE inhibitors or angiotensin II receptor blockers (ARBs) is beneficial in treating hypertension and heart failure.

## Critical Thinking Case-Based Questions

Q1. A 50-year-old woman, presented with complaints of persistent fatigue, dizziness, and swelling in her legs and feet. She had a history of chronic hypertension and has been on antihypertensive medication for several years. On examination, her blood pressure was 160/95 mm Hg. Laboratory tests revealed low serum potassium and high aldosterone levels.

Based on the given scenario, answer the following questions:
a. Which system is involved in this condition?
b. Explain the physiological role of the juxtaglomerular apparatus in regulating this system in this patient.
c. What are the potential treatments for managing hyperactivity of the said system?

## Multiple Choice Questions

Q1. What are the main components of the juxtaglomerular apparatus?
   a. Macula densa, Bowman's capsule, glomerulus
   b. Macula densa, JG cells, extraglomerular mesangial cells
   c. Proximal convoluted tubule, loop of Henle, distal convoluted tubule
   d. Glomerulus, efferent arteriole, collecting duct

Q2. What hormone is released by the granular cells of the juxtaglomerular apparatus?
   a. Aldosterone
   b. Renin
   c. Antidiuretic hormone (ADH)
   d. Angiotensin II

Q3. Where are the macula densa cells located?
   a. Along the afferent arteriole
   b. In the Bowman's capsule
   c. In the glomerulus
   d. Distal convoluted tubule

Q4. Which of the following statements regarding the juxtaglomerular apparatus is true?
   a. It is responsible for the filtration of blood
   b. It regulates blood pressure solely through the secretion of aldosterone
   c. It consists of the macula densa and proximal convoluted tubule
   d. It plays a role in the renin-angiotensin-aldosterone system

Q5. If the macula densa detects decreased sodium chloride concentration in the tubular fluid, what is the likely response?
   a. Release of aldosterone
   b. Constriction of the efferent arteriole
   c. Secretion of renin by JG cells
   d. Vasodilation of the afferent arteriole

Q6. A patient with low blood pressure is found to have increased renin levels in the bloodstream. Which component of the juxtaglomerular apparatus is most likely responsible for this?
   a. Macula densa
   b. JG cells
   c. Extraglomerular mesangial cells
   d. Bowman's capsule

Q7. How does angiotensin II affect renal blood flow?
   a. It causes vasodilation of the afferent arteriole
   b. It increases sodium reabsorption in the distal convoluted tubule
   c. It stimulates the release of aldosterone
   d. It causes vasoconstriction of the efferent arteriole

Q8. In response to decreased arterial pressure, how does the juxtaglomerular apparatus contribute to maintaining glomerular filtration rate (GFR)?
   a. By decreasing renin secretion
   b. By dilating the efferent arteriole
   c. By inhibiting angiotensin-converting enzyme (ACE)
   d. By decreasing sodium reabsorption in the proximal convoluted tubule

Q9. A patient presents with hypertension. Which component of the juxtaglomerular apparatus is likely dysregulated in this condition?
   a. Macula densa
   b. Juxtaglomerular cells
   c. Extraglomerular mesangial cells
   d. Bowman's capsule

Q10. A patient with renal artery stenosis is experiencing decreased renal blood flow. How might the juxtaglomerular apparatus respond to this situation?
   a. By releasing more aldosterone
   b. By constricting the afferent arteriole
   c. By inhibiting renin secretion
   d. By dilating the efferent arteriole

Q11. A pregnant woman develops pre-eclampsia, characterized by hypertension and proteinuria. Which aspect of the juxtaglomerular apparatus might be implicated in this condition?
   a. Macula densa
   b. Juxtaglomerular cells
   c. Extraglomerular mesangial cells
   d. Bowman's capsule

**Q12.** A patient with heart failure is prescribed an ACE inhibitor to manage blood pressure. How might this medication affect the juxtaglomerular apparatus?
a. By increasing renin secretion
b. By inhibiting angiotensin II production
c. By dilating the efferent arteriole
d. By promoting sodium reabsorption in the proximal convoluted tubule

**Q13.** A patient with diabetes insipidus has elevated levels of antidiuretic hormone (ADH). How might this condition affect the juxtaglomerular apparatus?
a. By decreasing renin secretion
b. By causing vasoconstriction of the efferent arteriole
c. By increasing sodium reabsorption in the distal convoluted tubule
d. By promoting dilation of the afferent arteriole

**Q14.** A patient with chronic kidney disease has impaired renal function and reduced glomerular filtration rate (GFR). How might the juxtaglomerular apparatus respond to compensate for this?
a. By decreasing renin secretion
b. By dilating the efferent arteriole
c. By inhibiting angiotensin-converting enzyme (ACE)
d. By promoting sodium reabsorption in the proximal convoluted tubule

**Q15.** A patient undergoing major surgery experiences a significant drop in blood pressure due to blood loss. How might the juxtaglomerular apparatus respond to this acute situation?
a. By releasing aldosterone
b. By constricting the efferent arteriole
c. By inhibiting renin secretion
d. By dilating the afferent arteriole

## ANSWERS
1. b   2. b   3. d   4. d   5. c   6. b   7. d   8. b   9. b   10. b   11. b   12. b   13. a   14. b
15. c

# Formation of Urine
## (Glomerular Filtration, Tubular Reabsorption and Secretion, Concentration of Urine)

**CHAPTER 59**

### COMPETENCY ADDRESSED
**PY7.3:** Describe the mechanism of urine formation involving processes of filtration, tubular reabsorption and secretion; concentration and diluting mechanism.

### LEARNING OBJECTIVES
**At the end of this chapter, the learner should be able to:**
- Describe the various processes involved in the formation of urine viz., glomerular filtration, tubular reabsorption and secretion and concentration of urine.

**Glomerular Filtration**
- Define glomerular filtration rate (GFR) precisely, mentioning the typical range and composition of glomerular filtrate.
- Describe the structures (filtration membrane) involved in glomerular filtration.
- Describe the physical factors that determine the GFR.
- Describe the physiological mechanism that regulates the GFR.
- Describe the measurement of the glomerular filtration rate.
- Apply the knowledge about GFR in various physio-clinical scenarios.

**Tubular Reabsorption and Secretion**
- Describe the role of various tubular segments in tubular reabsorption and secretion.
- Describe the factors regulating tubular reabsorption and secretion.
- Differentiate between obligatory and facultative reabsorption.
- Apply the knowledge to various physio-clinical scenarios.

**Concentration and Dilution of Urine**
- Describe the mechanism of concentration of urine through the countercurrent mechanism.
- Describe the factors leading to the formation of concentrated or dilute urine.
- Apply the knowledge to various physio-clinical scenarios.

The main function of the nephron is the excretion of nitrogenous waste products along with other nonexcretory functions.

The nephrons carry out three basic physiologic processes that determine the composition of urine and allow the kidneys to perform their homeostatic functions (**Fig. 59.1**):
1. **Glomerular filtration:** It is the first step and involves the glomerular capillaries filtering large amounts of fluid into Bowman's capsule.
2. **Tubular reabsorption** is the process in which fluid and solutes are reabsorbed from the filtrate and returned to the blood.
3. **Tubular secretion** is the process in which substances from the blood are secreted into the filtrate.

The urinary excretion rate of a substance is equal to the rate at which the substance is filtered minus its reabsorption rate plus the rate at which it is secreted from the peritubular capillary blood into the tubules.

**Urinary excretion rate** = Filtration rate − Reabsorption rate + Secretion rate

## GLOMERULAR FILTRATION

It is defined as the *ultrafiltration of plasma at the glomerulus*. It can also be defined as the rate of production of filtrate at the glomeruli from plasma per minute (**Fig. 59.2**).

It is an important measurement in the evaluation of kidney function. The glomerular filtration rate (GFR) in an adult is approximately *125 mL/min, or 180 L/day*.

The **filtration fraction** (the percentage of renal plasma flow that is filtered) averages **around 0.2**, meaning that **20% of the plasma passing through the kidney is filtered by the glomerular capillaries**.

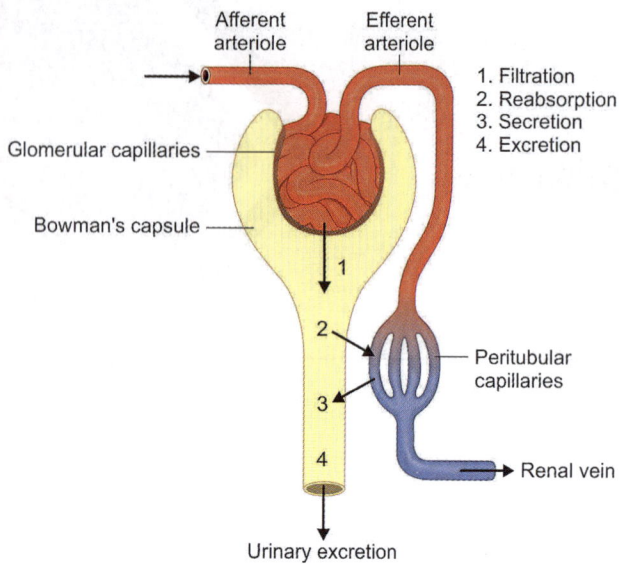

**Fig. 59.1:** Process of urine formation.

The filtration fraction is calculated as:

$$\text{Filtration fraction (FF)} = \frac{\text{GFR}}{\text{Renal plasma flow}}$$

$$\text{Renal plasma flow (RPF)} = \text{Renal blood flow (RBF)} \times (1 - \text{hematocrit})$$

The GFR averages about 20% of the RPF, whereas urine flow rate is <1% of the GFR. Consequently, >99% of the filtered fluid is often reabsorbed.

## Glomerular Capillary Membrane (Filtration Membrane)

It consists of three main layers:
1. **The capillary endothelium:** One of the characteristics of glomerular capillaries is high permeability. The capillary endothelium has *numerous fenestrae*, or microscopic pores, are thought to be **about 8 nm**. Endothelial cell proteins contain a staggering amount of **fixed negative charges** that **prevent plasma proteins** from passing through them.
2. **Basement membrane:** The endothelium is encircled by the basement membrane, which comprises a meshwork composed of *collagen and proteoglycan fibrillar* with big pores allowing water and small solutes to pass through. It carries proteoglycan-related significant **negative electrical charges** that also hinders the passage of negatively charged plasma proteins.
3. **Layer of epithelial cells (podocytes):** The final part of the glomerular membrane is a layer of epithelial cells (podocytes). These podocytes have long, foot-like processes (pedicels) and the crevices between the foot processes are called *slit pores* that allow only substances with a diameter of **<6–7 nm to pass**. The epithelial cells also **carries negative charge**.

All layers of the glomerular capillary wall act as a barrier to the filtration of plasma proteins while allowing for the fast filtration of water and the majority of plasma solutes.

## Composition of Glomerular Filtrate

The glomerular filtrate is quite similar to *ultrafiltrate of plasma* in composition. It has everything present in plasma except the plasma proteins. Most salts and organic compounds are present in glomerular filtrate in amounts that are comparable to those seen in plasma, along with other components. *Some low-molecular-weight substances, like calcium and fatty acids, cannot be freely filtered due of their partial binding to plasma proteins, hence are not filtered.*

## Physical Factors Determining GFR (Determinants of GFR)

The glomerular filtration rate is affected by two main factors:
1. The net filtration pressure
2. The glomerular capillary filtration coefficient ($K_f$)

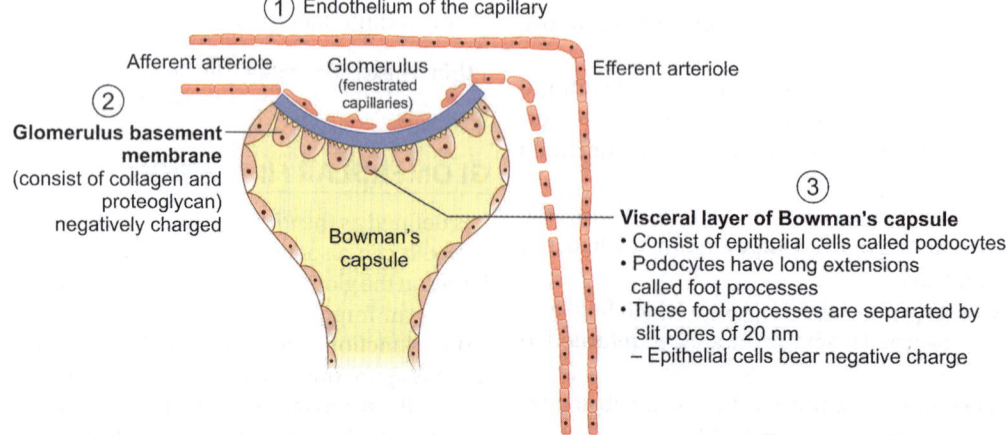

**Fig. 59.2:** Basic structure of glomerular capillary membrane and its major components.

It is represented as,

**GFR** = K$_f$ Net filtration pressure (NFP)

## Glomerular Capillary Filtration Coefficient (K$_f$)

It is a measure of the product of the hydraulic conductivity (the ease with which the fluid moves through the glomerular pores) and surface area of the glomerular capillaries.

*The GFR is directly proportional to K$_f$.*

The K$_f$ is affected by either decrease the glomerular surface area or hydraulic conductivity, which can occur in pathological conditions discussed in **Table 59.1**.

> *Give a physiological explanation for why persistent uncontrolled hypertension/diabetes mellitus results in reduced GFR.*
>
> Chronic uncontrolled hypertension may gradually reduce K$_f$ through thickening of the glomerular capillary basement membrane and, ultimately, through severely damaging the capillaries to the point of capillary function loss.

> *Describe the physiological cause of albuminuria when the GBM filtration barrier is not functioning adequately.*
>
> Albumin filtration is impeded by the layers of the glomerular capillary wall that are negatively charged. When the glomerular capillary membrane is damaged, the membrane loses its negative charge. Additionally, an increase in pore size causes albumin to be excreted in urine.

## Net Filtration Pressure

It is the resultant pressure developed at the filtration membrane. It is determined by the mathematical sum of various forces acting across the membrane **(Fig. 59.3)**. These forces are called as the Starling forces:

**Table 59.1:** Factors affecting the K$_f$ in various pathological conditions.

| Decreased K$_f$ | |
|---|---|
| **Decreased glomerular surface area** | **Decreased hydraulic conductivity** |
| Contraction of glomerular mesangial cells | Increased thickness of the glomerular capillary membrane |
| Decrease in functional glomerular capillaries | |
| Ageing | |
| **Increased K$_f$** | |
| **Increased glomerular surface area** | **Increased hydraulic conductivity** |
| Relaxation of glomerular mesangial cells | Damage to foot processes of the podocytes |
| | Loss of negative charge of the filtration membrane |

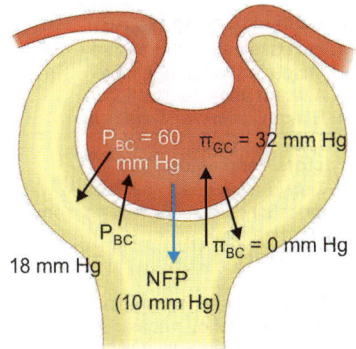

**Fig. 59.3:** Forces causing filtration by the glomerular capillaries (net filtration pressure).

- *Forces favoring filtration:*
  - Capillary hydrostatic pressure (P$_{GC}$ = 60 mm Hg)
  - Colloid osmotic pressure of bowman's capsule (π$_{BC}$ = 0 mm Hg)
- *Forces favoring reabsorption:*
  - Hydrostatic pressure of Bowman's capsule (P$_{BC}$ = 18 mm Hg)
  - Colloid osmotic pressure of glomerular capillaries (π$_{BC}$ = 32 mm Hg)

**NFP** = Sum of forces favoring filtration – Sum of forces favoring reabsorption
= (P$_{GC}$ + π$_{BC}$) – (P$_{BC}$ + π$_{GC}$) = (60 + 0) – (32 + 18) = 10 mm Hg

> *Why the colloid osmotic pressure in Bowman's capsule is 0 mm Hg?*
>
> As there is no plasma protein filtered at glomeruli, the COP in Bowman's capsule is zero.

> *What will happen to glomerular filtration rate if, the capillary hydrostatic pressure is 65 mm Hg, colloid osmotic pressure of the glomerular capillaries is 32 mm Hg, hydrostatic pressure in the Bowman's capsule is 18 mm Hg and colloid osmotic pressure of Bowman's capsule is 0 mm Hg. Comment on your findings.*
>
> *What will happen to GFR, if basement membrane loses its negative charge?*

Various factors controlling these forces are shown in **Figure 59.4**.

Glomerular hydrostatic pressure is the GFR factor that is most variable and under physiological control. The sympathetic nervous system, hormones, autacoids (vasoactive compounds secreted in the kidneys and acting locally), and other feedback controls that are inherent to the kidneys all have an impact on this variable.

## Autoregulation of Glomerular Filtration Rate and RBF

Despite of significant variations in arterial blood pressure, the kidneys' internal feedback mechanisms typically

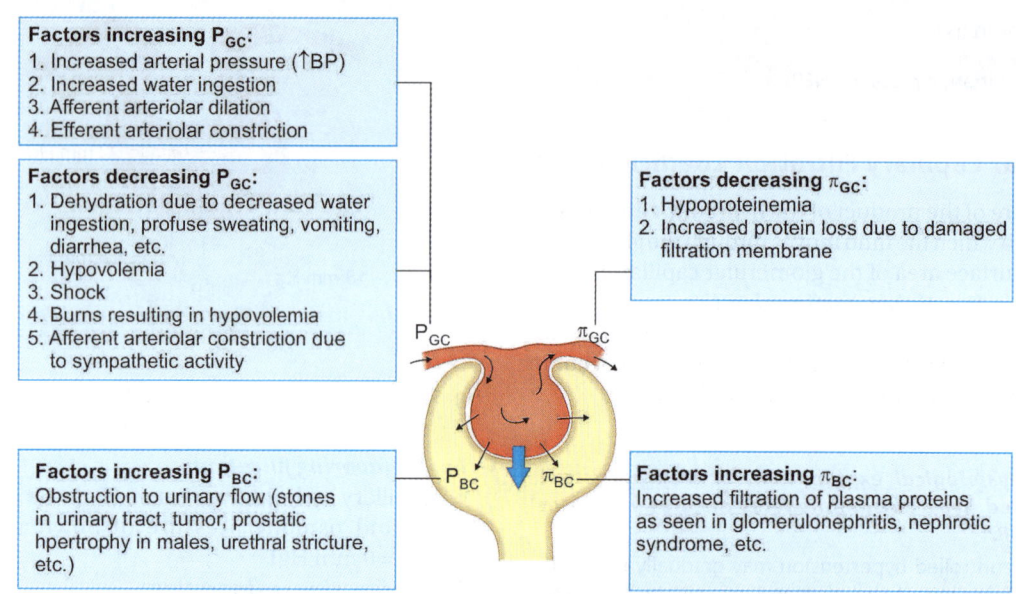

**Fig. 59.4:** Factors influencing forces that act for filtration in nephron.

maintain renal blood flow and GFR relatively constant within an autoregulatory range of **70–180 mm Hg**.

The term "Autoregulation" refers to this comparatively constant renal blood flow and GFR. The fundamental purpose of autoregulation in the kidneys is to keep the GFR reasonably stable and enable precise control of the excretion of water and solutes by the kidneys (**Fig. 59.5**). It autoregulates the RBF and GFR through two main mechanisms:
1. Tubuloglomerular feedback mechanism
2. Myogenic feedback mechanism

### Tubuloglomerular Feedback Mechanism

The tubuloglomerular feedback (TGF) mechanism is a critical regulatory system within the kidneys that helps maintain stable glomerular filtration rate (GFR) and systemic blood pressure. It involves a complex interplay between the juxtaglomerular apparatus (JGA), specifically the macula densa cells of the distal tubule, and the afferent arteriole of the nephron (**Flowchart 59.1** and **Fig. 59.6**).

### Myogenic Feedback Mechanism (Fig. 59.7)

Another process that contributes to maintaining a comparatively constant renal blood flow and GFR is the ability of individual blood vessels to adjust to stretching by contracting the vascular smooth muscle under increased arterial pressure, or the myogenic mechanism. This contraction also aids in preventing excessive increases in renal blood flow and the GFR as arterial pressure rises

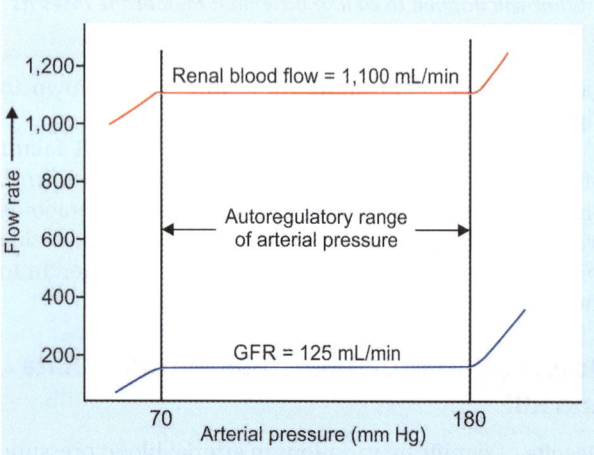

**Fig. 59.5:** Autoregulation in the kidney.

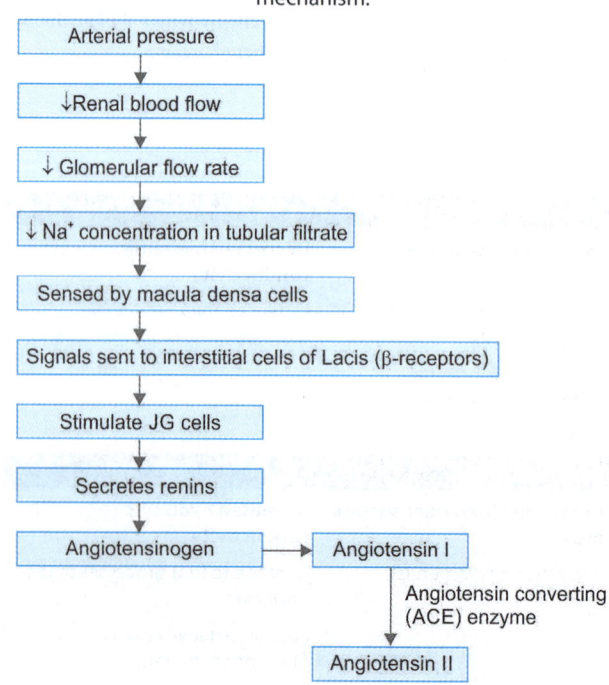

**Flowchart 59.1:** Steps involved in tubuloglomerular feedback mechanism.

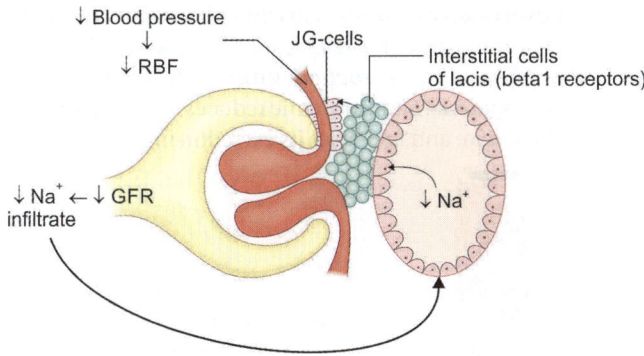

**Fig. 59.6:** Regulation of GFR through tubuloglomerular feedback mechanism.

**Table 59.2:** Hormones and autacoids that effect GFR.

| Hormone or autacoids | Effect on GFR | Mechanism |
|---|---|---|
| Norepinephrine, epinephrine | Decrease | Constricts afferent and efferent arterioles |
| Endothelin | Decrease | Released by kidney's injured vascular endothelial and induces renal vasoconstriction |
| Angiotensin II | Decrease | Angiotensin II selectively constricts efferent arterioles |
| Endothelial-derived nitric oxide | Increase | Nitric oxide produced by endothelial cells dilates blood vessels |
| Prostaglandins and bradykinin | Increase | Bradykinin and prostaglandins ($PGE_2$ and $PGI_2$) produce vasodilation. Additionally, they reduce the renal vasoconstrictor effects of angiotensin II and sympathetic nerves on afferent arterioles |

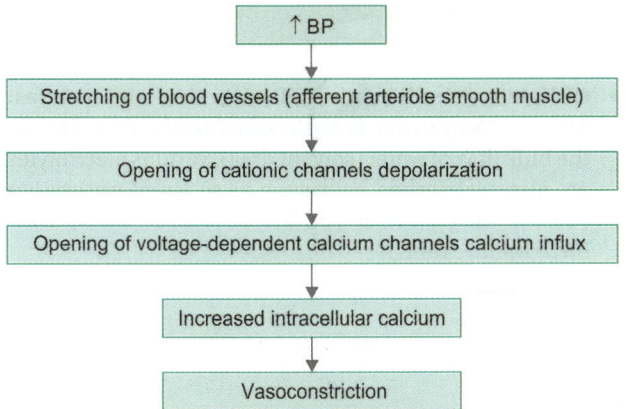

**Fig. 59.7:** Myogenic autoregulation of glomerular filtration rate (GFR).

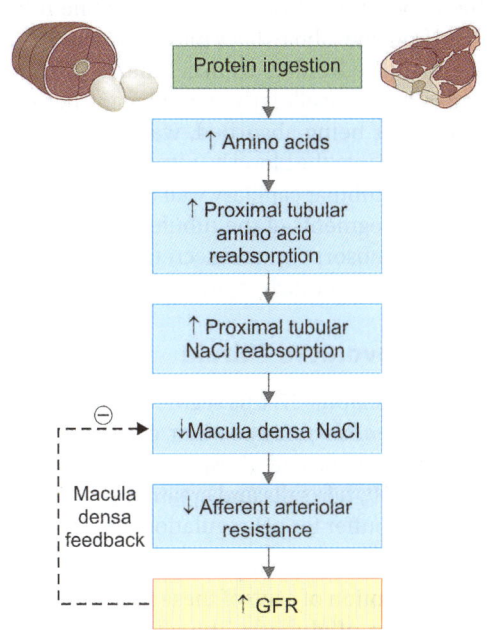

**Fig. 59.8:** Physiological justification for the rise in GFR following a high protein intake (A large amount of meat diet).

by raising vascular resistance. This contraction prevents excessive stretching of the vessel.

## Extrinsic Mechanism

**Neural mechanism:** The afferent and efferent arterioles, as well as practically all of arteries of kidneys are deeply innervated by sympathetic nerve fibers. Strong renal sympathetic nerve activation can constrict renal arteries, reduce renal blood flow, and lower GFR. But, the renal blood flow and GFR are not significantly affected by mild or moderate sympathetic activation.

**Hormones and autacoids** that influence the glomerular filtration rate are discussed in **Table 59.2**.

## Effect of High Protein Diet on Glomerular Filtration Rate (Glomerulotubular Balance) (Fig. 59.8)

Cotransport in the proximal tubules allows sodium and amino acids to be reabsorbed simultaneously. The increased amino acid reabsorption also stimulates sodium reabsorption. This decreased sodium transport to the macula densa caused by the enhanced sodium reabsorption causes a decrease in the resistance of the afferent arterioles via tubuloglomerular feedback. As a result of the increased renal blood flow and GFR brought on by the reduced afferent arteriolar resistance, sodium excretion can be kept close to normal while excretion of the waste products of protein metabolism, such as urea is increased.

- A patient is placed on nonsteroidal anti-inflammatory drugs (NSAIDs) for osteoarthritis. What effect would this have on GFR?
- A patient with Diabetes Mellitus is found to have a blood pressure of 146/94, during his outpatient visit. He is prescribed ACE-inhibitor for controlling his raised arterial pressure, what effect would this have on his GFR?

## Tubular Reabsorption and Secretion

The glomerular filtrate travels through the numerous renal tubule sections before being eliminated as urine. Along

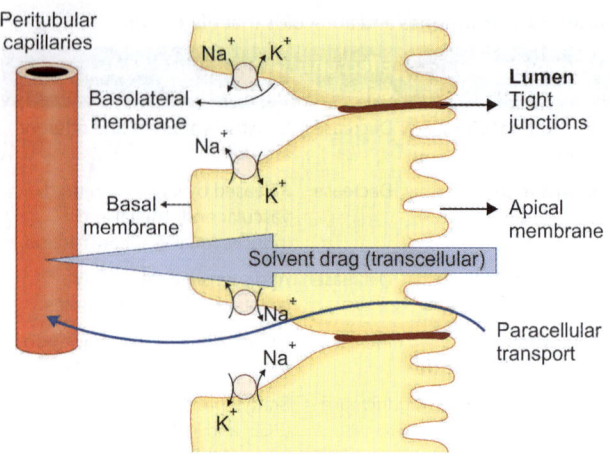

**Fig. 59.9:** Transcellular and paracellular transport.

this pathway, some substances are preferentially released from the blood into the tubular lumen, while others are reabsorbed from the tubules back into the blood. Substances can be transported either transcellularly (through cell membranes) or paracellularly (via the gaps between cell junctions). After being absorbed, water and solutes are then transported into the blood by ultrafiltration (bulk flow) through the peritubular capillary wall **(Fig. 59.9)**.

The various segments of the tubule play different roles in the tubular reabsorption and secretion.

Let's discuss the role of each segment in formation of urine.

## Proximal Convoluted Tubule

As discussed in chapter 57, this segment is responsible for:
- *Obligatory reabsorption* of water, electrolytes, glucose, amino acids, lactate and phosphate.
- Secretion of $H^+$, bile salts and creatinine.
- Bicarbonate buffer for pH regulation and $H^+$ secretion.

It is the main site for reabsorption of various substances. Lets the reabsorption of each of these in detail.
- **Reabsorption of glucose:** The glucose is reabsorbed *completely (100%)* by the secondary active cotransport by **sodium glucose-linked transporter (SGLT)**. The concentration gradient is created by the $Na^+$ $K^+$ ATPase pump. The glucose is then transported to the blood stream through the glucose transporter (GLUT) located on the basolateral membrane.

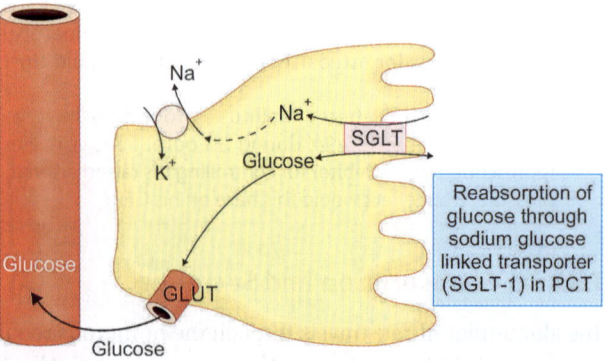

- **Reabsorption of amino acids and phosphate:** Even the filtered amino acids are *reabsorbed completely*. However, *phosphate is reabsorbed under the influence of parathormone*. Parathormone reduces the reabsorption of phosphate and increases its excretion in the urine.

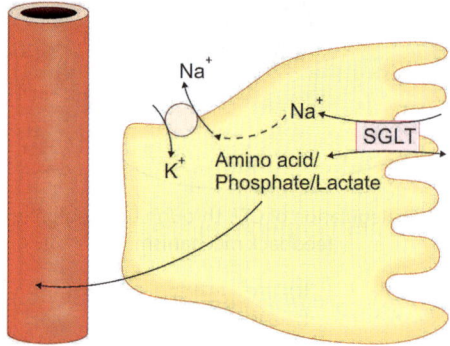

- **Obligatory reabsorption of water and electrolytes:** About **65% of water is reabsorbed in the PCT**. Due to the bulk flow of water (solvent drag), various electrolytes are also reabsorbed back such as *sodium, potassium (65%), magnesium (25%), calcium (65%) and bicarbonate ion.*

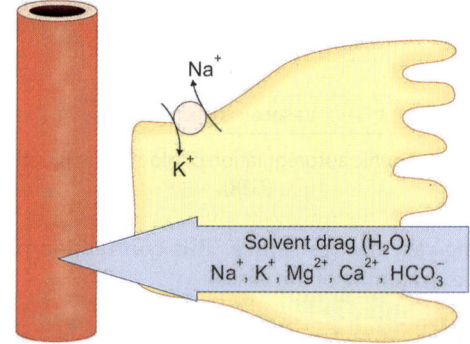

- **Secretion of $H^+$:** The bicarbonate buffer operational in the PCT is responsible for secretion of $H^+$ into the lumen. In early PCT, the $H^+$ secretion takes place through the $Na^+$-$H^+$ ATPase counter transport, whereas in late PCT $H^+$ATPase is responsible for $H^+$ secretion.

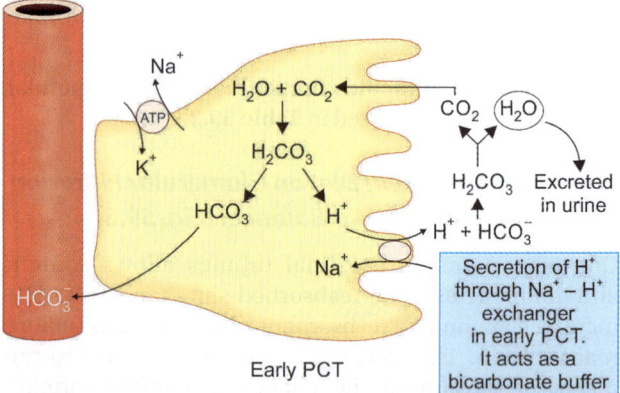

- **Osmolality of fluid in the PCT:** The osmolality of the fluid in the *PCT is 300 mOsm/L*, which is isotonic to the plasma.

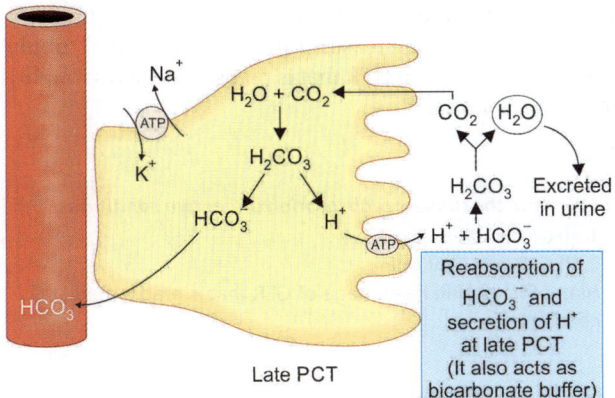

Reabsorption of $HCO_3^-$ and secretion of $H^+$ at late PCT (It also acts as bicarbonate buffer)

- It is impermeable to water and urea. As a result, the tube fluid is diluted, and this region is known as the "*diluting segment*".

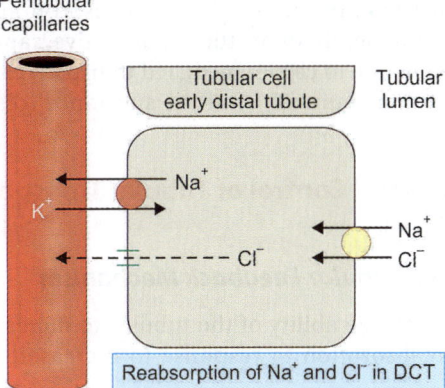

Reabsorption of $Na^+$ and $Cl^-$ in DCT

## Role of Loop of Henle in the Formation of Urine

This segment is important for the concentration of urine through the counter-current mechanism. It is discussed in detail in the section, concentration of urine.

Apart from the concentration of urine, the thick ascending limb of the loop of Henle is an important site for the *facultative reabsorption of $Ca^{2+}$, $Mg^{2+}$ and $HCO_3^-$*. Calcium reabsorption takes place under the influence of *parathyroid hormone*.

Another important cotransporter acting at this site is *$Na^+$ $K^+$ $2Cl^-$ cotransporter*, which is responsible for creating the medullary interstitial hyperosmolar gradient.

The fluid leaving this segment becomes hypotonic.

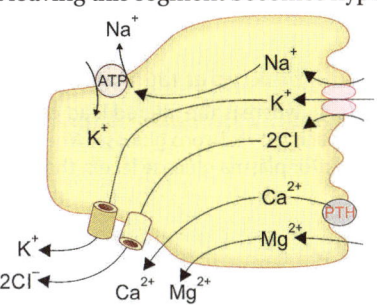

Reabsorption of $Na^+$, $K^+$, $Cl^-$ through Na–K–2Cl cotransporter at thick ascending limb of LOH. $Ca^{2+}$ and $Mg^{2+}$ reabsorption occurs under the influence of parathormone.

## Role of Distal Convoluted Tubule

The distal convoluted tubule plays an important role in three ways:
1. Reabsorption of $Na^+$ and $Cl^-$ through the *$Na^+Cl^-$ cotransporter*, where it reabsorbs around 5% of it.
2. Regulating the GFR and renal blood flow through the *tubuloglomerular* feedback mechanism, by sensing the $Na^+$ concentration in the filtrate and regulating the renin angiotensin mechanism.
3. The principal cells and *intercalated cells* in the late DCT are responsible for *regulation of $Na^+$ and $H^+$ concentration* in the body respectively.

## Role of Cortical Collecting Duct

The cortical collecting duct has two type of cells, which are similar to the ones present in the late DCT.
1. Principal cells (P-cells):

Reabsorption of $Na^+$ through epithelial sodium channels under the influence of aldosterone at P cells in late DCT and CCD. The $K^+$ secreted through the renal outer medullary potassium channel (ROMK)

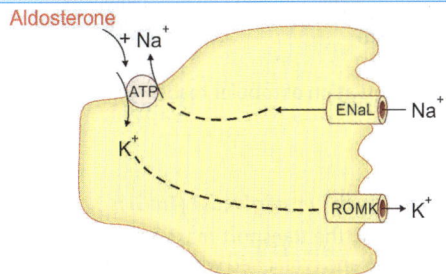

2. Intercalated cells (I-cells):

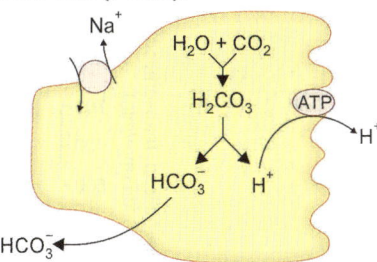

## Role of Medullary Collecting Duct

The medullary collecting duct reabsorbs >5% of the filtered water and sodium, yet it is extremely important in regulating the final urine output of water and solutes. The permeability of the medullary collecting duct to water is controlled by the level of ADH. High levels of ADH cause water to be actively reabsorbed, which reduces urine volume and concentrates the majority of solutes in the urine. The reabsorption of water here, under the influence of ADH is called the *facultative reabsorption*.

It is permeable to urea, so some of the tubular urea is reabsorbed into medullary interstitium. This helps to increase the osmolality in this area of the kidney.

**Transport maximum ($T_{max}$):** The reabsorption of any substance depends upon the reabsorptive capacity of the segment due to carrier mediated transport, called the transport maximum ($T_{max}$) of the substance (discussed below).

## Physiological Control of Tubular Transport (Fig. 59.10)

### Glomerulotubular Feedback Mechanism

It is the intrinsic ability of the tubules to increase their rate of reabsorption in response to increased tubular load. The total rate of reabsorption of solutes particularly sodium and water increases primarily in proximal tubule but the percentage of GFR that is reabsorbed stays roughly constant around 65%.

> *Calculate the tubular reabsorption under two conditions:*
> 1. If GFR is 125 mL/min
> 2. If GFR is 150 mL/min
>
> *Hint:* 65% of GFR. Percentage of GFR that is reabsorbed stays constant.

### Transport Maximum

It is the maximum capacity of the tubules to reabsorb substances. It is applicable to carrier mediated transport and is achieved due to saturation of carrier proteins.

The most important example for transport maximum to understand is for glucose (TmG). Usually, the filtered glucose in the tubular filtrate is completely reabsorbed in PCT through Sodium glucose linked to transport, where the filtered load of glucose is represented as:

$$GFR \times plasma\ glucose\ level = 125\ mL/min \times 1\ mg/mL$$

If the serum blood glucose level rises above 200 g/dL, the excess glucose begins to be excreted in the urine (glucosuria). However, the transport maximum for the glucose in 325 mg/min in females and 375 mg/min in males, which is the average value for all the nephrons.

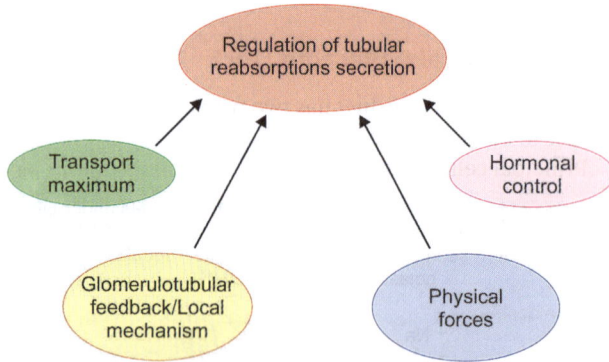

**Fig. 59.10:** Regulation of tubular reabsorption secretion.

> *If the transport maximum of glucose (TmG) is 325–375 mg/min, then why the glucosuria occurs at 180 mL/dL?*
>
> In the adult human, the transport maximum for glucose averages about 375 mg/min, whereas the filtered load of glucose is only about 125 mg/min and is reached when all nephrons have reached their maximal capacity to reabsorb glucose. When the amount of glucose being filtered rises above 375 mg/min due to significant increases in GFR and/or plasma glucose levels, the extra glucose is not reabsorbed and excreted into the urine.

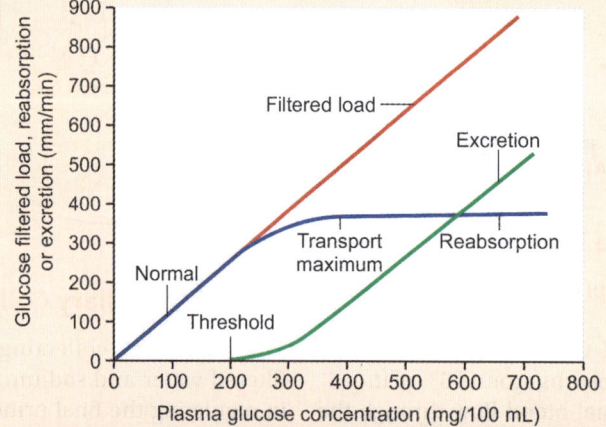

| Plasma level | Filtered load GFR × plasma glucose | $T_{max}$ = 375 mg/min | Effects |
|---|---|---|---|
| 80 mg/dL | 100 mg/min | Filtered load = $T_{max}$ | Whole of glucose is reabsorbed |
| 300 mg/dL | 375 mg/min | Filtered load = $T_{max}$ | Whole of glucose is reabsorbed |
| 310 mg/dL | 387 mg/min | Filtered load > $T_{max}$ | Glucose will appear in urine (Glycosuria) |

**Transport maximum for actively secreted substances:**
Creatinine = 16 mg/min
Para Aminohippuric acid (PAHA) = 80 mg/min

**Substances actively transported and do not exhibit transport maximum:**
**Sodium**: It shows **gradient time transport**, as the rate of transport depends upon the electrochemical gradient. The other factors which affect this transport are the permeability of tight junctions and interstitial physical forces. This effect is seen only in PCT, but in DCT, the sodium reabsorption under the effect of aldosterone also shows the transport maximum.

## Physical Factors Affecting Tubular Absorption and Secretion

The rate of reabsorption across the peritubular capillaries is controlled by hydrostatic and colloid osmotic forces. Reabsorption across the peritubular capillaries can be calculated as follows:

$$\text{Reabsorption} = K_f \times \text{net reabsorptive force}$$

The hydrostatic and colloid osmotic pressures that favour or oppose reabsorption across the peritubular capillaries are combined to form the net reabsorptive force.

**Why increase in filtration fraction increases peritubular reabsorption rate.**
Filtration fraction is defined as the ratio of GFR/RPF. A rise in GFR or a fall in RPF can both lead to an increase in filtration fraction. As the filtration fraction rises, more plasma is filtered through the glomerulus, increasing the protein concentration. As a result, the peritubular capillary colloidal osmotic pressure is increased, favoring reabsorption.

## Hormonal Control of Tubular Transport (Fig. 59.11)

The most significant hormones regulate tubular transport. They exert their primary effects on the renal tubule and have an impact on the excretion of solutes and water.

- **Aldosterone** acts on the *P-cells* of the cortical collecting tubule to stimulate renal sodium absorption and potassium secretion. It *activates the $Na^+$-$K^+$ ATPase pump* on the membrane's basolateral side and *enhances sodium permeability* on the membrane's luminal side via inserting *epithelial sodium channels (ENaC)*.
- **Angiotensin II** increases *sodium and water reabsorption* by stimulating aldosterone secretion, constricting the efferent arterioles, reducing peritubular capillary hydrostatic pressure and raising filtration fraction in the glomerulus.
- **Antidiuretic hormone** increases the *water permeability* of the distal tubule, collecting tubule, and collecting duct epithelia by inserting aquaporin channels on the luminal side of tubular epithelial cells, which in turn increases water absorption.
- **Atrial natriuretic peptide (ANP)** is secreted when specific cells of the cardiac atria are stretched as a result of plasma volume expansion and increased

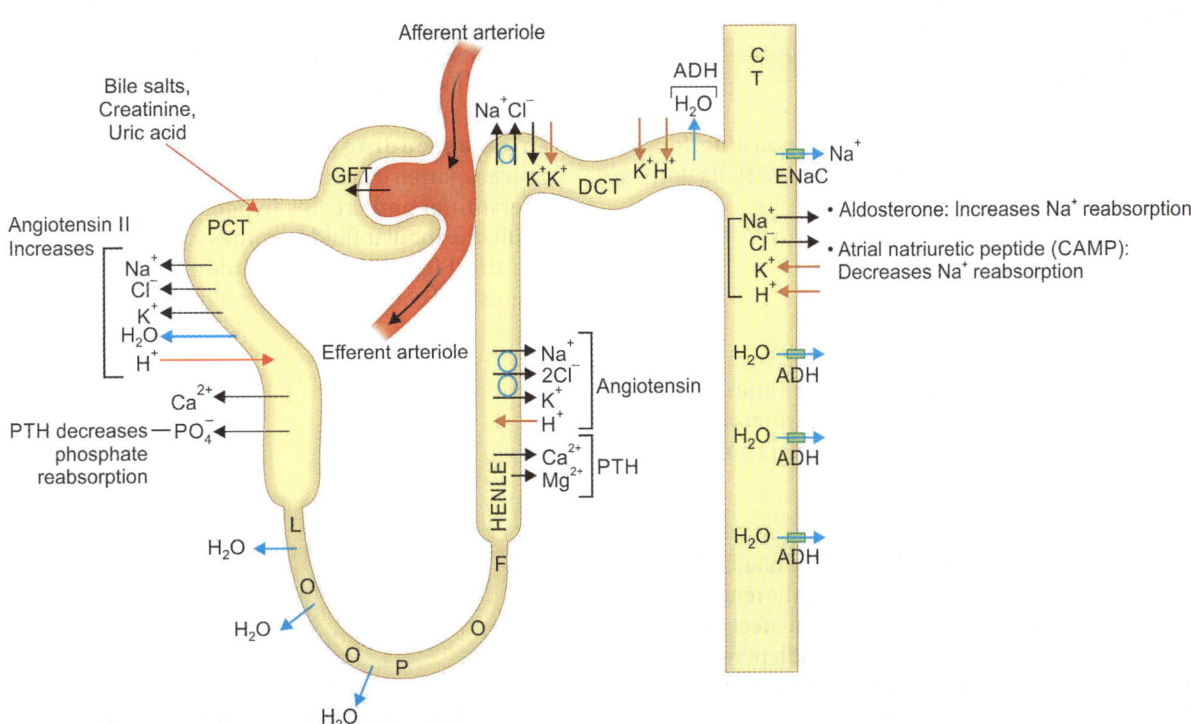

**Fig. 59.11:** Hormonal control of tubular reabsorption and secretion.

atrial blood pressure. Increased levels of this peptide, in turn directly inhibit reabsorption of sodium and water by the collecting ducts. In addition, it prevents the release of renin, which leads to the production of angiotensin II and a consequent decrease in renal tubular reabsorption. This decreased sodium and water reabsorption increases urinary excretion, which helps return the blood volume back toward normal.

## CONCENTRATION OF URINE

The kidneys control the osmolality and water balance of body fluids by excreting concentrated or diluted urine depending on physiological requirements. Water is retained in excess of solute when the urine is concentrated, and water is expelled from the body in excess of solute when the urine is dilute.

The osmolarity of the renal medulla and antidiuretic hormone (ADH) are necessary for the formation of concentrated or diluted urine.

### Renal Mechanisms for Excreting Concentrated/Dilute Urine

The kidneys form concentrated/dilute urine when the body is either dehydrated or water is constantly being lost from the body or if there is excessive accumulation of water in the body.

The various factors responsible for the formation of *concentrated urine with an osmolarity of up to 1,200–1,400 mOsm/L*, which is four to five times that of plasma:
1. Decreased water intake
2. Hyperosmolar renal medulla
3. Counter current mechanism
4. Decreased blood flow in vasa recta
5. Increased ADH production

Similarly these factors are also responsible for the formation *of dilute urine with osmolality as low as 30 mOsm/L*:
1. Increased water intake
2. Loss of hyperosmolar renal medulla
3. Increased blood flow in vasa recta
4. Decreased ADH production

Hence, we can understand that this mechanism is required to either conserve water in times of need/dehydration and excretes excess water, when water is not required. In a nutshell, it participates in water homeostasis.

### Hyperosmotic Renal Medulla

The hyperosmolar gradient of renal medulla is the main requirement for the water reabsorption in the renal medulla. This gradient is created by counter current mechanism and urea recycling. It creates the osmotic gradient required for water reabsorption to take place when there is a high level of ADH.

### Counter Current Mechanism

It is defined as a mechanism in which the *inflow and outflow are close to, opposite to and parallel to each other*, as seen in the **Figure 59.12**.

Counter current mechanism in our body:
- Loop of Henle and Vasa recta in renal medulla
- Intestinal villi
- Cutaneous circulation
- Testicular blood vessels

There are two components of the counter-current mechanism in kidney:
1. **Counter current multiplier system**, which creates the hyperosmolar gradient in the medullary interstitium. The loop of Henle of juxtamedullary nephrons participates in the countercurrent multiplier system.
2. **Counter current exchanger**, which maintains this hyperosmolar gradient by removing the excess water from the interstitium and returning it back to the bloodstream. This work is done by the vasa recta, a long U-pin shaped blood vessel, which is an extension of efferent arteriole.

#### Counter Current Multiplier System

As seen in the **Figures 59.13A and B**, there are three segments of loop of Henle (LOH):
1. **Thin descending limb of LOH**, which is freely permeable to water. This segment allows the movement of water from the tubule into medullary interstitium. As a result, the tubular fluid becomes hypertonic, as it descends deep into the medulla.
2. **Thin ascending limb of LOH** is **NOT** permeable to water. Hence it doesn't let the water to enter back into the tubule when it is leaving the medullary interstitium. This helps in maintaining the tonicity of the tubular filtrate.
3. **Thick ascending limb of LOH** has a $Na^+K^+2Cl^-$ co-transporter, which add the solute into the medullary interstitium and creates hyperosmolarity there. As a result, the tubular fluid becomes hypotonic.

See the **Figure 59.14** to understand the complete mechanism of counter current multiplier system

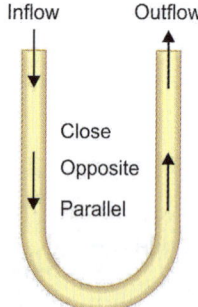

**Fig. 59.12:** Counter current mechanism.

PCT
DCT
Thick ascending limb of LDH (impermeable to water) adds solute to interstitium
Thin descending limb (permeable to water)
Thin ascending limb of LOH (Impermeable to waters)
A
B
300
400
600
800
1,000
1,200
1,400

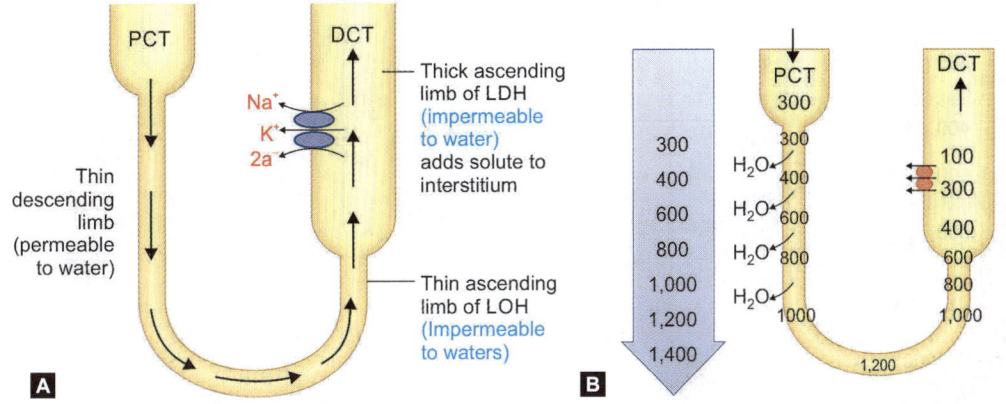

**Figs. 59.13A and B:** (A) Permeability of various segments of LOH; (B) Summary of counter current multiplier system.

PCT
DCT
1: Let us assume, the fluid in LOH is having concentration of 300 mOm/L
2: Thick ascending limb of LOH has active pumps which creates medullary hyperosmolar gradient. The fluid becomes hypotonic
3: The descending limb of LOH loses water and reaches equilibrium with interstitial fluids
4: The continuous flow of fluid from descending limb to ascending limb adds fresh solute to thick ascending limb which further increase the hyperosmotic medullary concentration gradient
5: The solute is constantly pumped into interstitium creating the hyperosmolarity
6: The medullary osmolarity eventually increases to 1,200–1,400 mOsm/L, creating the hyperosmolar gradient

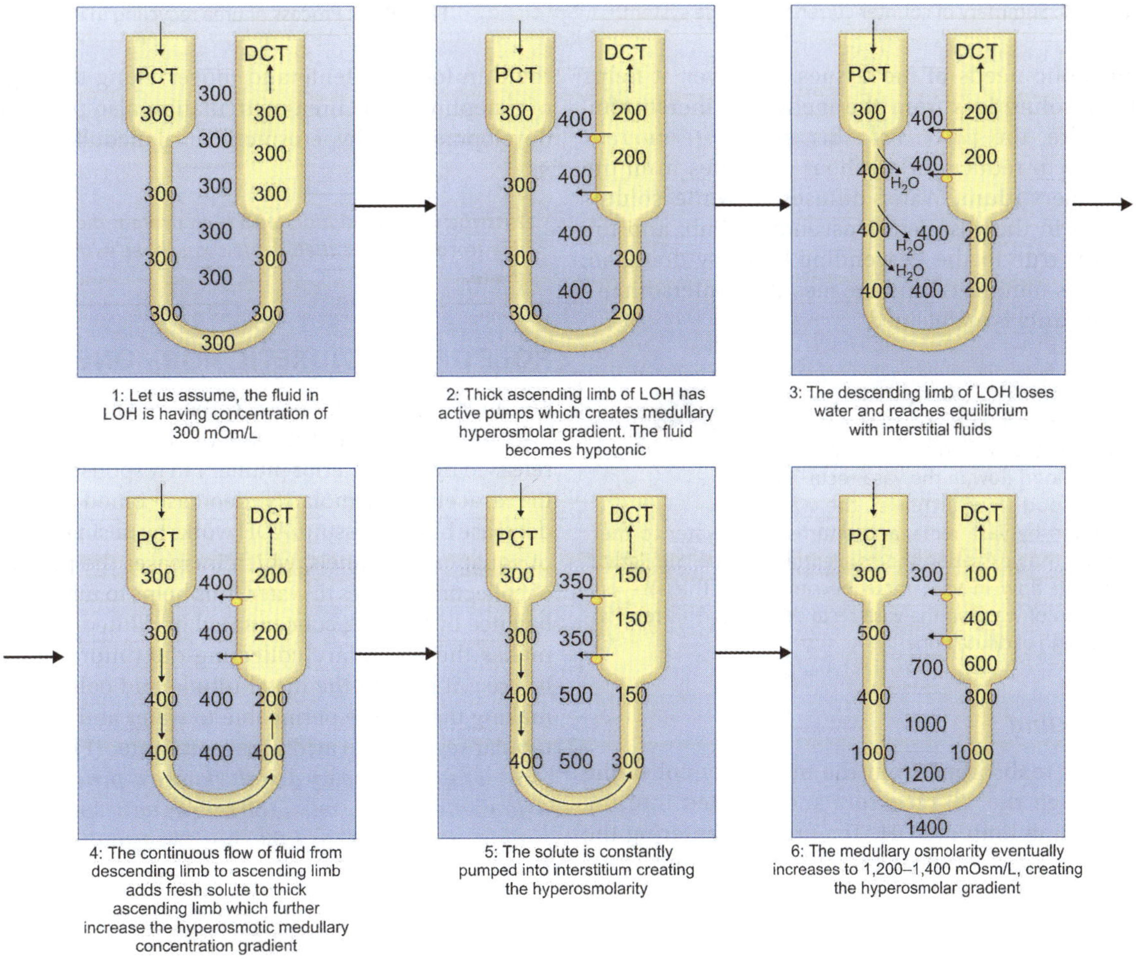

**Fig. 59.14:** Complete mechanism of counter current multiplier system.

### Counter Current Exchanger System (Fig. 59.15)

The vasa recta also form the hair pin bend around the LOH. It carries the excess water released by the LOH, back into the circulation. Since it doesn't let the hyperosmolar gradient get diluted due to the osmotic movement of water into medulla, it is also called the counter current exchanger and it maintains this gradient, as seen in the figure. The descending limb of vasa recta loses water due to the hyperosmolar gradient of renal medulla but the ascending limb takes away the water released by vasa recta as well as the descending limb of LOH.

**Special features that preserve hyperosmolarity of renal medulla:** The medullary blood flow, which is sluggish and low (>5% of the total renal blood flow), can only meet

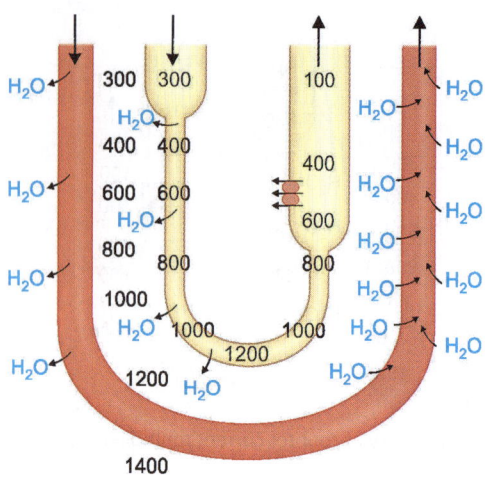

Fig. 59.15: Summary of counter current exchange system.

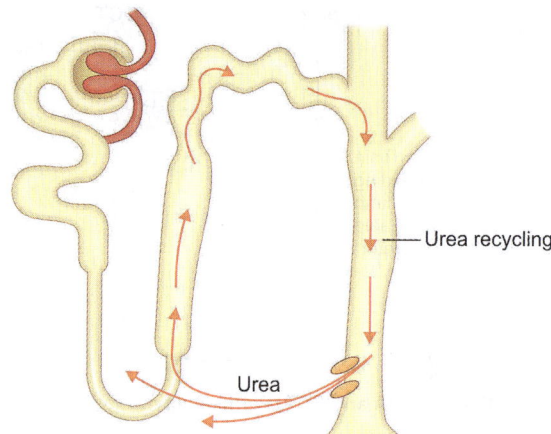

Fig. 59.16: Process of urea recycling in LOH.

the metabolic needs of the tissues. However, it helps to reduce solute loss from the medullary inerstitium. Furthermore, the *vasa recta act as countercurrent exchangers* to reduce the washout of solutes from the medulla inerstitium. Water diffuses in while solutes diffuse out in the vasa recti's ascending limb, and the opposite is true in the descending limb. By doing so, solute loss is minimized and the medullary interstitium's hyperosmolarity is maintained.

In the situations like dehydration, where the body needs to conserve water, there is decrease in renal blood flow which slows down the blood flow in the vasa recta. This sluggish blood flow increases the water reabsorption by vasa recta, and returns more water to the circulation, thus excreting the concentrated urine. Similarly, if the blood flow in vasa recta becomes fast, the rate of reabsorption of water in the vasa recta decreases. This results in the passage of dilute urine.

### Urea Recycling

The urea is reabsorbed from the medullary collecting ducts through the *V2 receptors* and secreted into the thin ascending limb of LOH. The urea, on entering the interstitium, increases the hyperosmolar gradient of the renal medulla. The process of urea recycling is shown in the **Figure 59.16**.

Urea *contributes about 40% to 50% of the osmolarity (500–600 mOsm/L) of the renal medullary interstitium* by passively moving from the inner medullary collecting ducts into the interstitium. The proximal tubule reabsorbs 40% to 50% of the filtered urea due to the reabsorption of water. As the tubular fluid passes through the descending LOH and collecting tubule, its urea concentration increases. Due to the high tubular fluid content of urea, it diffuses into the medullary interstitium as it enters the inner medullary collecting duct. A moderate amount of the urea that moves into the medullary interstitium eventually diffuses into the thin loop of Henle and moves along the segments of a nephron, this urea recirculation also promotes the development of a hyperosmotic renal medulla.

Describe why individuals with high protein diets are better able to concentrate their urine than those with low protein intake.

## ROLE OF ANTIDIURETIC HORMONE

The antidiuretic hormone is synthesized in the **supraoptic** and **paraventricular nuclei** of the hypothalamus, is released by the posterior pituitary in response to increases in extracellular osmolarity, decrease blood volume, and decrease blood pressure. ADH works by raising the number of aquaporin channels, which increases the permeability of collecting tubules to water. This helps to maintain water balance by forming concentrated or diluted urine. It also makes the medullary collecting duct more permeable to urea. It acts on the distal tubule and collecting ducts making them more permeable to water and allows these tubular segments to avidly reabsorb water **(Fig. 59.17)**.

*In a nut shell, every day the kidneys produce urine at a flow rate of 1 mL/min (180 mL/d) with specific gravity ranging from 1.005 to 1.030 and the osmolality ranging from 30 to 1200 mOsm/L.*

### Obligatory Urine Volume (OBV)

It refers to the *minimum amount of urine that must be excreted by the kidneys to eliminate waste products and maintain proper physiological function*. It represents the volume of urine necessary to clear solutes from the body without leading to the accumulation of toxins or electrolyte imbalances.

The obligatory urine volume can vary depending on factors such as dietary intake, metabolic rate, environmental conditions, and individual health status. Generally, it's estimated to be around *500 milliliters per day* in healthy

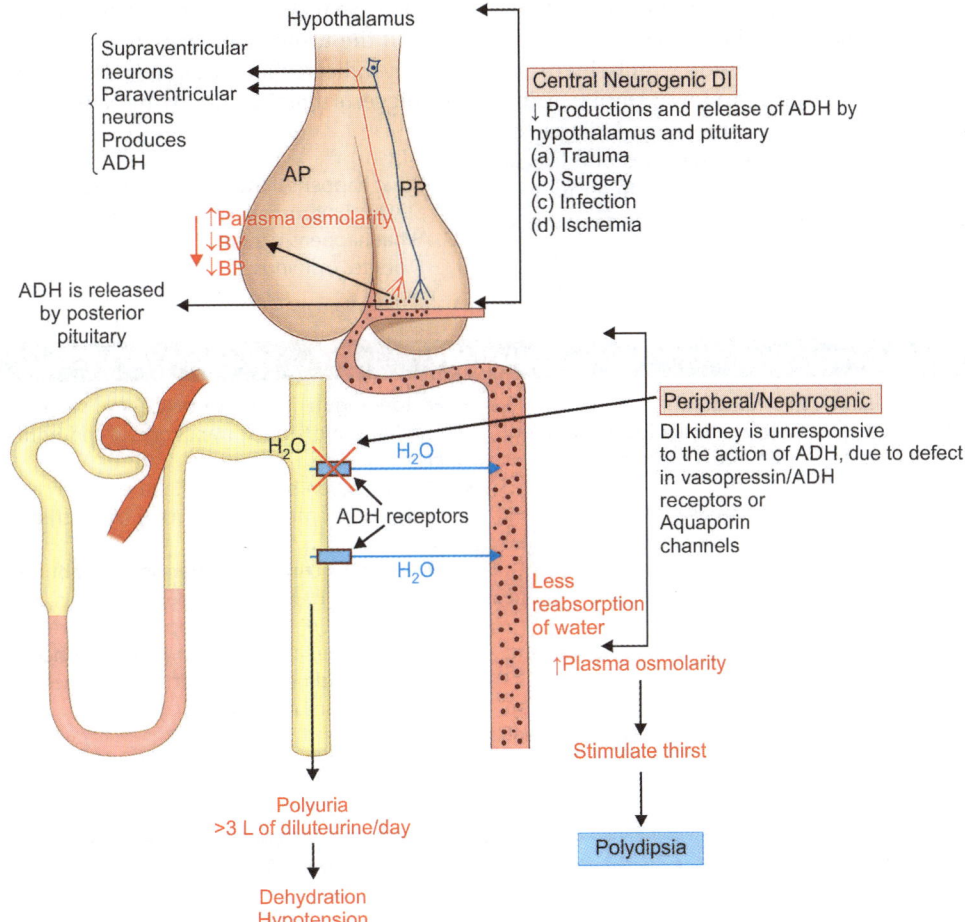

**Fig. 59.17:** Effects of antidiuretic hormone.

adults, although this can vary based on factors such as fluid intake, diet, and metabolic needs.

Maintaining an adequate urine volume is crucial for regulating body water balance, eliminating waste products (such as urea and creatinine), and controlling electrolyte concentrations in the body. Insufficient urine output can lead to dehydration and impaired kidney function, while excessive urine production can indicate conditions such as diabetes or excessive fluid intake.

**What is free water clearance? What is its physiological significance?**

Free water clearance ($C_{H_2O}$) is a term used to describe the ability of the kidneys to excrete free water while maintaining electrolyte balance.

It is a measure of the kidney's ability to concentrate or dilute urine, and it's particularly relevant in conditions affecting water balance in the body, such as diabetes insipidus, syndrome of inappropriate antidiuretic hormone (SIADH), or in certain kidney diseases.

Mathematically, free water clearance can be calculated using the formula:

$$C_{H_2O} = V(1 - U_{osm})/P_{osm}$$

Where:
$U_{Osm}$ is the osmolality of urine
$V$ is the urine flow rate
$P_{osm}$ is plasma osmolality

- **A positive free water clearance** indicates the excretion of free water, meaning that the kidneys are producing dilute urine and removing excess water from the body.
- **A negative free water clearance** suggests water retention or the production of concentrated urine.

## Diabetes Insipidus

Diabetes insipidus (DI) is the syndrome that results when there is a ADH/vasopressin deficiency or when the kidneys fail to respond to the hormone. It is characterized by excretion of large volumes of *dilute urine (polyuria), extreme thirst (polydipsia), and severe dehydration*.

### Pathophysiology

There are two different types:
1. **Central/neurogenic DI:** The secretion of ADH from the pituitary is insufficient.

2. **Nephrogenic DI:** The aquaporin channels are non-responsive/down regulated resulting in DI.

Water reabsorption is decreased, which leads to **polyuria**, the excessive excretion of low-osmolar urine volume, and an increase in blood osmolarity. A diagnosis can be made when urine osmolality decreases and **blood osmolality rises (>290 mOsm/L).** The specific gravity of urine is 1006 because the kidneys cannot concentrate it. When an ADH analogue is given, if urine osmolarity rises by 50% from the baseline value, this may show that the kidney is responsive to ADH. In other words, neurogenic DI is the cause. If the urine osmolarity does not significantly rise, this may indicate that the kidneys are not ADH-responsive. This suggests that the underlying cause of nephrogenic DI.

1. What happens if there is excessive secretion of ADH
   SIADH: Syndrome of inappropriate ADH secretion.
2. What happens if there is decrease secretion of ADH
   Diabetes Insipidus.

## SUMMARY

In this chapter we have learnt:
- Glomerular filtration rate (GFR) is meticulously defined, encompassing its typical range and the composition of glomerular filtrate.
- The filtration membrane, comprising fenestrated endothelium, basement membrane, and podocyte processes, plays a pivotal role in glomerular filtration.
- Physical factors such as hydrostatic pressure, colloid osmotic pressure, and filtration coefficient govern GFR.
- Physiological mechanisms, including autoregulation and hormonal control, tightly regulate GFR.
- Various tubular segments, including the proximal tubule, loop of Henle, distal tubule, and collecting duct, orchestrate tubular reabsorption and secretion.
- Factors regulating these processes, such as concentration gradients, membrane transporters, and hormonal influence, etc.
- The distinction between obligatory (essential for maintaining body function) and facultative (regulated based on body needs).
- The counter current mechanism is expounded upon as the mechanism behind urine concentration, facilitated by the arrangement of nephron loops and vasa recta.
- Factors influencing the formation of concentrated or dilute urine, including antidiuretic hormone (ADH) and renal medullary osmotic gradient.

## LET US SEE, HOW MUCH YOU HAVE LEARNT?

 *Review Questions*

Q1. Define glomerular filtration rate. Describe the factors affecting GFR.

Q2. Describe the methods used to measure glomerular filtration.

Q3. Give a physiological explanation for why persistent uncontrolled hypertension/diabetes mellitus results in reduced GFR.

Q4. Describe the physiological cause of albuminuria when the GBM filtration barrier is not functioning adequately.

Q5. Explain why, the proteins are not filtered across the glomerular basement membrane?

Q6. Explain why colloid osmotic pressure of Bowman's capsule is zero?

Q7. What will happen to glomerular filtration rate if, the capillary hydrostatic pressure is 65 mm Hg, colloid osmotic pressure of the glomerular capillaries is 32 mm Hg, hydrostatic pressure in the Bowman's capsule is 18 mm Hg and colloid osmotic pressure of Bowman's capsule is 0 mm Hg. Comment on your findings. What will happen to GFR, if basement membrane loses its negative charge?

Q8. What is glomerular capillary filtration coefficient? What is its clinical significance?

Q9. Explain how is GFR regulated? Explain the mechanism of autoregulation of renal blood flow and GFR.

Q10. What will happen to GFR in following conditions and why:
   a. In severe burns
   b. In severe dehydration
   c. Urethral stone, obstructing the urine flow
   d. Hypoproteinemia
   e. Increased water intake
   f. Constriction of afferent arteriole
   g. Constriction of efferent arteriole
   h. Dilation of afferent arteriole
   i. Dilation of efferent arteriole
   j. High blood pressure
   k. High protein diet

Q11. A patient is placed on nonsteroidal anti-inflammatory drugs (NSAIDs) for osteoarthritis. What effect would this have on GFR?

Q12. A patient with diabetes mellitus is found to have a blood pressure of 146/94, during his outpatient visit. He is prescribed ACE-inhibitor for controlling his raised arterial pressure, what effect would this have on his GFR?

Q13. Describe the role of PCT in formation of urine.

Q14. If the transport maximum of glucose (TmG) is 325–375 mg/min, then why the glucosuria occurs at 180 mL/dL?

Q15. How does thick ascending limb of loop of Henle participate in creating hyperosmolar medullary gradient?

Q16. What would happen, if the Na-K-2Cl pump in LOH stops functioning?
Q17. What would happen, if blood flow through vasa recta is increased?
Q18. What would happen to counter current mechanism in renal tissue hypoxia?
Q19. Describe the role of counter current multiplier and exchanger system in concentration of urine.
Q20. Describe the formation of dilute urine in a person, who had consumed 5 L of water.

## Multiple Choice Questions

Q1. A patient is diagnosed with kidney disease. Which of the following parameters would most accurately reflect the functionality of their kidneys?
   a. Glomerular filtration rate (GFR)
   b. Blood pressure
   c. Serum albumin levels
   d. Urine color

Q2. What is the typical range for glomerular filtration rate (GFR) in healthy adults?
   a. 30–50 mL/min
   b. 60–80 mL/min
   c. 90–120 mL/min
   d. 150–180 mL/min

Q3. If a patient's GFR is measured at 100 mL/min and their urine output per hour is 50 mL, what is their net filtration rate per hour?
   a. 50 mL/hr
   b. 75 mL/hr
   c. 100 mL/hr
   d. 150 mL/hr

Q4. A patient has been diagnosed with hypertension. How might this condition affect their glomerular filtration rate (GFR)?
   a. Increase GFR due to increased blood pressure
   b. Decrease GFR due to increased blood pressure
   c. No effect on GFR
   d. Increase GFR due to decreased blood pressure

Q5. Which of the following hormones is primarily responsible for regulating GFR by modulating arteriolar diameter?
   a. Insulin
   b. Renin
   c. Thyroxine
   d. Aldosterone

Q6. What are the main components of the glomerular filtrate?
   a. Water and large proteins
   b. Electrolytes and large proteins
   c. Water, electrolytes, glucose, and waste products
   d. Glucose and large proteins

Q7. If a patient's urine creatinine concentration is 100 mg/dL and their urine output is 2 L/day, what is their creatinine clearance rate?
   a. 50 mL/min
   b. 100 mL/min
   c. 200 mL/min
   d. 400 mL/min

Q8. A patient is admitted to the emergency department with dehydration. How might this condition affect their GFR?
   a. Increase GFR due to decreased blood volume
   b. Decrease GFR due to decreased blood volume
   c. Increase GFR due to increased blood volume
   d. No effect on GFR

Q9. Which of the following substances is typically used to estimate glomerular filtration rate (GFR) in clinical practice?
   a. Inulin
   b. Urea
   c. Sodium
   d. Calcium

Q10. What is the primary method of measuring glomerular filtration rate (GFR) in a clinical setting?
   a. Serum creatinine levels
   b. Blood urea nitrogen (BUN)
   c. Inulin clearance
   d. Urine protein levels

Q11. A patient consumes a high-sodium diet for an extended period. How might this diet affect their GFR?
   a. Increase GFR due to increased blood pressure
   b. Decrease GFR due to increased blood pressure
   c. Decrease GFR due to decreased blood pressure
   d. No effect on GFR

Q12. Which of the following physiological mechanisms directly regulates glomerular filtration rate (GFR) in response to changes in blood pressure?
   a. Renin-angiotensin-aldosterone system
   b. Thyroid hormone secretion
   c. Insulin sensitivity
   d. Parathyroid hormone release

Q13. Which of the following is NOT a component of the filtration membrane in the glomerulus?
   a. Endothelial cells
   b. Basement membrane
   c. Podocytes
   d. Mesangial cells

Q14. If a patient's GFR is measured at 120 mL/min and their urine output per hour is 80 mL, what is their net filtration rate per hour?
   a. 40 mL/hr
   b. 60 mL/hr
   c. 80 mL/hr
   d. 100 mL/hr

Q15. A patient is diagnosed with diabetes mellitus. How might this condition affect their glomerular filtration rate (GFR)?
   a. Increase GFR due to increased blood glucose levels
   b. Decrease GFR due to increased blood glucose levels
   c. Decrease GFR due to decreased blood glucose levels
   d. No effect on GFR

Q16. Which of the following factors would lead to a decrease in glomerular filtration rate (GFR)?
   a. Sympathetic nervous system activation
   b. Increased hydrostatic pressure in the glomerulus
   c. Vasodilation of the afferent arteriole
   d. Increased plasma protein concentration

Q17. What is the primary mechanism by which glomerular filtration rate (GFR) is regulated?
   a. Hormonal control
   b. Neural regulation
   c. Autoregulation
   d. Dietary intake

**Q18.** A patient is experiencing excessive loss of glucose in their urine. Which renal tubular segment is likely malfunctioning?
  a. Proximal convoluted tubule (PCT)
  b. Loop of Henle (LOH)
  c. Distal convoluted tubule (DCT)
  d. Collecting duct

**Q19.** Which of the following substances is primarily reabsorbed in the proximal convoluted tubule (PCT)?
  a. Glucose       b. Urea
  c. Potassium     d. Creatinine

**Q20.** If the glomerular filtration rate (GFR) is 120 mL/min and the renal plasma flow (RPF) is 600 mL/min, what is the filtration fraction?
  a. 0.2       b. 0.25
  c. 0.5       d. 0.8

**Q21.** A patient is prescribed a diuretic medication. How might this affect their urine volume and electrolyte levels?
  a. Increase urine volume and decrease electrolyte levels
  b. Decrease urine volume and increase electrolyte levels
  c. Increase urine volume without affecting electrolyte levels
  d. Decrease urine volume without affecting electrolyte levels

**Q22.** Which hormone stimulates sodium reabsorption in the distal convoluted tubule (DCT) and cortical collecting duct?
  a. Aldosterone
  b. Antidiuretic hormone (ADH)
  c. Parathyroid hormone (PTH)
  d. Atrial natriuretic peptide (ANP)

**Q23.** What is the primary site of water reabsorption in the nephron?
  a. Proximal convoluted tubule (PCT)
  b. Loop of Henle (LOH)
  c. Distal convoluted tubule (DCT)
  d. Collecting duct

**Q24.** If a patient's urine osmolality is 600 mOsm/kg and their serum osmolality is 300 mOsm/kg, what is their free water clearance?
  a. 300 mL/min       b. 600 mL/min
  c. 900 mL/min       d. 1200 mL/min

**Q25.** A patient is diagnosed with primary hyperaldosteronism. How might this condition affect their electrolyte balance and urine volume?
  a. Increase sodium reabsorption and decrease urine volume
  b. Decrease sodium reabsorption and increase urine volume
  c. Increase potassium reabsorption and decrease urine volume
  d. Decrease potassium reabsorption and increase urine volume

**Q26.** Which of the following substances is typically reabsorbed in the thick ascending limb of the loop of Henle?
  a. Water
  b. Sodium
  c. Urea
  d. Potassium

**Q27.** Which hormone is responsible for stimulating water reabsorption in the collecting ducts?
  a. Aldosterone
  b. Antidiuretic hormone (ADH)
  c. Parathyroid hormone (PTH)
  d. Atrial natriuretic peptide (ANP)

**Q28.** If a patient's tubular maximum for glucose reabsorption is 300 mg/dL and their blood glucose level is 400 mg/dL, how much glucose will be excreted in the urine?
  a. 100 mg/dL
  b. 200 mg/dL
  c. 300 mg/dL
  d. 400 mg/dL

**Q29.** A patient is experiencing hypokalemia. Which renal tubular segment might be involved in this electrolyte imbalance?
  a. Proximal convoluted tubule (PCT)
  b. Loop of Henle (LOH)
  c. Distal convoluted tubule (DCT)
  d. Collecting duct

**Q30.** Which of the following substances is typically secreted in the proximal convoluted tubule (PCT)?
  a. Sodium       b. Potassium
  c. Creatinine   d. Glucose

**Q31.** Which of the following is an example of obligatory reabsorption in the kidneys?
  a. Reabsorption of glucose in the PCT
  b. Reabsorption of urea in the DCT
  c. Reabsorption of potassium in the LOH
  d. Reabsorption of water in the collecting duct

**Q32.** If a patient's urine output is 1 L/day and their free water clearance is 300 mL/min, what is their urine osmolality?
  a. 100 mOsm/kg
  b. 200 mOsm/kg
  c. 300 mOsm/kg
  d. 400 mOsm/kg

**Q33.** A patient is prescribed a medication that blocks the action of aldosterone. How might this affect their electrolyte balance and blood pressure?
  a. Increase sodium reabsorption and decrease blood pressure
  b. Decrease sodium reabsorption and increase blood pressure
  c. Increase potassium reabsorption and decrease blood pressure
  d. Decrease potassium reabsorption and increase blood pressure

**Q34.** Which of the following hormones is responsible for promoting calcium reabsorption in the distal convoluted tubule (DCT)?
  a. Aldosterone
  b. Antidiuretic hormone (ADH)
  c. Parathyroid hormone (PTH)
  d. Atrial natriuretic peptide (ANP)

**Q35.** What is the term for the maximum rate at which a substance can be reabsorbed in the renal tubules?
  a. Tubular threshold
  b. Tubular maximum
  c. Glomerular filtration rate (GFR)
  d. Filtration fraction

Q36. If a patient's tubular maximum for a certain substance is 400 mg/dL and their blood concentration of that substance is 500 mg/dL, how much of that substance will remain in the urine?
a. 100 mg/dL
b. 200 mg/dL
c. 300 mg/dL
d. 400 mg/dL

Q37. A patient is experiencing excessive thirst and producing large volumes of dilute urine. Which hormone might be deficient in this patient?
a. Aldosterone
b. Antidiuretic hormone (ADH)
c. Parathyroid hormone (PTH)
d. Atrial natriuretic peptide (ANP)

Q38. Which of the following substances is typically reabsorbed in the thin descending limb of the loop of Henle?
a. Sodium
b. Urea
c. Glucose
d. Potassium

Q39. What is the primary function of the juxtaglomerular apparatus in the kidneys?
a. Regulation of blood pressure
b. Secretion of aldosterone
c. Filtration of blood
d. Regulation of GFR

Q40. If a patient's urine output is 2 L/day and their urine osmolality is 300 mOsm/kg, what is their daily obligatory urine volume?
a. 0.5 L/day
b. 1 L/day
c. 1.5 L/day
d. 2 L/day

Q41. A patient is diagnosed with primary hypothyroidism. How might this condition affect their renal function?
a. Increase sodium reabsorption and decrease urine volume
b. Decrease sodium reabsorption and increase urine volume
c. Increase potassium reabsorption and decrease urine volume
d. Decrease potassium reabsorption and increase urine volume

Q42. Which of the following substances is typically secreted in the distal convoluted tubule (DCT)?
a. Glucose
b. Sodium
c. Potassium
d. Urea

Q43. What is the term for the movement of substances from the blood into the renal tubules?
a. Reabsorption
b. Secretion
c. Filtration
d. Osmosis

Q44. If a patient's urine output is 1 L/day and their free water clearance is -200 mL/min, what is their urine osmolality?
a. 300 mOsm/kg
b. 400 mOsm/kg
c. 500 mOsm/kg
d. 600 mOsm/kg

Q45. A patient is prescribed a medication that blocks the action of antidiuretic hormone (ADH). How might this affect their urine concentration and volume?
a. Increase urine concentration and decrease volume
b. Decrease urine concentration and increase volume
c. Increase urine concentration and increase volume
d. Decrease urine concentration and decrease volume

Q46. Which of the following substances is typically reabsorbed in the proximal convoluted tubule (PCT) via paracellular transport?
a. Glucose
b. Sodium
c. Urea
d. Creatinine

Q47. What is the term for the movement of substances from the renal tubules back into the blood?
a. Reabsorption
b. Secretion
c. Filtration
d. Osmosis

Q48. If a patient's tubular maximum for sodium reabsorption is 200 mEq/L and their blood sodium concentration is 150 mEq/L, how much sodium will be excreted in the urine?
a. 50 mEq/L
b. 100 mEq/L
c. 150 mEq/L
d. 200 mEq/L

Q49. A patient is diagnosed with primary hyperparathyroidism. How might this condition affect their calcium reabsorption in the kidneys?
a. Increase calcium reabsorption
b. Decrease calcium reabsorption
c. Increase potassium reabsorption
d. Decrease potassium reabsorption

Q50. Which of the following substances is typically secreted in the proximal convoluted tubule (PCT)?
a. Glucose
b. Sodium
c. Potassium
d. Creatinine

Q51. Recall-Based Question: Which of the following substances is typically reabsorbed in the thick ascending limb of the loop of Henle?
a. Water
b. Sodium
c. Urea
d. Potassium

Q52. Calculation-Based Question: If a patient's urine output is 1 L/day and their free water clearance is -100 mL/min, what is their urine osmolality?
a. 300 mOsm/kg
b. 400 mOsm/kg
c. 500 mOsm/kg
d. 600 mOsm/kg

Q53. A patient is diagnosed with primary hyperaldosteronism. How might this condition affect their potassium excretion?
a. Increase potassium excretion
b. Decrease potassium excretion
c. Increase sodium excretion
d. Decrease sodium excretion

Q54. Which of the following substances is typically reabsorbed in the distal convoluted tubule (DCT) under the influence of aldosterone?
a. Glucose
b. Sodium
c. Potassium
d. Urea

Q55. Which of the following substances is typically reabsorbed in the collecting ducts under the influence of antidiuretic hormone (ADH)?
a. Glucose
b. Sodium
c. Water
d. Potassium

Q56. Calculation-Based Question: If a patient's tubular maximum for a certain substance is 400 mg/dL and their blood concentration of that substance is 300 mg/dL, how much of that substance will be reabsorbed?
a. 100 mg/dL
b. 200 mg/dL
c. 300 mg/dL
d. 400 mg/dL

Q57. A patient is prescribed a medication that blocks the action of parathyroid hormone (PTH). How might this affect their calcium reabsorption in the kidneys?
a. Increase calcium reabsorption
b. Decrease calcium reabsorption
c. Increase potassium reabsorption
d. Decrease potassium reabsorption

Q58. A hiker is stranded in a desert without access to water. How will their body adapt to maintain water balance and urine concentration?
a. Increase in urine volume and decrease in urine concentration
b. Decrease in urine volume and increase in urine concentration
c. Increase in urine volume and increase in urine concentration
d. Decrease in urine volume and decrease in urine concentration

Q59. Which part of the nephron plays a crucial role in concentrating urine through the countercurrent mechanism?
a. Proximal convoluted tubule (PCT)
b. Distal convoluted tubule (DCT)
c. Loop of Henle (LOH)
d. Collecting duct

Q60. If a person's urine osmolality is measured at 1200 mOsm/kg and their serum osmolality is 300 mOsm/kg, what is their urine concentration relative to plasma?
a. 1:1
b. 2:1
c. 3:1
d. 4:1

Q61. A patient is diagnosed with syndrome of inappropriate antidiuretic hormone (SIADH) secretion. How will this condition affect their urine concentration?
a. Increase urine concentration
b. Decrease urine concentration
c. No effect on urine concentration
d. Increase urine volume without affecting concentration

Q62. Which hormone is primarily responsible for regulating the concentration of urine by controlling water reabsorption in the collecting ducts?
a. Aldosterone
b. Antidiuretic hormone (ADH)
c. Parathyroid hormone (PTH)
d. Atrial natriuretic peptide (ANP)

Q63. What is the main mechanism by which the kidney concentrates urine?
a. Filtration
b. Reabsorption
c. Secretion
d. Countercurrent mechanism

Q64. If a person's urine volume is 1 liter and their urine osmolality is 800 mOsm/kg, what is their daily solute excretion?
a. 800 mOsm
b. 1,000 mOsm
c. 1,200 mOsm
d. 1,600 mOsm

Q65. A patient is experiencing dehydration due to excessive sweating. How will their urine concentration be affected?
a. Decrease in urine concentration
b. Increase in urine concentration
c. No change in urine concentration
d. Increase in urine volume without affecting concentration

Q66. Which part of the nephron is responsible for establishing the osmotic gradient in the renal medulla?
a. Proximal convoluted tubule (PCT)
b. Loop of Henle (LOH)
c. Distal convoluted tubule (DCT)
d. Collecting duct

Q67. Which of the following factors contributes to the formation of concentrated urine?
a. Low levels of antidiuretic hormone (ADH)
b. High levels of aldosterone
c. Low levels of aldosterone
d. High levels of atrial natriuretic peptide (ANP)

## ANSWERS

| | | | | | | |
|---|---|---|---|---|---|---|
| 1. a | 2. c | 3. a | 4. b | 5. b | 6. c | 7. b |
| 8. a | 9. a | 10. c | 11. b | 12. a | 13. d | 14. c |
| 15. a | 16. d | 17. c | 18. a | 19. a | 20. b | 21. a |
| 22. a | 23. d | 24. c | 25. a | 26. b | 27. b | 28. b |
| 29. c | 30. c | 31. a | 32. a | 33. b | 34. c | 35. b |
| 36. c | 37. b | 38. b | 39. d | 40. b | 41. b | 42. c |
| 43. b | 44. d | 45. b | 46. b | 47. a | 48. a | 49. a |
| 50. d | 51. b | 52. c | 53. a | 54. c | 55. c | 56. c |
| 57. b | 58. b | 59. c | 60. d | 61. a | 62. b | 63. d |
| 64. c | 65. b | 66. b | 67. a | | | |

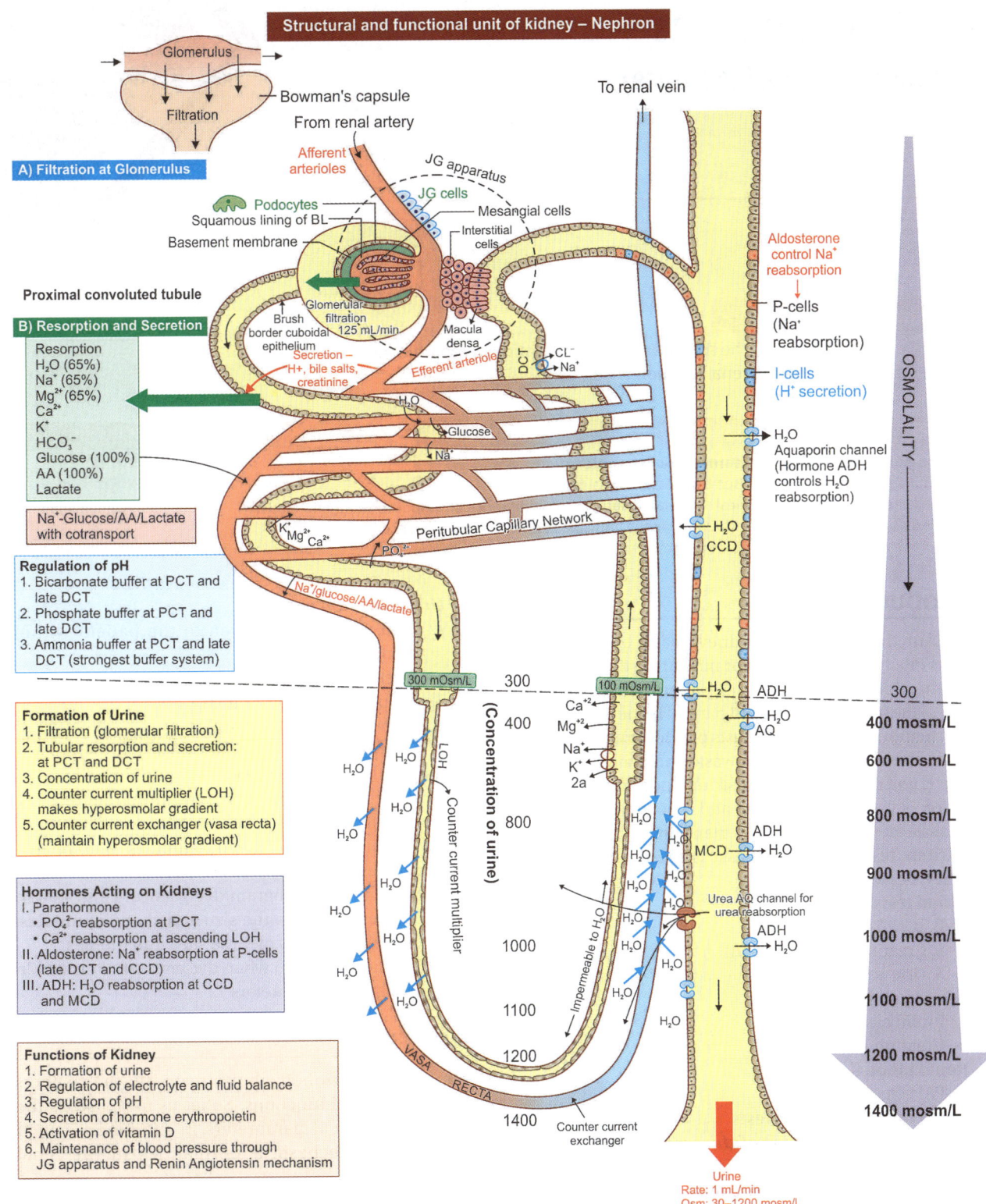

# Renal Function Tests
## (Including Plasma Clearance)

**CHAPTER 60**

### COMPETENCY ADDRESSED
PY7.4: Describe and discuss the significance and implication of renal clearance.
PY7.8: Describe and discuss renal function tests.

### LEARNING OBJECTIVES
**At the end of this chapter, the learner should be able to:**
- Enumerate the various tests used to assess the renal functions.
- Describe the utility, physiological significance and clinical significance of various renal function tests.
- Describe the significance of tests based on the principle of plasma/renal clearance.

## INTRODUCTION

Renal function tests assess kidney health by measuring various biochemical and cellular markers in the blood and urine. In addition, there are other battery of function tests to assess the function of different parts of kidney involved in the formation of urine. These tests provide crucial insights into the kidneys' ability to filter waste, maintain electrolyte balance, and regulate blood pressure. Understanding renal function is vital for diagnosing and managing conditions such as kidney disease and hypertension.

Various tests required to assess these functions are outlined below:
- **Blood tests**
  - B. urea 7-20 mg/dL
  - S. Creatinine 0.6–1.5 mg/dL
  - S. Uric acid levels
- **Tests to assess GFR**
  - Inulin clearance method
  - Creatinine clearance
- **Renal blood flow**:
  - PAH clearance
- **Renal tubular function tests**
  - ***Tubular reabsorption of glucose (TmG):*** Gives a fair index of proximal tubular function
  - ***Urine conc. test (Fishberg test)***
    - 200 mL of water given with diet at 8 PM
    - No fluid thereafter
    - Urine collected at midnight is discarded
    - Collect 3 samples in morning (8, 9 and 10 AM)
  - *Urine dilution test*
    - 1000 mL of water given to the patient within 20 minutes
    - Three samples are taken every hour and measure
      - Specific gravity (<1.003),
      - Urine volume (700 mL),
      - Urine osmolality (<1000 mosm)
- **Radiographic technique/IVP**
  - Organic $I_2$ containing compound injected I/V (Uropac)
  - Enter glomerulus → filtered → tubules → excreted
  - Time interval films are taken
    - First filter nephrogram dye gets concentrated in tubules, to assess the size and shape of tubules, increased density of these sites into tubules
    - Second film taken when dye gets concentrated in renal pelvis and ureters

## BLOOD TESTS

These tests mentioned above tests all the aspects involving the renal functions. So let us first discuss the various biochemical parameters in the blood, which can suggest some basic abnormalities in the renal function.

### Blood Urea (BUN)

**Normal values:** Typically, blood urea levels range from 7 to 20 mg/dL.

**Physiological significance:** Blood urea is a waste product formed from the breakdown of proteins in the liver. In a healthy individual, the kidneys efficiently filter urea from the blood, maintaining its levels within the normal range.

**Clinical significance:** In renal diseases, such as chronic kidney disease, the kidneys' ability to filter waste products like urea is impaired. This often leads to elevated blood urea levels, a condition known as *uremia*. However, it's important to note that BUN levels can be influenced by factors other than renal function, such as diet and hydration status.

Blood urea nitrogen (BUN) levels can rise due to various physiological and pathological conditions, including:

- **Dehydration:** Reduced fluid intake or excessive fluid loss (e.g., through vomiting, diarrhea, excessive sweating) can lead to dehydration, concentrating blood urea levels.
- **Impaired kidney function:** Conditions that affect kidney function, such as acute kidney injury (AKI) or chronic kidney disease (CKD), can result in decreased excretion of urea, leading to elevated BUN levels.
- **Heart failure:** In congestive heart failure, decreased blood flow to the kidneys can impair their ability to excrete urea, contributing to elevated BUN levels.
- **Gastrointestinal bleeding:** Blood loss from the gastrointestinal tract can result in increased absorption of nitrogenous compounds, including urea, leading to elevated BUN levels.
- **High protein diet:** Consuming a diet high in protein can increase the production of urea, leading to transient elevations in BUN levels.
- **Catabolic states:** Conditions associated with increased breakdown of protein, such as severe infections, trauma, burns, or certain cancers, can lead to elevated BUN levels due to increased urea production.
- **Certain medications:** Some medications, such as corticosteroids, tetracycline antibiotics, and diuretics, can affect kidney function or metabolism, potentially leading to elevated BUN levels.
- **Obstruction of urinary tract:** Obstruction of the urinary tract, such as by kidney stones or tumors, can impair urine flow and lead to decreased excretion of urea, contributing to elevated BUN levels.

## Serum Creatinine

**Normal values:** Normal serum creatinine levels vary depending on factors such as age, gender, and muscle mass. However, in adults, levels typically range from 0.6 to 1.3 mg/dL for males and 0.5 to 1.0 mg/dL for females.

**Physiological significance:** Creatinine is a waste product generated from the breakdown of creatine phosphate in muscles. In healthy individuals, the kidneys filter creatinine from the blood at a relatively constant rate, maintaining stable serum levels.

**Clinical significance:** In renal diseases, particularly CKD, the kidneys' ability to filter creatinine is compromised. As a result, serum creatinine levels rise, reflecting decreased renal function. Monitoring creatinine levels is crucial for assessing renal function, staging CKD, and determining the need for interventions such as dialysis or kidney transplantation. Serum creatinine levels can increase due to various conditions affecting kidney function and muscle metabolism mentioned below:

- **Acute kidney injury (AKI):** Any sudden decrease in kidney function, often due to conditions like severe dehydration, decreased blood flow to the kidneys (hypovolemia), or direct kidney damage (e.g., from toxins, drugs, or infections), can lead to elevated serum creatinine levels.
- **Chronic kidney disease (CKD):** CKD is characterized by gradual and progressive loss of kidney function over time. As kidney function declines, serum creatinine levels increase due to decreased filtration and excretion by the kidneys.
- **Urinary tract obstruction:** Obstruction of the urinary tract, such as by kidney stones, tumors, or enlarged prostate gland, can lead to impaired urine flow and subsequent elevation of serum creatinine levels.
- **Rhabdomyolysis:** Rhabdomyolysis is a condition characterized by rapid breakdown of skeletal muscle tissue, leading to the release of myoglobin and creatine kinase into the bloodstream. Elevated serum creatinine levels can occur as a result of muscle breakdown.
- **Severe muscle injury or trauma:** Conditions such as crush injuries, severe burns, or extensive surgery can cause significant muscle damage, resulting in elevated serum creatinine levels.
- **High protein diet:** Consumption of a diet high in protein can lead to increased creatinine production from muscle metabolism, resulting in transient elevation of serum creatinine levels.
- **Certain medications:** Some medications can affect kidney function or interfere with creatinine metabolism, leading to elevated serum creatinine levels. Examples include nonsteroidal anti-inflammatory drugs (NSAIDs), certain antibiotics (e.g., trimethoprim), and some chemotherapeutic agents.
- **Dehydration:** Dehydration can lead to decreased blood flow to the kidneys and reduced urine output, resulting in elevated serum creatinine levels due to decreased clearance by the kidneys.
- **Certain medical conditions:** Conditions such as severe heart failure, severe hypertension, and liver cirrhosis can lead to decreased renal perfusion and kidney dysfunction, contributing to elevated serum creatinine levels.
- **Aging:** As individuals age, there is a natural decline in kidney function, leading to a gradual increase in serum creatinine levels over time.

## Serum Uric Acid

**Normal values:** Normal serum uric acid levels typically range from 3.4 to 7.0 mg/dL in males and 2.4 to 6.0 mg/dL in females.

**Physiological significance:** Uric acid is a byproduct of purine metabolism. In healthy individuals, the kidneys excrete uric acid efficiently, preventing its accumulation in the blood.

**Clinical significance:** Renal dysfunction can lead to decreased excretion of uric acid, resulting in elevated serum levels. This predisposes individuals to conditions like hyperuricemia, which is associated with gout, kidney stones, and in severe cases, kidney damage due to uric acid crystal deposition. Serum uric acid levels can increase due to various factors and medical conditions, including:

- **Gout:** Gout is a type of arthritis characterized by the deposition of uric acid crystals in the joints, leading to inflammation and pain. Elevated serum uric acid levels are a key feature of gout.
- **Dietary factors:** Consumption of foods high in purines, such as red meat, organ meats (liver, kidney), seafood (anchovies, sardines), and certain types of alcohol (beer, spirits), can lead to increased production of uric acid and subsequently elevated serum levels.
- **Obesity:** Obesity is associated with increased production of uric acid and reduced excretion by the kidneys, leading to elevated serum uric acid levels.
- **Renal dysfunction:** Conditions that impair kidney function, such as chronic kidney disease (CKD), acute kidney injury (AKI), or obstructive nephropathy, can lead to decreased excretion of uric acid, resulting in elevated serum levels.
- **Metabolic syndrome:** Metabolic syndrome, a cluster of conditions including obesity, insulin resistance, high blood pressure, and dyslipidemia, is associated with elevated serum uric acid levels.
- **Certain medications:** Some medications can increase serum uric acid levels, including diuretics (especially thiazide diuretics), aspirin, cyclosporine, and niacin.
- **Genetic factors:** Genetic factors can predispose individuals to hyperuricemia and gout. Inherited conditions such as familial juvenile hyperuricemic nephropathy and Lesch-Nyhan syndrome can lead to elevated serum uric acid levels.
- **Dehydration:** Dehydration can lead to increased serum uric acid concentrations due to reduced urinary excretion of uric acid.
- **Certain medical conditions:** Conditions such as psoriasis, leukemia, lymphoma, and hemolytic anemia can be associated with increased cell turnover, leading to elevated serum uric acid levels.
- **Alcohol consumption:** Alcohol consumption, particularly beer and spirits, can increase serum uric acid levels by promoting the production of uric acid and reducing its excretion.

## TESTS TO ASSESS GLOMERULAR FILTRATION RATE (GFR)

These are the functional tests performed for the efficient and accurate assessment of glomerular filtration rate. The normal GFR is 125 mL/min.

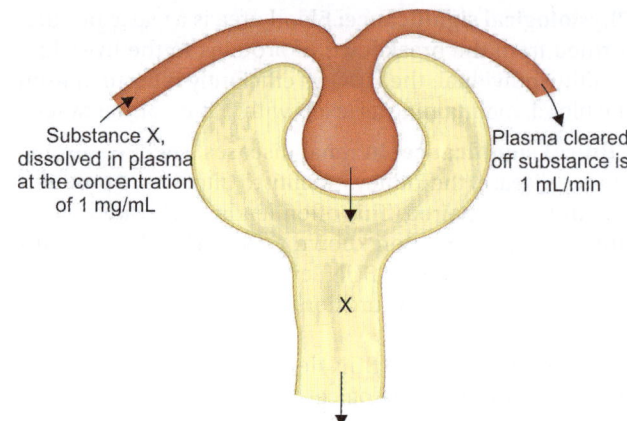

**Fig. 60.1:** Principle of plasma clearance.

These tests are based on the principle of *plasma clearance* (**Fig. 60.1**), which is defined as *"the amount of plasma cleared off a substance in one minute."*

> **Plasma Clearance can be Explained as**
> If the plasma carries a freely filterable substance, then the amount of plasma (mL), from which that substance is removed in 1 minute. It does not refer to amount to substance filtered in 1 minute, it measures the volume of plasma (ml) per minute.

Plasma clearance of various substances is shown in **Table 60.1**.

The principle of plasma clearance is used to measure:
- GFR by inulin clearance method and creatinine clearance method.
- Renal blood flow by Para-amino hippuric acid (PAH) clearance method.

### Inulin Clearance

It is a method used to estimate the glomerular filtration rate (GFR), which is a measure of the kidney's ability to filter blood. Inulin, a fructose polysaccharide, is infused intravenously and cleared solely by glomerular filtration without being reabsorbed or secreted by the renal tubules.

**Table 60.1:** Plasma clearance of various substances.

| Substance | Clearance (mL/min) |
|---|---|
| Glucose | 0 |
| Sodium | 0.9 |
| Chloride | 1.3 |
| Potassium | 12 |
| Phosphate | 25 |
| Urea | 75 |
| Inulin | 125 |
| Creatinine | 140 |
| PAH | 560 |

## Indications

- Assessment of kidney function in research studies.
- Validation of other GFR estimation methods.
- Evaluation of renal function in patients with suspected kidney disease, particularly when precise GFR measurement is needed.

## Properties of Inulin for Measuring GFR

- Inulin is freely filtered at the glomerulus
- It is neither reabsorbed nor secreted by the renal tubules
- It is minimally metabolized in the body
- It does not interfere with renal function
- Inulin is excreted unchanged in the urine, allowing for accurate measurement of its clearance.

## Procedure

- Obtain a baseline blood sample for inulin measurement and assess the patient's hydration status.
- Intravenous bolus dose of inulin is given to reach the desired inulin concentration, which is maintained by the infusion of inulin is initiated to achieve a steady-state plasma concentration ($P_{inulin}$).
- Timed urine collections are performed to measure urine volume (V) and inulin concentration in urine ($U_{inulin}$).
- Additional blood samples may be collected at specific time points to measure plasma inulin concentration.

Inulin clearance is calculated using the formula (**Fig. 60.2**):

$$\text{Inulin clearance} = \frac{U_{inulin} \times V}{P_{inulin}}$$

As seen in figure $U_{inulin}$ = 125 mg/mL, V = 1 mL/min and $P_{inulin}$ = 1 mg/mL
Then, 125 × 1/1 = 125 mL/min

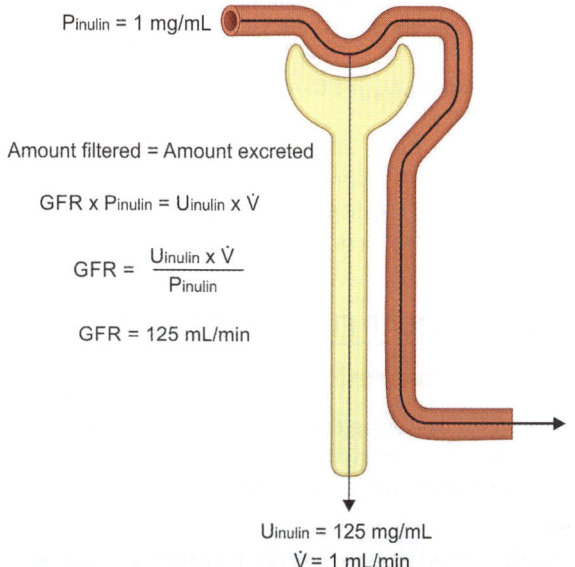

**Fig. 60.2:** Calculation of GFR.

## Limitations

- **Invasive procedure:** Inulin clearance requires intravenous infusion and timed urine collections, making it relatively invasive and impractical for routine clinical use.
- **Resource intensive:** The procedure requires specialized equipment and personnel for inulin infusion and urine collection, which may not be available in all healthcare settings.
- **Patient compliance:** Timed urine collections can be cumbersome for patients, potentially affecting the accuracy of results.
- **Cost:** Inulin is an expensive marker compared to other GFR estimation methods, limiting its widespread use in clinical practice.

## Creatinine Clearance Method

Creatinine clearance is a method used to estimate the glomerular filtration rate (GFR), which is a measure of kidney function. It involves the measurement of creatinine levels in both urine and blood to calculate the rate at which the kidneys are able to filter creatinine from the blood into the urine.

### Indications

- Assessment of kidney function, particularly in patients with suspected kidney disease or those at risk of kidney dysfunction.
- Monitoring kidney function over time, especially in patients with chronic kidney disease (CKD).
- Evaluation of drug dosing in patients with impaired kidney function, as creatinine clearance provides an estimate of renal clearance.

### Procedure

- A timed urine collection (e.g., over 24 hours) is performed to measure the total volume of urine produced.
- The concentration of creatinine in the collected urine sample is measured using laboratory techniques ($U_{Cr}$). The concentration of urinary creatinine is slightly more than the filtered creatinine because it is secreted into the proximal convoluted tubules of nephrons.
- A blood sample is obtained to measure the serum (blood) creatinine concentration ($P_{Cr}$). The plasma concentration of inulin is usually overestimated.
- Hence, the error in $U_{Cr}$ and $P_{Cr}$ cancel out each other, giving a reasonably accurate estimation.
- Creatinine Clearance = $(U_{Cr} \times V)/P_{Cr}$

*Adjustments: Creatinine clearance may be adjusted for factors such as body surface area (to obtain standardized values) or for incomplete urine collections.*

**Cockcroft-Gault Formula:**

$$\text{Creatinine clearance (mL/min)} = \frac{(140 - \text{age}) \times \text{weight (kg)}}{\text{Serum creatinine (mg/dL)} \times 72}$$

## Advantages

- Creatinine clearance is a widely available and relatively inexpensive method for estimating GFR.
- The procedure for collecting urine and blood samples for creatinine clearance measurement is relatively simple and can be performed in outpatient settings.
- Creatinine clearance provides an estimation of GFR, which is an important measure of kidney function.

## Limitations

- **Variability:** Creatinine clearance can vary based on factors such as muscle mass, diet, age, and sex, which may affect the accuracy of the measurement.
- **Timed urine collection:** Timed urine collections can be cumbersome for patients and may be prone to inaccuracies due to incomplete collections or variations in urine flow rate.
- **Creatinine production:** Creatinine is produced by muscle metabolism, so conditions affecting muscle mass or metabolism (e.g., malnutrition, muscle wasting) may affect creatinine clearance independent of kidney function.
- **Not as precise as inulin clearance:** Creatinine clearance may overestimate GFR, especially in patients with non-steady-state conditions, and is generally considered less accurate than inulin clearance for estimating GFR.

## ESTIMATION OF RENAL BLOOD FLOW

The renal blood flow is measured using the various methods like:
- Renal color Doppler ultrasonography
- Electromagnetic flowmeter
- PAH clearance

## PAH Clearance Method

Characteristics of substance used for measuring renal blood flow:
- Should not affect RBF
- Freely filtered
- Easy to measure the concentration of substance
- Nontoxic
- Not metabolized
- Not stored

Hence, the Para-amino-hippuric acid (PAH) is used for this purpose.

The PAH clearance test is done in a similar way, as done for inulin clearance test. But there is a slight difference that here we want to estimate the blood flow to the kidneys, which have two types of tissues, the nephrons and the interstitial cells.

Nephron, receive 90% of blood supply of renal artery, while 10% goes to the tissues. Hence, we can also say that the nephrons extract 90% of PAH from the blood it receives, which is freely filtered and freely secreted into the renal tubules.

*$P_{PAH}$ (Arterial concentration of PAH) = Amount of PAH entering the glomeruli (90%) + Amount of PAH entering the interstitial cells (10%), which return to circulation through the renal vein.*

From this, we can calculate the extraction ratio as

$$= \frac{\text{Arterial concentration of PAH} - \text{Venous concentration of PAH}}{\text{Arterial concentration of PAH}}$$

$$= \frac{100 - 10}{100} = 0.9$$

Hence, the 0.9 parts of PAH is extracted from the blood by the glomeruli.

In the end urinary PAH concentration is equal to the amount of PAH filtered at glomeruli and amount of PAH secreted into tubules.

*$U_{PAH}$ = Amount of PAH filtered at glomeruli + Amount of PAH secreted into tubules*

Since, we are able to measure only the amount of plasma that is filtered at the glomeruli, we can calculate only the effective renal plasma flow

$$ERPF = U_{PAH} \times V/P_{PAH}$$

The actual renal plasma flow (ARPF) can be calculated by dividing the ERPF by the extraction ratio. This will take into account the entire plasma flow through the kidney (including interstitial cells)

$$ARPF = ERPF/0.9$$

Since, we are able to calculate the ARPF, from ERPF, we can now find out the renal blood flow, by the formula

$$RBF \text{ (mL/min)} = \frac{100}{100 - \text{hematocrit}} \times ARPF = \frac{100}{100 - 45} \times ARPF = \frac{100}{55} \times ARPF$$

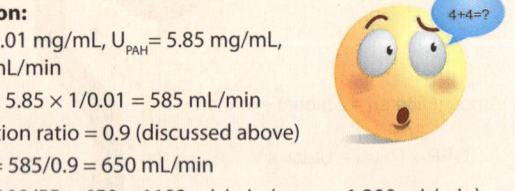

**Calculate the renal blood flow if, plasma concentration of PAH is 0.01 mg/mL, urine concentration of PAH is 5.85 mg/mL and urine flow rate is 1 mL/min.**

**Solution:**
$P_{PAH}$ = 0.01 mg/mL, $U_{PAH}$ = 5.85 mg/mL, V = 1 mL/min
ERPF = 5.85 × 1/0.01 = 585 mL/min
Extraction ratio = 0.9 (discussed above)
ARPF = 585/0.9 = 650 mL/min
RBF = 100/55 × 650 = 1182 mL/min (approx 1,200 mL/min)

## RENAL TUBULAR FUNCTION TESTS

### Tubular Reabsorption of Glucose

It is used for assessing the tubular maximum for glucose which involves measuring renal glucose handling, particularly in the proximal tubules of the kidneys.

**Method:**
- Fasting blood glucose level is measured in the morning
- A known amount of glucose solution is administered orally or intravenously. The dose typically used is

50 grams of glucose dissolved in water for an oral glucose tolerance test (OGTT).
- The blood glucose levels are measure at regular intervals after glucose administration. Common intervals include 30 minutes, 60 minutes, 90 minutes, and 120 minutes postadministration.
- The values of blood glucose concentration against time are plotted on the graph.
- The area under the curve (AUC) of the glucose levels over time is calculated. This represents the total amount of glucose filtered by the kidneys and not reabsorbed.
- The AUC is compared with the standard values to determine the tubular maximum for glucose.

### Interpretation

- If the patient's blood glucose levels *remain within normal limits* throughout the test, it suggests that the kidneys are effectively reabsorbing glucose up to their maximum capacity (tubular maximum).
- If blood glucose levels *exceed the renal threshold* (usually around 180 mg/dL or 10 mmol/L), it indicates that the kidneys have reached their maximum capacity to reabsorb glucose, and excess glucose is being excreted in the urine.

## Urine Concentration Test (Fishberg Test)

- The Fishberg concentration test is conducted by instructing the patient to consume 200 mL of water with their dinner at 8:00 PM. They are then advised not to consume any additional fluids after 8:00 PM.
- The urine collected at midnight is discarded to ensure that the bladder is empty before the test begins.
- Urine collection is initiated in the morning at 8:00 AM, and three consecutive urine samples are collected at 8:00 AM, 9:00 AM, and 10:00 AM. Accurate timing and collection of each sample are ensured.
- Each urine sample is analyzed for volume and concentration of solutes, particularly electrolytes and osmolality.
- Urine volume is measured accurately for each collection period, and urine concentration is assessed by measuring specific gravity or osmolality.
- The urine concentration and volume over the three collection periods are compared, and abnormal results, such as low urine concentration despite water deprivation, may indicate renal insufficiency or other renal disorders affecting urine concentration ability.
- The results are interpreted in the context of the patient's clinical history, medications, and underlying conditions that may affect renal function, and established guidelines are followed.

## Urine Dilution Test

The urine dilution test is a procedure conducted to assess the kidney's ability to dilute urine properly. It is performed by administering a specified volume of water to the patient and then measuring various parameters of the urine to evaluate its dilution capacity.

During the test, the patient is given a predetermined amount of water, typically 1000 mL, within a specific time frame, usually 20 minutes. Subsequently, urine samples are collected at regular intervals, typically every hour, to monitor the urine's dilution process.

Several parameters are measured during the test, including specific gravity, urine volume, and urine osmolality.

Normal specific gravity of diluted urine is between 1.001 to 1.003, volume >700 mL and osmolality <1000 mOSm.

The clinical significance of the urine dilution test lies in its ability to assess the kidney's ability to concentrate or dilute urine appropriately. Abnormal results may indicate underlying renal dysfunction, such as impaired renal tubular function or diabetes insipidus. By evaluating the kidney's ability to dilute urine, healthcare providers can diagnose and monitor various renal conditions, guide treatment decisions, and assess overall renal function.

## RADIOGRAPHIC TECHNIQUE/IVP (FIGS. 60.3 AND 60.4)

- An organic compound containing iodine as contrast media is injected intravenously.
- The compound enters the glomerulus, where it undergoes filtration and subsequently enters the tubules.
- The compound is excreted through the urinary system.
- Time interval films are taken during the procedure.
  - The first film captures the nephrogram, where the dye concentrates in the tubules. This film is used to assess the size and shape of the tubules. Increased density is observed at these tubular sites.
  - The second film is taken when the dye concentrates in the renal pelvis and ureters.

### Clinical Significance

- **Detection of abnormalities:** IVP helps detect various abnormalities in the urinary tract, including kidney stones, tumors, cysts, and structural abnormalities such as strictures or blockages in the ureters.
- **Evaluation of renal function:** By visualizing the excretion pattern of the contrast agent, IVP provides valuable information about renal function. Abnormalities in the excretion pattern may indicate impaired kidney function or obstruction.
- **Monitoring treatment response:** IVP can be used to monitor the response to treatment for urinary tract conditions. For example, it can assess the effectiveness of interventions such as the removal of kidney stones or the placement of ureteral stents.
- **Guidance for surgical planning:** IVP findings can guide surgical planning by providing detailed information about the anatomy and pathology of the urinary system. This helps surgeons determine the most appropriate

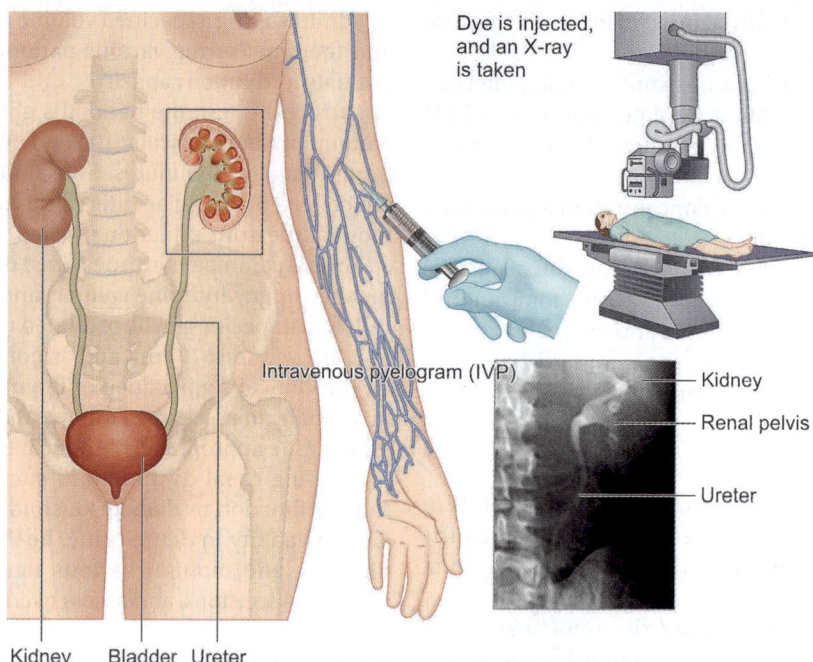

**Fig. 60.3:** Procedure of intravenous pyelogram.

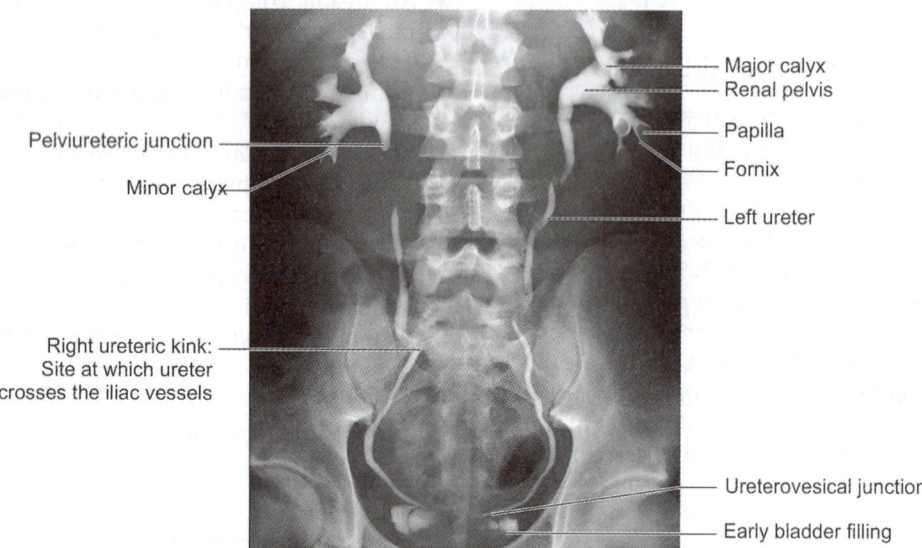

**Fig. 60.4:** Intravenous pyelogram.

approach for procedures such as nephrectomy or ureteral reconstruction.
- **Evaluation of hematuria:** IVP is often performed in patients with unexplained hematuria (blood in the urine) to identify the underlying cause, such as urinary tract stones or tumors.

## URINE ANALYSIS

- **Quantity:** 500–2500 mL/day
  - Increases after meals, after drinks and exposure to cold
  - Decreases with low water intake and excessive sweating
- **Color:** *Pale yellow due to UROCHROME.*
  **Abnormal urine color:**
  - Cloudy → strongly alkaline urine/excessive urates/infection
  - Smoky → hematuria >0.5 mL/L
  - Frothy → proteinuria
  - Milky → chyluria
  - Orange → excess urobilin
  - Brown → bilirubinuria
  - Red-dark brown → porphyrins/frank hematuria
  - Red-dark-brown–black → Hemoglobinuria/melanin (on standing)

- **Odor:** No odor ammoniacal on standing
- **Specific gravity:** 1.010

## Chemical

- **Glucose** – *nil*
- **Protein** – *nil*
    - Up to 150 mg of proteins are excreted daily in the urine.
        - 15 mg albumin
        - 25 mg Tamm Horsfall proteins (derived from cells of TAL)
        - Rest are derived from plasma proteins
        - Excretion >150 mg/day → proteinuria
- **Ketones** → *nil*;
    - Occurs in diabetic ketoacidosis, starvation, prolonged diarrhea and vomiting
- **pH** – *4.5–8*; acidic but becomes alkaline with
    - Postprandial alkaline tide
    - Alkali consumption
    - Impaired tubular acidification
    - UTI with urea splitting organisms
- **Bile pigments**: *nil;*
    - Bilirubinuria occurs in jaundice
- **Heme pigments**: *nil*
    - Appear in intravascular hemolysis
    - Crush injury to muscles
    - Myopathies which release heme from myoglobin
- **RBC** → *nil*

## Microscopic

- **Casts in urine:**
    - Cellular casts
        - Leucocyte casts → acute bacterial pyelonephritis
        - Red cell casts → acute glomerulonephritis
        - Tubular epithelial casts → ATN
    - Noncellular casts
        - Hyaline casts → Tamm Horsfall proteins, 1 cast/LPF is normal
        - Granular casts → <1 cast/LPF is normal
        - Broad Waxy casts → formed in renal failure in dilated nephrons.

### SUMMARY

In this chapter, we have studied the various tests used to assess the renal functions through various physical, biochemical, microscopic and functional analysis.
- We have learnt about the biochemical parameters present in blood like B. urea, S. creatinine and S. uric acid
- We have studied about the various function tests to study the GFR, RBF, tubular reabsorption, the concentrating and dilution capacity of nephrons.
- We have also learnt about the interpretation of urine analysis in healthy and diseased persons.

### LET US SEE, HOW MUCH YOU HAVE LEARNT?

 *Review Questions*

#### Long/Short Answer Questions

Q1. Define plasma clearance. What is the physiological and clinical significance of this test?
Q2. Describe the PAH clearance method to measure the renal blood flow.
Q3. Why the plasma clearance of glucose is zero?
Q4. How do renal function tests help diagnose kidney diseases or disorders?
Q5. What is inulin clearance test and its significance?

#### Explain Why? (Reasoning Questions)

Q1. Measuring serum creatinine levels is a useful indicator of glomerular filtration rate (GFR) and overall kidney function.
Q2. The clearance of inulin is considered the gold standard for measuring glomerular filtration rate (GFR).
Q3. Abnormalities in renal function tests, such as elevated creatinine or BUN, can indicate acute or chronic kidney disease.

 *Critical Thinking Case-Based Questions*

Q1. A 65-year-old man with a history of diabetes and hypertension, presented to his nephrologist with complaints of increasing fatigue, swelling in his ankles, and decreased urine output over the past few months. Laboratory tests revealed elevated serum creatinine and blood urea nitrogen (BUN) levels. His glomerular filtration rate (GFR) was significantly reduced, and a urinalysis showed proteinuria and microscopic hematuria. Based upon the scenario, answer the following questions:
  a. What is the probable diagnosis?
  b. Explain the physiological significance of renal function tests.
  c. How do elevated levels of serum creatinine and BUN correlate with impaired kidney function?

## Multiple Choice Questions

**Q1.** What is the primary purpose of renal clearance?
 a. To measure the amount of urine produced by the kidneys
 b. To measure the rate at which the kidneys remove a substance from the blood
 c. To assess the pH balance of urine
 d. To determine the concentration of electrolytes in urine

**Q2.** Which substance is commonly used to estimate renal clearance in clinical practice?
 a. Sodium chloride
 b. Creatinine
 c. Glucose
 d. Albumin

**Q3.** What does a high renal clearance value indicate?
 a. Impaired kidney function
 b. Efficient removal of a substance from the blood by the kidneys
 c. Excessive retention of water in the body
 d. Acidosis

**Q4.** What role does renal clearance play in pharmacokinetics?
 a. It helps predict drug metabolism in the liver
 b. It helps estimate the rate at which a drug is eliminated from the body by the kidneys
 c. It determines the onset of drug action
 d. It assesses drug absorption in the gastrointestinal tract

**Q5.** Which of the following is NOT a commonly used renal function test?
 a. Blood urea nitrogen (BUN)
 b. Serum creatinine
 c. Urinalysis
 d. Blood glucose

**Q6.** What does the glomerular filtration rate (GFR) measure?
 a. The rate at which urine is produced by the kidneys
 b. The rate at which blood is filtered by the kidneys
 c. The concentration of electrolytes in the blood
 d. The acidity of urine

**Q7.** Which condition is often associated with an elevated serum creatinine level?
 a. Dehydration
 b. Hyperglycemia
 c. Kidney failure
 d. Hypothyroidism

**Q8.** How does a urinalysis help assess renal function?
 a. By measuring the volume of urine produced
 b. By detecting the presence of abnormal substances in urine
 c. By assessing blood glucose levels in urine
 d. By measuring the pH of urine

**Q9.** In the inulin clearance test, if the plasma inulin concentration is 0.25 mg/mL, urine inulin concentration is 35 mg/mL, and urine flow rate is 1 mL/min, what is the estimated GFR?
 a. 100 mL/min
 b. 140 mL/min
 c. 175 mL/min
 d. 200 mL/min

**Q10.** In the PAH clearance test, if the plasma PAH concentration is 0.02 mg/dL, urine PAH concentration is 14 mg/dL, and urine flow rate is 1 mL/min, what is the estimated renal blood flow?
 a. 1,050 mL/min
 b. 1,150 mL/min
 c. 1,250 mL/min
 d. 1,350 mL/min

**Q11.** What is the clearance of a substance when its concentration in the plasma is 10 mg/dL, its concentration in the urine is 100 mg/dL, and urine flow is 2 mL/min?
 a. 2 mL/min
 b. 10 mL/min
 c. 20 mL/min
 d. 200 mL/min

### ANSWERS

**1.** b **2.** b **3.** b **4.** b **5.** d **6.** b **7.** c **8.** b **9.** b **10.** c **11.** c

# Physiological Basis of Diuretics and Renal Disorders

**CHAPTER 61**

**COMPETENCY ADDRESSED**

PY7.7: Describe artificial kidney, dialysis and renal transplantation.

**LEARNING OBJECTIVES**

At the end of this chapter, the learner should be able to:
- Define the physiological basis of the use of diuretics in various medical diseases.
- Describe the physiological basis of clinical features and management of acute renal failure.
- Describe the physiological basis of clinical features and management of chronic renal failure.
- Describe the physiological basis of artificial kidney or process of dialysis.
- Describe the rationale for renal transplant for a patient of chronic renal failure with end stage renal disease.

## DIURETICS

Diuretics are the drugs which increase the rate of urine volume output along with the excretion of solutes especially sodium and chloride.

### Indications for the Use of Diuretics

- **Hypertension:** Diuretics are frequently used as first-line agents in the treatment of hypertension (high blood pressure). They help reduce blood volume and lower blood pressure by promoting the excretion of sodium and water from the body.
- **Edema:** Diuretics are used to manage edema, which is the abnormal accumulation of fluid in the body's tissues. This can occur due to conditions such as heart failure, liver cirrhosis, kidney disease, or peripheral vascular disease.
- **Heart failure:** Diuretics are often prescribed to patients with heart failure to reduce fluid overload and alleviate symptoms such as shortness of breath and leg swelling. They help decrease the workload on the heart by reducing venous return and preload.
- **Kidney disease:** In certain cases of kidney disease, such as nephrotic syndrome or acute kidney injury, diuretics may be used to manage fluid retention and electrolyte imbalances.
- **Hypercalcemia:** Loop diuretics, such as furosemide, can be used to promote the excretion of calcium in the urine and lower elevated blood calcium levels in conditions such as hyperparathyroidism or hypercalcemia of malignancy.
- **Ascites:** Diuretics are sometimes used in the management of ascites, which is the accumulation of fluid in the abdominal cavity often seen in patients with liver cirrhosis.
- **Prevention of kidney stone formation:** Thiazide diuretics, such as hydrochlorothiazide, may be prescribed to prevent the formation of calcium-containing kidney stones by reducing urinary calcium excretion.
- **Glaucoma:** Carbonic anhydrase inhibitors, which are a type of diuretic, can be used to lower intraocular pressure in patients with open-angle glaucoma or ocular hypertension.
- **Adjunctive therapy in hyperkalemia:** Loop diuretics may be used as adjunctive therapy in the management of hyperkalemia (elevated blood potassium levels) to promote potassium excretion in the urine.
- **Cerebral edema:** In cases of cerebral edema, such as traumatic brain injury or cerebral infarction, osmotic diuretics like mannitol may be used to reduce intracranial pressure and improve cerebral perfusion.

### Mechanism of Action of Diuretics

It involves altering the renal handling of electrolytes, particularly $Na^+$, leading to increased urine production. It is discussed in detail in **Flowchart 61.1**.

**Flowchart 61.1:** Mechanism of action of diuretics.

```
Inhibition of sodium reabsorption
(Diuretics primarily act by inhibiting the reabsorption of Na+ in different segments of the renal tubules.
By blocking sodium reabsorption, diuretics prevent the reabsorption of water, resulting in increased
urine production and decreased extracellular fluid volume)
                    ↓
Increased sodium loss
(The inhibition of sodium reabsorption by diuretics leads to an increase in sodium excretion in the urine.
As sodium is excreted, water follows passively due to osmotic forces, resulting in increased urine output)
                    ↓
Decreased water reabsorption
(Since sodium reabsorption is coupled with water reabsorption in the renal tubules, the inhibition of
sodium reabsorption by diuretics also leads to decreased water reabsorption.
This results in increased water loss in the urine)
                    ↓
Change in tubular filtrate composition
(By altering the reabsorption of sodium and other electrolytes, diuretics cause changes in
the composition of the tubular filtrate. This altered composition affects the osmolarity and electrolyte
balance of the urine, leading to increased urine volume and changes in electrolyte excretion)
```

## Classification Depending upon Site of Action (Fig. 61.1)

### Acting on SITE I (PCT)

> **Which type of diabetes (diabetes mellitus or diabetes insipidus) would result in more diuresis?**
> Diabetes mellitus would result in more diuresis due to osmotic diuresis affecting the PCT and obligatory reabsorption of water whereas diabetes insipidus affect only the facultative reabsorption.

- **Osmotic diuretics (glycerol, sucrose, glucose, mannitol)**
  - Increased osmotically active substances
  - Retain water and increases the urinary volume
  - Changes the composition of tubular filtrate
  - The diabetic patients experience diuresis due to increases glucose in the tubules.
  - Mannitol is used in the treatment of *cerebral edema* for the same reason.
- **Carbonic anhydrase inhibitors (acetazolamide)**
  - The enzyme carbonic anhydrase is inhibited
  - This prevents secretion of H+ and reabsorption of $HCO_3^-$
  - Hence, the Na+ reabsorption is inhibited due to stoppage of Na+-H+ counter transport
  - *Metabolic acidosis* is a main complication, as it results in retention of H+
  - It is used to *lower the intraocular tension*.

### Acting on SITE II (From PCT to LOH)

**Loop diuretics [frusemide (Lasix), ethacrynic acid, bumetanide]**
- It is the most potent diuretic
- It acts on thick ascending limb and blocks *Na+-K+-2Cl-*
- It also disturbs the hyperosmolality of medullary interstitium resulting in the formation of dilute urine.
- Increases the solute load of tubules, and decreases water reabsorption
- Hence causes diuresis
- This diuretic results in intense K+ loss causing hypokalemia
- It is widely used in *treatment of water retention, cardiac failure, pulmonary edema, renal failure, ascites*, etc.

### Acting on SITE III (Early DCT)

**Thiazides (Chlorothiazide, hydrochlorothiazide)**
- *Blocks Na+-Cl- cotransport* in the cells of early DCT
- Increases solute load in the tubule
- Increased water loss
- It is first line of treatment in *hypertension* for decreasing the afterload.

### Acting on SITE IV (Late DCT and Collecting Ducts)

- **Aldosterone antagonist (spironolactone)**
  - It acts on *late DCT and collecting ducts*
  - It *blocks the Na+-K+ ATPase pump* present on basolateral membrane
  - Prevent reabsorption of Na+ and secretion of K+
  - Prevents K+ loss; hence called as potassium *sparing diuretics*
  - It is frequently used as an adjuvant to the loop diuretics to minimize the K+ loss.
- **Directly acting diuretics (triamterene, amiloride)**
  - Directly combine with apical epithelial sodium channels on collecting duct (ENaC) resulting in blockage of reabsorption of Na+.
  - It is also a K+ sparing diuretic, hence conserves potassium.

## ACUTE RENAL FAILURE (ARF)/ACUTE KIDNEY INJURY (AKI)

It is a syndrome which occurs due to *sudden and rapid fall in GFR* which leads to *accumulation of various*

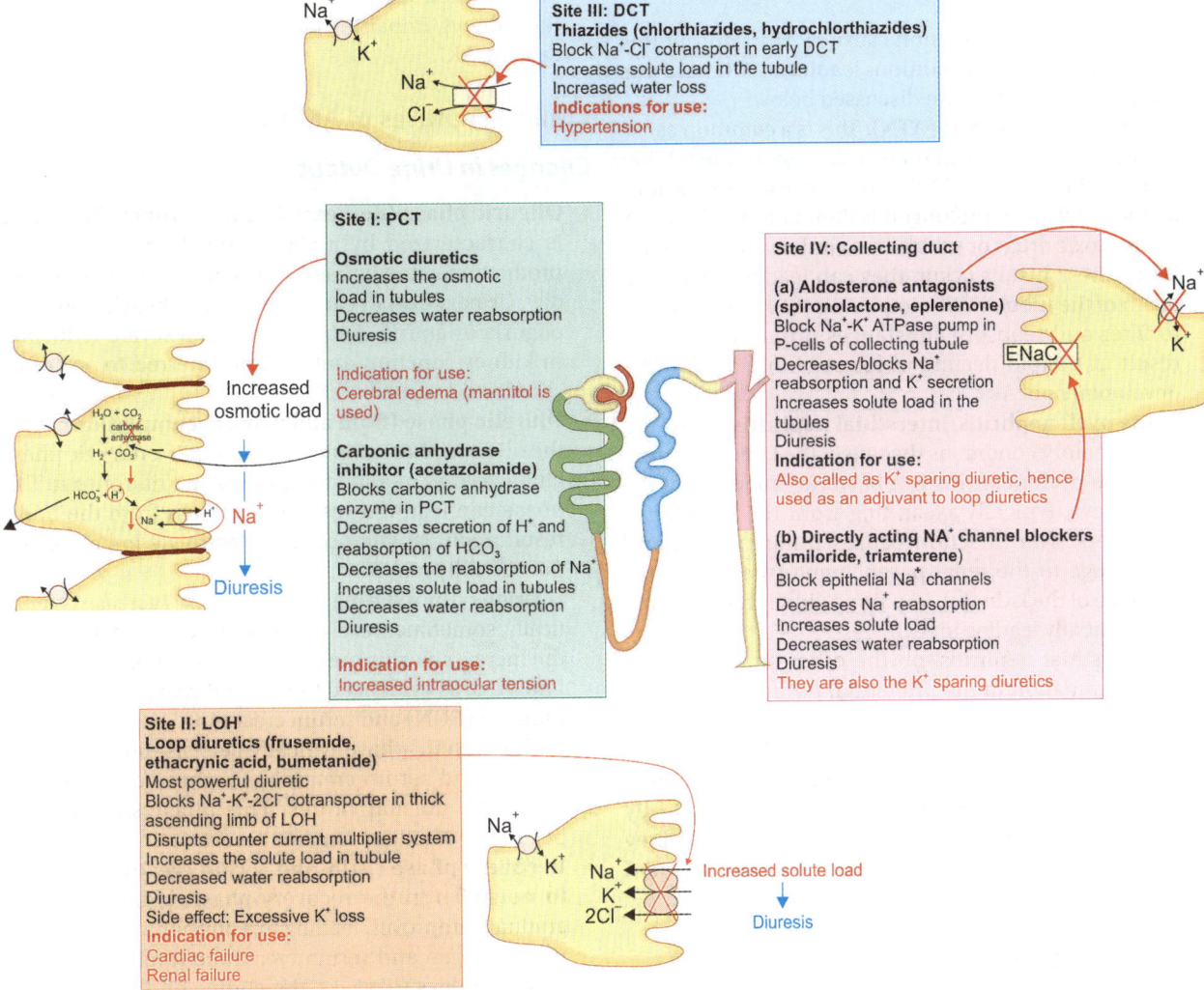

**Fig. 61.1:** Different diuretics and their site of action.

*nitrogenous waste products*, imbalance in pH and electrolyte disturbances.

## Causes of ARF/AKI

### Prerenal Causes

It is the most common cause of ARF, making up to *55% of all the causes*. Various conditions leading to ARF are:
- **Hypovolemia:** When there is a decrease in blood volume, such as in severe dehydration, hemorrhage, or fluid loss from burns; the kidneys receive less blood flow. This reduced blood flow can lead to decreased filtration and impaired kidney function. Without sufficient blood volume, the kidneys struggle to maintain proper filtration and electrolyte balance, potentially leading to AKI.
- **Cardiac failure:** In cases of heart failure, the heart's ability to pump blood effectively is compromised. This can result in decreased blood flow to the kidneys, leading to AKI. Additionally, heart failure can cause fluid buildup in the body, which can further contribute to renal dysfunction by increasing pressure in the kidneys and impairing their ability to filter properly.
- **Renal artery stenosis:** This condition involves narrowing of one or both renal arteries that supply blood to the kidneys. When the blood flow to the kidneys is restricted due to stenosis, it can lead to reduced oxygen and nutrient delivery to the kidney tissues. Over time, this can cause ischemia (lack of blood flow) and damage to the kidneys, potentially resulting in AKI.
- **Peripheral vasodilation (as in anaphylactic shock/sepsis):** In conditions like anaphylactic shock or severe sepsis, there is widespread vasodilation throughout the body's blood vessels. This leads to a significant drop in blood pressure and reduced perfusion to vital organs, including the kidneys. The kidneys rely on adequate blood pressure and perfusion to maintain their function. When blood pressure drops too low due to vasodilation, it can lead to AKI due to inadequate renal blood flow.

## Intrarenal

It is the second most common cause of AKI, contributing *40% of causes*. Various conditions leading to ARF/AKI due to the diseases of kidney are discussed below:

- **Acute tubular necrosis (ATN):** This is a common cause of AKI and occurs when there is damage to the tubular cells of the kidneys. ATN can be caused by various factors, including prolonged ischemia to the kidneys, nephrotoxic drugs or substances, and severe infections. When these insults occur, they can lead to injury and death of the tubular cells, impairing the kidney's ability to filter and reabsorb substances properly. This can result in a rapid decline in kidney function and the development of AKI.
- **Acute pyelonephritis/interstitial nephritis:** These are inflammatory conditions that affect the kidney tissue.
  - Acute pyelonephritis is a bacterial infection of the kidneys, typically ascending from the bladder or ureters. The infection causes inflammation and damage to the renal parenchyma (the functional tissue of the kidneys), impairing kidney function and potentially leading to AKI.
  - Interstitial nephritis, on the other hand, involves inflammation of the interstitial tissue between the kidney tubules. This inflammation can be caused by various factors, including medications (such as antibiotics or NSAIDs), infections, or autoimmune diseases. Interstitial nephritis can lead to AKI by disrupting the normal functioning of the kidney tubules and interfering with urine production and excretion.

## Postrenal Causes

These are least common but most treatable causes, making up to *5% of all the causes*. Various clinical conditions resulting in postrenal AKI, are discussed below:

- **Stone in the ureter or neck of the bladder:** When a stone forms in the ureter) or becomes lodged in the neck of the bladder, it can obstruct urine flow. This obstruction can lead to a buildup of urine in the kidney, causing pressure to build up in the renal pelvis and impairing kidney function. The increased pressure can compress the kidney tissue and interfere with blood flow to the kidney, leading to decreased filtration and the development of AKI. Additionally, if the obstruction is severe or prolonged, it can cause backflow of urine into the kidneys, further contributing to kidney damage and dysfunction.
- **Narrowing of the urethra:** Narrowing or strictures in the urethra can also cause obstructive uropathy and lead to AKI. Urethral strictures can be caused by various factors, including scar tissue formation from previous infections or surgeries, inflammation, or congenital abnormalities. When the urethra is narrowed, urine flow out of the bladder is restricted, leading to urinary retention and buildup of pressure in the bladder and urinary tract. This increased pressure can back up into the kidneys, impairing kidney function and potentially causing AKI.

## Clinical Features of ARF/AKI

### Changes in Urine Output

- **Oliguric phase (decreased urine output):** This phase is characterized by a significant decrease in urine production, often defined as less than 400 milliliters per day. Urinary output can be severely reduced, leading to oliguria or anuria. Anuria indicates a severe reduction in kidney function and is often referred to as "renal shutdown."
- **Diuretic phase (fluid and urine accumulation):** After the oliguric phase, some patients enter a diuretic phase characterized by a sudden increase in urine output. This phase can lead to excessive fluid loss from the body, resulting in dehydration and electrolyte imbalances if not carefully managed.

  Urine output during this phase may increase dramatically, sometimes reaching several liters per day. Despite the increased urine output, kidney function may still be impaired, as evidenced by elevated levels of blood urea nitrogen (BUN) and serum creatinine.

  The diuretic phase typically persists until the levels of BUN and serum creatinine begin to decrease and approach normal values. This phase signifies the beginning of kidney function recovery.
- **Recovery phase (BUN and serum creatinine return to normal):** In the recovery phase, kidney function gradually improves, leading to a normalization of blood urea nitrogen and serum creatinine levels. This phase may take days to weeks, depending on the severity of the initial insult and the patient's overall health status.

### Other Clinical Features

- **Restlessness/anxiety/cramps:** These symptoms can result from electrolyte imbalances, such as hyperkalemia and metabolic acidosis. The altered levels of potassium and acid-base balance can affect nerve and muscle function, leading to neuromuscular irritability and manifestations like restlessness, anxiety, and muscle cramps.
- **Hyponatremia (dilutional):** In AKI, the kidneys may lose their ability to properly regulate sodium levels in the body. This can lead to dilutional hyponatremia, where there is an excess of water relative to sodium in the blood. The impaired excretion of water and sodium retention contribute to this dilutional effect.
- **Hypocalcemia:** The kidneys play a crucial role in maintaining calcium balance in the body by regulating its reabsorption and excretion. In AKI, impaired kidney function can lead to decreased activation of vitamin D, which is necessary for calcium absorption in the gut. Additionally, there may be increased phosphorus levels,

which further lower serum calcium levels through complex interactions.
- **Hyperkalemia (retention of K⁺):** Normally, the kidneys are responsible for excreting excess potassium from the body. In AKI, however, kidney function is impaired, leading to decreased potassium excretion and retention of potassium in the bloodstream. Hyperkalemia can have serious cardiac effects, including arrhythmias and cardiac arrest.
- **Metabolic acidosis (retention of H⁺):** The kidneys play a central role in maintaining acid-base balance by excreting hydrogen ions (H⁺) and reabsorbing bicarbonate ions ($HCO_3^-$). In AKI, the kidneys may lose this ability, resulting in the retention of hydrogen ions and the accumulation of metabolic acids, leading to metabolic acidosis.
- **Hypertension:** AKI can lead to hypertension due to volume overload from fluid retention, activation of the renin-angiotensin-aldosterone system (RAAS), and impaired sodium excretion. However, in some cases, AKI can also cause hypotension due to decreased cardiac output and peripheral vasodilation.
- **Edema (due to retention of fluid):** Impaired kidney function in AKI can lead to fluid retention and sodium retention, resulting in the development of edema. The kidneys are responsible for maintaining fluid balance in the body, and when this function is compromised, excess fluid can accumulate in the interstitial spaces, leading to edema.
- **Anemia:** AKI can contribute to the development of anemia through various mechanisms, including decreased production of erythropoietin, shortened red blood cell lifespan due to uremic toxins, and blood loss from gastrointestinal bleeding or other complications.
- **Platelet dysfunction:** In AKI, uremia and other metabolic disturbances can affect platelet function. Uremic toxins may directly impair platelet function, leading to defects in platelet adhesion and aggregation. Additionally, AKI can cause qualitative and quantitative platelet abnormalities, resulting in an increased risk of bleeding despite a moderate decrease in platelet count.

## Management

- ARF is reversible if proper treatment is started well in time
- Cause should be found out and removed
- Dialysis is required in acute stage

# CHRONIC RENAL FAILURE (CRF)/CHRONIC KIDNEY DISEASE (CKD)

(For case-based learning scenario, refer to early clinical exposure for clinical physiology)

Chronic kidney disease (CKD) is a *progressive* and *irreversible* condition characterized by the *gradual loss of kidney function* over time. It is typically defined by abnormalities in kidney structure or function, such as abnormalities in urine or blood tests, or imaging studies, that persist for at least 3 months. CKD is classified into different stages based on the level of kidney function, as measured by the glomerular filtration rate (GFR), and the presence of kidney damage.

The stages of CKD, according to the National Kidney Foundation, are as follows:
- **Stage 1:** Kidney damage with normal or increased GFR (GFR ≥90 mL/min/1.73 m²)
- **Stage 2:** Mild reduction in GFR (GFR 60–89 mL/min/1.73 m²)
- **Stage 3:** Moderate reduction in GFR (GFR 30–59 mL/min/1.73 m²)
  - *Stage 3a* (GFR 45–59 mL/min/1.73 m²)
  - *Stage 3b* (GFR 30–44 mL/min/1.73 m²).
- **Stage 4:** Severe reduction in GFR (GFR 15–29 mL/min/1.73 m²)
- **Stage 5:** Kidney failure (GFR <15 mL/min/1.73 m²) or end-stage renal disease (ESRD).

## Causes of CKD

- **Diabetes:** Diabetes mellitus, particularly type 1 and type 2 diabetes, is one of the leading causes of CKD. High blood sugar levels over time can damage the small blood vessels in the kidneys, impairing their function.
- **Hypertension:** Chronic hypertension is another major cause of CKD. High blood pressure can damage the small blood vessels in the kidneys and cause scarring, reducing kidney function.
- **Glomerulonephritis:** Glomerulonephritis refers to inflammation of the glomeruli, the tiny filtering units in the kidneys. Chronic glomerulonephritis can lead to scarring and impaired kidney function.
- **Polycystic kidney disease (PKD):** PKD is an inherited disorder characterized by the growth of cysts in the kidneys. Over time, these cysts can enlarge and lead to kidney damage and CKD.
- **Autoimmune diseases:** Certain autoimmune diseases, such as lupus nephritis and vasculitis, can cause inflammation and damage to the kidneys, leading to CKD.
- **Obstructive uropathy:** Conditions that obstruct urine flow, such as kidney stones, enlarged prostate, or urinary tract tumors, can cause damage to the kidneys over time, leading to CKD.
- **Recurrent kidney infections:** Chronic or recurrent kidney infections, particularly if left untreated, can cause scarring and damage to the kidneys, leading to CKD.
- **Interstitial nephritis:** Interstitial nephritis is inflammation of the kidney's tubules and surrounding structures. It can be caused by medications, infections, autoimmune diseases, or other factors and can lead to CKD if left untreated.
- **Congenital abnormalities:** Some individuals may be born with structural abnormalities of the kidneys or

urinary tract that can predispose them to CKD later in life.
- **Other factors:** Other factors that can contribute to CKD include obesity, smoking, aging, exposure to toxins or heavy metals, and certain medications, such as nonsteroidal anti-inflammatory drugs (NSAIDs) and some antibiotics.

## Pathophysiology

Pathophysiology of CKD is discussed in **Figure 61.2**.

## Clinical Features of CKD

- **Isosthenuria:** Isosthenuria refers to the *inability of the kidneys to adequately concentrate or dilute urine*. This occurs because the damaged nephrons in CKD lose their ability to respond to changes in water and electrolyte balance, resulting in urine with a fixed osmolality close to that of plasma.
- **Edema:** Edema is a common manifestation of CKD due to *fluid retention* resulting from impaired kidney function. The kidneys are unable to effectively excrete excess fluid and sodium, leading to fluid accumulation in the body's tissues.
- **Hypertension:** CKD often leads to hypertension due to various factors, including volume overload, activation of the renin-angiotensin-aldosterone system, and impaired sodium excretion by the kidneys.
- **Anemia:** *Decreased production of erythropoietin* by the damaged kidneys leads to anemia in CKD. Erythropoietin is a hormone produced by the kidneys that stimulates red blood cell production in the bone marrow. Without adequate erythropoietin, there is a decrease in red blood cell production, leading to anemia.
- **Restlessness:** Restlessness can result from various factors associated with CKD, including *electrolyte imbalances, metabolic acidosis, and uremia*.
- **Urinous breath:** Uremic toxins that accumulate in the body due to impaired kidney function can lead to a characteristic *urinous or ammonia-like odor* on the breath.
- **Secondary hyperparathyroidism and renal osteodystrophy:** CKD can lead to secondary hyperparathyroidism due to hypocalcemia and impaired vitamin D activation. Overactivity of the parathyroid glands results in increased secretion of parathyroid hormone (PTH), leading to *bone resorption and the development of renal osteodystrophy*.

## Blood Investigations

- **Increased blood urea and serum creatinine levels** are hallmark laboratory findings in CKD, reflecting impaired kidney function and decreased glomerular filtration rate (GFR).
- **Electrolyte imbalances:** CKD can disrupt electrolyte balance, leading to abnormalities such as hyponatremia, hypocalcemia, hypermagnesemia, hyperkalemia, and hyperphosphatemia
- **Metabolic acidosis:** Impaired kidney function in CKD results in the accumulation of metabolic acids and the inability to excrete hydrogen ions, leading to metabolic acidosis.
- **Platelet dysfunction:** CKD can cause platelet dysfunction, resulting in defects in platelet adhesion and aggregation, which may increase bleeding time.

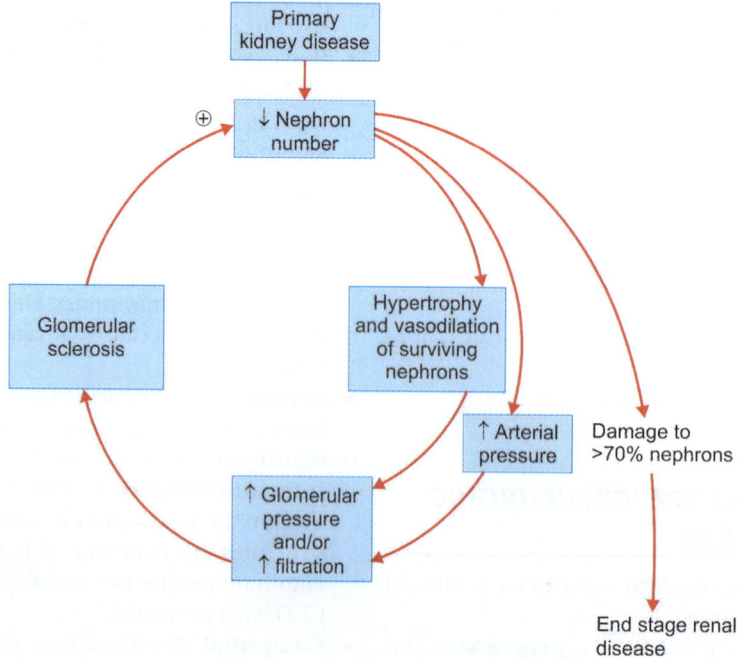

**Fig. 61.2:** Pathophysiology of CKD.

## Management of CKD

Since there is a *progressive loss of the nephrons in CKD*, the mainstay of the management stays with dialysis and renal transplant, if a compatible kidney donor is available.

## DIALYSIS/ARTIFICIAL KIDNEY

It is a process by which various metabolic nitrogenous waste products are removed from the body by artificial means.

### Principle

Process of simple diffusion across the semipermeable membrane and the unwanted waste products are removed **(Fig. 61.3)**.

### Types

Hemodialysis, peritoneal dialysis.

### *Hemodialysis*

In hemodialysis, blood is circulated outside the body through a machine called a *dialyzer*, which acts as an artificial kidney.

#### Components

- **Blood delivery system:** This includes vascular access, which can be in the form of an arteriovenous fistula, arteriovenous graft, or central venous catheter. The access site allows blood to be withdrawn from the body and returned after passing through the dialyzer.
- **Dialyzer:** Also known as an artificial kidney, the dialyzer is the central component of the hemodialysis machine. It contains thousands of tiny hollow fibers made of a *semipermeable membrane (cellophane membranes)* that allows for the exchange of solutes and fluids between the blood and dialysate.
- **Dialysate:** This is the fluid that circulates on the other side of the semipermeable membrane within the dialyzer. *The composition of the dialysate is carefully controlled to mimic the composition of normal plasma, except for specific waste products like urea, creatinine, phosphates, urates, and sulfates, which are removed from the blood during dialysis*.

#### Procedure

- A vascular access site, typically in the form of an arteriovenous fistula, arteriovenous graft, or central venous catheter, is established to allow blood to be withdrawn from the body and returned after passing through the dialyzer.
- The patient's blood is pumped from the vascular access site into the dialyzer at a controlled rate, usually between 300 and 450 milliliters per minute.
- Heparin, a medication that prevents blood clotting, is often administered to the patient to prevent clotting within the dialyzer and blood tubing.

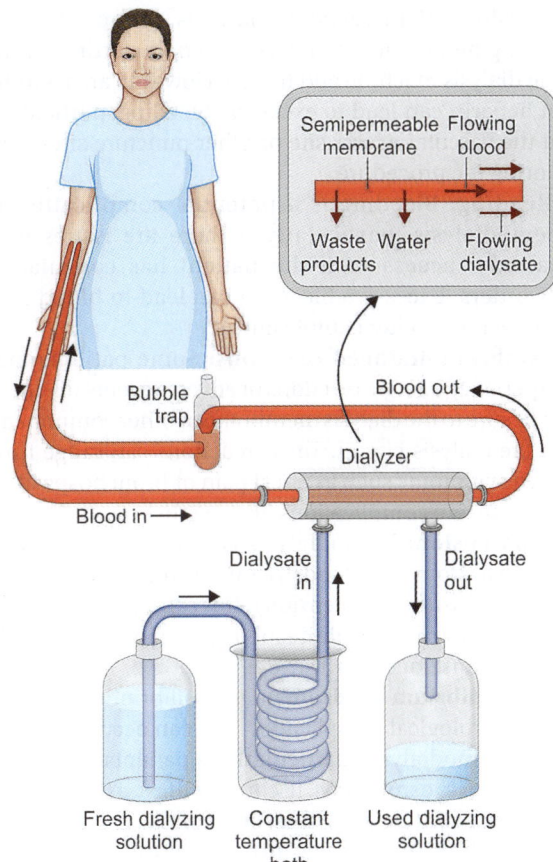

**Fig. 61.3:** Principle of dialysis.

- As the blood flows through the dialyzer, waste products and excess fluids are removed from the blood across the semipermeable membrane, while essential substances are retained in the bloodstream.
- After passing through the dialyzer, the purified blood is returned to the patient's circulation through the vascular access site.
- Hemodialysis sessions typically last between *3 and 6 hours* and are usually performed thrice a week in a dialysis center. The frequency and duration of dialysis sessions may vary depending on the patient's condition and prescribed treatment regimen.

#### Complications

- **Infection:** Infection at the site of vascular access, such as an arteriovenous fistula or catheter insertion site, is a common complication of hemodialysis. It can lead to local inflammation, systemic infection (sepsis), and potentially serious complications if not promptly treated.
- **Sepsis:** Sepsis is a life-threatening condition that can occur when an infection spreads throughout the bloodstream. Hemodialysis patients are at increased risk of developing sepsis, particularly if they have vascular access-related infections or if the dialysis equipment is not properly maintained and sterilized.

- **Overdose of heparin:** Heparin is commonly used during hemodialysis to prevent blood clotting within the dialysis machine and tubing. However, an overdose of heparin can lead to excessive bleeding, particularly at the vascular access site or other puncture sites used during the procedure.
- **Bleeding:** Bleeding is a potential complication of hemodialysis, particularly if there are issues with vascular access or if the patient has coagulation disorders. Excessive bleeding can lead to blood loss, anemia, and other complications.
- **Membrane-induced reactions:** Some patients may experience allergic reactions or adverse events related to exposure to the dialysis membrane or other components of the dialysis circuit. These reactions can range from mild symptoms such as chest pain or bronchospasm to more severe complications like anaphylaxis.
- **Hypotension:** Hemodialysis can lead to rapid fluid removal from the bloodstream, resulting in a drop in blood pressure (hypotension). This can cause symptoms such as dizziness, lightheadedness, nausea, and even loss of consciousness if severe.
- **Disequilibrium syndrome:** Disequilibrium syndrome is a neurological complication that can occur during or after hemodialysis, particularly in patients with rapid changes in osmolality. It can manifest as headache, nausea, vomiting, dizziness, or seizures.
- **Electrolyte imbalance and arrhythmias:** Sudden changes in electrolyte levels, such as sodium, potassium, and calcium, during hemodialysis can lead to electrolyte imbalances and potentially life-threatening cardiac arrhythmias if not properly managed.

## *Peritoneal Dialysis*

In peritoneal dialysis (PD), a dialysate solution is infused into the peritoneal cavity through a catheter. The solution is left in the abdomen for a specified dwell time (usually 20–60 minutes), during which waste products and excess fluids diffuse across the peritoneal membrane. After the dwell time, the used dialysate is drained out, and fresh dialysate is infused for the next cycle. This process can be repeated multiple times throughout the day and can also be done overnight, allowing for continuous dialysis over 24–40 hours.

### Complications of Peritoneal Dialysis

Peritonitis is a common and serious complication of peritoneal dialysis, where the peritoneal cavity becomes infected. This can lead to *abdominal pain, fever, cloudy dialysate, and systemic symptoms* if not promptly treated with antibiotics.

### Hemodialysis vs Peritoneal Dialysis

- Disequilibrium syndrome, characterized by neurological symptoms like headache and dizziness, is *less common in peritoneal dialysis* compared to hemodialysis. This is because the fluid and solute removal in PD is gradual and more continuous, leading to fewer rapid changes in osmolality.
- Unlike hemodialysis, where heparin is often used to prevent clotting in the dialysis circuit, peritoneal dialysis *does not require anticoagulation*. Therefore, patients on PD are not at risk of heparin-induced side effects such as bleeding or heparin-induced thrombocytopenia.
- Peritoneal dialysis does not involve rapid changes in fluid and electrolyte balance like hemodialysis, *reducing the risk of electrolyte imbalances and associated cardiac arrhythmias.*
- Peritoneal dialysis does not involve the use of a semipermeable membrane like hemodialysis, so there is *no risk of hypersensitivity reactions to the dialysis membrane.*

## RENAL TRANSPLANTATION

It is considered the treatment of choice for many patients with end-stage renal disease (ESRD) because it offers the best chance for long-term survival and improved quality of life compared to dialysis. However, there are specific indications for renal transplantation, as well as legal and ethical issues that must be considered.

Indications and prerequisites for renal transplantation:

- **End-stage renal disease (ESRD):** Renal transplantation is indicated for patients with irreversible kidney failure who require dialysis for survival.
- **Adequate physical and psychosocial health:** Candidates for renal transplantation should be in relatively good physical health and have adequate cardiovascular function to undergo surgery. Additionally, they should have appropriate psychosocial support systems in place to help with the post-transplant recovery process.
- **No absolute contraindications:** While certain medical conditions may make transplantation more challenging, there are generally no absolute contraindications to renal transplantation. However, careful assessment and management of comorbidities are necessary to optimize transplant outcomes.
- **Suitable donor availability:** Availability of suitable living or deceased donors is also an important consideration for renal transplantation. Living donors may be related or unrelated to the recipient and must undergo thorough evaluation to ensure donor safety and compatibility.

### Legal and Ethical Issues

- **Organ procurement and allocation:** Legal frameworks govern organ procurement and allocation to ensure fair and equitable distribution of donor organs. This includes criteria for determining priority on transplant waiting lists based on factors such as medical urgency, tissue matching, and time on the waiting list.
- **Informed consent:** Both donors and recipients must provide informed consent before undergoing transplantation. This involves a comprehensive

understanding of the risks, benefits, and alternatives to transplantation, as well as the implications for post-transplant care and lifestyle.
- **Ethical considerations:** Ethical considerations surrounding renal transplantation include equity in access to transplantation, organ donation, allocation of scarce resources, and ensuring respect for donor autonomy and recipient autonomy.
- **Immunosuppressive therapy:** After transplantation, recipients require lifelong immunosuppressive therapy to prevent rejection of the donor organ. Legal and ethical considerations include ensuring access to necessary medications, managing potential side effects and complications, and addressing nonadherence to medication regimens.
- **Financial and insurance issues:** Renal transplantation can be costly, and financial considerations may impact access to transplantation and post-transplant care. Legal and ethical frameworks aim to ensure equitable access to transplantation regardless of financial status and to protect recipients from financial hardship related to transplant-related expenses.

## SUMMARY

- Diuretics are medications that increase urine production, used in conditions like heart failure and hypertension. They work by targeting different parts of the kidney to promote sodium and water excretion. Understanding their physiological basis involves knowing kidney anatomy and how it regulates fluid balance. Different diuretic classes have unique mechanisms and are chosen based on the underlying condition and patient factors.
- AKI is a sudden decline in kidney function, leading to waste accumulation and electrolyte imbalances. Its basis lies in disruptions to kidney blood flow, filtration, and tubular function. Clinical signs include low urine output, electrolyte disturbances, and fluid overload. Management involves treating the cause, correcting imbalances, and sometimes using dialysis.
- CKD is a gradual loss of kidney function over time, leading to various complications. It stems from structural and functional kidney changes like scarring and damage. Clinical features include hypertension, anemia, and bone disorders. Management aims to slow progression, control symptoms, and may include dialysis or transplantation.
- Dialysis is a treatment to remove waste and fluids when kidneys fail. It uses a semipermeable membrane to filter blood and remove toxins. Dialysis is vital for patients with severe kidney dysfunction and is typically done several times a week.

## LET US SEE, HOW MUCH YOU HAVE LEARNT?

 *Review Questions*

### Long/Short Answer Questions

Q1. Define diuretics. What is the mechanism of action of?
   a. Osmotic diuretics
   b. Loop diuretics
   c. Potassium sparing diuretic
Q2. Why mannitol is used in a patient of cerebral edema?
Q3. What is the physiological basis of anemia in a patient of CKD?
Q4. Why a patient of CKD gets fractures of his bones easily?
Q5. What is dialysis? What are the indications, procedure and complications of hemodialysis?
Q6. What medicolegal precautions should be observed for a patient posted for renal transplantation?

### Explain Why? (Reasoning Questions)

Q1. Loop diuretics are effective in treating edema associated with heart failure and renal disorders.
Q2. Potassium-sparing diuretics are often prescribed in combination with loop diuretics.
Q3. Patients with CKD are at increased risk of developing metabolic acidosis and how this relates to renal dysfunction.
Q4. NSAIDs can exacerbate renal dysfunction in patients with conditions such as CKD or heart failure.

 *Critical Thinking Case-Based Questions*

Q1. Subhash, a 60-year-old man, presented to ER with complaints of swelling in his legs, difficulty breathing, and fatigue. He had a history of uncontrolled hypertension. Despite being on multiple medications, including diuretics, he had noticed worsening symptoms over the past few weeks. Examination revealed bilateral pedal edema, jugular venous distension, and crackles in the lung bases. His serum electrolytes showed low potassium levels.
   Based on the given scenario, answer the following questions:
   a. What is the probable diagnosis?
   b. Explain the physiological basis of diuretics in managing fluid balance.

c. What mechanisms might contribute to this patient's symptoms of pedal edema and jugular venous distension?

d. What potential complications might arise from diuretic therapy?

## Multiple Choice Questions

**Q1.** A 65-year-old patient with congestive heart failure presents with worsening dyspnea and lower extremity edema. Which of the following diuretics would be most appropriate for initial management to reduce fluid overload?
  a. Furosemide (loop diuretic)
  b. Hydrochlorothiazide (thiazide diuretic)
  c. Spironolactone (potassium-sparing diuretic)
  d. Mannitol (osmotic diuretic)

**Q2.** A 50-year-old male with a history of diabetes and hypertension is admitted to the hospital with acute kidney injury. Laboratory tests reveal elevated serum creatinine and blood urea nitrogen (BUN), along with oliguria. Which of the following best describes the underlying pathophysiological mechanism of AKI in this patient?
  a. Tubular obstruction due to kidney stones
  b. Reduced renal blood flow leading to ischemic injury
  c. Glomerular inflammation causing nephrotic syndrome
  d. Autoimmune attack on renal tubules

**Q3.** A 60-year-old female with a long-standing history of poorly controlled hypertension and proteinuria is diagnosed with stage 3 chronic kidney disease. Which of the following physiological changes is most likely to contribute to the progression of CKD in this patient?
  a. Glomerular hyperfiltration
  b. Tubulointerstitial fibrosis
  c. Decreased renin-angiotensin-aldosterone system activity
  d. Increased erythropoietin production

**Q4.** A 70-year-old man with end-stage renal disease (ESRD) undergoing hemodialysis develops hypotension and dizziness during his dialysis session. Which of the following physiological mechanisms is the most likely cause of his symptoms?
  a. Rapid removal of potassium ions
  b. Hypovolemia due to ultrafiltration
  c. Excessive secretion of antidiuretic hormone (ADH)
  d. Hyperkalemia due to inadequate dialysate potassium concentration

**Q5.** A 55-year-old woman with ESRD is being evaluated for renal transplantation. Which of the following physiological principles best explains the rationale for renal transplant as a treatment option for her?
  a. Restoration of glomerular filtration rate (GFR)
  b. Reduction of proteinuria and urinary sediment
  c. Correction of electrolyte imbalances
  d. Improvement of tubular reabsorption efficiency

**Q6.** Akash, a 45-year-old man, was admitted to the hospital with symptoms of weakness, fatigue, and decreased urine output. His medical history revealed that he recently underwent a blood transfusion for severe anemia secondary to chronic kidney disease. However, shortly after the transfusion, he developed acute kidney injury (AKI). Laboratory tests show elevated serum creatinine and urea levels, along with signs of hemolysis. Which of the following physiological mechanisms best explains the clinical features of AKI observed in Akash following the incompatible blood transfusion?
  a. Tubular obstruction due to hemoglobinuria
  b. Ischemic injury to renal tubules from decreased blood flow
  c. Glomerular inflammation leading to nephrotic syndrome
  d. Direct toxic effect of incompatible blood on kidney tubules

**Q7.** Mr Patel, a 60-year-old man with a history of chronic kidney disease (CKD) stage 4, presents to his nephrologist with complaints of bone pain and muscle weakness. He has been undergoing hemodialysis three times a week for the past year due to declining kidney function. Despite adherence to his dialysis regimen and phosphate-binding medications, he continues to experience worsening bone symptoms.
Which of the following physiological mechanisms is most likely contributing to the bone manifestations observed in Mr Patel's condition?
  a. Increased parathyroid hormone (PTH) secretion
  b. Excessive vitamin D supplementation
  c. Accelerated bone resorption due to hypercalcemia
  d. Impaired osteoblast function

### ANSWERS
**1.** a    **2.** b    **3.** b    **4.** b    **5.** a    **6.** a    **7.** a

# Urinary Bladder and its Applied Physiology

**62 CHAPTER**

**COMPETENCY ADDRESSED**

**PY7.6:** Describe the innervations of urinary bladder, physiology of micturition and its abnormalities.
**PY7.9:** Describe cystometry and discuss the normal cystometrogram.

**LEARNING OBJECTIVES**

**At the end of this chapter, the learner should be able to:**
- Describe the functional anatomy of urinary bladder.
- Describe the innervation of urinary bladder.
- Describe the micturition reflex.
- Describe the physiology of neurogenic bladder.

## FUNCTIONAL ANATOMY OF URINARY BLADDER

The urinary bladder is a hollow, smooth muscle chamber consisting of two main parts: the body and the neck. The body serves as the primary reservoir for urine, while the neck is a funnel-shaped extension that connects with the urethra. The detrusor muscle, the smooth muscle of the bladder, contracts to increase bladder pressure during urination, facilitating the emptying process. The detrusor muscle cells are interconnected, allowing for coordinated contraction of the entire bladder **(Fig. 62.1)**.

Located on the posterior wall of the bladder, above the bladder neck, is a triangular area called the trigone. This area serves as a landmark, with smooth mucosa, distinguishing it from the folded mucosa elsewhere in the bladder. The ureters enter the bladder at the upper angles of the trigone, while the bladder neck opens into the posterior urethra at its lowermost apex.

Each ureter courses obliquely through the detrusor muscle before entering the bladder and then passes beneath the bladder mucosa before emptying into the bladder. The bladder neck, also known as the posterior urethra, is composed of detrusor muscle interlaced with elastic tissue and contains the internal sphincter muscle, which maintains tone to prevent urine flow until bladder pressure exceeds a critical threshold.

Beyond the posterior urethra, the urethra traverses the urogenital diaphragm, which houses the external sphincter of the bladder. Unlike the smooth muscle of the bladder, the external sphincter is a voluntary skeletal muscle under conscious control, allowing individuals to regulate urination voluntarily, even when involuntary mechanisms attempt to empty the bladder.

### Urinary Sphincters Guarding the Urinary Bladder

Urinary sphincters, diligent sentinels of the bladder's domain, regulate the flow with precision, ensuring retention and release in perfect harmony. They are discussed in **Flowchart 62.1**.

### Innervation of Urinary Bladder (Figs. 62.2 and 62.3)

- **Sensory innervation of bladder:**
  - Pelvic splanchnic nerves S2, S3 and S4
  - Hypogastric plexus (T11–L2)
  - Sensory fibers run in fasciculus gracilis to spinal pontine and supra pontine centers
  - Sensation of bladder pain is carried by anterolateral column
- **Motor innervation of bladder:**
  - Sympathetic motor fibers (T10–L2) via hypogastric nerves–relaxes bladder
  - Parasympathetic motor innervation from sacral detrusor nerves S2, S3 and S4–voiding
  - Somatic motor innervation from sacral pudendal nucleus S2, S3 and S4

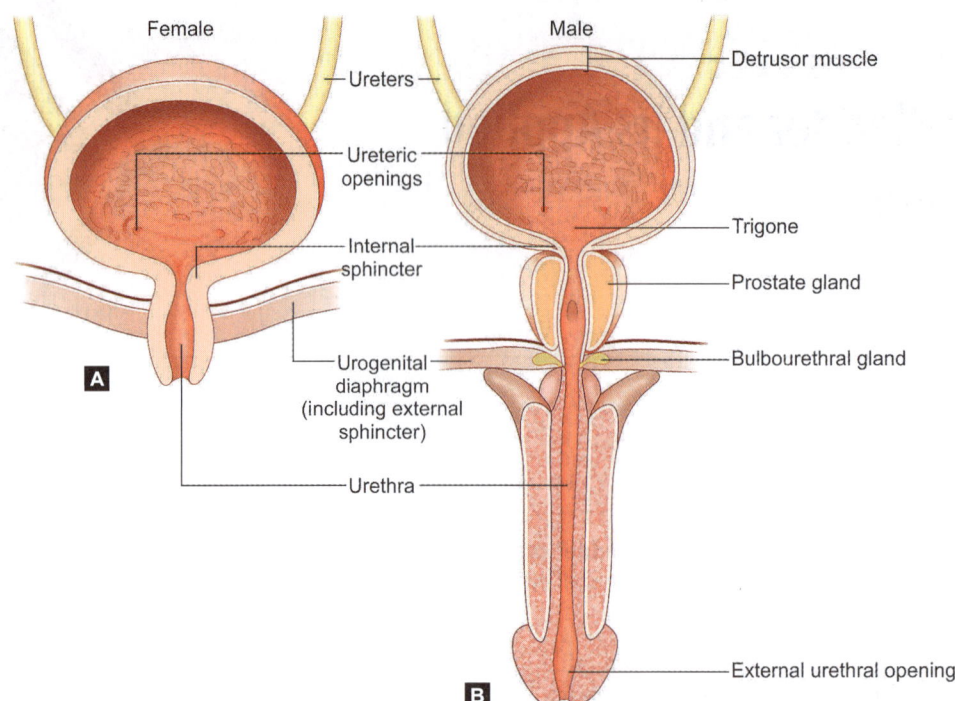

**Fig. 62.1:** Functional anatomy of urinary bladder: (A) Female; (B) Male.

**Flowchart 62.1:** Urinary sphincters and their role in bladder regulation.

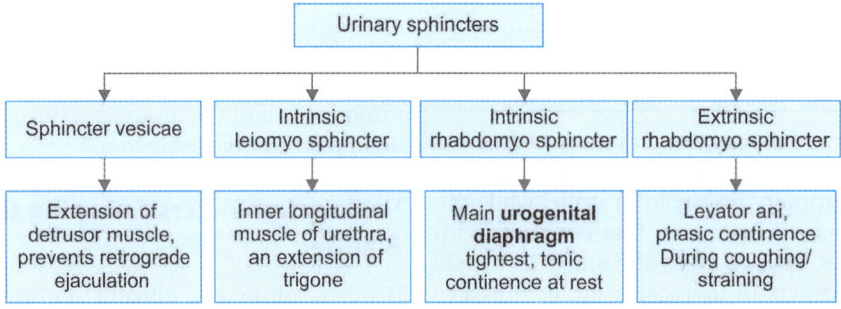

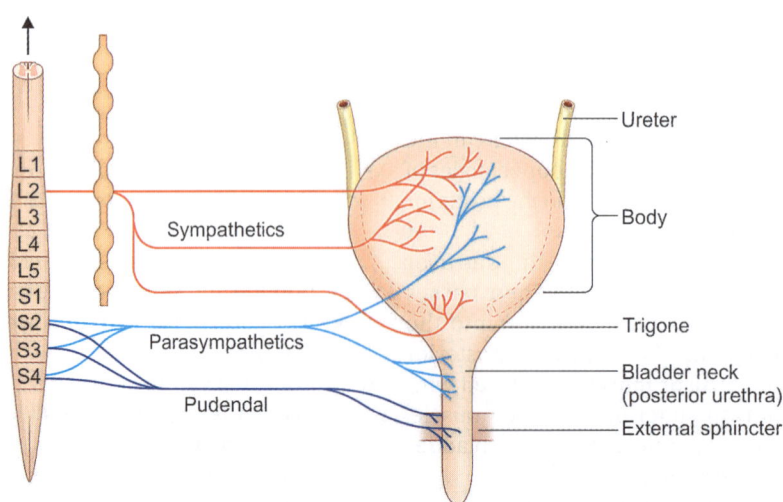

**Fig. 62.2:** Innervation of urinary bladder.

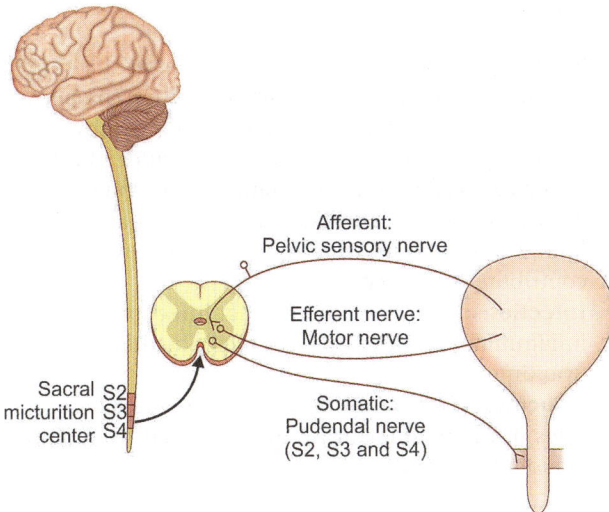

**Fig. 62.3:** Sacral micturition pathway.

## Micturition Reflex

It is a single complete cycle of
- Progressive and rapid rise in pressure
- Period of sustained pressure
- Return of pressure to basal tone of bladder

The micturition reflex is a spinal cord reflex that controls the emptying of the bladder **(Fig. 62.4)**. Its key components include afferent pathways via the pelvic nerves, a center known as the sacral micturition center, and efferent pathways through the parasympathetic pelvic nerves. *This reflex allows for the coordinated contraction of the bladder and relaxation of the urinary sphincters to facilitate urine release.*

## Role of Higher Centers

However, higher centers in the brain also play a crucial role in regulating the micturition reflex. These higher centers include facilitatory areas in the pons and hypothalamus, as well as inhibitory areas in the midbrain. They exert final control over micturition, maintaining partial inhibition of the reflex except when desired.

> **The reflex:**
> - Afferent: Pelvic nerves
> - Center: Sacral micturition center
> - Efferent: Parasympathetic pelvic nerves
>
> **Higher centers:**
> - Facilitatory area in pons and hypothalamus
> - Inhibitory area in mid brain
> - Exert a final control of micturition
>   - Keep the micturition reflex partially inhibited except when desired
>   - Can prevent micturition even if reflex occurs
>   - Can facilitate SMC, to initiate a reflex

These higher centers can prevent micturition even if the reflex occurs, allowing individuals to consciously delay urination when necessary. They can also facilitate the sacral micturition center to initiate the reflex when appropriate, ensuring efficient bladder emptying while maintaining control over the process. This complex interplay between spinal cord reflexes and higher brain centers ensures effective urinary control and prevents unwanted voiding.

## URODYNAMIC STUDIES (CYSTOMETRY AND RADIOGRAPHIC TECHNIQUE)

Urodynamic studies, such as cystometry, are valuable tools in assessing bladder function and diagnosing various urinary disorders:

## Objectives of Urodynamic Study

- **Accommodation:** Assessing the bladder's ability to expand and hold urine without significant increases in pressure.
- **Total bladder capacity:** Determining the maximum volume of urine the bladder can hold.
- **Bladder contractions:** Identifying involuntary contractions of the bladder muscles.
- **Voluntary bladder control:** Evaluating the patient's ability to initiate and control bladder emptying voluntarily.
- **Unstable bladder activity:** Detecting abnormal bladder contractions or overactivity that can lead to urinary urgency or incontinence.
- **Bladder sensations:** Assessing the patient's perception of bladder fullness and urge to void.

## Types

- **Voiding cystometry:** Measures bladder function during the storage and voiding phases, assessing detrusor muscle activity and pressure changes.

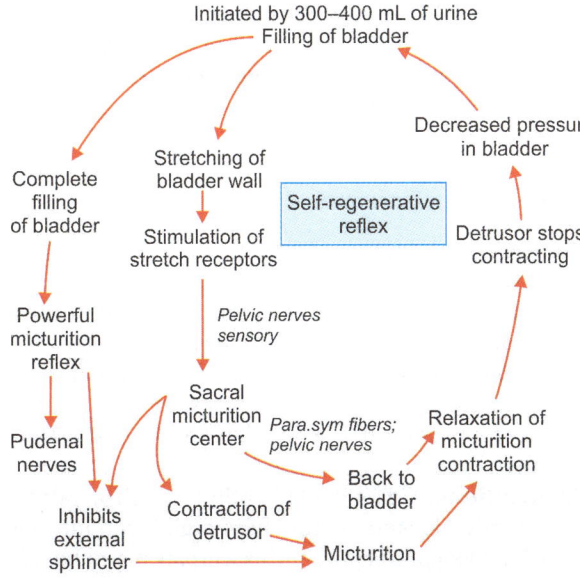

**Fig. 62.4:** Micturition reflex (self-regenerative reflex).

- **Static cystometry:** Focuses solely on the storage phase, evaluating bladder capacity and pressure without assessing voiding.

## Procedure

- The patient is catheterized to empty the bladder completely before the procedure.
- The bladder is filled with sterile water or saline in small increments, typically 50 mL at a time.
- Simultaneously, intravesical pressure and bladder volume are recorded at each increment of fluid injection.
- The relationship between intravesical pressure and bladder volume is graphically plotted to assess bladder function and detect abnormalities.
- Urodynamic studies provide valuable information for diagnosing conditions such as urinary incontinence, neurogenic bladder dysfunction, and bladder outlet obstruction. They help guide treatment decisions and monitor the effectiveness of interventions aimed at improving bladder function and urinary symptoms **(Fig. 62.5)**.

## NEUROGENIC BLADDER

Neurogenic bladder refers to dysfunction of the bladder due to neurological damage or disease. Conditions such as spinal cord injury, multiple sclerosis, or stroke can disrupt the normal neural pathways involved in bladder control. This disruption can lead to various bladder dysfunctions, including urinary retention, urinary incontinence, or a combination of both. Various types of bladder dysfunctions are described below:

## Atonic Bladder

An atonic bladder, also known as a de-afferented bladder, sensory paralytic bladder, or tabetic bladder, refers to a condition characterized by *loss of sensation of bladder fullness and impaired detrusor muscle function,* leading to urinary retention and overflow incontinence.

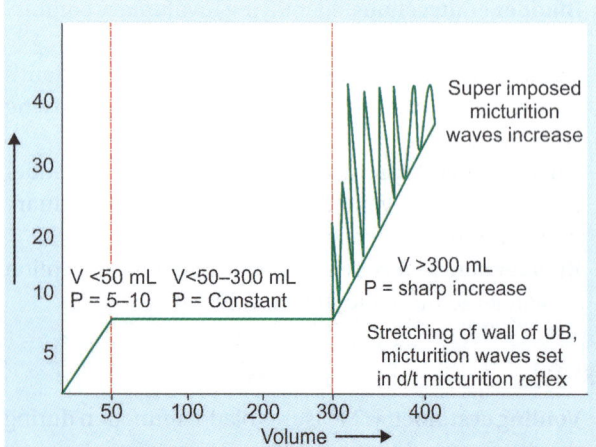

**Fig. 62.5:** Pressure changes in the bladder.

## Causes

- **Neurological damage:** Damage to the nerves that supply the bladder, often due to conditions such as spinal cord injury, multiple sclerosis, or diabetic neuropathy.
- **Sensory loss:** Loss of sensation of bladder fullness, which can result from nerve damage or dysfunction.
- **Medications:** Certain medications, such as anticholinergics or opioids, can impair bladder function and contribute to urinary retention.
- **Infections:** Chronic urinary tract infections or other inflammatory conditions can affect bladder function over time.
- **Structural abnormalities:** Rarely, structural abnormalities of the bladder or urethra can lead to impaired bladder function.

## Clinical Features

- **Urinary retention:** Inability to fully empty the bladder, leading to increased residual urine volume.
- **Overflow incontinence:** Dribbling of urine due to bladder overdistension and involuntary leakage.
- **Loss of sensation:** Patients may not feel the sensation of bladder fullness or the urge to urinate.
- **Increased residual volume:** Measurement of residual urine volume after voiding may reveal elevated levels.
- **Increased intravesical pressure:** Bladder pressure may rise due to incomplete emptying and bladder distension.

Overall, an atonic bladder results in significant functional impairment and can lead to complications such as urinary tract infections, bladder stones, and renal damage if left untreated. Management typically involves bladder retraining, intermittent catheterization, medications to improve bladder contractility, and addressing any underlying causes contributing to the condition.

## Motor Paralytic Bladder

A de-deafferented bladder, also known as a motor paralytic bladder, is a condition characterized by *dysfunction of the motor fibers innervating the bladder,* resulting in impaired bladder contractility and inability to initiate micturition.

## Causes

- **Neurological damage:** Damage to the motor nerves that supply the bladder, often due to conditions such as spinal cord injury, cauda equina syndrome, poliomyelitis, nerve damage during pelvic surgery.
- **Neurogenic bladder:** Disorders affecting the nervous system, such as multiple sclerosis or spinal cord tumors, can disrupt motor nerve function and lead to bladder paralysis.
- **Medications:** Certain medications, such as alpha-adrenergic blockers or anticholinergics, can interfere with bladder contractility and exacerbate motor bladder dysfunction.

- **Trauma:** Pelvic trauma or injury to the spinal cord can damage motor nerve fibers and impair bladder function.

## Clinical Features

- **Inability to initiate micturition:** Patients are unable to voluntarily initiate the process of urination, leading to urinary retention.
- **Weak urinary stream:** When able to void, patients may experience a weak urinary stream due to decreased bladder contractility.
- **Urinary hesitancy:** Difficulty starting the urine stream despite feeling the urge to urinate.
- **Incomplete emptying:** Despite efforts to void, the bladder may not completely empty, leading to increased residual urine volume.
- **Bladder distension:** Over time, chronic urinary retention can lead to bladder distension and increased bladder capacity.

Management of a de-efferented bladder typically involves interventions aimed at improving bladder emptying and reducing urinary retention. This may include intermittent catheterization, pharmacotherapy to enhance bladder contractility, and addressing any underlying neurological conditions contributing to the dysfunction. In severe cases, surgical options such as bladder augmentation or urinary diversion may be considered. Early diagnosis and management are essential to prevent complications such as urinary tract infections and renal damage.

## Decentralized Bladder

An autonomous bladder, also known as a decentralized bladder, refers to a condition characterized by *dysfunction of both afferent (sensory) and efferent (motor) pathways involved in bladder control*. This results in impaired bladder sensation and contractility, leading to urinary dysfunction.

## Causes

- **Spinal cord disorders:** Conditions affecting the spinal cord, such as tumors, spina bifida, or traumatic injuries, can disrupt the communication between the bladder and the central nervous system.
- **Neurological damage:** Damage to the micturition centers in the brain or spinal cord can disrupt the neural pathways involved in bladder control.
- **Neurogenic bladder:** Various neurological conditions, including multiple sclerosis, Parkinson's disease, or stroke, can affect bladder function and lead to autonomous bladder dysfunction.

## Features of Autonomous Bladder

- **Automatic bladder function:** Due to disruption of neural pathways, bladder function becomes automatic and uncontrolled by conscious effort. Patients may experience urinary urgency and frequency without being able to voluntarily inhibit voiding.
- **Atonic bladder symptoms:** Similar to features seen in atonic bladder dysfunction, patients may experience urinary retention, overflow incontinence, and dribbling of urine due to impaired detrusor muscle function and loss of bladder sensation.
- **Increased residual volume:** Measurement of residual urine volume after voiding may reveal elevated levels, indicating incomplete bladder emptying.
- **Urinary tract infections:** Chronic urinary retention and incomplete bladder emptying increase the risk of urinary tract infections, which can further exacerbate bladder dysfunction.
- **Bladder distension:** Chronic bladder overdistension due to impaired contractility can lead to bladder wall hypertrophy and decreased bladder compliance.

Management of an autonomous bladder typically involves a multidisciplinary approach aimed at optimizing bladder function and minimizing complications. This may include intermittent catheterization to empty the bladder, pharmacotherapy to improve bladder contractility, and addressing any underlying neurological conditions contributing to the dysfunction. Regular monitoring and follow-up are essential to prevent complications such as urinary tract infections and renal damage.

## Reflex Bladder

A reflex or automatic bladder refers to a condition characterized by the *loss of higher neural controls over bladder function, leading to uncontrolled and involuntary bladder emptying* mediated by local spinal reflex pathways.

## Causes

- **Spinal cord lesions:** Lesions or injuries to the spinal cord above the level of the spinal micturition center, such as spinal cord injury or spinal cord tumors, can disrupt descending neural pathways responsible for voluntary bladder control.
- **Neurological disorders:** Certain neurological conditions, including transverse myelitis or spinal cord infarction, can impair higher brain centers' control over bladder function.
- **Spinal shock:** Following spinal cord injury, a period of spinal shock may occur, during which reflex activity is temporarily suppressed. Subsequently, as neurons regain excitability, local spinal reflexes may become hyperactive, leading to unannounced bladder emptying.

## Features of Reflex/Automatic Bladder

- **Loss of higher controls:** Patients lose voluntary control over bladder function due to disruption of descending neural pathways from higher brain centers.
- **Spinal reflex pathways:** With intact afferent and efferent pathways and spinal cord reflex circuits, local micturition reflexes become predominant in regulating bladder function.
- **Unannounced bladder emptying:** Patients may experience uncontrolled and involuntary bladder

emptying without warning, leading to urinary urgency and incontinence.
- **Spinal shock:** Initially, following spinal cord injury, a period of spinal shock may occur, during which reflex activity is suppressed, leading to urinary retention. Subsequently, as spinal reflexes become hyperactive, uncontrolled bladder emptying may occur.
- **Neurogenic bladder dysfunction:** Reflex bladder dysfunction is a form of neurogenic bladder dysfunction characterized by uncontrolled reflexive bladder contractions in the absence of voluntary control.

Management of reflex or automatic bladder involves strategies to optimize bladder emptying and minimize urinary incontinence. This may include bladder training, timed voiding, and the use of medications to relax the bladder and reduce involuntary contractions. In severe cases, intermittent catheterization or surgical interventions to regulate bladder function may be necessary. Regular monitoring and follow-up are essential to prevent complications such as urinary tract infections and renal damage.

## Uninhibited Bladder

An uninhibited bladder is a condition characterized by *loss of inhibition from higher neural centers, leading to frequent and relatively uncontrolled micturition*.

### Causes

- **Head injury/trauma:** Traumatic brain injury or head trauma can disrupt neural pathways responsible for inhibiting bladder function, leading to uninhibited bladder contractions.
- **Loss of inhibition:** Damage to the brain or spinal cord can result in the loss of inhibitory signals from higher brain centers, which normally regulate bladder function.

### Features of Uninhibited Bladder

- **Frequent micturition:** Patients experience frequent urination due to uncontrolled bladder contractions.
- **Uncontrolled urination:** Micturition occurs relatively uncontrolled, leading to urgency and sometimes urge incontinence.
- **Interrupted inhibitor signals:** Inhibitory signals from higher brain centers are interrupted, allowing facilitatory impulses to keep the sacral micturition center excitable.
- **Excitation of micturition reflex:** Even small amounts of urine entering the bladder can excite the micturition reflex, leading to the expulsion of urine and increased frequency of micturition.

Management of an uninhibited bladder involves strategies aimed at reducing urinary frequency and urgency, as well as preventing episodes of urge incontinence. This may include bladder training techniques, timed voiding schedules, behavioral therapies, and pharmacological interventions to relax bladder muscles and reduce uninhibited contractions. In severe cases, interventions such as botulinum toxin injections into the bladder or surgical procedures may be considered to modulate bladder function and improve urinary control. Regular monitoring and follow-up are essential to assess treatment effectiveness and prevent complications such as urinary tract infections.

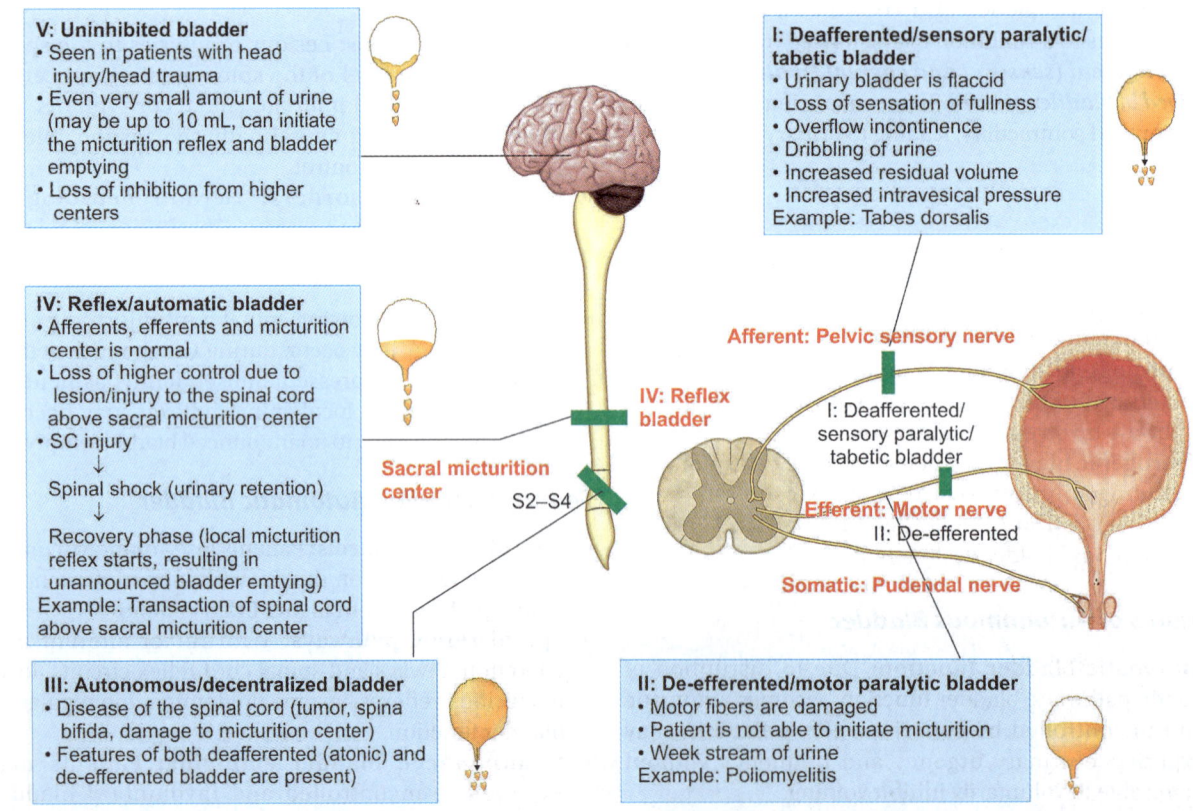

## SUMMARY

- The urinary bladder is a muscular sac located in the pelvic cavity responsible for storing urine before it is expelled from the body. Its main components include the body, which serves as the reservoir for urine, and the neck, which connects to the urethra. The bladder wall is composed of smooth muscle known as the detrusor muscle, and the trigone is a triangular area formed by the openings of the ureters and urethra. The urethra serves as the exit route for urine from the bladder.
- The bladder receives both autonomic and somatic innervation. Autonomic nerves regulate bladder function, with parasympathetic fibers promoting bladder contraction (via the pelvic nerves) and sympathetic fibers facilitating bladder relaxation (via the hypogastric nerves). Somatic innervation via the pudendal nerve controls the external urinary sphincter, allowing for voluntary control over urination.
- The micturition reflex is a complex neurological process that controls the initiation and completion of urination. It involves afferent signals from stretch receptors in the bladder wall, which convey information about bladder filling to the spinal cord. Efferent signals then trigger detrusor muscle contraction and relaxation of the urinary sphincters, leading to coordinated bladder emptying.
- Neurogenic bladder refers to dysfunction of the bladder due to neurological damage or disease. Conditions such as spinal cord injury, multiple sclerosis, or stroke can disrupt the normal neural pathways involved in bladder control. This disruption can lead to various bladder dysfunctions, including urinary retention, urinary incontinence, or a combination of both. Management of neurogenic bladder often involves a combination of medical therapies, behavioral interventions, and sometimes surgical procedures to optimize bladder function and minimize complications.

## LET US SEE, HOW MUCH YOU HAVE LEARNT?

### Review Questions

#### Long/Short Answer Questions

Q1. Describe the autonomous bladder.
Q2. Describe the atonic bladder.
Q3. What is cystometry? What are its indications?
Q4. Describe the micturition reflex.

#### Explain Why? (Reasoning Questions)

Q1. The detrusor muscle of the urinary bladder contracts during the voiding phase of micturition.
Q2. The sensation of bladder fullness increases as the bladder fills with urine, and how this sensation is conveyed to the central nervous system.
Q3. Patients with spinal cord injuries often develop neurogenic bladder dysfunction.

### Critical Thinking Case-Based Questions

Q1. Rakesh, a 35-year-old male, was involved in a severe road traffic accident resulting in significant trauma to his spine. Upon arrival at the emergency department, he is found to have sustained a transection of the spinal cord at the L4-L5 level.

*Presenting complaints:*
- **Urinary retention:** He reports an inability to pass urine since the accident.
- **Loss of bladder sensation:** Rakesh mentions that he has not felt the urge to urinate since the accident.
- **Bladder distension:** On examination, his lower abdomen appears distended, and palpation reveals a palpable bladder.

*Clinical findings:*
- **Neurological examination:** Rakesh demonstrates signs of lower limb paralysis and sensory loss below the level of the spinal cord injury.
- **Bladder palpation:** The bladder is palpable and distended, indicating urinary retention.
- **Absent reflexes:** Deep tendon reflexes in the lower limbs are absent, consistent with the level of spinal cord injury.

Based on above scenario answer the following questions:
a. What is your probable diagnosis?
b. Describe the type of bladder dysfunction that is present in Rakesh.

### Multiple Choice Questions

Q1. What is the primary function of the detrusor muscle in the urinary bladder?
   a. Relaxation during urination
   b. Contraction during urination
   c. Sensation of bladder fullness
   d. Control of urinary sphincters

Q2. Which type of nerve fibers are responsible for transmitting signals of bladder fullness to the brain?
   a. Sympathetic fibers
   b. Motor fibers
   c. Afferent fibers
   d. Efferent fibers

Q3. Which neurological condition can disrupt the normal function of the micturition reflex?
   a. Stroke
   b. Osteoarthritis
   c. Hypertension
   d. Psoriasis

Q4. What is the role of parasympathetic nerves in bladder function?
   a. Relaxation of the bladder
   b. Contraction of the bladder
   c. Voluntary control of urination
   d. Sensation of bladder fullness

Q5. Which nerve controls the external urinary sphincter, allowing for voluntary control over urination?
   a. Pelvic nerve
   b. Hypogastric nerve
   c. Pudendal nerve
   d. Sacral nerve

Q6. What neurological consequence would likely occur following a spinal cord injury at the L4-L5 level?
   a. Loss of bladder sensation
   b. Increased bladder contractility
   c. Loss of detrusor muscle function
   d. Increased urinary sphincter tone

Q7. Which term describes the involuntary expulsion of urine due to disruption of higher brain center control over bladder function?
   a. Uninhibited bladder
   b. Atonic bladder
   c. Neurogenic bladder
   d. Reflex bladder

Q8. What is the primary symptom of a patient with a neurogenic bladder due to spinal cord injury?
   a. Urinary retention
   b. Frequent micturition
   c. Weak urinary stream
   d. Loss of bladder sensation

Q9. Which spinal cord level is most commonly affected in a patient with urinary dysfunction following a road traffic accident?
   a. Cervical spine
   b. Thoracic spine
   c. Lumbar spine
   d. Sacral spine

Q10. What is the initial management strategy for a patient with urinary retention following a spinal cord injury?
   a. Bladder training
   b. Intermittent catheterization
   c. Pharmacotherapy
   d. Surgical intervention

Q11. Hina, a 45-year-old woman, presents to the urology clinic complaining of urinary incontinence and difficulty emptying her bladder completely. Upon further evaluation, she undergoes cystometry.

What diagnostic test is most appropriate for evaluating Hina's bladder function and assessing for conditions such as detrusor muscle dysfunction and urinary retention?
   a. Cystoscopy
   b. Uroflowmetry
   c. Cystometry
   d. Renal ultrasound

Q12. Mahesh, a 60-year-old man, has been diagnosed with an atonic bladder following a spinal cord injury. He experiences urinary retention and requires regular bladder emptying to prevent complications.

Which of the following management strategies is most appropriate for Mahesh's atonic bladder?
   a. Bladder training
   b. Anticholinergic medications
   c. Intermittent catheterization
   d. Alpha-blocker medications

Q13. Suman, a 30-year-old woman, sustained a traumatic brain injury in a car accident. Since the accident, she has been experiencing frequent and uncontrolled episodes of urination, often without warning.

What term best describes Suman's bladder dysfunction characterized by loss of higher brain center control over bladder function?
   a. Atonic bladder
   b. Autonomous bladder
   c. Neurogenic bladder
   d. Uninhibited bladder

Q14. Jai Kumar, a 55-year-old man, is being evaluated for bladder dysfunction. During the assessment, the healthcare provider explains the micturition reflex to him.

What physiological process is primarily responsible for initiating the micturition reflex and triggering bladder contraction during urination?
   a. Sympathetic nervous system activation
   b. Parasympathetic nervous system activation
   c. Somatic nervous system activation
   d. Central nervous system inhibition

Q15. Leela, a 40-year-old woman, is undergoing urodynamic testing to evaluate her bladder function. During cystometry, she experiences the sensation of bladder fullness and the urge to urinate.

What component of bladder function is primarily assessed during cystometry, which involves measuring bladder pressure and volume changes in response to filling?
   a. Bladder sensation
   b. Bladder compliance
   c. Detrusor muscle contractility
   d. Urinary sphincter tone

### ANSWERS

1. b  2. c  3. a  4. b  5. c  6. a  7. a  8. a  9. c  10. b  11. c  12. c  13. d  14. b
15. c

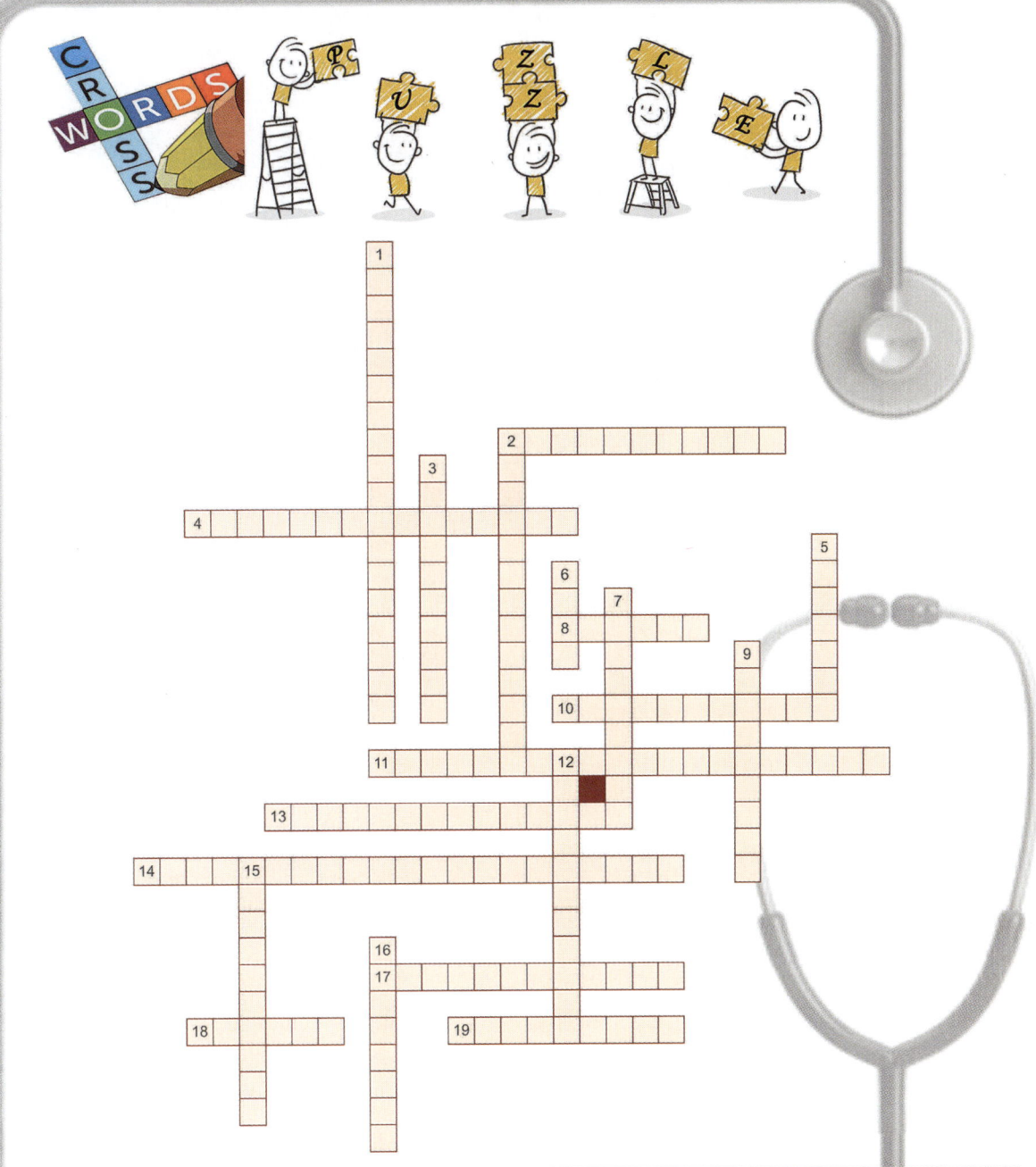

### Across
2. Component of RAAS, causing renal retention of salt and water
4. Measure of the volume of plasma from which a substance is completely removed per unit time
8. Condition with elevated blood urea levels
10. Hormone released by the posterior pituitary gland to regulate water reabsorption
11. The process by which the kidneys filter blood, removing excess wastes and fluids
13. Aldosterone antagonist preventing $K^+$ secretion
14. Minimum volume of urine that must be excreted to eliminate waste products
17. Inability of the kidneys to adequately concentrate or dilute the urine
18. Polysaccharide indicator used to assess the GFR and renal blood flow
19. Most powerful diuretic acting on Loop of Henle

### Down
1. Rate at which solute-free water is excreted by the kidneys
2. Loss of sensation of bladder fullness and impaired detrusor muscle function
3. Increases GFR and produces vasodilatation
5. Structural and functional unit of the kidney
6. Located on basolateral membrane for transport of glucose
7. Small openings in the capillary endothelium
9. Structure responsible for the counter current exchange mechanism in the kidney
12. Part of the nephron responsible for creating the medullary osmotic gradient crucial for urine concentration
15. Double layer structure responsible for filtration of blood in the kidney
16. Process by which various waste products are removed from the body by artificial means

# SECTION 8

# ENDOCRINE PHYSIOLOGY

## Section Outline

**Chapter 63:** Endocrine System and Hormones
**Chapter 64:** Physiology of Bone and Calcium Regulation
**Chapter 65:** Physiology of Hypothalamus
**Chapter 66:** Physiology of Pituitary Gland
**Chapter 67:** Thyroid Gland
**Chapter 68:** Physiology of Adrenal Gland
**Chapter 69:** Glucose Homeostasis: Role of Endocrine Pancreas
**Chapter 70:** Physiology of Thymus and Pineal Gland
**Chapter 71:** Metabolic Syndrome (A Self-Directed Learning Module)

# Endocrine System and Hormones

**CHAPTER 63**

### COMPETENCY ADDRESSED
**PY8.6:** Describe and differentiate the mechanism of action of steroid, protein and amine hormones.

### LEARNING OBJECTIVES
**At the end of this chapter, the learner should be able to:**
- Define the endocrine gland, hormone.
- Classify the hormones on the basis of their chemical structure.
- Describe the mechanism of action of each of the hormones.
- Describe the basis and changes in primary, secondary and tertiary endocrinal disorders.

**Endocrine glands** are the ductless glands that pour their secretions into the bloodstream, away from the target organ **(Fig. 63.1)**. The chemical secreted by these glands are called hormones.

## HORMONES

They are the chemical messengers, synthesized and secreted into blood by endocrine glands, to influence the target organs. Various endocrine glands and their hormones are tabulated in **Table 63.1**.

## CLASSIFICATION OF HORMONES

Based on the chemical structure, the hormones are classified in **Table 63.2**.

## MECHANISM OF HORMONE ACTION

### Hormones Acting on Intracellular Receptors

The Lipophilic/lipid soluble hormones, which can cross the cell membrane, act on intracellular receptors.
- The thyroid hormone bind to the intranuclear receptors and binds to the thyroid hormone response element situated on the DNA, which leads to the transcription of mRNA and new protein synthesis.
- The steroid hormone bind to the intracytoplasmic receptors and binds to the steroid hormone response element situated on the DNA, which leads to the transcription of mRNA and new protein synthesis.

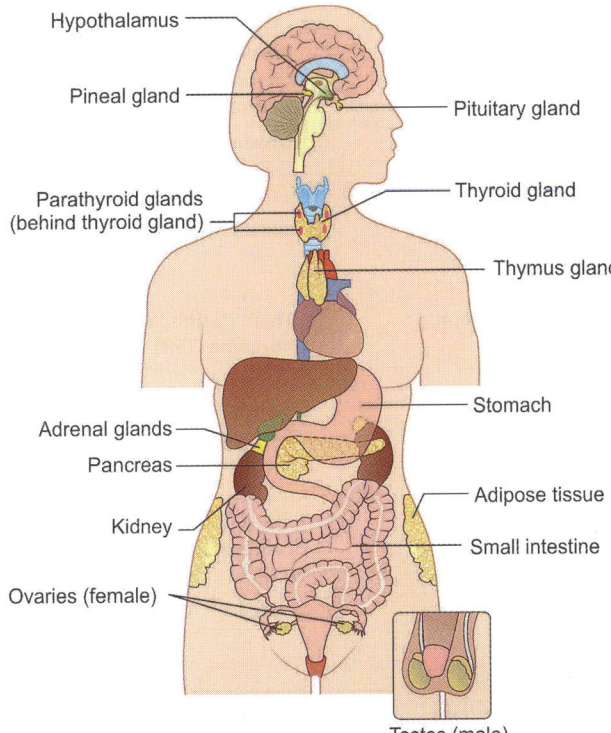

**Fig. 63.1:** Endocrine system of human body.

**Table 63.1:** Endocrine glands and their secretions with functions and mechanism of action.

| Endocrine gland | Part of gland secreting the hormone | Hormones | Functions | Type of hormone | Mechanism of action |
|---|---|---|---|---|---|
| Hypothalamus | Paraventricular nucleus | Thyrotropin-releasing hormone (TRH) | Stimulates the secretion of TSH and prolactin from anterior pituitary gland | Peptide hormone | G protein coupled PLC/IP3, DAG pathway |
| | | Corticotropin releasing hormone (CRH) | Stimulates the secretion of ACTH from anterior pituitary gland | Peptide hormone | G protein coupled PLC/IP3, DAG pathway |
| | | Somatostatin (Growth hormone inhibiting hormone) | Inhibits the release of GH from anterior pituitary | Peptide hormone | G protein coupled PLC/IP3, DAG pathway |
| | | Oxytocin | Stimulates milk ejection from breast and uterine contractions | Peptide hormone | G protein coupled PLC/IP3, DAG pathway |
| | Arcuate nucleus | Growth hormone releasing hormone (GHRH) | Stimulates the secretion of GH from anterior pituitary gland | Peptide hormone | G protein coupled PLC/IP3, DAG pathway |
| | | Prolactin inhibiting hormone (PIH)/Dopamine | Inhibits the release of prolactin | Amine hormone | G protein coupled adenylyl cyclase/cAMP pathway |
| | | Gonadotrophin releasing hormone (GnRH) | Stimulates the secretion of FSH and LH from anterior pituitary gland | Peptide hormone | G protein coupled PLC/IP3, DAG pathway |
| | Supraoptic nucleus | Vasopressin/antidiuretic hormone (ADH) | Increases water reabsorption by kidneys, causes vasoconstriction and increases blood pressure | Peptide hormone | G protein coupled adenylyl cyclase/cAMP pathway |
| | Other hormones | Prolactin releasing factor Neuropeptide Y | Stimulates the release of prolactin | Peptide hormone | G protein coupled adenylyl cyclase/cAMP pathway |
| | | Orexins | Regulates wakefulness, feeding reward and thermogenesis | Peptide hormone | G protein coupled PLC/IP3, DAG pathway |
| Anterior pituitary gland | Somatotrophs | Growth hormone (GH) | Stimulates protein synthesis and growth of all somatic cells | Peptide hormone | Enzymatic receptor through Janus kinase (JAK-STAT pathway) |
| | Thyrotrophs | Thyroid stimulating hormone (TSH) | Stimulates synthesis of T3 and T4 from thyroid gland | Peptide hormone | G protein coupled adenylyl cyclase/cAMP pathway |
| | Gonadotrophs | Follicle stimulating hormone (FSH) | • Stimulates the development of follicles in ovaries in females<br>• Spermatogenesis in males | Peptide hormone | G protein coupled adenylyl cyclase/cAMP pathway |
| | | Luteinizing hormone (LH) | • Stimulates the ovulation in females Maintains corpus luteum till implantation<br>• Secretion of testosterone in males | Peptide hormone | G protein coupled adenylyl cyclase/cAMP pathway |
| | Lactotrophs | Prolactin | Stimulates the formation of milk (Galactopoiesis) during lactation | Peptide hormone | Tyrosine kinase linked receptor |
| | Corticotrophs | Adrenocorticotropin hormone (ACTH) | Stimulates synthesis of mineralocorticoids and glucocorticoids from adrenal gland | Peptide hormone | G protein coupled adenylyl cyclase/cAMP pathway |

*Contd...*

Contd...

| Endocrine gland | Part of gland secreting the hormone | Hormones | Functions | Type of hormone | Mechanism of action |
|---|---|---|---|---|---|
| Posterior pituitary gland | Paraventricular nucleus of hypothalamus | Oxytocin (Synthesized in hypothalamus, stored and released from post. Pituitary) | Stimulates milk ejection from breast and uterine contractions | Peptide hormone | G protein coupled PLC/IP3, DAG pathway |
| | Supraoptic nucleus of hypothalamus | Antidiuretic hormone (ADH) (Synthesized in hypothalamus, stored and released from post. Pituitary) | Increases water reabsorption by kidneys, causes vasoconstriction and increases blood pressure | Peptide hormone | G protein coupled adenylyl cyclase/cAMP pathway |
| Thyroid | Chief cells | Triiodothyronine (T3), thyroxine (T4) | Increases the rates of chemical reactions in most cells, thus increasing body metabolic rate | Amine hormone | Intranuclear receptors with new protein synthesis |
| | Parafollicular cells | Calcitonin | Promotes deposition of calcium in the bones and decreases extracellular fluid calcium ion concentration | Peptide hormone | G protein coupled adenylyl cyclase/cAMP pathway |
| Parathyroid gland | Chief cells | Parathormone | Increases serum calcium level | Peptide hormone | G protein coupled adenylyl cyclase/cAMP pathway |
| Pancreas | Alpha cells | Glucagon | Increases synthesis and release of glucose from the liver into the body fluids | Peptide hormone | G protein coupled adenylyl cyclase/cAMP pathway |
| | Beta cells | Insulin | Promotes glucose entry in many cells, and in this way controls carbohydrate metabolism | Peptide hormone | Tyrosine kinase enzyme receptors |
| | Delta cells | Somatostatin | Inhibits release of insulin and glucagon | Peptide hormone | G protein coupled adenylyl cyclase/cAMP pathway |
| Adrenal cortex | Zona glomerulosa | Mineralocorticoids (Aldosterone) | Increases renal sodium reabsorption, potassium secretion, and hydrogen ion secretion | Steroid hormone | Intracytoplasmic receptors with new protein synthesis |
| | Zona fasciculata | Glucocorticoids | Has multiple metabolic functions for controlling metabolism of proteins, carbohydrates, and fats; also has anti-inflammatory effects | Steroid hormone | Intracytoplasmic receptors with new protein synthesis |
| | Zona reticularis | Sex steroids (Androgen and estrogen) and glucocorticoids to some extent | Promotes the development of secondary sexual characters at puberty | Steroid hormone | Intracytoplasmic receptors with new protein synthesis |
| Adrenal medulla | Enlarged and specialized sympathetic ganglion, post ganglionic fibers are embedded in it to form lumps of chromaffin cells<br>• Epinephrine secreting type (90%)<br>• Nor epinephrine secreting type (10%) | • Epinephrine<br>• Nor epinephrine | Action is similar to activation of sympathetic nervous system | Amine hormone | • α-receptor: PLC/IP3, DAG pathway<br>• β2-receptor: G protein coupled adenylyl cyclase/cAMP pathway |

Contd...

*Contd...*

| Endocrine gland | Part of gland secreting the hormone | Hormones | Functions | Type of hormone | Mechanism of action |
|---|---|---|---|---|---|
| Ovaries | Granulosa cells of ovarian follicle, corpus luteum | Estrogen | Promotes growth and development of female reproductive system, female breasts, and female secondary sexual characteristics | Steroid hormone | Intracytoplasmic receptors with new protein synthesis |
| Ovaries | Corpus luteum, placenta, ovarian follicle | Progesterone | Stimulates secretion of "uterine milk" by the uterine endometrial glands and promotes development of secretory apparatus of breasts | Steroid hormone | Intracytoplasmic receptors with new protein synthesis |
| Testes | Leydig cells | Testosterone | Promotes development of male reproductive system and male secondary sexual characteristics steroid | Steroid hormone | Intracytoplasmic receptors with new protein synthesis |
| Other | Kidney | Erythropoietin | Increases erythrocyte production | Peptide hormone | Cytokine receptor by JAK STAT pathway |
| Other | Kidney | Renin | Catalyses conversion of angiotensinogen to angiotensin I (acts as an enzyme) | Peptide hormone | Mitogen activated kinase (MAP kinases) |
| Other | Kidney | 1,25-DHCC (Active form of vitamin D3) | Increases intestinal absorption of calcium and bone mineralization | Steroid hormone | Intracytoplasmic receptors with new protein synthesis |
| Other | Liver | IGF-I and II (Insulin-like growth factor) | Modulates the effect of growth hormone | Peptide hormone | Tyrosine kinase enzyme receptors |
| Other | Heart | Atrial natriuretic peptide (ANP) | Increases sodium excretion by kidneys reduces blood pressure | Peptide hormone | cGMP Pathway |
| Other | Pineal | Melatonin | Stimulates the sleep wake cycles | Peptide hormone | G protein coupled adenylyl cyclase/cAMP pathway |
| Other | GIT | Gastrin | Stimulates hydrogen chloride secretion by parietal cells | Peptide hormone | G protein coupled PLC/IP3, DAG pathway |
| Other | GIT | Secretin | Stimulates pancreatic acinar cells to release bicarbonate and water | Peptide hormone | G protein coupled adenylyl cyclase/cAMP pathway |
| Other | GIT | Gastric inhibitory peptide (GIP) | Inhibits the gastric motility. Stimulates the secretion of insulin from beta cells of pancreas | Peptide hormone | G protein coupled adenylyl cyclase/cAMP pathway |
| Other | GIT | Cholecystokinin (CCK) | Stimulates gallbladder contraction and release of pancreatic enzymes | Peptide hormone | G protein coupled adenylyl cyclase/cAMP pathway |
| Other | GIT | Motilin | Stimulates intestinal motility and induces hunger contractions and migrating motor complexes | Peptide hormone | G protein coupled PLC/IP3, DAG pathway |
| Other | Placenta | Progesterone, estrogen (During pregnancy) | Maintains the pregnancy and prepares the maternal body for pregnancy | Steroid hormone | Intracytoplasmic receptors with new protein synthesis |

*Contd...*

Contd...

| Endocrine gland | Part of gland secreting the hormone | Hormones | Functions | Type of hormone | Mechanism of action |
|---|---|---|---|---|---|
| | | hCG | Promotes growth of corpus luteum and secretion of estrogens and progesterone by corpus luteum | Peptide hormone | G protein coupled adenylyl cyclase/cAMP pathway |
| | | Human placental lactogen (HPL) | Probably helps promote development of some fetal tissues, as well as the mother's breasts | Peptide hormone | Cytokine receptor by JAK-STAT pathway |
| | | Relaxin | Relaxes the pelvic ligaments of mother for easy delivery of baby | Peptide hormone | G protein coupled adenylyl cyclase/cAMP pathway and MAP kinase pathway |
| | Adipose tissue | Leptin | Inhibits appetite, stimulates thermogenesis | Peptide hormone | Cytokine receptor by JAK-STAT pathway |

**Table 63.2:** Types of hormones and their properties.

| | Amine hormones | Peptide hormones | Steroid hormones |
|---|---|---|---|
| Examples | • **Iodinated** → Thyroxine<br>• **Noniodinated**<br>  ▪ Epinephrine<br>  ▪ Nor-epinephrine<br>  ▪ Dopamine<br>  ▪ Serotonin | • **Insulin family**<br>  *Insulin, IGF-I*<br>• **GH family**<br>  *GH, prolactin, HPL*<br>• **Glycoprotein**<br>  *LH, FSH, TSH, hCG*<br>• **Secretin family**<br>  *Secretin, glucagon, VIP, GIP*<br>• **Others**<br>  *ANP, calcitonin, CCK, ADH, ACTH, PTH* | • **Adrenal cortex**<br>  *Mineralocorticoids, glucocorticoids*<br>• **Gonadal hormones**<br>  *Estrogen, progesterone, testosterone*<br>• **1,25-DHCC** |
| Precursor | Tyrosine/tryptophan/phenylalanine | Amino acids | Cholesterol |
| Synthesis | • Thyroxine: Tyr<br>• Dopamine: Tyr and Phe<br>• Epinephrine and nor epinephrine: Tyr and Phe<br>• Serotonin: Tryptophan | Preprohormone *(in RER)* → pro hormone → hormone (*explained below*) | Synthesized from cholesterol |
| Storage | • Thyroxine → stored in colloid<br>• Catecholamines → Stored in granules inside the cells | Packed by Golgi app. To form secretory granules | Hormones present in cytosol, bound to proteins |
| Release/Secretion | Secreted by $Ca^{2+}$ mediated exocytosis **(Fig. 63.2)** | • Regulated pathway<br>  *External stimulus triggers the release of hormone*<br>• Constitutive pathway<br>  *Release of hormone from endoplasmic reticulum and GA along with other hormones* | On stimulation, becomes free from intracellular proteins and are transported outside the cell by diffusion |
| Transported in blood | • Thyroxine → mainly bound to globulin (Thyroid binding globulin) and albumin, very little free<br>• Catecholamines → freely soluble in plasma | Freely soluble in plasma; transported in a dissolved form | • Mainly bound to globulin (corticoid binding globulin) and albumin<br>• Dopamine: Very little free |
| Metabolism and excretion In liver and kidney | • Thyroxine → slowly metabolized and excreted<br>• Catecholamines → rapidly metabolized and excreted | Rapidly metabolized and excreted | Slowly metabolized and excreted |

Contd...

Contd...

|  | Amine hormones | Peptide hormones | Steroid hormones |
|---|---|---|---|
| Mechanism of hormone action | • Thyroxine → act via intracellular, intranuclear receptors<br>• Catecholamines → Act via receptors on plasma membrane | Act via receptors on plasma membrane | Act via intracellular, intracytoplasmic receptors |
| Response | • Thyroxine → slow<br>• Catecholamines → fast | Fast | Slow |
| Regulation | • **Feedback mechanism:** Positive and negative feedback mechanism.<br>• **Neural regulation:** Control of higher centers and ANS<br>• **Rhythmic control:**<br>　▪ Pulsatile: Few min. to hours (GH)<br>　▪ Diurnal: Occurring for several hours (day-night cycle) (ACTH)<br>　▪ Periodical: Lasting for many days (Hormones of menstrual cycle)<br>　▪ Developmental: Occurring in different phases of development (Pubertal H)<br>　▪ Seasonal: Occurring in different seasons; seen in birds<br>• **Humoral control**<br>　▪ Hormonal: Hormone mediated release of other hormone<br>　▪ Glucagon → Release of insulin<br>　▪ Chemical: Chemical mediated release of other hormone<br>　▪ Hypokalemia inhibition of insulin secretion | | |

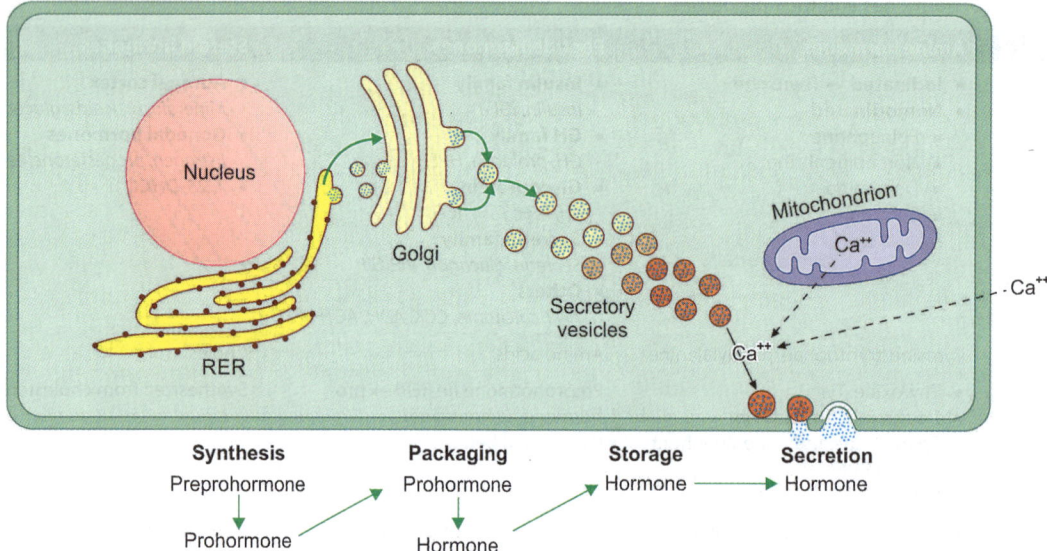

**Fig. 63.2:** $Ca^{2+}$ mediated synthesis of protein hormone.

## Hormones Acting on Receptors of Plasma Membrane

(*Catecholamines and peptide hormones* act on receptors of plasma membrane because they are hydrophilic and cannot cross the cell membrane).

These chemical messengers (called as first messenger), especially peptide hormones, require another chemical messenger to bring about their physiological response (second messenger).

- Most of the hormones secreted by hypothalamus act via G protein coupled receptors through IP3/DAG. Just remember the exceptions
- Most of the hormones secreted by anterior pituitary gland act via G protein coupled receptors through adenylyl cyclase/cAMP. Just remember the exceptions
- All steroid hormones act through intracytoplasmic receptors

The main signaling pathways involved in hormone action are:
- **G protein coupled receptors acting through**
  - ***Phospholipase C/IP$_3$ and DAG pathway***:
    - *TRH*
    - *CRH*
    - *GnRH*
    - *Oxytocin*

- ♦ α-adrenergic receptors
- ♦ Gastrin
- ■ **Adenylyl cyclase/cAMP pathway**
  - ♦ ACTH
  - ♦ FSH, LH
  - ♦ ADH
  - ♦ Parathormone
  - ♦ Calcitonin
  - ♦ β-adrenergic receptors
  - ♦ Glucagon
  - ♦ GI hormones except Gastrin
  - ♦ Angiotensin II
  - ♦ hCG
  - ♦ Somatostatin
  - ♦ TSH
- **Receptors acting through enzyme linked cytokine receptors**
  - ■ *Growth hormone (Janus kinase enzyme/JAK-STAT pathway)*
  - ■ *Insulin (Tyrosine kinase)*
  - ■ *IGF1, IGF2 (Tyrosine kinase)*
  - ■ *Erythropoietin (Janus kinase enzyme/JAK-STAT pathway)*
  - ■ *Fibroblast growth factor*
  - ■ *Growth hormone*
  - ■ *Hepatocyte growth factor*
  - ■ *Leptin*
  - ■ *Prolactin*
  - ■ *Vascular endothelial growth factor*

These mechanisms are discussed in detail in Chapter 3 on cell signaling and transduction.

## PRINCIPLES OF ENDOCRINAL DISORDERS

### Disorders of Secretion

The main disorders of endocrine glands can be due to either overfunctioning (hypersecretion) and decreased functioning (hyposecretion).

- **Hypersecretion:** Excessive secretion of hormone by gland
- **Hyposecretion:** Decreased secretion of hormone by gland

### Disorders of Target Cell Responsiveness (Receptor Sensitivity)

Another form of endocrinal dysfunction is abnormal responsiveness of hormone receptor **(Table 63.3)**. It is described below:

- **Hyporesponsiveness:** Also called **Down regulation/unresponsive/insensitive receptors** with normal/increased hormone levels.
- **Hyper-responsiveness:** Also called **up regulation/highly responsive receptors** with normal/decreased hormone levels.

Based on the level of gland involvement, the endocrinal disorders are classified as:

- **Primary endocrinal disorder:** Disorder of the hormone secreting gland.
- **Secondary endocrinal disorder:** Increased/decreased stimulation of gland to produce hormones by its tropic hormones. The disorder lies at the levels of pituitary gland or the main regulating factor.

**Table 63.3:** Disorders of hypo and hypersecretion of endocrine hormones.

| Gland | Hormone | Hyposecretion | Hypersecretion |
|---|---|---|---|
| **Pituitary** | **Growth hormone** | Dwarfism | • Gigantism (in children)<br>• Acromegaly (in adults) |
| | **All hormones** | Pan hypopituitarism | - |
| | **ADH** | Diabetes Insipidus | SIADH |
| **Thyroid** | **Thyroxine** | • Hypothyroidism<br>• Cretinism (Children)<br>• Myxedema (Adults) | • Hyperthyroidism<br>• Thyrotoxicosis<br>• Graves disease (Auto immune) |
| **Parathyroid** | **Parathormone** | • Hypoparathyroidism<br>• Hypo calcemic tetany | Hyperparathyroidism |
| **Adrenal cortex** | **Glucocorticoids** | Adrenocortical insufficiency (Addisons disease) | Cushing's syndrome |
| | **Mineralocorticoids** | Occurs along with adrenal insufficiency | Conn's syndrome |
| | **Sex steroids** | x | • Virilization syndrome<br>• Adrenogenital syndrome<br>• *Precocious puberty in males and pseudohermaphroditism in females* |
| **Adrenal medulla** | **Epinephrine** | x | Pheochromocytoma |
| **Endocrine pancreas** | **Insulin** | Diabetes mellitus | Chronic hypoglycemia (Insulinoma) |
| | **Glucagon** | Rare | Glucagonoma (Tumor of alpha cells) |

- **Tertiary endocrinal disorder:** Increased/decreased stimulation of gland to produce hormones by its tropic hormones which are further regulated by peripheral hormonal concentrations through feedback control. The disorder lies at the levels of hypothalamus in hypothalamic pituitary gland axis.

### How to differentiate between primary secondary and tertiary endocrinal disorders:

|  | Primary disorder | Secondary disorder | Tertiary disorder | Receptor sensitivity |
|---|---|---|---|---|
| **Hyperfunctioning:** | | | | |
| Gland hormone level | Increased | Increased | Increased | Decreased |
| Pituitary hormone level | Decreased | Decreased | Increased | Decreased |
| Hypothalamic hormone level | Decreased | Increased | Increased | Decreased |
| **Hypofunctioning:** | | | | |
| Gland hormone level | Decreased | Decreased | Decreased | Increased |
| Pituitary hormone level | Increased | Decreased | Decreased | Increased |
| Hypothalamic hormone level | Increased | Increased | Decreased | Increased |

## SUMMARY

- Endocrine glands are specialized organs that secrete hormones directly into the bloodstream, regulating various bodily functions and maintaining homeostasis.
- Hormones, the chemical messengers of the endocrine system, are classified based on their chemical structure into several categories:
  - **Peptide hormones:** Comprised of chains of amino acids, peptide hormones include insulin, growth hormone, and oxytocin. These hormones exert their effects by binding to specific receptors on cell surfaces, initiating intracellular signaling cascades.
  - **Steroid hormones:** Derived from cholesterol, steroid hormones such as cortisol, estrogen, and testosterone are lipid-soluble. They can diffuse through cell membranes and bind to intracellular receptors, modulating gene expression and protein synthesis.
  - **Amino acid derivative hormones:** These hormones, such as epinephrine (adrenaline), norepinephrine, and thyroid hormones (thyroxine and triiodothyronine), are derived from amino acids. They typically act through cell surface receptors and intracellular signaling pathways.
- Each hormone exerts its effects through distinct mechanisms of action:
  - **Peptide hormones:** Peptide hormones bind to cell surface receptors, triggering secondary messenger systems like cyclic adenosine monophosphate (cAMP) or phosphoinositide pathway, leading to physiological responses within the cell.
  - **Steroid hormones:** Steroid hormones diffuse through the cell membrane and bind to intracellular receptors, forming hormone-receptor complexes that modulate gene transcription and protein synthesis.
  - **Amino acid derivative hormones:** These hormones also act via cell surface receptors, initiating signaling cascades that regulate cellular functions, such as metabolism, cardiovascular activity, and stress response.
- The chapter further explores the basis and changes in primary, secondary, and tertiary endocrine disorders:
  - **Primary endocrine disorders:** Arise from dysfunction within the endocrine gland itself, leading to abnormal hormone production. Examples include primary adrenal insufficiency (Addison's disease) and primary hypothyroidism.
  - **Secondary endocrine disorders:** Result from inadequate stimulation or inhibition of an endocrine gland by regulatory mechanisms outside the gland. For instance, secondary hypothyroidism occurs due to deficient secretion of thyroid-stimulating hormone (TSH) from the pituitary gland.
  - **Tertiary endocrine disorders:** Involve dysfunction in the hypothalamus, affecting the regulation of hormone production by the pituitary gland. Disorders like tertiary adrenal insufficiency stem from impaired secretion of corticotropin-releasing hormone (CRH) from the hypothalamus.

## LET US SEE, HOW MUCH YOU HAVE LEARNT?

### Long/Short Answer Questions

Q1. Describe the mechanism of action of:
  a. Steroid hormones
  b. Thyroid hormones
  c. Peptide hormones

Q2. What is the difference between primary and secondary endocrinal disorders? How will you differentiate from the hormone assay?

### Multiple Choice Questions

Q1. What is the primary function of endocrine glands?
  a. Produce and release hormones
  b. Store nutrients
  c. Regulate body temperature
  d. Filter blood

Q2. Which of the following hormones is classified as a peptide hormone?
  a. Cortisol
  b. Thyroxine
  c. Insulin
  d. Testosterone

Q3. Steroid hormones exert their effects by:
  a. Binding to cell surface receptors
  b. Activating secondary messenger systems
  c. Diffusing through cell membranes and binding to intracellular receptors
  d. Stimulating neurotransmitter release

Q4. The mechanism of action of peptide hormones typically involves:
  a. Direct modulation of gene transcription
  b. Diffusion through cell membranes
  c. Binding to intracellular receptors
  d. Activation of secondary messenger systems

Q5. Which category of hormones includes epinephrine and norepinephrine?
  a. Peptide hormones
  b. Steroid hormones
  c. Amino acid derivative hormones
  d. Protein hormones

Q6. Primary endocrine disorders arise from:
  a. Dysfunction within the endocrine gland itself
  b. Inadequate stimulation of the endocrine gland
  c. Dysfunction in the hypothalamus
  d. Overstimulation of the endocrine gland

Q7. Secondary endocrine disorders result from:
  a. Dysfunction within the endocrine gland itself
  b. Inadequate stimulation of the endocrine gland
  c. Dysfunction in the hypothalamus
  d. Overstimulation of the endocrine gland

Q8. Tertiary endocrine disorders involve dysfunction in:
  a. The endocrine gland itself
  b. Inadequate stimulation of the endocrine gland
  c. Dysfunction in the hypothalamus
  d. Overstimulation of the endocrine gland

Q9. Which disorder is an example of tertiary endocrine dysfunction?
  a. Addison's disease
  b. Cushing's syndrome
  c. Tertiary hypothyroidism
  d. Hyperthyroidism

Q10. What is the primary role of hormone-receptor complexes formed by steroid hormones?
  a. Activation of secondary messenger systems
  b. Inhibition of gene transcription
  c. Modulation of gene transcription
  d. Stimulation of neurotransmitter release

### ANSWERS

1. a    2. c    3. c    4. d    5. c    6. a    7. b    8. c    9. c    10. c

# Physiology of Bone and Calcium Regulation

## 64 CHAPTER

### COMPETENCY ADDRESSED
**PY8.1:** Describe the physiology of bone and calcium metabolism.
**PY8.2:** Describe the synthesis, secretion, transport, physiological actions, regulation and effect of altered (hypo and hyper) secretion of the parathyroid gland.

### LEARNING OBJECTIVES
**At the end of this chapter, the learner should be able to:**
- Describe the physiological role of calcium in our body.
- Describe the role of various hormones in regulating the serum calcium levels.
- Describe bone physiology in terms of the structure of bone, cells in bone and their function.
- Describe the clinical importance of hypocalcemia and hypercalcemia.
- Describe the etiopathogenesis, clinical features (signs and symptoms), diagnosis and management of clinical hypocalcemia and hypercalcemia.
- Differentiate between osteoporosis and osteopenia.

## PHYSIOLOGY OF CALCIUM REGULATION

Calcium is an important electrolyte in our body, present everywhere, i.e., in all cells, plasma bones. Calcium is required for many routine physiological processes:
- **Muscle contraction:** It acts the coupler for excitation and contraction of muscle contraction. It also results in the initiation of muscle contraction.
- Electrical transmission of impulse.
- Release of synaptic vesicles from glands/synaptic knobs. It results in interaction between the snare proteins for docking.
- Action potential of cardiac and smooth muscles.
- It provides tensile strength to bone by mineralization of osteoid.
- It acts as cofactor in clotting mechanism. It is classified as clotting factor IV.
- It acts as second messenger for signal transduction pathways in PLC/IP3, DAG pathway and calcium-calmodulin complex.

**Normal serum calcium level ranges from 9–11 mg%.** The majority (85%) of calcium is present in the bones, 14–15% in cells and <1% is present in the extracellular fluid **(Fig. 64.1)**. The calcium present in ECF is further present in three forms:

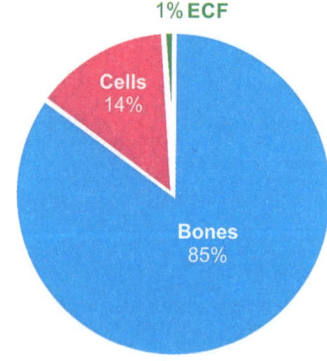

**Fig. 64.1:** Distribution of calcium in the body.

1. **Bound with plasma proteins:** This calcium is non-diffusible and nonionized. Hence, it is not available for physiological functions. It constitutes around 41% of calcium present in ECF.
2. **Diffusible and nonionized calcium:** It constitutes 9% of calcium in ECF but it is also not available for physiological functions.
3. **Diffusible ionized calcium** forms 50% of the total calcium present in ECF. It is responsible for the physiological actions of calcium. It can cross the capillary membrane.

It makes up for half the concentration of plasma calcium levels.

## The Bone: Structure, Bone Formation and Its Role in Maintaining Calcium Pool

We have seen that the majority of calcium in our bodies is present in our bones. So, it is important to learn the structure and physiology of bone (**Fig. 64.2**).

The bone is made up of both organic and inorganic constituents. The organic part is made up of a proteinaceous osteoid matrix comprising collagen and proteoglycans and the inorganic is made up of salts comprising calcium, magnesium and phosphorus. These salts make flat plate-like crystals of calcium hydroxyapatite.

The mechanism of formation of bone and composition is shown in the **Figure 64.3**. Various cells of bone are shown in **Table 64.1**.

## Osteocytic Membrane Pump

The *extensive network of long, filmy processes extending from osteocyte to osteocyte throughout the bone structure connects with the surface osteocytes and osteoblasts.* This extensive system is called the *osteocytic membrane system*, forming a membrane which separates bone and extracellular fluid. The space between the osteocytic membrane and the bone is filled with *bone fluid*. The osteocytic membrane pumps calcium ions from the bone fluid into the extracellular fluid, creating a calcium ion concentration in the bone fluid.

When activity of *osteocytic pump is activated, the bone fluid calcium concentration falls* even lower, and calcium phosphate salts are then released from the bone causing bone resorption. This effect is called *osteolysis*, and it occurs without resorption of the bone's fibrous and gel matrix. When the pump is inactivated, the bone fluid calcium concentration rises to a higher level and calcium phosphate salts are redeposited in the matrix.

## Mechanism of Action of Bone Resorption by Osteoclasts

The mechanism of osteolysis by action of osteoclasts is shown in **Figure 64.4**.

*Why the postmenopausal women develop osteoporosis?*
Estrogen stimulates OPG production. Hence, the decreased levels of estrogen in postmenopausal women increases osteoclastic activity, resulting in osteoporosis. Hence,

**Table 64.1:** Various cells present in the bone and their function.

| Cell | Peculiarities | Function |
|---|---|---|
| Osteocyte | These are the bone cells present in the bone and are most abundant | • Participate in the formation of an osteocytic membrane pump<br>• Maintain the calcium level in bone fluid<br>• Stimulate bone remodeling |
| Osteoblast | They are the bone-forming cells. They have parathyroid hormone receptors | Calcium deposition of the bones |
| Osteoclast | They are bone resorption cells as they have enzymes and acids that dissolve the bone. These cells don't have parathyroid hormone receptors | Bone resorption |

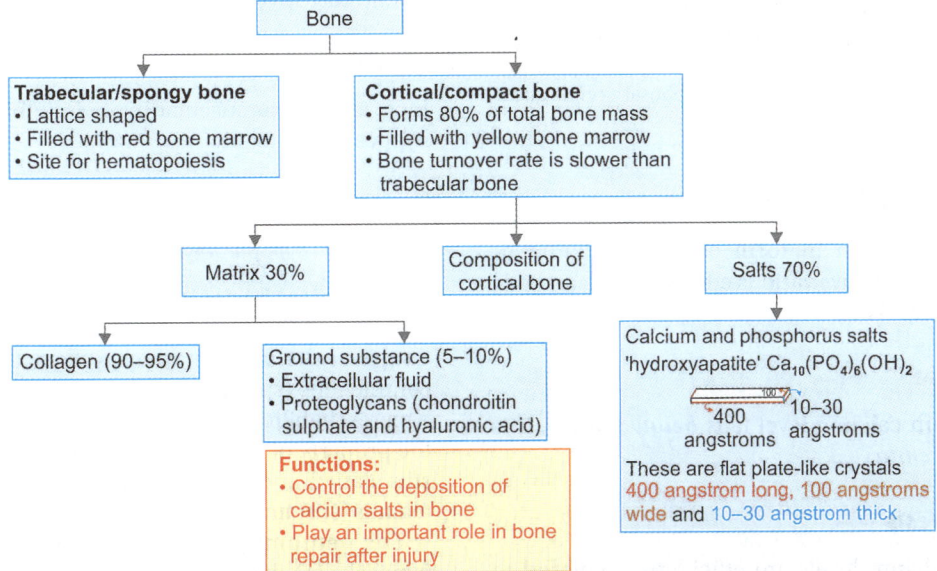

**Fig. 64.2:** Types and composition of bone.

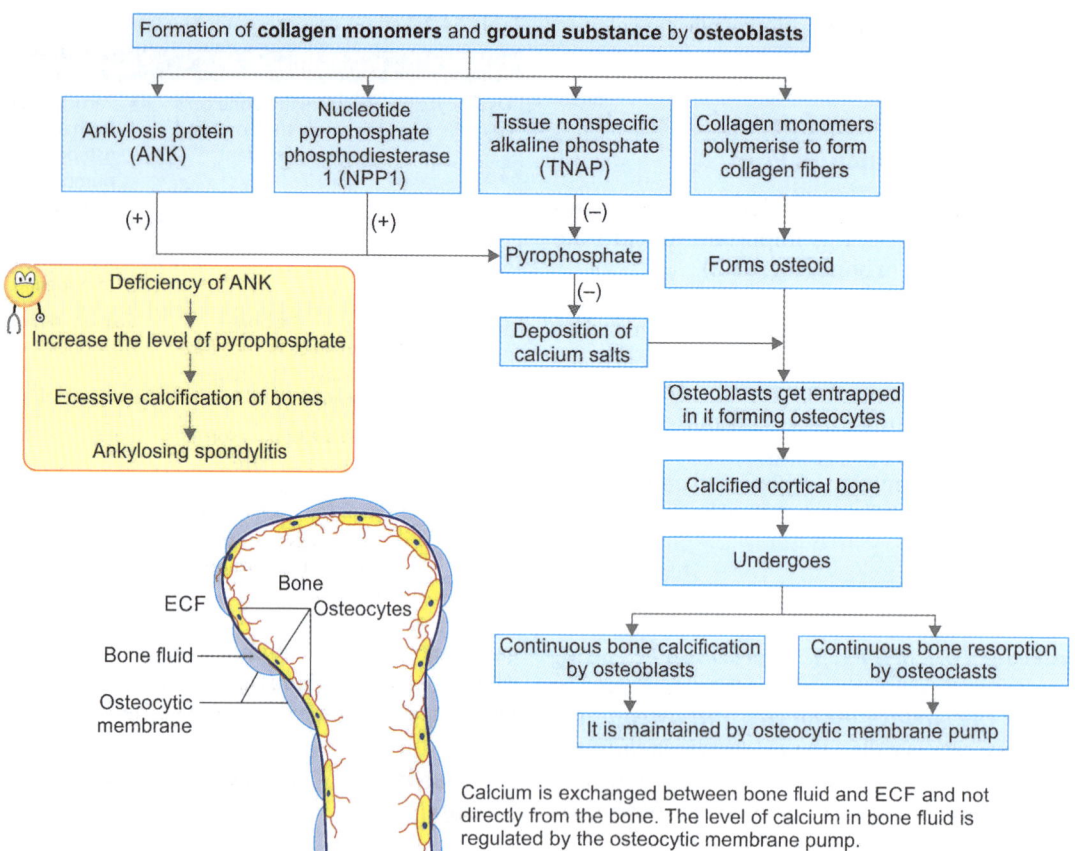

Fig. 64.3: Formation of bone.

estrogen provides a protective effect against osteoporosis in premenopausal women.

*Why do excessive glucocorticoids result in osteoporosis?*

Glucocorticoids also promote osteoclast activity and bone resorption by increasing RANKL production and decreasing the formation of OPG. The balance of OPG and RANKL produced by osteoblasts plays a major role in determining osteoclast activity and bone resorption resulting in osteoporosis.

**Clinical correlation:** Drugs that mimic the action of OPG by blocking the interaction of RANKL with its receptor appear to be useful for treating bone loss in postmenopausal women and in some patients with bone cancer.

## CALCIUM DYSREGULATION

Calcium dysregulation in form of hypocalcemia or hypercalcemia which have various effects on human body as shown in **Figure 64.5**.

### Hypocalcemia

The fall in serum calcium level falls *below 9 mg%*, it is called *hypocalcemia*.

### Etiopathogenesis

Usually, the calcium levels are efficiently regulated in our body. But the hypocalcemia can occur in any of the conditions mentioned below:

- **Hypoparathyroidism**
  - Due to surgical removal of parathyroid glands (along with thyroid glands)
  - Autoimmune hypoparathyroidism
- **Vitamin D3** deficiency resulting in decreased absorption of $Ca^{2+}$ from gut
  - End stage renal disease
  - End stage liver disease

### Clinical Features

- Increased neuromuscular hyperexcitability resulting in hypocalcemic tetany

**Explain the physiological basis of neuromuscular hyperexcitability in hypoparathyroidism/hypocalcemia.**

**Physiological basis:** It is clinically very important to understand that *fall in serum calcium levels below 6 mg% results in tetany*, which is characterized by tetanic contractions (spasm) of muscle due to neuromuscular hyperexcitability. This condition derives its name from the property of skeletal muscle in which the repetitive stimulation above the tetanizing frequency results in tetanus (sustained contraction) **(Fig. 64.6)**.

The neuromuscular hyperexcitability caused by hypocalcemia has two probable explanations:
1. **By decrease in the stearic hinderance to the influx $Na^+$ at the time of depolarization** of muscle. During

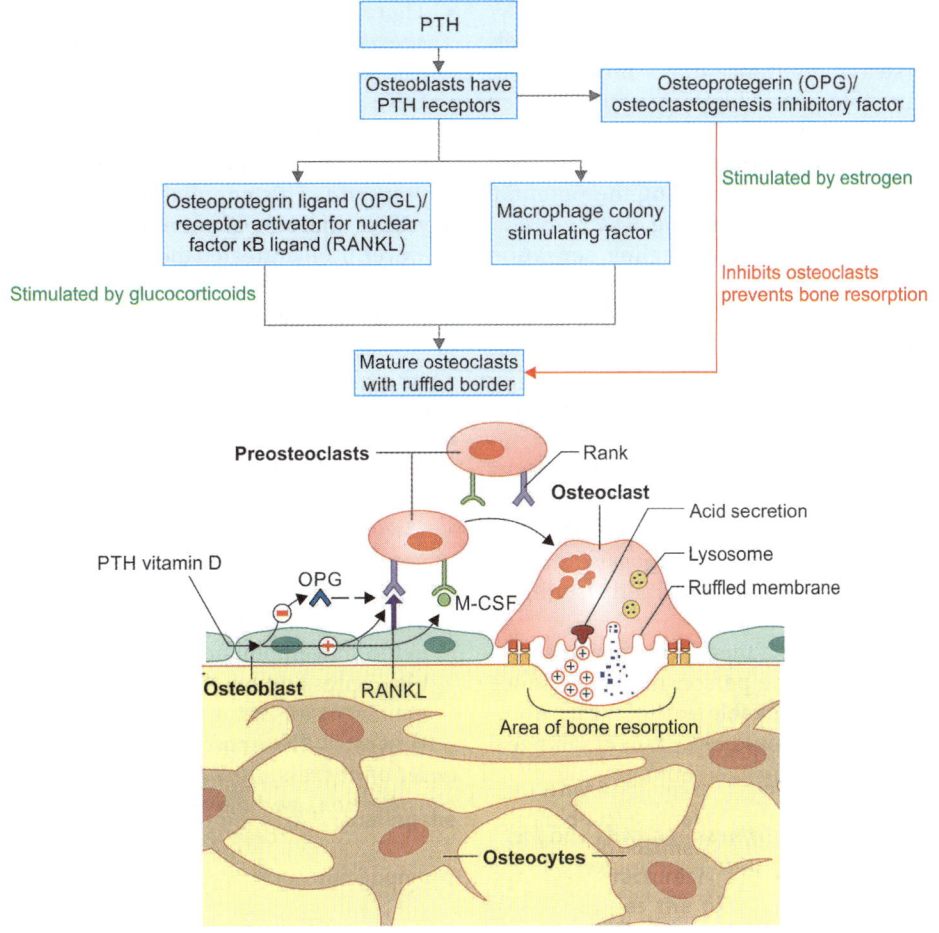

**Fig. 64.4:** Mechanism of osteolysis.

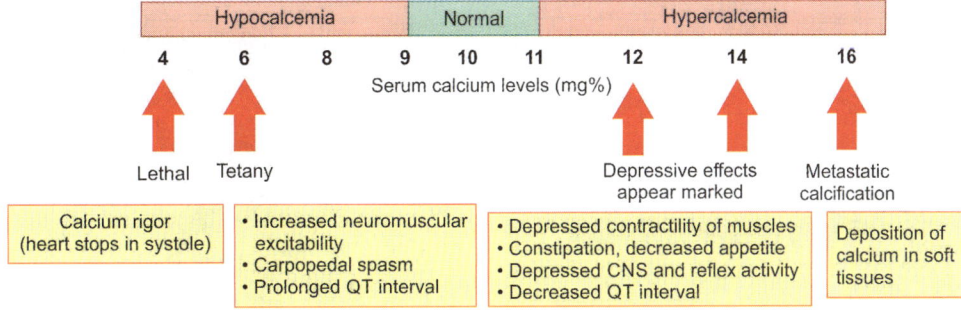

**Fig. 64.5:** Effects of hypocalcemia and hypercalcemia.

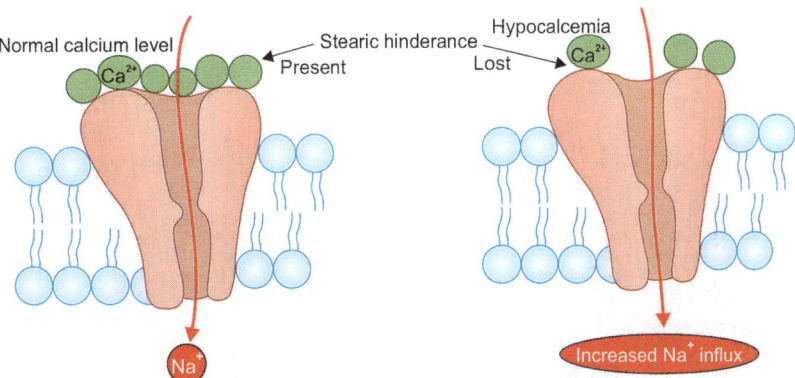

**Fig. 64.6:** Decreased stearic hinderance during hypocalcemia resulting in increased neuromuscular hyperexcitability.

normal concentration of calcium in ECF, the Ca$^{2+}$ binds the exterior of ACh gated sodium channels resulting in stearic hindrance to Na$^+$ influx. But in hypocalcemia, this stearic hindrance is decreased resulting in massive Na$^+$ influx.

2. **It raises the resting membrane potential** of muscles to close the threshold by decreasing the potential difference across the membrane **(Fig. 64.7)**.

- **Parasthesias:** Altered sensation/tingling sensation occurring due to neuronal hyperexcitability.
- **Circumoral numbness:** The patient complains of decreased sensation or paresthesia around the lips. This is usually the first sign of hypocalcemia.
- **Cramps:** The skeletal muscles may have cramps and sustained contraction or spasms in the muscles.
- **Tetany:** Tetanus is the property of skeletal muscle, where there is summation of contraction, if there is an increased frequency of stimulation, muscles show neuromuscular hyperexcitability. In hypocalcemia, the muscles undergo fusion of contractions and resulting in sustained contraction called *tetany*.
- **Followed by convulsions:** If there is further decrease in the S. calcium levels, the person may experience convulsions due to hyperexcitable state of the neurons.
- **Laryngeal stridor:** There could be spasm of laryngeal muscles resulting in difficulty in breathing.
- Dystonia and psychosis
- The patient has a feeling of *stiffness* in *hands* and *feet*
- He also complains of *colicky pain* in abdomen

- There is *bronchoconstriction* resulting in *bronchospasm:* In later stages can lead to laryngeal stridor and can cause death due to asphyxia.
- **ECG:** Shows *prolonged QT interval* (delayed conduction) due to prolonged ST segment **(Fig. 64.8)**.

Clinically, the patient presents with *circumoral paresthesia*. This complaint should alarm the treating physician, that his patient might be having hypocalcemia. However, if left untreated the patient can develop muscular spasms in the upper and lower limbs called *Carpopedal spasm* **(Fig. 64.9)**. Due to the typical posture of the hand in this spasm, it is also called *obstetrician tip hand*. There is *flexion at the wrist, adduction of the thumb, flexion at metacarpophalangeal joints and extension of interphalangeal joints.*

However, if the physician suspects hypocalcemia, it can be confirmed eliciting bedside signs:

- **Chvostek sign (Fig. 64.10):** In this, tapping on a facial nerve results in twitching of the facial muscles of the same side.
- **Trousseau sign (Fig. 64.11):** In this, when the pressure in the sphygmomanometer cuff is raised above systolic blood pressure for 3 to 5 minutes, the latent tetany is manifested resulting in a carpopedal spasm.

However, *hypercalcemia of 12 mg% results in the onset of depression contractility of muscles, anorexia, constipation, and depressed CNS activity and reflexes*. Even in the cardiac muscle, it causes *decreased QT*

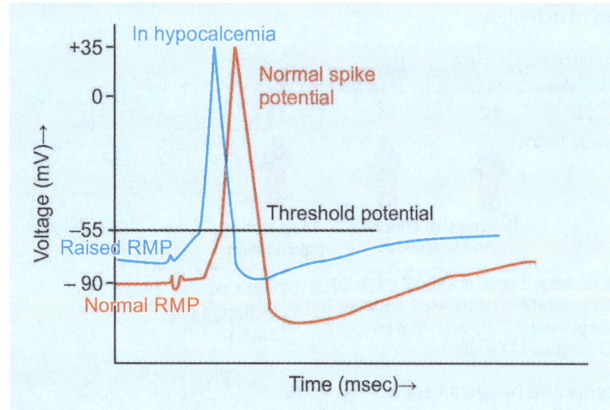

**Fig. 64.7:** Increased RMP close to threshold also increases the neuromuscular hyperexcitability.

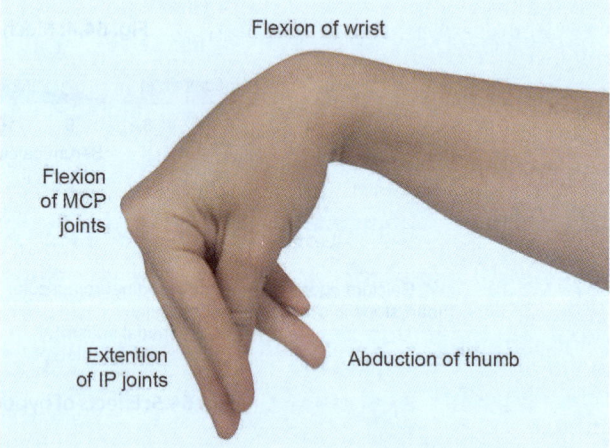

**Fig. 64.9:** Carpopedal spasm.

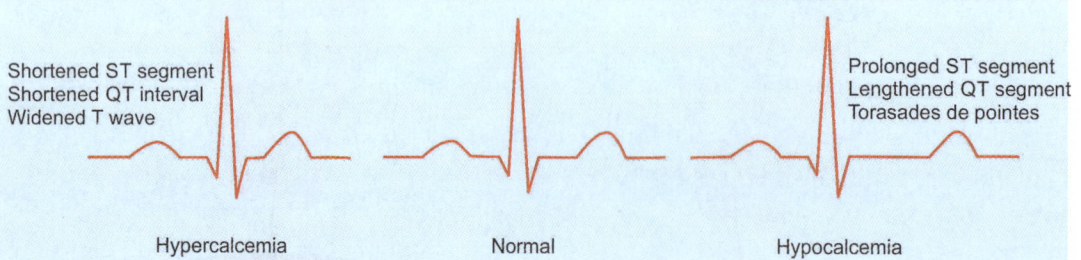

**Fig. 64.8:** ECG changes in hypoparathyroidism.

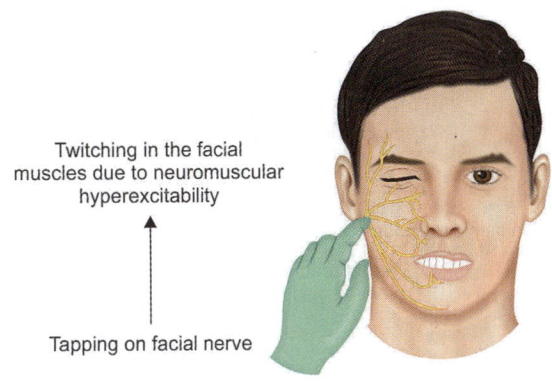

**Fig. 64.10:** Chvostek's sign.

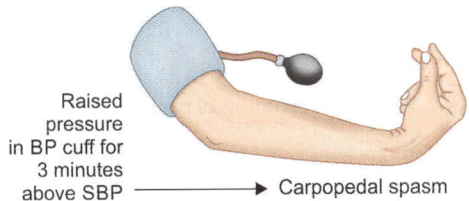

**Fig. 64.11:** Trousseau's sign.

*interval*. These effects become marked at serum calcium levels of 15 mg%.

Here we can see that calcium needs very close regulation and even minor alterations can result in serious effects. There is a very fine balance in calcium intake and excretion (**Fig. 64.12**) which is further regulated by three important calcium regulating hormones viz. *Parathormone, vitamin D3 and calcitonin*. We require to consume at least 1000 mg of calcium daily to maintain the calcium balance of our body.

## Management of Hypocalcemia

- Slow injection calcium gluconate is given over 10 minutes, incase of emergency.
- Oral calcium is administered for maintenance of calcium levels.
- ***Injection PTH not given, leads to increased calcium levels by the bone resorption. Also, the injection PTH results in the formation of antibodies against PTH.***

> **Why injection calcium gluconate is given over 10 minutes instead of the bolus dose?**
> A bolus dose of calcium gluconate will result in sudden stoppage of heart during systole, also called as calcium rigor.

## HORMONAL CONTROL OF CALCIUM LEVEL (FIG. 64.13)

As discussed above, three main hormones regulating serum calcium levels, along with their physiological role are mentioned in **Table 64.2**.

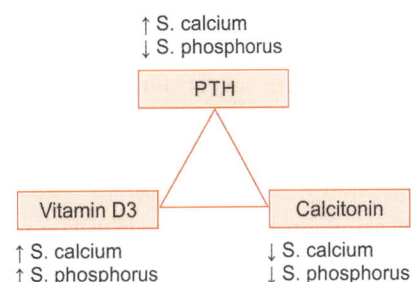

**Fig. 64.13:** Hormonal regulation of calcium.

**Table 64.2:** Hormonal control of calcium levels.

| Hormone | Source | Functions |
|---|---|---|
| Parathormone | Parathyroid gland | Increases S. calcium level by:<br>• Increasing bone resorption<br>• Stimulating vitamin D3 resulting in increased absorption of calcium from GIT<br>• Increases the excretion of phosphate in urine |
| Vitamin D3 | Formed in the skin and activated in the liver and kidney | • It stimulates the absorption of calcium from GIT<br>• Decreases renal calcium and phosphorus secretion |
| Calcitonin | Parafollicular cells of the thyroid gland | It lowers the serum calcium and phosphorus levels |

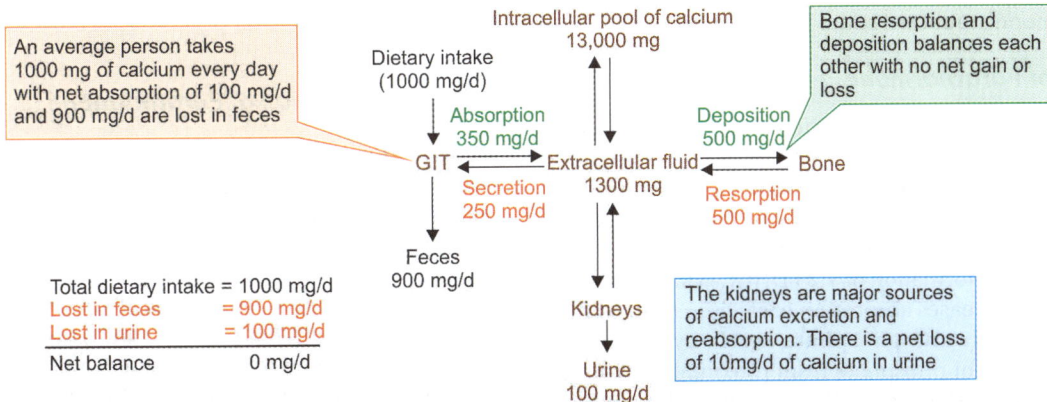

**Fig. 64.12:** Calcium balance in the body.

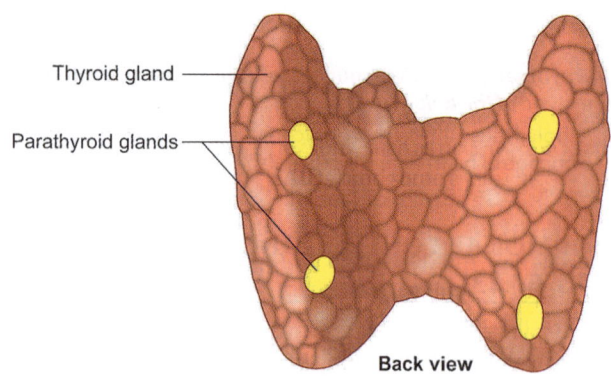

**Fig. 64.14:** Parathyroid glands embedded in the posterior surface of the thyroid gland.

Before going into the role of various hormones in regulation of calcium levels, let us first discuss the Parathyroid gland and parathormone.

## Parathyroid Gland and Parathormone

Parathyroid glands are concerned with calcium regulation. It secretes parathormone, a polypeptide hormone, which is responsible for resorption of calcium from the bones resulting in increased calcium levels in the blood.

### Physiological Anatomy

There are *four small parathyroid glands* embedded in the posterior surface of the thyroid gland (**Fig. 64.14**). Two of these are embedded in superior pole and two in inferior pole of thyroid gland.

Histologically, it has two types of cells:
1. *Chief cells* that secrete *parathormone*
2. *Oxyphil cells*, which are *depleted chief cells*

The plasma levels of parathormone range between *10–55 pg/mL*, with a half-life of *10 minutes*. The hormones rapidly *metabolized in liver*.

### Synthesis

Like other peptide hormones the parathormone, the precursor molecule is preprohormone which is formed in the endoplasmic reticulum. The steps in the synthesis of parathormone are shown in the **Figure 64.15**.

### Actions of Parathormone

- PTH directly acts on bone, increases bone resorption and mobilize calcium.
- **Increases plasma calcium levels by:**
  - Increasing the reabsorption of calcium in distal convoluted tubule (DCT) of kidneys.
  - Increasing formation of 1,25 DHCC (vitamin D) and hence, increases absorption of calcium from GIT.
- **Decreases plasma phosphate levels** by decreasing reabsorption of phosphate from proximal convoluted tubule (PCT) of the kidney. Hence, it is phosphaturic in nature.

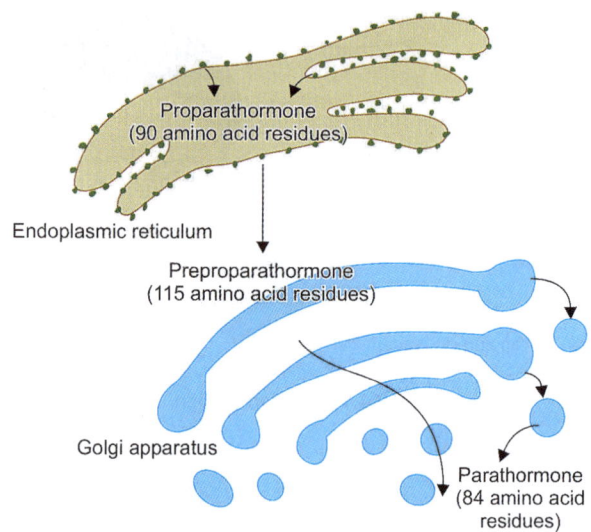

**Fig. 64.15:** Synthesis of parathormone.

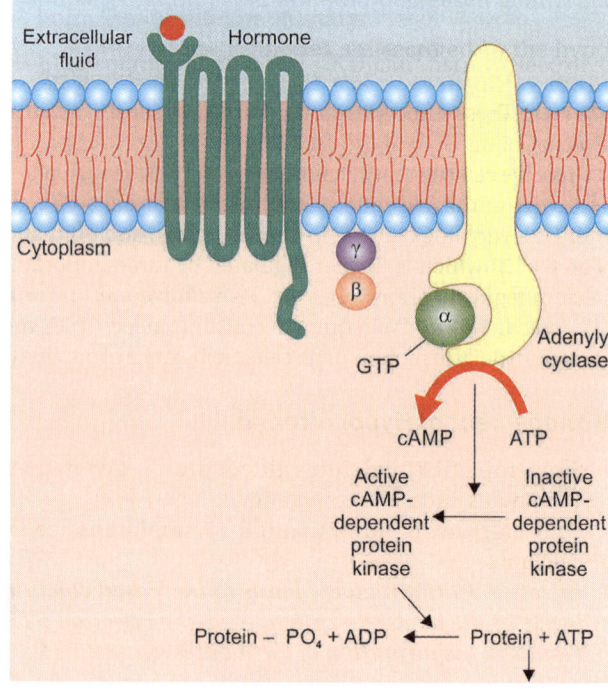

**Fig. 64.16:** Mechanism of action of PTH through adenylyl cyclase.

### Mechanism of Action of Parathormone

Parathormone activates adenylyl cyclase and increases cAMP. Hence, the response occurs due to the phosphorylation of proteins (**Fig. 64.16**).

> **What will happen to S. calcium and phosphate levels when infusion of PTH is given to a lab animal?**
> The infusion of PTH increases the S. calcium levels, but it reaches the plateau in around 4 hours, whereas the S. phosphorus levels decrease much rapidly, i.e., within 1–2 hours.

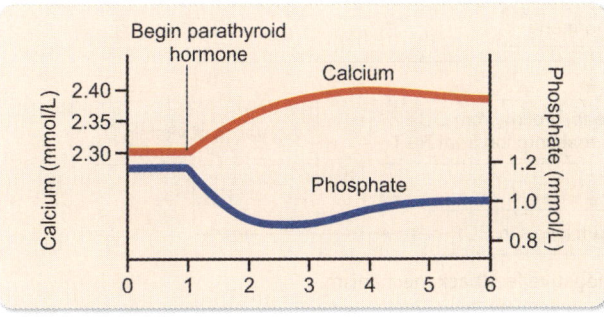

### Onset of Action

- **Rapid phase (which begins in minutes to hours):** Activation of already existing osteocytes to increase release of calcium and phosphate from bones (**Flowchart 64.1**).

  *The bone resorption takes place from areas around the osteocytes in the bone matrix and the osteoblasts along the bone surface.* It activates osteocytic membrane pump, decreasing calcium in bone fluid and increasing bone resorption (**Fig. 64.17**).

- **Slow phase:** When PTH remains elevated for a long time it results in bone resorption through the osteoclasts. These *osteoclasts do not have PTH receptors*, but are stimulated by these signals received from osteocytes and osteoblasts through the

**Flowchart 64.1:** Action of PTH on calcium concentration.

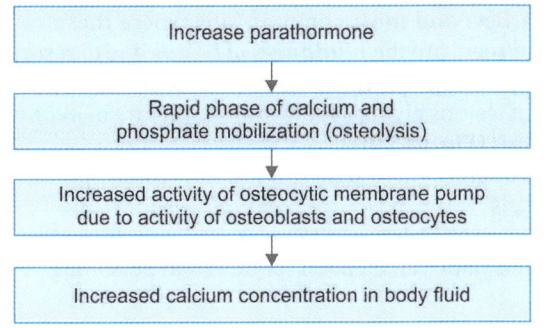

**Flowchart 64.2:** Effects of hypocalcemia on bones.

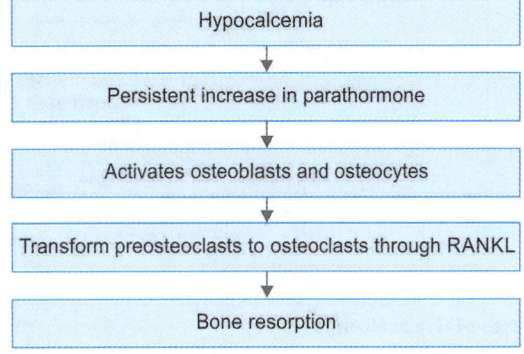

RANKL proteins (discussed in the chapter of calcium homeostasis) (**Flowchart 64.2**).

Hence, the long-term elevation of parathormone results in increase the osteoclastic activity along with the increased activity of osteoblasts to take the weekend bones, but the net result is mobilization of calcium from the bones into the extracellular fluid. This could even result in the development of large cavities in the bones filled with multinucleated osteoclasts.

### Regulation of PTH Secretion

**Calcium is the prime regulator of PTH secretion**, i.e., the concentration of calcium in the extracellular fluid regulates the parathyroid hormone secretion. An increase in the calcium levels decreases the PTH secretion through *negative feedback mechanism* which operates via **G protein coupled calcium sensing receptor** present in the parathyroid gland which operates through **phospholipase C, IP3 and DAG mechanism (Fig. 64.18)**.

## Abnormalities of the Parathyroid Gland

### Hypoparathyroidism

It is a clinical condition resulting in low serum calcium levels due to decreased secretion of parathyroid hormone.

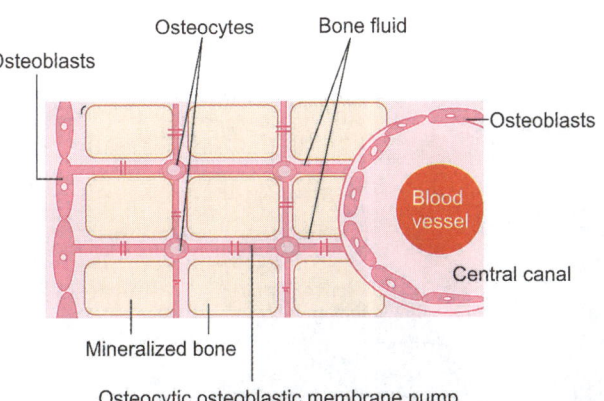

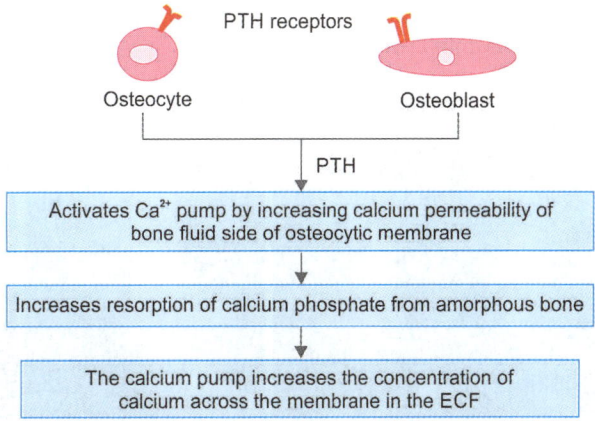

**Fig. 64.17:** Rapid phase of onset of action of PTH.

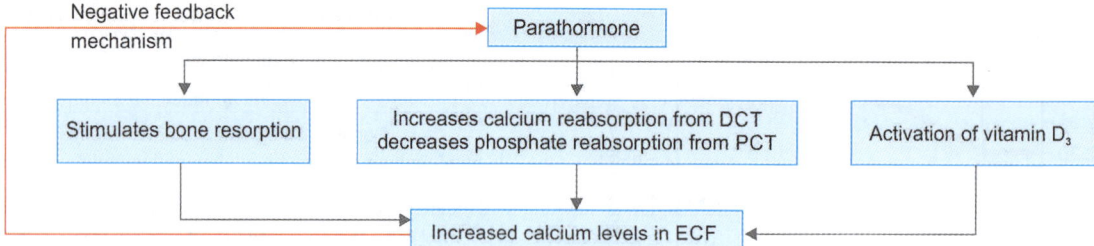

**Fig. 64.18:** Regulation of PTH by negative feedback mechanism.

**Causes of Hypocalcemia**
- Hypoparathyroidism
- Rickets
- Osteomalacia
- Alkalosis
- Pregnancy and lactation

### Etiopathogenesis

- **Acquired causes:** It occurs due to removal of parathyroid glands along with thyroidectomy (removal of thyroid gland) due to any reason.
- **Hereditary causes:**
  - *Di George syndrome:* Due to defective development of parathyroid gland and thymus
  - Autoimmune polyglandular failure

### Clinical Features

The clinical presentation of hypoparathyroidism is primarily due to hypocalcemia.

## Hyperparathyroidism

It refers to increased activity of the parathyroid glands resulting in increased calcium resorption from the bones and raised serum calcium levels.

### Etiopathogenesis

- Primary hyperparathyroidism
  - Increased activity of parathyroid gland
    - Tumor
    - Pregnancy and lactation
- Secondary hyperparathyroidism
  - Due to pathology somewhere else
    - Chronic renal failure
    - Vitamin D deficiency

### Clinical Features

- **Hypercalcemia:** There is raised serum calcium level up to 12 mg% due to increased bone resorption.
- **Hypophosphatemia:** There is decreased serum phosphate level [<2.5 mg% (normal level 12 mg%)] due to increase excretion of phosphate from kidneys.
- **Renal stones:** Hypercalcemia results in the formation of calcium stones in the kidney.
- **Peptic ulcer:** The calcium ions stimulates the release of gastric acid secretion and hence, results in the formation of peptic ulcers.
- **Increased bone resorption:** This results in the formation of the cavities in the bones which appear as cyst on the X-ray. These cavities or cysts heal with fibrosis, hence, called *osteitis fibrosa cystica* (**Fig. 64.19A**). These fibrosed cavity is appear as swelling on the surface of bone, mimicking a tumor hence, called *brown tumor* (**Fig. 64.19B**), which is a misnomer. The earliest and most common site, where these cavities are seen, are the *phalanges of hands* due to resorption of phalanges (**Fig. 64.19C**). The skull shows punched out lesions giving a radio graphic picture of *pepper pot skull* (**Fig. 64.19D**).
- Sudden marked dehydration and coma "parathyroid crisis".
- If serum Calcium >17 mg%, it leads to widespread metastatic calcification "parathyroid poisoning".

### Signs and Symptoms

- Tiredness, malaise and weakness
- **Renal features:** Renal colic, polyuria, hematuria and hypertension.

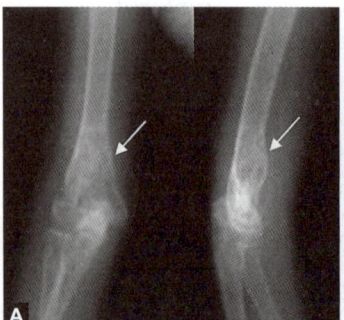 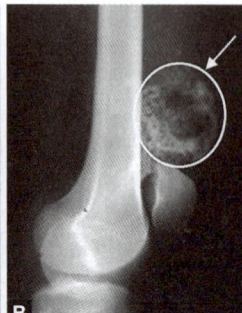 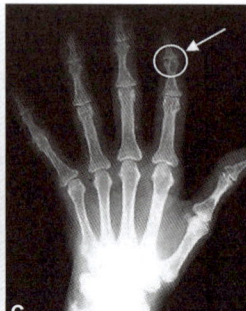 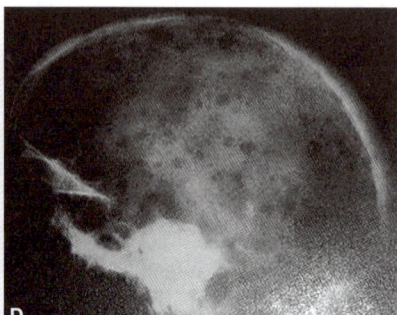

**Figs. 64.19A to D:** (A) Osteitis fibrosa cystica; (B) Brown tumor; (C) Cavities in phalanges; (D) Pepper pot skull.

- **Bones:** Bone pain, mainly affects cortical bone and leads to formation of bone cysts and locally destructive areas "Brown's Tumor".
- **Abdominal pain**
- **Ectopic calcification:** Deposition of calcium in soft tissues.
- **Corneal calcification:** Deposition of calcium in cornea.

## Lab Findings

- **Hypercalcemia:** Serum calcium is above 12 g/dL
- **Hypophosphatemia**

## Treatment

- Increased fluid intake
- Avoid increased calcium and vitamin D intake.

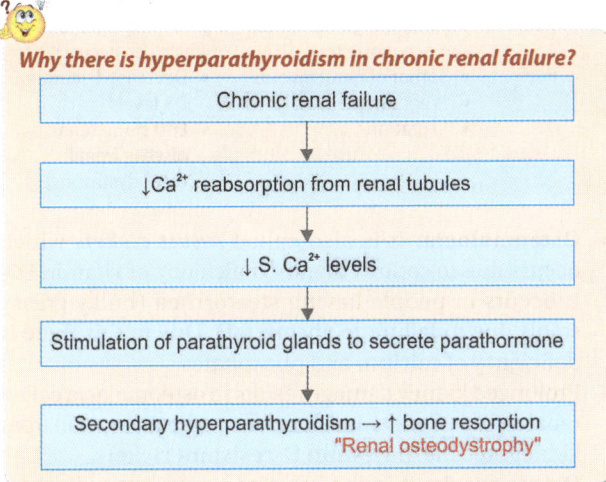

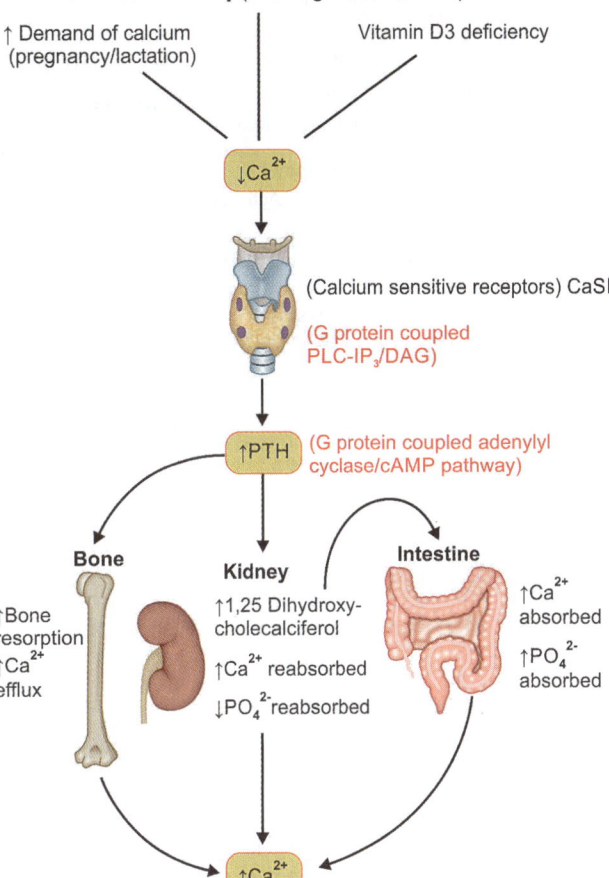

Fig. 64.20: Role of PTH in hypocalcemia.

concentration back to normal. An increased S. calcium level decreases the secretion of parathormone and decreased formation of active form of vitamin D3 (**Fig. 64.21**).

*What would happen to vitamin D3 levels in a patient in end stage kidney disease?*

The kidneys are required for the activation of vitamin D3. In the absence of functional kidneys, the active form of vitamin D3 which is the most potent form, is not formed resulting in the deficiency of vitamin D3.

*Why a patient with hyperparathyroidism get renal stones?*

Whenever there is hypercalcemia, it gets filtered from the kidney. The crystals of calcium phosphate tend to precipitate in the kidney, forming calcium phosphate stones. Also, calcium oxalate stones develop because even normal levels of oxalate cause calcium precipitation at high calcium levels. Most of renal stones are soluble in alkaline media, hence, the tendency for formation of renal calculi is considerably greater in alkaline urine than in acid urine. *For this reason, acidotic diets and acidic drugs are frequently used to treat renal calculi.*

### Role of Parathormone in Hypocalcemia

See **Figure 64.20**.

### Role of Vitamin D3 in Calcium Homeostasis

It is very interesting to note that the *serum calcium level is the prime regulator for release of these hormones*.

Decreased S. calcium stimulates the production of parathormone and increases the formation of 1,25-dihydroxycholecalciferol. It increases the calcium

### Calcitonin

It is the peptide hormone secreted by the parafollicular cells of the thyroid gland. This hormone decreases the level of calcium and phosphorus in the blood. Hence, the increased serum calcium level act as the potent stimulus for the release of the calcitonin.

The physiological effects of calcitonin are not well defined but however has been to shown to have a weak effect on serum calcium levels. Its effects are potentially opposite to the effects of parathormone. It inhibits bone resorption and increases calcium excretion in urine.

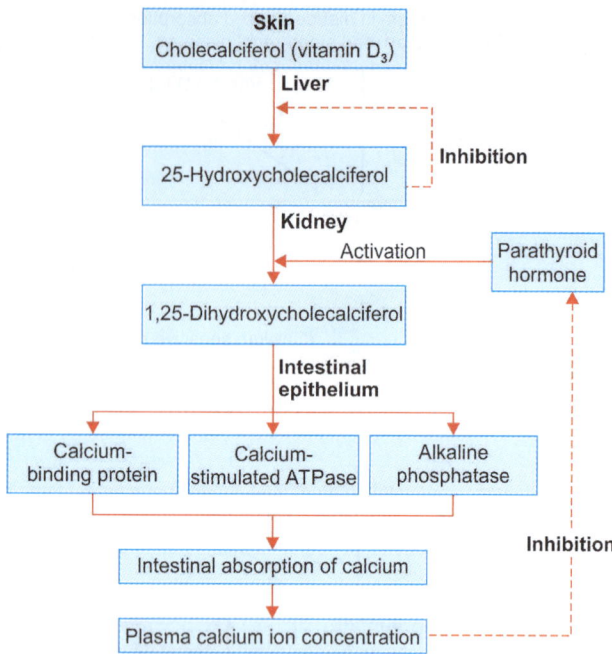

**Fig. 64.21:** Formation and action of vitamin D3.

**Table 64.3:** Endocrinal disorders related to parathormone, vitamin D3 (calcitriol).

| | Primary endocrine disorder | Secondary endocrine disorder |
|---|---|---|
| Hypoparathyroidism | Decreased activity of parathyroid gland resulting in low PTH, which can occur due to:<br>• Surgical removal of parathyroid glands along with thyroidectomy<br>• Autoimmune destruction of parathyroid glands (polyglandular failure)<br>• DiGeorge syndrome: Defective development of parathyroid glands | Increased serum calcium levels due to:<br>• Excessive quantities of calcium in the diet<br>• Increased dietary intake of vitamin D<br>• Increased bone resorption caused by factors other than PTH (disuse of bones) |
| Hyperparathyroidism | Increased activity of parathyroid gland which can occur due to:<br>• Tumor of parathyroids<br>• Pregnancy<br>• Lactation | Increased activity of parathyroid gland which can occur due to:<br>• Decreased vitamin D3 levels<br>• End stage renal disease (renal osteodystrophy) |

## Functions of Calcitonin

- It is required for **skeletal development** and bone remodeling in growing children.
- **Prevents excessive loss of calcium** from the bones of mother during pregnancy and lactation.
- Pharmacologically, it is used as a **treatment for Paget's disease** of bone to reduce serum calcium and phosphorus levels. Paget's disease is characterized by an imbalance in the osteoclastic and osteoblastic activity resulting in bone pain, fractures, arthritis, deformities, nerve compression, and hearing loss. Calcitonin can slow down abnormal bone remodeling and reduce symptoms.
- It also acts as a *biomarker*; as it is **raised in inflammatory disorders**.

Various disorders of PTH and calcitriol are tabulated in **Table 64.3**.

## Vitamin D3 Deficiency

The deficiency of vitamin D3 results in rickets in children and osteomalacia in adults.

- **Rickets:** It is characterized by *decrease serum vitamin D3 resulting in hypocalcemia and hypophosphatemia in children.*

  The parathormone causes bone resorption and raises serum calcium levels hence, results in only slight decrease in calcium levels whereas phosphate levels are further depressed due to the phosphaturic effect of parathormone. Chronic rickets result in secondary hyperparathyroidism resulting in weak bones and increased osteoblastic activity. The osteoblasts lay down large quantity of osteoid which remains uncalcified resulting in the formation of weaker bones.

- **Osteomalacia:** It is also called *adult rickets* which occurs due to serious dietary deficiency of vitamin D3. It occurs in people having steatorrhea (bulky greasy stools due to failure to absorb fat). Due to this there is deficiency of calcium and phosphates.
- Prolonged kidney damage results in osteomalacia called renal rickets. Congenital deficiency of reabsorption from kidneys results in **vitamin D-resistant rickets.**
- **Osteoporosis:** It is the most common bone disorder seen in adults especially in old age. There is *diminished organic bone matrix* rather than from poor bone calcification. The osteoblastic activity in the bone is usually less than normal. The main causes of osteoporosis are as follows:
  - There is *lack of physical stress on the bones* because of physical inactivity.
  - The patient is having *severe malnutrition* to the extent that sufficient protein matrix cannot be formed.
  - *Lack of vitamin C,* which is necessary for secretion of intercellular substances by all cells, including formation of osteoid by the osteoblasts.
  - *The postmenopausal women lack estrogen secretion.* The estrogens decrease the number and activity of osteoclasts (discussed above), hence, predisposes to osteoporosis.
  - In old age, growth hormone and other growth factors are reduced significantly along with reduction in protein anabolic, so bone matrix cannot be deposited adequately.
  - The patients of *Cushing syndrome*, have massive quantities of glucocorticoids secreted in this disease. This causes decreased deposition of protein throughout the body and increased catabolism of protein. This depresses the osteoblastic activity.

## SUMMARY

- Serum calcium levels are important for many physiological processes, such as muscle contraction, nerve impulse, blood clotting and bone formation.
- Serum calcium levels are tightly regulated within a normal range by a complex homeostatic mechanism involving the skeleton, the kidney, and the intestine.
- The major hormones that are responsible for maintaining normal serum calcium levels are parathyroid hormone (PTH) and vitamin D. These hormones control serum calcium levels on a long-term basis.
- PTH is secreted by the parathyroid glands in response to low serum calcium levels. It increases serum calcium levels by stimulating osteoclasts, which break down bone to release calcium into the bloodstream. PTH also inhibits osteoblasts, which deposit bone and reduce calcium in the bloodstream. PTH also increases calcium reabsorption in the kidney and calcium absorption in the intestine. PTH release is inhibited by rising serum calcium levels.
- Vitamin D is produced in the skin by exposure to sunlight or obtained from the diet. It is activated in the liver and kidney to form calcitriol, the active form of vitamin D. Calcitriol acts on the intestine to increase calcium absorption from the diet. Calcitriol also acts on the bone and kidney to regulate calcium metabolism. Calcitriol synthesis is stimulated by low serum calcium levels and inhibited by high serum calcium levels.
- Calcitonin is another hormone that is involved in calcium homeostasis, but its role is less significant than PTH and vitamin D. Calcitonin is secreted by the thyroid gland in response to high serum calcium levels. It lowers serum calcium levels by inhibiting osteoclasts and increasing calcium excretion in the kidney. Calcitonin release is stimulated by low serum calcium levels.
- Abnormalities in the hormonal control of serum calcium levels can lead to disorders of calcium metabolism, such as hypercalcemia or hypocalcemia, which can have serious consequences for health and well-being.

## LET US SEE, HOW MUCH YOU HAVE LEARNT?

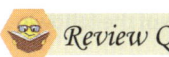

### *Review Questions*

### *Short Answer Type Questions*

Q1. Enumerate the functions of calcium in our body.
Q2. Describe the role of various hormones in regulating the serum calcium levels.
Q3. Describe the role of the osteocytic membrane pump in regulating serum calcium levels.
Q4. What are the normal calcium levels? Define hypocalcemia and hypercalcemia?
Q5. What happens to neuromuscular excitability, if serum calcium falls below 9 mg/dL?
Q6. Describe the etiopathogenesis, clinical features (signs and symptoms), diagnosis and management of clinical hypocalcemia/hypoparathyroidism.
Q7. What happens to serum calcium levels in a person with end-stage renal disease?
Q8. Why do postmenopausal women have a higher tendency to get fractures?
Q9. Why does the patient of Cushing's syndrome have osteoporotic bones?
Q10. What happens to serum calcium levels, if a patient hyperventilates?
Q11. Why do we prescribe calcitonin for Paget's disease?

### *Structured Long Answer Questions*

Q1. Describe the synthesis and mechanism of action of parathormone. Describe the effect of hyperparathyroidism on bones.
Q2. Describe the hormonal control of calcium levels in blood in terms of:
- Enumerate various hormones involved in calcium homeostasis
- Describe the functions of each hormone
- 'There is interdependence of these hormones in calcium regulation'. Justify your statement.

Q3. How does calcium homeostasis affect the function of the nervous system and the muscular system?

### *Critical Thinking Case-Based Questions*

Q1. A 45-year-old woman presents to the emergency department with muscle cramps, tingling in her fingers and around her mouth, and anxiety. She had a total thyroidectomy for papillary thyroid cancer 3 months ago and has been taking levothyroxine 100 mcg daily. She denies any fever, chest pain, shortness of breath, or other symptoms. On physical examination, she is alert and oriented, with a blood pressure of 140/90 mm Hg, a pulse of 90 beats per minute, and a respiratory rate of 18 breaths per minute. She has dry skin and brittle nails. She exhibits positive Chvostek's sign and Trousseau's sign. Her electrocardiogram shows a prolonged QT interval. Her laboratory results are as follows:

- Serum calcium: 6.8 mg/dL (normal range: 8.5–10.2 mg/dL)

- Serum phosphorus: 5.6 mg/dL (normal range: 2.5–4.5 mg/dL)
- Serum magnesium: 1.8 mg/dL (normal range: 1.7–2.4 mg/dL)
- Serum parathyroid hormone (PTH): <5 pg/mL (normal range: 10–65 pg/mL)
- Serum 25-hydroxyvitamin D: 20 ng/mL (normal range: 30–100 ng/mL)

Based on the given case history, answer the following questions:
a. What is the most likely diagnosis for this patient?
b. What is the physiological role of the parathyroid hormone (PTH) in regulating calcium and phosphorus levels in the body?

## Multiple Choice Questions

**Q1.** Which hormone primarily regulates calcium metabolism in the body?
  a. Insulin
  b. Glucagon
  c. Parathyroid hormone
  d. Thyroid hormone

**Q2.** Where is parathyroid hormone synthesized?
  a. Adrenal glands
  b. Thyroid gland
  c. Parathyroid glands
  d. Pancreas

**Q3.** Which of the following is NOT a function of parathyroid hormone (PTH)?
  a. Increasing intestinal absorption of calcium
  b. Increasing renal reabsorption of calcium
  c. Stimulating bone resorption
  d. Decreasing blood phosphate levels

**Q4.** What effect does calcitonin have on blood calcium levels?
  a. Increases blood calcium levels
  b. Decreases blood calcium levels
  c. Has no effect on blood calcium levels
  d. Increases calcium absorption in the intestines

**Q5.** Which of the following conditions is characterized by an overproduction of parathyroid hormone?
  a. Hyperthyroidism
  b. Hypothyroidism
  c. Hyperparathyroidism
  d. Hypoparathyroidism

**Q6.** What is the primary role of vitamin D in calcium metabolism?
  a. To increase renal excretion of calcium
  b. To decrease calcium absorption in the intestines
  c. To increase calcium absorption in the intestines
  d. To decrease renal reabsorption of calcium

**Q7.** A 55-year-old woman presents with muscle weakness and bone pain. Laboratory tests show elevated serum calcium and low serum phosphate levels. Which condition is most likely affecting her?
  a. Hyperparathyroidism
  b. Hypoparathyroidism
  c. Osteoporosis
  d. Osteomalacia

**Q8.** A patient with chronic kidney disease develops hypocalcemia. Which physiological mechanism is most likely responsible for this condition?
  a. Increased parathyroid hormone secretion
  b. Decreased vitamin D activation
  c. Increased calcium reabsorption in the kidneys
  d. Decreased calcitonin secretion

**Q9.** A young male patient presents with symptoms of tetany and muscle cramps. His blood tests reveal low calcium levels and high phosphate levels. Which of the following is the most likely diagnosis?
  a. Hyperparathyroidism
  b. Hypoparathyroidism
  c. Primary hyperaldosteronism
  d. Cushing's syndrome

**Q10.** How does the parathyroid hormone (PTH) increase blood calcium levels?
  a. By decreasing calcium absorption in the intestines
  b. By increasing calcium reabsorption in the kidneys
  c. By decreasing bone resorption
  d. By increasing phosphate reabsorption in the kidneys

**Q11.** What is the primary reason for bone demineralization in patients with chronic hyperparathyroidism?
  a. Excessive secretion of calcitonin
  b. Increased osteoclastic activity
  c. Reduced vitamin D synthesis
  d. Decreased intestinal absorption of calcium

**Q12.** Which of the following is not a common sign or symptom of rickets?
  a. Bowed legs or knock knees
  b. Bone pain and tenderness
  c. Poor growth and development
  d. Joint swelling and inflammation

**ANSWERS**
1. c    2. c    3. d    4. b    5. c    6. c    7. a    8. b    9. b    10. b    11. b    12. d

# Physiology of Hypothalamus

**CHAPTER 65**

### COMPETENCY ADDRESSED
**PY8.2:** Describe the synthesis, secretion, transport, physiological actions, regulation, and effect of altered (hypo and hyper) secretion of pituitary gland, thyroid gland, parathyroid gland, adrenal gland, pancreas and **hypothalamus**.

### LEARNING OBJECTIVES
**At the end of this chapter, the learner should be able to:**
- Enumerate the various nuclei of hypothalamus.
- Describe the neuro endocrine functions of hypothalamus.
- Describe the physio-clinical significance of activity and defects in various hypothalamic nuclei.

Hypothalamus is the master endocrine gland and the head autonomic ganglia. Apart from these two major functions, it forms an integral part of limbic system which controls the emotions of an individual.

## FUNCTIONAL ANATOMY

Hypothalamus is a small triangular structure weighing only 4 grams, located below the thalamus and above the pituitary gland **(Fig. 65.1)**. It forms the floor and inferolateral walls of the third ventricle.

**Hypothalamic nuclei (Fig. 65.2):** Based on their location, the hypothalamic nuclei are divided into two main groups:

1. Lateral group of nuclei **(Fig. 65.3)**
   - Lateral hypothalamus
   - Periventricular nuclei
2. Medial group of nuclei
   - Anterior group
     - Anterior hypothalamus
     - Suprachiasmatic nucleus
     - Preoptic nucleus
     - Supraoptic nucleus
     - Paraventricular nucleus

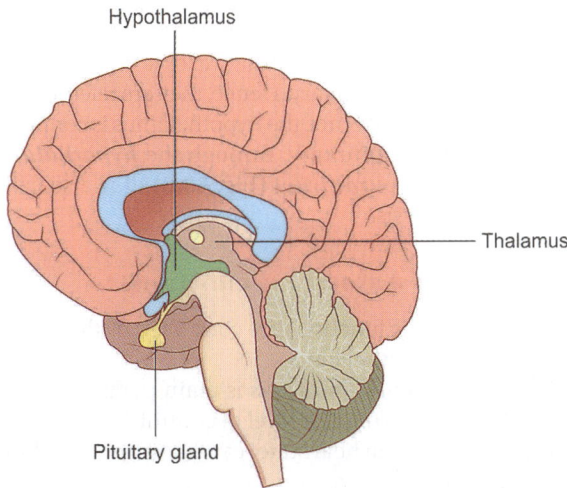

**Fig. 65.1:** Location of hypothalamus.

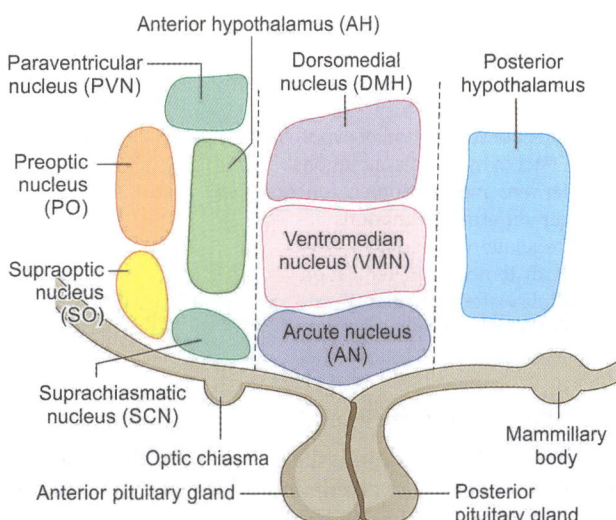

**Fig. 65.2:** Hypothalamic nuclei.

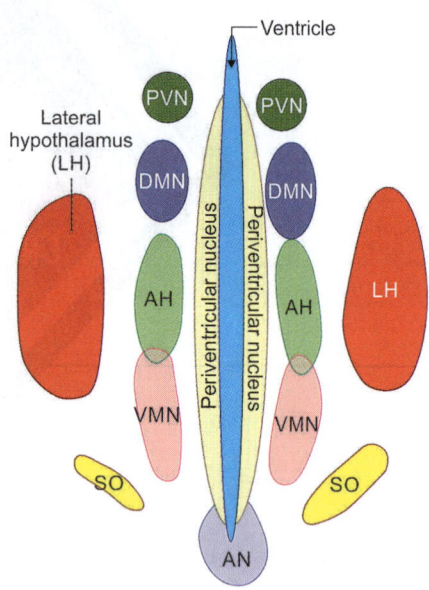

**Fig. 65.3:** Coronal section showing lateral nuclear group.

- Median group
  - Arcuate nucleus
  - Ventromedial nucleus
  - Dorsomedial nucleus
- Posterior group
  - Posterior hypothalamus
  - Mamillary bodies

## FUNCTIONS OF HYPOTHALAMUS (SEE FIG. 65.7)

As discussed above, hypothalamus is main control center for the release of all the hormones, autonomic and emotional functions of body. Let's discuss all these functions one by one.

**Functions of hypothalamus**

**Endocrine functions**
- Regulation of anterior pituitary hormones by Hypothalamo-pituitary–gland axis
- Synthesis of hormones secreted from posterior pituitary

**Autonomic functions**
- Regulation of cardiovascular functions

**Behavioral effects**
- Effect of stimulation of hypothalamic nuclei
- Effect of hypothalamic lesions
- Reward and punishment function

**Other vegetative functions**
- Regulation of feeding
- Body temperature regulation
- Body water regulation
- Regulation of circadian rhythm

### Endocrine Functions

The hypothalamus controls the secretions of almost all the hormones of the body. It communicates with the anterior and posterior pituitary differently.

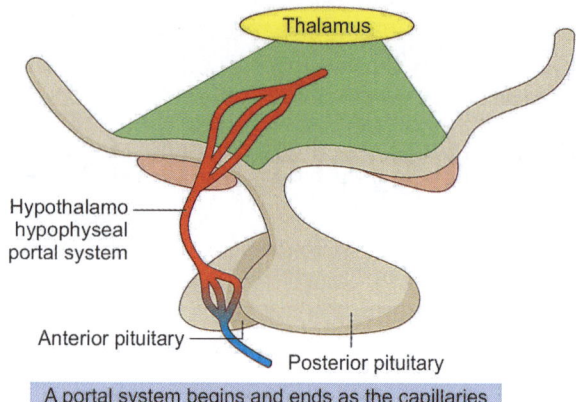

**Fig. 65.4:** Hypothalamo-hypophyseal portal system.

1. The anterior pituitary gland receives the regulating hormones from hypothalamus through the portal system called *hypothalamo-hypophyseal portal system* (**Fig. 65.4**).

   Lets first see, how hypothalamus controls the hormones of anterior pituitary.

   Six regulatory hormones are secreted by the hypothalamus, viz.
   a. Growth hormone releasing hormone (GHRH) secreted by periventricular nuclei
   b. Growth hormone inhibitory hormone (GHIH)/somatostatin secreted by periventricular and arcuate nuclei
   c. Thyroid releasing hormone (TRH) secreted by periventricular nuclei
   d. Corticotropin releasing hormone (CRH) secreted by paraventricular nuclei
   e. Gonadotropin releasing hormone (GnRH) secreted by preoptic nuclei
   f. Prolactin inhibiting hormone (PIH)/Dopamine secreted by arcuate nuclei

   These hormones stimulate/inhibit the secretion of hormones secreted by the anterior pituitary gland. The hormonal modulation by these regulatory factors on hypophyseal hormones in shown in the **Figure 65.5**.

2. Oxytocin and antidiuretic hormone (vasopressin) are secreted by posterior pituitary gland are basically synthesized in the supraoptic and paraventricular nuclei of hypothalamus. These hormones move to the terminal buttons of these neurons through axoplasmic streaming, into the posterior pituitary. Hence, they are released from posterior pituitary. Since the hypothalamus is connected to the posterior pituitary, through the *hypothalamo-hypophyseal neural tract* (**Fig. 65.6**), it is also called neurohypophysis.

### Regulation of Autonomic Functions

Various autonomic functions are controlled by the anterior and posterior hypothalamus.
- The *anterior hypothalamus* is main parasympathetic ganglia acting as highest level of control.
  - It decreases the heart rate, cardiac output and blood pressure.

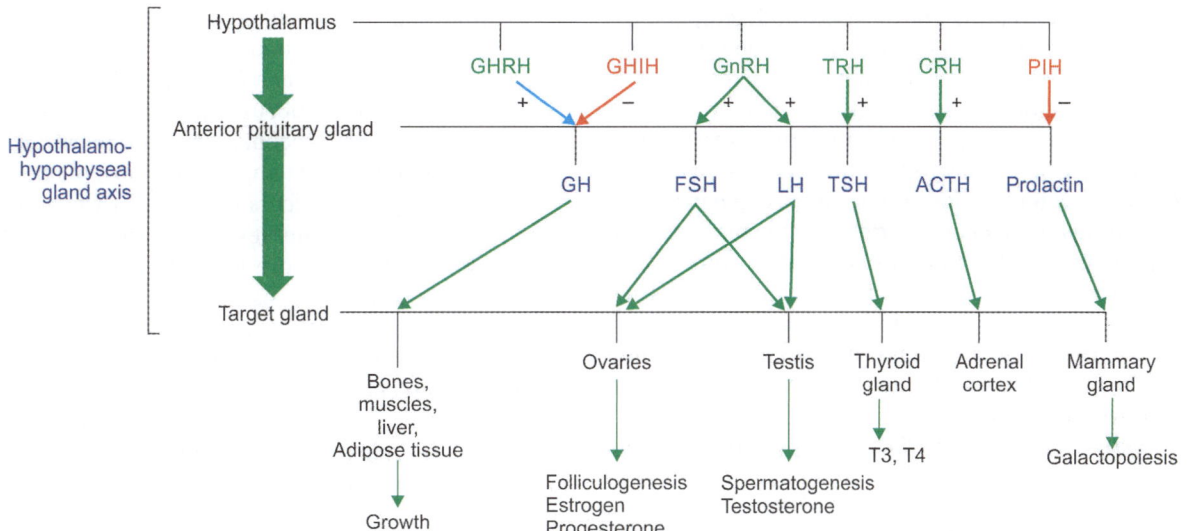

**Fig. 65.5:** Hypothalamo-hypophyseal-gland axis for regulation of release of hormones.

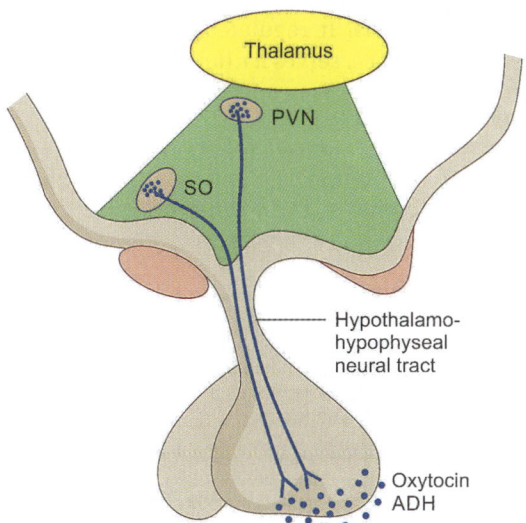

**Fig. 65.6:** Hypothalamo-hypophyseal neural tract.

- It increases the GI motility and secretions.
- It regulates the hypothalamic set point for temperature regulation. *The lesions of anterior hypothalamus results in hyperthermia.* The temperature regulation is discussed below.
- The *posterior hypothalamus* is main sympathetic ganglia acting as highest level of control.
  - It increases the heart rate, cardiac output and blood pressure.
  - It decreases the GI motility and secretions.
  - It regulates the body temperature. *The lesions of posterior hypothalamus results in cold bloodedness/poikilothermia.*

## Other Vegetative Functions of Hypothalamus

### Regulation of Feeding

- The *lateral hypothalamus* acts as the feeding center, controlling the hunger. It also controls *thirst and emotional drive*. Damage to this area results in loss of desire to eat. This condition is called as *anorexia*. It can sometimes cause fatal starvation.
- The *ventromedial nucleus acts as satiety center*. Stimulation of this center can stop the feeding behavior of the animal but its damage can result in a voracious appetite of the animal. This can cause morbid obesity in animal/person, called as *hypothalamic obesity*.
- Some other centers associated with feeding are *arcuate nucleus*, affecting the appetite and *mammillary bodies* responsible for controlling feeding reflexes like licking of lips, swallowing, etc.

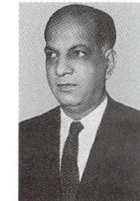

Dr BK Anand, an eminent Indian physiologist who had discovered the hypothalamic 'feeding center' in 1951.

### Body Temperature Regulation

The normal core body temperature of humans ranges from 97°F (36°C) to 99.5°F (37.5°C), with an average core body temperature between 98.0 to 98.6°F. The *anterior hypothalamus and preoptic area have heat and cold sensitive neurons*.

- The firing rate of heat sensitive neurons increases manifolds (2–10 times) with an rise of 10°C in body temperature.
- The firing rate of cold sensitive neurons increases with the fall in body temperature.

*How does our body sense the temperature?*
Temperature sensitive receptors present in the skin carry the impulses to the higher centers of brain.

*How does our body respond/adapt to ambient environmental temperature?*

- **During high temperature exposure:**
  - *Vasodilation of cutaneous blood vessels* occurs due to inhibition of posterior hypothalamus (sympathetic).

- **Increased sweating** with the rise in body temperature. We all know that evaporation causes cooling. Hence, every 1°C rise in body temperature increase loss of body heart by 10 times through evaporation of sweat.
- Inhibition of heat producing mechanisms like shivering or processes involving thermogenesis.
- **Response of body to low temperature exposure:**
  - **Cutaneous vasoconstriction** due to stimulation of posterior hypothalamus resulting in vasoconstriction.
  - **Piloerection** (contraction of arrector pili muscles due to sympathetic stimulation—goose bumps) on the skin. It is an important mechanism of conservation of heat in animals, where the air gets trapped in hair, providing insulation.
  - **Increased heat production** by body (thermogenesis): thyroxine secretion, sympathetic excitation heat production resulting in increased BMR and shivering resulting in heat production.
    - *Shivering:* Posterior hypothalamic nuclei have an area called the **primary motor center for shivering**, which gets inhibited by anterior hypothalamus but stimulated by cold signals from skin and spinal cord. Shivering causes heat production by the body.
    - *Chemical thermogenesis:* It is also called chemical thermogenesis, occurring due to oxidation of food stuffs by catecholamines and releasing heat to maintain body temperature. Most of chemical thermogenesis occurs in brown fat which is rich in sympathetic nerves and mitochondria. This stimulates the expression of thermogenin and hence, thermogenesis.

Set point for temperature control: It is the critical core body temperature of *about 37.1°C*, regulates the heat gain or loss mechanisms in order to maintain a body temperature close to set point. The various mechanisms involved in the regulation of body are discussed in unit 11 on integrated physiology.

## Body Water Regulation

The hypothalamus plays a vital role in regulation of the water homeostasis. It regulates the water intake and excretion and hence, serves it's function.

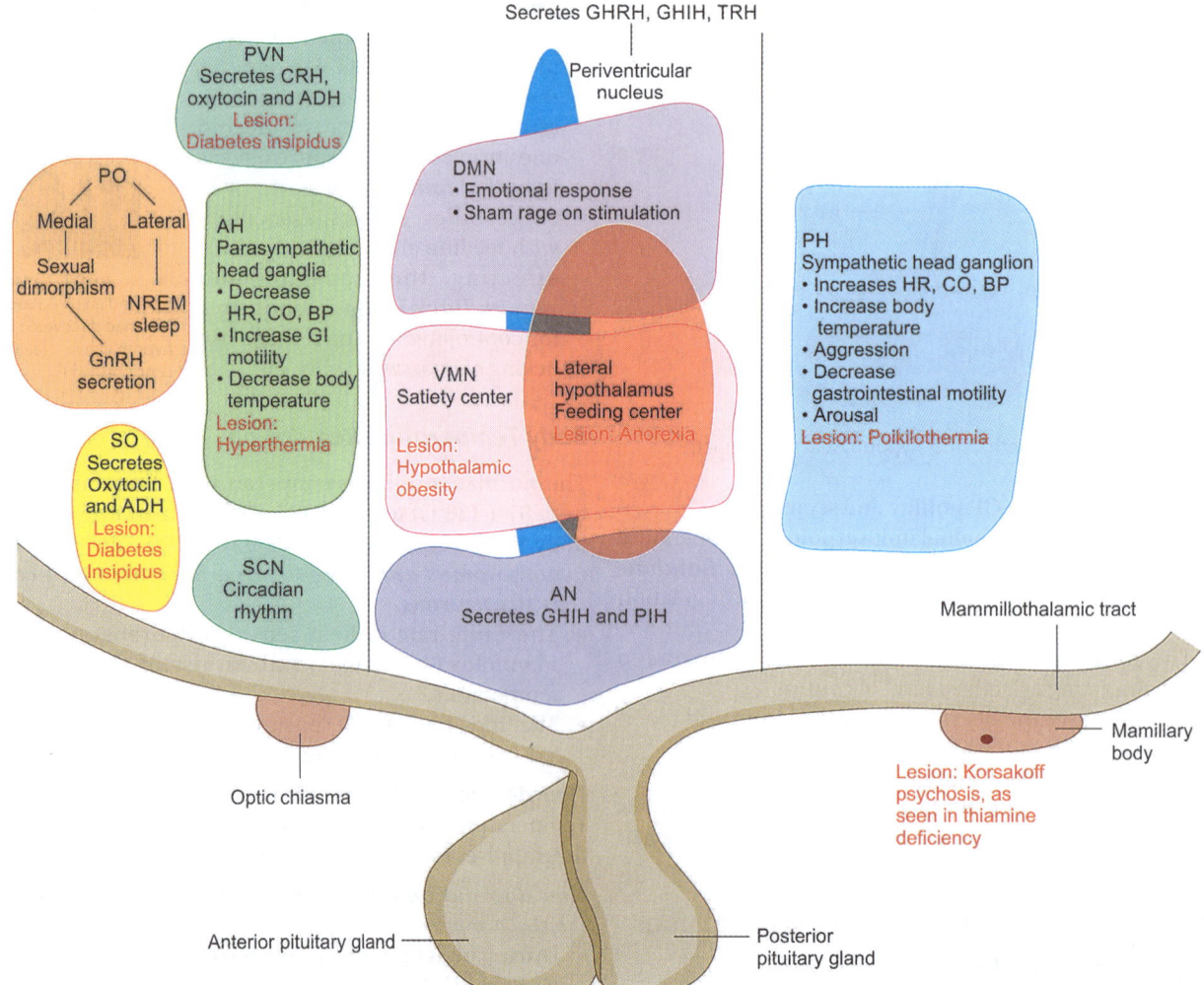

**Fig. 65.7:** Hypothalamic nuclei with their functions and lesions.

- The thirst center is located in the lateral hypothalamus which increases the water intake in response to various thirst mechanisms of body like blood tonicity, volume, etc.
- The *supraoptic and paraventricular nuclei* secrete antidiuretic hormone which regulate the excretion of water from the renal tubules.

### Regulation of Circadian Rhythm

The circadian rhythm is best understood as the master or biological clock which controls our sleep wake cycles, secretion of hormones, etc. The *suprachiasmatic nucleus* lying just above the optic chiasma, gets the input from retinohypothalamic tract and regulates the circadian rhythm. Of late this has greatly attracted many scientists into the field of chronobiology.

### Behavioral Functions

Hypothalamus is an important part of the limbic system and hence, shows some significant behavioral effects.
- Stimulation of *lateral hypothalamus* affects the general activity of animal. It can cause *aggressive behavior* leading to overt rage and fighting. However, stimulation of VMN nucleus causes tranquility. Both these nuclei are well known for controlling the feeding behavior of an animal. We can remember it by a simple fact that when a person is hungry, he becomes agitated and angry but a well fed person is calm!
- The periventricular nuclei located adjacent to third ventricle, is usually responsible for secretion of various regulatory hormones for pituitary gland. Stimulation of these nuclei leads to fear and punishment reactions.

### SUMMARY

- Hypothalamus is the master autonomic and endocrine gland, located just below the thalamus and above the pituitary gland.
- It has many nuclei, which are divided into anterior, medial, posterior and lateral groups, based on their location.
- The anterior and posterior hypothalamus serves as the autonomic ganglia.
- The hypothalamus controls the secretion of hormones of anterior pituitary by secreting the releasing or inhibiting hormones from periventricular nuclei, arcuate nuclei, preoptic nuclei. These regulatory hormones reach the anterior pituitary through hypothalamo hypophyseal portal system.
- The hormones secreted from posterior pituitary are infact synthesized in paraventricular and supraoptic nucleus of hypothalamus and released from posterior pituitary through hypothalamo hypophyseal neural tract.
- The release of these hormones is regulated by the negative feedback mechanism affecting the hypothalamo hypophyseal gland axis, as studied in homeostasis.

### LET US SEE, HOW MUCH YOU HAVE LEARNT?

 *Review Questions*

#### Long/Short Answer Questions

Q1. Enumerate the hypothalamic nuclei. Describe their function in detail.
Q2. Describe the role of hypothalamus in temperature regulation.
Q3. Describe the role of hypothalamus in water homeostasis.
Q4. What would happen to a person, if the lateral hypothalamus is stimulated?
Q5. What would happen, if there is a lesion in the posterior hypothalamus?
Q6. Why do the obstetricians prescribe dopamine inhibitors for milk formation in a woman with failure of lactation after delivery?
Q7. What is the role of master clock in our daily routine? How can this be useful in preventing various lifestyle related diseases?

#### Explain Why? (Reasoning Questions)

Q1. Damage to the hypothalamus can lead to disruptions in body temperature regulation.
Q2. Lesions in the hypothalamus can affect appetite and lead to disorders such as obesity or anorexia.
Q3. The hypothalamus plays a crucial role in the stress response by regulating the release of corticotropin-releasing hormone (CRH).

 *Critical Thinking Case-Based Questions*

Q1. A 32-year-old woman, reported to OPD with complaints of persistent fatigue, weight gain, and feeling unusually cold. She also reported irregular menstrual cycles and decreased libido. On physical examination, she had dry skin and a slowed heart rate. Blood tests revealed low levels of thyroid hormones (T3 and T4) and elevated thyroid-stimulating hormone (TSH). An MRI of the brain showed a small mass in the region of the hypothalamus.

Based upon the given case scenario, answer the following questions:
a. Explain the role of the hypothalamus in regulating endocrine function.
b. Discuss how a hypothalamic mass could lead to this patient's clinical presentation.
c. Write a note on regulation of hypothalamus.

## Multiple Choice Questions

Q1. A 58-year-old man, known hypertensive, was brought to the neuro ICU, with intracranial hemorrhage affecting the hypothalamic area around the third ventricle. He is most likely to have problem with:
   a. Temperature regulation
   b. Secretion of regulatory hormones
   c. Disturbed circadian rhythm
   d. Behavior resulting in aggression and rage

Q2. A patient presents with symptoms of excessive thirst and frequent urination. Which hormone produced by the hypothalamus is likely to be involved in the regulation of water balance?
   a. Cortisol
   b. Thyroid-stimulating hormone (TSH)
   c. Antidiuretic hormone (ADH)
   d. Growth hormone (GH)

Q3. A patient complains of feeling excessively hot and sweating profusely. Dysfunction in which hypothalamic hormone might be responsible for these symptoms?
   a. Thyrotropin-releasing hormone (TRH)
   b. Gonadotropin-releasing hormone (GnRH)
   c. Corticotropin-releasing hormone (CRH)
   d. Thyroid-stimulating hormone (TSH)

Q4. A patient presents with symptoms of fatigue, weight gain, and cold intolerance. Dysfunction in which hypothalamic hormone might lead to these symptoms?
   a. Dopamine
   b. Growth hormone-releasing hormone (GHRH)
   c. Thyrotropin-releasing hormone (TRH)
   d. Somatostatin

Q5. A patient is diagnosed with insufficient milk production after childbirth. Dysfunction in which hypothalamic hormone might contribute to this condition?
   a. Oxytocin
   b. Gonadotropin-releasing hormone (GnRH)
   c. Prolactin-inhibiting hormone (PIH)
   d. Growth hormone-releasing hormone (GHRH)

Q6. A patient exhibits symptoms of delayed puberty, including lack of secondary sexual characteristics. Dysfunction in which hypothalamic hormone might be involved?
   a. Prolactin-inhibiting hormone (PIH)
   b. Corticotropin-releasing hormone (CRH)
   c. Gonadotropin-releasing hormone (GnRH)
   d. Thyrotropin-releasing hormone (TRH)

Q7. A patient presents with symptoms of excessive stress, including elevated blood pressure and cortisol levels. Dysfunction in which hypothalamic hormone might contribute to these symptoms?
   a. Somatostatin
   b. Dopamine
   c. Vasopressin
   d. Corticotropin-releasing hormone (CRH)

Q8. A patient exhibits symptoms of acromegaly, such as enlarged hands and feet. Dysfunction in which hypothalamic hormone might contribute to this condition?
   a. Growth hormone-releasing hormone (GHRH)
   b. Gonadotropin-releasing hormone (GnRH)
   c. Corticotropin-releasing hormone (CRH)
   d. Thyrotropin-releasing hormone (TRH)

Q9. A patient presents with symptoms of polyuria and polydipsia. Dysfunction in which hypothalamic hormone might be responsible for these symptoms?
   a. Corticotropin-releasing hormone (CRH)
   b. Prolactin-inhibiting hormone (PIH)
   c. Vasopressin
   d. Growth hormone-releasing hormone (GHRH)

Q10. A patient is diagnosed with infertility due to irregular menstrual cycles. Dysfunction in which hypothalamic hormone might contribute to this condition?
   a. Somatostatin
   b. Dopamine
   c. Prolactin-inhibiting hormone (PIH)
   d. Gonadotropin-releasing hormone (GnRH)

Q11. A patient exhibits symptoms of excessive growth, including tall stature and enlarged facial features. Dysfunction in which hypothalamic hormone might contribute to this condition?
   a. Thyrotropin-releasing hormone (TRH)
   b. Growth hormone-releasing hormone (GHRH)
   c. Corticotropin-releasing hormone (CRH)
   d. Prolactin-inhibiting hormone (PIH)

Q12. A patient presents with symptoms of amenorrhea and hot flashes. Dysfunction in which hypothalamic hormone might contribute to these symptoms?
   a. Thyrotropin-releasing hormone (TRH)
   b. Vasopressin
   c. Gonadotropin-releasing hormone (GnRH)
   d. Corticotropin-releasing hormone (CRH)

Q13. A patient exhibits symptoms of low blood pressure and dehydration. Dysfunction in which hypothalamic hormone might contribute to these symptoms?
   a. Growth hormone-releasing hormone (GHRH)
   b. Thyrotropin-releasing hormone (TRH)
   c. Vasopressin
   d. Prolactin-inhibiting hormone (PIH)

Q14. A patient presents with symptoms of gigantism. Dysfunction in which hypothalamic hormone might contribute to this condition?
   a. Thyrotropin-releasing hormone (TRH)
   b. Gonadotropin-releasing hormone (GnRH)
   c. Growth hormone-releasing hormone (GHRH)
   d. Corticotropin-releasing hormone (CRH)

Q15. A patient exhibits symptoms of hyperprolactinemia, including lactation in the absence of pregnancy.

Dysfunction in which hypothalamic hormone might contribute to this condition?
a. Vasopressin
b. Gonadotropin-releasing hormone (GnRH)
c. Prolactin-inhibiting hormone (PIH)
d. Thyrotropin-releasing hormone (TRH)

Q16. A patient presents with symptoms of cushingoid features, such as moon face and central obesity. Dysfunction in which hypothalamic hormone might contribute to this condition?
a. Corticotropin-releasing hormone (CRH)
b. Growth hormone-releasing hormone (GHRH)
c. Thyrotropin-releasing hormone (TRH)
d. Dopamine

Q17. A patient exhibits symptoms of anorexia and weight loss. Dysfunction in which hypothalamic hormone might contribute to these symptoms?
a. Thyrotropin-releasing hormone (TRH)
b. Corticotropin-releasing hormone (CRH)
c. Growth hormone-releasing hormone (GHRH)
d. Somatostatin

Q18. A patient presents with symptoms of low libido and erectile dysfunction. Dysfunction in which hypothalamic hormone might contribute to these symptoms?
a. Thyrotropin-releasing hormone (TRH)
b. Vasopressin
c. Gonadotropin-releasing hormone (GnRH)
d. Corticotropin-releasing hormone (CRH)

Q19. A patient exhibits symptoms of hyponatremia and fluid retention. Dysfunction in which hypothalamic hormone might contribute to these symptoms?
a. Prolactin-inhibiting hormone (PIH)
b. Vasopressin
c. Corticotropin-releasing hormone (CRH)
d. Growth hormone-releasing hormone (GHRH)

Q20. A patient presents with symptoms of hyperthyroidism, including weight loss and heat intolerance. Dysfunction in which hypothalamic hormone might contribute to these symptoms?
a. Thyrotropin-releasing hormone (TRH)
b. Prolactin-inhibiting hormone (PIH)
c. Growth hormone-releasing hormone (GHRH)
d. Corticotropin-releasing hormone (CRH)

Q21. A patient exhibits symptoms of hirsutism and irregular menstrual cycles. Dysfunction in which hypothalamic hormone might contribute to these symptoms?
a. Somatostatin
b. Dopamine
c. Gonadotropin-releasing hormone (GnRH)
d. Thyrotropin-releasing hormone (TRH)

Q22. A patient presents with symptoms of infertility and oligomenorrhea. Dysfunction in which hypothalamic hormone might contribute to these symptoms?
a. Vasopressin
b. Growth hormone-releasing hormone (GHRH)
c. Thyrotropin-releasing hormone (TRH)
d. Corticotropin-releasing hormone (CRH)

Q23. A patient exhibits symptoms of hypothyroidism, including weight gain and cold intolerance. Dysfunction in which hypothalamic hormone might contribute to these symptoms?
a. Prolactin-inhibiting hormone (PIH)
b. Growth hormone-releasing hormone (GHRH)
c. Corticotropin-releasing hormone (CRH)
d. Thyrotropin-releasing hormone (TRH)

Q24. A patient presents with symptoms of hyperprolactinemia, including galactorrhea. Dysfunction in which hypothalamic hormone might contribute to these symptoms?
a. Somatostatin
b. Dopamine
c. Prolactin-inhibiting hormone (PIH)
d. Gonadotropin-releasing hormone (GnRH)

Q25. A patient exhibits symptoms of low energy and decreased muscle mass. Dysfunction in which hypothalamic hormone might contribute to these symptoms?
a. Growth hormone-releasing hormone (GHRH)
b. Vasopressin
c. Corticotropin-releasing hormone (CRH)
d. Thyrotropin-releasing hormone (TRH)

Q26. A patient presents with symptoms of increased appetite and weight gain. Dysfunction in which hypothalamic hormone might contribute to these symptoms?
a. Corticotropin-releasing hormone (CRH)
b. Prolactin-inhibiting hormone (PIH)
c. Thyrotropin-releasing hormone (TRH)
d. Somatostatin

Q27. Which hypothalamic nucleus is primarily responsible for regulating body temperature?
a. Suprachiasmatic nucleus
b. Paraventricular nucleus
c. Ventromedial nucleus
d. Preoptic nucleus

Q28. Which hypothalamic nucleus is involved in regulating circadian rhythms and the sleep-wake cycle?
a. Arcuate nucleus
b. Suprachiasmatic nucleus
c. Dorsomedial nucleus
d. Lateral hypothalamic area

Q29. Which hypothalamic nucleus plays a crucial role in controlling hunger and satiety?
a. Arcuate nucleus
b. Paraventricular nucleus
c. Ventromedial nucleus
d. Dorsomedial nucleus

Q30. Damage to which hypothalamic nucleus might lead to disturbances in water balance and thirst regulation?
a. Arcuate nucleus
b. Suprachiasmatic nucleus
c. Lateral hypothalamic area
d. Supraoptic nucleus

Q31. The nucleus responsible for the synthesis and release of oxytocin and vasopressin is the:
a. Suprachiasmatic nucleus
b. Arcuate nucleus
c. Lateral hypothalamic area
d. Supraoptic nucleus

Q32. Damage to which hypothalamic nucleus might disrupt the regulation of body weight and energy balance?
a. Suprachiasmatic nucleus
b. Arcuate nucleus
c. Paraventricular nucleus
d. Ventromedial nucleus

Q33. Which hypothalamic nucleus is involved in controlling the release of gonadotropin-releasing hormone (GnRH) and thereby regulating reproductive functions?
  a. Ventromedial nucleus
  b. Lateral hypothalamic area
  c. Arcuate nucleus
  d. Preoptic nucleus

Q34. The nucleus responsible for regulating the release of growth hormone-releasing hormone (GHRH) and somatostatin, thus influencing growth and metabolism, is the:
  a. Paraventricular nucleus
  b. Arcuate nucleus
  c. Ventromedial nucleus
  d. Dorsomedial nucleus

Q35. Damage to which hypothalamic nucleus might impair the regulation of the autonomic nervous system, including heart rate and blood pressure?
  a. Dorsomedial nucleus
  b. Paraventricular nucleus
  c. Suprachiasmatic nucleus
  d. Lateral hypothalamic area

## ANSWERS

| 1. a | 2. c | 3. a | 4. c | 5. c | 6. c | 7. d | 8. a | 9. c | 10. d | 11. b | 12. c | 13. c | 14. c |
| 15. c | 16. a | 17. b | 18. c | 19. b | 20. a | 21. c | 22. d | 23. d | 24. b | 25. a | 26. d | 27. d | 28. b |
| 29. a | 30. d | 31. d | 32. d | 33. d | 34. b | 35. b | | | | | | | |

# Physiology of Pituitary Gland

**CHAPTER 66**

### COMPETENCY ADDRESSED
**PY8.2:** Describe the synthesis, secretion, transport, physiological actions, regulation and effect of altered (hypo and hyper) secretion of **pituitary gland**, thyroid gland, parathyroid gland, adrenal gland, pancreas and hypothalamus.

### LEARNING OBJECTIVES
**At the end of this chapter, the learner should be able to:**
- Enumerate the various hormones secreted by anterior, intermediate and posterior pituitary gland.
- Describe the synthesis, secretion, mechanism of action, regulation and functions of growth hormone.
- Describe the related clinical effects of hypo- and hypersecretion of the growth hormone in children and adults.
- Describe the synthesis, secretion, mechanism of action, regulation, functions of hormones of posterior pituitary.

## FUNCTIONAL ANATOMY

Pituitary gland is a small **pea sized gland** located in the **sella turcica of the base of skull**, just below the hypothalamus. The optic chiasma is present anterior to the pituitary gland and the mammillary body is present posteriorly **(Fig. 66.1)**.

Embryologically, the anterior pituitary gland is derived from the invagination of pharyngeal Rathke's pouch whereas the posterior pituitary is an outgrowth of hypothalamic neural tissue. Hence, both the anterior and posterior pituitary glands are histologically different.

The *anterior pituitary gland* is made up of epithelioid cells and have different types of distinct cells having specific functions (Fig. 66.2):
- **Somatotrophs (30-40%):** These cells secrete growth hormone. These cells stain with acidic dyes, hence, called acidophils
- **Corticotrophs (20%):** Secrete adrenal corticotropic hormone (ACTH)
- **Gonadotrophs (3-5%):** Secrete follicle stimulating hormone (FSH) and Luteinizing hormone (LH)
- **Thyrotrophs (3-5%):** Secretes thyroid stimulating hormone (TSH)
- **Lactotrophs (3-5%):** Secretes prolactin (Prl)

### FACT CHECK
The pituitary tumors secreting large quantities of GH are called *acidophilic tumors.*

The posterior pituitary gland has **Magnocellular neurons** located in **supraoptic** and **paraventricular** nucleus of the hypothalamus. The hormones (Oxytocin and ADH) are synthesized in the cell bodies of these nuclei and released from the posterior pituitary gland.

## HORMONES OF PITUITARY GLAND

The various hormones secreted by the pituitary gland and their functions are summarized in **Table 66.1**.

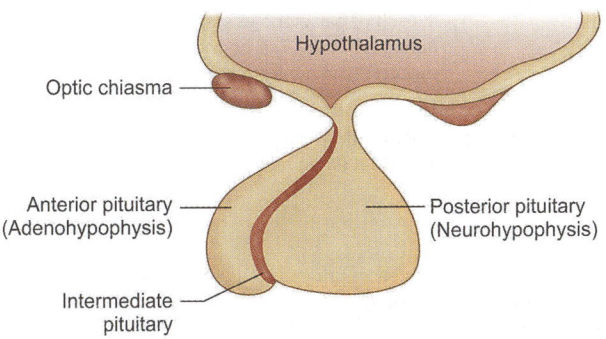

**Fig. 66.1:** The pituitary gland.

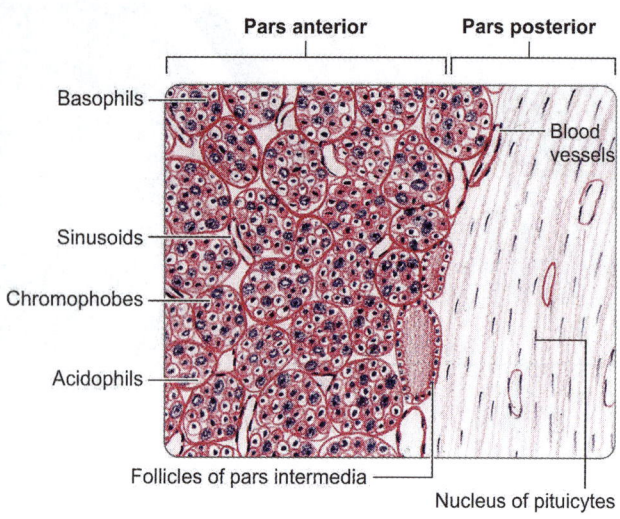

**Fig. 66.2:** Histology of pituitary gland.

The anterior pituitary receives various regulatory hormones from hypothalamus through hypothalamo-hypophyseal-portal system **(Fig. 66.3)** whereas the posterior pituitary is connected to hypothalamus through the hypothalamo-hypophyseal-neural tract **(Fig. 66.4)**. These are discussed in detail in Chapter 65.

## GROWTH HORMONE

It is the peptide hormone secreted by the somatotrophic cells of anterior pituitary gland.

### Physiological Actions of Growth Hormone (Table 66.2)

Growth hormone is the only hormone, secreted by the liver which acts directly on the target tissues (bone, muscle, adipose tissue and metabolism).

**Table 66.1:** Pituitary hormones and their features.

| Hormone | Type of hormone | Target gland | Mechanism of action | Function |
|---|---|---|---|---|
| **Anterior pituitary gland** | | | | |
| Growth hormone | Peptide hormone with 191 amino acids | Bone, cartilages, muscles, liver and adipose tissue | JAK STAT pathway | • Stimulates body growth<br>• Stimulates secretion of insulin-like growth factor-1<br>• Stimulates lipolysis<br>• Inhibits actions of insulin on carbohydrate and lipid metabolism |
| Adrenal corticotropic hormone | Peptide hormone with 39 amino acids | Adrenal cortex | G protein coupled adenylyl cyclase cAMP pathway | Stimulates production of glucocorticoids and androgens by the adrenal cortex |
| Follicle stimulating hormone | Glycoprotein with 2 subunits (α and β) | Ovaries in women and sertoli cells in men | G protein coupled adenylyl cyclase cAMP pathway | • Stimulates the maturation of ovarian follicles in women and spermatogenesis in men. It increases the sensitivity of follicular cells and Leydig cells to LH<br>• It results in secretion of estrogen from ovaries |
| Luteinizing hormone | Glycoprotein with 2 subunits (α and β) | Ovaries in women and Leydig cells in men | G protein coupled adenylyl cyclase cAMP pathway | • Ovulation in women<br>• Luteinizes the corpus luteum during luteinizing phase for endometrial development for implantation<br>• Also, it results in secretion of progesterone and estrogen from ovaries<br>• In males, it results in the secretion of testosterone |
| Thyroid stimulating hormone | Glycoprotein with 2 subunits (α and β) | Thyroid gland | G protein coupled adenylyl cyclase cAMP pathway | Stimulates the thyroid follicles to produce thyroxine and T3 |
| Prolactin | Peptide hormone with 198 amino acids | Breasts | | It results is galactopoiesis (synthesis of milk in breast during lactation). This hormone usually remains suppressed in nonlactating women and men |
| **Posterior pituitary gland** | | | | |
| Oxytocin | Polypeptide with 9 amino acids | Smooth muscle of full-term pregnant uterus, myoepithelial cells of breasts | G protein coupled adenylyl cyclase cAMP pathway | • Parturition reflex<br>• Milk let down reflex |
| ADH | Polypeptide with 9 amino acids | Cortical and medullary collecting ducts of kidney | G protein coupled adenylyl cyclase cAMP pathway results in synthesis of aquaporins which are inserted in the apical membrane to increase the permeability of water, hence, reabsorption of water | Decreases urine output and conserves water in the body |

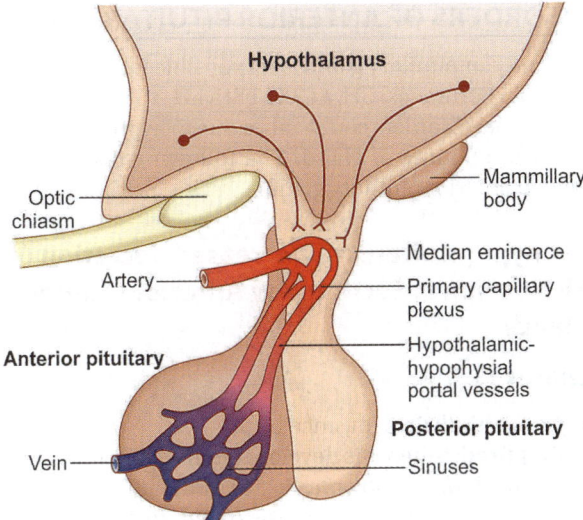

**Fig. 66.3:** Hypothalamo-hypophyseal-portal system.

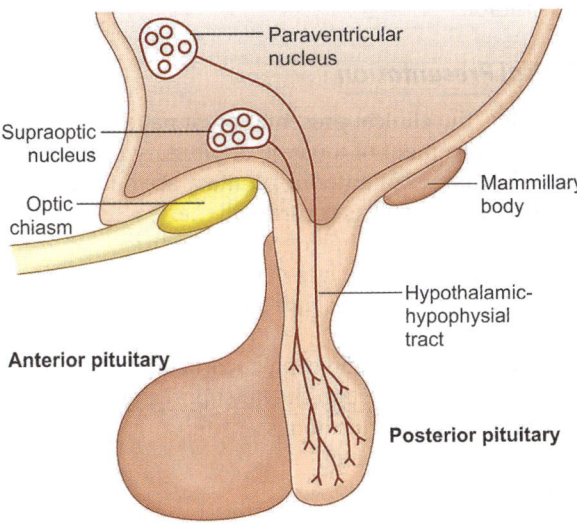

**Fig. 66.4:** Hypothalamo-hypophyseal-neural tract.

**Table 66.2:** Physiological actions of growth hormone.

| Promotes linear growth |
|---|
| • Stimulates bone and cartilage growth |
| • Stimulates the growth of muscles |
| **Metabolic effects** |
| • Carbohydrate metabolism: Produces hyperglycemia |
| • *Protein metabolism:* Increases formation of new proteins, decreases protein catabolism. It exerts protein sparing effect for energy |
| • *Lipid metabolism:* Enhances fat utilization for energy. Causes lipolysis |
| **Synergistic effects with other hormones** |
| • Stimulates growth along with insulin |
| • Exerts its effects through somatomedins (Insulin like growth factor-1? IGF-1) |

### Linear Growth

It directly acts on the bones, cartilage and muscles to promote the linear growth of an individual. It does so by the following actions:
- It causes **growth of all the tissues** of the body, which are capable of growing.
- It promotes the **differentiation** of various cells.
- Increases **deposition of protein by osteogenic and chondrocytic cells**, hence, promoting linear bone growth. It also results in differentiation of **chondrocytes into osteocytes, hence, affecting the bone growth.** GH strongly stimulates the osteoblasts, hence, the bone constantly becomes thicker during the life time under the influence of GH.

### Metabolic Effects of Growth

- Effect on carbohydrate metabolism:
  - ▪ **Decreased uptake of glucose** by tissues (skeletal muscle and fat)
  - ▪ **Increased production of glucose** by liver (glycogenolysis and gluconeogenesis)
  - ▪ It increases the blood glucose level (**hyperglycemia**)
  - ▪ It results in **increased insulin secretion (hyperinsulinemia)**
  - ▪ All the above effects are **diabetogenic**, as they result in the **'insulin resistance'** and cause pituitary diabetes in individuals with hypersecretion of GH
- Effect on protein metabolism:
  - ▪ It promotes **deposition of proteins** in tissues.
  - ▪ It enhances the **transport of amino acids inside the cells**, through the cell membrane. *This action is similar to insulin*.
  - ▪ It **increases new protein synthesis** by ribosomes in the cytoplasm.
  - ▪ GH increases the **transcription of DNA** to form new mRNA for new protein synthesis.
  - ▪ GH **decreases the protein catabolism** and spares the proteins for energy generation. It is called '**protein sparing effect**' of GH.
- Effect on lipid metabolism:
  - ▪ It increases **the fat utilization for energy**. It enhances the conversion of fatty-acids to acetyl CoA and its subsequent utilization for energy production.
  - ▪ GH results in **fat mobilization**.
  - ▪ The combined effect of protein anabolism and fat catabolism results in **increase in lean body mass**.
  - ▪ It exerts the **ketogenic effect** by excessive utilization of fats and increasing the levels of acetoacetic acid in liver. These ketone bodies are released into body fluids resulting in ketosis. Excessive mobilization of fats from adipose tissues may cause fatty liver.

### Action through Somatomedins (Insulin like Growth Factor-1/IGF-1)

There are 4 types of somatomedins but *IGF-1/Somatomedin C is most important*. The growth effects of

GH are mediated through IGFs rather than direct effects on bones and peripheral tissues.

Deficiency of IGF-1 in children, with normal or raised levels of GH, results in dwarfism. *The African Pygmy* people are short statured because they have a *congenital deficiency of IGF-1*. However, the *Levi-Laron dwarfs* have a mutation of *GH receptor*. In both these type of dwarfs, the GH is normal or elevated.

## Regulation of Secretion of GH

The GH secretion is pulsatile, showing 8–10 pulses in 24 hours. The GH secretion is primarily under the control of hypothalamus through the secretion of GHRH and GHIH (Somatostatin). It is increased by all the factors which are associated with increased stress in an individual.

- Starvation associated with protein deficiency
- Hypoglycemia
- Low fatty acids in blood
- Exercise
- Excitement
- Trauma
- Gherlins
- Amino acids like arginine

All these factors are directly or indirectly associated with increased stress, which increases the GH and increases blood sugar level and exploits the diabetogenic potential of GH/metabolic effects of GH.

> **What is the effect of kwashiorkor (severe protein energy malnutrition) on GH?**
>
> The plasma GH levels are very high in patients with kwashiorkor but they gradually decrease in these patients after the treatment, showing that the starvation/protein deficiency stimulates the GH secretion. This rise is seen as an attempt to deposit the proteins in the tissues, which are otherwise deficient **(Fig. 66.5)**.

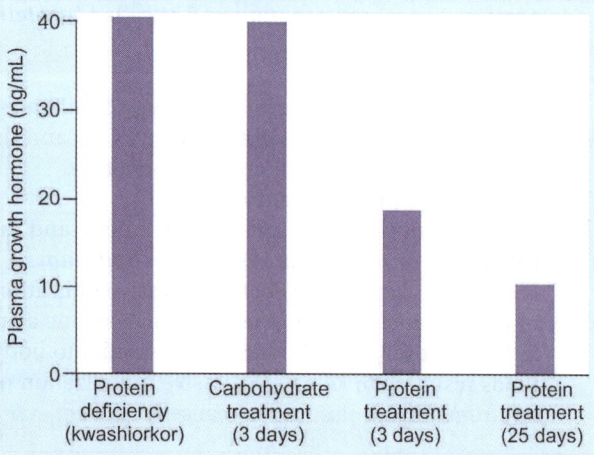

**Fig. 66.5:** Relation of plasma GH level with protein levels.

## DISORDERS OF ANTERIOR PITUITARY GLAND

The anterior pituitary gland is responsible for the secretion of 6 main hormones: GH, ACTH, FSH, LH, TSH and PRL. The endocrine disorders could either due to hypofunctioning/hyperfunctioning of gland. The following disorders are seen in anterior pituitary gland:

## Panhypopituitarism (Decreased Secretion of All Hormones Secreted by Anterior Pituitary Gland)

### Causes

- **Congenital:** Present since birth
- **Acquired:** When it is developed during lifetime:
  - *Sheehan's syndrome:* Postpartum pituitary necrosis. There is ischemic necrosis of pituitary gland due to excessive blood loss during delivery resulting in extremely compromised blood flow in pituitary.
  - When the pituitary gland is damaged by the pituitary tumor.

### Clinical Presentation

**In adults:** The clinical presentation of patient depending on the involvement of the type of pituitary cells. Usually, all the hormones of anterior pituitary are decreased and hence, produces effects accordingly, i.e.,

- Person is lethargic due to hypothyroidism
- Weight gain due to of lack of fat mobilization by growth, adrenocorticotropic, adrenocortical, and thyroid hormones
- Depressed production of glucocorticoids
- Loss of sexual function due to suppressed secretion of the gonadotropic hormones

### Management

Administration of adrenocortical and thyroid hormones reverses all the functions except the sexual functions.

### In Children

Panhypopituitarism in children results in dwarfism due to deficiency of growth hormone. These children also fail to attain puberty due to absence of FSH and LH. If there is only isolated deficiency of GH, the sexual functions may be preserved. Hence, the deficiency of GH results in dwarfism, which is referred as *'pituitary dwarfs'*.

The treatment of these type of GH deficiency is by giving human GH (hGH), which was earlier extracted from human pituitary glands but is now commercially prepared from *E. coli* bacteria by recombinant DNA technology. The substitution, if done early in life, can completely cure the dwarfism.

**Dwarfs:** Individuals with short stature:
- **Pituitary dwarfs:** Deficiency of growth hormone in children resulting in short stature. Mental development is normal. They are also called as intelligent dwarfs.
- **African Pygmy dwarfs:** Deficiency of IGF-1. GH can be normal or even elevated.
- **Levi-Laron dwarfs:** Mutation of growth hormone receptors. GH can be normal or even elevated.
- **Thyroid dwarfs:** Deficiency of thyroid hormone in infancy and childhood. These children have mental retardation and infantile proportions.

**Flowchart 66.1:** Metabolic effects of GH.

Persistent hyperglycemia
↓
Continuous stimulation of beta cells of pancreas to produce insulin
↓
Pancreatic beta cell exhaustion
↓
Development of diabetes mellitus

## Hypersecretion of Growth Hormone (Gigantism)

The hypersecretion of growth hormone before adolescence can result in excessive growth of tissues resulting in *Gigantism*. The child attains a tall stature because the epiphyseal closure has not taken place. The main cause of this disease is tumor of acidophils (somatotrophs).

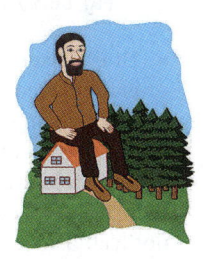

### Clinical Features

- Tall stature **(Fig. 66.6)**
- Body proportions are maintained
- Due to metabolic effects of GH:
  - Increased blood sugar levels (***hyperglycemia***)

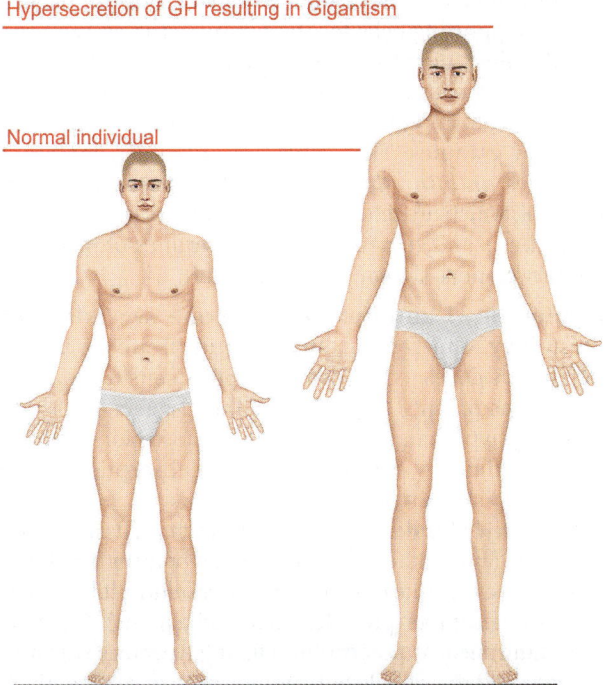

**Fig. 66.6:** Gigantism.

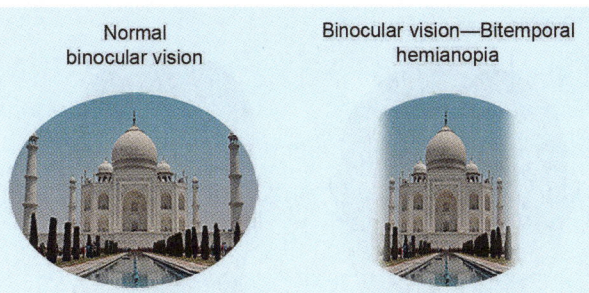

**Fig. 66.7:** Bitemporal hemianopia.

- The patients usually develop diabetes mellitus due to beta cell exhaustion **(Flowchart 66.1)** called *'pituitary diabetes'*.
- The acidophilic tumor compresses the optic chiasma producing the compression of nasal fibers arising from retina (for temporal vision) resulting in *Bitemporal hemianopia* **(Fig. 66.7)**.

The patient with gigantism due to pituitary tumor can eventually result in hypopituitarism due to destruction of pituitary gland due to growing tumor. This can result in death in early adulthood. If the pituitary tumor is diagnosed early in childhood, the neurosurgical removal of tumor can cure the disease.

## Acromegaly

If the *growth hormone secretion increases in the adults*, i.e., after the closure of epiphysis, it can lead to acromegaly. The word acromegaly means the enlargement of the acral parts of the body. Here the person cannot grow in the height but there is the growth of cartilaginous parts, hands, feet, soft tissues, membranous bones, etc., resulting the growth of acral parts. This imparts typical *'acromegalic facies'* to the patient.

### Clinical Features

- **Acromegalic facies:** The patient has a typical facial presentation due to growth of membranous bones resulting in protrusion of lower jaw (prognathism), Forehead bossing due to prominent supraorbital ridges, enlargement of nose, bulldog scalp (excessive skin folds of the scalp), enlarged tongue **(Fig. 66.8)**.

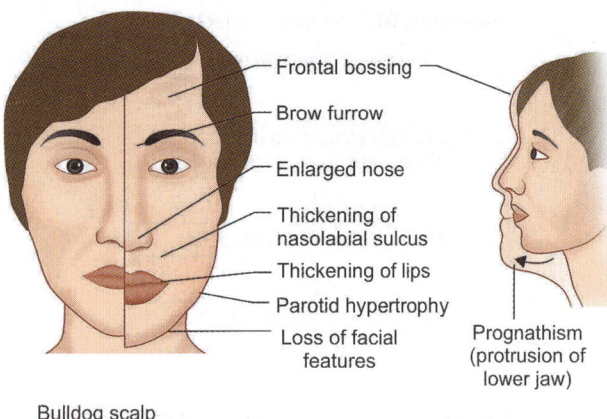

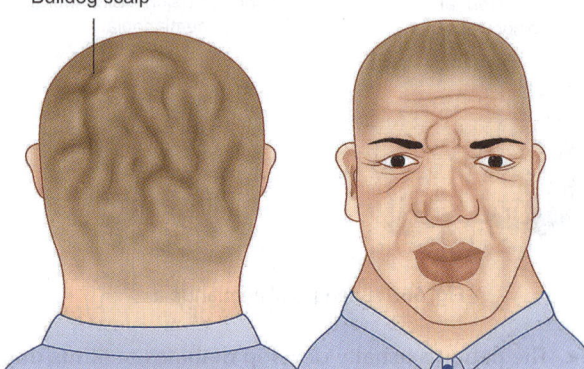

**Fig. 66.8:** Acromegalic facies and bulldog scalp.

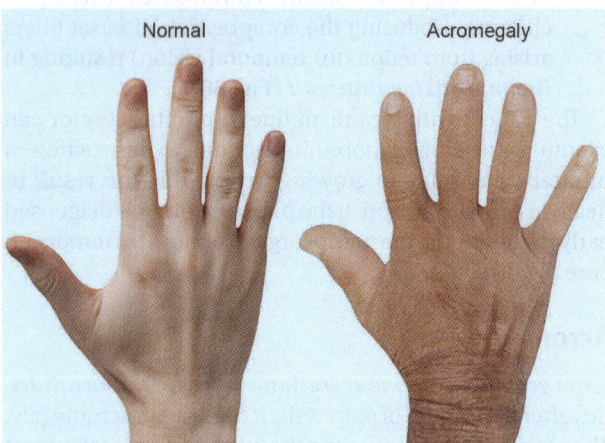

**Fig. 66.9:** Difference in normal and acromegalic hand.

- **Growth of acral parts of body:**
  - Enlargement and thickening of fingers and toes **(Fig. 66.9)**
  - Growth of vertebra resulting in kyphosis (hunched back) **(Fig. 66.10)**
- **Metabolic disturbances:** These occur due to high level of GH in the body resulting in:
  - There is hyperglycemia which stimulates beta cells to produce inulin. This results in persistent hyperinsulinemia leading to insulin resistance and beta cell exhaustion. This results in development of diabetes mellitus in patients with acromegaly.

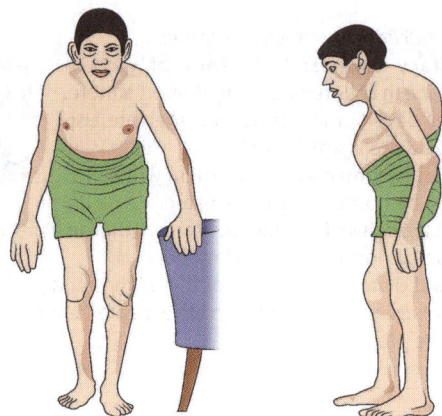

**Fig. 66.10:** Kyphosis in a patient of acromegaly.

- Due to excessive fat mobilization and lipolysis, there is increased utilization of fat for energy production. The person feels in high energy state.
- There is increased protein deposition in the muscles.
- **Visual field defects:** Bitemporal hemianopia due to compression caused by enlarged pituitary gland on optic chiasma.
- **Other features:**
  - Joint pains (arthralgias)
  - Organomegaly (hepatomegaly and increased kidney size)
  - Edema
  - Carpel tunnel syndrome, etc.

## HORMONES OF POSTERIOR PITUITARY GLAND

The posterior pituitary gland, also called as *neurohypophysis*, is made of *glial like cells called pituicytes*. These pituicytes are the supporting cells for the neurons arising from the hypothalamic supraoptic and paraventricular nuclei. These neural tracts pass to the posterior pituitary through the pituitary stalk and end as the terminal knobs containing secretory granules. These secretory granules contain 2 hormones, *antidiuretic hormone (ADH)/vasopressin and oxytocin*, which are released on the capillary surface.

Synthesis and secretion of the hormones of posterior pituitary gland is shown in **Figure 66.11**.

**Regulation of antidiuretic hormone secretion:** In physiology, the regulation of antidiuretic hormone secretion is governed by osmoreceptors sensing changes in blood osmolality **(Fig. 66.12)**. This triggers a cascade involving hypothalamic neurons and posterior pituitary release, ultimately controlling water reabsorption in the kidneys to maintain fluid balance.

- *Increased plasma osmolarity*: The increased osmolarity of body fluids either due to decreased body fluid volume or excessive solute due to ingestion results in stimulation of osmoreceptors (present near hypothalamus). This pulls the fluid out of osmoreceptor cell, which decreases its size. They send the signals to hypothalamus to secrete ADH. Hence, tonicity of body fluids, act as a powerful feedback mechanism for ADH secretion from hypothalamus.

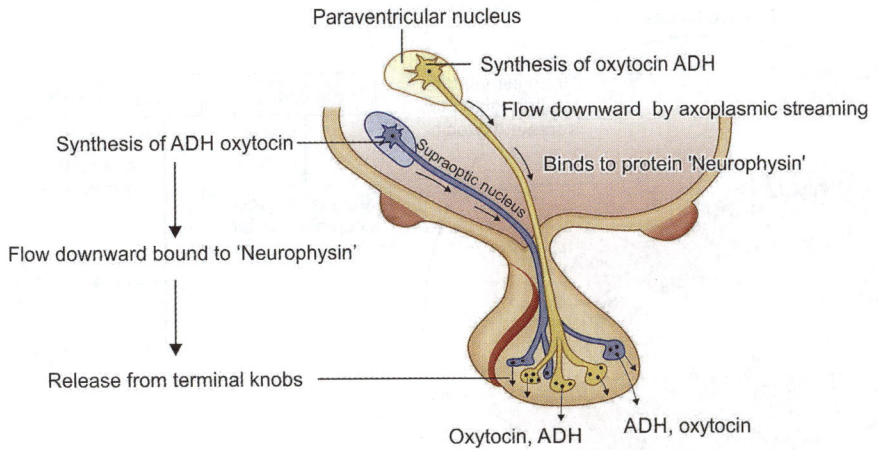

Fig. 66.11: Synthesis and release of hormones from posterior pituitary gland.

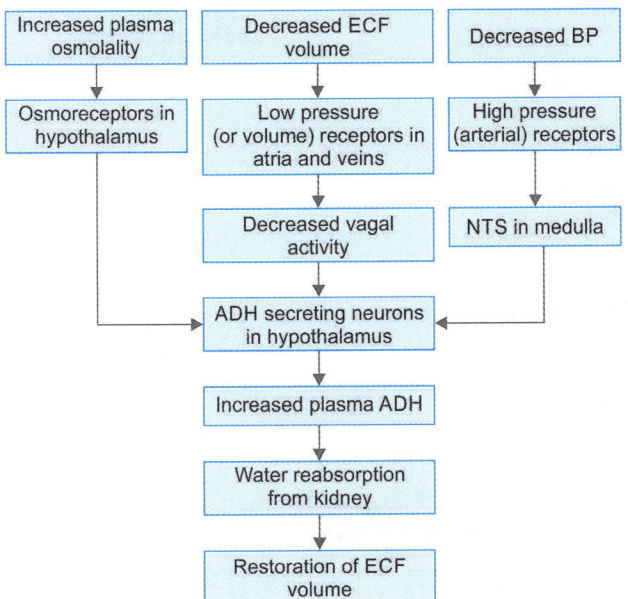

Fig. 66.12: Regulation of ADH secretion.

**Osmoreceptors**: These are small areas near hypothalamus, which lie outside blood brain barrier. Located in **organum vasculosum**. It is a highly vascular structure lying in the anteroventral wall of third ventricle **(AV3V region)**. Lesion of AV3V results in impaired ADH secretion. However, stimulation with angiotensin II or electrical stimulation increases ADH secretion.

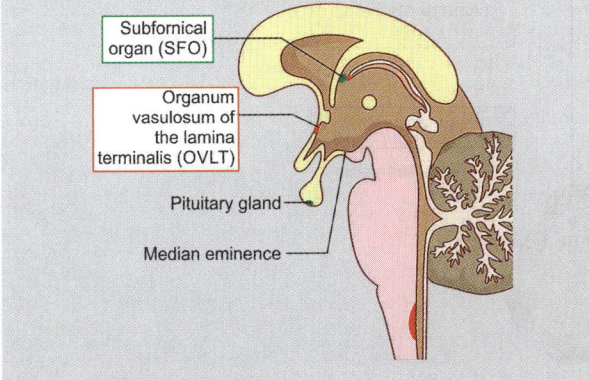

- ***Decreased blood volume (hypovolemia):*** When blood volume decreases by 15–25 %, there is strong stimulation of ADH secretion by 50 times the normal.
  The increased blood volume stretches the atrial walls which sends signals to brain and inhibit the secretion of ADH. However, hypovolemia, decreases the firing rate of atrial stretch receptors and result in decreased stimulation of brain area and strongly increases the ADH secretion.
- ***Decreased blood pressure (hypotension):*** Similar to the above-mentioned mechanism, the inhibition of atrial stretch receptors results in secretion of ADH.

> ADH is primarily formed in supraoptic nuclei and oxytocin in paraventricular nuclei.

## Functions

- **In low concentration:** Antidiuretic effect and water conservation by kidneys.
- **In high concentration:** Arteriolar constriction through out the body exerting its vasopressor effect. Hence, it is also called vasopressin.

## DIABETES INSIPIDUS (DI)

It is defined as excessive diuresis/loss of water from kidneys due to failure of facultative reabsorption of water from kidney discussed in Chapter 60.

## Types of DI

Based on the basic etiology, it is of two types:
1. **Neurogenic DI:** The secretion of ADH from hypothalamus/neurohypophysis is decreased. The decreased production of ADH results in decreased synthesis of aquaporins in collecting ducts of kidney and hence, decreases the water reabsorption.
2. **Nephrogenic DI:** The secretion of ADH from hypothalamus and neurohypophysis is normal but the ADH receptors in renal collecting ducts is defective.

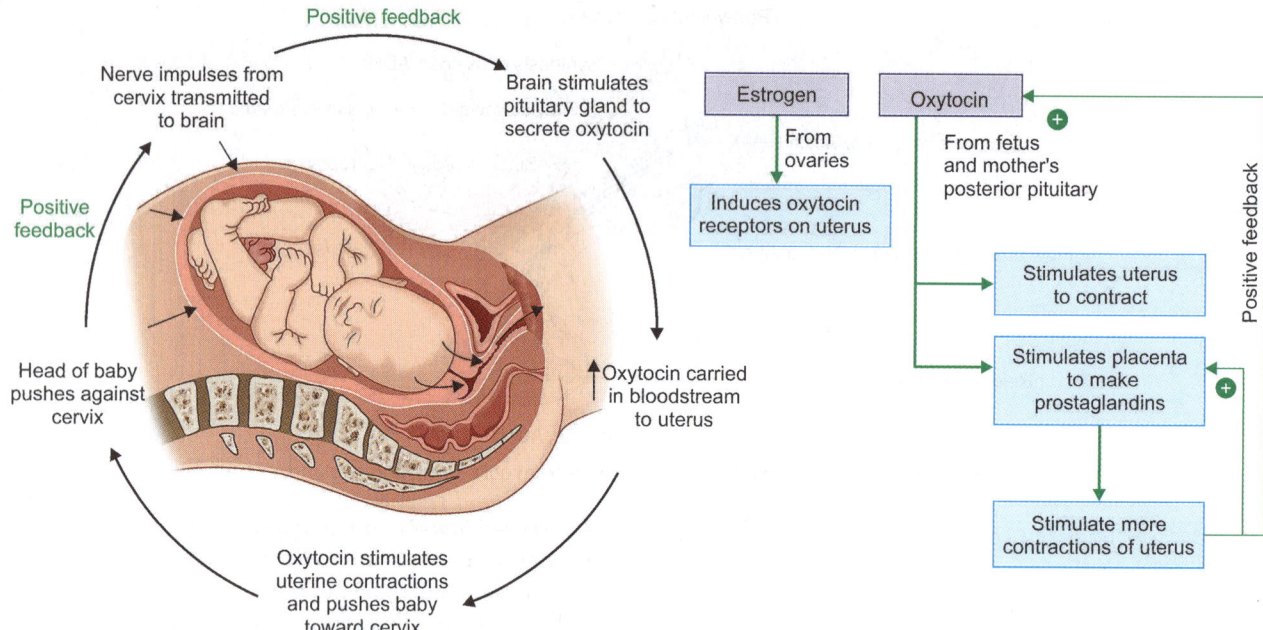

Fig. 66.13: Parturition reflex (Ferguson reflex).

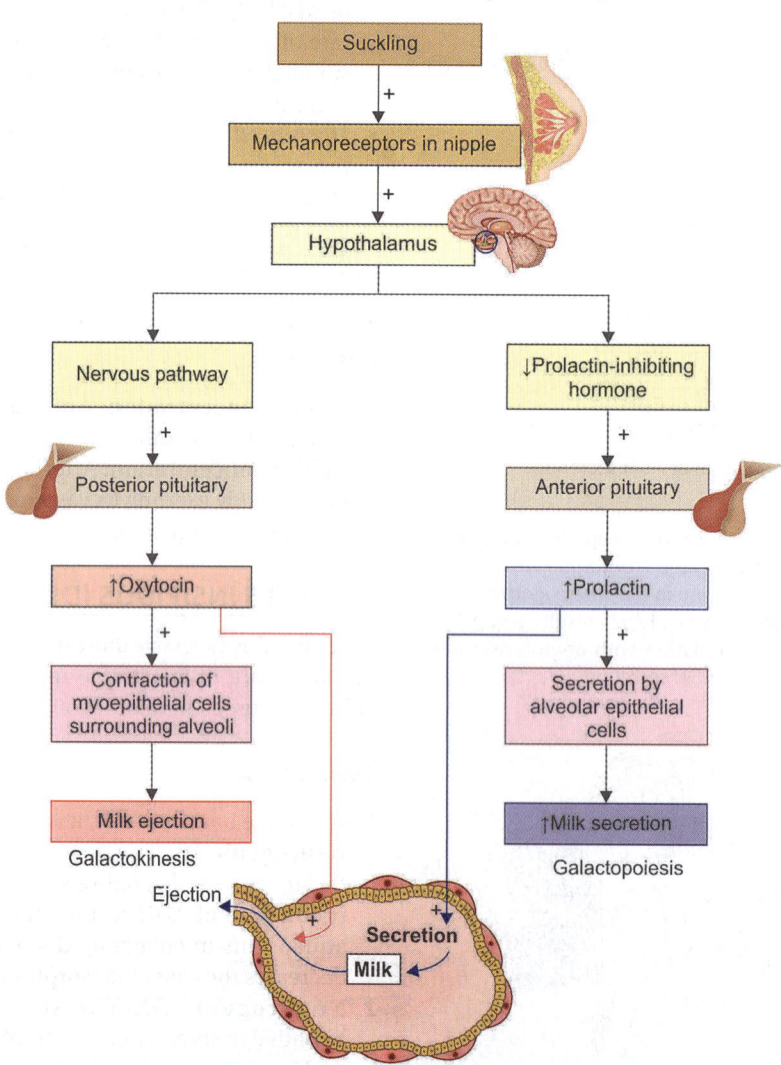

Fig. 66.14: Milk let-down reflex.

Hence, the available ADH is not able to act on the renal tubule to cause water reabsorption resulting in diuresis.

## OXYTOCIN

This hormone, commonly called as love hormone, is responsible of uterine contraction of a full term pregnant uterus resulting in birth of the baby (parturition reflex, discussed below). It is also responsible for contraction of myoepithelial cells of the breast resulting in galactokinesis (milk let down, explained below). It has been postulated, that oxytocin is responsible for social interactions, bonding between two individuals, mother-child nurturing relationship. It is believed to increase during cuddling and hugging. Its role in addiction, autism, etc., is under scientific exploration.

### Parturition Reflex (Ferguson Reflex)

It is a positive feedback mechanism involving oxytocin, resulting in the birth of the baby at the term **(Fig. 66.13)**.

### Milk Let Down Reflex (Fig. 66.14)

The suckling at the nipples by the baby sends the signals to the hypothalamus of the mother, resulting in decreased levels of dopamine secretion from hypothalamus (prolactin inhibiting factor) which further increases the release of Prl from anterior pituitary, to increase the milk formation and secretion (galactopoiesis). However, the suckling also stimulates the paraventricular nucleus to secrete oxytocin from neurohypophysis. This results in the contraction of myoepithelial cells surrounding the alveoli of the mammary glands containing milk. This squeezes the milk into the mouth of the baby, called galactokinesis.

## SUMMARY

- The pituitary gland has 3 lobes, anterior, intermediate and posterior. The anterior pituitary secretes six hormones, viz, growth hormone, prolactin, thyroid-stimulating hormone, adrenocorticotropic hormone, follicle-stimulating hormone, luteinizing hormone; while posterior pituitary secretes antidiuretic hormone, and oxytocin. The intermediate lobe is rudimentary in humans, though it is developed in some lower animals.
- Growth hormone (GH) is synthesized and secreted by the anterior pituitary gland. GH has direct metabolic effects on tissues by binding to cells and has indirect effects by stimulating cells in the liver to produce insulin-like growth factors (IGFs or somatomedins). GH affects almost every tissue in the body, especially skeletal muscle and cartilage cells. The overall effects, arising from an interplay between GH and IGF-1, are important for skeletal growth, muscle strength, bone density, and cardiac function. GH secretion is regulated by the hypothalamus, which secretes growth hormone-releasing hormone (GHRH) and growth hormone-inhibiting hormone (GHIH or somatostatin) into the hypophyseal portal venous blood surrounding the pituitary.
- GH deficiency in children results in short stature due to slow bone and muscle maturation and delayed puberty. GH excess in children causes gigantism, characterized by excessive linear growth, and in adults, it causes acromegaly, which is characterized by overgrowth of hand bones, feet bones, jaw bones, malfunctioning of gonads, enlargement of viscera, tongue, lungs, heart, liver, spleen, and endocrine gland like thyroid, adrenal, etc.
- The posterior pituitary gland stores and releases two hormones: oxytocin and antidiuretic hormone (ADH or vasopressin). Oxytocin facilitates uterine contractions during labor, allows for milk letdown during breastfeeding, promotes social bonding, and moderates testosterone levels. ADH stimulates water reabsorption by kidneys and hence, plays a crucial role in water homeostasis and regulating the blood volume, plasma tonicity and blood pressure.

## LET US SEE, HOW MUCH YOU HAVE LEARNT?

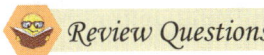
Review Questions

### Long/Short Answer Questions

Q1. Enumerate the hormones secreted by the anterior pituitary gland. Describe the actions of growth hormone.

Q2. Describe the physiological basis of the following in the patient of acromegaly:
   a. Large hands and feet
   b. Bossing of frontal bone of skull
   c. Prognathism
   d. Kyphosis
   e. Development of diabetes mellitus

Q3. What would happen to ADH levels, if a patient is having severe dehydration due to diarrhea and vomiting?

Q4. What would happen, if blood supply to the pituitary gland is stopped for a few hours, especially after the hyper hemodynamic state, as seen during pregnancy?

Q5. Why does children with severe protein energy malnutrition have high level of growth hormone in plasma?

Q6. What is association of growth hormone and insulin in promoting growth of an individual?

Q7. What is IGF-1? What is the physiological significance of IGF-1 in growth?

Q8. What is the difference in thyroid and pituitary dwarfs?

### Explain Why? (Reasoning Questions)

**Q1.** Excessive secretion of growth hormone (GH) in children leads to gigantism, while in adults it leads to acromegaly.

**Q2.** Damage to the posterior pituitary gland can result in diabetes insipidus.

**Q3.** The pituitary gland is often referred to as the "master gland" in the endocrine system.

**Q4.** An increase in prolactin secretion from the anterior pituitary gland can cause galactorrhea and menstrual disturbances in women.

### Critical Thinking Case-Based Questions

**Q1.** A 35-year-old woman presents to the emergency department with a headache, visual disturbances, and menstrual irregularities. She has a history of infertility and has been trying to conceive for the past year. On examination, she has bitemporal hemianopia and galactorrhea. MRI of the brain reveals a pituitary macroadenoma.

Based on the above case scenario, answer the following questions:
a. Why this patient is experiencing menstrual irregularities and infertility?
b. What is the physiological basis of bitemporal hemianopia in this patient?
c. Why this patient is presenting with galactorrhea?

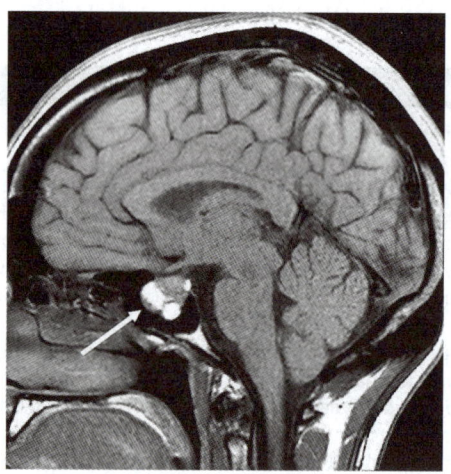

### Fill in the Blanks

1. The African Pygmies have deficiency of _____
2. The Levi-Laron dwarfs have mutation of _____
3. The synthetic hGH is obtained from _____
4. Parturition reflex is a typical example of _____ feedback mechanism.
5. A subcutaneous injection of _____ can be helpful in reducing the levels of GH, in a patient with high secretion of GH.

### Multiple Choice Questions

**Q1.** A 12-year-old child presents with short stature, delayed skeletal maturation, and proportionate body parts. The child's parents are of average height. Which of the following conditions is most likely responsible for the child's presentation?
Based on the scenario, what is the most likely diagnosis for the child's condition?
a. Acromegaly  b. Gigantism
c. Dwarfism  d. Hypothyroidism

**Q2.** A 45-year-old adult presents with enlargement of the hands, feet, and facial features. The patient reports a gradual increase in shoe and ring size over the past few years. Imaging studies reveal a pituitary adenoma. Which of the following conditions is most likely causing the patient's symptoms?
Based on the scenario, what is the most likely diagnosis for the patient's condition?
a. Dwarfism  b. Gigantism
c. Acromegaly  d. Hypopituitarism

**Q3.** A 16-year-old adolescent presents with accelerated growth, large hands and feet, and coarse facial features. The adolescent's parents are of average height. Imaging studies reveal a pituitary adenoma. Which of the following conditions is most likely responsible for the adolescent's presentation?
Based on the scenario, what is the most likely diagnosis for the adolescent's condition?
a. Dwarfism  b. Acromegaly
c. Gigantism  d. Hypothyroidism

Q4. A 30-year-old woman presents with features of acromegaly, including enlarged hands, feet, and facial features. She reports having experienced these symptoms since adolescence. Imaging studies reveal a pituitary adenoma. What complication of acromegaly should the healthcare provider be particularly concerned about in this patient?
Based on the scenario, which complication of acromegaly is the patient at increased risk for?
   a. Diabetes insipidus
   b. Osteoporosis
   c. Cardiovascular disease
   d. Hypothyroidism

Q5. A 9-year-old child presents with accelerated growth, increased height, and advanced bone age. The child's parents are both of average height. Which of the following conditions should be considered in the differential diagnosis?
Based on the scenario, what condition should be considered in the differential diagnosis for the child's presentation?
   a. Hypothyroidism
   b. Cushing's syndrome
   c. Gigantism
   d. Dwarfism

Q6. Which hormone is primarily responsible for stimulating the secretion of cortisol from the adrenal cortex?
   a. Thyroid-stimulating hormone (TSH)
   b. Growth hormone (GH)
   c. Adrenocorticotropic hormone (ACTH)
   d. Prolactin

Q7. Which part of the pituitary gland is responsible for producing antidiuretic hormone (ADH)?
   a. Anterior pituitary
   b. Posterior pituitary
   c. Pars intermedia
   d. Pars tuberalis

Q8. What is the primary function of follicle-stimulating hormone (FSH) in males?
   a. Stimulating ovulation
   b. Initiating spermatogenesis
   c. Stimulating breast milk production
   d. Regulating thyroid hormone secretion

Q9. Which hormone is responsible for stimulating milk production in the mammary glands?
   a. Thyroid-stimulating hormone (TSH)
   b. Prolactin
   c. Adrenocorticotropic hormone (ACTH)
   d. Luteinizing hormone (LH)

Q10. What is the primary function of growth hormone (GH) in children?
   a. Regulating metabolism
   b. Stimulating bone and tissue growth
   c. Controlling blood sugar levels
   d. Regulating water balance

Q11. A patient presents with symptoms of excessive thirst and urination. Lab results show low levels of antidiuretic hormone (ADH). Which part of the pituitary gland may be dysfunctional in this case?
   a. Anterior pituitary
   b. Posterior pituitary
   c. Pars intermedia
   d. Pars tuberalis

Q12. A pregnant woman experiences lactation suppression despite childbirth. Which hormone might be deficient in this case?
   a. Thyroid-stimulating hormone (TSH)
   b. Prolactin
   c. Adrenocorticotropic hormone (ACTH)
   d. Luteinizing hormone (LH)

Q13. A child exhibits delayed growth and short stature. Which hormone deficiency might be responsible for this condition?
   a. Follicle-stimulating hormone (FSH)
   b. Thyroid-stimulating hormone (TSH)
   c. Growth hormone (GH)
   d. Prolactin

Q14. A female patient presents with irregular menstrual cycles and difficulty conceiving. Which hormone imbalance might be causing these symptoms?
   a. Follicle-stimulating hormone (FSH) excess
   b. Thyroid-stimulating hormone (TSH) deficiency
   c. Prolactin excess
   d. Adrenocorticotropic hormone (ACTH) deficiency

Q15. A patient exhibits symptoms of adrenal insufficiency, including fatigue and weight loss. Which hormone deficiency might be causing these symptoms?
   a. Thyroid-stimulating hormone (TSH)
   b. Growth hormone (GH)
   c. Adrenocorticotropic hormone (ACTH)
   d. Prolactin

Q16. A newborn infant presents with ambiguous genitalia. Which hormone imbalance might be responsible for this condition?
   a. Follicle-stimulating hormone (FSH) deficiency
   b. Thyroid-stimulating hormone (TSH) excess
   c. Prolactin excess
   d. Gonadotropin-releasing hormone (GnRH) deficiency

Q17. A patient presents with symptoms of acromegaly, including enlarged hands and feet. Which hormone excess might be causing these symptoms?
   a. Growth hormone (GH)
   b. Adrenocorticotropic hormone (ACTH)
   c. Thyroid-stimulating hormone (TSH)
   d. Prolactin

Q18. A pregnant woman develops diabetes insipidus during pregnancy. Which hormone deficiency might be responsible for this condition?
   a. Growth hormone (GH)
   b. Adrenocorticotropic hormone (ACTH)
   c. Thyroid-stimulating hormone (TSH)
   d. Antidiuretic hormone (ADH)

Q19. A patient presents with symptoms of hyperthyroidism, including weight loss and heat intolerance. Which pituitary hormone might be involved in regulating thyroid function?
   a. Prolactin
   b. Adrenocorticotropic hormone (ACTH)
   c. Thyroid-stimulating hormone (TSH)
   d. Growth hormone (GH)

Q20. A patient presents with symptoms of Cushing's syndrome, including weight gain and hypertension. Which hormone excess might be causing these symptoms?
   a. Prolactin
   b. Thyroid-stimulating hormone (TSH)
   c. Adrenocorticotropic hormone (ACTH)
   d. Growth hormone (GH)

Q21. A child presents with symptoms of precocious puberty, including early development of secondary sexual characteristics. Which hormone excess might be responsible for this condition?
   a. Follicle-stimulating hormone (FSH)
   b. Luteinizing hormone (LH)
   c. Growth hormone (GH)
   d. Adrenocorticotropic hormone (ACTH)

Q22. A patient presents with symptoms of polyuria and polydipsia. Lab results show low levels of antidiuretic hormone (ADH). Which part of the pituitary gland may be dysfunctional in this case?
   a. Anterior pituitary
   b. Posterior pituitary
   c. Pars intermedia
   d. Pars tuberalis

Q23. A child exhibits delayed growth and short stature. Which hormone deficiency might be responsible for this condition?
   a. Follicle-stimulating hormone (FSH)
   b. Thyroid-stimulating hormone (TSH)
   c. Growth hormone (GH)
   d. Prolactin

Q24. A female patient presents with irregular menstrual cycles and difficulty conceiving. Which hormone imbalance might be causing these symptoms?
   a. Follicle-stimulating hormone (FSH) excess
   b. Thyroid-stimulating hormone (TSH) deficiency
   c. Prolactin excess
   d. Adrenocorticotropic hormone (ACTH) deficiency

Q25. A patient exhibits symptoms of adrenal insufficiency, including fatigue and weight loss. Which hormone deficiency might be causing these symptoms?
   a. Thyroid-stimulating hormone (TSH)
   b. Growth hormone (GH)
   c. Adrenocorticotropic hormone (ACTH)
   d. Prolactin

Q26. A 30-year-old female presents with amenorrhea, galactorrhea, and visual disturbances. She also reports headaches. MRI reveals a pituitary adenoma compressing the optic chiasma. Which hormone excess is most likely causing her symptoms?
   a. Growth hormone (GH)
   b. Prolactin
   c. Adrenocorticotropic hormone (ACTH)
   d. Thyroid-stimulating hormone (TSH)

Q27. A 20-year-old male presents with symptoms of delayed puberty, including lack of secondary sexual characteristics and small testicular size. He also reports decreased sense of smell. MRI reveals a small pituitary gland. Which hormone deficiency might be responsible for his condition?
   a. Follicle-stimulating hormone (FSH)
   b. Luteinizing hormone (LH)
   c. Thyroid-stimulating hormone (TSH)
   d. Growth hormone (GH)

Q28. A 45-year-old male presents with symptoms of central obesity, hypertension, and diabetes mellitus. Lab results show elevated cortisol levels. MRI reveals a pituitary adenoma. Which hormone excess is most likely causing his symptoms?
   a. Growth hormone (GH)
   b. Prolactin
   c. Adrenocorticotropic hormone (ACTH)
   d. Thyroid-stimulating hormone (TSH)

Q29. A newborn presents with micropenis and undescended testes. Lab results show low levels of testosterone. MRI reveals an absent or hypoplastic pituitary gland. Which hormone deficiency is most likely responsible for this condition?
   a. Follicle-stimulating hormone (FSH)
   b. Luteinizing hormone (LH)
   c. Growth hormone (GH)
   d. Thyroid-stimulating hormone (TSH)

Q30. A 25-year-old female presents with symptoms of hyperthyroidism, including weight loss, palpitations, and heat intolerance. Lab results show elevated levels of thyroid hormones. MRI reveals a pituitary adenoma. Which hormone excess is most likely causing her symptoms?
   a. Growth hormone (GH)
   b. Prolactin
   c. Adrenocorticotropic hormone (ACTH)
   d. Thyroid-stimulating hormone (TSH)

## ANSWERS

1. c   2. c   3. c   4. c   5. c   6. c   7. b   8. b   9. b   10. b   11. b   12. b   13. c   14. c
15. c   16. d   17. a   18. d   19. c   20. c   21. b   22. b   23. c   24. c   25. c   26. b   27. b   28. c
29. b   30. d

# Thyroid Gland

## 67 CHAPTER

### COMPETENCY ADDRESSED
**PY8.2:** Describe the synthesis, secretion, transport, physiological actions, regulation and effect of altered (hypo and hyper) secretion of pituitary gland, **thyroid gland**, parathyroid gland, adrenal gland, pancreas and hypothalamus.
**PY8.4:** Describe function tests: **Thyroid gland**; adrenal cortex, adrenal medulla and pancreas.

### LEARNING OBJECTIVES
**At the end of this chapter, the learner should be able to:**
- Describe the functional anatomy of the thyroid gland.
- Describe this synthesis, release, transport, mechanism of action, regulation and actions of thyroid hormone.
- Describe the clinical conditions related to abnormal secretion (hypo and hyperthyroidism) in terms of physiological basis of clinical feature and their management.

## FUNCTIONAL ANATOMY OF THYROID GLAND

Thyroid gland is situated in the neck below the larynx in midline **(Fig. 67.1A)**. It is the largest endocrine gland weighing around 10 to 30 grams. Anatomically, it has two loads connected by an isthmus hence, giving it a butterfly like shape. It is highly vascular and it becomes functional in early fetal life.

Microscopically, it is made-up of follicles made-up of single layer of cuboidal epithelium which are filled with colloid and glycoprotein called thyroglobulin along with the thyroid hormones **(Fig. 67.1B)**. Some interspersed para follicular (C-cells) are also present along with thyroid follicles which secrete another hormone called calcitonin.

## HORMONES OF THYROID GLAND

There are three main hormone secreted by the thyroid gland:
1. Thyroxine ($T_4$)
2. Triiodothyronine ($T_3$)
3. Calcitonin—secreted from para follicular cells

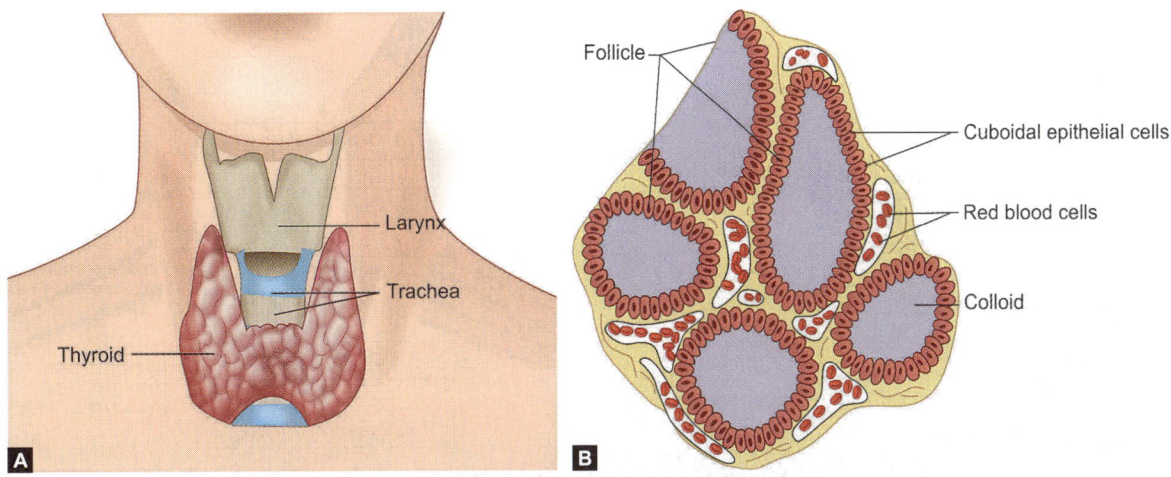

**Figs. 67.1A and B:** (A) Thyroid gland location; (B) Microanatomy of thyroid gland.

## FUNCTIONS

Primarily the thyroid hormones are concerned with tissue metabolism which regulates the basal metabolic rate, oxygen consumption of the tissues and finally resulting in the growth and development of the individual. However, the detailed functions of the thyroid hormones are later in the chapter.

Calcitonin secreted by the thyroid gland is responsible for the calcium homeostasis which is discussed separately in chapter.

## BIOSYNTHESIS OF THYROID HORMONE

The various steps for the biosynthesis of thyroid hormone are enumerated below **(Fig. 67.2)**:
- Iodide trapping
- Oxidation of I$^-$ to form I$_2$ (Rate limiting step)
- Synthesis and secretion of thyroglobulin
- Iodination of tyrosine (Organification of TGB)
- Coupling reaction
- Release of thyroid hormones

### Iodide Trapping

The iodine from the food is concentrated in the thyroid gland, hence, called iodide trapping. The Na$^+$-K$^+$ ATPase pump create concentration gradient which results in activation of *Na$^+$-I-symport*. Hence, the iodide is concentrated up to 30–250 times inside the thyroid gland for the synthesis of thyroxine. 20% of the absorbed iodide is taken up by the thyroid gland. *This step is regulated by TSH*, secreted by anterior pituitary gland. This iodide is transported in the colloid through an apical counter transporter molecule called **pendrin**, in exchange with Cl$^-$. Normal requirement of iodide –150 micrograms/day.

### Oxidation of I$^-$ to I$_2$

I$^-$ is oxidized by peroxide to I$_2$, present at the apical border. It is an **obligatory step,** which is necessary for thyroid hormone synthesis.

## Synthesis and Secretion of Thyroglobulin (Tg)

It is synthesized within the endoplasmic reticulum of the follicular cell, packed in Golgi apparatus and released into the colloid. Tg is a glycoprotein (carbohydrate moiety by GA and protein moiety by ER) formed by 123-Tyrosine amino acid residues. Iodination of tyrosine residues forms thyroid hormones.

> **TSH dependent steps**
> - Iodide trapping
> - Organification
> - Coupling reaction
> - Release of hormones

## Organification of Tg

Iodination of tyrosine residue in Tg takes place resulting in the formation of MIT (monoiodotyrosine) and DIT (Diiodotyrosine). Iodination of tyrosine residues takes place under the influence of TSH

*MIT → DIT occurs in the presence of peroxide*

## Coupling Reaction

- MIT + DIT → T3
- DIT + DIT → T4
- DIT + MIT → Reverse T3 (RT3) (very little)
- T3 and T4 remain attached to Tg molecule in the storage in colloid. They are released when they are secreted
- This also takes place under the influence of TSH

> **Thyroid secretes**
> - T4: 80 μg/day
> - T3: 4 μg/day
> - RT3: 2 μg/day

> **Plasma levels of T3 and T4**
> - Plasma T4: 8 μg/dL
> - Free plasma T4: 2 ng/dL
> - Plasma T3: 0.15 μg/dL
> - Free plasma T3: 0.3 ng/dL

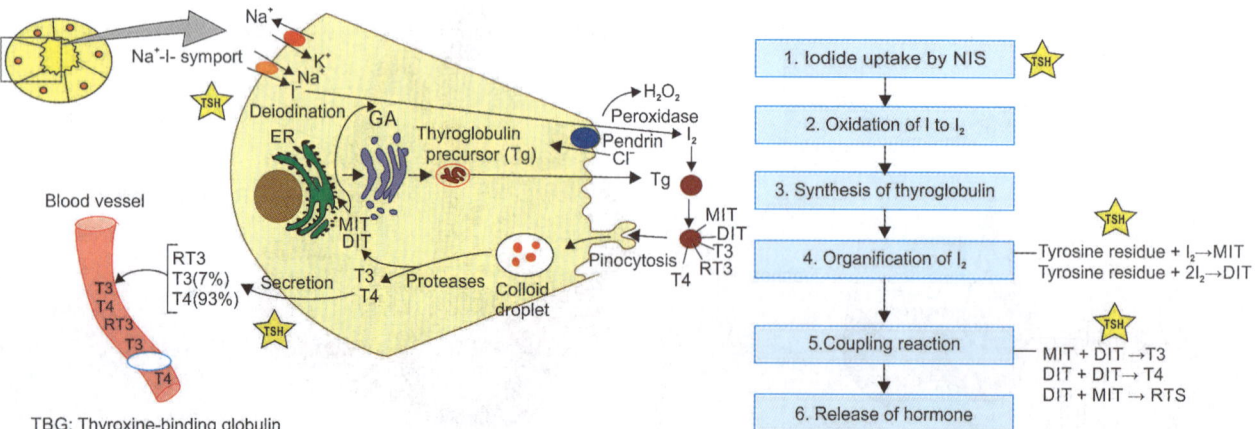

**Fig. 67.2:** Biosynthesis of thyroid hormone.

### Release of Thyroid Hormones

- T3 and T4 attached to Tg are taken up by follicular cells by pinocytosis
- The colloid droplets are broken down by the lysosomal enzymes
- Peptide bonds are broken to release MIT and DIT by enzyme Deiodinase
- $I^-$ and amino acids returned to recirculation to form new thyroid hormone.

## TRANSPORT IN BLOOD

About 99% of thyroxine and triiodothyronine are transported in the blood bound to a plasma proteins primarily thyroxine binding globulin (TBG) and slightly with thyroxine-binding prealbumin and albumin. Since most of the thyroxine is in the bound form, it is released slowly to the tissues. The **half-life** of **thyroxine** is around **6 days** while of **T3** is **one day**. The bound form of the hormone does not have any physiological actions but once released as free form (free T3 and free T4) the hormone shows its metabolic effects and participates in the feedback regulation. In the tissues, the **T3 is five times more active than T4**. Hence, most of the T3 is formed in the peripheral tissues by peripheral conversion from T4.

## MECHANISM OF ACTION OF THYROID HORMONES

The thyroid hormones have a slow onset of action and have a long latent. It can be attributed to the binding of thyroxine with plasma proteins and the slow release into the tissue cells. The thyroid hormones bind to the intracellular intranuclear receptors, as they can easily cross the cell membrane being lipophilic in nature. The mechanism of action is shown in the **Figure 67.3**.

## ACTIONS OF THYROID HORMONE

### Genomic Actions

- **Metabolic rate:** Thyroid hormones increase the basal metabolic rate and increase the activity of various organ systems like the heart and the central nervous system. Due to increased BMR, there is a calorigenic action of thyroid hormones, i.e., it increases the body temperature.
  *Physiological basis*: Thyroxine increases the number and activity of mitochondria, which in turn increases the production of ATP. This further increases the activity of $Na^+ K^+$ ATPase pump, which increases the BMR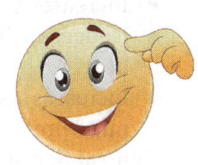
- **Effect on growth and development:** It regulates the growth in growing children. It is responsible for growth of bones along with growth hormone. Hyperthyroid children tend to grow faster but eventually results in early closure of epiphysis.
- **Effect on metabolism:**
  - *Carbohydrate metabolism:* Stimulates carbohydrate metabolism
    - Rapid glucose uptake by cells
    - Increased glycolysis
    - Increased gluconeogenesis
    - Increased rate of absorption from GIT
    - Increases insulin secretion
    - Increased cellular metabolic enzymes by thyroid hormone
  - *Fat metabolism:* Stimulates fat metabolism
    - Mobilization of fats from adipose tissue

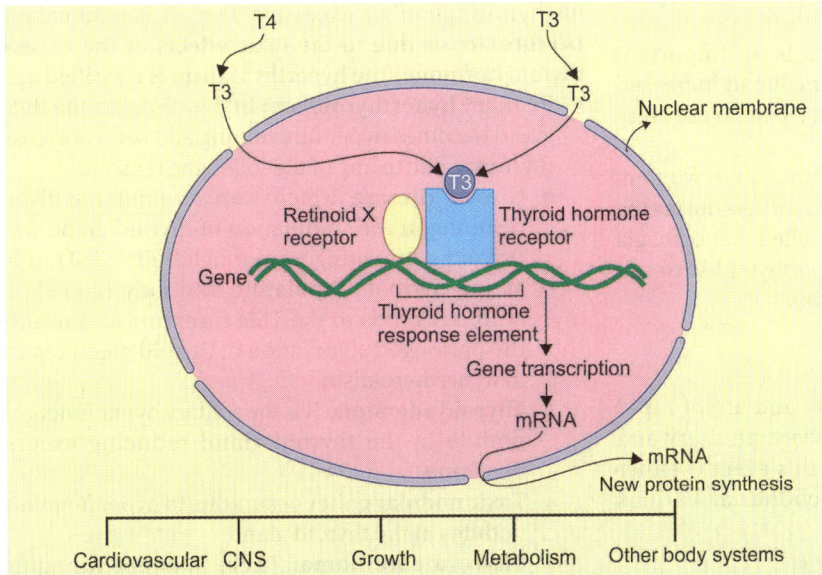
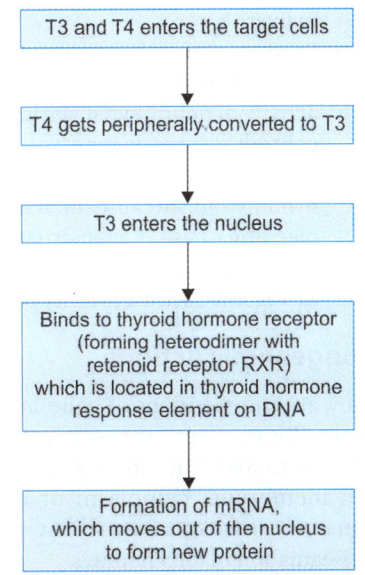

**Fig. 67.3:** Mechanism of action of thyroid hormones.

- Increases free fatty acids in plasma
- Decreases cholesterol, phospholipids, triglycerides
- Deposition of fats in liver
  - *Protein metabolism:*
    - At normal levels of thyroid hormone, it results in protein anabolism
    - In excessive secretion of thyroid hormones, it results in protein catabolism
- **Cardiovascular system:**
  - Increases responsiveness of heart to catecholamines
  - Increases heart rate
  - Increases blood flow and cardiac output
  - Hence, positive chronotropic and inotropic effect on heart
  - Increases systolic and diastolic blood pressure; widens pulse pressure and raises mean arterial pressure.
- **Central nervous system:**
  - Increases rapidity of cerebration
  - Shows an excitatory effect on nervous system
  - An important effect of thyroid hormone is to promote growth and development of brain during fetal life. Hence, the deficiency of thyroid hormone in fetal life and infancy leads to mental retardation.
  - Excessive thyroid hormone causes tiredness and insomnia due to the constant activation of neural synapses. However, hypothyroidism is associated with hypersomnia or excessive sleeping.
- **Other body systems:**
  - Increases gastrointestinal motility
  - Increases rate of respiration by increasing the oxygen utilization
  - TH is required for normal reproduction
  - Stimulates pancreas to produce insulin
  - Activates parathyroid gland by affecting bone metabolism
  - Increases the production of glucocorticoids due to increased metabolism of glucocorticoids by thyroxine in liver.
  - Produces muscle tremor, which is an important sign of hyperthyroidism. It occurs due to increased activity of neural synapses in spinal cord in the areas controlling muscle tone.
  - It is required for normal sexual function in women, hypothyroidism causes increased blood loss during the bleeding phase of menstruation called menorrhagia and polymenorrhea. However, hyperthyroidism result in oligomenorrhea (Scanty periods).

## Nongenomic Actions

They are independent of gene activity and are of rapid onset. These effects are seen in the heart, pituitary and adipose tissues. The site of action for this effect is either cell membrane, cytoplasm or mitochondria. Various nongenomic actions are as follows:
- Regulation of ion channels
- Oxidative phosphorylation
- Activation of intracellular second messengers

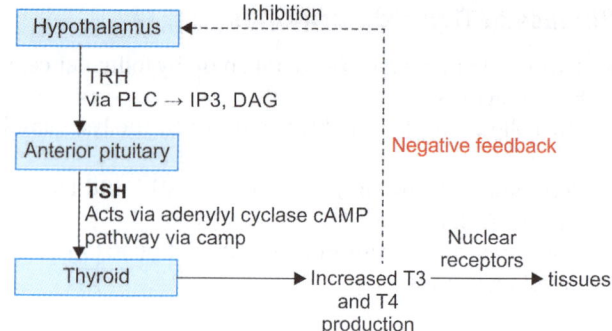

**Fig. 67.4:** Hypothalamic–pituitary–thyroid axis.

## METABOLISM OF THYROID HORMONES

The thyroid hormones get metabolized in liver and kidneys, where they are conjugated with glucuronide and excreted through kidneys. They also enters enterohepatic circulation through bile.

## REGULATION OF THYROID HORMONE SECRETION

It is primarily regulated by the negative feedback mechanism of hypothalamic–pituitary–thyroid axis **(Fig. 67.4)**.

## DISORDERS OF THYROID GLAND

The thyroid gland when functioning normally is called euthyroid, but in conditions where the gland is producing more hormone it is labeled hyperthyroidism and when less amounts of thyroxine are produced the condition is called hypothyroidism.

### Hyperthyroidism

It is defined as the overproduction of thyroxine either due to the overactivity of the thyroid gland or by overstimulation of thyroid gland by excessive TSH. It is also called as *thyrotoxicosis* due to the toxic effects of the excessive thyroid hormone. The hyperthyroidism is classified as:
- **Primary hyperthyroidism:** In this disorder, the thyroid gland becomes hyper functioning add secrets excessive thyroxine due to any of the following reasons:
  - **Graves' disease**, which is an autoimmune disorder resulting in the stimulation of thyroid gland by the thyroid stimulating immunoglobulin (TSI) or long acting thyroid stimulating antibody (LATS). This antibody binds to the TSH receptors and results in the prolonged stimulation of thyroid gland resulting in hyperthyroidism.
  - **Thyroid adenoma:** It is the solitary hyper functioning nodule in the thyroid gland reducing excessive thyroxine.
  - **Toxic nodular goiter** occurs due to hyper functioning nodules in the thyroid gland.
  - **Thyroid carcinoma:** There is hyper functioning multiple nodules with abnormal malignant cells producing excessive thyroxine.

- **Secondary hyperthyroidism:** This disorder is seen when the pituitary secretes excessive TSH and stimulates the thyroid gland to produce more thyroxine.

### Physiological Basis of Clinical Features of Hyperthyroidism

- **Increased basal metabolic rate:** The excessive thyroxine increases the number and activity of the mitochondria hence, increases these cellular metabolism and the activity of various pumps and ion channels, increasing the basal metabolic rate.
- **Increased appetite:** The increased basal metabolic rate increases the cellular metabolism resulting stimulation of the feeding center hence, increases the appetite.
- **Loss of weight:** Despite of the fact the person is eating more there is muscle wasting and weight loss because excessive thyroxine results in protein catabolism and decreases the muscle mass.
- **Heat intolerance:** Excessive cellular metabolism produces more heat in the tissues resulting in the heat intolerance.
- **Exophthalmos/proptosis:** There is bulging of the eyeballs as if the patient is staring at you. This is called as exophthalmos due to the *swelling of retro orbital connective tissues*, which pushes the eyeballs the words outside. This causes *stretching of the optic nerve*. The eyelids do not cover the eyeballs and the person is unable to blink. The eyeballs remain uncovered and become prone to dryness and ulceration.

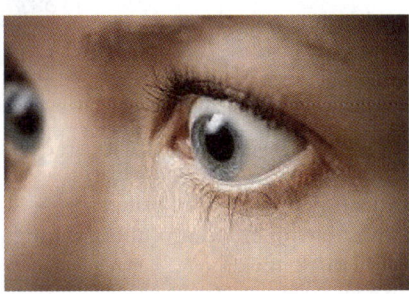

- **Cardiovascular effects:** Due to the stimulatory effect of thyroxine on the heart there is increase in the heart rate, cardiac output and the blood pressure.
- **Effects on respiratory system:** The patient experiences difficulty in breathing (Dyspnea).
- **Effects on gastrointestinal tract:** Since thyroxine stimulates the gastrointestinal secretions and motility, it results in diarrhea.
- **Effect on central nervous system:** It increases the activity of the synapses hence, resulting in *hyperreflexia, fine tremors, nervousness, restlessness, fatigability and difficulty in sleeping (insomnia)*.
- The skin of the patient remains **warm and moist** due to cutaneous vasodilation.
- Thyrotoxic myopathy → muscular weakness due to increased protein catabolism.

**Table 67.1:** Laboratory findings in primary vs. secondary hyperthyroidism.

| | Primary hyperthyroidism | Secondary hyperthyroidism |
|---|---|---|
| T3, T4 | Raised | Raised |
| TSH | Decreased (due to negative feedback mechanism) | Increased (due to overproduction from pituitary) |
| Additional tests | • TSI/LATS present in Graves' disease<br>• FNAC/biopsy for multinodular goiter | |
| Radiological investigation | Radioactive iodine uptake studies for hyperfunctioning nodule | X-ray skull for pituitary adenoma |

### Lab Findings

Laboratory findings in primary and secondary hyperthyroidism is shown in **Table 67.1**.

### Treatment

- **Thyroid hormone level lowering drugs**
    - Thiocyanates and perchlorates: Inhibit I⁻ trapping
    - Propyl thiouracil and carbimazole: Inhibit iodination and coupling reaction
- Steroids in Graves' disease
- Surgery to remove hyper functioning nodule
- Thyroidectomy for malignant lesions

## Hypothyroidism

It is defined as the *decreased production of thyroxine* either due to the hypo functioning of the thyroid gland or by suppression of thyroid gland by decreased TSH. It is called as *myxedema in adults* and *cretinism in children*. The hypothyroidism is classified as:

- **Primary hypothyroidism:** In this disorder, the thyroid gland becomes hypo functioning add secrets less thyroxine due to any of the following reasons:
    - Endemic goiter
    - Autoimmune thyroiditis (Hashimoto's thyroiditis)
    - Iatrogenic (postsurgical, radio $I_2$ exposure)
    - Drugs (iodine excess, lithium)
    - Congenital disorders (inborn errors of thyroid synthesis, abnormal thyroid gland)
    - Deficiency of I⁻ trapping mechanism
    - Deficiency of peroxidase enzyme
    - Deficiency of deiodinase enzyme
- **Secondary hypothyroidism:** This disorder is seen when the pituitary secretes less TSH and suppresses the thyroid gland and produces less thyroxine, as seen in pituitary failure.
- **Tertiary hypothyroidism:**
    - Hypothalamic failure
    - Decreased TRH and hence, decreased TSH
- **Other causes:** Peripheral resistance of the receptors

## Myxedema

Hypothyroidism in adults is called as myxedema. It derives its name from myxomatous nonpitting edema. The patients with hypothyroidism present with the following clinical features and the physiological basis for the same are given along with:

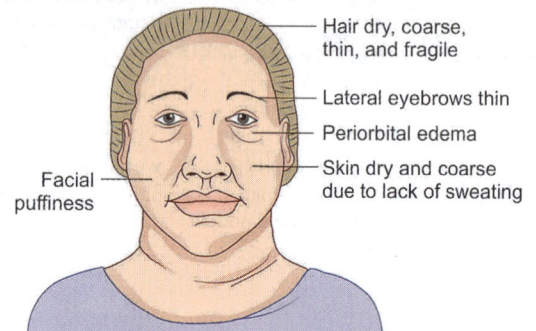

### Physiological Basis of Clinical Features

**General symptoms:**

- *Decreased basal metabolic rate* due to decreased cellular metabolism.
- Cool peripheral extremities due to decreased heat production due to decreased metabolism. This also results in *cold intolerance*.
- There is *decreased appetite* due to slow down of cellular metabolism but it results in a *weight gain*.
- The gelatinous thickening of vocal cords result in *husky and slow voice*, also called *Smoker voice*.

**Metabolism:**

- Decreased protein metabolism
- Decreased carbohydrate metabolism, resulting in decreased glucose uptake by the cells and decreased glucose utilization.
- Decreased fat metabolism. There is decrease in free fatty acids but increase in S. cholesterol levels and triglyceride levels.

**Subcutaneous tissue:** There is *accumulation of glycosaminoglycans in subcutaneous tissue which results in gelatinous nonpitting pretibial myxedema*. This also result in compression in the tight subcutaneous compartment and cause carpel tunnel syndrome. There is fluid effusions into body spaces.

**SKIN:** The skin becomes *dry, coarse* and has a *yellowish tint (carotenemia)*. Facial features show edematous appearance, puffy face, edematous eyelids. There is *thinning of hair and hair loss*. Loss of lateral one third eyebrows may also occur (madarosis).

> Carotenemia occurs due to accumulation of circulating β-carotene in hypothyroid patients. Thyroid hormones result in induction of liver enzyme and metabolize β-carotene.

**CVS:** There is decreased responsiveness of heart to catecholamines, resulting in *bradycardia, decreased stroke volume, increased cholesterol* levels and increased chances of atherosclerosis.

**CNS:** Difficulty in concentration on work, *decreased cerebration* resulting in *poor memory, tiredness, weakness, slow mentation, hypersomnia*.

There are paresthesia and delayed reflexes *"Hung Up Ankle Reflex"*.

**Reproductive system**

- Menorrhagia: Increased blood loss during periods
- Increased incidence of miscarriages
- Prolactin levels are increased
- Libido decreases in both men and women

## Cretinism

The *hypothyroidism in children* is called cretinism, which can occur at any time from fetal life, infancy and childhood. If mother is euthyroid, baby is normal at birth but hypothyroidism manifests later during infancy. But if even mother is hypothyroid, the baby is affected in utero and severely affected at the time of birth. A cretin baby shows the following clinical features:

- Persistence of physiological jaundice
- Hoarse cry
- Feeding problems
- Sleeps most of the time
- Noisy breathing, nasal obstruction, apnea
- Constipation
- Delayed milestones
- Facial features
  - Puffy face
  - Swollen eyelids
  - Widely separated eyes
  - Narrow palpebral fissure
  - Broad nose with depressed bridges
  - Open mouth with broad protuberant tongue
  - Short and thick neck
- Signs and symptoms
  - Coarse, sparse and brittle hair
  - Skin is dry, scaly, thick and pale yellow due to carotenemia
  - Slow growth
  - Child appears **short, stocky, large head** as compared to trunk
  - Retains infantile characters
  - "Mentally retarded dwarfs" as compared to pituitary dwarfs which are intelligent
  - Bradycardia
  - Refractory anemia
  - Slow tendon reflexes

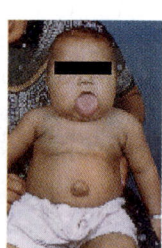

**Wolff-Chaikoff effect and the Jod-Basedow phenomenon:** The Wolff-Chaikoff effect, named after Jan Wolff and Israel Lyon Chaikoff who discovered it in the 1940s, refers to the *transient inhibition of thyroid hormone synthesis* in response to a *high concentration of iodide in the bloodstream*. When the body is exposed to excessive amounts of iodide, such as through dietary intake or contrast agents used in medical imaging, the thyroid gland temporarily reduces its production of thyroid hormones, primarily thyroxine (T4) and triiodothyronine (T3). This effect *helps prevent the overproduction of thyroid hormones*, maintaining thyroid function within a narrow range. Once iodide levels normalize, the Wolff-Chaikoff effect dissipates, and thyroid hormone synthesis resumes its normal activity.

**The Jod-Basedow phenomenon**, named after Eugen Jod and Karl Adolph von Basedow, refers to the induction of hyperthyroidism in individuals with endemic goiter or latent Graves' disease following an abrupt increase in iodine intake. Like the Wolff-Chaikoff effect, the Jod-Basedow phenomenon involves the influence of iodine on thyroid function. However, while the Wolff-Chaikoff effect causes transient hypothyroidism due to iodine excess, the Jod-Basedow phenomenon triggers the onset of hyperthyroidism in susceptible individuals. This phenomenon underscores the complex relationship between iodine intake and thyroid function and highlights the importance of monitoring iodine supplementation, especially in populations with pre-existing thyroid disorders.

## Diagnosis

Diagnosis is done by laboratory investigations mainly which are tabulated in **Table 67.2**.

**Table 67.2:** Laboratory findings in primary and secondary hypothyroidism.

|  | Primary hypothyroidism | Secondary hypothyroidism |
|---|---|---|
| T3, T4 | Decreased | Decreased |
| TSH | Increased (due to less negative feedback mechanism) | Decreased (due to decreased production from pituitary) |

- Increased cholesterol levels
- X-ray:
  - Absence of distal femoral epiphysis
  - Large fontanelles
  - Wide sutures of skull
  - Enlarged sella turcica
- Low voltage ECG

### Treatment

- Thyroxine replacement
- Early diagnosis and replacement in infants

The features of cretinism (thyroid dwarfism) are different from pituitary dwarfism. They are summarized in Table.

## Endemic Goiter

- *Enlargement of thyroid gland*
- Can be normal, hypo or hyper thyroid disorder
- Not a neoplasm
- Most commonly associated with hypothyroidism
- Endemic because it due to decreased availability of iodine in that region

| Characteristic | Thyroid dwarfism (Cretinism) | Pituitary dwarfism |
|---|---|---|
| Etiology | Congenital hypothyroidism due to iodine deficiency or thyroid gland abnormalities | Congenital or acquired deficiency of growth hormone (GH) secretion or action |
| Primary hormonal defect | Reduced production or secretion of thyroid hormones (T3 and T4) | Reduced production or secretion of growth hormone (GH) |
| Growth retardation | Severe short stature with disproportionate body proportions (short limbs, large head, short neck) | Short stature with disproportionate body proportions (e.g., short limbs) |
| Cognitive development | Profound intellectual disability is common | Intellectual development may be normal unless there is early onset and severe deficiency |
| Physical features | Coarse facial features, protruding tongue, umbilical hernia, and delayed dentition | Proportional body with normal facial features |
| Developmental milestones | Delayed or absent milestones (e.g., sitting, walking) | Delayed but not typically absent milestones |
| Associated features | Developmental delays, goiter (if due to iodine deficiency), and other symptoms of hypothyroidism | Delayed bone age, delayed puberty, hypoglycemia, and other symptoms of growth hormone deficiency |

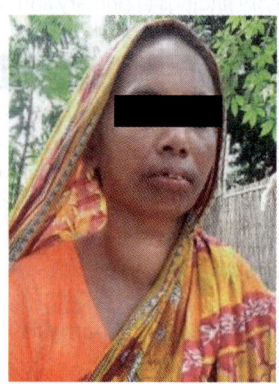

**Why there is enlargement of the thyroid gland in endemic goiter?**

In endemic goiter, there is dietary deficiency of Iodine which result in decreased concentration of iodine in colloid. This results in decreased synthesis of thyroid hormone. This further leads to loss of negative feedback to pituitary, which increases the level of TSH. TSH stimulates the thyroid gland to produce thyroglobulin (Tg). Continued production of Tg increases the volume of colloid, hence, enlarging the size of thyroid gland.

## THYROID FUNCTION TESTS

- **Radioactive iodine uptake:** Hyperfunctioning nodules take up the radioactive iodine and appear as hot areas on radiographic scans.
- **Hormone concentrations:** Serum concentration (bound and free form) of T3, T4, free T3 and free T4 levels
- **Tests for feedback control:**
  - **TRH stimulating tests:** Injection TRH results in the activation of hypothalamic pituitary thyroid axis.
  - **Thyroid suppression tests:** Administration of exogenous triiodothyronine results in the activation of negative feedback cycle and suppresses the TSH levels. It is used to distinguish between toxic multinodular goiter from nontoxic goiter.
- **Nonspecific tests:**
  - Measurement of basal metabolic rate
  - Serum cholesterol levels
  - Systolic ejection time
- **Tests for thyroid damage:**
  - Serum thyroid globulin levels
  - Autoantibodies: Levels of thyroid stimulating immunoglobulin (TSI).

## SUMMARY

- The thyroid gland is located in the neck, just below the Adam's apple. It consists of two lobes connected by a thin tissue called the isthmus. The gland is made up of follicular cells, which produce thyroid hormones, primarily thyroxine (T4) and triiodothyronine (T3). These hormones are essential for regulating metabolism, growth, and development.
- Thyroid hormones are synthesized from the amino acid tyrosine and iodine. Thyroglobulin, a protein produced by the follicular cells, serves as a precursor for thyroid hormone synthesis.
- Thyroid hormones are stored in colloid-filled follicles within the thyroid gland. When stimulated by thyroid-stimulating hormone (TSH) from the pituitary gland, follicular cells release T3 and T4 into the bloodstream.
- Once released, thyroid hormones bind to transport proteins such as thyroxine-binding globulin (TBG), transthyretin, and albumin, which transport them through the bloodstream to target tissues.
- Thyroid hormones enter target cells and bind to thyroid hormone receptors located in the nucleus. This binding initiates gene transcription, leading to changes in protein synthesis and metabolic activity within the cell.
- The synthesis and release of thyroid hormones are primarily regulated by a negative feedback loop involving the hypothalamus, pituitary gland, and thyroid gland. Thyroid-releasing hormone (TRH) from the hypothalamus stimulates the release of TSH from the pituitary gland, which, in turn, stimulates thyroid hormone production. Elevated levels of thyroid hormones inhibit the release of TRH and TSH, maintaining homeostasis.
- **Hypothyroidism:** Hypothyroidism occurs when the thyroid gland does not produce enough thyroid hormones. This can result in symptoms such as fatigue, weight gain, cold intolerance, and dry skin. The most common cause is autoimmune thyroiditis (Hashimoto's disease). Treatment involves hormone replacement therapy with synthetic thyroid hormones.
- **Hyperthyroidism:** Hyperthyroidism is characterized by excessive production of thyroid hormones. Symptoms may include weight loss, rapid heartbeat, tremors, and heat intolerance. Graves' disease, an autoimmune disorder, is the most common cause. Treatment options include antithyroid medications, radioactive iodine therapy, and surgery.

## LET US SEE, HOW MUCH YOU HAVE LEARNT?

 *Review Questions*

### Long/Short Answer Questions

Q1. Describe the synthesis of thyroid hormone.
Q2. Enumerate the steps in thyroid synthesis, regulated by TSH.
Q3. Describe the mechanism of action of TSH and thyroxine.
Q4. What would happen, if a person consumes an iodine deficient diet?

Q5. What would happen, if a person consumes a diet with iodine excess?
Q6. Why there is an enlarged thyroid gland in colloid goiter, even when the patient has hypothyroidism?
Q7. What would happen, if the thyroid gland produces excessive thyroid hormone?
Q8. Describe the regulation of thyroid hormone secretion.
Q9. Differentiate between thyroid and pituitary dwarf.
Q10. What is cretinism? Describe the clinical features and their physiological basis.
Q11. What is the cause of exophthalmos in thyrotoxicosis?

## Explain Why? (Reasoning Questions)

Q1. Hyperthyroidism results in symptoms such as weight loss, increased heart rate, and heat intolerance.
Q2. Iodine is essential for the synthesis of thyroid hormones.
Q3. The thyroid gland enlarges in conditions like Graves' disease.

### Critical Thinking Case-Based Questions

Q1. A 55-year-old woman presents to the clinic with complaints of fatigue, weight gain, and feeling cold all the time. She reports that these symptoms have been gradually worsening over the past several months. She also mentions experiencing constipation, dry skin, and hoarseness of voice. On further inquiry, she denies any recent illnesses or significant stressors in her life. Investigations reveal elevated levels of thyroid-stimulating hormone (TSH) and low levels of free thyroxine (T4), consistent with primary hypothyroidism, elevated cholesterol levels anemia, (normocytic normochromic anemia). Based on this history given, answer the following questions:
   a. What is your probable diagnosis?
   b. Explain why this patient is having weight gain, cold intolerance, constipation, dry skin, hoarseness of voice?
   c. Usually the patients with this disease have non-pitting pretibial edema. Explain why?
   d. Why these patients have yellowish tint of skin?

### Multiple Choice Questions

Q.1 A 45-year-old female presents with weight gain, fatigue, and cold intolerance. Laboratory tests reveal elevated thyroid-stimulating hormone (TSH) levels and low free thyroxine (T4) levels. What is the most likely diagnosis?
   a. Hyperthyroidism
   b. Graves' disease
   c. Hashimoto's thyroiditis
   d. Hypothyroidism

Q2. Which of the following is the primary precursor for thyroid hormone synthesis?
   a. TSH           b. Tyrosine
   c. Thyroglobulin d. Triiodothyronine (T3)

Q3. In which cellular organelle does the synthesis of thyroid hormones primarily occur?
   a. Golgi apparatus
   b. Endoplasmic reticulum
   c. Mitochondria
   d. Thyroid follicles

Q.4 A 30-year-old male presents with weight loss, palpitations, and tremors. Laboratory tests reveal low TSH levels and elevated free T4 levels. What is the most likely diagnosis?
   a. Hypothyroidism      b. Hashimoto's thyroiditis
   c. Hyperthyroidism     d. Thyroid storm

Q5. What is the primary regulator of thyroid hormone secretion?
   a. Thyroid-stimulating hormone (TSH)
   b. Thyroid-releasing hormone (TRH)
   c. Thyroxine-binding globulin (TBG)
   d. Triiodothyronine (T3)

Q6. Which of the following conditions is characterized by an autoimmune attack on the thyroid gland, leading to hypothyroidism?
   a. Graves' disease         b. Thyroid storm
   c. Hashimoto's thyroiditis d. Thyroid adenoma

Q7. A patient presents with a diffuse goiter, exophthalmos, and symptoms of hyperthyroidism. What is the most likely diagnosis?
   a. Hashimoto's thyroiditis
   b. Thyroid storm
   c. Graves' disease
   d. Toxic multinodular goiter

Q8. Which of the following investigations is most appropriate for diagnosing hyperthyroidism?
   a. Thyroid ultrasound
   b. Thyroid function tests (TFTs)
   c. Thyroid uptake scan
   d. Fine-needle aspiration biopsy (FNAB)

Q9. Which of the following symptoms is NOT typically associated with hypothyroidism?
   a. Weight gain
   b. Heat intolerance
   c. Cold intolerance
   d. Fatigue

Q10. A patient with hyperthyroidism is treated with radioactive iodine therapy. What is the mechanism of action of this therapy?
   a. Destruction of thyroid follicles
   b. Inhibition of thyroid hormone synthesis
   c. Blockade of thyroid hormone release
   d. Stimulation of thyroid hormone receptors

Q11. A patient presents with symptoms of hypothyroidism, including myxedema and bradycardia. What is the most appropriate initial treatment?
   a. Levothyroxine
   b. Methimazole
   c. Propranolol
   d. Radioactive iodine

Q12. Which of the following is NOT a symptom of thyrotoxicosis?
   a. Weight loss
   b. Tremors
   c. Bradycardia
   d. Exophthalmos

Q13. Which of the following is a potential complication of untreated hyperthyroidism?
   a. Myxedema coma
   b. Thyroid storm
   c. Cretinism
   d. Hashimoto's thyroiditis

Q14. A patient with hyperthyroidism is found to have elevated levels of thyroid peroxidase antibodies (TPOAb). What autoimmune condition is most likely present?
   a. Graves' disease
   b. Hashimoto's thyroiditis
   c. Toxic multinodular goiter
   d. Thyroid adenoma

## ANSWERS

1. d   2. b   3. d   4. c   5. a   6. c   7. c   8. b   9. b   10. a   11. a   12. c   13. b   14. b

# Physiology of Adrenal Gland

## 68 CHAPTER

> **COMPETENCY ADDRESSED**
>
> **PY8.2:** Describe the synthesis, secretion, transport, physiological actions, regulation and effect of altered (hypo and hyper) secretion of pituitary gland, thyroid gland, parathyroid gland, **adrenal gland**, pancreas and hypothalamus.
> **PY8.4:** Describe function tests: Thyroid gland; **adrenal cortex, adrenal medulla** and pancreas.

**LEARNING OBJECTIVES**

At the end of this chapter, the learner should be able to:
- Discuss functional anatomy of adrenal gland.
- Biosynthesis of adrenal gland hormones.
- Discuss the physiological actions of adrenal gland hormones.
- Discuss the pharmacological actions of corticosteroid.
- Explain the regulation adrenal gland hormone secretion.
- Explain what happens if there is decreased/hypo-secretion of adrenal gland hormone.
- Explain what happens if there is increased/hyper-secretion of adrenal gland hormone.

## PHYSIOLOGICAL ANATOMY OF ADRENAL GLAND

The pair of adrenal glands are situated on the upper poles of kidney, hence, also called suprarenal glands. These glands have an outer cortex and inner medulla. Embryologically, the medulla comes from neural crest whereas the adrenal cortex is formed from intermediate mesoderm (**Fig. 68.1**). The adrenal cortex has three layers:
1. Zona glomerulosa secretes aldosterone (mineralocorticoids)
2. Zona fasciculata secretes cortisol and corticosterone (glucocorticoids)
3. Zona reticularis secretes sex hormones/androgens.

**Adrenal medulla:** Secretes epinephrine. It is discussed in detail in Autonomic Nervous System.

## Biosynthesis of Hormones of Adrenal Gland (Fig. 68.2)

Adrenal cortex cells first convert LDL cholesterol to pregnenolone using enzyme cholesterol desmolase in the mitochondria of adrenal cells under the effect of ACTH and

**GFR:**
**G**lomerulosa
**F**asciculata
**R**eticularis

Angiotensin II. It is the *rate limiting step*. Pregnenolone is converted to aldosterone in zona glomerulosa by the enzyme aldosterone synthase, cortisol in zona fasciculata, and adrenal androgens in zona reticularis.

*Explain why zona glomerulosa does not make sex steroids or corticosteroids?*

The zona glomerulosa does not make sex steroids or corticosteroids because it lacks the enzymes 11β-hydroxylase and 17α-hydroxylase, which are required for the synthesis of these hormones.

## Secretion and Transport of Adrenocortical Hormones

After the synthesis these hormones are secreted into the blood stream and are transported in free and bound forms:
- Cortisol:
  - Free form: 5–10%
  - Bound form: 90–95%, bound to *transcortin* or *cortisol binding globulin*.
- Aldosterone:
  - Free form: 40%
  - Bound form: 60% bound to plasma proteins.

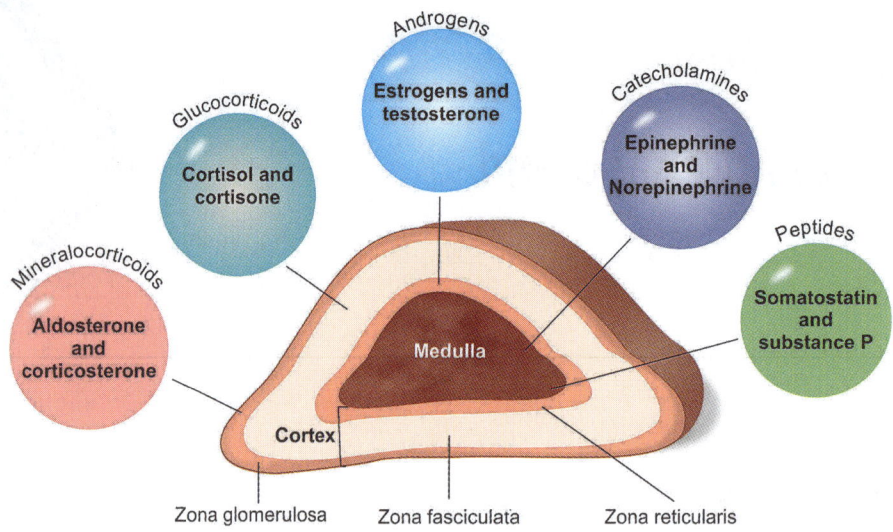

**Fig. 68.1:** Anatomy of adrenal gland and their hormones.

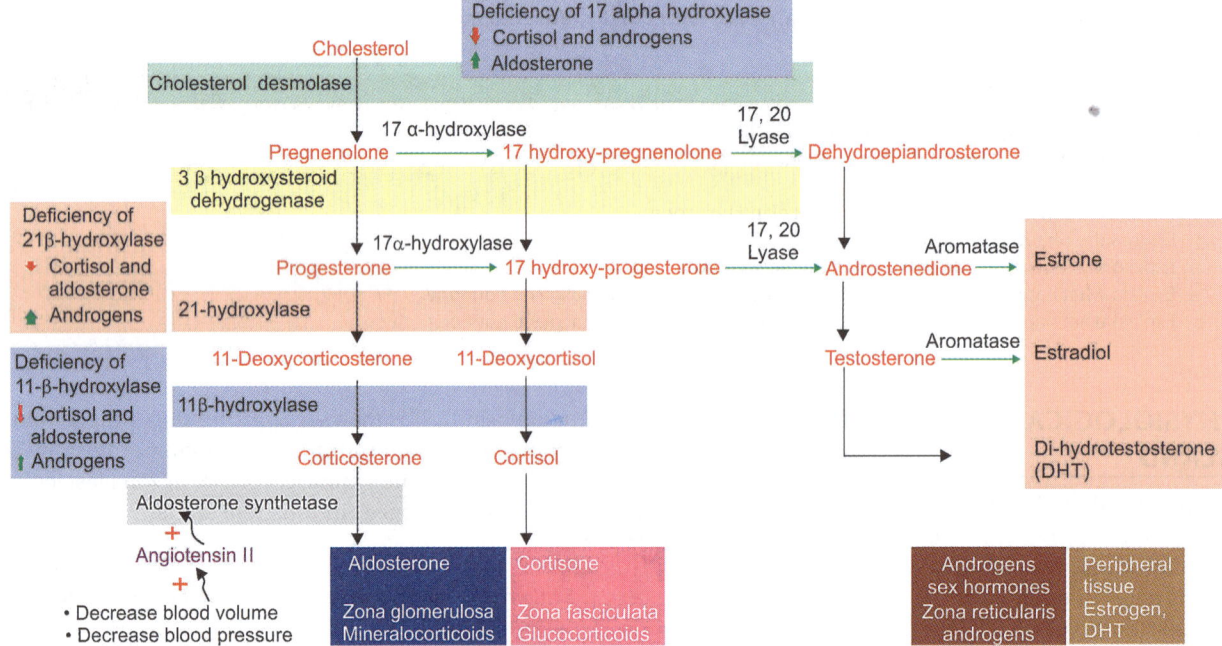

**Fig. 68.2:** Biosynthesis of hormones released by adrenal gland.

## Metabolism and Excretion of Adrenocortical Hormones

These hormones are metabolized in liver, where they are conjugated with glucuronic acid and form inactive conjugated hormones. 25% of this inactivated hormone gets excreted into bile and then through feces, whereas 75% of the inactivated hormone is filtered and excreted through urine. Hence, in liver failure the levels of these hormones will rise in the blood.

## MINERALOCORTICOIDS (ALDOSTERONE)

Since the aldosterone is primarily concerned with the regulation of minerals (sodium and potassium), it is referred to as mineralocorticoid.

## Physiological Effects of Aldosterone (Fig. 68.3)

It is the natural mineralocorticoid in humans. It acts on the *principal cells (P-cells)* of the distal convoluted tubules and collecting ducts. It crosses the cell membrane and *binds to the receptors present in the cytoplasm* and activate the genes that results in the *reabsorption of sodium and water and secretion of potassium ions*. It *activates sodium potassium ATPase pump* and an increase the number of *potassium channels* in the luminal membrane. It also *acts on intercalated cells (I-cells)* of the collecting ducts and *stimulates secretion of $H^+$ and $HCO_3^-$ reabsorption*.

- It increases the reabsorption of sodium chloride and the secretion of potassium in the sweat and salivary gland ducts.

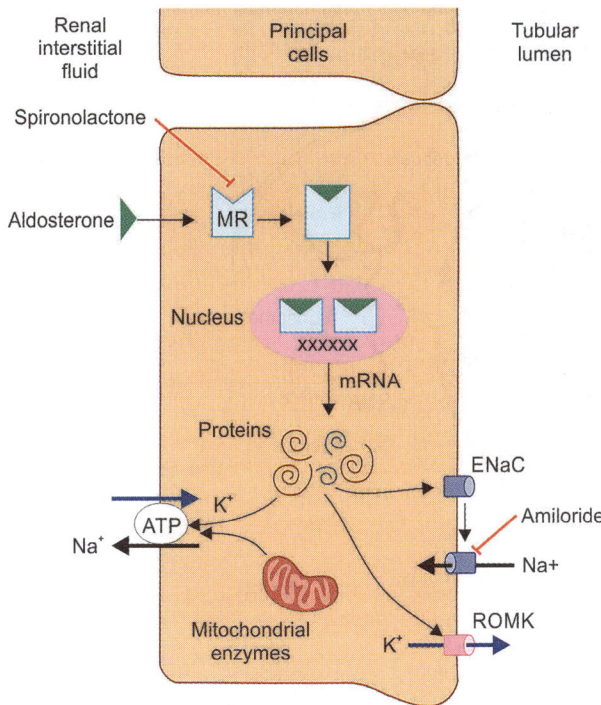

**Fig. 68.3:** Effects of aldosterone.

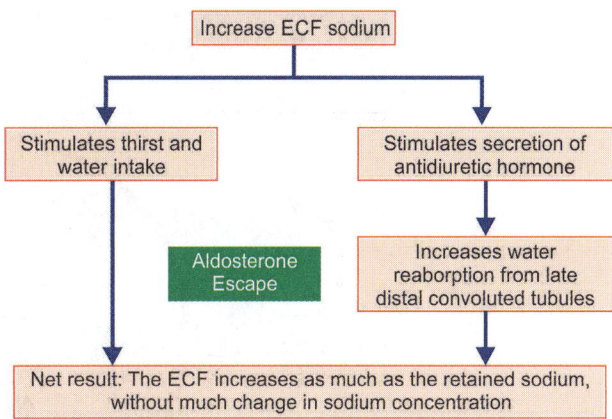

**Fig. 68.4:** Effects of increased ECF sodium and aldosterone escape.

- It also greatly enhances the colon's capacity to absorb sodium, reducing sodium loss in the stool.

## Regulation of Aldosterone Secretion

The most potent *stimulus* for controlling aldosterone release is an *increase in extracellular potassium ion and angiotensin II concentration*. Increased sodium ion concentration and an *increase in atrial natriuretic hormone* released by the stretched heart are factors that *reduce aldosterone secretion*.

- Stimuli that increase aldosterone secretion: *K⁺, angiotensin II*
- Stimuli that decrease aldosterone secretion: *Na⁺, ANP*

## Effects of Hypersecretion of Aldosterone

*Hypernatremia, hypokalemia, muscle weakness and alkalosis are among the clinical signs of an oversecretion of aldosterone* in a patient. Aldosterone increases the rate at which salt and water are reabsorbed by the renal tubules, hence, it *increases*
- *Blood volume*
- *Extracellular fluid volume*
- *Arterial pressure*

Mineralocorticoid deficiency causes severe renal sodium chloride wasting and hyperkalemia

But the majority of patients appear to have normal sodium levels because of **aldosterone escape (Fig. 68.4)**.

In these patients, blocking the aldosterone receptor will be helpful.

## Effects of Hyposecretion of Aldosterone

Aldosterone hyposecretion results in hyponatremia and increased sodium excretion, which lowers extracellular fluid volume, arterial pressure, and cardiac output.

*Explain the physiological basis of muscle weakness in hypersecretion of aldosterone.*

A high aldosterone level causes hypokalemia, which lowers the ECF potassium and increases its concentration gradient leading to increased efflux of the ion. RMP becomes more negative (hyperpolarized) and it takes more time to reach the threshold. As a result, the muscles' excitability is reduced.

## GLUCOCORTICOID (CORTISOL, CORTICOSTERONE)

### Mechanism of Action

The cortisol being lipid soluble can easily cross the cell membrane and binds to the intracellular cytoplasmic receptors. The hormone receptor complex thus formed, binds to the hormone response element situated on DNA and forms the new mRNA and new proteins. Hence, the steroids take longer to bring about their functions **(Fig. 68.5)**.

### Physiological Effects of Cortisol (Fig. 68.6)

- **Effect on carbohydrate metabolism:** Cortisol acts on glucose metabolism to cause *hyperglycemia* (diabetogenic hormone). Hyperglycemia is caused by increasing the synthesis of enzymes involved in *glycogenolysis* and *gluconeogenesis*. It *antagonizes the actions of insulin* and decreases the cellular uptake and utilization of glucose by adipose tissue to increase the availability of glucose for the brain, red blood cells, and skeletal muscles.

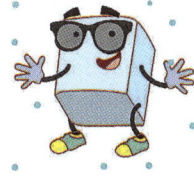

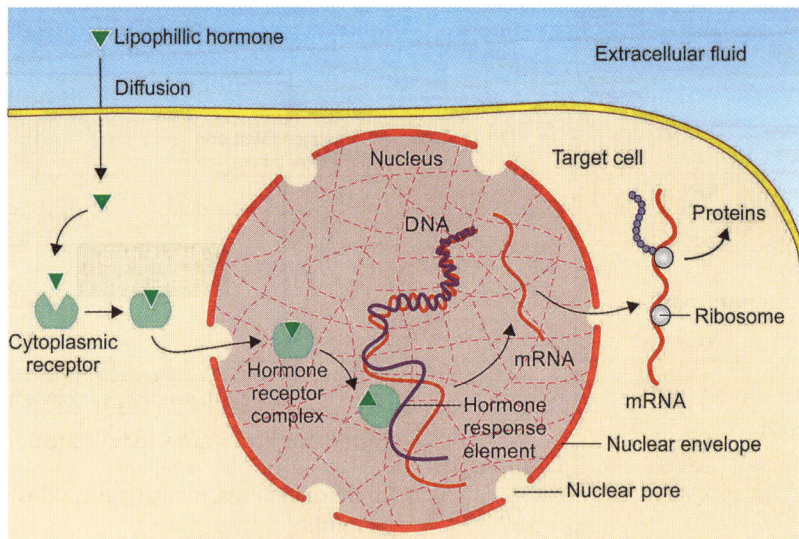

**Fig. 68.5:** Mechanism of action of glucocorticoids.

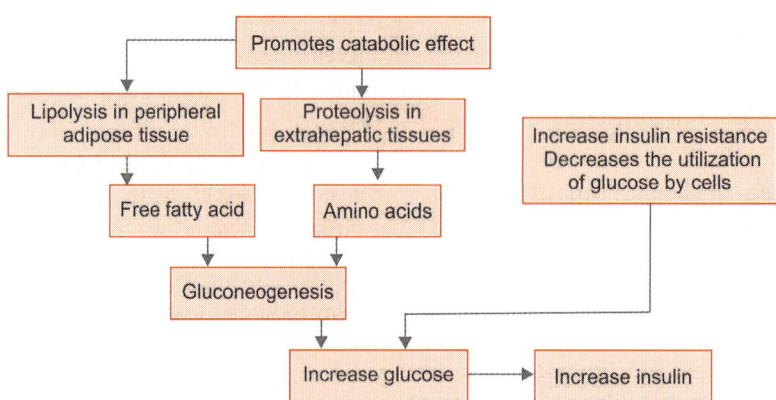

**Fig. 68.6:** Effects of cortisol on carbohydrates, fats and proteins.

Prolonged exposure to high amounts of glucocorticoids can result in *'adrenal diabetes'*.

- **Effect on protein metabolism:** Glucocorticoids *increases the rate of protein breakdown* in most tissues (extra-hepatic tissues, mainly muscle), which increases amino acid concentration in plasma. Glucocorticoid increases transport of amino acid in liver and also enhances the liver enzymes required for protein synthesis, which in turn increases the synthesis of liver proteins and plasma proteins. As a result, cortisol reduces tissue protein store by mobilizing amino acids from nonhepatic tissues.
- **Effect on fat metabolism:** It results in the *redistribution and mobilization of fat*. It increases the concentration of free fatty acids in the plasma by releasing fat from adipose tissue. It promotes the use of fat for energy and lowers the use of glucose for energy. This leads to the formation of large amount of ketone bodies. Additionally, it results in a loss of fat in the extremities and a deposition of fat to the face and upper trunk.
- **Effect on water metabolism:** It *reduces vasopressin/ADH level* and increases excretion of water, glomerular filtration rate (GFR), and renal plasma flow.
- **Effect on mineral metabolism:** It *decreases blood calcium* level by inhibiting its absorption from intestine and increasing excretion through urine causing spontaneous fractures, deformities and decrease linear growth. It enhances the retention of sodium and to a lesser extent, increase excretion of potassium.
- **Effect on blood cells:** It *decreases the number of circulating eosinophils* (eosinopenia) by increasing their destruction in the spleen and lungs (RE system). It also *lowers the number of basophils* in the circulation and *increases the number of neutrophils, platelets and red blood cells*. It decreases the circulating lymphocytes count and the size of the lymph nodes and thymus. It *decreases the secretion of the cytokine IL-2* leads to reduces proliferation of lymphocytes.
- **Permissive action of cortisol:** Permissive function of hormones means one hormone exerts its full effect only in the presence of another hormone. *Glucocorticoids is essential for the constrictor, lipolytic, and bronchodilator effect of catecholamines*. It is also required for calorigenic effect of glucagon.

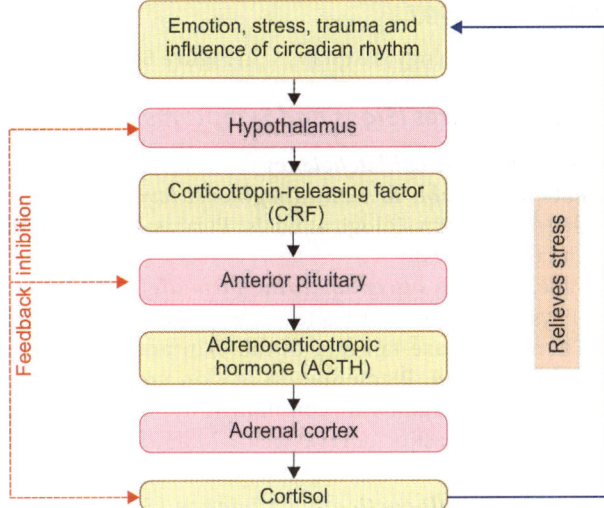

**Fig. 68.7:** Cortisol regulating the stress and its feedback mechanism on hypothalamus and anterior pituitary.

- **Antistress effect of cortisol (Fig. 68.7):** Glucocorticoids and ACTH are needed to withstand any type of stress (Physical/Mental). It has a permissive effect, maintaining the vascular reactivity to catecholamines. It causes the rapid mobilization of FFA and amino acids from cellular reserves, allowing the body to use them for energy and glucose synthesis. *Although cortisol is known to mobilize labile proteins, it does not mobilize fundamental proteins that are necessary for cellular function, such as neurons and muscle contractile proteins.*
- **Effect on bone:** Glucocorticoids **stimulate bone resorption** by promoting osteoclastic activity. It also decreases bone formation and mineralization by inhibiting bone osteoblastic activity and protein catabolism in the bone.
- **Effect on muscle:** It causes *muscle weakness* by increasing protein catabolism in muscles.
- **Effect on nervous system:** It is essential for the normal functions of nervous system.
- **Effect on stomach:** It *increases gastric acid secretion* and blood flow to the gastric mucosa.
- **Effect on reproductive system:** It decreases the secretion of GnRH and affects the secretion of sex steroids.
- **Other effects:** It help mobilize amino acids from the mother's tissues to be used for synthesis of fetal tissues. It stimulates growth of the ductal system of the breast. It increases the maturation of surfactant in the lungs.

## Pharmacological Effects of Androgens

- **Effect on vascular reactivity:** It increases sensitivity of arterioles to the action of norepinephrine and epinephrine (through permissive action) and upregulates the arteriole $\alpha_1$ receptor. Blood pressure rises as a result of vasoconstriction.

***Explain why is glucocorticoid given in severe shock?***
Glucocorticoid can increase the sensitivity of the blood vessels to the vasoconstrictor effects of catecholamines, and also inhibit the production of nitric oxide, which is a potent vasodilator. This can help increase the blood pressure and the tissue oxygenation.

- **Anti-inflammatory effect of cortisol:** It exerts immediate effect of inhibiting inflammatory response to tissue injury by stabilizing lysosomal membrane inhibiting release of proteolytic enzymes, leukotrienes and prostaglandins this decreasing permeability of capillaries and preventing loss of plasma into the tissues. It also decreases migration of leucocytes into the inflamed area and phagocytosis of the damaged cells. It also increases the rate of healing by mobilizing amino acids and FFA to use them to repair the damaged tissue and cellular energy.
- **Antifever effect:** It reduces the *release of interleukin-I* from white blood cells and reduces fever.
- **Antiallergic effect of cortisol:** It suppresses allergic reactions by blocking histamine release from mast cells and basophils.
- **Effect on immunity:** It suppresses immune response and **decrease the number of T-lymphocytes and antibodies (immunosuppressive effects).** This helps in preventing immunological rejection of transplanted tissues and organs.

## Regulation of Cortisol Secretion

Cortisol secretion is controlled by ACTH that is secreted from anterior pituitary. It is released in a diurnal circadian pattern, with the highest levels released at around 8 AM and its lowest levels between midnight and 4 AM. Synthesis and secretion of ACTH is associated with secretion of melanocyte stimulating hormone (MSH) by pituitary. When the rate of secretion of ACTH is high, formation of MSH also increases.

## Negative Feedback Mechanism

Cortisol exerts inhibitory effect on the hypothalamus and anterior pituitary to decrease ACTH secretion **(Fig. 68.8).** It exerts negative feedback on the secretion of corticotropin-releasing hormone (CRF) from hypothalamus and adrenocorticotropic hormone (ACTH) from anterior pituitary.

***Explain why hyperpigmentation in hypoadrenalism (adrenal insufficiency)-Addison's disease?***
When cortisol secretion is depressed, the normal negative feedback to the hypothalamus and anterior pituitary is also depressed. This allows excessive release of ACTH as well as MSH. MSH stimulates the formation of the black pigment melanin, that gets deposited in the skin and mucus membrane.

**Explain why pregnant women have high total plasma cortisol levels without symptoms of glucocorticoids excess?**

Estrogen increases the liver's ability to synthesize corticosteroid binding globulin (CBG). As a result, during pregnancy, the level of CBG rises, more cortisol is bound, and initially, the free cortisol decreases. As a result, cortisol and ACTH secretion are stimulated, and a new equilibrium is created with elevated bound cortisol and normal free cortisol levels.

**Explain why patients with nephrosis have low total plasma cortisol without symptoms of glucocorticoid deficiency?**

Patients with nephrosis have low total plasma cortisol without symptoms of glucocorticoid deficiency because the low total cortisol is mainly due to the loss of cortisol-binding globulin (CBG) in the urine.

## DISORDERS OF ADRENOCORTICAL HORMONES

### Hyposecretion of Adrenocortical Hormones (Hypoadrenalism/Adrenal Insufficiency/Addison's Disease)

**Adrenal insufficiency:** Disorders of the adrenal cortex resulting in hyposecretion of essential steroid hormones (glucocorticoids, mineralocorticoids and androgens).

### Pathophysiology

The pathophysiology is explained in **Figure 68.8**.

### Clinical Features (Signs and Symptoms)

#### Due to glucocorticoid deficiency
- Patient is **unable to maintain glucose level** in between the meals: (Physiological basis: Permissive action of glucocorticoids)
- Patient is highly **susceptible to the harmful effects of stress**. (Physiological basis: Antistress effect of glucocorticoids)
- There is diffuse tanning of the skin and the **spotty pigmentation**. Pigmentation of skin creases on the hands and the gums are common. (Physiological basis: Excessive release of ACTH as well as MSH). Pigmentation is seen only in primary adrenal insufficiency.

#### Due to mineralocorticoid deficiency (Seen only in primary adrenal insufficiency)
- Loss of sodium and water from the body (hyponatremia), which **lowers ECF and BP**, causing orthostatic hypotension, loss of weight, tiredness. It also causes brain cell swelling and neurological symptoms like headache, nausea, lethargy; disorientation.
- Small heart because hypotension decreases the work of the heart.
- Accumulation of potassium in the body (hyperkalemia)
- Desire to eat salt (salt craving).

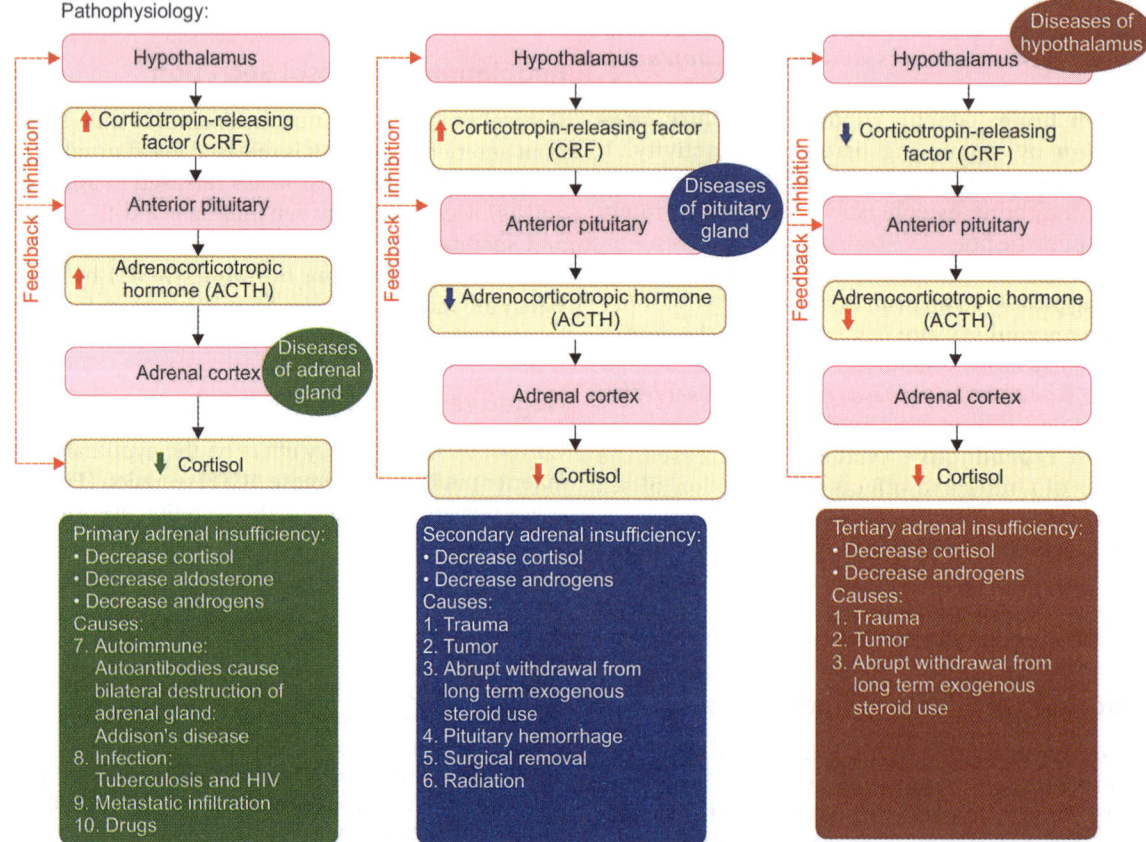

**Fig. 68.8:** Pathophysiology of adrenal insufficiency.

*Explain why is there no aldosterone deficiency and hyperkalemia in secondary and tertiary adrenal insufficiency?*

The primary regulator of aldosterone release from the adrenal cortex are potassium levels and angiotensin II (RAAS). Secondary and tertiary adrenal insufficiency is characterized by decreased ACTH secretion and aldosterone secretion from the zona glomerulosa of the adrenal cortex is ACTh-independent. As a result, aldosterone production is maintained in these two situations and electrolyte imbalance is avoided. in addition, there is no hyperpigmentation.

**Addisonian crisis:** It is also known as an adrenal crisis. It is a life-threatening condition that occurs due to acute adrenal insufficiency. This typically happens when the adrenal glands suddenly stop producing enough cortisol and, sometimes, aldosterone.

*Clinical features:*
- Severe fatigue
- Dehydration
- Low blood pressure
- Abdominal pain
- Confusion.

It can be triggered by stress, infections, trauma, surgery, or suddenly stopping corticosteroid medications. Prompt medical attention is crucial as untreated cases can lead to shock, coma, or even death.

*Treatment:*
- Immediate administration of intravenous fluids
- Corticosteroids (such as hydrocortisone)
- Correction of electrolyte imbalances.

Patients with known adrenal insufficiency should carry emergency information and medications at all times to prevent and manage crises effectively. Regular medical follow-ups and adherence to treatment regimens are essential to prevent recurrence.

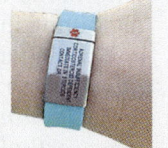

# Hypersecretion of Adrenocortical Hormones (Hyperadrenalism)

**Cushing syndrome:** It is a hormonal disorder caused due to prolonged exposure of the body's tissues to high level of the hormone "cortisol".

## Pathophysiology

Physiological basis of the pathology of the Cushing syndrome is explained in **Figure 68.9**.

## Clinical Features (Signs and Symptoms) (Fig. 68.10)

- *Buffalo hump, truncal obesity, and thin extremities* (Physiological basis: Redistribution and mobilization of fat from extremities with deposition of fat in the upper back, abdomen and face), giving the lemon on sticks appearance.
- Rounded *Moon shaped face* (Physiological basis: Facial obesity and retention of salt and water)
- *Hypertension* (Physiological basis: Permissive effect and mineralocorticoid effect of cortisol)

*What is Cushing disease?*
When Cushing syndrome is due to excess secretion of ACTH by anterior pituitary it is called Cushing disease.

- *Increase blood glucose level* causing adrenal diabetes (Physiological basis: Effect of cortisol on carbohydrate metabolism)
- *Severe weakness* (Physiological basis: Because of proteolysis, there is loss of muscle protein)
- The patient is **highly susceptible to infections** (Physiological basis: Suppressed immune system)

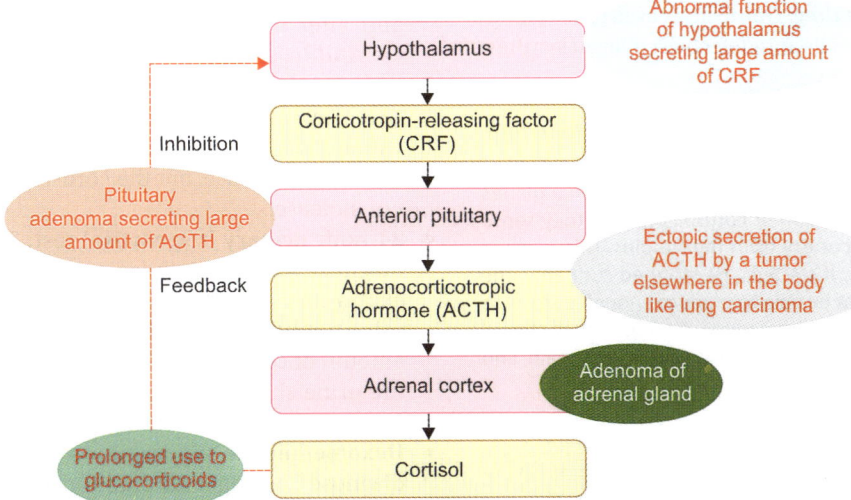

**Fig. 68.9:** Pathophysiology of Cushing syndrome.

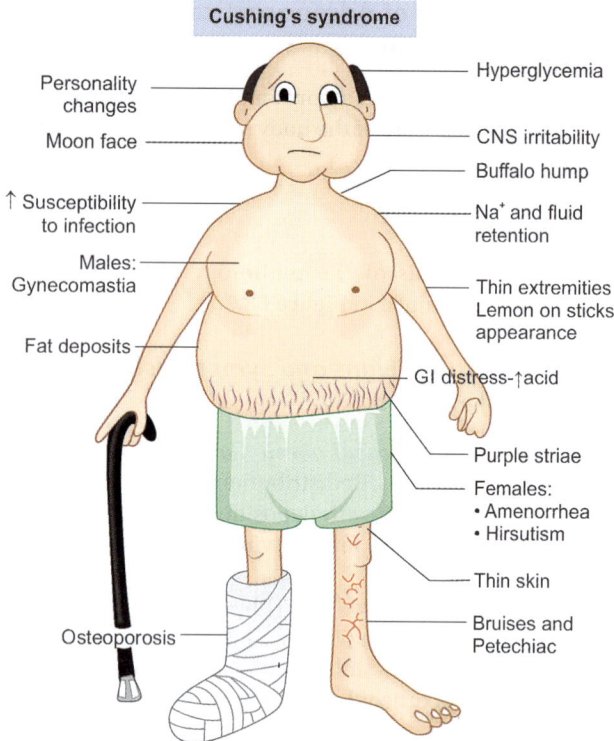

**Fig. 68.10:** Clinical features of Cushing syndrome.

- Large *purplish abdominal stria* (Physiological basis: Because of excess protein catabolism, the skin and subcutaneous tissues are thin and tear easily)
- *Osteoporosis* and weakness of bone (Physiological basis: Glucocorticoids stimulate bone resorption by promoting osteoclastic activity. It also decreases bone formation and mineralization by inhibiting bone osteoblastic activity and protein catabolism in the bone. Also see Chapter 64).
- Increased **CNS stimulation** and result in mental disorders that can include **overeating, sleeplessness, excitement**, and even overt toxic psychoses.
- *Weakness* (Physiological basis: Potassium depletion).
- *Delayed wound healing:* Due to decreased functioning of immune mediator cells and defective collagen synthesis.

> **Why the steroids are tapered off, after their long-term administration?**
>
> When steroids are taken for a long time, the adrenal glands reduce their own production of cortisol, because they sense that there is enough cortisol from the steroids. This is called adrenal suppression1. If steroids are stopped suddenly, the adrenal glands may not be able to produce enough cortisol to meet the body's needs, which can cause symptoms of steroid withdrawal, such as fatigue, weakness, nausea, joint pain, and low blood pressure.

### Hyperaldosteronism

Hyperaldosteronism occurs due to the excess production of aldosterone from the adrenal gland. Primary hyperaldosteronism is the excess aldosterone production either by an adrenal adenoma **(Conn syndrome)** or bilateral adrenal hyperplasia producing excess aldosterone. These patients present with **hypertension and hypokalemia**. Secondary hyperaldosteronism occurs due to **excessive activation of the renin-angiotensin-aldosterone system (RAAS)**, due to renin-producing tumor, renal artery stenosis, or any conditions heart failure, renal failure, liver failure, dehydration, which decreases blood flow to the kidney.

## ADRENAL FUNCTION TESTS

Adrenal function tests are tests that measure the levels and functions of the hormones produced by the adrenal glands. Some of the common adrenal function tests are:

- **ACTH stimulation test:** This test is used to diagnose *primary adrenal insufficiency* (Addison's disease) or secondary adrenal insufficiency. It involves giving an injection of synthetic ACTH, a hormone that stimulates the adrenal glands to produce cortisol, and measuring the blood cortisol levels before and after the injection. *Normally, the cortisol levels should rise after the injection, but in people with adrenal insufficiency, the cortisol levels remain low or do not increase enough.*
- **Insulin tolerance test:** This test is used to diagnose secondary adrenal insufficiency or tertiary adrenal insufficiency. It involves giving an injection of insulin, a hormone that lowers the blood sugar levels, and measuring the blood cortisol and ACTH levels before and during the test. *Normally, low blood sugar levels should trigger the pituitary gland to produce more ACTH, which in turn stimulates the adrenal glands to produce more cortisol.* However, in people with secondary or tertiary adrenal insufficiency, the cortisol and ACTH levels do not rise enough or at all.
- **CRH stimulation test:** This test is used to *differentiate between secondary and tertiary adrenal insufficiency*. It involves giving an injection of CRH, a hormone that stimulates the pituitary gland to produce ACTH, and measuring the blood cortisol and ACTH levels before and after the injection. *Normally, the ACTH and cortisol levels should rise after the injection, but in people with secondary adrenal insufficiency, the ACTH levels are low or do not increase,* while in people with tertiary adrenal insufficiency, the ACTH levels are normal or increase, but the cortisol levels are low or do not increase.
- **24-hour urinary free cortisol test:** This test is used to diagnose *Cushing syndrome*, a condition caused by excess cortisol in the body. It involves collecting all the urine produced in a 24-hour period and measuring the amount of cortisol in it. Normally, the cortisol levels in the urine should be low, but in people with Cushing syndrome, the cortisol levels are high.
- **Dexamethasone suppression test:** This test is used to diagnose Cushing syndrome and to determine its cause. It involves giving a dose of dexamethasone, a synthetic glucocorticoid that suppresses the production of

cortisol, and measuring the blood cortisol levels before and after the dose. *Normally, the cortisol levels should decrease after the dose, but in people with Cushing syndrome, the cortisol levels remain high or do not decrease enough.* Depending on the dose and the response of cortisol, the cause of Cushing syndrome can be identified as either pituitary, adrenal, or ectopic.

- **Aldosterone and renin tests:** These tests are used to diagnose primary aldosteronism, a condition caused by excess aldosterone in the body. Aldosterone is a hormone that regulates the balance of sodium and potassium in the blood and affects the blood pressure. Renin is an enzyme that stimulates the production of aldosterone. These tests involve measuring the blood levels of aldosterone and renin, and calculating the ratio between them. Normally, the ratio should be low, but in people with primary aldosteronism, the ratio is high.
- **DHEA sulfate test:** This test is used to measure the level of DHEA sulfate, a weak androgen hormone produced by the adrenal glands. DHEA sulfate is involved in the development of sexual characteristics and the production of other sex hormones. *This test can help diagnose adrenal tumors, adrenal hyperplasia, or adrenal insufficiency.*

## SUMMARY

- The adrenal medulla secretes catecholamines. More epinephrine is released into the bloodstream than norepinephrine. The adrenal cortex secretes sex hormones, mineralocorticoids, and glucocorticoids
- The principal regulators of mineralocorticoid secretion are $K^+$ level and angiotensin II, while ACTH controls the secretion of glucocorticoids and sex hormones.
- Both ACTH and MSH can be released excessively when cortisol output is low. MSH stimulates the synthesis of melanin, a dark pigment that is deposited in the skin and mucous membranes.
- Aldosterone induces the secretion of potassium ions and the reabsorption of sodium and water by its action on the principal cells (P-cells) of the collecting ducts and distal convoluted tubules. It also increases the secretion of $H^+$ and $HCO_3^-$ reabsorption by acting on the intercalated cells (I-cells) of the collecting ducts.
- Glucocorticoid is a lipolytic, proteolytic, and diabetogenic hormone. It has antifever, anti-inflammatory, antiallergic, and anti-immune properties. It increases sensitivity of arterioles to the action of norepinephrine and epinephrine.
- Cushing syndrome a hormonal disorder caused due to prolonged exposure of the body's tissues to high level of the hormone cortisol. Cushing disease is the term used when Cushing syndrome results from excessive anterior pituitary ACTH output.
- Sudden stoppage of glucocorticoids therapy can cause suppression of HPA axis and precipitate adrenal insufficiency.

## LET US SEE, HOW MUCH YOU HAVE LEARNT?

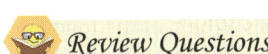

*Review Questions*

### Long/Short Answer Questions

Q1. Why a patient of mineralocorticoids/aldosterone insufficiency experiences salt craving?

Q2. Give the physiological basis of following symptoms in a patient of Cushing's syndrome:
   a. Delayed wound healing
   b. Purple striae
   c. Osteoporosis
   d. Dry skin
   e. Centripetal fat distribution/buffalo hump
   f. Hyperlipidemia

Q3. Why do we need to taper down the dose of corticosteroids after a long-term administration?

Q4. What would happen to a patient taking corticosteroids for almost a year?

Q5. What will happen to the level of adrenocortical hormones in the patients of liver failure?

### Explain Why? (Reasoning Questions)

Q1. Chronic overproduction of cortisol by the adrenal cortex leads to Cushing's syndrome.

Q2. Aldosterone secretion from the adrenal cortex is crucial for maintaining blood pressure and electrolyte balance.

Q3. Adrenal medulla hypersecretion of catecholamines can cause episodes of hypertension, palpitations, and anxiety, as seen in pheochromocytoma.

Q4. Congenital adrenal hyperplasia (CAH) results from enzyme deficiencies affecting cortisol synthesis.

 *Critical Thinking Case-Based Questions*

Q1. Ajay, a 40-year-old man, presented to the clinic with complaints of persistent fatigue, muscle weakness, weight loss, and darkening of his skin, especially in the creases of his palms and around his joints. He also reported episodes of dizziness upon standing. Laboratory tests revealed low blood pressure, hyponatremia (low sodium), hyperkalemia (high potassium), and low cortisol levels. An ACTH stimulation

test showed a suboptimal response. Further imaging studies suggested adrenal gland atrophy. Based on the above case scenario, answer the following questions:
a. Explain the physiological role of the adrenal gland in hormone production and regulation.
b. Discuss how adrenal insufficiency could lead to Ajay's clinical presentation.
c. Enumerate the main hormones produced by the adrenal gland.

## Multiple Choice Questions

Q1. Which of the following is the most common cause of moon facies?
a. Prolonged steroid usage
b. Antibodies to the adrenal cortex
c. Grave's disease
d. Pituitary microadenoma causing excess ACTH

Q2. A 47-year-old man arrives with four to six times-daily episodes of increased heart rate associated with sitting and facial flushing. He has no signs in between episodes. The diagnosis made for him was phaeochromocytoma, a cancer of the adrenal medulla. How does the tumor affect the amount of blood sugar?
a. Decrease serum glucose and increase insulin secretion
b. Increase serum glucose and decrease insulin secretion
c. Decrease serum glucose and increase insulin resistance
d. Increase serum glucose and decrease insulin resistance

Q3. A 48-year-old guy travels across the country by car, and when his vehicle breaks down, he ends as stuck in Pali, Rajasthan. He is left without water or nourishment for more than 72 hours. Which area of the adrenal gland releases a hormone in reaction to the person's level of hydration?
a. Zona fasciculata
b. Zona glomerulosa
c. Adrenal medulla
d. Zona reticularis

Q4. A 33-year-old female who is obese and has a history of asthma was using corticosteroids in the past. She had been on hypertension medication for 5 years. She complained of an irregular menstrual cycle and widespread weakness. Her face is round and red, and her neck has a hump:

a. Cushing disease
b. Conn's disease
c. Cushing syndrome
d. Addison's disease

Q5. 42-year male patient was found to have thin extremities and fat redistributed at abdomen and upper back. He has reddish purple striae on skin and his blood glucose level. Which of the following is the most likely cause for this condition?
a. Increased glucocorticoid
b. Increased growth hormone
c. Increased insulin
d. Increased glucagon

Q6. You are a medical student doing a clinical rotation in endocrinology. You are asked to see a 35-year-old woman who has been referred by her primary care physician for evaluation of possible Cushing syndrome. She complains of weight gain, especially around her abdomen and face, thinning of her hair, irregular periods, and easy bruising. She also has a history of hypertension and diabetes mellitus. On physical examination, you notice that she has a round face with facial plethora, a buffalo hump, and purple striae on her abdomen. You suspect that she has Cushing syndrome and order some tests to confirm your diagnosis. Which of the following tests is the most appropriate initial screening test for above mentioned syndrome?
a. 24-hour urinary free cortisol
b. Serum cortisol level
c. Low-dose dexamethasone suppression test
d. High-dose dexamethasone suppression test

### ANSWERS

**1.** a  **2.** b  **3.** b  **4.** c  **5.** a  **6.** c

# Glucose Homeostasis: Role of Endocrine Pancreas

## CHAPTER 69

### COMPETENCY ADDRESSED

**PY8.2:** Describe the synthesis, secretion, transport, physiological actions, regulation and effect of altered (hypo and hyper) secretion of pituitary gland, thyroid gland, parathyroid gland, adrenal gland, **pancreas** and hypothalamus.
**PY8.4:** Describe function tests: Thyroid gland, adrenal cortex, adrenal medulla and **pancreas**.

### LEARNING OBJECTIVES

**At the end of this chapter, the learner should be able to:**
- Enumerate the various hormones secreted by endocrine pancreas.
- Describe the synthesis, storage, release, regulation and actions of insulin.
- Describe the effect of lack of insulin on metabolism.
- Describe the physiology of secretion of glucagon and somatostatin.

The pancreas is a unique organ having the dual mode of secretion, i.e., the secretion of enzymes in the pancreatic juice for digestion which is secreted by the pancreatic acinar cells called **exocrine pancreas**; and another is the secretion of hormones (Insulin, glucagon and somatostatin) from the specialized cells called **Islets of Langerhans** dispersed in between the pancreatic acini, called **endocrine pancreas**. The islets of Langerhans has three type of cells namely alpha cells which secretes glucagon, beta cells which secretes insulin and delta cells which secrete somatostatin.

| Exocrine pancreas | Endocrine pancreas |
|---|---|
| • Has acinar cells with ducts<br>• Secrete enzymes in pancreatic juice | • Islets of Langerhans scattered in between pancreatic acini<br>• Secretes hormones from these Islets:<br>  ■ α cells—Glucagon<br>  ■ β cells—Insulin<br>  ■ δ cells—Somatostatin |

## INSULIN

It was first isolated by Banting and Best in 1922 and identified as a polypeptide hormone secreted by *β-cells of islets of Langerhans*.

## Synthesis

Synthesis of insulin happens in RER of beta cells of islets of Langerhans of pancreas **(Fig. 69.1)**.

$$\underset{\text{(Mol Wt. 11500 Da)}}{\substack{\text{Endoplasmic}\\\text{reticulum}\\\text{preproinsulin}}} \rightarrow \underset{\text{(9000 Da)}}{\substack{\text{Golgi}\\\text{apparatus}\\\text{proinsulin}}} \rightarrow \substack{\text{Secretory}\\\text{granules}\\\text{insulin +}\\\text{C-peptide}}$$

C-peptide assay is useful in assessing beta cell function in exogenous insulin intake. C peptide and insulin are packed in secretory granules and secreted in equimolar quantities. Some of proinsulin is also secreted along with insulin. **Proinsulin and C peptide have no insulin-like effect.**
**C-peptide** binds to G protein-coupled membrane receptor and activates $Na^+$-$K^+$ ATPase and nitric oxide synthase.
**Q. What would happen to C peptide levels in patients with type I diabetes mellitus?**
C-peptide decreases when the endogenous secretion of insulin decreases.

## Storage, Release, Metabolism of Insulin

The formed insulin is **stored in the β-cells** till it gets stimulated by raised blood glucose level, to release the

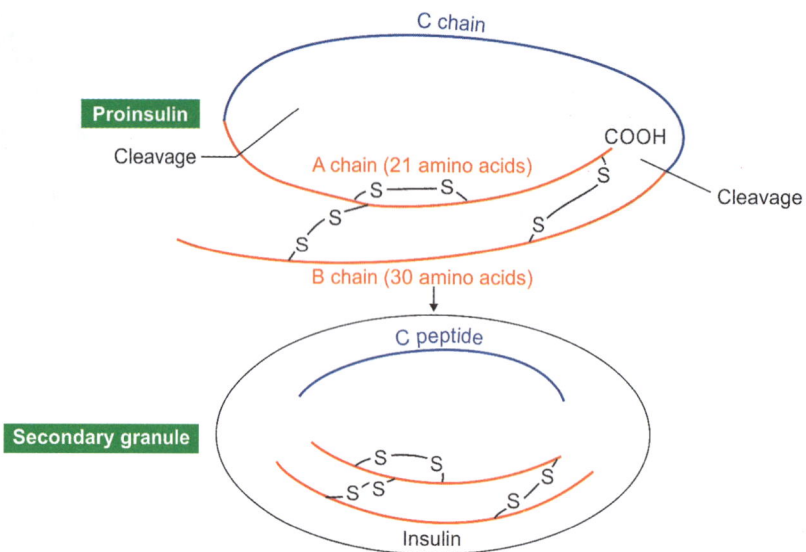

**Fig. 69.1:** Synthesis of insulin.

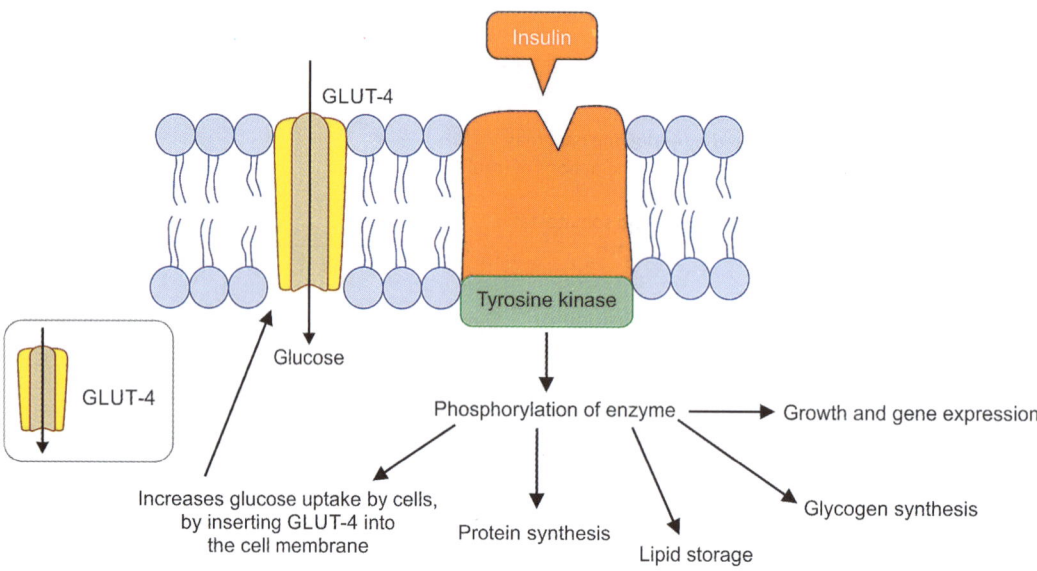

**Fig. 69.2:** Effects of action of insulin.

insulin into blood stream which reaches the target cells where it acts through membrane receptors with tyrosine kinase activity. It has *short half life of 6 minutes*. It gets metabolized by liver and excreted through kidney.

## Actions of Insulin (Fig. 69.2)

### Rapid Actions

- Glucose uptake by the target cell due to activation of GLUT 4 *(Target cells acting through GLUT 4 are skeletal and cardiac muscle cells, adipose tissue and other cells. There are 7 glucose transporter proteins (GLUT 1 to GLUT 7), out of which GLUT 4 is present in insulin sensitive cells and GLUT 2 is present on the beta cells.* **Brain does not need insulin for glucose uptake.**

- Rapid uptake of amino acids and potassium by insulin sensitive cells:

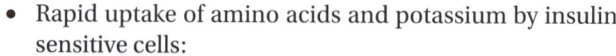
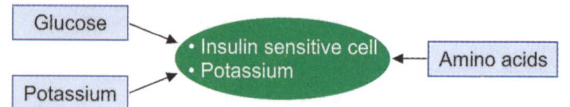

### Intermediate Actions

- Increased protein synthesis
- Decreased protein breakdown
- Glycogen synthesis
- inhibition of gluconeogenesis

### Delayed Actions

Increases mRNA for lipogenesis.

## Effects of Insulin

Insulin plays a crucial role in metabolism of carbohydrates, fat and protein metabolism. The effects of insulin are discussed in **Table 69.1**.

## Release of Insulin from Beta Cells

The release of insulin from pancreatic beta cells is a tightly regulated process crucial for maintaining blood glucose homeostasis (**Flowchart 69.1** and **Fig. 69.3**). This orchestrated secretion responds to fluctuating glucose levels, facilitating cellular uptake and storage, thus safeguarding metabolic equilibrium.

## Regulation of Insulin Secretion

- Plasma glucose is the prime regulator
- Amino acids like arginine and leucine stimulate insulin secretion
- **Hormone:**
    - Increasing the plasma glucose level stimulate insulin secretion like: Growth hormone, Glucagon, Glucocorticoids, etc.
    - Secreted from GIT: Enteroglucagon, Gastrin, CCK, etc.
- **Neural:**
    - Sympathetic: Decrease secretion of insulin secretion (mainly thru alpha rec.)
    - Parasympathetic: Increase the insulin secretion
- **Drugs:** Oral hypoglycemics increase the insulin secretion

## DIABETES MELLITUS

The syndrome caused by the deficiency of insulin is called as diabetes mellitus.

Criteria for diagnosing DM:
- Fasting blood glucose level: ≥126 mg/dL on 2 separate occasions
- Postprandial glucose level: ≥200 mg/dL at 2 hours

## Classification

**Primary DM:**
- Autoimmune (Type I DM):
    - **Insulin dependent DM (Type I IDDM)**
    - Noninsulin dependent DM (Type I NIDDM)
- Nonautoimmune (Type II DM):
    - Insulin dependent DM (Type II IDDM)
    - **Noninsulin dependent DM (Type II NIDDM)**

**Secondary DM:** Due to any other cause
- Pituitary diabetes (due to persistent hyperglycemia caused by excessive secretion of growth hormone)
- Adrenal diabetes (due to hyperglycemic effect of glucocorticoids)

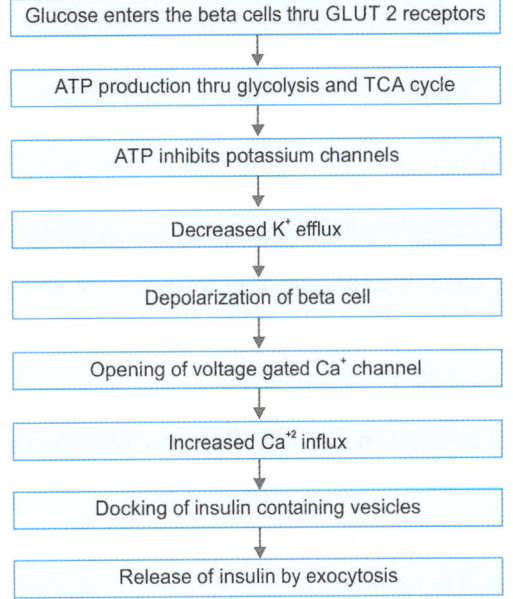

**Flowchart 69.1:** Secretion of insulin from beta cells on glucose entry.

**Table 69.1:** Effects of insulin on major metabolic pathways.

| Carbohydrate metabolism | Fat metabolism | Protein metabolism |
| --- | --- | --- |
| Increased glucose uptake by insulin sensitive cells and liver | Excess glucose is converted into fat and stored in adipose tissue | Increased uptake of amino acid in muscle |
| **Decreases plasma glucose levels** | **Activates lipoprotein lipase,** which splits triglycerides in the blood into free fatty acids, which are stored in adipose tissue | Increased synthesis of new protein |
| Increased utilization of glucose by **Glycolysis** | **Inhibits hormone sensitive lipase,** which splits stored TGs into FFA and releases into blood | Decreased protein breakdown |
| Conversion of extra glucose into glycogen by **Glycogenesis** | | Decreased uptake of AA by liver, **prevents gluconeogenesis** |
| Decreased synthesis of glucose from fat and amino acids **(Inhibition of Gluconeogenesis)** | | |
| **Summary** | | |
| *Decreases plasma glucose levels and stores in the form of glycogen and fat for use when glucose levels fall in blood* | *Excess glucose is stored as fat. It also promotes fat storage in adipose tissue and decreases FFA levels in blood* | *Protein sparing action with increased protein synthesis and decreased breakdown* |

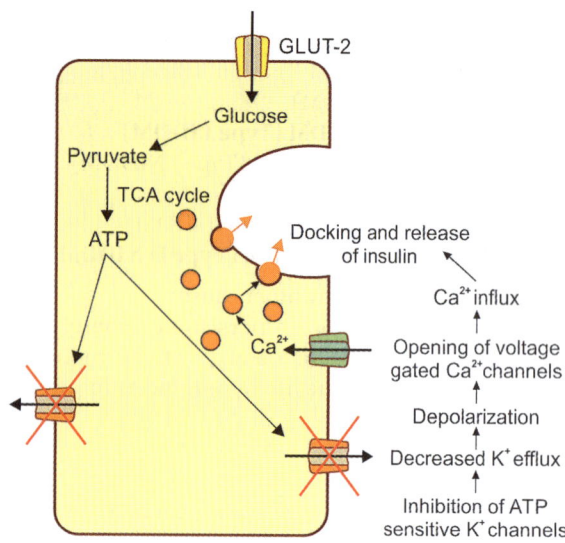

**Fig. 69.3:** Release of insulin from beta cells.

## Cause/Etiology

- Autoimmune: Antibodies to beta cells (Type I IDDM)
- Genetic: As seen in type II NIDDM; due to HLA DR4
- Infections: Certain viral infections like measles and mumps results in damage to beta cells, hence, result in type I diabetes mellitus
- Persistent hyperglycemia due to other causes (secondary) Increase in hyperglcemic hormone → increased secretion of insulin → exhaustion of beta cells → failure of beta cells to produce insulin → DM
- Inflammation of pancreas

## Effect of Insulin Lack (Deficiency of Insulin) on Metabolism

Deficiency of insulin leads to imbalance in metabolism which can cause different pathologic events. These are discussed in **Table 69.2**.

## Pathogenesis of Diabetes Mellitus (Flowchart 69.2)

In diabetes mellitus, the absence or insufficient production of insulin disrupts glucose regulation. Without insulin, glucose cannot enter cells for energy, leading to hyperglycemia. This prolonged high blood sugar damages blood vessels and organs, causing complications like neuropathy, nephropathy, and retinopathy.

## Clinical Features

### Chief Complaints

- Excessive thirst, increased frequency of micturition, increased hunger (polydipsia, polyuria and polyphagia)
- Weight loss due to increased protein catabolism
- Increased susceptibility to infections due to hyperglycemia
- Delayed wound healing

### On Examination/Investigations

- Hyperglycemia (FBS >126 g/dL)
- Glucosuria (passage of glucose in urine, renal threshold for glucose is 180 g/dL)
- Increased glycosylated Hb (HbA1C > 6 gm%)
- **Ketosis:** Due to β-oxidation of fats as the cells are starving and are unable to use the glucose present in the blood.
- **Acidosis:** Due to lactic acidosis and ketosis.
- **Hyperkalemia:** Due to lack of insulin, the potassium uptake of cells is markedly reduced and hence, presents as hyperkalemia.

Clinical features of type 1 and type 2 diabetes mellitus are compared in **Table 69.3**.

## Stages of DM

- **Prepotential DM:** Asymptomatic stage with strong genetic predisposition. Hyperplasia of beta cells.

**Table 69.2:** Effects of insulin deficiency on major metabolic pathways.

| Carbohydrate metabolism | Fat metabolism | Protein metabolism |
|---|---|---|
| Decreased glucose uptake by insulin sensitive cells and liver | Excess glucose is not converted into fat and stored fat is mobilized from adipose tissue into blood stream | Decreased uptake of amino acid in muscle |
| *Increases plasma glucose level* (Hyperglycemia) | **Inhibits lipoprotein lipase,** which splits triglycerides in the blood into free fatty acids, which are stored in adipose tissue → Increases FFA in blood | Decreased synthesis of new protein |
| Decreased utilization of glucose by **Glycolysis** | **Stimulates hormone sensitive lipase,** which splits stored TGs into FFA and releases into blood → Increases FFA in blood | Increased protein breakdown |
| Decreased conversion of extra glucose into glycogen by **Glycogenesis** | | Increased uptake of AA by liver, **results in gluconeogenesis** |
| Increased synthesis of glucose from fat and amino acids **(Stimulation of Gluconeogenesis)** | | |
| **Summary** | | |
| *Increases plasma glucose levels (Hyperglycemia) and decreases stores in the form of glycogen and fat because of incapability of cells to use glucose* | *Increases FFA in blood → promotes atherosclerosis and formation of ketone bodies (Acetoacetic acid and β-OH butyric acid) → ACIDOSIS* | *Protein breakdown to produce glucose → Increased plasma glucose levels (hyperglycemia)* |

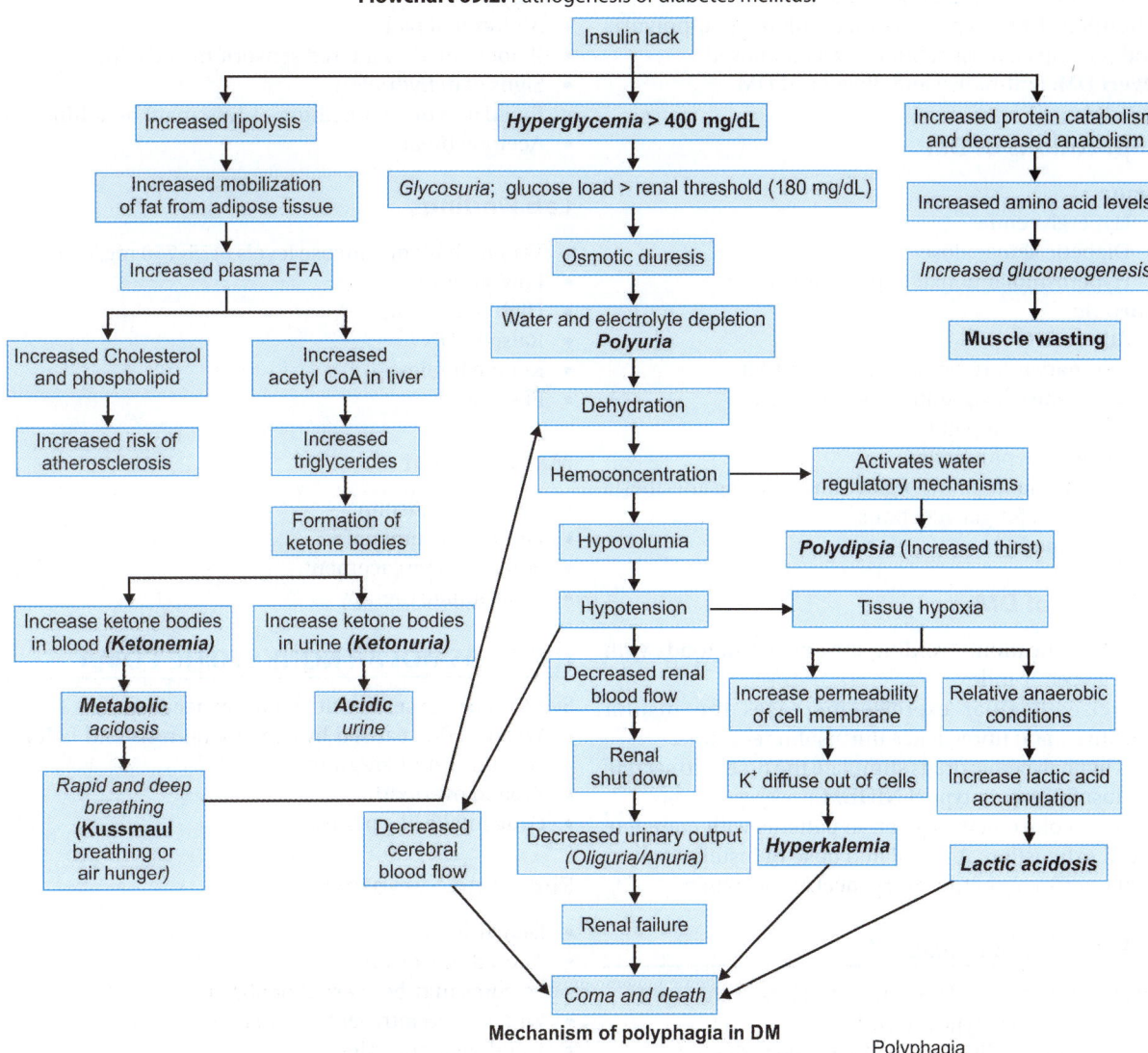

Flowchart 69.2: Pathogenesis of diabetes mellitus.

Table 69.3: Differences between type 1 and type 2 diabetes mellitus.

|  | Type I IDDM | Type II NIDDM |
| --- | --- | --- |
| **Age of onset** | <40 years | >40 years |
| **Weight** | Normal/wasted | Overweight/obese |
| **Etiology** | Autoimmune, little genetic preponderance | Genetic |
| **Onset** | Sudden | Gradual |
| **Beta cells** | Destroyed | Normal |
| **Insulin secretion** | Decreased | Normal; decreases gradually |
| **Receptors** | Normal/upregulation of receptors | Down regulation/receptor insensitivity |
| **Acute complication** | Diabetic ketoacidosis | Nonketotic hyperosmolar coma |
| **Treatment** | Insulin | • Exercise, lifestyle modification, weight loss<br>• Oral hypoglycemic drugs |

- **Latent DM:** Asymptomatic + glucosuria in stress
- **Chemical DM:** Hyperglycemia, polyphagia, polyuria and polydipsia present but not yet diagnosed
- **Overt DM:** Full-blown and diagnosed DM

## Complications of DM

- **Acute**
  - Hyperglycemia
  - Diabetic ketoacidosis
  - Hyperosmolar nonketonuric coma
- **Chronic**
  - Atherosclerosis
  - Coronary artery syndrome → silent MI
  - Gangrene of extremities → foot ulcers
  - Diabetic retinopathy
  - Diabetic nephropathy
  - Diabetic neuropathy → glove and stocking anesthesia
  - Increased fungal infections
  - Dermopathy

## Treatment of DM

- Diet modification: Avoiding the sugar and foods with high glycemic index.
- Exercise: Regular exercise increases the insulin sensitivity and upregulates the insulin receptors.
- Oral hypoglycemic drugs stimulate the β-cells to secrete the insulin, esp. in type II NIDDM.
- Insulin replacement is given in patients with complete β-cell exhaustion. A calculated dose of insulin is given subcutaneously before every meal in the patient.

## DIABETIC KETOACIDOSIS

- Occurs due to lack of insulin and excess of glucagon
- Most common in type I IDDM
- Pathogenesis is discussed in **Flowchart 69.3**.

### Signs and Symptoms

- Anorexia
- Nausea and vomiting
- Polyuria
- Abdominal pain
- If not treated → altered sensorium and coma
- Signs of dehydration
- Rapid and deep breathing → Kussmaul breathing
- Acetone breath

### Lab Findings

- Very high blood glucose levels (475–750 mg/dL)
- Low sodium
- High potassium
- Raised BUN
- Ketone bodies ++
- FFA raised

### Management

- Infusion of insulin
- Fluid replacement
- Potassium replacement
- Bicarbonate therapy

## HYPEROSMOLAR NONKETOTIC COMA

Syndrome of excessive dehydration because of:
- Water deficit caused by osmotic diuresis and failure to consume enough water.
- Protein overload
- Drug intake like phenytoin, etc.

### Signs and Symptoms

- Dehydration
- Altered sensorium
- Seizures may be present or absent
- Widespread intravascular coagulation
- Bleeding tendencies +

### Lab Findings

- Hyperglycemia (1000 mg/dL)
- BUN very high

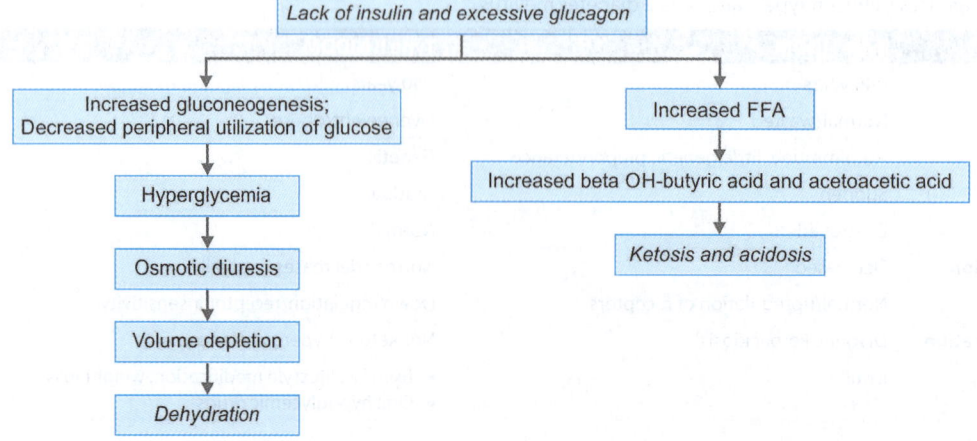

**Flowchart 69.3:** Effects of lack of insulin and excessive glucagon on ketosis and acidosis.

- Raised creatinine
- Hypernatremia
- Hyperkalemia
- Hyperosmolarity
- Raised FFA, but less than diabetic ketoacidosis
- Ketone bodies

## Management

- Intravenous fluids
- Potassium replacement is required earlier in this scenario
- Bicarbonate treatment if acidosis present
- Antibiotics for infection

## Role of Potassium in Treatment of DKA

In the treatment of diabetic ketoacidosis (DKA), potassium plays a crucial role in correcting electrolyte imbalances. Insulin therapy drives potassium back into cells, leading to hypokalemia, which can be exacerbated by dehydration and acidosis. Therefore, potassium supplementation is essential to prevent dangerous cardiac arrhythmias and restore normal potassium levels, aiding in the resolution of DKA **(Flowchart 69.4)**.

# GLUCAGON

- Polypeptide hormone secreted by α-cells of pancreas
- Hormone of energy release (Catabolic hormone) → Increases blood sugar levels, called as hyperglycemic hormone

## Mechanism of Action

Acts via G protein coupled membrane receptors which activate adenylyl cyclase and synthesis cAMP as second messenger.

## Actions

Raises blood sugar level by:
- Stimulating glycogenolysis in liver (Breakdown of glycogen stored in liver)
- Stimulating gluconeogenesis
- Stimulating mobilization of fat from the adipose tissue and increasing the lipolysis → increased production of ketone bodies.
- Stimulates the secretion of GH, insulin and pancreatic somatostatin.

**Regulation:** Plasma glucose is the main regulator of glucagon secretion.

**Flowchart 69.4:** Potassium playing crucial role in DKA.

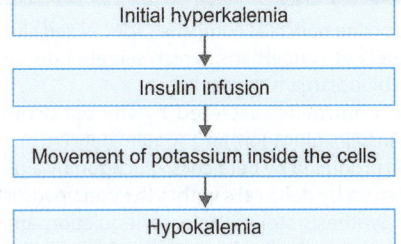

# SOMATOSTATIN

- Polypeptide hormone secreted by δ-cells of pancreas

| Found in | Function |
|---|---|
| Brain | Neurotransmitter |
| Hypothalamus | GHIH |
| Endocrine pancreas | Inhibits secretion of insulin and glucagon |
| GIT | Inhibitor GI hormone |

- Mechanism of action: Acts through G—protein coupled receptors by inhibiting adenylyl cyclase and decreasing cAMP

## Actions

- Locally within islets → decreases secretion of insulin and glucagon
- Decreases motility of stomach, duodenum and gallbladder
- Decreases the secretion and absorption in GIT

## Effects

- Extends the period of time over which the food nutrients are assimilated in the blood
- By decreasing the insulin and glucagon secretion → decreasing the utilization of absorbed nutrients by tissues and prevents rapid exhaustion of food → making it available for longer period of time.

## Factors Affecting Release of Somatostatin

- Increased blood glucose
- Increased amino acids
- Increased free fatty acids
- Increased conc. of GI hormone

The other hormones which increase the blood sugar level are called as diabetogenic hormones, which are Glucagon, Growth hormone, Glucocorticoids, Thyroxine, Catecholamines.

## SUMMARY

- The endocrine pancreas comprises specialized clusters of cells called islets of Langerhans, which secrete hormones directly into the bloodstream.
- The main hormones secreted by the endocrine pancreas include insulin, glucagon, and somatostatin.
- Insulin is produced by beta cells, glucagon by alpha cells, and somatostatin by delta cells within the pancreatic islets.
- **Insulin:** Synthesis, storage, release, regulation, and actions:
  - Insulin is synthesized as a preprohormone in beta cells of the pancreas and undergoes processing to become proinsulin, which is then cleaved into insulin and C-peptide.
  - Newly synthesized insulin is stored in granules within beta cells until needed.
  - Insulin release is triggered by elevated blood glucose levels, amino acids, gastrointestinal hormones (e.g., incretins), and neural inputs (e.g., vagal stimulation).
  - Insulin acts on various tissues, including muscle, liver, and adipose tissue, to promote glucose uptake, glycogen synthesis, lipogenesis, and protein synthesis, thereby lowering blood glucose levels.
- Insulin deficiency, as seen in conditions such as type 1 diabetes mellitus, leads to dysregulation of glucose metabolism.
- In the absence of insulin, glucose uptake by peripheral tissues is impaired, resulting in hyperglycemia.
- Lipolysis in adipose tissue is increased, leading to elevated levels of free fatty acids and ketone bodies, which can result in ketoacidosis.
- Protein breakdown is also increased, contributing to muscle wasting and metabolic disturbances.
- Glucagon, produced by alpha cells, is released in response to low blood glucose levels and stimulates glycogenolysis, gluconeogenesis, and lipolysis, thereby raising blood glucose levels.
- Somatostatin, produced by delta cells, acts as a paracrine and endocrine hormone, inhibiting the secretion of both insulin and glucagon, as well as regulating gastrointestinal motility and secretion.

## LET US SEE, HOW MUCH YOU HAVE LEARNT?

### Review Questions

#### Long/Short Answer Questions

Q1. Describe the synthesis, mechanism of action and functions of insulin.
Q2. What would happen to carbohydrate metabolism, if there is deficiency of insulin?
Q3. What would happen to lipid metabolism, if there is deficiency of insulin?
Q4. What would happen to protein metabolism, if there is deficiency of insulin?
Q5. Why a patient of diabetes mellitus experiences polydipsia, polyuria and polyphagia?
Q6. Enumerate the diabetogenic hormones.
Q7. What are the functions of glucagon?
Q8. What are the functions of somatostatin?
Q9. Differentiate between type 1 IDDM and type 2 NIDDM.
Q10. Why do we administer potassium to a patient of diabetic ketoacidosis after the initial treatment, even when there is initial hyperkalemia at presentation?
Q11. Why a patient of diabetic ketoacidosis has air hunger?

#### Explain Why? (Reasoning Questions)

Q1. Insulin secretion is crucial for lowering blood glucose levels after a meal.
Q2. Glucagon is essential during fasting to maintain blood glucose levels.
Q3. Insulin resistance to elevated blood glucose levels despite normal or high levels of insulin.
Q4. Somatostatin helps regulate glucose homeostasis.
Q5. Type 1 diabetes mellitus results in hyperglycemia and ketoacidosis due to autoimmune destruction of pancreatic beta cells.

### Critical Thinking Case-Based Questions

Q1. Sujata, a 55-year-old woman, presented to OPD with complaints of excessive thirst, frequent urination, and unexplained weight loss over the past few months. She also reported feeling fatigued and having blurred vision. A blood test revealed a fasting blood glucose level of 280 mg/dL and elevated HbA1c levels. Further investigation showed low levels of C-peptide. Sujata had no significant family history of diabetes but mentions that she had a viral infection a few months ago.

Based on the given clinical scenarios, answer the following questions:
a. Explain the role of the endocrine pancreas in glucose homeostasis.
b. Discuss how dysfunction in this system can lead to Sujata's clinical presentation.
c. What are the potential long-term complications of poorly controlled blood glucose levels?

## Multiple Choice Questions

Q1. A 30-year-old patient with type 1 diabetes mellitus presents with symptoms of hypoglycemia. Which hormone would be expected to be elevated in this scenario?
 a. Insulin
 b. Glucagon
 c. Somatostatin
 d. Cortisol

Q2. A 45-year-old patient with insulin resistance is started on a new medication that increases insulin sensitivity. Which of the following is the most likely mechanism of action of this medication?
 a. Inhibition of insulin synthesis
 b. Stimulation of insulin release
 c. Inhibition of glucagon release
 d. Stimulation of glucose uptake by peripheral tissues

Q3. A patient presents with symptoms of hyperglycemia, polyuria, and polydipsia. Laboratory tests reveal elevated blood glucose levels and low insulin levels. What is the most likely diagnosis?
 a. Type 1 diabetes mellitus
 b. Type 2 diabetes mellitus
 c. Diabetic ketoacidosis
 d. Gestational diabetes mellitus

Q.4. During a fasting state, which of the following hormones is primarily responsible for maintaining blood glucose levels?
 a. Insulin
 b. Glucagon
 c. Somatostatin
 d. Cortisol

Q.5. A patient with diabetes mellitus experiences an episode of hypoglycemia. Which of the following hormones would be expected to be elevated in response to this hypoglycemic episode?
 a. Insulin
 b. Glucagon
 c. Somatostatin
 d. Growth hormone

Q.6. A 35-year-old woman with gestational diabetes is treated with insulin injections to manage her blood glucose levels. Which of the following hormones is responsible for stimulating insulin release in response to a meal?
 a. Glucagon
 b. Somatostatin
 c. Gastrin
 d. Incretins (GLP-1 and GIP)

Q.7. A patient presents with symptoms of hypoglycemia, including confusion and sweating. The patient's blood glucose level is found to be low. Which hormone is responsible for counter-regulating the effects of insulin and raising blood glucose levels in this situation?
 a. Insulin
 b. Glucagon
 c. Somatostatin
 d. Cortisol

Q.8. A 50-year-old patient with chronic pancreatitis develops diabetes mellitus due to damage to pancreatic beta cells. Which of the following hormones would be expected to be deficient in this patient?
 a. Insulin
 b. Glucagon
 c. Somatostatin
 d. Amylin

Q.9. A patient presents with symptoms of diabetes insipidus, including excessive thirst and polyuria. Which of the following hormones is primarily responsible for regulating water balance?
 a. Insulin
 b. Glucagon
 c. Vasopressin (antidiuretic hormone)
 d. Aldosterone

Q10. A patient with type 2 diabetes mellitus is treated with a medication that inhibits glucagon release from pancreatic alpha cells. What would be the expected effect of this medication on blood glucose levels?
 a. Increase
 b. Decrease
 c. No change
 d. Variable

Q11. A patient with type 1 diabetes mellitus experiences an episode of diabetic ketoacidosis (DKA). Which of the following hormones is responsible for stimulating ketogenesis in the liver during DKA?
 a. Insulin
 b. Glucagon
 c. Somatostatin
 d. Cortisol

Q12. A 60-year-old patient presents with symptoms of hypoglycemia. The patient has a history of pancreatic surgery for a tumor. Which hormone is most likely deficient in this patient?
 a. Insulin
 b. Glucagon
 c. Somatostatin
 d. Amylin

Q13. A patient with type 1 diabetes mellitus experiences a sudden onset of confusion and weakness. Which hormone deficiency is most likely responsible for these symptoms?
 a. Insulin
 b. Glucagon
 c. Somatostatin
 d. Amylin

Q14. A 40-year-old patient presents with symptoms of hyperglycemia, including fatigue and blurred vision. Laboratory tests reveal elevated blood glucose levels and low levels of insulin. What is the most likely diagnosis?
 a. Type 1 diabetes mellitus
 b. Type 2 diabetes mellitus
 c. Diabetic ketoacidosis
 d. Hyperosmolar hyperglycemic state (HHS)

Q15. A patient with type 2 diabetes mellitus is treated with a medication that inhibits hepatic glucose production. Which of the following hormones would be expected to be targeted by this medication?
 a. Insulin
 b. Glucagon
 c. Somatostatin
 d. Cortisol

Q16. A patient presents with symptoms of hyperglycemia, polyuria, and polydipsia. Laboratory tests reveal elevated blood glucose levels and normal insulin levels. What is the most likely diagnosis?
 a. Type 1 diabetes mellitus
 b. Type 2 diabetes mellitus
 c. Gestational diabetes mellitus
 d. Latent autoimmune diabetes in adults (LADA)

Q17. A patient with type 1 diabetes mellitus experiences an episode of hypoglycemia. Which of the following hormones would be expected to be decreased in response to this hypoglycemic episode?
a. Insulin
b. Glucagon
c. Somatostatin
d. Cortisol

Q18. A 55-year-old patient with poorly controlled type 2 diabetes mellitus is started on a new medication that inhibits glucose reabsorption in the kidneys. Which of the following hormones would be expected to be elevated as a compensatory response to this medication?
a. Insulin
b. Glucagon
c. Somatostatin
d. Vasopressin (antidiuretic hormone)

Q19. A patient with diabetes mellitus experiences an episode of hypoglycemia. Which of the following hormones is responsible for stimulating glycogenolysis in the liver to raise blood glucose levels?
a. Insulin
b. Glucagon
c. Somatostatin
d. Cortisol

Q20. A 50-year-old patient with type 2 diabetes mellitus is treated with a medication that inhibits glucagon-like peptide-1 (GLP-1) degradation. Which of the following physiological effects would be expected from this medication?
a. Decreased insulin secretion
b. Increased glucagon secretion
c. Delayed gastric emptying
d. Enhanced peripheral glucose uptake

Q21. A patient presents with symptoms of hypoglycemia, including palpitations and sweating. Which hormone is responsible for stimulating gluconeogenesis in the liver to raise blood glucose levels?
a. Insulin
b. Glucagon
c. Somatostatin
d. Cortisol

Q22. A 60-year-old patient with type 2 diabetes mellitus is treated with a medication that inhibits glucagon release from pancreatic alpha cells. Which of the following physiological effects would be expected from this medication?
a. Decreased blood glucose levels
b. Increased blood glucose levels
c. No change in blood glucose levels
d. Increased insulin sensitivity

Q23. A patient with diabetes mellitus experiences an episode of hypoglycemia. Which of the following hormones is responsible for stimulating lipolysis in adipose tissue to raise blood glucose levels?
a. Insulin
b. Glucagon
c. Somatostatin
d. Cortisol

Q24. A 40-year-old patient with type 2 diabetes mellitus is treated with a medication that enhances insulin sensitivity in peripheral tissues. Which of the following hormones would be expected to be increased as a compensatory response to this medication?
a. Insulin
b. Glucagon
c. Somatostatin
d. Growth hormone

Q25. A patient with type 1 diabetes mellitus experiences an episode of hypoglycemia. Which of the following hormones is responsible for stimulating glycogen synthesis in the liver to raise blood glucose levels?
a. Insulin
b. Glucagon
c. Somatostatin
d. Epinephrine

**ANSWERS**

1. b  2. d  3. a  4. b  5. b  6. d  7. b  8. a  9. c  10. b  11. b  12. b  13. a  14. b
15. b  16. b  17. a  18. d  19. b  20. d  21. d  22. a  23. d  24. d  25. d

# Physiology of Thymus and Pineal Gland

## CHAPTER 70

**COMPETENCY ADDRESSED**

PY8.3: Describe the physiology of thymus and pineal gland.

**LEARNING OBJECTIVES**

At the end of this chapter, the learner should be able to:
- Discuss physiologic anatomy of the thymus gland.
- Discuss the physiological functions of the gland.
- Explain what happens if thymus gland is removed.
- List the clinical significance of the gland.
- Discuss physiologic anatomy of the pineal gland.
- Describe the hormones released by the gland.
- Describe the physiological functions of melatonin.
- Explain the regulation of melatonin.
- Explain what happens when melatonin levels are low or high?
- Describe the clinical significance of melatonin.

## THYMUS

### PHYSIOLOGICAL ANATOMY

It is a flat, encapsulated primary lymphoid organ located in the anterior superior mediastinum, right behind the sternum. It is bilobed and has two subcomponents: the cortex and the medulla **(Fig. 70.1)**. This organ is most active during childhood, attains its maximum size at puberty and involutes and replaced by fat by early adulthood. Thymic involution is suggested to be caused by the increased level of androgens present in the blood stream during puberty.

### Functions

- **Hormone secreted by thymus:** Thymus secretes *thymosin* that helps the development of T-lymphocytes.
- **Site for T-cell differentiation and maturation:** It is an essential component of the immune system. The immature T-cells migrate form the bone marrow to thymus for maturation and differentiation. In the thymus, T cells multiply and differentiate into different types of T cells. The immature T cells do not have T cells receptors on their surfaces, nor do they CD4 and CD8. The chemicals released by the thymus stimulate T-cells to produce T cell receptors (TCR), CD4 and CD8. CD4 and CD8 receptors bind with two molecules under thymic epithelial cells:
  1. CD8 binds with MCH class I molecules.
  2. CD4 binds with MCH class II molecules.
- **Immune tolerance:** The recognition of self antigens during the course of development is called as immune tolerance. The immune tolerance develops by two mechanisms:
  1. *Positive selection* in thymus that results in development of T cells that recognize foreign antigen

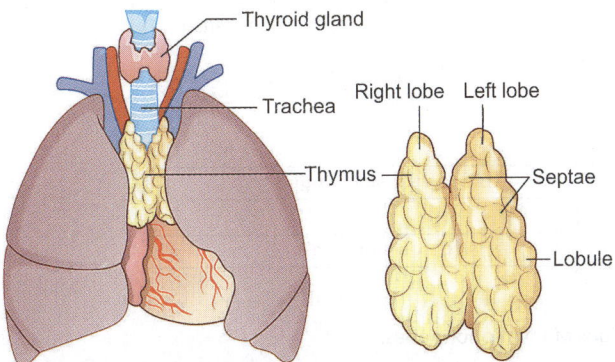

**Fig. 70.1:** Anatomy of thymus.

presented by the MHC antigens in the cortex of the thymus. The T cell receptors which bind strongly with foreign antigen and weakly with self antigen are retained in lymphocytic pool and helps in building up immunity.

2. **Negative selection** results in elimination of cells by apoptosis, of the T cells, which fail to recognize the self antigens and binds strongly with MHC antigens presenting them. This selection prevents the development of autoimmune response.

## FACTORS AFFECTING THYMUS

- **Insulin** is known to play an essential role in thymic growth.
- **Glucocorticoids** decrease the circulating lymphocyte count and the size of the lymph nodes and thymus by inhibiting lymphocyte mitotic activity.

## CLINICAL SIGNIFICANCE (FIG. 70.2)

- *Failure of the tolerance mechanism causes autoimmune diseases*. There is loss of immune tolerance of own cells, which causes autoimmune disease like rheumatic heart disease, myasthenia gravis, etc. *Hence, thymectomy is a part of treatment in myasthenia gravis.*
- As humans age, and their thymus regresses, they have an increased susceptibility for disease. The decrease in thymus size and function leads to decreased circulating T cells.
- Effects of removal of thymus gland: The thymus gland is necessary for the maturation and development of T-cells. If this gland is removed, the number of T cells decreases, limiting their ability to fight many infections.

A person can live without thymus gland but the effects of not having a thymus gland depend on how old the person was when it was removed.

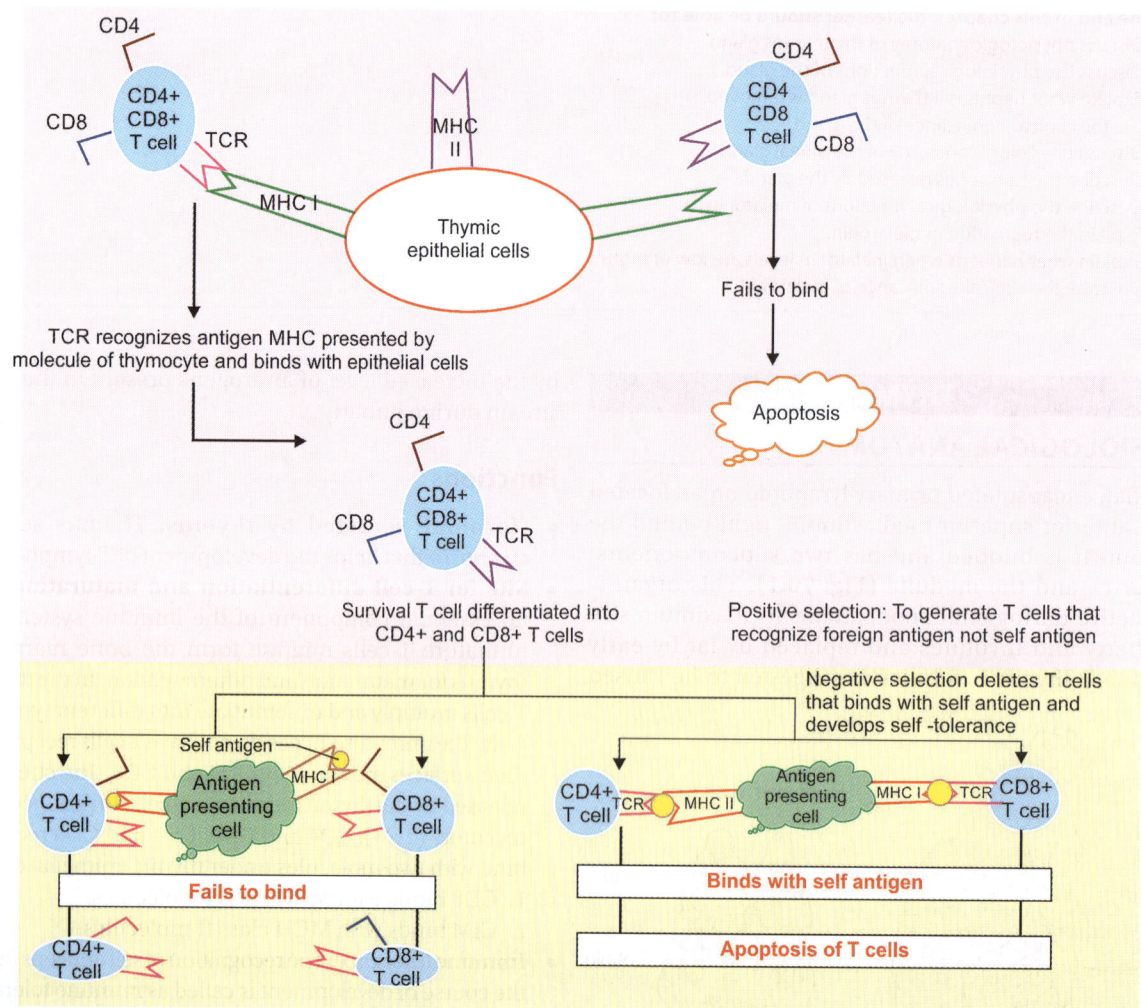

**Fig. 70.2:** Mechanism of actions of thymic hormones.

# PINEAL GLAND

## PHYSIOLOGIC ANATOMY OF PINEAL GLAND

The pineal gland is a pine cone-shaped unpaired endocrine gland located in the posterior aspect of the cranial fossa in the brain. It is called the third eye as retina has a direct connection with it. The pineal gland is also known as the epiphysis cerebri, innervated by the sympathetic fibers. The neurons in pineal gland are sensitive to epinephrine. It has abundant blood supply and is highly vascularized. It is also a circumventricular organ which lacks blood brain barrier.

## PHYSIOLOGY OF PINEAL GLAND

Pineal gland contains specialized neurons called pinealocytes with endocrine functions. It is controlled by suprachiasmatic nucleus of hypothalamus, responsible for regulating the circadian rhythm (the internal biological clock that regulate sleep-wake cycle and other physiological processes). Hence, the main function of pineal gland is concerned with maintaining the sleep wake cycle of an individual.

## FUNCTION OF PINEAL GLAND

It produces hormone, *melatonin* in response to amount of light exposure. When the light levels are low, such as during the night, it produces more melatonin as compared to when the light levels are high, such as during the day. Melatonin secretion is regulated by norepinephrine that is secreted by sympathetic fibers that innervate the pineal gland. Hence, the production of melatonin is responsible for induction of sleep at night.

## MECHANISM OF SECRETION OF MELATONIN (FIG. 70.3)

The nervous pathway involves the passage of light signals from the eyes to the suprachiasmatic nucleus (SCN) of the hypothalamus and then to the pineal gland, activating pineal secretion. During the daytime, light stimulates the retinohypothalamic (RHT) pineal pathway. The retinal ganglion cells activate the suprachiasmatic nucleus (SCN) through the optic nerve. SCN via a complex network inhibits the superior cervical ganglion (SCG) causing sympathetic nervous system inhibition, preventing melatonin release from the pituitary into the circulation. However, at night, lack of activation of SCN causes sympathetic nervous system stimulation, causing melatonin release by the pineal gland, inducing sleepiness.

> Pineal gland produces and secretes melatonin in response to changes in light exposure.

## FUNCTIONS OF MELATONIN

- **Regulation of circadian rhythms:** The primary function of melatonin is to regulate circadian rhythm which is the internal biological clock that regulates *sleep-wake cycle* and other physiological processes. It helps regulate our

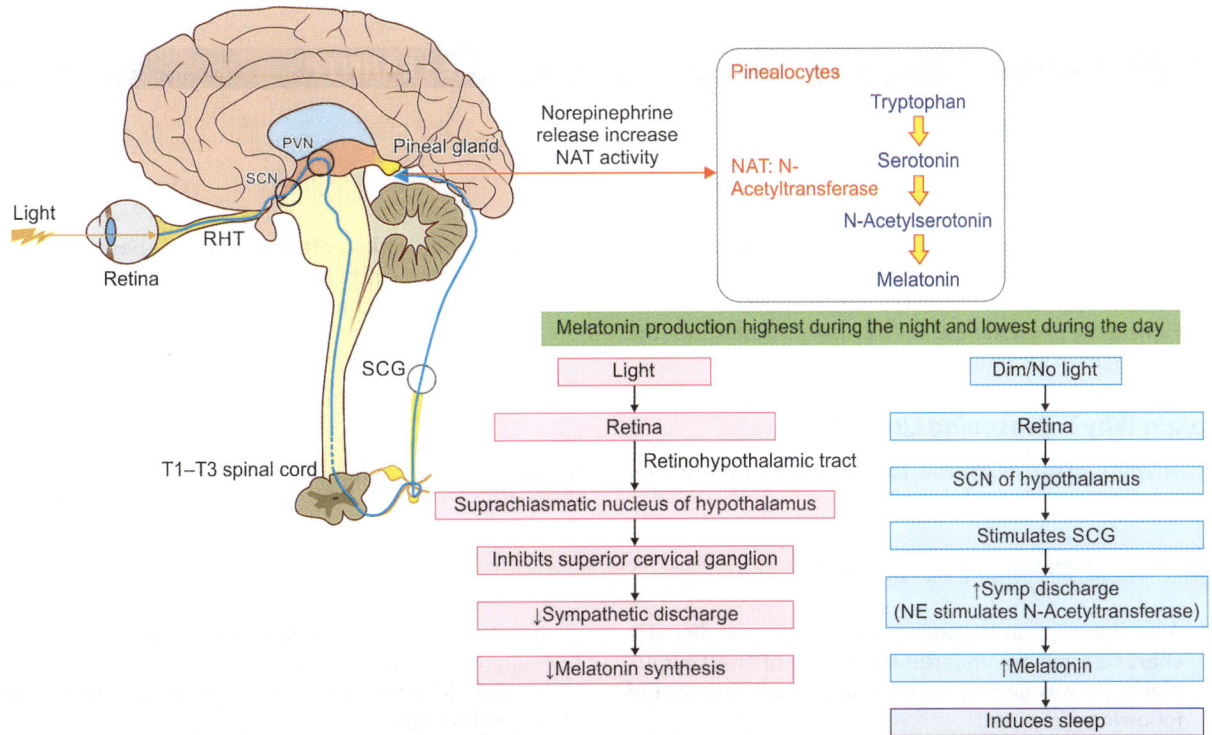

**Fig. 70.3:** Mechanism of secretion of melatonin.

levels of alertness and tiredness by synchronizing our biological clock with the day-night cycle.
- **Sleep induction:** Melatonin is a major factor in the induction of sleep. It assists in letting the body know when it's time to go to sleep. As melatonin levels rise in the evening, it makes you feel drowsy and facilitates the onset of sleep.
- **Antioxidant properties:** Melatonin has antioxidant properties and can help protect cells and tissues from oxidative stress and neurodegeneration caused by free radicals.
- **Immune system support:** Melatonin play a role in modulating the immune system, helping the body defend against infections and diseases.
- **Regulation of reproductive hormones:** It is antigonadotrophic. It decreases the secretion of FSN and LH from anterior pituitary. When the pineal gland is removed in these rodents, it was found that there was an increase in concentrations of FSH and LH.

## CLINICAL SIGNIFICANCE

- Calcification of pineal gland is common.
- **Disturbance of pineal gland secretion:** Low melatonin levels in elderly persons have shown sleep pattern disturbances.
- **Jet lag:** Disturbance of the sleep-wake cycle is seen when traveling across multiple time zones. It takes several days for circadian rhythm to adjust to a new light-dark cycle of their new location. Melatonin help regulating circadian rhythm.
- Melatonin is effective in sleep onset insomnia.
- Tumor or cyst of pineal gland blocks the duct that allows the cerebrospinal fluid (CSF) to circulate, which causes increase in intracranial pressure.

**Aging:** Due to the age-related decrease in melatonin production, older adults may have difficulty falling asleep. Supplementing with melatonin can help control sleep problems associated with ageing.

## SUMMARY

- Thymus secretes thymosin that helps the maturation and differentiation of T-lymphocytes.
- The organ is largest and most active during the newborn and preadolescent stages, and by early adulthood, it has involuted and been replaced by fat.
- Positive selection in thymus that results in differentiation of T cells that recognize foreign antigen.
- Negative selection results in self-tolerance to prevent formation of autoantibodies against our own cells.
- Removal of thymus gland suppresses T-cell immunity and results in immunodeficiency.
- Pineal gland secretes the hormone, melatonin that help regulating circadian rhythm and sleep-wake cycle.
- It is referred as the "hormone of darkness" because its production is stimulated by darkness and inhibited by light.
- The release of melatonin is primarily influenced by the suprachiasmatic nucleus in the brain.
- The primary function of melatonin is to regulate circadian rhythm and sleep-wake cycle.
- Melatonin production decreases with age.

## LET US SEE, HOW MUCH YOU HAVE LEARNT?

### Review Questions

#### Long/Short Answer Questions
- Q1. What are the effects of removal of thymus gland?
- Q2. Explain the physiological basis of using melatonin in the treatment of jetlag.
- Q3. Explain the physiological basis of using melatonin in the treatment of insomnia.
- Q4. Why do shift workers often experience obesity, diabetes, and increased risk of accidents? Their circadian rhythms are disturbed by changes in sleep/wake times.

#### Explain Why? (Reasoning Questions)
- Q1. Thymus gland is crucial for the development and maturation of T lymphocytes.
- Q2. Melatonin secretion plays a role in regulating sleep-wake cycles.

### Critical Thinking Case-Based Questions

- Q1. A newborn infant is diagnosed with a genetic disorder characterized by underdevelopment of the thymus gland. He was getting frequent infections. Answer the following questions:
    a. What is the physiological basis of newborn having frequent infections?
    b. What is the primary function of the thymus in the immune system?
    c. How does the thymus changes during puberty and adulthood?

## Multiple Choice Questions

**Q1.** A person without thymus would not be able to:
a. Reject a tissue transplant
b. Receive a tissue transplant
c. Develop an inflammatory response
d. Produce antibodies

**Q2.** A gland called 'Clock of ageing' that gradually reduces and degenerates in ageing is called:
a. Thyroid
b. Thymus
c. Parathyroid
d. Pituitary

**Q3.** Which of the following hormone is responsible for cell mediated immunity?
a. Thyroid
b. Adrenaline
c. Thymosin
d. Parathyroid

**Q4.** Incorrect about thymus gland:
a. Lobular in structure
b. Located in ventral side of heart and aorta
c. Important for development of immune system
d. It degenerates in old age

**Q5.** Which of the following four glands is correctly matched with the accompanying description?
a. Thyroid—hyperactivity in young children causes cretinism
b. Thymus—starts undergoing atrophy after puberty
c. Parathyroid—secrete parathormone which promotes movement of calcium ions from blood into bone during calcification
d. Pancreas—delta cells of the islets of Langerhans secrete a hormone which stimulates glycolysis

**Q6.** What is the primary function of thymus and at what stage of development does the thymus begins to function?
a. Producing hormone, Embryonic
b. Filtering blood, Neonatal
c. Developing immune cells, Fetal
d. Regulating digestion, Adulthood

**Q7.** A newborn infant is diagnosed with a genetic disorder characterized by underdevelopment of the thymus gland. He was getting frequent infections. Which of the following is a consequence of this condition?
a. Reduced risk of infection
b. Impaired T cell development
c. Enhanced immune response
d. Improved vaccination response

**Q8.** A patient presents with muscle weakness and fatigue, particularly in the facial muscles. Thymic imaging reveals a thymic tumor. Which autoimmune condition is most likely associated with this presentation?
a. Multiple sclerosis
b. Diabetes
c. Myasthenia gravis
d. Rheumatoid arthritis

**Q9.** A 5-year-old boy presents with a history of recurrent infections, particularly viral infections. On examination, the patient has a small, underdeveloped thymus gland. What is the most likely explanation for the recurrent infections in this patient?
a. Impaired positive selection of T cells
b. Excessive negative selection of T cells
c. Overactive thymus gland
d. Defective bone marrow
e. High levels of circulating B cells

**Q10.** The release of melatonin is primarily influenced by the:
a. Pituitary gland
b. Adrenal gland
c. Suprachiasmatic nucleus in the brain
d. Thymus gland

**Q11.** What happens to melatonin production as people age?
a. It remains constant throughout life
b. It increases with age
c. It decreases with age
d. It becomes erratic and unpredictable

**Q12.** What is the term for the condition in which an individual's internal clock is out of sync with their external environment, such as in shift workers?
a. Circadian desynchronization
b. Melatonin imbalance
c. Nocturnal dysfunction
d. Chronotype mismatch

**Q13.** Melatonin sometimes used as a supplement to help with:
a. Increasing alertness during the day
b. Promoting sleep
c. Reducing heart rate
d. Enhancing memory and cognition

**Q14.** A 17-year-old girl with a 2-month history of insomnia. She says she tries to maintain good sleep hygiene and avoid caffeinated beverages after noon. She has no significant medical history and takes no medications. She denies any tobacco or any drug. Vitals are normal. Her provider recommends an over-the-counter supplement due to minimal side-effects and no addictive potential. This supplement contains a hormone that is produced and released by which of the following:
a. Medulla
b. Pineal gland
c. Hypothalamus
d. Cerebellum

**Q15.** Artificial light, extended work-time and reduced sleep-time disrupts the activity of:
a. Thymus
b. Pineal gland
c. Adrenal gland
d. Posterior pituitary gland

**Q16.** What is the role of melatonin in sleep cycles?
a. It helps the brain transition into wakefulness
b. It keeps the brain from becoming overactive during the REM stage of sleep
c. It is released during the transition between stage I and stage 2 sleep
d. It triggers the onset of sleep

### ANSWERS

1. b  2. b  3. c  4. b  5. b  6. c  7. b  8. c  9. a  10. c  11. c  12. a  13. b  14. b
15. b  16. c

# Metabolic Syndrome
## (A Self-Directed Learning Module)

**CHAPTER 71**

> **COMPETENCY ADDRESSED**
> PY8.5: Describe the metabolic and endocrine consequences of obesity and metabolic syndrome, stress response. Outline the psychiatry component pertaining to metabolic syndrome.

> **LEARNING OBJECTIVES**
> At the end of this chapter, the learner should be able to:
> - Define metabolic syndrome and its components.
> - Identify the causes and clinical features of metabolic syndrome.
> - Describe the physiological basis of clinical features.
> - Explain the pathogenesis of metabolic syndrome.
> - Discuss lifestyle modifications and management strategies for metabolic syndrome.
> - Recognize associated complications and their implications.
> - Outline the psychiatry component pertaining to metabolic syndrome.

**CASE SCENARIO**

A 35-year-old woman, presents to her primary care physician with complaints of fatigue, increased thirst, frequent urination, and difficulty losing weight despite efforts to diet and exercise. On examination, she is found to have a body mass index (BMI) of 32 kg/m², elevated blood pressure (140/90 mm Hg), and fasting blood glucose of 120 mg/dL. Further investigation reveals dyslipidemia with elevated triglycerides and low HDL cholesterol. Sarah expresses concerns about her health and struggles with her self-esteem due to her weight.

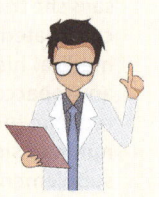

## INTRODUCTION TO METABOLIC SYNDROME

Metabolic syndrome is a cluster of metabolic abnormalities that significantly increase the risk of developing cardiovascular disease, type 2 diabetes mellitus, and other serious health conditions. These abnormalities often occur together and are linked to insulin resistance. The syndrome is diagnosed based on a combination of clinical criteria, including *obesity, hypertension, dyslipidemia, insulin resistance (hyperinsulinemia) and glucose intolerance*.

The metabolic syndrome is usually seen in patients with a strong genetic predisposition or having a poor eating habits with sedentary life style.

## DIAGNOSTIC CRITERIA

There are several sets of diagnostic criteria for metabolic syndrome, including those from organizations like the International Diabetes Federation (IDF), the National Cholesterol Education Program Adult Treatment Panel III (NCEP-ATP III), and the American Heart Association/National Heart, Lung, and Blood Institute (AHA/NHLBI). Common criteria include:

- **Obesity:** Defined by waist circumference or BMI. For example, the IDF criteria specify central obesity as waist circumference ≥94 cm (37 inches) in men and ≥80 cm (31.5 inches) in women. Excessive accumulation of body fat, particularly visceral adiposity, which contributes to insulin resistance and inflammation. Central obesity, characterized by increased waist circumference, is a key feature of metabolic syndrome.

- **Hypertension:** Elevated blood pressure, typically defined as systolic blood pressure ≥130 mm Hg or diastolic blood pressure ≥85 mm Hg, or receiving treatment for hypertension. Elevated blood pressure, resulting from various factors including increased sympathetic activity, sodium retention, endothelial dysfunction, and altered renal function. Hypertension further exacerbates cardiovascular risk in individuals with metabolic syndrome.

- **Dyslipidemia:** Abnormal lipid profile, often characterized by elevated triglycerides (≥150 mg/dL) and/or reduced high-density lipoprotein (HDL) cholesterol (≤40 mg/dL in men, ≤50 mg/dL in women). Imbalance in lipid levels, characterized by elevated triglycerides, decreased HDL cholesterol, and often accompanied by small, dense low-density lipoprotein (LDL) particles. Dyslipidemia contributes to atherosclerosis and cardiovascular disease risk.
- **Insulin resistance:** Often assessed indirectly through fasting plasma glucose or insulin levels, or through measures such as the homeostatic model assessment of insulin resistance (HOMA-IR). Reduced responsiveness of tissues to insulin action, leading to impaired glucose uptake by muscle and adipose tissue, increased hepatic glucose production, and dysregulated lipid metabolism. Insulin resistance is a central pathophysiological feature of metabolic syndrome.
- **Glucose intolerance:** Elevated fasting glucose (≥100 mg/dL) or impaired glucose tolerance (2-hour postprandial glucose ≥140 mg/dL) or previously diagnosed type 2 diabetes. Impaired glucose regulation, including elevated fasting glucose levels and/or impaired glucose tolerance. Glucose intolerance reflects underlying insulin resistance and predisposes individuals to type 2 diabetes mellitus.

## PATHOPHYSIOLOGY

### Role of Adipose Tissue in Inflammation and Insulin Resistance

Adipose tissue is not merely an energy storage depot but also an active endocrine organ that secretes various bioactive molecules called **adipokines**. In obesity, especially visceral adiposity, there is an increased secretion of proinflammatory adipokines such as **tumor necrosis factor-alpha (TNF-α), interleukin-6 (IL-6), and leptin**, while anti-inflammatory adipokines like adiponectin are decreased.

The chronic low-grade inflammation associated with excess adipose tissue contributes to the development of insulin resistance. Proinflammatory cytokines impair insulin signalling pathways in target tissues, such as skeletal muscle, liver, and adipocytes, leading to decreased glucose uptake and dysregulated lipid metabolism.

### Impact of Dyslipidemia on Cardiovascular Health

Dyslipidemia in metabolic syndrome is characterized by elevated triglycerides, decreased high-density lipoprotein (HDL) cholesterol, and often an increase in small, dense low-density lipoprotein (LDL) particles.
- Elevated triglycerides contribute to atherogenic dyslipidemia, promoting the formation of atherosclerotic plaques in blood vessels.
- Low levels of HDL cholesterol are associated with impaired reverse cholesterol transport, leading to decreased clearance of cholesterol from peripheral tissues and increased risk of atherosclerosis.
- Small, dense LDL particles are more susceptible to oxidation and have a greater propensity to infiltrate arterial walls, initiating the inflammatory process and promoting plaque formation.

### Mechanisms Underlying Hypertension in Metabolic Syndrome

Multiple factors contribute to hypertension in metabolic syndrome, including increased sympathetic nervous system activity, sodium retention, endothelial dysfunction, and altered renin-angiotensin-aldosterone system (RAAS) activity.
- Adipose tissue-derived factors such as leptin and adiponectin influence sympathetic tone and vascular function, contributing to hypertension.
- Insulin resistance leads to endothelial dysfunction and impaired nitric oxide-mediated vasodilation, promoting vasoconstriction and hypertension.
- Dysregulation of the RAAS, with increased angiotensin II levels and aldosterone secretion, promotes sodium retention and vascular remodeling, further exacerbating hypertension.

### Insulin Resistance and its Contribution to Hyperglycemia

Insulin resistance refers to impaired cellular response to insulin, particularly in muscle, liver, and adipose tissue. In response to insulin resistance, pancreatic beta cells initially compensate by secreting more insulin (hyperinsulinemia) to maintain normal blood glucose levels. Over time, beta cell function declines, leading to inadequate insulin secretion relative to insulin resistance.

Hyperinsulinemia and defective insulin action result in impaired glucose uptake by peripheral tissues, increased hepatic glucose production, and dysregulated lipolysis, contributing to hyperglycemia and the development of type 2 diabetes mellitus.

## LIFESTYLE MODIFICATIONS AND MANAGEMENT

### Dietary Interventions

- Emphasis should be placed on adopting a balanced diet that includes a variety of nutrient-dense foods such as fruits, vegetables, whole grains, lean proteins, and healthy fats.
- Calorie restriction may be necessary for individuals who are overweight or obese to achieve weight loss and improve metabolic parameters.
- Focus on reducing intake of refined carbohydrates, sugary beverages, saturated and trans fats, and processed foods high in added sugars and sodium.

- Encourage portion control and mindful eating practices to promote satiety and prevent overconsumption.

### Regular Physical Activity and Exercise Recommendations

- Regular physical activity is essential for improving insulin sensitivity, promoting weight loss, and reducing cardiovascular risk.
- Recommend at least 150 minutes of moderate-intensity aerobic exercise or 75 minutes of vigorous-intensity aerobic exercise per week, along with muscle-strengthening activities on two or more days per week.
- Encourage a variety of activities that individuals enjoy, such as walking, jogging, cycling, swimming, dancing, or strength training exercises.
- Incorporate physical activity into daily routines, such as taking the stairs instead of the elevator, walking or biking to work, or participating in recreational sports.

### Smoking Cessation and Moderation of Alcohol Intake

- Smoking cessation is crucial for reducing cardiovascular risk and improving overall health. Provide support and resources to help individuals quit smoking, such as counseling, nicotine replacement therapy, or prescription medications.
- Advise moderation or avoidance of alcohol consumption, as excessive alcohol intake can contribute to weight gain, hypertension, dyslipidemia, and liver dysfunction. Encourage individuals to adhere to recommended limits for alcohol consumption or abstain altogether if appropriate.

### Pharmacological Interventions

- In addition to lifestyle modifications, pharmacological interventions may be necessary to target specific components of metabolic syndrome and reduce cardiovascular risk.
- Medications commonly used in the management of metabolic syndrome include:
  - Antihypertensive agents (e.g., angiotensin-converting enzyme inhibitors, angiotensin II receptor blockers, calcium channel blockers, diuretics) to control blood pressure.
  - Lipid-lowering medications (e.g., statins, fibrates, niacin, ezetimibe) to improve lipid profiles and reduce cardiovascular risk.
  - Antidiabetic medications (e.g., metformin, sulfonylureas, thiazolidinediones, glucagon-like peptide-1 receptor agonists, sodium-glucose co-transporter 2 inhibitors) to improve glycemic control and insulin sensitivity.
  - Weight-loss medications (e.g., orlistat, liraglutide) may be considered in individuals who have not achieved adequate weight loss with lifestyle interventions alone.
- Pharmacological therapy should be individualized based on the patient's specific metabolic profile, comorbidities, and risk factors, and initiated and monitored by a healthcare professional.

## ASSOCIATED COMPLICATIONS

### Cardiovascular Disease

- **Atherosclerosis:** Metabolic syndrome predisposes individuals to the development of atherosclerosis, a condition characterized by the buildup of plaque within the arteries. This plaque consists of cholesterol, fatty substances, cellular waste products, calcium, and fibrin. Over time, atherosclerosis can lead to narrowing and hardening of the arteries, impairing blood flow to vital organs such as the heart, brain, and extremities.
- **Myocardial infarction (heart attack):** Atherosclerosis increases the risk of coronary artery disease, which can result in the formation of blood clots (thrombosis) and subsequent blockage of blood flow to the heart muscle. This can lead to myocardial infarction, or heart attack, which is a serious and potentially life-threatening condition.
- **Stroke:** Atherosclerosis affecting the arteries supplying the brain increases the risk of cerebrovascular events such as ischemic stroke or transient ischemic attacks (TIAs). These occur when blood flow to part of the brain is interrupted, leading to neurological deficits or damage.

### Type 2 Diabetes Mellitus

- Insulin resistance, a hallmark of metabolic syndrome, predisposes individuals to the development of type 2 diabetes mellitus. Over time, the pancreas may become unable to compensate for insulin resistance by producing sufficient insulin, leading to hyperglycemia and the onset of diabetes.
- Type 2 diabetes mellitus is associated with a range of complications, including cardiovascular disease, neuropathy, nephropathy, retinopathy, and lower limb amputations.

### Nonalcoholic Fatty Liver Disease (NAFLD)

- Nonalcoholic fatty liver disease encompasses a spectrum of liver conditions ranging from simple hepatic steatosis (accumulation of fat in the liver) to nonalcoholic steatohepatitis (NASH), which involves inflammation and liver cell damage.
- Metabolic syndrome is a major risk factor for NAFLD, with insulin resistance, dyslipidemia, and obesity contributing to hepatic lipid accumulation and inflammation.
- NAFLD can progress to advanced liver disease, including fibrosis, cirrhosis, and hepatocellular carcinoma (liver cancer), particularly in individuals with additional risk factors such as excessive alcohol consumption or viral hepatitis.

### Sleep Apnea

- Sleep apnea is a sleep disorder characterized by repeated interruptions in breathing during sleep, leading to fragmented sleep patterns and inadequate oxygenation of tissues.
- Obesity, particularly central adiposity, is a major risk factor for obstructive sleep apnea. Excess adipose tissue in the neck and throat can obstruct the upper airway, leading to episodes of apnea or hypopnea.
- Sleep apnea is associated with daytime fatigue, impaired cognitive function, cardiovascular complications (such as hypertension and arrhythmias), and an increased risk of motor vehicle accidents.

### Increased Risk of Certain Cancers

Metabolic syndrome is associated with an increased risk of several types of cancer, including colorectal cancer, breast cancer (in postmenopausal women), endometrial cancer, and liver cancer.

The mechanisms underlying the association between metabolic syndrome and cancer risk are complex and multifactorial, involving factors such as chronic inflammation, insulin resistance, dysregulated adipokine secretion, and alterations in sex hormone metabolism.

## PSYCHIATRY COMPONENT

### Psychological Impact of Obesity and Metabolic Syndrome

- Individuals with obesity and metabolic syndrome often experience a significant psychological burden related to their condition. This may include feelings of shame, guilt, embarrassment, and frustration about their weight and health status.
- The stigma associated with obesity can lead to social discrimination, negative body image, and impaired quality of life. It may also contribute to avoidance of healthcare settings and reluctance to seek help for related health concerns.
- The chronic nature of metabolic syndrome and the challenges associated with making and sustaining lifestyle changes can lead to feelings of hopelessness and despair.

### Association with Depression, Anxiety, and Low Self-esteem

- Metabolic syndrome is associated with an increased risk of psychiatric disorders such as depression, anxiety, and low self-esteem.
- Obesity and metabolic abnormalities can have a direct impact on brain function and mood regulation through various biological mechanisms, including inflammation, hormonal dysregulation, and altered neurotransmitter activity.
- Psychosocial factors, such as social isolation, financial stress, and interpersonal difficulties, may also contribute to the development or exacerbation of mental health disorders in individuals with metabolic syndrome.
- Depression and anxiety can further worsen metabolic parameters through behaviors such as poor dietary choices, physical inactivity, and medication non-adherence.

### Importance of Holistic Approach to Patient Care, Including Addressing Mental Health Concerns

- A holistic approach to patient care is essential for effectively managing metabolic syndrome and improving overall health outcomes. This approach recognizes the interconnectedness of physical, psychological, and social factors influencing health and well-being.
- Healthcare providers should routinely assess and address the mental health needs of individuals with metabolic syndrome, including screening for depression, anxiety, and other psychiatric symptoms.
- Incorporating strategies to enhance self-esteem, coping skills, and resilience can help individuals better manage the challenges associated with their condition and improve adherence to lifestyle modifications and treatment plans.
- Collaborative care models involving interdisciplinary teams, including primary care providers, mental health professionals, dietitians, and exercise physiologists, can optimize patient outcomes by addressing both physical and mental health concerns.
- Education and support programs that promote self-care, stress management, and positive health behaviors can empower individuals with metabolic syndrome to take an active role in their health and well-being.

### Conclusion of Module

Metabolic syndrome is a complex condition with significant metabolic, endocrine, and psychiatric implications. By understanding its pathophysiology, clinical manifestations, and management strategies, healthcare professionals can provide comprehensive care to patients like Sarah, addressing both their physical and mental health needs.

> **Case-based Learning Activities**
> - Analyze the case and identify the components of metabolic syndrome she exhibits.
> - Discuss the physiological mechanisms underlying her clinical features.
> - Develop a comprehensive lifestyle modification plan for her, considering her dietary habits, physical activity level, and psychosocial factors.
> - Explore the potential complications she may face if her metabolic syndrome is left unmanaged.
> - Reflect on the impact of metabolic syndrome on Her's mental health and devise strategies to address her concerns and improve her overall well-being.

## LET US SEE, HOW MUCH YOU HAVE LEARNT?

 *Multiple Choice Questions*

**Q1.** Which of the following is NOT a component of metabolic syndrome?
  a. Obesity
  b. Hypertension
  c. Hyperthyroidism
  d. Dyslipidemia

**Q2.** Mr X, a 45-year-old man, presents to his physician with complaints of abdominal obesity, elevated blood pressure, and high fasting blood glucose levels. Based on these findings, which of the following conditions is X, most likely at risk for?
  a. Osteoporosis
  b. Metabolic syndrome
  c. Hypothyroidism
  d. Cushing's syndrome

**Q3.** Which physiological mechanism contributes to insulin resistance in individuals with metabolic syndrome?
  a. Increased adiponectin secretion
  b. Enhanced glucose uptake by muscle cells
  c. Chronic low-grade inflammation
  d. Reduced triglyceride levels in the blood

**Q4.** Mukesh, a 50-year-old man, has been diagnosed with metabolic syndrome. Which lifestyle modification is most appropriate for Mukesh to manage his condition?
  a. Smoking cessation
  b. Increasing saturated fat intake
  c. Decreasing physical activity
  d. Consuming a diet high in refined carbohydrates

**Q5.** A 55-year-old man with metabolic syndrome, has a history of heavy alcohol consumption. Which of the following complications he is at increased risk for?
  a. Hypertension
  b. Nonalcoholic fatty liver disease
  c. Type 1 diabetes mellitus
  d. Asthma

**Q6.** Which mental health disorder is commonly associated with metabolic syndrome?
  a. Obsessive-compulsive disorder (OCD)
  b. Bipolar disorder
  c. Depression
  d. Schizophrenia

**Q7.** Seema, a 40-year-old woman with metabolic syndrome, reports feelings of sadness, hopelessness, and fatigue during her recent clinic visit. Which mental health condition should her healthcare provider screen for?
  a. Anxiety disorder
  b. Bipolar disorder
  c. Depression
  d. Attention deficit hyperactivity disorder (ADHD)

**Q8.** Which of the following is NOT an associated complication of metabolic syndrome?
  a. Stroke
  b. Rheumatoid arthritis
  c. Nonalcoholic fatty liver disease
  d. Increased risk of certain cancers

**Q9.** Mahesh Babu, a 60-year-old man with metabolic syndrome, complains of disrupted sleep, loud snoring, and daytime fatigue. What condition should his healthcare provider evaluate him for?
  a. Depression
  b. Sleep apnea
  c. Anxiety disorder
  d. Insomnia

**ANSWERS**

**1.** c  **2.** b  **3.** c  **4.** a  **5.** b  **6.** c  **7.** c  **8.** b  **9.** b

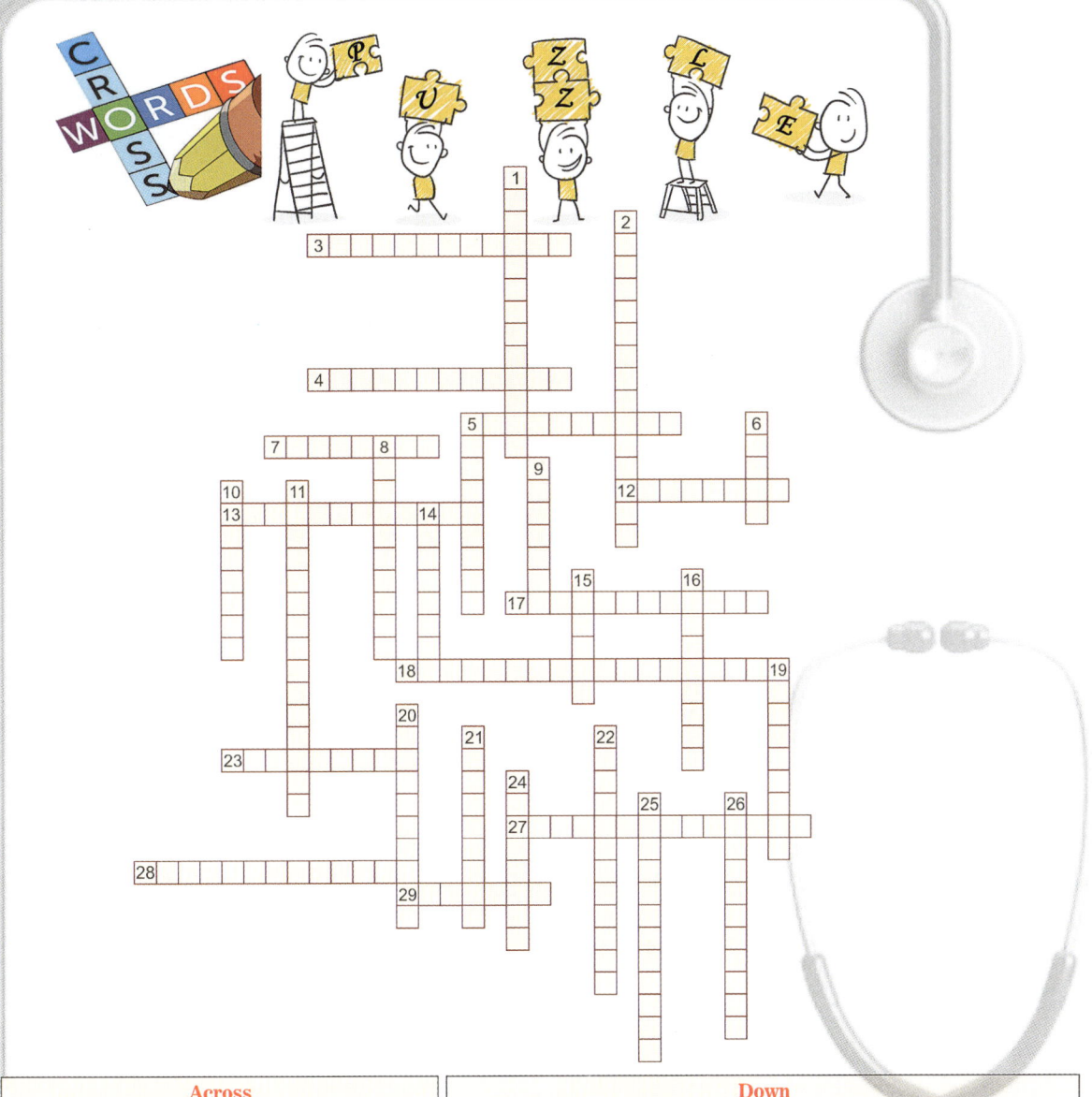

### Across

3. This hormone stimulates vitamin D resulting in increased absorption of Ca from GIT
4. Polypeptide hormone secreted by δ-cells of pancreas
5. Result of hypersecretion of growth hormone in adults
7. Hormone that is also known as love hormone responsible for uterine contractions
12. Hormone that helps in differentiation and maturation of T-lymphocytes
13. Result of lesions that affect anterior hypothalamus
17. Disorder due to vitamin D3 deficiency causing diminished bone matrix
18. Decreased secretion of all hormones secreted by anterior pituitary gland
23. Type of breathing (rapid and deep) seen in diabetic patients
27. Result of lesions that affect posterior hypothalamus
28. Glycoprotein present in the colloid of the follicles of thyroid gland
29. Hormone that is essential for thymic growth

### Down

1. Highly vascular small areas located in organum vasculosum
2. Prolonged hyperglycemia due to high amounts of glucocorticoids
5. Enzyme that helps in conversion of estradiol from testosterone
6. Organ that don't need insulin for glucose uptake
8. Cells that secrete parathormone by parathyroid glands
9. Disease due to decreased hypocalcemia and hypophosphatemia in children
10. Sign of twitching of facial muscles of the same side by tapping, seen in hypocalcemia
11. Neural tract between hypothalamus and posterior pituitary
14. Hypofunctioning of the thyroid gland in adults
15. Proinflammatory adipokine that increases in visceral obesity
16. Psychosis occurring due to thiamine deficiency due to damage to mammillothalamic tract
19. Hormone produced by pineal gland in response to amount of light exposure
20. Hormone secreted by parafollicular cells of thyroid gland
21. Electrolyte that plays crucial role in correcting imbalances in treatment of diabatic ketoacidosis
22. Abnormal lipid profile, often characterized by elevated triglycerides
24. Chemical released by hypothalamus inhibiting prolactin secretion from anterior pituitary
25. Cells of pituitary gland that secrets growth hormone
26. Another name for cortisol binding globulin

# SECTION 9

# REPRODUCTIVE PHYSIOLOGY

## Section Outline

**Chapter 72:** Reproductive Physiology and Endocrinology
**Chapter 73:** Sex Determination and Sex Differentiation of Embryo
**Chapter 74:** Life Cycle of Reproductive Physiology
**Chapter 75:** Reproductive Physiology in Males
**Chapter 76:** Reproductive Physiology in Females
**Chapter 77:** Physiology of Pregnancy and Lactation
**Chapter 78:** Contraception

# Reproductive Physiology and Endocrinology

**72 CHAPTER**

### COMPETENCY ADDRESSED
**PY9.5:** Describe and discuss the physiological effects of sex hormones.

### LEARNING OBJECTIVES
**At the end of this chapter, the learner should be able to:**
- Describe the basics of the reproductive system.
- Enumerate the hormones associated with reproductive physiology.
- Describe the synthesis, secretion, mechanism of action, and regulation of various reproductive hormones in males and females.

## INTRODUCTION

The reproductive physiology deals with the functioning of male and female reproductive systems resulting in procreation and continuation of species. In this unit, we shall be learning about the embryonic development, differentiating into the either sex in terms of sex determination and differentiation. We will also learn about various chromosomal aberrations occurring during the sex differentiation. The physiological changes occurring in both the genders during adolescence will also be discussed in this unit. The functional anatomy of male and female tract along with gametogenesis and physiological role during reproductive period of life is also discussed in detail.

The reproductive period in both the genders begins at adolescence or puberty, which marks the various physical, functional and hormonal changes occurring in the growing children. These changes are discussed in detail in Chapter 74.

In this chapter, we will discuss the role of various hormones, participating in the hypothalamo-pituitary-gonadal axis, maintaining the normal functioning of the reproductive system in either gender.

## HYPOTHALAMO-PITUITARY-GONADAL AXIS

As discussed earlier, the hypothalamus communicates with the anterior pituitary through hypothalamo-hypophyseal portal system which carries the hypothalamic hormones to the anterior pituitary **(Fig. 72.1)**.

## REPRODUCTIVE HORMONES

Reproductive hormones are not just secreted by ovaries and testis, rather hypothalamus, pituitary gland and adrenal gland secret hormones that affects the reproductive physiology. All these hormones with their sources, mechanism of action and functions are discussed in **Table 72.1**.

*Why the postmenopausal women become more prone to the following?*

- **Osteoporosis:** The estrogen stimulates the osteoprotegerin (OPG), which is also called as the osteoclastogenesis inhibitory factor. It binds to RANKL and blocks the receptors, thus inhibiting the differentiation from pro-osteoclasts to mature osteoclasts. Hence, it prevents the bone resorption and osteoporosis. When the estrogen levels decrease (as seen in postmenopausal women), this protective effect of estrogen is lost and the bones tend to get demineralized predisposing them to easy fractures. (PS: Excessive glucocorticoids inhibit OPG and results in osteoporosis).
- **Atherosclerosis:** The estrogen increases the LDL receptors in the liver and increases the metabolism of LDL cholesterol. In postmenopausal women the estrogen levels are low, which decreases the LDL metabolism and increases the circulating LDL cholesterol. This predisposes the postmenopausal women to atherosclerosis. Hence we can say that estrogen has the cardioprotective effect.

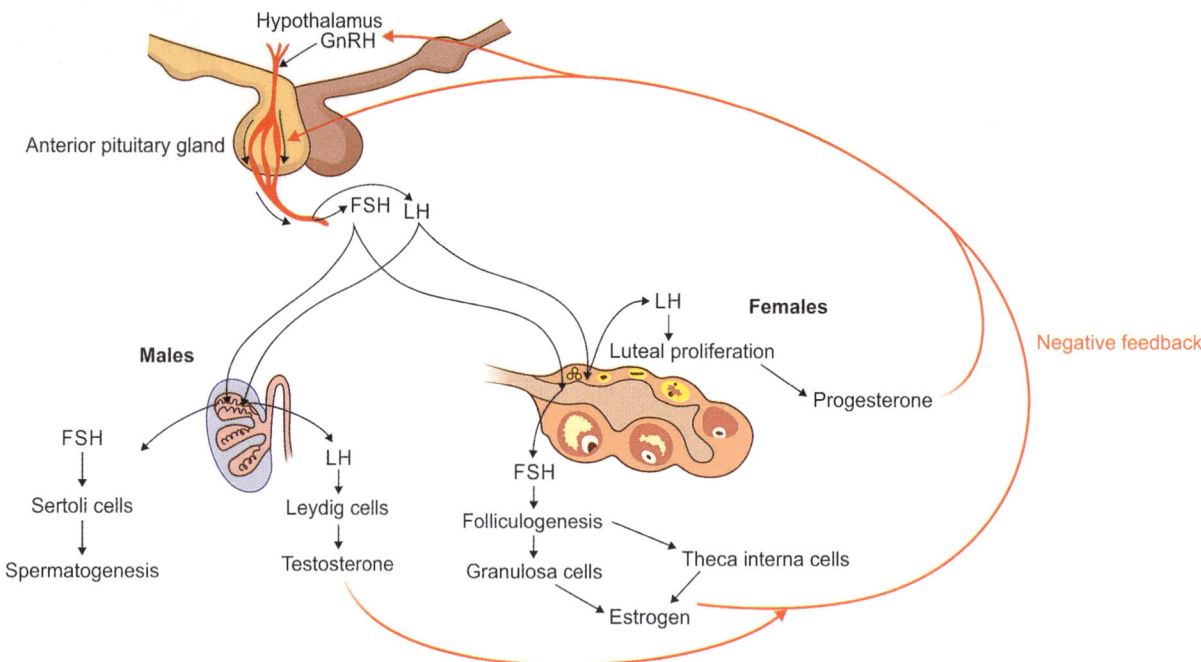

**Fig. 72.1:** Hypothalamo-pituitary-gonadal axis.
(FSH: follicle-stimulating hormone; LH: luteinizing hormone; GnRH: gonadotropin-releasing hormone)

**Table 72.1:** Reproductive hormones and their features.

| Hormone | Source | Mechanism of action | Functions |
|---|---|---|---|
| **Hypothalamic hormones** | | | |
| Gonadotropin-releasing hormone (GnRH) | Secreted from **arcuate nuclei** of hypothalamus, secreted in pulses of 1–3 hours. It primarily affects the LH secretion | PLC/IP3, DAG pathway | Stimulates the secretion of gonadotropins (FSH and LH) from the anterior pituitary |
| **Pituitary hormones** | | | |
| Follicle stimulating hormone (FSH) (Glycoprotein hormone; molecular weight: 30,000) | **Protein hormone** secreted from the gonadotrophs of anterior pituitary gland | Adenylyl cyclase/cAMP pathway | **Males:**<br>• Stimulation of Sertoli cells (spermatogenesis)<br>• Increased no. of LH receptors<br>• Increased secretion of inhibin<br>**Females:**<br>• Stimulation of granulosa cells → estrogen<br>• Increased no. of LH receptors<br>• Increased secretion of inhibin<br>• Stimulates growth of ovarian follicle |
| Luteinizing hormone (LH) (Glycoprotein hormone; molecular weight: 30,000) | | | **Males:**<br>• Stimulation of **Leydig cells** to produce **testosterone**<br>**Females:**<br>• Ovulation<br>• Formation of corpus luteum<br>• Stimulation of progesterone synthesis<br>• Maintenance of corpus luteum |
| **Gonadal hormones** | | | |
| In males (from testis) | | | |
| Testosterone (Steroid hormone) Plasma levels >3 ng/mL | Steroid hormone secreted from interstitial Leydig cells of testis | Intracytoplasmic receptors and synthesis of new proteins | • In embryonic life, testosterone is responsible for **sex differentiation of fetus to male**. Absence of testosterone results in development of female fetus |

*Contd...*

Contd...

| Hormone | Source | Mechanism of action | Functions |
|---|---|---|---|
| | **What will happen to sperm count and testosterone level in person with prolonged X-ray exposure/ heat exposure?**<br><br>The Sertoli cells are sensitive to prolonged X-ray exposure or heat. Hence, results in decreased sperm count. The Leydig cells are resistant to these factors, which results in normal testosterone levels.<br><br>Hence, a person with prolonged exposure to X-ray or heat develops sterility, not impotence. | | • In fetal life, testosterone results in **testicular descent** in the scrotal sacs. Deficiency of testosterone results in undescended testis<br>• **Spermatogenesis:** Formation of sperms<br>• Appearance of **secondary sexual characters** like the appearance of beard, axillary hair, change in the pitch of voice due to laryngeal growth, male pattern of hair distribution<br>• Thickening of bones and **bone growth**<br>• It is responsible for the **growth of the pelvis** to android shape, i.e., long funnel-shaped pelvis with narrow outlet; in contrast to gynecoid pelvis (broad) in females<br>• Increases the **muscle growth**<br>• The **skin becomes thick** and more prone to **acne**<br>• It **increases** the basal metabolic rate (**BMR**)<br>• Due to increased BMR, it results **in increased formation of red blood cells**<br>• It affects the fluid volume by causing fluid retention and **expansion of extracellular fluid volume** (ECF volume)<br>• It leads to recession of hairline, resulting in male pattern of baldness (**androgenic alopecia**)<br>• Therapeutically, it **prevents osteoporosis** in elderly men<br>• High doses of testosterone in children can **hasten up the epiphyseal closure** |
| In female (from ovaries) | | | |
| **Estrogen (Steroid hormone)** | **In nonpregnant state (Estradiol):**<br>(Most abundant and most potent)<br>• Granulosa cells<br>• Corpus luteum<br>**In pregnancy (Estriol):**<br>• Placenta<br>**Other sites (Estrone):**<br>• Postmenopausal women<br>• Adipose tissue<br>• Brain<br><br>The estrogen is also produced in males. Though the source is unknown, it is believed to be secreted from Sertoli cells, by the peripheral conversion of testosterone | Intracytoplasmic ERα and ERβ receptors and synthesis of new proteins | • Stimulates the growth of ovary and ovarian follicles, **'follicular development'**<br>• Stimulates smooth muscle contraction of fallopian tubes, hence **increases tubal motility**. Also increases ciliary activity of tubes<br>• **Uterus:**<br>  ▪ **Increase in size** of uterus<br>  ▪ **Proliferation** of uterine **endometrium** during follicular phase<br>  ▪ Increase in **uterine blood flow**<br>  ▪ Increase in **activity and excitability** of uterine muscles<br>  ▪ Increases its **sensitivity to oxytocin**<br>• **Cervical mucus:** Abundant, **clear, watery mucus**. Its effects are more pronounced at the time of ovulation for easy penetration of sperm<br>• **Vagina:**<br>  ▪ Prepubertal-cuboidal<br>  ▪ Pubertal and postpubertal-stratified (more resistant to trauma and infection)<br>• **Breast development:**<br>  ▪ Growth of breast<br>  ▪ Growth of ducts<br>  ▪ Deposition of fat in breast<br>• **Effect on secondary sexual characteristics:**<br>  ▪ Feminine body structure with **narrow shoulders and wide hips**<br>  ▪ **Wide carrying angle**<br>  ▪ **Fat deposition** at hips, thighs and breasts<br>  ▪ Voice remains **high pitched**<br>  ▪ **Less hair on body** and more on scalp |

Contd...

Contd...

| Hormone | Source | Mechanism of action | Functions |
|---|---|---|---|
| | | | • *Soft and smooth texture of skin* with increased vascularity and increased warmth<br>• Inhibits acne formation<br>• Female pattern of pubic hair triangle with base upward and apex downwards<br>• **Effect on endocrine organs**<br>  ▪ *Inhibits LH secretion* (negative feedback)<br>  ▪ *Inhibits FSH secretion*<br>  ▪ *Stimulates prolactin secretion*<br>  ▪ Promotes **synthesis of angiotensinogen** from liver. Thus, it **activates renin-angiotensin** system<br>  ▪ *Increases formation of thyroxine binding globulin*<br>  ▪ *Stimulate androgen secretion* from adrenal cortex<br>• **Effect on musculoskeletal system:**<br>  ▪ Prevents osteoporosis by inhibiting osteoclasts<br>  ▪ Causes epiphyseal closure → determines the height of female<br>• **Effect on water and electrolytes:** Promotes salt and water retention<br>• **Effect on lipid profile:** Cholesterol lowering action → prevents atherosclerosis<br>• **Effect on brain:** It safeguards neurons, enhances synaptic plasticity, and influences mood, cognition, and sexual behavior. Neurotransmitter regulation, structural changes, and neurogenesis are among its mechanisms, impacting learning, memory, and emotional regulation |
| **Progesterone (Steroid hormone)** | • Puberty-ovary, corpus luteum<br>• Pregnancy-placenta<br><br>*The level rises after ovulation as it is required for the maintenance of pregnancy. But if pregnancy does not occur-progesterone level decreases-leading to menstruation and shedding of endometrium* | Intracytoplasmic receptors and synthesis of new proteins | • **Effect on uterus**<br>  ▪ Induces secretary changes in endometrium (primed by estrogen)<br>  ▪ Prepare the uterus for implantation of the fertilized ovum<br>  ▪ Decreases the contraction of the uterine smooth muscle<br>  ▪ Prevent the expulsion of the implanted ovum<br>• **Cervical mucus**<br>  ▪ Thick mucus forms 'cervical mucus plug'<br>  ▪ Impermeable to sperm<br>  ▪ Prevents the ascending infections to the growing fetus<br>• **Effect on the breast**<br>  ▪ Development of lobules and alveoli of the breast<br>  ▪ Alveoli cells become secretory in nature<br>  ▪ Inhibit lactation during pregnancy<br>• **Effect on hypothalamo-pituitary axis**<br>  ▪ Negative feedback mechanism<br>  ▪ Decreases LH secretion<br>  ▪ Prevents ovulation<br>• **Other actions**<br>  ▪ Thermogenic<br>  ▪ Anti-inflammatory<br>  ▪ Decreases maternal immune response<br>  ▪ Prevent endometrial and breast cancer<br>  ▪ Natriuretic and diuretic by blocking aldosterone on kidney tubules |
| *Common hormones in both the genders* | | | |
| **Relaxin (Protein hormone)** | • Corpus luteum<br>• Placenta<br>• Uterus<br>• Breast | | • Relaxes pubic symphysis, pelvic joints and ligaments<br>• Causes softening and dilatation of uterine cervix<br>• Inhibits uterine contractions |

*Contd...*

Contd...

| Hormone | Source | Mechanism of action | Functions |
|---|---|---|---|
| | • Prostate gland in males | | • Promotes development of mammary glands<br>• In males, it facilitates sperm motility and penetration of ovum |
| Inhibin (Protein hormone) | Granulosa cells in ovaries in females | | To provide feedback signal to inhibit FSH secretion from anterior pituitary |
| Androgens | Ovaries and adrenal gland | Intracytoplasmic receptors and synthesis of new proteins | • Stimulate the growth of pubic and axillary hair<br>• Promote growth of skeletal muscle<br>• Help in maintaining sexual desire (libido)<br>• Responsible for acne in women |

## Synthesis of Hormones Responsible for Reproductive Physiology

The main precursor for the synthesis of various steroid hormones is cholesterol. **Figure 72.2** shows the schematic representation of synthesis of hormones from cholesterol. Apart from this, theca cells and granulosa cells plays important role in synthesis of reproductive hormones (**Fig. 72.3**).

## MECHANISM OF ACTION

Acts via intracytoplasmic receptors (steroid receptors). **Figure 72.4** shows the mechanism of action of steroid hormones through steroid receptors.

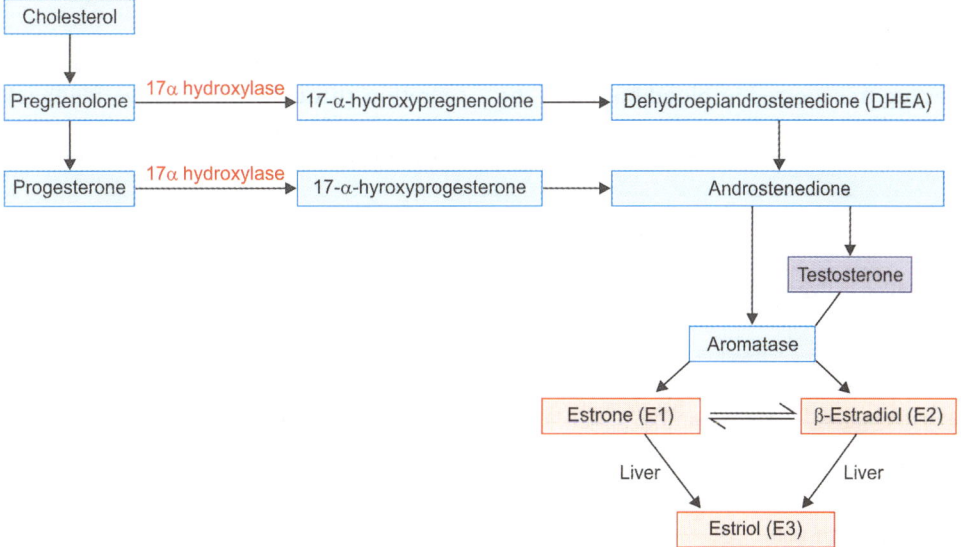

**Fig. 72.2:** Formation of male and female steroid hormones.

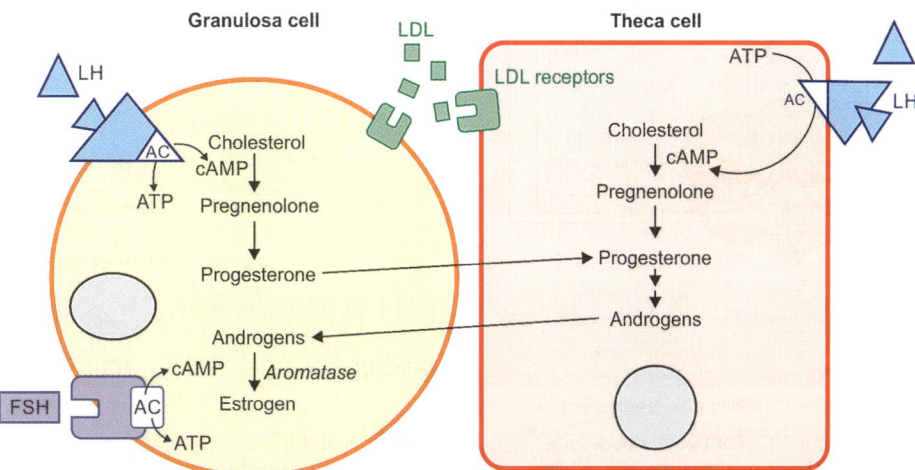

**Fig. 72.3:** Interaction of the granulosa cells and theca cells. FSH and LH receptors act via adenylyl cyclase (AC) cAMP pathway and stimulate steroidogenesis in follicular cells. Formation of estrogen in granulosa cells takes place due to the aromatase activity.

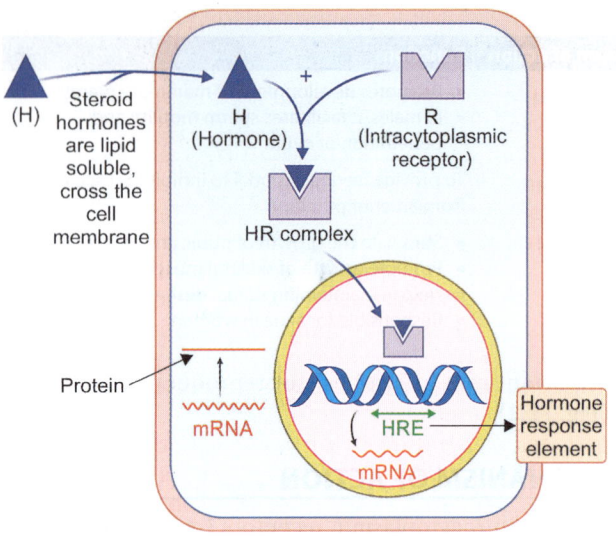

**Fig. 72.4:** Steroid receptors are the main site of action of steroid hormones.

## TRANSPORT AND METABOLISM

These hormones are transported in blood bound to the plasma proteins, albumin and specific testosterone, estrogen and progesterone binding proteins.

Like other steroid hormones, the reproductive hormones get conjugated to form glucuronides and sulfates in liver. Let's quickly have a look on each one of them:

- **Testosterone:** After release, 97% of testosterone binds with plasma albumin and beta globulin (sex hormone binding protein). Most of the circulating testosterone gets fixed to the tissues (prostate) in the form of *dihydrotestosterone (DHT)*. The unfixed free testosterone is rapidly metabolized by the liver into *androsterone* and *dehydroepiandrosterone* and conjugated as glucuronide and sulfate.
- **Estradiol:** Liver also converts the active form, estradiol into less potent *estriol*. Hence, during liver failure/decreased activity, the patient develops *hyperestrinism* (excessive amount of circulating estradiol).
- **Progesterone:** The end product of progesterone metabolism is *pregnanediol*. The metabolized hormone is excreted in the bile and in the urine.

## REGULATION OF SECRETION OF HORMONES (FIG. 72.5)

All these steroid reproductive hormones regulate their secretion through the negative feedback homeostatic mechanism. However, in female there is positive feedback mechanism occurring at the time of ovulation.

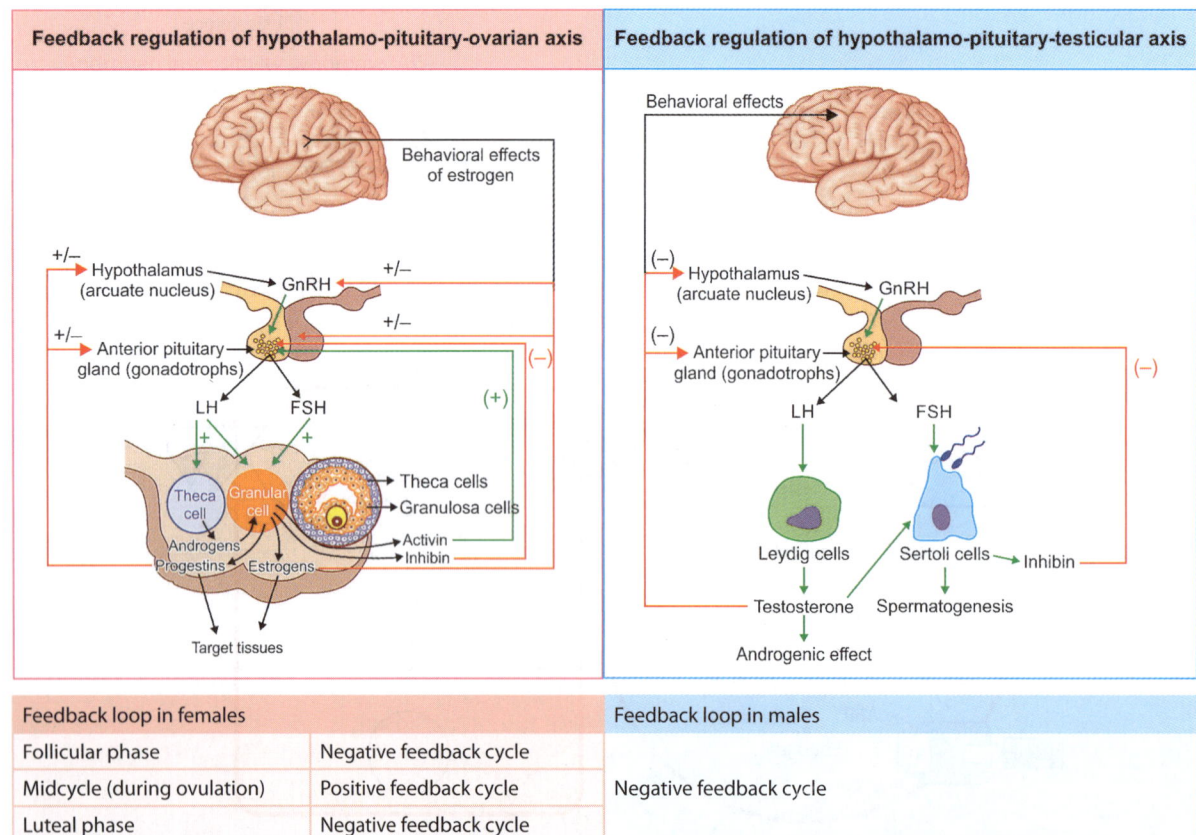

**Fig. 72.5:** Feedback regulation of male and female hormones with their feedback loop.

## SUMMARY

- In this chapter, we have learnt the significance of key organs such as the gonads (testes in males and ovaries in females), as well as accessory reproductive organs like the fallopian tubes, uterus, and external genitalia. The roles of these organs in gamete production, fertilization, and pregnancy are underscored, setting the stage for a comprehensive exploration of reproductive physiology and hormone regulation. The key hormones associated with reproductive physiology, include gonadotropin-releasing hormone (GnRH), follicle-stimulating hormone (FSH), luteinizing hormone (LH), estrogen, progesterone, testosterone, and others.

- Furthermore, the synthesis, secretion, mechanisms of action, and regulation of these reproductive hormones in both males and females are elucidated. The intricate processes of hormone production, their targets, and the feedback mechanisms governing their release are explored in detail.

## LET US SEE, HOW MUCH YOU HAVE LEARNT?

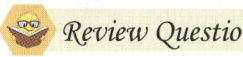

### *Review Questions*

#### *Long/Short Answer Questions*

Q1. Describe the synthesis, mechanism of action, functions and regulation of:
  a. Testosterone
  b. Estrogen
  c. Progesterone

Q2. Write a note on feedback regilation of hypothalamo-pituitary-ovarian axis.

Q3. Write a note on feedback regilation of hypothalamo-pituitary-testicular axis.

#### *Explain Why? (Reasoning Questions)*

Q1. Premenopausal women are protected from the atherosclerosis.

Q2. The postmenopausal women become more prone to osteoporosis.

Q3. What would happen to the sperm count of a person working near the hot furnace?

### *Multiple Choice Questions*

Q1. Which of the following is not an essential organ of the male reproductive system?
  a. Testes         b. Penis
  c. Ovaries        d. Epididymis

Q2. Which hormone stimulates the development of ovarian follicles in females?
  a. Luteinizing hormone (LH)
  b. Follicle-stimulating hormone (FSH)
  c. Testosterone
  d. Estrogen

Q3. What is the primary hormone secreted by the corpus luteum after ovulation?
  a. Testosterone
  b. Progesterone
  c. Estrogen
  d. Gonadotropin-releasing hormone (GnRH)

Q4. In males, which hormone is responsible for stimulating the production of sperm cells?
  a. Testosterone
  b. Follicle-stimulating hormone (FSH)
  c. Luteinizing hormone (LH)
  d. Progesterone

Q5. Which hormone is responsible for the development of male secondary sexual characteristics?
  a. Estrogen
  b. Progesterone
  c. Testosterone
  d. Follicle-stimulating hormone (FSH)

Q6. Which hormone is responsible for triggering ovulation in females?
  a. Luteinizing hormone (LH)
  b. Follicle-stimulating hormone (FSH)
  c. Estrogen
  d. Progesterone

Q7. What is the primary function of the fallopian tubes in the female reproductive system?
  a. Sperm production     b. Fertilization
  c. Menstruation         d. Hormone secretion

Q8. Which hormone is responsible for the development and maintenance of the uterine lining during the menstrual cycle?
  a. Progesterone         b. Testosterone
  c. Estrogen             d. Luteinizing hormone (LH)

Q9. What is the name of the structure where sperm mature and are stored in the male reproductive system?
  a. Vas deferens         b. Epididymis
  c. Seminal vesicles     d. Prostate gland

Q10. In females, which hormone is primarily responsible for the development of secondary sexual characteristics such as breast growth?
  a. Progesterone         b. Testosterone
  c. Estrogen             d. Luteinizing hormone (LH)

**ANSWERS**

1. c    2. b    3. b    4. b    5. c    6. a    7. b    8. a    9. b    10. c

# Sex Determination and Sex Differentiation of Embryo

**CHAPTER 73**

> **COMPETENCY ADDRESSED**
>
> **PY9.1:** Describe and discuss sex determination; sex differentiation and their abnormalities and outline psychiatry and practical implication of sex determination.

>  **LEARNING OBJECTIVES**
>
> At the end of this chapter, the learner should be able to:
> - Describe the determination of sex.
> - Describe the process of sex differentiation.
> - Describe the abnormalities related to sex determination and differentiation.

## SEX DETERMINATION

Sex determination is the genotype of the fetus, whether male or female, determined by presence of sex chromosomes, 'X' and 'Y' (**Fig. 73.1**). Each human adult has 46 chromosomes including the sex chromosomes. These 46 chromosomes comprise of 44 (22 pair) of autosomes and 2 (1 pair) of sex chromosomes, also called as *diploid chromosomes*.

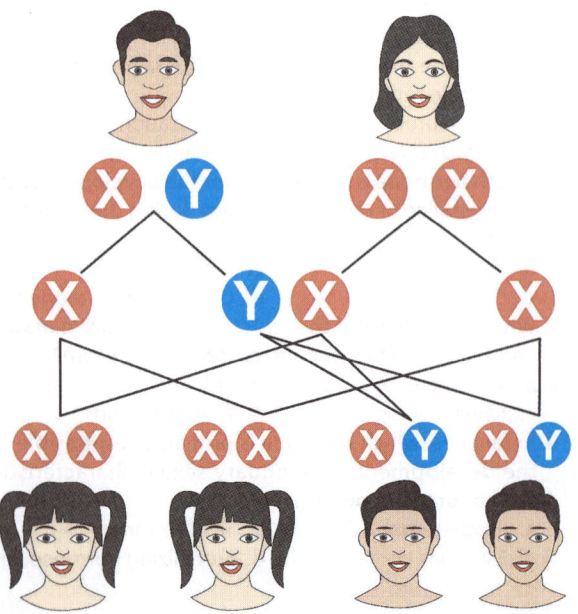

**Fig. 73.1:** Sex determination based on principles of inheritance. The sex chromosomes indicate the genotypic male or female offspring.

- Females: 44 autosomes and 2X chromosomes.
- Males: 44 autosomes and XY chromosomes.

Please note: Sperms and ova are mature male and female gametes respectively. They have half the number of chromosomes, i.e., 22 autosomes and one sex chromosome (Ovum: 22+X, Sperm 22+X or 22+Y.)

> **Barr Body**
>
> During embryonic development, one of the X chromosomes of somatic cells in female embryo becomes inactive. The inactive X chromosome of each somatic cell forms a condensed mass called as Barr body or sex chromatin. It is seen near the nuclear membrane of the cell.
>
>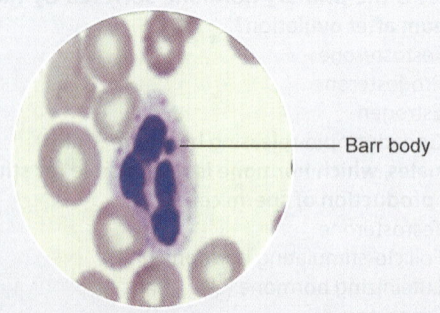
>
> **Significance of Barr body**
> - **Helps in identification of sex genotype:** Since Barr bodies are present only in somatic cells of females, genotype can be identified by cytological tests by testing cells from buccal mucosal cells, vaginal mucosal cells, polymorphonuclear cells (neutrophils) or epithelial cells of epidermis.

- **Identification of abnormal genotype:** Cell having two or more Barr bodies is considered to be abnormal cell having more than normal X chromosomes.
- Absence of Barr body helps in **diagnosis of Turner syndrome (XO)**, i.e., absence of second X chromosome.

## SEX DIFFERENTIATION

Sex differentiation occurs after sex determination in the embryo. It refers to all the changes, which happen in fetus, for the development of genital organs according to the genotypically determined sex. Hence, the sex differentiation represents the phenotypic sex of the fetus.

**Stages of sex differentiation**
The stages can be broadly classified as:
- Gonadal differentiation
- Genital differentiation

## Gonadal Differentiation

It includes formation of gonads, i.e., ovaries in females and testes in males, according to genotype of the embryo. Gonads develop at genital ridge or the urogenital ridge, present on each side of adrenal gland. Primordial germ cells migrate to genital ridge and proliferate leading to formation of bipotential/primordial/primitive gonads, which are identical in males and females up to 6 weeks.

Further development depends upon the genotype which is discussed in **Table 73.1**.

## Genital Differentiation (Phenotype Sex Differentiation)

Differentiation of internal genitalia, urethra and external genitalia.

## Differentiation of Internal Genitalia

It occurs from neutral sex anlagen-6th week of gestation.
Primordia of internal genitalia-paired set of Wolffian (male) ducts and paired set of Mullerian (female) ducts. By 7th week of gestation, embryo has both male and female primordial ducts **(Table 73.2)**.

**Table 73.1:** Development of male and female genotype.

| Male genotype | Female genotype |
|---|---|
| • Bipotential gonads differentiate into testes at 6th week, under the effect of Y chromosome. Y chromosome has genes for testicular differentiation and formation of MIS (Mullerian duct inhibitory substance) <br> • Testicular differentiation goes on from 3rd to 5th week of gestation <br> • At about 35th week, testes descend through inguinal canal into the scrotum | • If the genotype is female, by about 10th week of gestation, ovarian differentiation begins on bipotential gonads <br> • Ovarian differentiation occurs due to absence of TDF (Testes determining factor). At 11–12 weeks, meiosis occur in oogonia to form the oocyte |

**Table 73.2:** Genital development of male and female internal organs.

| Male | Female |
|---|---|
| • Male genotype (44+XY): Secretion of testosterone and MIS (Mullerian Inhibiting substance) <br> • Testosterone: Formation of epididymis, vas deferens and seminal vesicles <br> • MIS: Regression of Mullerian ducts by apoptosis | • Female genotype (44+XX): Absence of MIS <br> • Mullerian ducts proliferate and form uterine tubes, uterus, upper 2/3 of vagina by 8 weeks <br> • Wolffian ducts degenerate |

Hence, natural tendency for the fetus is to develop female phenotype, because absence of testis initiates development of female genitalia.

### Differentiation of External Genitalia

External genitalia develop from common anlagen. They are bipotential till 8th week of gestation.

In male fetus due to presence of testosterone-external genitalia have male characteristics by 5th month of gestation-prostrate, prostatic urethra, penile of urethra, shaft of penis, glans penis, scrotum.

In female fetus due to absence of any hormone, female external genitalia developurethra, labia minora and majora, clitoris.

> **The Practical Implication**
>
> **The preconception and prenatal diagnostic techniques act, 1994 (PCPNDT ACT, 1994)**
> This act was passed by Government of India in 1994 to regulate the genetic counselling centers, genetic laboratories, genetic clinics, prenatal diagnostic techniques which prohibits the prenatal sex determination of the fetus. According to this law, any person (parents, medical geneticist, gynecologist, radiologist or any other registered medical practitioner) found indulged in prenatal sex determination, shall be charged under the non-bailable, cognizable and noncompoundable offence with heavy monetary and legal punishment.

**Figure 73.2** shows the differentiation and development of genitalia from gonadal ridges in males and females.

## DISORDERS OF SEXUAL DEVELOPMENT

These can occur due to:
- Defect in sex chromosomes
- Hormonal abnormalities

### Defect in Sex Chromosomes-Chromosomal Abnormalities

Chromosomal abnormalities result from defects in chromosomes. It can be either deletion, mutation or other causes. **Table 73.3** enumerates various chromosomal abnormalities with their features and genotypes.

### Hormonal Abnormalities

For male development, androgens by fetal testes are required.

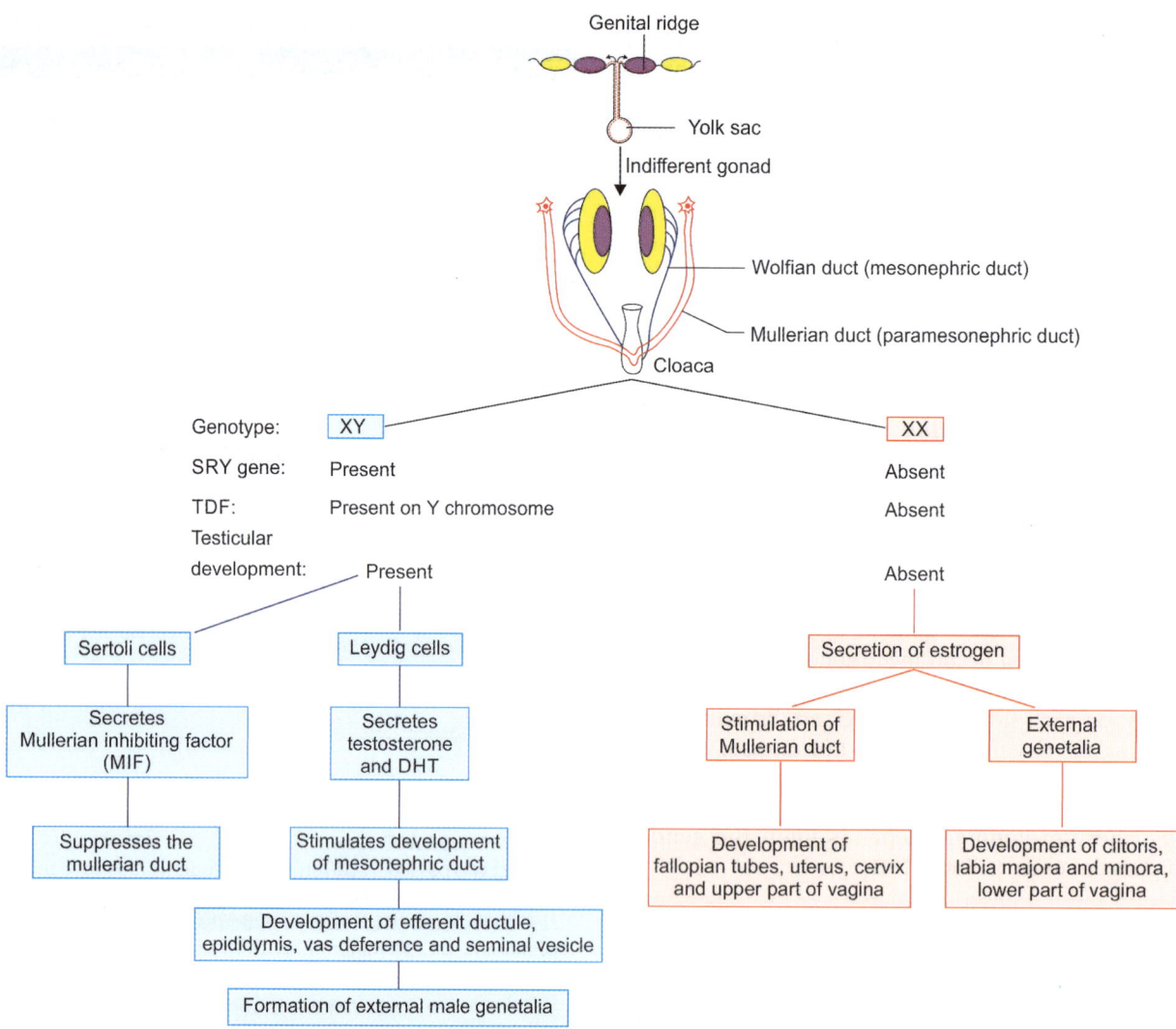

**Fig. 73.2:** Sex differentiation from the genital ridge.

**Table 73.3:** Chromosomal abnormalities.

| Chromosomal abnormality | Cause | Genotype | Characteristics features |
|---|---|---|---|
| **Trisomy** | Nondisjunction of sex chromosomes: Pair of chromosome do not separate during meiotic division. Resulting gamete has 24 chromosomes (instead of 23). After fertilization, zygote will have 47 chromosomes (3 sex chromosomes instead of 2)<br><br>Down's syndrome (mongolism)—autosomal chromosomal trisomy of 21 chromosome | XXX (Super female) | Poor sexual development, less menstruation, mental retardation |
|  |  | XXY (Klinefelter syndrome) | • Most common<br>• Normal male external and internal genitalia, tall and obese<br>• Poor development of testis and seminiferous tubules (seminiferous dysgenesis), sterility, gynecomastia, poorly developed secondary sexual characteristics-sparse pubic and body hair, small penis and testes<br>• Low testosterone<br>• High LH, FSH, estradiol<br>• Positive sex chromatin test |
| **Monosomy** | Both chromosomes of a pair go to one gamete. Other gamete has only 22 chromosomes and after fertilization, zygote will have 45 chromosomes | Female phenotype 44+XO (Turner's syndrome) | • Turner's syndrome: Incidence 1 in 2500 females<br>• Female phenotype due to absence of Y chromosome<br>• Normal external and internal genitalia<br>• Delayed puberty-amenorrhea or less menstruation, infertility<br>• Ovarian dysgenesis<br>• Mental retardation |

*Contd...*

Contd...

| Chromosomal abnormality | Cause | Genotype | Characteristics features |
|---|---|---|---|
| | | | • Dwarfism: Webbed neck, ptosis, low hair line, small jaw, low set ears-epicanthus, coarctation of aorta |
| | | Male phenotype 44+YO | Very lethal: Intrauterine death of fetus |
| Triploidy | Sometimes gametes have diploid chromosomes, hence, resultant zygotes will have 46 + 23 = 69 chromosomes | — | Born dead |
| More than three sex chromosomes | | XXXY, XXXXY, XXYY, XXXX | Severe mental retardation |
| • Translocation<br>• Deletion<br>• Duplication<br>• Inversion | Abnormalities in number of chromosomes during crossing over process | | |
| Mosaicism | Due to transverse splitting of centromere resulting in two dissimilar chromosomes | | |

However, if genetic female is exposed to androgen during 8th to 13th week of gestation, male like development occurs.

> If the mother has androgen secreting adrenal tumor during pregnancy, the female fetus develops into phenotypic male, despite of female genotype, due to presence of testosterone.

## Pseudo Hermaphroditism

It means individual having genotype (gonads) of one sex and genitalia of other sex.

It can be:
- **Female pseudohermaphroditism:**
  - Genotype: Female XX.
  - Gonads and internal genitalia are of female type; but at prepubertal age, there is masculinization of female causing development of penis and masculine type hair growth. There is increased levels of testosterone and androgens.
- **Male pseudohermaphroditism:** Person is genetically male (XY) but have feminization.
  - *Androgen resistance:* The person has infertility with testicular feminizing syndrome (external genitalia female type but with blind vagina). There is no female internal genitalia. The nervous system and hypothalamus develop as females with primary amenorrhea.
  - Abnormal testicular development.
  - Congenital deficiency of 17-alpha hydroxylase.

## True Hermaphroditism

Gonads of both sexes are present-extremely rare condition. Ovary on one side and testes on other side. As a result, there is wide variation in internal and external genitalia. Various combinations are possible resulting in varied characteristics features.

## CHROMOSOMAL ANOMALY

### Down's Syndrome

**Definition:** Down syndrome, also known as trisomy 21, is a chromosomal anomaly characterized by the presence of an extra copy of chromosome 21. This additional genetic material leads to developmental delays, intellectual disability, and distinctive physical features.

**Chromosomal anomaly:** Down syndrome is caused by an error in cell division called nondisjunction, which results in an extra chromosome 21. While most people have 46 chromosomes (23 pairs), individuals with Down syndrome have 47 chromosomes, with three copies of chromosome 21 instead of the usual two.

**Clinical features (Fig. 73.3):** The clinical features of Down syndrome can vary widely among individuals, but some common characteristics include:
- Distinctive facial features such as upward slanting eyes, a flat facial profile, and a small nose.
- Low muscle tone (hypotonia) and poor muscle strength, which can affect motor skills and coordination.
- Intellectual disability ranging from mild to moderate, impacting learning and cognitive abilities.
- Developmental delays in speech and language skills, as well as motor milestones such as sitting, crawling, and walking.
- Increased risk of certain medical conditions such as congenital heart defects, hearing loss, vision problems, gastrointestinal issues, and thyroid disorders.
- Short stature and slower growth compared to typically developing individuals.

### Klinefelter Syndrome

Klinefelter syndrome, also known as 47,XXY or XXY syndrome, is a chromosomal disorder that affects males. It occurs when there is at least one extra X chromosome

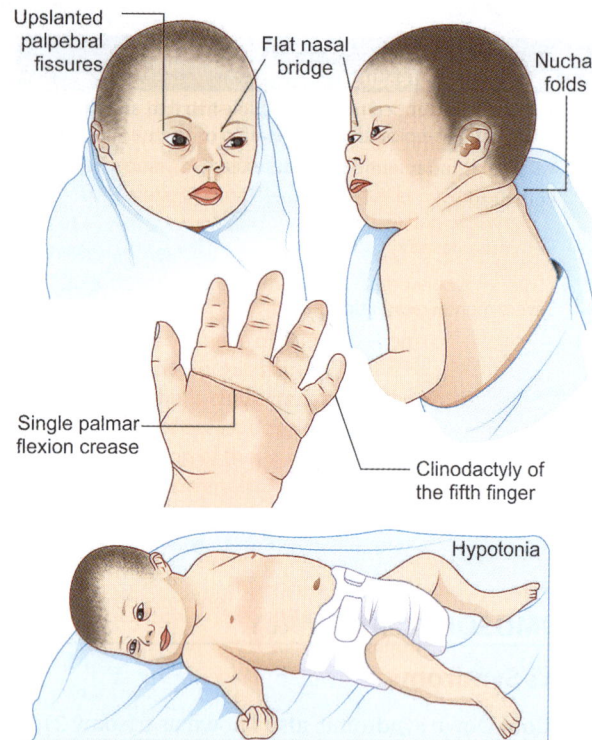

**Fig. 73.3:** Clinical features of Down syndrome.

in addition to the usual XY chromosome configuration. Typically, males have one X and one Y chromosome (46,XY), but individuals with Klinefelter syndrome have an extra X chromosome, resulting in a total of 47 chromosomes (XXY).

**Clinical features of Klinefelter syndrome (Fig. 73.4):**
- **Infertility:** Klinefelter syndrome is the most common genetic cause of male infertility. The presence of an extra X chromosome can lead to reduced sperm production (oligospermia) or complete absence of sperm (azoospermia).
- **Hypogonadism:** Individuals with Klinefelter syndrome often have underdeveloped testes, leading to lower testosterone levels. This can result in delayed or incomplete puberty, reduced muscle mass, decreased facial and body hair growth, and breast development (gynecomastia).
- **Physical characteristics:** Some physical features associated with Klinefelter syndrome include
  - Tall stature, long limbs
  - Decreased muscle tone (hypotonia)
  - Wider hips, and a narrower shoulder-to-hip ratio.
  - Additionally, individuals may have smaller-than-average testes and an increased risk of certain health conditions such as osteoporosis and varicose veins.

**Learning and developmental challenges:** While intelligence is typically within the normal range, individuals with Klinefelter syndrome may experience learning difficulties, language delays, and problems with attention and executive function skills.

**Psychosocial implications:** Klinefelter syndrome can impact self-esteem and social interactions, particularly during adolescence when differences in physical development may become more apparent. Early diagnosis and appropriate support can help individuals with Klinefelter syndrome navigate these challenges and lead fulfilling lives

## Turner's Syndrome

Turner syndrome, also known as 45,X or monosomy X syndrome, is a chromosomal disorder that affects females. It occurs when one of the two X chromosomes is either completely or partially missing, resulting in a total of 45 chromosomes instead of the usual 46 (45,X).

**Clinical features of Turner syndrome (Fig. 73.5):**
- **Short stature:** One of the most characteristic features of Turner syndrome is short stature, with affected individuals typically being shorter than average. Growth

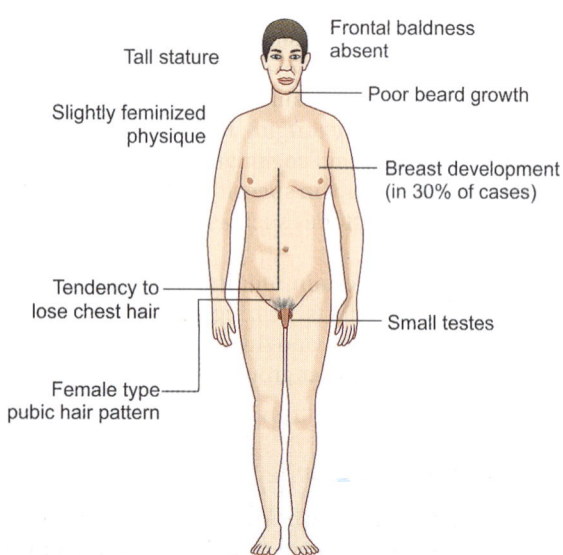

**Fig. 73.4:** Clinical features of Klinefelter syndrome.

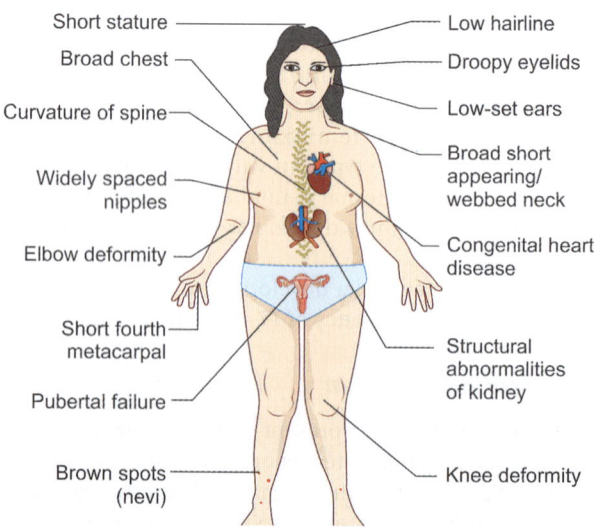

**Fig. 73.5:** Clinical features of Turner syndrome.

may be slower during childhood, and adult height is often significantly below average.
- **Gonadal dysgenesis:** Individuals with Turner syndrome have underdeveloped or absent ovaries, leading to ovarian insufficiency and infertility. This can result in delayed or absent puberty, amenorrhea (absence of menstruation), and infertility.
- **Physical characteristics:** Other physical features associated with Turner syndrome may include a webbed neck (extra folds of skin on the neck), low hairline at the back of the neck, drooping eyelids (ptosis), widely spaced nipples, and a shield-shaped chest with widely spaced nipples.
- **Lymphedema:** Some individuals with Turner syndrome may experience lymphedema, which is swelling caused by a buildup of lymph fluid. Lymphedema typically affects the hands and feet and may be present at birth or develop later in childhood.
- **Cardiovascular abnormalities:** Turner syndrome is associated with an increased risk of certain heart defects, including coarctation of the aorta (narrowing of the aorta), bicuspid aortic valve, and other structural abnormalities of the heart.
- **Hormonal imbalances:** Turner syndrome can lead to hormonal imbalances, including decreased production of estrogen. This may result in symptoms such as osteoporosis (weak bones), early menopause, and an increased risk of certain health conditions such as diabetes and thyroid disorders.

## SUMMARY

This chapter explores the intricacies of sex determination and differentiation, shedding light on their biological processes and potential abnormalities. It begins by elucidating the mechanisms of sex determination, emphasizing the role of genetic and hormonal factors in determining an individual's sex.

Furthermore, the chapter delves into the process of sex differentiation, detailing how genetic sex (determined at conception) influences the development of reproductive organs and secondary sexual characteristics during prenatal and postnatal stages. It discusses the differentiation of gonads into ovaries or testes, as well as the development of external genitalia and other sexual characteristics.

Moreover, the chapter addresses abnormalities of sex determination and differentiation, such as disorders of sex development (DSD) and intersex variations, exploring their genetic, hormonal, and anatomical complexities.

## LET US SEE, HOW MUCH YOU HAVE LEARNT?

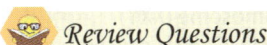

### Long/Short Answer Questions

Q1. Describe the process of sex differentiation from the genital ridge of the embryo.
Q2. Explain what would happen to the fetus, if the mother with genetically female fetus develops the androgen secreting tumor.
Q3. Write short notes on:
   a. Down syndrome
   b. Klinefelter syndrome
   c. Turner syndrome
Q4. What is the significance of Barr body?

### Explain Why? (Reasoning Questions)

Q1. The presence of the SRY gene on the Y chromosome is critical for male sex determination in an embryo.
Q2. The development of the Müllerian ducts into female reproductive structures requires the absence of anti-Müllerian hormone (AMH) and androgens.

 *Critical Thinking Case-Based Questions*

Q1. Rekha and Vijay, a couple from a rural area in India, were expecting their first child. During a routine prenatal check-up at 20 weeks, the ultrasound revealed ambiguous genitalia. Genetic testing showed the baby has a 47,XXY karyotype, indicating Klinefelter syndrome. The doctor explained that this chromosomal disorder affects sex differentiation and referred them to a specialist in pediatric endocrinology for further evaluation and management. Based upon the given scenario, answer the following questions:
   a. Explain the physiological mechanisms of sex determination and sex differentiation in embryos.
   b. Enumerate other chromosomal abnormalities.
   c. What are the genetic and hormonal factors involved in sex determination and differentiation in embryos?
   d. What are the clinical features of Klinefelter syndrome?

## Multiple Choice Questions

Q1. What primarily determines an individual's genetic sex?
 a. Presence of the SRY gene on the Y chromosome
 b. Presence of two X chromosomes
 c. Absence of the SRY gene on the X chromosome
 d. Presence of the AR gene on the X chromosome

Q2. Which of the following is NOT a typical feature of androgen insensitivity syndrome (AIS)?
 a. Development of male external genitalia
 b. Presence of XY chromosomes
 c. Inability to respond to androgens
 d. Development of female secondary sexual characteristics

Q3. Which hormone is responsible for the differentiation of the external genitalia into male structures during embryonic development?
 a. Estrogen
 b. Progesterone
 c. Testosterone
 d. Follicle-stimulating hormone (FSH)

Q4. Turner syndrome is characterized by:
 a. Presence of an extra X chromosome (XXY)
 b. Presence of only one X chromosome (XO)
 c. Presence of an extra Y chromosome (XYY)
 d. Presence of two X chromosomes and one Y chromosome (XXY)

Q5. Which of the following is a common cause of ambiguous genitalia in newborns?
 a. Congenital adrenal hyperplasia (CAH)
 b. Klinefelter syndrome
 c. Androgen insensitivity syndrome (AIS)
 d. Turner syndrome

Q6. Which hormone is primarily responsible for the differentiation of the internal reproductive organs (e.g., uterus, fallopian tubes) in females during embryonic development?
 a. Estrogen
 b. Progesterone
 c. Testosterone
 d. Mullerian inhibiting substance (MIS)

Q7. Complete androgen insensitivity syndrome (CAIS) is characterized by:
 a. Partial response to androgens
 b. Inability to respond to androgens
 c. Presence of XY chromosomes
 d. Development of ambiguous genitalia

Q8. The presence of the SRY gene on the Y chromosome leads to:
 a. Development of female external genitalia
 b. Development of male external genitalia
 c. Development of both male and female external genitalia
 d. No impact on external genitalia development

Q9. Which of the following is a characteristic feature of Klinefelter syndrome?
 a. Presence of only one X chromosome (XO)
 b. Presence of two X chromosomes and one Y chromosome (XXY)
 c. Presence of an extra Y chromosome (XYY)
 d. Presence of an extra X chromosome (XXY)

Q10. Congenital adrenal hyperplasia (CAH) is caused by:
 a. Deficiency of adrenal androgens
 b. Overproduction of adrenal androgens
 c. Deficiency of estrogen
 d. Overproduction of estrogen

**ANSWERS**

1. a   2. a   3. c   4. b   5. a   6. d   7. b   8. b   9. b   10. b

# Life Cycle of Reproductive Physiology

**74**
CHAPTER

### COMPETENCY ADDRESSED

**PY9.2:** Describe and discuss puberty: Onset, progression, stages; early and delayed puberty and outline adolescent clinical and psychological association.
**PY9.7:** Describe and discuss the effects of the removal of gonads on physiological functions.
**PY9.11:** Discuss the hormonal changes and their effects during perimenopause and menopause.

###  LEARNING OBJECTIVES

**At the end of this chapter, the learner should be able to:**
- Onset of puberty in both the gender, in terms of development of genitalia, reproductive hormones and other systemic changes.
- Progression and stages of puberty in both the genders
- Applied aspects related to the onset of puberty in terms of early and delayed puberty
- The psychological changes associated with onset of puberty
- The effect of removal of gonads in both the genders, before and after the attainment of puberty
- Hormonal changes and their effects during perimenopause and menopause.

## PUBERTY (ADOLESCENCE)

It is a normal phase of development that occurs when a child's body transits into adult body and endocrine and gametogenic functions of gonads have developed to the point where reproduction is possible.

In neonatal period, the male testis secrete testosterone which is required for sex differentiation of fetus and the testicular descent. But after birth, the levels of testosterone, decrease to a minimum, till the adolescence. It occurs due to very less amount of gonadotropins (FSH, LH) are secreted by anterior pituitary, in prepubertal boys. On the other hand, the absence of testis development factor (TDF) in female fetus, the testosterone is not secreted in utero, which results in the development of female fetus and sex differentiation under the effect of estrogen. The levels of FSH and LH remain quite low in female children also, till the attainment of puberty.

At puberty because of increased release of GnRH from hypothalamus causing secretion of gonadotropins from pituitary glands, hence resulting in the hormonal, physical and systemic changes in the adolescents.

The age of onset of puberty in boys 9–14 years and in girls is 8–13 years.

## Stages of Puberty

In females, the stages of puberty are described as:
- **Thelarche:** Development of breasts
- **Pubarche:** Development of axillary hair and pubic hair
- **Menarche:** First menstrual period

## TANNER'S CLASSIFICATION/SEXUAL MATURITY RATING

Tanner's classification, also known as the Tanner stages or Tanner scale, is a widely used method to assess the stages of sexual development during puberty. It categorizes physical changes into five stages, ranging from prepubertal to adult (**Fig. 74.1** and **Table 74.1**). The sexual maturity rating (SMR) is a component of Tanner's classification, specifically focusing on the development of secondary sexual characteristics such as breast development in females and genital development in males.

## Growth Spurt

The adolescent boys and girls undergo a growth spurt during puberty due to increased level of sex steroids

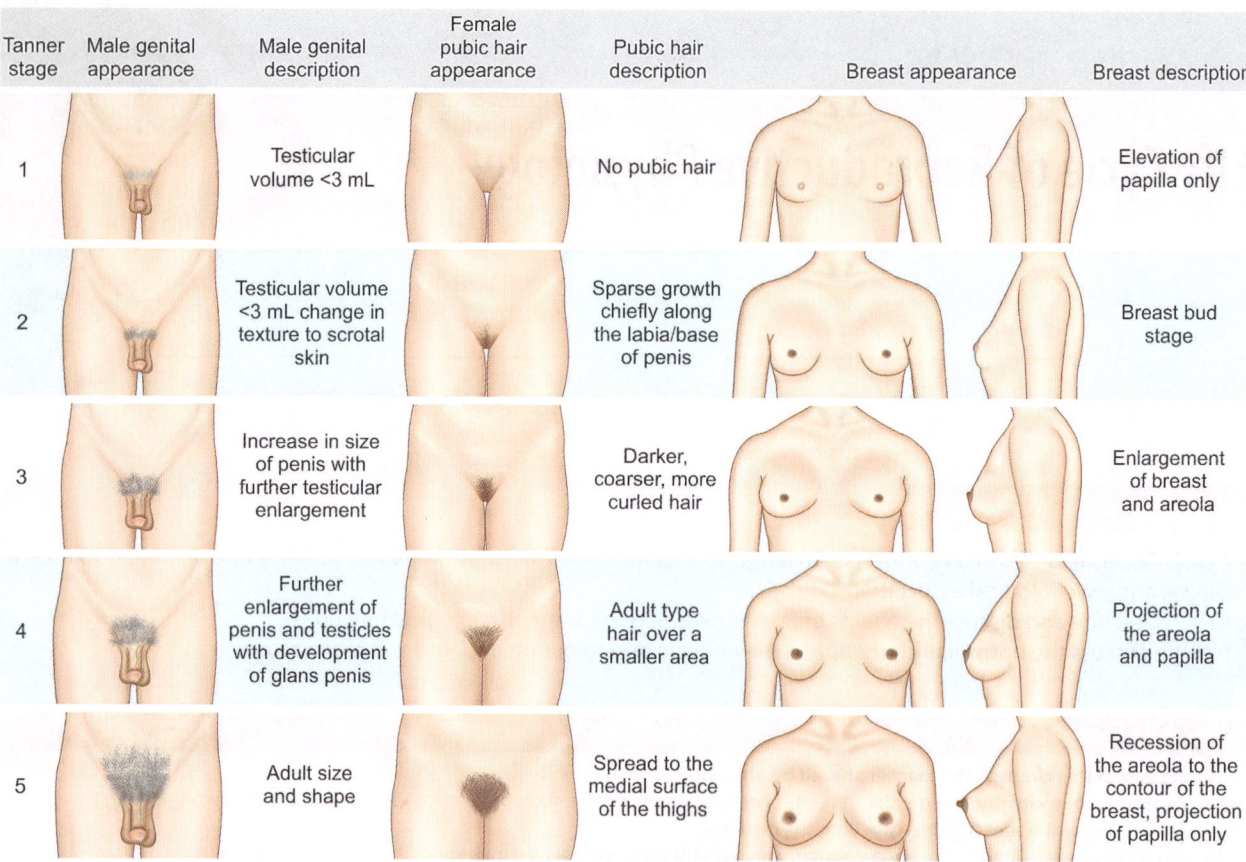

**Fig. 74.1:** Tanner's classification of sexual maturity in males and females.

**Table 74.1:** Stages of puberty in males and females.

| Stage of puberty | Bone age (years) F-Female M-Male | Females | Males |
|---|---|---|---|
| 1 | Up to 7.5 | Childhood—preadolescent | Childhood—preadolescent |
| 2 | F: 10.5 M: 12 | Thelarche—appearance of 'breast bud'. It is the first sign of puberty in girls | Enlargement of male genitalia-testes |
| 3 | F: 11.5 M: 14 | • Pubarche—appearance of pubic and axillary hair<br>• Increase in height, enlargement of breasts | Enlargement of penis, growth of pubic and axillary hair |
| 4 | F: 13 M: 15.5 | • Enlargement of the areola<br>• Menarche—beginning of menstruation | • Growth of internal and external adult genitalia<br>• Increase in height |
| 5 | F: 14 M: 16.5 | Formation of adult genitalia'<br>Appearance of secondary sexual characteristics:<br>• Broad hips, narrow shoulders, converging thighs, female distribution of fat-breasts, hips<br>• Appearance of pubic (concave upwards) and axillary hair<br>• High pitched voice<br>• Increase in size of clitoris, labia majora and labia minora<br>• Increase in size of uterus, vagina<br>• Appearance of acne<br>• Interest in opposite sex | Formation of adult genitalia'<br>• Appearance of secondary sexual characteristics—muscular body, broad shoulders<br>• Increase in hair on body specially on axilla, face, chest, pubic area (triangle with downward base)<br>• Enlargement of larynx, deep coarse voice<br>• Increase in penis, seminal vesicle, prostrate and bulbourethral glands<br>• Appearance of acne<br>• Interest in opposite sex |

resulting in increased secretion of growth hormones and insulin like growth factor-I (IGF-I). The increased secretion of these hormones results in linear growth due to skeletal and muscular growth, growth of immune system and metabolic changes in the adolescents.

## Adrenarche

The zona reticularis of adrenal cortex, secrete adrenal androgens, referred as adrenarche. It occurs just before the onset of puberty at around 6–8 years of age. It is responsible for development of secondary sexual characters or pubarche. It leads to the appearance of axillary and pubic hair, oily skin and appearance of acne in both boys and girls.

## DISORDERS OF ADOLESCENCE

### Precocious Puberty (Early Puberty)

It is defined as the early appearance of secondary sexual characters very early in the childhood; around 8 years of age in girls and 9 years in boys. It is broadly classified as:
- **Central precocious puberty:** It occurs due to early activation of hypothalamo-hypophysial-gonadal axis. It is mostly seen in girls and is idiopathic. However, it could be associated with certain pathologies like neoplasms (gonadotropin secreting tumors), genetic causes, etc.
- **Peripheral precocious puberty:** It occurs due to the excessive secretion of sex steroids, while the hypothalamo-hyposeal-gonadal axis is not activated. It is associated with McCune Albright syndrome, excessive levels of exogenous sex steroids, testotoxicosis.

### Delayed Puberty

Delayed puberty is defined as lack of appearance of physical signs of puberty in boys up to 14 years of age and 13 years in girls. It is also called as delayed puberty when there is difference of more than 4 years in first and last sign of puberty in both the sexes, i.e., first sign of testicular development till complete development in boys and from thelarche to menarche in girls.

#### Causes
- Hypogonadotropic hypogonadism
- Hypergonadotropic hypogonadism
- Hypopituitarism
- Chromosomal abnormalities
- Hypothalamic dysfunction due to secondary causes
- **Hypogonadotropic hypogonadism**
  - Deficiency of GnRH, LH, or FSH, due to damage to the hypothalamus or pituitary gland from surgery, tumor, infection or injury.
  - Genetic defects, severe stress, and long-term use of opioids or glucocorticoids can also be a cause.
  - Nutritional problems and iron overload may also cause hypogonadotropic hypogonadism.
  - Constitutional delay of growth and puberty is a transient state of hypogonadotropic hypogonadism associated with prolongation of the childhood growth phase, delayed skeletal maturation, delayed pubertal growth spurt, and low IGF-1 secretion.
- **Hypergonadotropic hypogonadism** is the failure of the gonads to produce sex hormones. FSH and LH are elevated due to minimal negative feedback on the hypothalamic-pituitary-gonadal axis.
- **Hypopituitarism** is a lack of release of hormones from the pituitary gland.

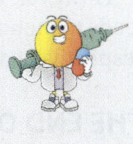

*Kallman syndrome* is a specific disorder falling under *hypopituitarism* where neurons in the developing brain fail to migrate, resulting in *anosmia*, the absence of a sense of smell, and a *lack of GnRH cells* in the hypothalamus.

- **Chromosomal abnormalities** are a cause of delayed puberty shared by both males and females.

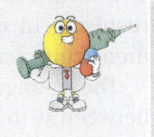

In females, *Turner syndrome (45 XO)* is a common cause of ovarian failure resulting from a missing or incomplete X chromosome.
A common chromosomal disorder in males with delayed puberty is *Klinefelter syndrome (47 XXY)*.

#### Other Causes
- Hypothyroidism
- Cystic fibrosis
- Sickle cell disease
- Celiac disease
- Diabetes mellitus
- Poor nutrition
- Long-term glucocorticoid use

## CASTRATION/GONADECTOMY (REMOVAL OF GONADS)

The surgical removal of either testes in males or ovaries in females is called as gonadectomy. It is also called castration. It is mostly done to avoid tumor risk in certain conditions.

### Gonadectomy is performed in any of these conditions:
- Disorders of sex development (DSD) which has tumor risk. There is the possibility of hormone production discordant to the gender, children and adolescents.
- Partial gonadal dysgenesis.
- Complete androgen insensitivity syndrome (CAIS): 46 XY karyotype, in which normal testes are present but with female gender assignment. Hence, the genetic male is phenotypically female and is raised as a female. This syndrome is linked to gonadal tumors, so gonadectomy is recommended immediately upon diagnosis. It also requires hormonal replacement therapy, psychological and genetic counseling.

### Effect of Castration on Physiological Effects

If the castration is done in either sex before puberty, it results in the absence of gonadal maturation. However, secondary sexual characters appear as the adrenal androgens are normal. The levels of sex steroids remain low resulting in sterility and impotence in males and the absence of menarche in females.

However, if the gonadectomy is done after puberty. It leads to menopause and andropause in females and males respectively due to complete gonadal removal.

## THE END OF REPRODUCTIVE PERIOD (MENOPAUSE AND ANDROPAUSE)

### Menopause

The decline of female sex hormones, particularly estrogen, resulting in cessation of ovarian activity and cyclical menstrual changes are called *menopause*.

The average age of menopause is 51, however it occurs between 40 to 50 years. Since, the ovarian function comes to an end with menopause, natural pregnancy is not possible after menopause.

There is reduction in circulating estrogen results in reduced negative feedback on gonadotropin hormones, secreted by anterior pituitary (FSH and LH). Hence, the levels of FSH, LH rise, indicating lower levels of sex steroids. The period just before the menopause is called *perimenopausal period*. The women in this period show many changes due to the waxing and waning activity of the ovaries and fluctuations in the levels of sex steroids.

### Changes During Perimenopause and Menopause

Various changes occur in women during perimenopausal women characterized by:
- Hot flushes and sweating
- Mood swings
- Thinner and dry vaginal lining
- Sleep disturbances
- Prone to osteoporosis
- Increased risk of cardiovascular diseases

### Andropause

Menopause in women is a universal phenomenon, which is well described and timed process. In contrast, men experience a gradual and slow decline in testosterone secretion often termed as andropause or male climacteric or late-onset hypogonadism (LOH). However, the true andropause/gonadal failure occurs only in men who have undergone surgical or medical castration.

It is characterized by:
- Erectile dysfunction
- Decreased muscle mass and strength
- Increased body fat
- Decreased bone mineral density
- Osteoporosis
- Decreased vitality
- Depressed mood
- Low serum testosterone level

## SUMMARY

- This chapter thoroughly explores puberty, gonadal function, and menopause, shedding light on their physiological and psychological implications across the lifespan.
- The chapter begins by elucidating the onset, progression, and stages of puberty, emphasizing the intricate hormonal changes driving physical and sexual maturation. It examines factors influencing puberty timing, such as genetics, environment, and nutrition, discussing variations like early and delayed puberty and their clinical significance.
- Furthermore, it delves into the clinical and psychological associations of adolescence, addressing the challenges and opportunities during this transitional period. It explores physical changes, emotional turbulence, and social pressures experienced by adolescents, underscoring supportive environments and access to healthcare in promoting adolescent health.
- Moreover, the chapter explores gonadal physiology and effects of gonad removal on health and hormonal balance, if done before and after the puberty.
- Finally, it examines hormonal changes and effects during perimenopause and menopause, marking the end of female reproductive phase. It discusses declining estrogen and progesterone levels, and associated symptoms such as hot flashes and mood changes. Additionally, it explores management strategies for menopausal symptoms and long-term health implications.

## LET US SEE, HOW MUCH YOU HAVE LEARNT?

 *Review Questions*

Q1. Describe the physical, hormonal and emotional changes occurring in girls at the time of puberty.
Q2. Describe the physical, hormonal and emotional changes occurring in boys at the time of puberty.
Q3. What would happen, if the gonads are removed (castration) in a child before puberty?
Q4. What would happen, if the gonads are removed (castration) in a child after the puberty is attained?
Q5. What is precocious puberty? Describe the types and effects of precocious puberty.
Q6. What is menopause? What physiological changes occur at menopause in the women?

## Multiple Choice Questions

**Q1.** You are a healthcare provider counseling a family concerned about their daughter's delayed puberty. Given the information from the chapter, what could be a potential cause of delayed puberty in this case?
a. Early onset of menstruation
b. Genetic factors
c. Poor nutrition
d. Environmental pollution

**Q2.** An adolescent girl presents with irregular menstrual cycles and mood swings. Which hormone imbalance is most likely contributing to her symptoms?
a. Elevated estrogen levels
b. Decreased progesterone levels
c. Elevated testosterone levels
d. Decreased follicle-stimulating hormone (FSH) levels

**Q3.** A 15-year-old boy is referred for evaluation of gynecomastia (enlarged breasts). Which condition is commonly associated with gynecomastia during adolescence?
a. Turner syndrome
b. Klinefelter syndrome
c. Down syndrome
d. Androgen insensitivity syndrome

**Q4.** A 17-year-old male athlete presents with delayed puberty and decreased muscle mass. Which hormone deficiency is most likely responsible for his symptoms?
a. Testosterone
b. Estrogen
c. Growth hormone
d. Follicle-stimulating hormone (FSH)

**Q5.** A 10-year-old girl presents with early onset of pubic hair growth and breast development. What is the most likely cause of her early puberty?
a. Genetic factors
b. Environmental exposure to endocrine-disrupting chemicals
c. Chronic illness
d. Nutritional deficiency

**Q6.** A 13-year-old boy is diagnosed with precocious puberty. Which hormonal abnormality is most likely responsible for his early sexual maturation?
a. Elevated estrogen levels
b. Elevated testosterone levels
c. Decreased luteinizing hormone (LH) levels
d. Decreased follicle-stimulating hormone (FSH) levels

**Q7.** A 45-year-old woman presents with irregular menstrual periods and hot flashes. What is the most likely hormonal change associated with her symptoms?
a. Increased estrogen levels
b. Decreased estrogen levels
c. Increased progesterone levels
d. Decreased luteinizing hormone (LH) levels

**Q8.** A 52-year-old woman complains of vaginal dryness and mood swings. Which hormone replacement therapy would be most appropriate for managing her symptoms?
a. Estrogen-only therapy
b. Progesterone-only therapy
c. Combined estrogen and progesterone therapy
d. Testosterone therapy

**Q9.** A 30-year-old woman with Turner syndrome presents with amenorrhea and infertility. What is the most likely cause of her reproductive issues?
a. Hypothalamic dysfunction
b. Ovarian dysgenesis
c. Hyperprolactinemia
d. Polycystic ovary syndrome (PCOS)

**Q10.** A 25-year-old woman undergoes bilateral oophorectomy (removal of ovaries). What hormone replacement therapy should be initiated post-surgery?
a. Estrogen-only therapy
b. Progesterone-only therapy
c. Combined estrogen and progesterone therapy
d. Testosterone therapy

**Q11.** A 60-year-old woman complains of night sweats and difficulty sleeping. What is the most likely hormonal change associated with her symptoms?
a. Increased estrogen levels
b. Decreased estrogen levels
c. Increased progesterone levels
d. Decreased follicle-stimulating hormone (FSH) levels

**Q12.** A 20-year-old male is diagnosed with hypogonadism and delayed puberty. Which hormone replacement therapy would be most appropriate for managing his condition?
a. Testosterone therapy
b. Estrogen therapy
c. Progesterone therapy
d. Growth hormone therapy

**Q13.** A 45-year-old woman with menopausal symptoms seeks advice on hormone replacement therapy. What is the most common indication for hormone replacement therapy during menopause?
a. Prevention of osteoporosis
b. Prevention of cardiovascular disease
c. Relief of menopausal symptoms
d. Prevention of breast cancer

**Q14.** Pubarche refers to the onset of
a. Breast development in females
b. Testicular enlargement in males
c. Pubic hair growth in both sexes
d. Menstruation in females

**Q15.** Which hormone is primarily responsible for initiating pubarche?
a. Estrogen
b. Progesterone
c. Testosterone
d. Follicle-stimulating hormone (FSH)

**Q16.** At what age does pubarche typically occur in females?
a. 8–9 years  b. 10–11 years
c. 12–13 years  d. 14–15 years

**Q17.** Which of the following is NOT a characteristic of pubarche?
a. Appearance of axillary hair

b. Deepening of the voice
c. Growth of pubic hair
d. Development of body odor

**Q18. What is the primary indication of pubarche in males?**
a. Growth spurt
b. Appearance of facial hair
c. Increase in muscle mass
d. Enlargement of the testes

**Q19. Menarche refers to the:**
a. Onset of breast development
b. Appearance of axillary hair
c. First occurrence of menstruation
d. Growth of pubic hair

**Q20. Adrenarche is characterized by the:**
a. Onset of breast development
b. Activation of the adrenal glands
c. First occurrence of menstruation
d. Development of secondary sexual characteristics

**Q21. What is the primary hormone involved in adrenarche?**
a. Estrogen
b. Progesterone
c. Testosterone
d. Follicle-stimulating hormone (FSH)

**Q22. Thelarche refers to the:**
a. Onset of breast development
b. Appearance of axillary hair
c. First occurrence of menstruation
d. Growth of pubic hair

**Q23. Tanner's classification is used to assess:**
a. Bone age
b. Body mass index (BMI)
c. Pubertal development
d. Cognitive development

**Q24. Tanner stage 2 in males is characterized by:**
a. Absence of pubic hair
b. Sparse, fine pubic hair
c. Enlargement of testes and scrotum
d. Presence of axillary hair

**Q25. Which Tanner stage signifies the completion of pubertal development?**
a. Tanner stage 4
b. Tanner stage 3
c. Tanner stage 5
d. Tanner stage 2

## ANSWERS

1. c   2. b   3. b   4. a   5. b   6. b   7. b   8. c   9. b   10. c   11. b   12. a   13. c   14. c
15. c   16. b   17. b   18. b   19. c   20. b   21. c   22. a   23. c   24. c   25. c

# Reproductive Physiology in Males

## 75
CHAPTER

### COMPETENCY ADDRESSED
**PY9.3:** Describe male reproductive system: Functions of testis and control of spermatogenesis and factors modifying it and outline its association with psychiatric illness.
**PY9.5:** Describe and discuss the physiological effects of sex hormones.
**PY9.9:** Interpret a normal semen analysis report including (a) sperm count, (b) sperm morphology and (c) sperm motility, as per WHO guidelines and discuss the results.

### LEARNING OBJECTIVES
**At the end of this chapter, the learner should be able to:**
- Describe functional anatomy of male reproductive system.
- Describe histological anatomy of the testis and the functions of various testicular cells.
- Describe synthesis and physiological effects of male sex hormones.
- Describe the stages, factors affecting and regulation of spermatogenesis.
- Describe and analyze the report of semen sample in terms of sperm count, sperm morphology, sperm morphology as per WHO guidelines.

## FUNCTIONAL ANATOMY OF MALE REPRODUCTIVE SYSTEM (FIGS. 75.1A TO C)

The primary male reproductive organ are the pair of testis, which are housed in the scrotal sacs. Each testis is composed of up to 900 seminiferous tubules which are highly coiled structures. The sperms, formed in the seminiferous tubules enter a long tube called epididymis which finally opens into vas deferens. The vas deferens enlarges to form the ampulla of vas deference before entering the prostate gland. The contents from both the ampullae and seminal vesicles pass to ejaculatory duct, through the prostate gland into the urethra. The large number of urethral glands and bulbourethral glands (Cowper's glands) add the mucus to the ejaculate near the origin of urethra.

> **The male reproductive tract consists of:**
> - **Glands:** A pair of testes, seminal vesicles, bulbourethral glands, prostrate.
> - **Ducts:** Epididymis, vas deference, ejaculatory ducts, urethra.
> - **Supporting structures:** Spermatic cords, scrota, penis.

## MICROSCOPIC ANATOMY OF TESTIS (FIG. 75.2)

The cross section of seminiferous tubule shows 2–3 layers of immature germ cells called spermatogonia. At puberty, these spermatogonia begin to undergo mitotic division, proliferate and differentiate. There are two type of cells present in the testis:

### Sertoli Cells

These cells are large with abundant cytoplasm. They surround the developing spermatogonia towards the central human of the tubule.

### *Functions of Sertoli Cells*

- **Forms blood testes barrier:**
  - Limits the transport of many substances from blood to seminiferous lumen.
  - Protects the spermatogenic cells from toxic substances and circulating antibodies present in blood.
  - Helps in maintain of seminiferous luminal fluid concentration.

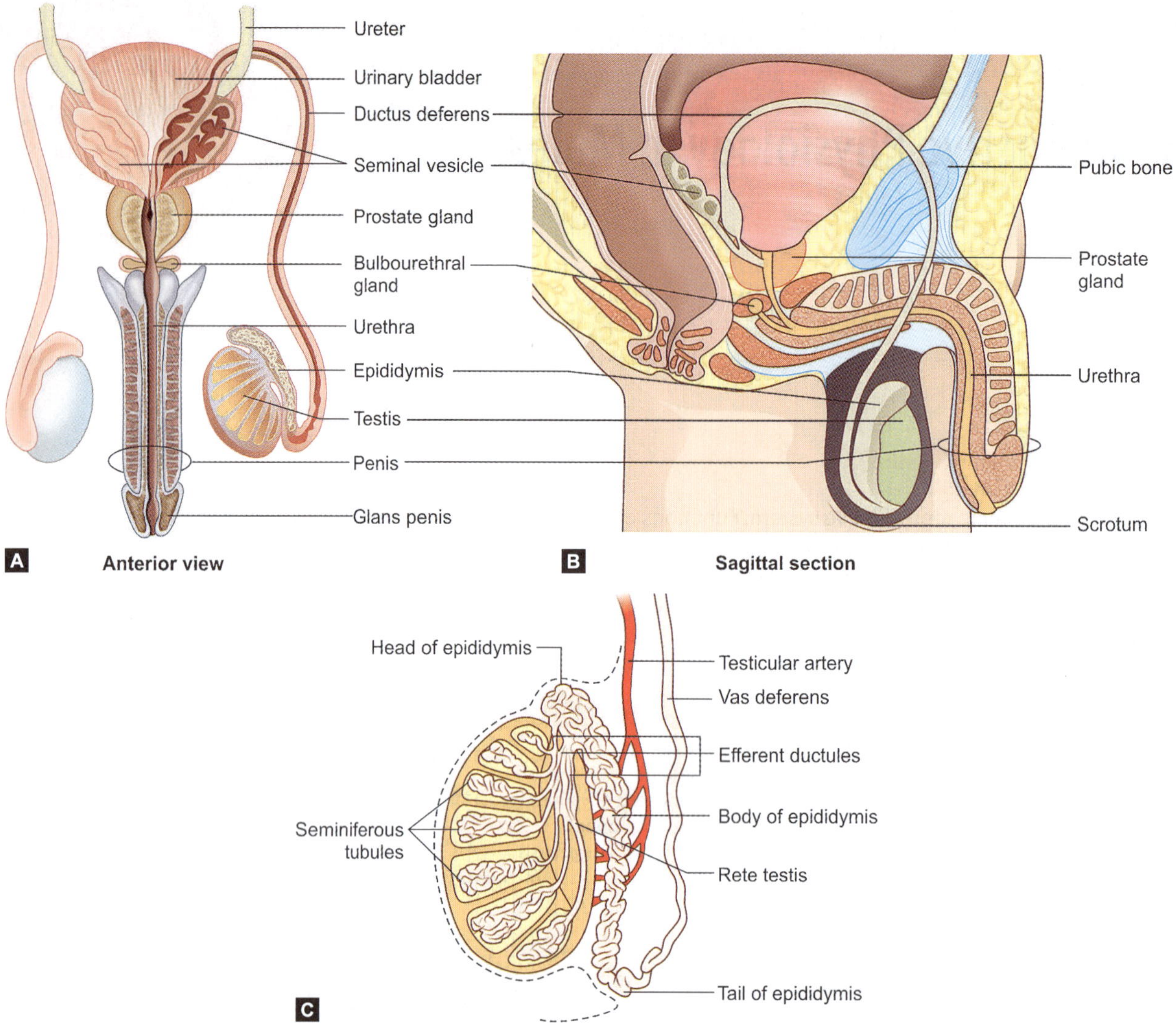

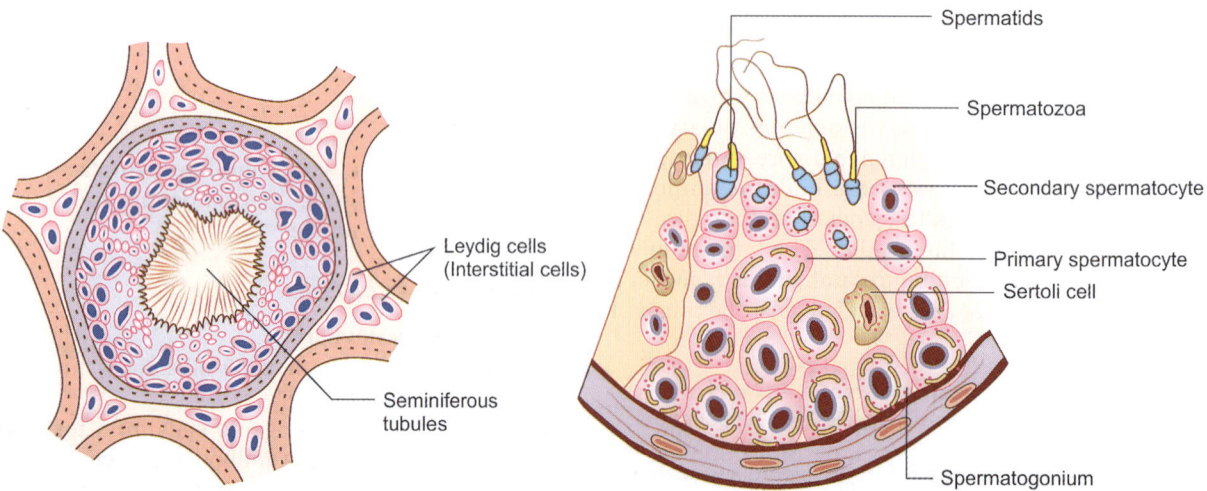

**Figs. 75.1A to C:** (A) Anterior view of male reproductive system; (B) Sagittal view; (C) Structure of testis.

**Fig. 75.2:** Microscopic structure of testis showing Sertoli and Leydig cells.

- Provides **support and nutrition** to spermatogenic cells and removes waste products.
- They **secrete**:
  - **Androgen binding protein:** It helps in maintaining high concentrations of testosterone in lumen of seminiferous tubules as it has high affinity for testosterone.
  - Secrete the **estrogen** in males
  - **Mullerian inhibitory substance (MIS),** which helps in regression of Mullerian duct in fetus and help in male sexual development.
  - **Inhibin:** Inhibits spermatogenesis before puberty by regulating FSH secretion.
  - It also secretes transport proteins like **transferrin** and **ceruloplasmin**.

## Leydig Cells

These cells are the interstitial cells, present in the interstitial septa. The main function of these cells is the production of the male hormone, testosterone. The hormone is responsible for the development of the testicular germinal epithelium and hence the spermatogenesis.

## FUNCTIONS OF TESTES

- Spermatogenesis
- Synthesis and secretion of androgenic hormone-testosterone.

## Formation of Sperms (Spermatogenesis)

Spermatogenesis is the formation of sperms in the *seminiferous tubules* of the testis of the males **(Fig. 75.3)**. Germinal epithelial cells of the seminiferous tubules are known as spermatogonia which form the sperms through different stages **(Table 75.1)**.

> **Changes in the Spermatogonia during Spermiogenesis**
> - Loss of some cytoplasm.
> - Reorganization of chromatin material to form a compact head.
> - Collecting the remaining cytoplasm and cell membranes at one end of the cell to form a tail.
> - The entire period of spermatogenesis from germinal cell to sperm **takes about 74 days** and **each spermatogonia cell gives rise to 64 sperm cells**.

### Regulation of Spermatogenesis

- **Hormonal regulation of spermatogenesis:**
  - *Testosterone:* Secreted by interstitial cells of Leydig of testis. It is essential for *growth* and *division of germinal cells* in forming sperm.
  - *Luteinizing hormone (LH):* Stimulates cells of Leydig to secrete testosterone.
  - *Follicle stimulating hormone (FSH):* Stimulates cells of Sertoli helping in the conversion of spermatids to sperms. It also inserts the LH receptors into the spermatogonia.

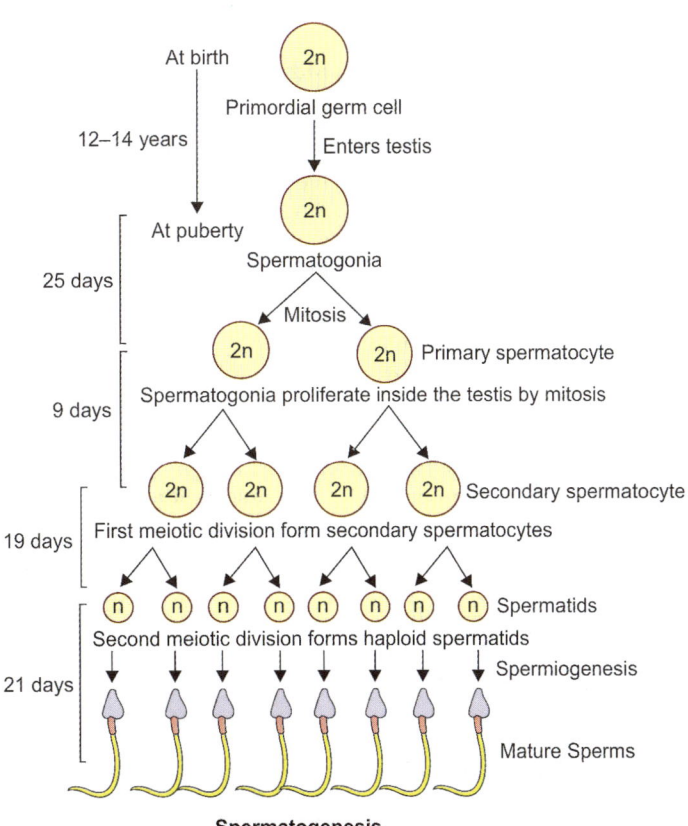

**Fig. 75.3:** Steps showing spermatogenesis.

Table 75.1: Stages of spermatogenesis.

| I | Stage of proliferation | Primordial spermatogonia located immediately adjacent to the basement membrane of the germinal epithelium **divide four times** to **form spermatogonia**, and migrate centrally and lie enveloped by Sertoli cells throughout other stages |
|---|---|---|
| II | Stage of growth | Spermatogonia enlarge to form primary spermatocytes, having diploid cells (46 or 23 pair of chromosomes), within a period of 24 days |
| III | Stage of maturation | |
| | 1st meiotic division | • Primary spermatocyte divides to form two secondary spermatocytes<br>• When primary spermatocyte divides into secondary spermatocyte, each pair of chromosomes separates out so that each secondary spermatocyte contains 23 chromosomes (each chromosome containing two chromatids) |
| | 2nd meiotic division | • Within 2 to 3 days, secondary spermatocyte divides to form four spermatids<br>• Two chromatids of each of 23 chromosomes split apart forming two sets of 23 chromosomes. During division one set passes into one daughter spermatid and another set into another daughter spermatid |
| IV | Stage of transformation (Spermiogenesis) | • Within a few weeks, matured spermatozoa are formed from spermatids via metamorphosis, called spermiogenesis is characterized by absence of cell division<br>• Spermatids only mature and are physically reshaped by enveloping Sertoli cells to form spermatozoa (sperms) |

- *Estrogen:* Formed from testosterone by the Sertoli cells (when stimulated by FSH) and is essential for spermatogenesis.
- *Growth hormone:* Promotes early division of spermatogonia. In its absence the spermatogenesis is severely deficient.
- *Inhibin:* If spermatogenesis proceeds rapidly, cells of Sertoli release hormone inhibin (glycoprotein) which has a strong effect on inhibiting the secretion of FSH and also a slight effect on hypothalamus to inhibit secretion of GnRH.
- Other factors:
  - *Temperature:* Normal spermatogenesis occurs at temperature 1–2 degree lower than normal body temperature. This is achieved by location of testes outside the body in scrotum.
  - *Infectious diseases:* Like mumps cause degeneration of seminiferous tubules thereby decreasing spermatogenesis.
  - *Stress* may reduce testosterone levels and spermatogenesis.

Failure of testes to descend from abdomen into the scrotum is known as cryptorchidism (undescended testes). If testes remain in abdominal cavity for a long-time, tubular epithelium degenerate due to higher temperature, and testes become totally nonfunctional.

## STRUCTURE OF SPERM

Spermatid elongates into a spermatozoon having head and tail (**Fig. 75.4**).

- The head is composed of condensed nucleus within thin cytoplasmic cell membrane. Outside the head, there is a thick cap called *acrosome* formed mainly from Golgi apparatus containing a number of enzymes like *hyaluronidase* and *other proteolytic enzymes,* which *play role in fertilization*. Acrosome enzymes help in **causing penetration of sperm through granulosa and zona pellucida of the ovum to cause fertilization.**
- Tail of the sperm is called the **flagellum**. It has three main components:
  1. Central skeleton called axoneme made of 9+2 microtubules.
  2. Thin covering of axoneme
  3. Collection of mitochondria surrounding axoneme.
  
  **Function of flagellum:** Back and forth movement of tail causes motility for the sperm. Energy is supplied by ATP from mitochondria. Normal sperm can move in a straight line at a velocity of 1 to 4 mm/min.

### Maturation of the Sperm (Fig. 75.5)

Both the testis form around 120 million sperms/day. These sperms are nonflagellate, nonmotile and incapable of fertilizing the ovum. These sperms then enter the 6-meter-long epididymis and undergo maturation during this stay, which could be as long as 1 month or shorter, depending on the number of ejaculates. Within 18 to 24 hours into epididymis, the sperms become flagellate and motile but

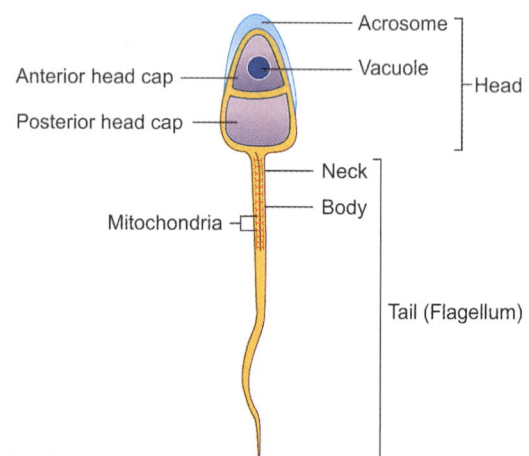

Fig. 75.4: Structure of sperm.

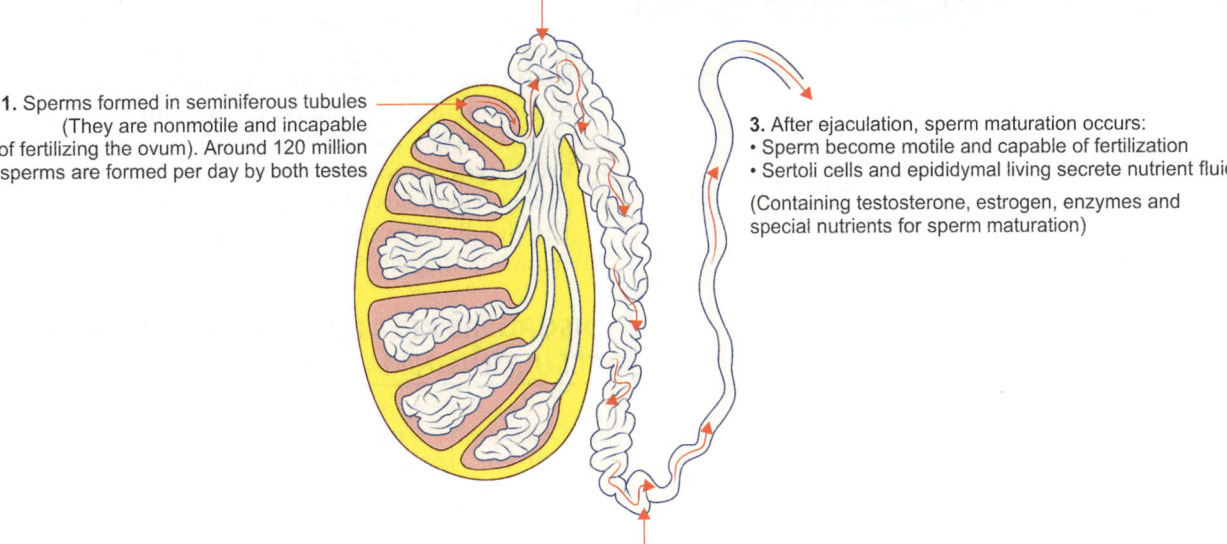

**Fig. 75.5:** Maturation of sperm in testes.

still are incapable of fertilization as they are inhibited by certain substances in the epididymis.

Most of the sperms are stored in epididymis and a few in vas deferens. The sperms in epididymis are fertile but inactivated. They are activated at the time of ejaculation when the nutrient fluid secreted by Sertoli cells and lining of epididymis is added in the ejaculate. This fluid is rich in hormones (testosterone, estrogen), enzymes and nutrients. The sperm becomes very active in female genital tract owing to increase in temperature. The life span of a sperm in testis is many weeks, whereas in the female genital tract is 1–2 days. Motile and fertile sperms show flagellated movement at a rate of 1 to 4 mm/min.

## SEMINAL VESICLE

The seminal vesicles secrete a *mucoid material* rich in **fructose, citric acid, prostaglandins and fibrinogen**, into the ejaculatory duct.

### Functions:
- It **increases the bulk of semen**
- It provides **nutrition** to the sperm
- Prostaglandins **aids in fertilization** of ovum by reacting with cervical mucus and making it more receptive to sperm motility. It also increases the reverse peristalsis in fallopian tubules, which allows the sperm to reach the upper end of fallopian tubes within 5 minutes.

## PROSTATE GLAND

The prostate glands secrete **thin, milky fluid rich in calcium, citrate ion, phosphate, clotting factor and profibrinolysin.** It is secreted at the same time, when the vas deference pushes the sperms into the ejaculatory duct.

### Functions:
- It adds to the **bulk** of semen
- The **alkaline pH** of prostatic fluid aids in the fertilization by two ways:
  1. By **neutralizing the acidic pH of the fluid** in the vas deferens which keeps the sperms inhibited in inactive state.
  2. By **neutralizing the acidic vaginal pH** and creating the favorable atmosphere for sperm motility and fertility. **The sperms exhibit maximum motility at a pH of 6.0–6.5.**

## SEMEN

### Composition of Semen

The seminal volume is formed by following main constituents:
- Fluid and sperms ejaculated from vas deferens (10%).
- **Seminal fluid (60%):** Gives the mucoid consistency to semen.
- **Prostatic fluid (30%):** Gives milky appearance to the semen.
- Mucus secreted by bulbourethral glands.
- **Clotting enzyme:** It is present in the prostatic fluid. This results in the formation of the fibrin coagulum due to the activation of the fibrinogen. It hold the semen deep in the vagina, close to the uterine cervix.
- **Hormones:** Testosterone and estrogen.
- **Other substances:** Fructose, citric acid, prostaglandins etc.

**Table 75.2:** WHO guidelines for semen analysis (2022).

|  | Normal values |
|---|---|
| Volume | ≥1.5 mL |
| pH | 7.2–8.0 |
| Appearance | Opalescent |
| Liquefaction time | Maximum 40 minutes |
| Concentration of sperms | Minimum 15 million/mL or ≥39 million/ejaculate |
| Sperm motility | ≥32% |
| Total motility | ≥40% |
| Morphology | ≥4% normal |
| Leukocytes | <1 million/mL |

**Table 75.2** discusses the normal values of various parameter of semen.

## Fate of Semen in the Vagina

The thick coagulum of semen in deeper vagina, keeps the sperm entrapped and nonmotile for first few minutes of ejaculation. After 15–30 minutes, the prostatic profibrinolysin results in the *liquefaction* of the coagulum. In this phase, the sperms get activated and show active motility. After ejaculation, maximum life span of sperm is 24 to 48 hours at body temperature.

> **Sperm Banks**
> The donor sperms can be stored in the sperm banks at –100°C for years and can be thawed and used as replacement for patients with male infertility.

## Capacitation of Spermatozoa

Various *changes taking place in sperms, in female genital tract*, which enables it to fertilize the ovum is known as capacitation of the sperms. It takes 1 to 10 hours for changes to occur.

These changes can be summarized as:
- Fluid present in the fallopian tubes and uterus washes out inhibitory factors suppressing sperm activity.
- The cholesterol vesicles present in the seminal fluid strengthens the acrosomal membrane. However, in the female genital tract, the sperms swim away from the cholesterol vesicles, which results in the weakening of the acrosomal wall.
- Membrane of sperm becomes permeable to calcium which increases motility and facilitates release of enzymes from acrosome, hence facilitating the sperm penetration into the zona pellucida.

*Capacitation of the sperm is an important step, before the fertilization.* In its absence, the fertilization does not take place.

### Acrosome Reaction

The acrosome of the sperm has the large amount of hyaluronidase and the proteolytic enzymes.
- **Hyaluronidase enzyme:** It depolymerizes the hyaluronic acid polymers which holds together the granulosa cells of ovum.
- **Proteolytic enzyme:** Results in the digestion of the structural proteins adhering to the ovum.

The details of male sexual act and fertilization are discussed in Chapter 77.

## DISORDERS RELATED TO SPERMATOGENESIS, RESULTING IN MALE INFERTILITY

> Oligozoospermia—reduced sperm count
> Asthenozoospermia—reduced sperm motility
> Teratozoospermia—reduced percentage of sperm with normal morphology.
> Oligoasthenoteratozoospermia—combination of above.
> Azoospermia—absence of sperm in the ejaculate.

### Bilateral Orchitis

Many viral diseases like mumps, can result in the inflammation of the seminiferous tubular epithelium. This adversely affects spermatogenesis and hence results in male sterility/infertility. Also, children born with congenital degeneration of testicular epithelium can develop sterility in adulthood.

### Effect of Increased Temperature

Spermatogenesis require a slightly lower temperature (around 2°C) than the body temperature. But if, the person is exposed to higher environmental temperature due to his occupation or any other reason may result in decreased sperm count. The scrotal sacs play an important role in maintaining the temperature of the testes during summers and winters resulting in controlled cooling. In winter the scrotal muscles contract and pull the testes close to body to maintain the temperature.

### Cryptorchidism

During the embryonic life, the testes develop in the abdominal cavity and descend into the scrotal sac through the inguinal canal at about 3 weeks to 1 month before the birth. Sometimes, the testis fail to descend into the scrotum and remain in abdomen or inguinal canal. These undescended testes are incapable of making the sperms and result in sterility. However, if this condition is diagnosed in childhood, the testis could be surgically positioned into the scrotum, before the onset of puberty.

The main reason for undescended testes is abnormal secretion of testosterone by fetal testes. So, these patients may not show good results in terms of sperm production.

## Decreased Sperm Count

Normally around 3.5 mL of semen is ejaculated during a single sexual act. Each milliliter of semen contains around 120 million sperms (range of 35 million to 400 million sperms per mL). If the sperm count falls below 20 million/mL, the person is likely to be infertile.

## Abnormal Sperm Morphology and Motility

The normal sperm morphology and motility is required for fertilization. The abnormal sperm shapes, shown in **Figure 75.6** render an individual infertile. The normal sperm motility after capacitation is forward moving with whiplash movement of the flagellum. In case the sperms show nondirectional movement or abnormal flagellar movement, will also result in infertility.

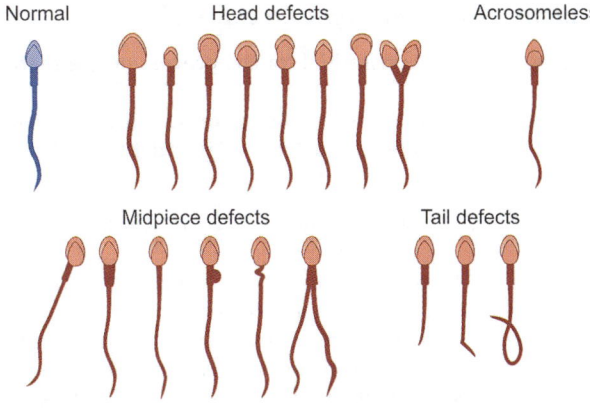

**Fig. 75.6:** Different sperm morphological abnormalities.

## SUMMARY

- This chapter provides a comprehensive overview of the functional and histological anatomy of the male reproductive system, focusing on the testes and the synthesis of male sex hormones. It also delves into the intricate process of spermatogenesis and the evaluation of semen samples.
- The chapter begins by detailing the functional anatomy of the male reproductive system, including the testes, epididymis, vas deferens, and accessory glands. It highlights the roles of these structures in sperm production, storage, and transport, as well as in the synthesis and secretion of seminal fluid.
- Furthermore, the histological anatomy of the testes is explored, elucidating the structure and functions of various testicular cells such as Sertoli cells, Leydig cells, and germ cells. The synthesis and physiological effects of male sex hormones, particularly testosterone, are discussed in relation to reproductive and nonreproductive functions.
- Moreover, the chapter provides a comprehensive overview of spermatogenesis, detailing the stages of sperm development from spermatogonia to mature spermatozoa. It examines the factors influencing spermatogenesis, including hormonal regulation, temperature regulation, and nutritional factors.
- Additionally, the chapter analyzes the evaluation of semen samples, focusing on parameters such as sperm count, sperm morphology, and sperm motility according to World Health Organization (WHO) guidelines. It discusses the significance of these parameters in assessing male fertility and reproductive health, as well as the implications of abnormalities in semen analysis.
- Overall, this chapter offers valuable insights into the intricate processes of male reproductive physiology, from the anatomical structures involved in sperm production to the evaluation of semen quality. It serves as a comprehensive resource for understanding male reproductive health and fertility assessment.

## LET US SEE, HOW MUCH YOU HAVE LEARNT?

### Review Questions

#### Long/Short Answer Questions

Q1. Describe the functions of Sertoli cells.
Q2. Describe the functions of Leydig cells.
Q3. Describe the process of maturation of sperms in testis.
Q4. Describe the functions of seminal and prostatic fluid in the semen.
Q5. Describe the normal composition and functions of each component in the semen.
Q6. What would happen to sperm count in a patient with undescended testis?
Q7. Write short notes on:
 a. Capacitation
 b. Acrosome reaction
Q8. Describe the changes occurring in the semen in the female vagina.

## Explain Why? (Reasoning Questions)

Q1. Testosterone is essential for the process of spermatogenesis.
Q2. Deficiency in follicle-stimulating hormone (FSH) can lead to reduced sperm production and infertility in males.
Q3. How conditions like cryptorchidism (undescended testes) can impair fertility?
Q4. Proper temperature regulation of the testes is crucial for effective spermatogenesis.

## Critical Thinking Case-Based Questions

Q1. Ravi, a 34-year-old man, visited a fertility clinic with his wife after trying to conceive for over a year without success. His medical history was unremarkable, but a semen analysis revealed a low sperm count (oligospermia) and poor sperm motility. Blood tests showed low levels of testosterone and elevated levels of follicle-stimulating hormone (FSH) and luteinizing hormone (LH). Further examination indicated small testes.

Based upon the given history, answer the following questions:
a. Explain the physiological processes involved in spermatogenesis.
b. Discuss the role of male hormones in this process, and discuss how hormonal imbalances could lead to Ravi's clinical presentation of infertility.
c. Enumerate other disorders related to male infertility.

## Multiple Choice Questions

Q1. What is the primary function of Leydig cells in the testes?
 a. Sperm production
 b. Synthesis of testosterone
 c. Sperm storage
 d. Seminal fluid secretion

Q2. Which structure is responsible for the storage and maturation of spermatozoa?
 a. Seminiferous tubules
 b. Epididymis
 c. Vas deferens
 d. Prostate gland

Q3. What type of cells form the blood-testis barrier and provide support to developing germ cells?
 a. Leydig cells
 b. Spermatogonia
 c. Sertoli cells
 d. Myoid cells

Q4. Which hormone stimulates the production of testosterone by Leydig cells?
 a. Luteinizing hormone (LH)
 b. Follicle-stimulating hormone (FSH)
 c. Estrogen
 d. Prolactin

Q5. What is the primary function of Sertoli cells in spermatogenesis?
 a. Synthesis of testosterone
 b. Secretion of seminal fluid
 c. Support and nourishment of germ cells
 d. Storage of mature spermatozoa

Q6. Which of the following is NOT a stage of spermatogenesis?
 a. Spermiogenesis
 b. Spermatocytogenesis
 c. Spermatogenesis
 d. Spermiocytogenesis

Q7. What is the approximate duration of spermatogenesis in humans?
 a. 30 days
 b. 60 days
 c. 90 days
 d. 120 days

Q8. Which parameter of semen analysis assesses the concentration of spermatozoa in a semen sample?
 a. Sperm motility
 b. Sperm count
 c. Sperm morphology
 d. Seminal fluid volume

Q9. What is the normal range of sperm count according to WHO guidelines?
 a. >10 million sperm per mL
 b. >15 million sperm per mL
 c. >20 million sperm per mL
 d. >30 million sperm per mL

Q10. What does abnormal sperm morphology indicate in semen analysis?
 a. Low sperm count
 b. Reduced sperm motility
 c. Structural defects in sperm cells
 d. Increased seminal fluid volume

Q11. What is the function of the seminal vesicles in semen production?
 a. Sperm storage
 b. Sperm maturation
 c. Synthesis of testosterone
 d. Secretion of seminal fluid components

Q12. Which hormone stimulates the contraction of smooth muscle in the male reproductive system during ejaculation?
 a. Testosterone
 b. Estrogen
 c. Oxytocin
 d. Prolactin

Q13. What is the primary function of the prostate gland in semen production?
 a. Sperm storage
 b. Neutralization of acidic vaginal pH
 c. Secretion of alkaline fluid
 d. Synthesis of testosterone

Q14. What is the function of the Cowper's (bulbourethral) glands in semen production?
   a. Sperm storage
   b. Secretion of seminal fluid
   c. Synthesis of testosterone
   d. Regulation of testicular temperature

Q15. What is the role of fructose in seminal fluid?
   a. Energy source for sperm motility
   b. Alkaline buffer to neutralize vaginal acidity
   c. Antimicrobial agent to prevent infection
   d. Structural component of sperm cells

Q16. A couple has been trying to conceive for over a year without success. They decide to undergo fertility testing, and the male partner provides a semen sample for analysis. The results show a sperm count of 10 million sperm per mL. What is the most likely interpretation of this finding?
   a. Normal sperm count according to WHO guidelines
   b. Borderline low sperm count, requiring further evaluation
   c. High sperm count, indicating optimal fertility
   d. Absence of sperm in the semen sample

Q17. A 35-year-old male presents with concerns about his fertility. He underwent semen analysis, which revealed normal sperm count and motility but abnormal sperm morphology according to WHO guidelines. What is the most appropriate next step in management?
   a. Initiate hormone replacement therapy
   b. Perform genetic testing for chromosomal abnormalities
   c. Repeat semen analysis to confirm findings
   d. Recommend assisted reproductive techniques such as intracytoplasmic sperm injection (ICSI)

## ANSWERS

1. b    2. b    3. c    4. a    5. c    6. d    7. c    8. b    9. c    10. c    11. d    12. c    13. c    14. b
15. a    16. b    17. d

# Reproductive Physiology in Females

**76 CHAPTER**

> **COMPETENCY ADDRESSED**
>
> **PY9.4:** Describe female reproductive system: (a) functions of ovary and its control; (b) menstrual cycle—hormonal, uterine and ovarian changes.

>  **LEARNING OBJECTIVES**
>
> **At the end of this chapter, the learner should be able to:**
> - Describe the functional anatomy of the female reproductive tract.
> - Describe the process of oogenesis in terms of stages factors affecting it and regulation.
> - Describe the menstrual cycle in terms of:
>   – Ovarian changes
>   – Hormonal changes
>   – Endometrial changes
>   – Cervical mucus changes
> - Describe the process of ovulation, factors affecting it and the indicators of ovulation.

## FUNCTIONAL ANATOMY OF FEMALE REPRODUCTIVE SYSTEM

The main organs of human female reproductive system include ovaries, fallopian tubes, uterus, and vagina. The **Figure 76.1** shows various parts of the female genital tract. The main functions of the various parts of the human female reproductive tract are given below:

**Ovaries:** The ovaries have the female germ cells which forms the female gamete (ovum) during each monthly sexual cycle (menstrual cycle).

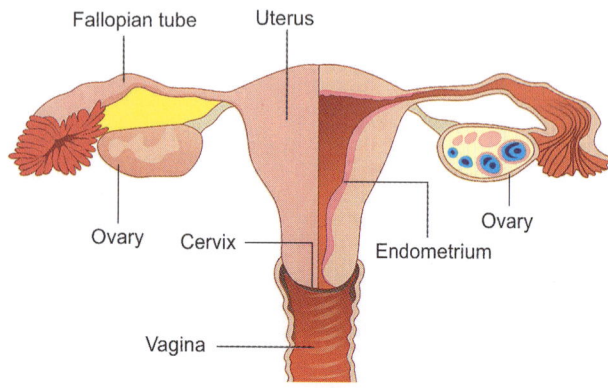

**Fig. 76.1:** Female reproductive system.

**Fallopian tubes:** They are the muscular tubes which provides the pathway for the ovum to travel from the ovary towards the uterine cavity. The fallopian tube acts as the site for fertilization of the ovum by sperms.

**Uterus:** The uterus prepares itself every month to receive the fertilized ovum, during the reproductive period of the life. If the ovum doesn't get fertilized it sheds the endometrial lining to prepare for the next monthly cycle.

## OOGENESIS (FORMATION OF OVUM) (FIG. 76.2)

During embryonic life, the primordial germ cells reach the germinal epithelium and differentiate into **oogonia** or **primordial ova**. These primordial ova are then surrounded by the epithelioid like cells, derived from ovarian stroma, called *granulosa cells*. The primordial ova surrounded by the granulosa cells is called a *primordial follicle*. This ovum, is still immature and is called a *primary oocyte*. During the **fifth month of fetal life**, the oogonia start the **first meiotic division**, but it is **arrested in prophase I until puberty**. **At birth**, there are 1 to 2 million ova present in the ovary at **stage of primary oocytes**. The first meiotic division is completed at puberty, where each primary oocyte divides into a large ovum (secondary oocyte) and a small

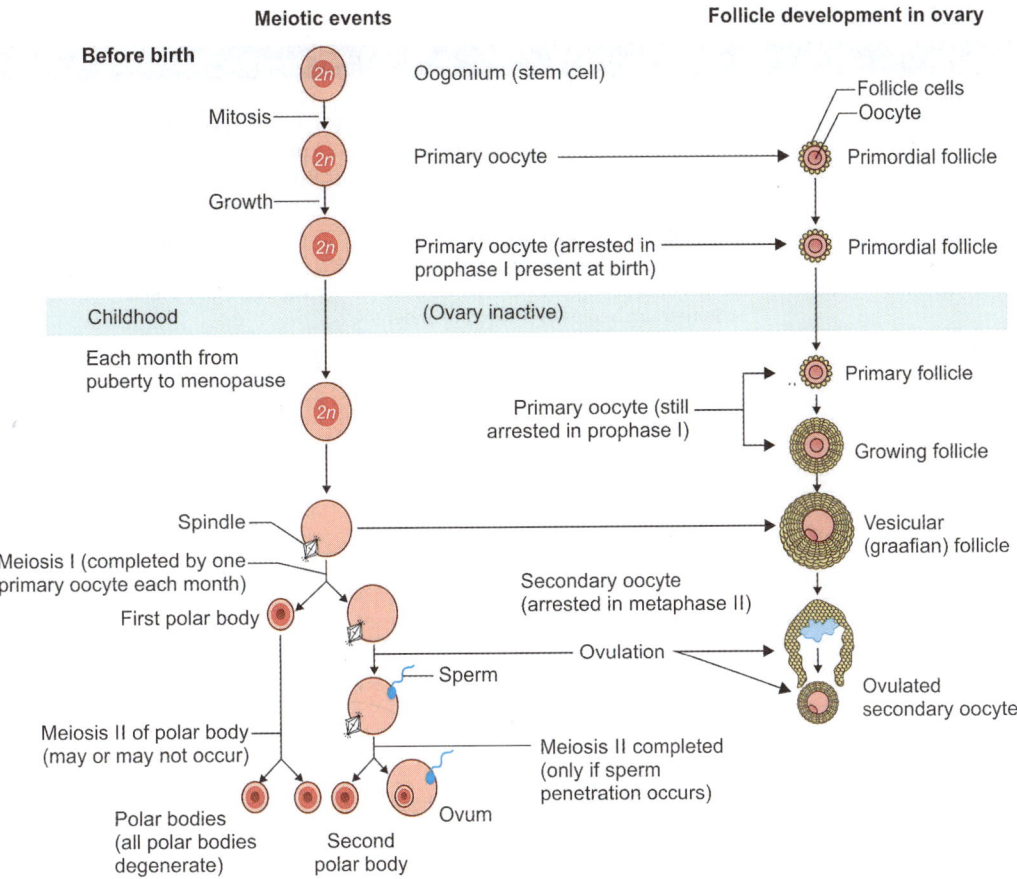

**Fig. 76.2:** Stages of formation of ovum.

polar body with haploid number (23) of chromosomes in each. The ovum then undergoes *second meiotic division*, which **arrests in metaphase II**, until fertilization of ovum. This **second meiotic division gets completed only during fertilization** and a second polar body is released along with the formation of zygote.

## THE FEMALE SEXUAL CYCLE (MENSTRUAL CYCLE)

The regular monthly changes in the ovary, the lining of the uterus (endometrium), occur during the reproductive period of females (i.e., from menarche to menopause).

*Menarche* is the onset of the first menstrual cycle at puberty, usually between 10 to 14 years of age, due to a progressive increase in the secretion of FSH and LH, beginning at the age of 8-12 years. The end of reproductive life in women is marked by **menopause**, usually occurring between 40-50 years of life. This period is marked by **a gradual decline** in **ovarian activity** and **female sex hormones**.

The duration of each female sexual cycle is 26-32 days (average 28 days). Depending on the various hormonal, ovarian and endometrial changes it is divided into two main phases as shown in **Table 76.1**. Complete menstrual cycle with its hormonal control is shown in **Figure 76.3**.

## Follicular Development in Ovary

### The Primordial Follicle

We have seen earlier that at birth, the child has **primordial follicle** in the ovaries, which has the primary oocyte surrounded by a single layer of granulosa cells. During childhood, till puberty, the granulosa cells provide nurture the oocyte and also secretes the **oocyte maturation inhibiting factor**, which keeps the primary oocyte in the stage of *meiotic arrest at prophase I*.

### Formation of Primary Follicle

But when the anterior pituitary of the child begins to secrete FSH and LH at puberty, the ovaries begin to grow resulting in the moderate enlargement of ovum initially. Every month, the cyclical increase in the levels of FSH and LH stimulates the growth of many follicles. The growing follicles add up additional layers of granulosa cells and transform to form **primary follicles**.

### Formation of Secondary Follicle

Before we study the structure and formation of secondary follicle, we must understand the role of pituitary hormones

Table 76.1: Phases of menstrual cycle.

| | From day 1 to day 14 | From day 14 to day 28 |
|---|---|---|
| On the basis of ovarian changes | It is called the **preovulatory or follicular phase,** due to the follicular development of the primary, secondary follicle and antral follicle leading to ovulation | Since the ovulation has already taken place, this phase is called **postovulatory or luteal phase.** After ovulation, the follicle proliferates and secretes a large quantity of *progesterone* and *estrogen* |
| On the basis of uterine changes | The endometrium is shed during the initial 1–5 days resulting in the bleeding phase of the menstrual cycle. After the 5th day, the endometrium begins to proliferate under the effect of estrogen secreted by the antral follicle. Hence called **the proliferative phase** | The endometrium further proliferates and produces abundant secretions, hence called **the secretory phase** |
| Main Hormone | Estrogen | Progesterone |

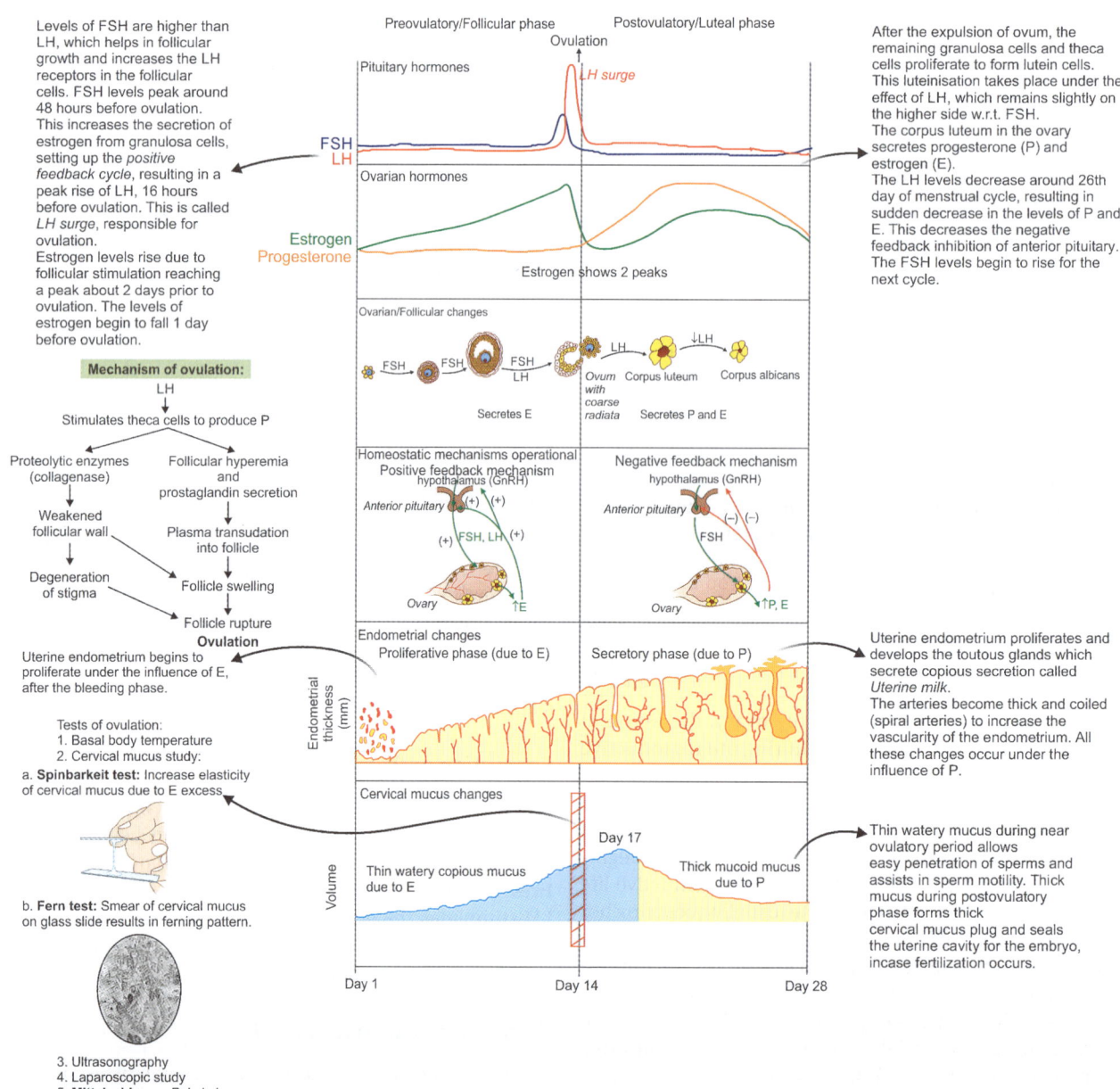

Fig. 76.3: Menstrual cycle and hormonal control of it.

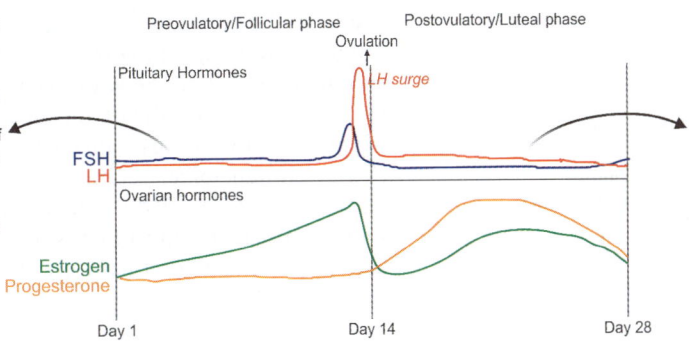

Levels of FSH are higher than LH, which helps in follicular growth and increases the LH receptors in the follicular cells. FSH levels peak around 48 hours before ovulation. This increases the secretion of estrogen from granulosa cells, setting up the *positive feedback cycle*, resulting in a peak rise of LH, 16 hours before ovulation. This is called *LH surge*, responsible for ovulation.
Estrogen levels rise due to follicular stimulation reaching, a peak about 2 days prior to ovulation. The levels of estrogen begin to fall 1 day before ovulation.

After the expulsion of ovum, the remaining granulosa cells and theca cells proliferate to form lutein cells. This luteinization takes place under the effect of LH, which remains slightly on the higher side w.r.t. FSH.
The corpus luteum in the ovary secretes progesterone (P) and estrogen (E). The LH levels decrease around 26th day of menstrual cycle, resulting in sudden decrease in the levels of P and E. This decreases the negative feedback inhibition of anterior pituitary. The FSH levels begin to rise for the next cycle.

**Fig. 76.4:** Role of FSH and LH in preovulatory and postovulatory phases.

in folliculogenesis (the details of gonadotropins are given in the chapter on reproductive hormones) **(Fig. 76.4)**.

- **Role of follicle stimulating hormone:** The FSH, is secreted by the anterior pituitary gland. During the first half of the female sexual cycle (Day 1 to day 14 of a 28-day cycle; where day 1 refers to the first day of the bleeding phase of the menstrual cycle), the levels of FSH rise and are slightly higher than the levels of luteinizing hormone (LH). The FSH:
  - **Stimulates the growth of 6–12 follicles** each month, where the follicles grow in size and add up the additional layers of the granulosa cells, up to the antral stage.
  - It also stimulates the **addition of** a second type of cells to the follicle called the **theca cells**.
  - FSH along with estrogen promotes the LH receptors on granulosa cells which results in a synergistic effect of LH and FSH on follicular development.
- **Role of luteinizing hormone:** During the first half of menstrual cycle the level of LH is slightly less than FSH, but it shows an increase, as it progresses towards day 14. The estrogen secreted by follicular cells along with LH results in the proliferation of follicular theca cells and results in the secretion of estrogen (positive feedback cycle).

### Structure of Secondary Follicle

- **Granulosa cells:** They are the multiple layers of epithelioid cells.
- **Theca cells** are epithelioid cells forming the outer layer of the secondary follicle.
- **Zona pellucida:** The granulosa cells secrete glassy material containing mucopolysaccharides forming a thick layer between oocyte and granulosa cells.

### Formation of Tertiary/Antral Follicle

- **Early antral follicle:**
  - *Theca cells:* Early theca cells of secondary follicle differentiate into theca interna and theca externa.
    - *Theca interna:* Epithelioid cells, similar to granulosa cells. They secrete sex steroids hormones, estrogen and progesterone.
    - *Theca externa:* Develop into a highly vascular connective tissue capsule of developing follicle and provides mechanical support from outside. Theca cells receive blood, lymphatic and nerve supply.
  - *Granulosa cells:* They proliferate in last few days of follicular development. They are avascular. They acquire FSH receptors. They secrete estrogen and fill up the antral cavity with the follicular fluid. Further maturation of the follicle is FSH dependent.
- **Late graafian/antral follicle:** This stage is reached only in the occurs in postpubertal ovary. Only a single follicle with abundant FSH receptors become the dominant follicle called the *"graafian follicle"*. The nondominant follicles undergo degeneration called atresia.

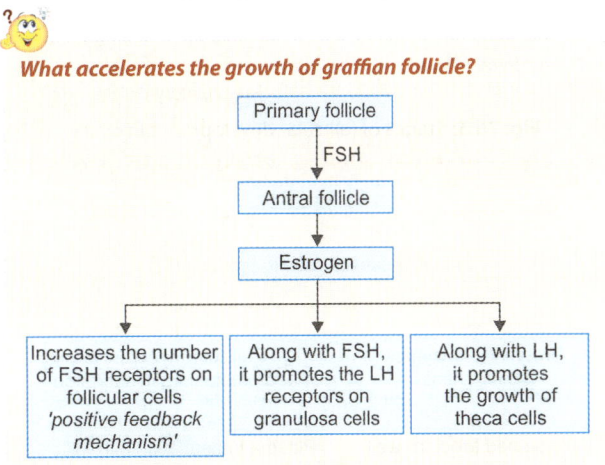

This follicle has a large antrum filled with follicular fluid, rich in estrogen, progesterone, FSH, LH, prolactin, androstenedione, growth factors, inhibin, activins, GnRH, CRH, opioid peptide and oxytocin. This follicle becomes preovulatory follicle.

Summary of stages of follicular development is shown in **Figure 76.5**.

### Ovulation

Extrusion of ovum from the mature graafian follicle at day 14 of the menstrual cycle occur. The mechanism of ovulation is postulated below **(Fig. 76.6)**:

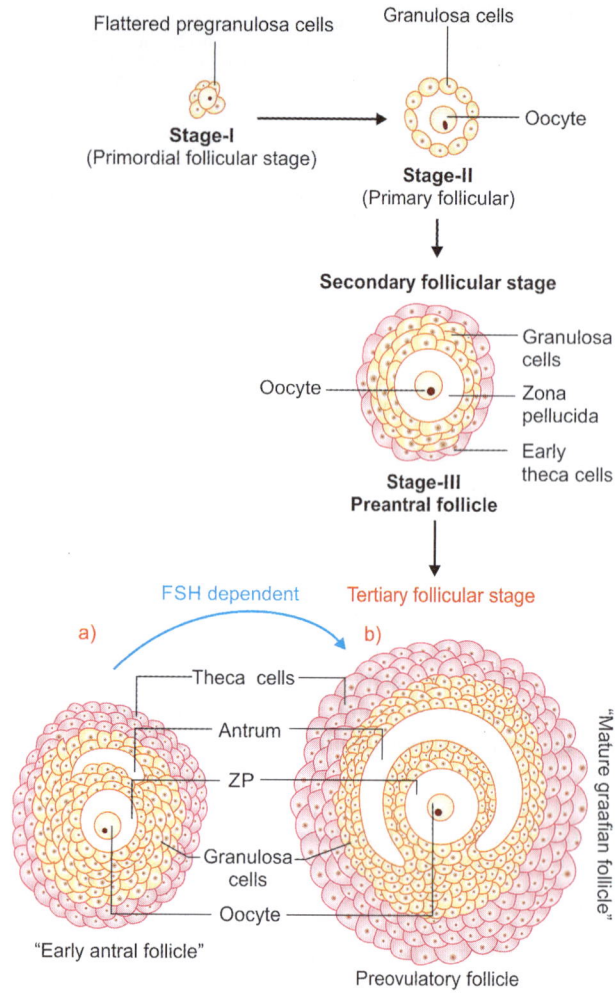

**Fig. 76.5:** Stages of follicular development in ovary.

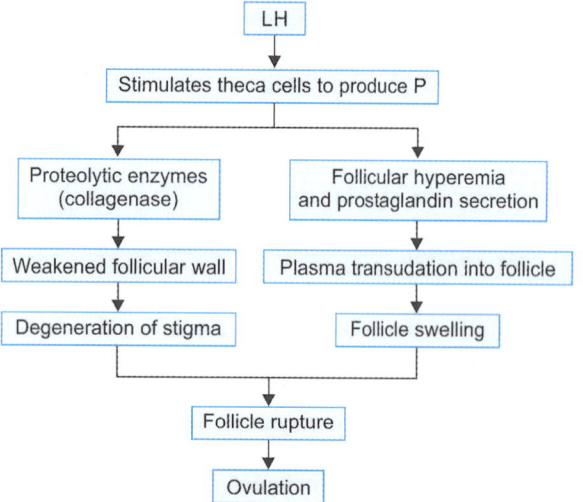

**Fig. 76.6:** Mechanism of ovulation.

A few hours before ovulation, the proteolysis of the basement membrane occurs close to the surface of the ovary, along with the rapid swelling of the follicle. This results in the protrusion of a stigma like a nipple. In a few minutes, fluid begins to ooze from the nipple resulting in rupture of follicle along with release of viscous fluid. The viscous fluid carries the ovum surrounded by a thousand of small granulosa cells, called corona radiata.

The remnant follicle, comprising of some granulosa cells and theca cells forms the *lutein cells*. These cells enlarge and get filled with lipid inclusions giving them a yellow appearance called *luteinization*. The corpus luteum is well vascularized.

- The **granulosa cells** in the corpus luteum actively form the hormones mainly **progesterone** and less **estrogen**.
- **Theca cells** mainly form the **androgens, androstenedione and testosterone**. These hormones are converted into estrogen by aromatase in the granulosa cells.

The ovum is released and taken up by the fallopian tube. Depending upon fertilization, the released ovum can have either fate:

- *If fertilization occurs*, due to penetration of the ovum by sperm, there is completion of 2nd meiotic division resulting in the formation of a zygote. The zygote gets implanted in the endometrium of the uterine cavity and results in the secretion of *human chorionic gonadotropin (hCG)* from the chorionic trophoblasts. The hCG luteinizes the corpus luteum and converts it into the *corpus luteum of pregnancy*. This secrets the progesterone for the first trimester, till the placenta takes over the endocrine function.
- *If fertilization does not occur*, as happens in most of the monthly cycles, oocyte begins to degenerate within 24–48 hours. The ruptured follicle gets filled with blood called *corpus hemorrhagicum*, in which cells of the follicle proliferate and replace blood with luteal cells, rich in lipids called *corpus luteum* (discussed above). This corpus luteum degenerates in 13 days, becomes necrotic 'luteolysis'. The corpus luteum becomes avascular and fibrous called *corpus albicans*. The lutein cells also secrete a small amount of inhibin, which inhibits FSH secretion from anterior pituitary. Low levels of FSH and LH result in involution of corpus luteum. This degeneration occurs in about 12 days, i.e., on 26th day of menstrual cycle. Sudden cessation of estrogen, progesterone and inhibin secretion by corpus luteum removes the negative feedback from anterior pituitary. This increases the FSH and LH levels, hence initiating the follicular development for the next cycle.

## Functions of Corpus Luteum

- Secretes the steroidal hormones during luteal phase (progesterone, estrogen, inhibin and androgens)
- Provides endocrinal environment for implantation of ovum
- Maintains early part of pregnancy by secreting progesterone, till placenta becomes functional

### Indicators of Ovulation

- **Basal body temperature:** The basal body temperature, rises just after ovulation due to the thermogenic effect of progesterone. Hence, continuous monitoring of early morning basal body temperature recording.
- **Mittelschmerz:** There is mid cycle pain in lower abdomen, at the time of ovulation, due to rupture of follicle.
- **Vaginal discharge:** Thin, copious and watery discharge; under the influence of estrogen.
- **Spinnbarkeit test:** Cervical mucus can be stretched like a thread up to 10 cm or more, under the influence of estrogen, around the ovulation.
- **Fern test:** Appearance of fern-like pattern on smear of cervical mucus on the slide; under the influence of estrogen.
- **Laparoscopic examination:** Direct observation of ovarian follicles through laparoscopic examination.
- **Plasma LH levels:** To study the duration LH surge, for the confirmation of ovulation.

## UTERINE CHANGES

The uterine cycle is divided into three phases **(Fig. 76.7)**:
1. Bleeding phase
2. Proliferative phase

These two phases correspond with the follicular phase of the ovarian cycle (predominant hormone estrogen)
- **Secretory phase,** corresponds with the luteal phase (predominant hormone-progesterone).
- **Bleeding phase:** Starts with day 1 of menstrual cycle. There is bleeding per vaginum, due to sloughing of the endometrium and blood vessels.
- **Proliferative phase:** Begins after the bleeding phase. The endometrial lining is thin in the beginning. There is proliferation of the endometrium, endometrial glands and the blood supply of the endometrium. The endometrium is prepared for implantation. Changes occur due to high estrogen content.
- **Secretory phase:** It begins after ovulation due to increased progesterone content. Estrogen shows small secondary increase. Endometrium becomes thick and endometrial glands become thick, tortuous and starts secreting the uterine secretions known as uterine milk. Spiral arteries become enlarged, coiled and torturous. These uterine changes occur to provide nourishment to the developing embryo. If pregnancy doesn't occur, there is decrease in the progesterone levels, resulting in reduced blood supply to the endometrium. There is focal necrosis of endometrium, leading to sloughing off of the endometrium and hence the bleeding phase.

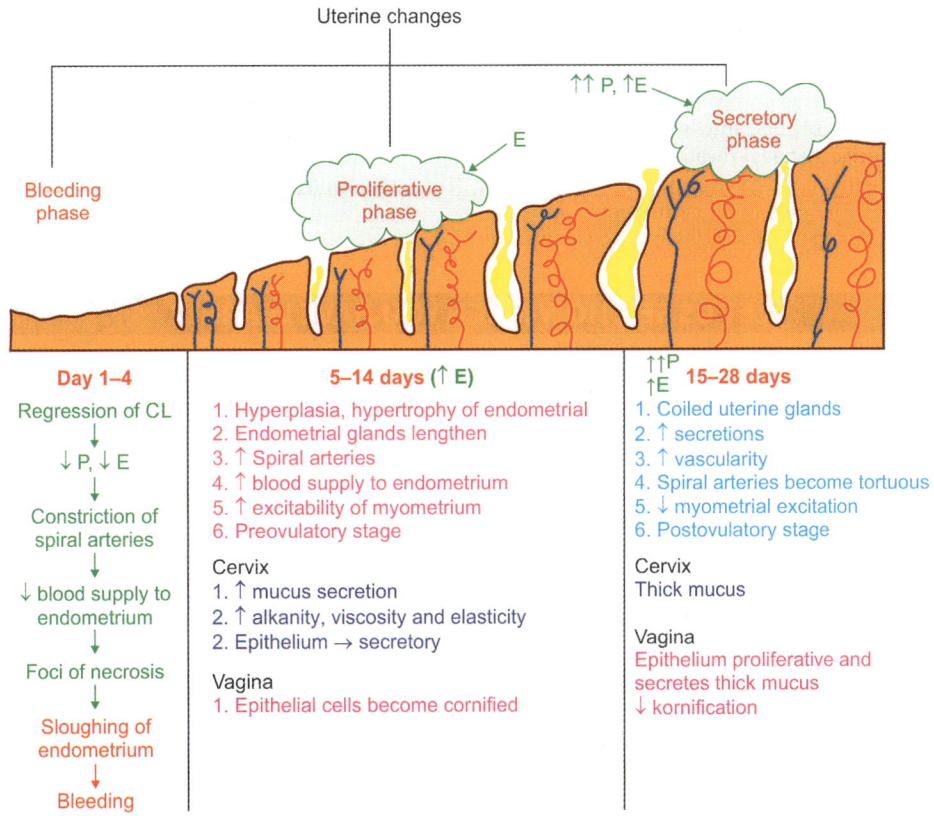

**Fig. 76.7:** Uterine changes in menstrual cycle.

## SUMMARY

- The female reproductive tract consists of several organs that work together to facilitate reproduction.
  - *Ovaries:* Paired organs located on either side of the uterus, responsible for producing eggs (ova) and hormones like estrogen and progesterone.
  - *Fallopian tubes (oviducts):* Two tubes that extend from the ovaries to the uterus, providing a pathway for eggs to travel from the ovaries to the uterus. Fertilization typically occurs in the fallopian tubes.
  - *Uterus:* A hollow, muscular organ where a fertilized egg implants and develops into a fetus during pregnancy.
  - *Cervix:* The lower portion of the uterus that connects to the vagina. It produces cervical mucus that changes in consistency throughout the menstrual cycle.
  - *Vagina:* A muscular canal that connects the cervix to the external genitalia. It serves as the birth canal during childbirth and also facilitates menstruation.
- Oogenesis refers to the process of egg cell development in the ovaries. It occurs in several stages:
  - *Oogonium stage:* During fetal development, oogonia (primordial germ cells) proliferate via mitosis.
  - Oogonia undergo mitotic divisions to form primary oocytes, which become arrested in prophase I of meiosis until puberty.
  - Each month, one or more primary oocytes resume meiosis due to hormonal stimulation, resulting in the release of a secondary oocyte from the ovary during ovulation.
  - If the secondary oocyte is fertilized by a sperm cell, it completes meiosis II to form a mature ovum (egg) and a second polar body.
  - Factors affecting oogenesis include hormonal regulation (gonadotropins such as FSH and LH), age, and certain medical conditions or environmental factors.
- The menstrual cycle is divided into several phases, each characterized by specific changes in ovarian hormones, ovarian follicles, the endometrium, and cervical mucus:
  - *Ovarian changes:* The menstrual cycle begins with the follicular phase, during which follicles in the ovary mature under the influence of follicle-stimulating hormone (FSH). Ovulation occurs around mid-cycle when a mature follicle ruptures and releases an egg.
  - *Hormonal changes:* Follicle development is primarily regulated by FSH and luteinizing hormone (LH), which stimulate estrogen production by the ovaries. After ovulation, LH surge triggers the release of the egg and stimulates the formation of the corpus luteum, which produces progesterone.
  - *Endometrial changes:* In the menstrual cycle, the endometrium undergoes cyclic changes in response to estrogen and progesterone. Following ovulation, the endometrium thickens and becomes more vascularized to prepare for embryo implantation. If fertilization does not occur, estrogen and progesterone levels decline, leading to endometrial shedding (menstruation).
  - *Cervical mucus changes:* Cervical mucus changes in consistency throughout the menstrual cycle, becoming thinner and more slippery around ovulation to facilitate sperm transport.
- Ovulation is the release of a mature egg from the ovary into the fallopian tube, where it can be fertilized by sperm. It is influenced by various factors:
  - *Hormonal regulation:* Ovulation is triggered by a surge in luteinizing hormone (LH) from the anterior pituitary gland, which occurs around mid-cycle.
  - *Follicular development:* Ovulation is preceded by the maturation of ovarian follicles under the influence of follicle-stimulating hormone (FSH).
  - *Factors affecting ovulation:* Factors such as stress, hormonal imbalances, and certain medical conditions (e.g., polycystic ovary syndrome) can affect ovulation.
  - *Indicators of ovulation:* Common indicators of ovulation include changes in cervical mucus consistency, basal body temperature (which typically rises after ovulation), and ovulation predictor kits that detect the surge in LH.

## LET US SEE, HOW MUCH YOU HAVE LEARNT?

 *Review Questions*

### Long/Short Answer Questions

Q1. Describe the process of ovulation and its regulation.
Q2. Draw a well labeled self-explanatory diagram showing the changes in hormones, ovarian follicle and uterine endometrium.
Q3. Describe the tests for ovulation.
Q4. Describe the mechanism of ovulation.

### Explain Why? (Reasoning Questions)

Q1. The basal body temperature rises at the time of ovulation.
Q2. The surge in luteinizing hormone (LH) mid-cycle triggers ovulation and the release of an egg from the ovarian follicle.
Q3. The shedding of the uterine lining occurs if fertilization does not take place.

## Critical Thinking Case-Based Questions

**Q1.** Maya, a 28-year-old woman, visited her gynecologist with concerns about irregular menstrual cycles and difficulty conceiving. She reported menstrual cycles varying in length from 25 to 35 days and was unsure about the timing of ovulation. Maya had been trying to conceive for over a year without success. She had no significant medical history, and her partner's fertility had been confirmed normal.

Based on the given case scenario, answer the following questions:
a. Explain the physiological phases of the menstrual cycle and the process of ovulation.
b. Discuss how irregularities in these processes could contribute to Maya's difficulty in conceiving.
c. What diagnostic tests could be performed to assess ovulation?

## Multiple Choice Questions

**Q1.** Which hormone is responsible for stimulating the development of ovarian follicles?
a. Estrogen
b. Follicle-stimulating hormone (FSH)
c. Luteinizing hormone (LH)
d. Progesterone

**Q2.** During which phase of the menstrual cycle does ovulation typically occur?
a. Menstrual phase
b. Proliferative phase
c. Secretory phase
d. Ovulatory phase

**Q3.** What is the primary function of the corpus luteum?
a. Produce estrogen
b. Produce progesterone
c. Trigger ovulation
d. Stimulate follicular development

**Q4.** Which structure connects the ovaries to the uterus?
a. Fallopian tubes
b. Cervix
c. Endometrium
d. Vagina

**Q5.** Which hormone is responsible for thickening the endometrium in preparation for embryo implantation?
a. Estrogen
b. Follicle-stimulating hormone (FSH)
c. Luteinizing hormone (LH)
d. Progesterone

**Q6.** What is the main function of cervical mucus during the menstrual cycle?
a. Nutrient supply to the egg
b. Protection against pathogens
c. Facilitation of sperm transport
d. Hormone production

**Q7.** Which phase of oogenesis involves the release of a secondary oocyte from the ovary?
a. Oogonium stage
b. Primary oocyte stage
c. Ovulation
d. Fertilization

**Q8.** What is the fate of the secondary oocyte if fertilization does not occur?
a. It becomes a mature ovum
b. It degenerates
c. It forms the embryo
d. It implants in the endometrium

**Q9.** Which hormone surge triggers ovulation?
a. Follicle-stimulating hormone (FSH)
b. Estrogen
c. Luteinizing hormone (LH)
d. Progesterone

**Q10.** What is the primary function of the uterus?
a. Ovulation
b. Fertilization
c. Embryo implantation
d. Sperm production

**Q11.** A woman is experiencing thick, sticky cervical mucus. What phase of her menstrual cycle is she most likely in?
a. Menstrual phase
b. Proliferative phase
c. Ovulatory phase
d. Secretory phase

**Q12.** Which hormone would you expect to be elevated in a woman during the secretory phase of her menstrual cycle?
a. Estrogen
b. Follicle-stimulating hormone (FSH)
c. Luteinizing hormone (LH)
d. Progesterone

**Q13.** A woman's basal body temperature has risen. What phase of her menstrual cycle is she likely in?
a. Menstrual phase
b. Proliferative phase
c. Ovulatory phase
d. Secretory phase

**Q14.** If a woman's progesterone levels are low during the secretory phase, what effect might this have on her endometrium?
a. Thickening
b. Shedding
c. Implantation
d. Ovulation

**Q15.** A woman's cervical mucus is thin and stretchy. What phase of her menstrual cycle is she likely in?
a. Menstrual phase
b. Proliferative phase
c. Ovulatory phase
d. Secretory phase

**Q16.** A woman is experiencing abdominal pain on one side of her lower abdomen. Which phase of her menstrual cycle is she most likely in?
a. Menstrual phase
b. Proliferative phase
c. Ovulatory phase
d. Secretory phase

**Q17.** A woman's progesterone levels remain elevated beyond the typical secretory phase. What could this indicate?
a. Menstruation
b. Pregnancy
c. Menopause
d. Ovulation

**Q18.** A woman's cervical mucus is thick and sticky, and her basal body temperature is low. What phase of her menstrual cycle is she likely in?
a. Menstrual phase
b. Proliferative phase
c. Ovulatory phase
d. Secretory phase

**Q19.** A woman's progesterone levels are low during the secretory phase, and her endometrium is shedding. What is the most likely explanation for these findings?
a. Menstruation
b. Pregnancy
c. Ovulation
d. Menopause

**Q20.** What is the stage of the oocyte at the time of fertilization?
 a. Primary oocyte
 b. Secondary oocyte
 c. Ovum
 d. Zygote

**Q21.** At what point does the secondary oocyte complete meiosis II to become a mature egg?
 a. Before fertilization
 b. During fertilization
 c. After implantation
 d. After ovulation

**Q22.** Which stage of follicular development is characterized by the presence of a fluid-filled cavity called an antrum?
 a. Primordial follicle
 b. Primary follicle
 c. Secondary (antral) follicle
 d. Graafian (mature) follicle

**Q23.** What is the final stage of follicular development before ovulation occurs?
 a. Primordial follicle
 b. Primary follicle
 c. Secondary (antral) follicle
 d. Graafian (mature) follicle

**Q24.** Which of the following is a function of follicle-stimulating hormone (FSH)?
 a. Stimulate the development of ovarian follicles
 b. Trigger ovulation
 c. Thicken the endometrium
 d. Inhibit progest

## ANSWERS

| 1. b | 2. d | 3. b | 4. a | 5. d | 6. c | 7. c | 8. b | 9. c | 10. c | 11. a | 12. d | 13. c | 14. b |
| 15. c | 16. c | 17. b | 18. a | 19. a | 20. b | 21. b | 22. c | 23. d | 24. a | | | | |

# Physiology of Pregnancy and Lactation

**77**
CHAPTER

### COMPETENCY ADDRESSED

**PY9.8:** Describe and discuss the physiology of pregnancy, parturition and lactation and outline the psychology and psychiatry-disorders associated with it.

### LEARNING OBJECTIVES

**At the end of this chapter, the learner should be able to:**
- Process of fertilization, implantation and pregnancy.
- Physiology of pregnancy.
- Physiological changes in the mother during pregnancy.
- Role of placenta in the maintenance of pregnancy-secretion of placental hormones.
- Process of parturition-parturition reflex.
- Physiological basis of lactation-milk let down reflex.

## PHYSIOLOGY OF CONCEPTION

The conception of the fetus occurs after the male and female gametes fuse to form the embryo. The female gamete (egg) is released from the ovary and is picked up by the ampullary part of the fallopian tube, where it then travels to the fallopian tube.

### Male and Female Sexual Act

The male and female sexual act (Physiology of Coitus), is important for depositing to sperms in the female genital tract. But for the ease of understanding, we will discuss them one by one. First of all let's take up the male sexual act.

The *male sexual act* begins with the psychic or physical stimulation of the male, especially the glans penis. The complete act has four stages:
1. Penile erection
2. Emission
3. Ejaculation
4. Resolution

### Penile Erection

The *pelvic parasympathetic nerves* arising from *sacral segment* of spinal cord innervate the penis. The erection is purely controlled by the parasympathetic nervous system. These nerves carry the neurotransmitters acetylcholine, nitric oxide (NO) and vasoactive intestinal peptide (VIP)—out of these, the nitric oxide plays an important role in penile erection.

Nitric oxide acts via the *guanylyl cyclase cGMP pathway* and results in vasodilation of the penile arteries. The increased blood flow in the corpora cavernosa and corpora spongiosum of the penis makes it hard and elongated, termed as an erection. Penile erection is also accompanied by lubrication from the urethral glands to reduce friction between the male and female parts during intercourse. The majority of the lubricating fluid is, however, secreted by the female.

### Emission

When the male penis is stimulated during the act, the vas deferens contracts and pours its contents into the internal urethra. Here, other fluids are also released from prostate gland and seminal vesicles. Hence the fluid from vas deferens, prostatic fluid and seminal fluid together form the semen in the internal urethra. This stage is termed as emission. The male feels the accumulation of semen in the internal urethra. This entire stage is controlled by pelvic *sympathetic nerves* arising from *T12-L2 spinal segments*.

### Ejaculation

The emission as well as ejaculation occurs due to the *Sympathetic stimulation*. The hypogastric and sacral nerves arise from *T12 to L1 spinal segments*. The penile stimulation results in the rhythmic contractions in the penile muscles. This results in the contraction of ischiocavernosus and bulbocavernosus muscles and the release of semen into the external urethra. This results is deposition of semen into the vagina of the female genital tract. The rhythmical contractions associated with emission and ejaculation are associated with *male orgasm* or *climax*.

The other effects of the sympathetic activation during emission and ejaculation, appears during this phase like increase in heart rate and respiratory rate.

### Resolution

Once the ejaculation takes place, the male undergoes the resolution phase where sexual desire is lost for next 1–2 minutes. The penile erection wanes off and it shrinks back to its normal size.

The *female sexual act*, has been summarized below:
Quite like the male sexual act, the female sexual act begins with the psychic and physical stimulation of female external genitalia and clitoris.

Sensory signals are carried by pudendal nerve and sacral plexus from clitoris to sacral segments of spinal cord and also to cerebrum.

The female sexual act also has three main stages:
1. Female erection and lubrication
2. Female orgasm
3. Resolution

### Female Erection and Lubrication

The female erectile tissue extends from the introitus to the clitoris. Female erection is also controlled by the parasympathetic nerves carrying ACh, NO, and VIP. The NO results in increased blood flow to the erectile tissue resulting in tightening and engorgement of the introitus. This results in producing tightness around the penis and producing the massaging action of both the penis and vagina. The parasympathetic nerves also stimulate the Bartholin glands to secrete mucus for lubrication of the genital tract.

### Female Orgasm

At the peak of the sexual stimulation, along with psychic stimulation the signals from cerebrum initiate local reflexes and cause orgasm. It is analogous to male emission and ejaculation. During orgasm, the perineal muscles contract rhythmically which increase the motility of her fallopian tubes. Hence female orgasm and aids in the fertilization process by enhancing the motility of the sperms. Also it keeps the cervix dilated for about 30 minutes after the orgasm.

The sympathetic activation during orgasm results in increased heart rate and respiratory rate.

### Resolution

The cerebral activation during the orgasm result in the intense muscle tension in the body. After the orgasm, the tension is released resulting in relaxation called resolution.

## Fate of Gametes

### The Ovum

The ovum is released from the ovary in the secondary oocyte stage with 23 unpaired chromosomes into the abdomen on the at 14th day of a 28-day menstrual cycle. After ovulation, the ovum, along with hundreds of granulosa cells called *corona radiata*, enters one of the fallopian tubes to reach the uterine cavity. The cilia present in the fallopian tube aid in the movement of the ovum towards the uterine end of the tube under the influence of estrogen.

### The Sperms

We have already discussed in our previous chapter that life span of spam in female genital tract is only 24–48 hours. Hence, these sperms have to complete the fertilization process in a limited period of time.

It is interesting to note that the ejaculate deposits around half a billion sperms m the female vagina. After the ejaculate liquefies, the sperms deposited in the female vagina begin to ascend upwards in female genital tract, towards the egg in the fallopian tube. During this journey many sperms get trapped or get activated by female system. The sperms ascend upward along the uterine wall and only a few thousand succeed in reaching the ampulla of fallopian tube.

## Fertilization of Ovum

The ejaculated sperms ascend upwards towards the fallopian tubes and reaches the ampullae. The transport of these sperms is facilitated by the peristaltic movement of tubes due to the prostaglandins present in semen and oxytocin secreted from female posterior pituitary gland. Fertilization takes place in the ampullae of the fallopian tubes.

Before fertilization, the sperm has to undergo some changes as mentioned below:
- **Capacitation:** Various changes occurring in spermatozoa in the female genital tract are called capacitation of spermatozoa. *If these changes do not occur in spermatozoa, they are not able to fertilize the ovum.* These changes can be summarized as follows:
  - The *fluid* present in uterine cavity and fallopian tubes **washes the inhibitory factors present in the semen**.
  - The sperm deposited in vagina swims upwards in the uterine cavity where they **lose their excessive cholesterol present in semen**. The membrane covering the acrosome weakens.
  - **Increased calcium influx** in the sperm and **increasing the flagellar motility** giving it **powerful**

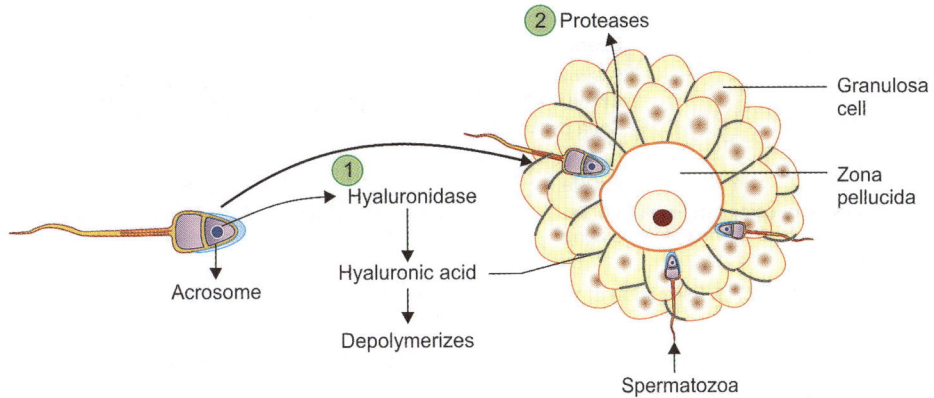

**Fig. 77.1:** Acrosome reaction by hyaluronidases and proteases.

*whiplash motion* instead of weak undulating movement.
- **Acrosome reaction:** The acrosome present in the head of the sperm has large quantities of hyaluronidase and proteolytic enzymes.

These enzymes facilitate the penetration of sperm into the ova. The *hyaluronidase enzyme depolymerizes the intercellular cement*, hyaluronic acid, holding the granulosa cells. The proteolytic enzymes digest the structural elements holding on the ovum **(Fig. 77.1)**.

When the sperm reaches the ovum, the spermatozoa penetrates through the layers of granulosa cells and ***reach the zona pellucida***. The zona pellucida has specific sperm binding receptors *(ZP receptors)*. The proteolytic enzyme present in the acrosome **dissolves the zona pellucida** beneath head. The zona pellucida is penetrated and a pathway is created which carries the genetic material of the sperm inside the oocyte. The haploid genomes of both the gametes fuse to form a diploid zygote. This process is called as fertilization.

We had studied earlier at the *meiotic division of oocyte is at metaphase arrest, which gets completed at the time of fertilization.*

## Polyspermy Block

Out of half a billion sperms deposited female vagina, only one sperm fertilizes the ovum. It is very interesting to note that when a sperm fuses with the zona pellucida, it brings about certain changes in the ovum which are responsible for the polyspermy block. These changes are summarized below:
- **Internalization of sperm binding ZP receptors:** Due to the internalization ZP receptors, the other sperms cannot bind to the zona pellucida.
- **Cortical reaction (Fig. 77.2):** Once the zona pellucida is dissolved, the cortical reaction sets in. There are numerous vesicles below the zona pellucida containing the cortical granules whenever the one pellucida is penetrated, these cortical granules are released in abundance. This is termed as cortical reaction.

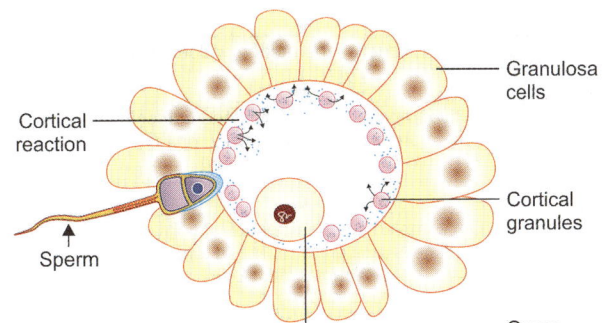

**Fig. 77.2:** Cortical reaction.

The cortical reaction *results in the hardening of the jelly like zona pellucida*, making it unfavorable for further penetration by the sperms.

> What is capacitation what are the various changes occurring in spermatozoa during capacitation?
> What is acrosome reaction?
> What is polyspermy block?

## PREGNANCY

Till now, we have studied a physiology of conception. From here onwards, we will study about the fate of fertilized ovum and physiology of pregnancy.

The second meiotic division of the gets completed after fertilization, forming the mature ovum and a second polar body. The mature ovum consists of haploid number (22 unpaired + X chromosome) called *female pronucleus*. The *male pronucleus* containing 22 + X or Y chromosome in the sperm fuses with female pronucleus to form fertilized ovum or zygote **(Fig. 77.3)**.

It undergo several divisions and forms morula, blastula and blastocyst. The blastocyst reaches the uterine cavity on around 4–5 days after fertilization. It gets implanted on the posterior uterine wall (most common site) and forms the chorionic villi by 5–7 days after ovulation. Before

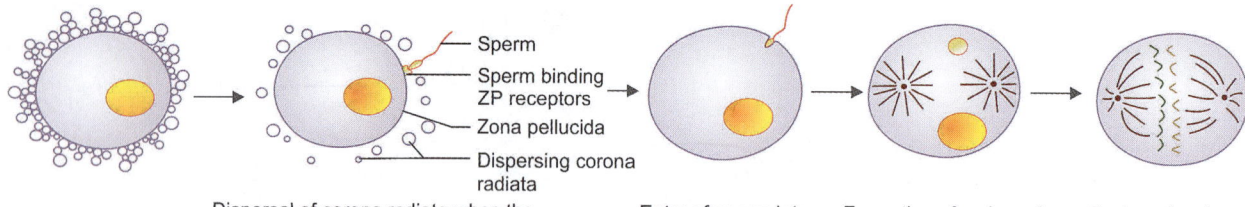

Fig. 77.3: Formation of zygote after fusion of male and female gametes.

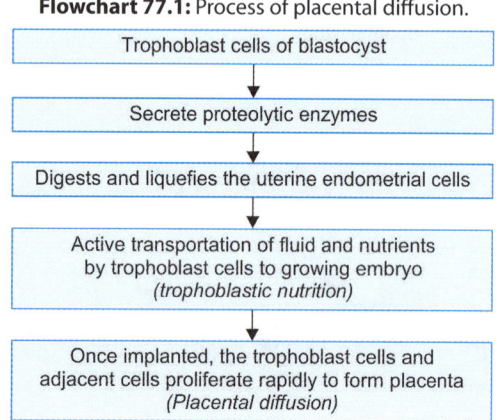

Flowchart 77.1: Process of placental diffusion.

implantation, the blastocyst receives its nutrition from uterine milk.

## Implantation

The trophoblast cells developing on the surface of the blastocyst, secrete proteolytic enzymes which digest and liquefy the uterine endometrial cells. The trophoblast cells transport the nutrients to the growing embryo for first trimester (up to 12–13 weeks) through the trophoblastic nutrition. Once the implantation is complete, the trophoblastic cells proliferate rapidly to form placenta (placental diffusion) **(Flowchart 77.1)**.

## Fetoplacental Circulation

Fetoplacental circulation is the vital exchange system between the fetus and placenta, facilitating the transfer of nutrients, oxygen, and waste products. This circulation is essential for fetal growth and development during pregnancy (**Flowchart 77.2** and **Fig. 77.4**).

### Diffusion of Oxygen Through Placental Membrane

See **Figure 77.5**.

### Diffusion of Carbon Dioxide Through Placental Membrane

Carbon dioxide is highly diffusible gas and readily diffuses across the placental membranes It is continuously formed in fetus due to active metabolism resulting in small increase

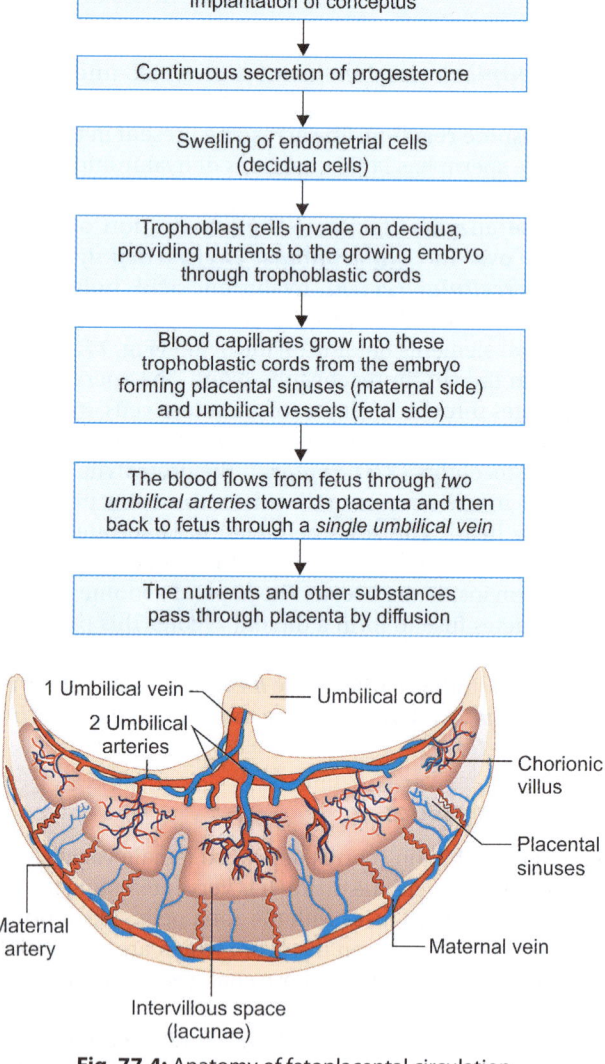

Fig. 77.4: Anatomy of fetoplacental circulation.

in $PCO_2$ (about 2–3 mm Hg), which is sufficient for this diffusion to occur.

### Diffusion of Nutrients Through the Placental Membrane

The growing fetus requires essential nutrients for growth and development. The ***glucose*** gets easily transported

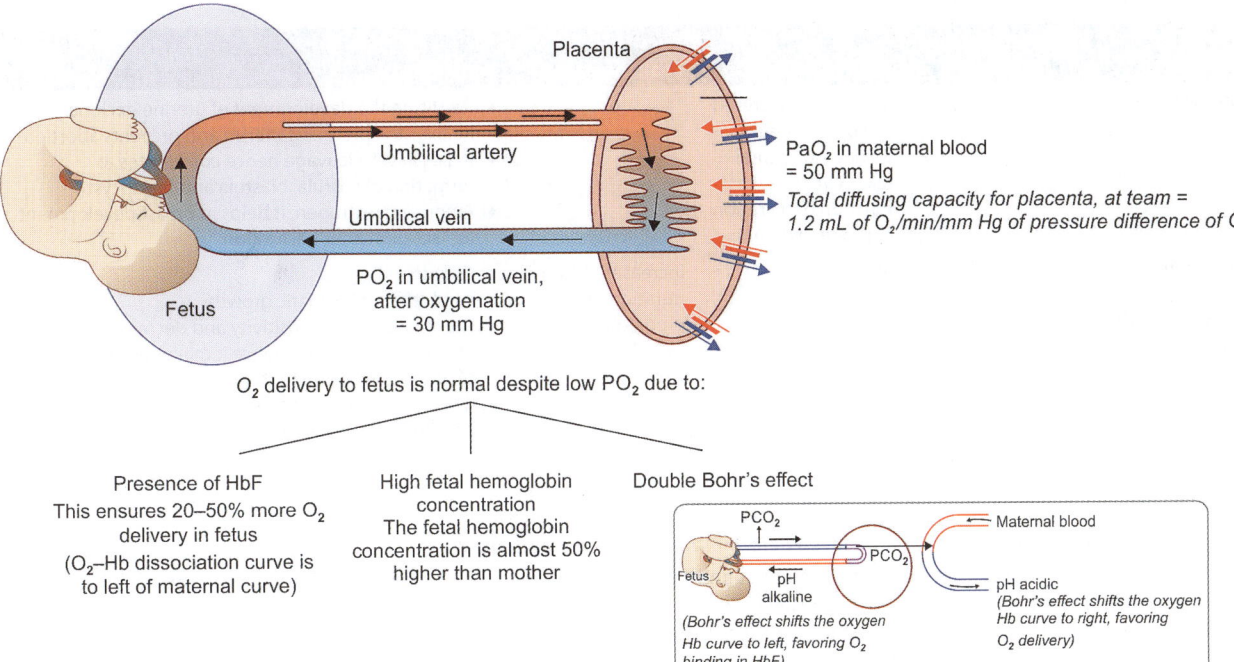

**Fig. 77.5:** Exchange and diffusion of oxygen through placental membrane.

across the placental membranes by the *facilitated diffusion*, as the fetal requirement of glucose is almost same as the mother. Fatty acids being lipid soluble, are easily transported across the placental membranes. The other nutrients like amino acids, electrolytes and minerals are easily transported from mother to the growing fetus.

### Diffusion of Excretory Products Through the Placental Membrane

The concentration of excretory products like nonprotein nitrogens (urea, creatinine) is high in fetal blood as compared to maternal blood. Hence, they tend to diffuse rapidly through the placental membrane. The urea tends to diffuse more easily as compared to creatinine.

## PLACENTAL HORMONES

During pregnancy, the placenta takes over the endocrine function for secreting enough hormones for the maintenance of pregnancy and growth of the fetus. It secretes various hormones like **(Table 77.1)**:

- Estrogen
- Progesterone
- Human chorionic gonadotropin (hCG)
- Human chorionic somatomammotropin (hCS)/human placental lactogen (hPL)

> A term pregnancy is of 40 weeks duration, which is divided into 3 trimesters.
> First trimester: Week 1-week 16, second trimester: Week 17-week 28, third trimester: Week 29-week 40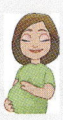

**Table 77.1:** Placental hormones and their features.

| Hormone | Secreted by/source | Onset of secretion | Peak increase | Functions |
|---|---|---|---|---|
| **hCG (structural similarity with LH)** | Syncytial trophoblast cells | 8–9 days after ovulation, if fertilization takes place | 10–12 weeks of pregnancy. Declines by 16–20 weeks of pregnancy | • Prevents involution of corpus luteum<br>• It luteinizes the corpus luteum to secrete large quantities of Progesterone for first trimester of pregnancy<br>• It stimulates male fetal testes to produce testosterone |
| **Estrogen** | Syncytial trophoblast cells | Initially, it is secreted by corpus luteum. But later placenta takes over the function of secretion of estrogen | It reaches its peak (30 times higher) near the term of pregnancy | • Enlargement of maternal uterus<br>• Enlargement of mother's breast<br>• Growth of breast ductal system<br>• Enlargement of mothers external genitalia<br>• Relaxes pelvic ligaments for the easy passage of baby during parturition |

*Contd...*

Contd...

| Hormone | Secreted by/source | Onset of secretion | Peak increase | Functions |
|---|---|---|---|---|
| Progesterone | | Initially, it is secreted by corpus luteum. But later placenta takes over the function of secretion of progesterone | | • Results in the development of uterine decidua<br>• Relaxes the pregnant uterus, and prevents abortion<br>• It aids in cell cleavage hence contributes to formation of morula, blastula and blastocyst<br>• Along with estrogen, it helps in breast development for lactation after parturition |
| hCS/hPL (structural similarity with GH) | Placenta | 5th week of pregnancy | Increases with duration of pregnancy | • Growth of breasts<br>• Weak effect of somatic growth<br>• Decreases insulin sensitivity and decreases glucose utilization in mother. Hence it makes large quantity of glucose available for fetus<br>• Release of free fatty acids from maternal fat stores, providing alternate source of energy for mother |

**What will happen if corpus luteum is removed before 7th week of the pregnancy?**
Since the placenta is not mature to secrete enough quantities of progesterone and estrogen for maintenance of pregnancy, removal of corpus luteum in the first trimester would result in spontaneous abortion.

**What is the role of fetus, in the formation of placental hormones?**
The fetus plays a very important role in steroidogenesis (formation of steroid hormones) during pregnancy, hence the fetus and placenta are jointly referred as *fetoplacental unit.*
The fetal adrenal cortices enlarge and secrete dehydroepiandrosterone (DHEA) during pregnancy. This DHEA is converted to estradiol, estrone and estriol by placenta and transported to maternal blood.

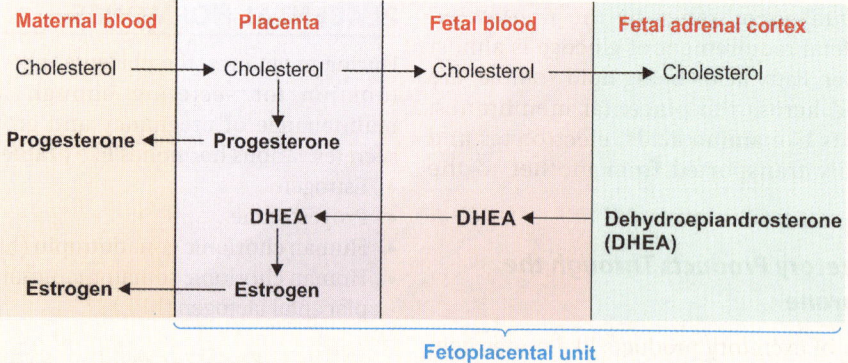

### Role of hCG in Pregnancy (Fig. 77.6)

We have already studied in the menstrual cycle, that if the fertilization takes place, the corpus luteum becomes the '*corpus luteum of pregnancy*' and continues to secrete the progesterone for first trimester of the pregnancy.

**Explanation for the formation of corpus luteum of pregnancy:** The hormone hCG secreted by chorionic villi, has structural similarities with the luteinizing hormone (LH), secreted by anterior pituitary gland. In case the ovum is not fertilized, the LH is responsible for luteinizing the corpus luteum for the period after ovulation. After which the level of 14 drops resulting in drop in the levels of progesterone and estrogen. This results in the withdrawal bleeding during the bleeding phase of menstrual cycle.

However, in case the ovum is fertilized, the hCG luteinizes the corpus luteum instead of LH. Hence, the corpus proliferates further and continues to secrete progesterone and estrogen for the entire length of first trimester or till placenta takes over the function of hormone synthesis.

The levels of hCG decline after the first trimester resulting in regression of corpus luteum.

#### Pregnancy test

The pregnancy test is based on the presence of hCG in urine during first trimester of the pregnancy.

*Principle:* It is based on the antigen-body reaction
The test is performed on a card impregnated/coated with anti-hCG antibody. The card is placed in a plastic case with a well and a window. The well is used to put a few drops of urine whereas the window is used to read the results. After adding urine into the well, and waiting for sometime, there line appears in the window.

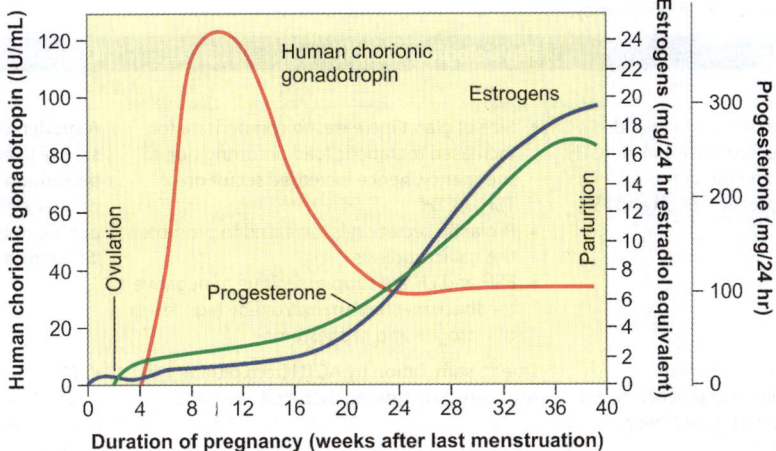

**Fig. 77.6:** Levels of hCG as compared to other placental hormones through pregnancy.

*Reading the result:*
1. A **single red line appearing at C** (control) indicates the absence of antigen (hcG) in urine, and hence **Negative test result** for pregnancy.

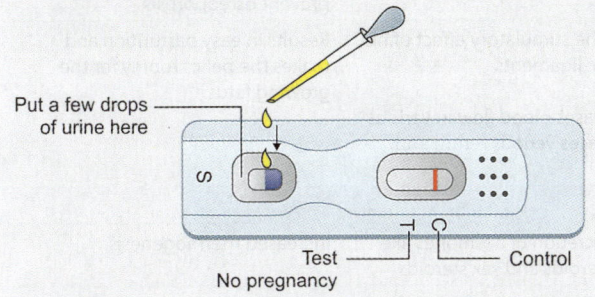

2. **Two red lines** appearing at C (control) and T (test) indicated presence of hcG in urine. Hence, yields **Positive test result for pregnancy**, i.e., the lady is pregnant.

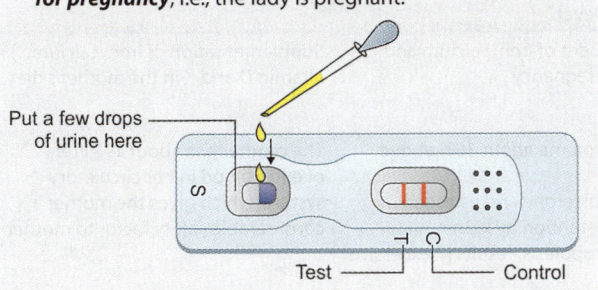

## Physiological Changes in Mother During Pregnancy

During pregnancy, females undergo various physiological changes ranging from hormonal to cardiovascular system which can affect the overall health of the mother. These physiological changes are discussed in **Table 77.2**.

> *Why some women develop hypertension during pregnancy (pregnancy induced hypertension, PIH)?*
> About 5% women experience PIH, i.e., sudden increase in arterial pressure during pregnancy along with proteinuria called as pre-eclampsia/toxemia of pregnancy. It occurs due to:
> - Excessive salt and water retention
> - Excessive weight gain by mother
> - Development of maternal edema
> - Hypertension
> - Arterial vasospasm in kidneys, brain and liver
> - Decreased GFR due to thickened basement membrane
> - Proteinuria
>
> Cause: Insufficient blood supply to placenta results in release of substances (cytokines like Tumor necrosis factor-α and interleukin-6) from placenta. These substances result in dysfunction of maternal vascular endothelium.
> Extreme degree of pre-eclampsia is called as eclampsia.

## Role of Placenta During Pregnancy

The placenta plays a very important role during the pregnancy
- It provides a physical and immunological barrier between the mother and the growing fetus.
- It provides the nutrition to the growing fetus.
- It maintains the oxygen delivery to the fetus through the double Bohr's effect.
- The feto-placental unit results in the steroidogenesis for maintenance of pregnancy.

## Amenorrhea During Pregnancy

Amenorrhea during pregnancy occurs due to the suppression of menstrual cycles by high levels of hormones like progesterone and human chorionic gonadotropin (hCG), which maintain the uterine lining and support the developing fetus **(Flowchart 77.3)**.

## PARTURITION

The process of delivery of the baby is called Parturition.

As seen in the **Figure 77.7**, the maternal and fetal factors play an important role in delivery of the baby at the term, called Parturition.

**Table 77.2:** Physiological changes in pregnancy.

| | Change | Physiological basis | Clinical importance |
|---|---|---|---|
| ***Hormonal changes*** | | | |
| Pituitary gland | • Increased size of gland<br>• Increased secretion of ACTH, TSH and prolactin<br>• Suppression of LH and FSH | • Size of gland increases to compensate for increased metabolic load occurring due to pregnancy, hence increased secretion of TSH, ACTH<br>• Prolactin secretion is increased to promote the galactopoiesis<br>• FSH and LH are suppressed due to negative feedback mechanism exerted by high levels of estrogen and progesterone | A sudden decrease in the blood supply to enlarged pituitary after parturition results in postpartum pituitary ischemia resulting in panhypopituitarism. This is called **'Sheehan's syndrome'** |
| Adrenal glands | • Moderate increase in secretion of glucocorticoids<br>• Aldosterone secretion doubles | Due to stimulation by ACTH from pituitary, in response to increased metabolic demand | • Mobilizes amino acids for growth of fetus<br>• Excessive retention of sodium and water |
| Thyroid gland | Increase size of gland | Stimulated by hCG, TSH and human chorionic thyrotropin | |
| Parathyroid glands | • Enlarges during pregnancy<br>• Increased secretion of parathormone<br>Results in increase S. calcium levels | • Increases bone resorption in mother<br>• Stimulates bone formation in fetus<br>• Further increases in lactation | The recommended daily allowance of calcium increases during pregnancy and lactation; hence supplementation is advised to prevent osteoporosis |
| Gonads (Relaxin) | Secreted by corpus luteum of ovary and placenta | • Secreted under the stimulatory effect of hCG<br>• Relaxes the pelvic ligaments<br>• Softens cervix<br>• Vasodilator, increases blood flow in various tissues and increases venous return and cardiac output | Results in easy parturition and makes the pelvis roomy for the growing fetus |
| ***Metabolism*** | | | |
| Basal metabolic rate (BMR) | Increases about 15% during later half of pregnancy | Due to increased secretion of hormones like thyroxine, corticosteroids and sex steroids | Increased thermogenesis |
| Weight Gain | Average weight gain is about 11 kg, occurring in last trimester | Increase in food intake due to increased desire of food due to<br>• Increased demand<br>• High hormonal level | |
| Nutrition | • Hypochromic anemia<br>• Calcium deficiency | Increased requirement of iron, calcium and vitamin D during pregnancy | Supplementation of iron, calcium, vitamin D and K in the mother's diet |
| ***Circulatory changes*** | | | |
| Blood flow | • Blood flow through the placenta up to 625 mL/min<br>• Increase in cardiac output to 30–40% by 27 weeks of pregnancy | Increase in blood volume about 30% above normal due to:<br>• Secretion of aldosterone and estrogen<br>• Increased fluid retention by kidney<br>• Increased erythropoiesis, results in excessive fluid volume | The mother has about 1–2 liters of extra blood in her circulatory system, which gives the mother a considerable safety factor to mother |
| Maternal respiration | • Increased minute ventilation of mother of about 50%<br>• Growing uterus presses the diaphragm, so that lung expansion decreases. Hence, respiratory rate increases to maintain the ventilation | • Increased BMR<br>• Increased oxygen utilization by mother<br>• Increased progesterone increases the sensitivity of respiratory center to carbon dioxide | |
| Maternal kidney function | Increase urine formation | Due to increased fluid intake and increased load of excretory products:<br>• Increased reabsorptive capacity of sodium, chloride, and water up to 50% due to increased production of salt- and water-secreting hormones (aldosterone and placental hormone)<br>• Increased renal blood flow and glomerular filtration rate up to 50% due to vasodilation due to nitric oxide and relaxin | Results in salt and water retention during pregnancy |

**Flowchart 77.3:** Series of events causing amenorrhea during pregnancy.

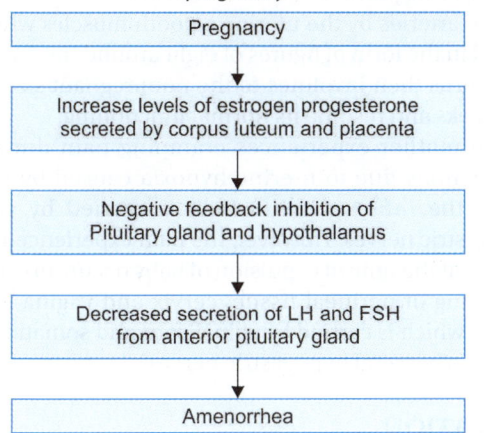

## Maternal Factors

- The full-term fetus stretches the uterine walls and increases their contractility.
- The fetal head when stretches the cervix/there is cervical irritation, the myogenic reflexes stimulate the fundus of the uterus.
- The levels of estrogen rise markedly at term, increasing the estrogen-to-progesterone ratio. Raised estrogen increases uterine contractility by increasing the gap junctions between uterine smooth muscles and upregulating the oxytocin receptors.
- The cervical stretching stimulates the supraoptic nucleus and paraventricular nucleus of the hypothalamus resulting in the release of oxytocin from the posterior pituitary gland.
- The high levels of oxytocin stimulate myogenic contraction by acting on the highly sensitive increased number of oxytocin receptors.

## Fetal Factors

- The release of oxytocin from fetal pituitary and cortisol from fetal adrenal cortex results in additional uterine stimulation.
- The prostaglandins also result in uterine stimulation.

## Parturition Reflex

The stretching of cervix due to the fetal descent stimulates the hypothalamus to release oxytocin from posterior

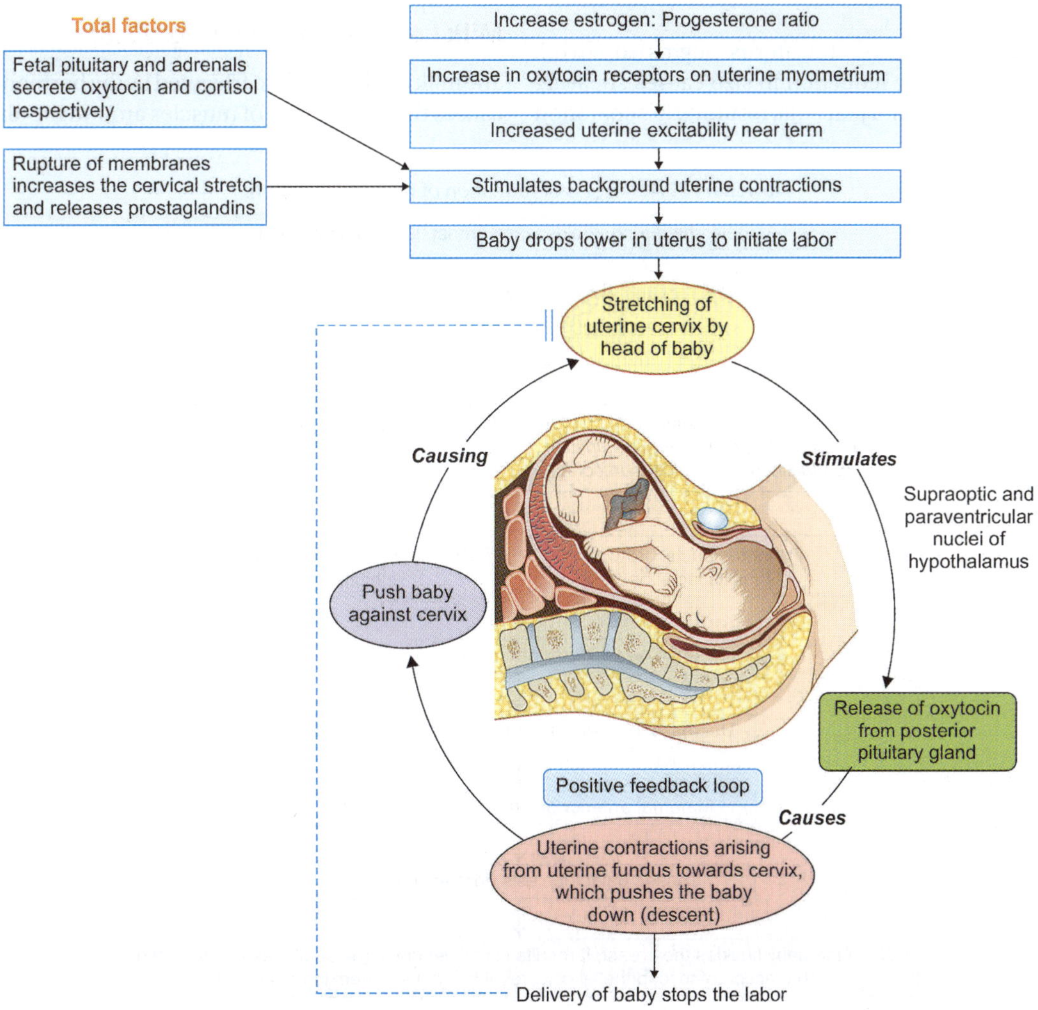

**Fig. 77.7:** Parturition reflex.

pituitary. The oxytocin hormone, increases the uterine contractility resulting in rhythmic fundic contractions called as *labor*. These labor contractions start from uterine fundus and progress towards the cervix, pushing the baby down towards the cervix, further increasing the stretch on the cervix. This process of uterine contraction and cervical stretching increase the force of uterine contraction hence progressively increasing the duration and intensity of these contractions *(positive feedback mechanism)*. The other mechanism eliciting the positive feedback effect is the progressive increase in the rate of secretion of oxytocin from the posterior pituitary gland. The labor contractions along with the bearing down effort by the mother during contractions, results in pushing the baby down and expulsion of baby. Once the baby is expelled, the positive feedback stops and the uterine contractions cease.

> **What will happen, if the mother has more than 500 mL of bleeding after delivery?**
> Loss of more than 500 mL of blood is called **Postpartum Hemorrhage (PPH)**. In this the mother goes into hypovolemic shock. It is a rare but serious complication. This needs active management by the medical team.

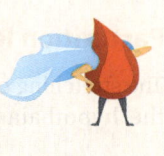

In next 30–45 minutes, the uterus begins to shrink and reduce in size. The reduction in size causes shearing between uterine walls and placenta, resulting in separation of placenta and its delivery. A mother loses nearly 350 mL of blood during parturition. The blood loss is controlled from uterine arteries by the uterine smooth muscles which are placed in the form of figures of eight around these arteries. The uterus then involutes to the nonpregnant size over a few weeks and resume its normal functioning.

The mother experiences cramping pain during the contractions due to uterine hypoxia caused by cramps called the *labor pains*, which is carried by visceral hypogastric nerves. However, the pain experienced by the mother at the time of expulsion of baby occurs to excessive stretching of perineal tissue, cervix and vagina is more severe, which is carried by spinal cord and somatic nerves instead of visceral hypogastric nerves.

## LACTATION

Lactation is regulated by a complex interplay of hormones, primarily prolactin and oxytocin. Prolactin stimulates milk production in the mammary glands, while oxytocin triggers the ejection of milk (let-down reflex) from the alveoli into the ducts, facilitating breastfeeding. The process is sustained by regular feeding sessions, which maintain milk supply and demand equilibrium **(Flowchart 77.4)**.

### Milk Let Down Reflex (Fig. 77.8)

The milk let-down reflex, triggered by the hormone oxytocin, causes the contraction of muscles around the alveoli in the

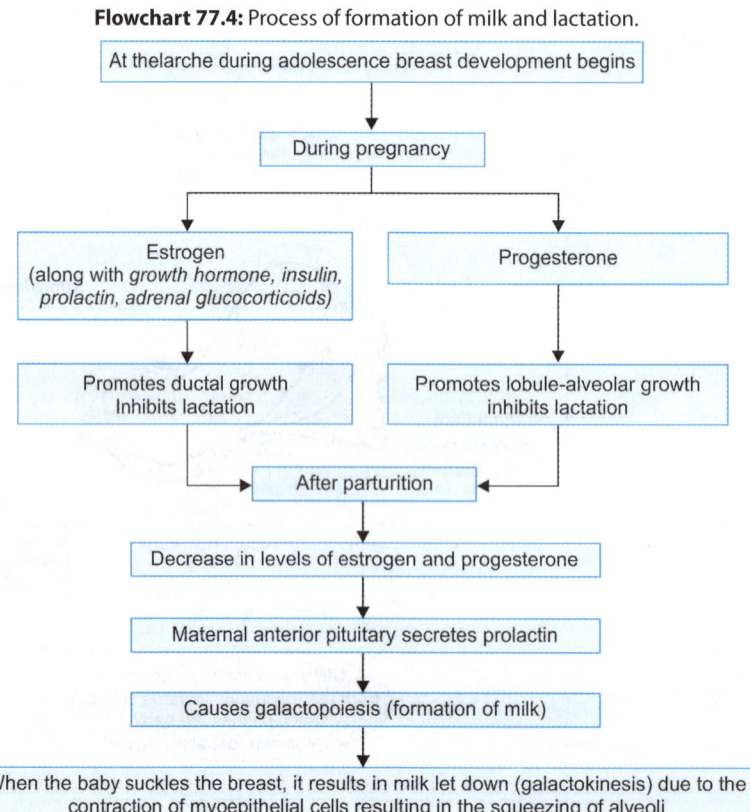

**Flowchart 77.4:** Process of formation of milk and lactation.

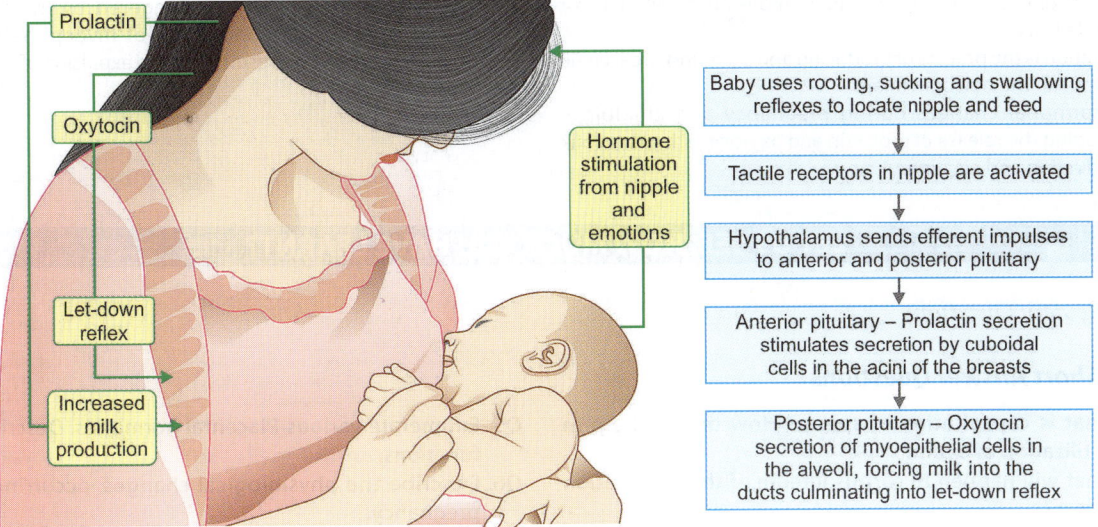

Fig. 77.8: Milk let down reflex.

breast, pushing milk into the ducts and making it available for breastfeeding. This reflex is stimulated by factors such as the sound, sight, or thought of the baby, facilitating efficient milk extraction during nursing sessions.

## Lactational Amenorrhea

The ovarian cycle is suppressed in lactating mothers for a few months called lactational amenorrhea. The reason for this can be explained as the inhibition of gonadotropins (FSH and LH) secreted by the anterior pituitary gland due to raised prolactin levels **(Fig. 77.9)**. Hence ovulation is inhibited, conferring contraceptive protection to lactating mother. However, if mother is not consistent in lactating, she may resume her ovarian activity resulting in loss of this contraceptive function.

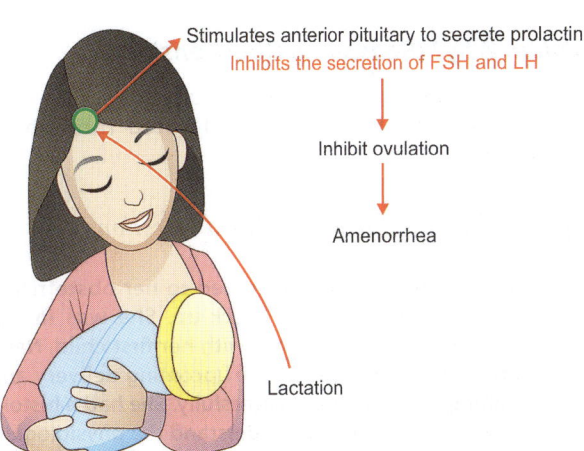

Fig. 77.9: Lactation causing temporary amenorrhea.

### SUMMARY

- Fertilization occurs when a sperm cell penetrates the zona pellucida of the secondary oocyte, resulting in the formation of a zygote.

  After fertilization, the zygote undergoes several mitotic divisions, forming a blastocyst.

  Implantation occurs when the blastocyst attaches to the endometrium of the uterus, followed by invasion and embedding of the trophoblast into the endometrial lining.
- Pregnancy is characterized by the growth and development of the embryo/fetus within the uterus.

  Hormonal changes, particularly rising levels of estrogen and progesterone, play a crucial role in maintaining pregnancy by suppressing ovulation, thickening the endometrium, and inhibiting uterine contractions.
- Pregnancy induces numerous physiological adaptations in the mother's body to support fetal growth and development.

  These changes include increased blood volume, cardiac output, respiratory rate, and renal blood flow.

  Hormonal fluctuations also lead to alterations in metabolism, weight gain, and changes in the musculoskeletal system to accommodate the growing fetus.
- The placenta is a temporary organ formed during pregnancy that serves as the interface between the maternal and fetal circulatory systems. It facilitates nutrient and gas exchange, removes waste products, and produces hormones essential for pregnancy maintenance.

  Placental hormones include human chorionic gonadotropin (hCG), estrogen, progesterone, and human placental lactogen (hPL), which support fetal growth and regulate maternal physiology.
- Parturition, or childbirth, is the process by which the fetus is expelled from the uterus at the end of pregnancy.

  It is initiated by a complex series of hormonal and physiological changes, including increased production of oxytocin and prostaglandins, which stimulate uterine contractions and cervical dilation. The parturition reflex involves the coordinated

actions of the uterus, cervix, and hormones to facilitate labor and delivery.
- Lactation is the process of producing and secreting breast milk to nourish the newborn infant.
  Hormonal changes during pregnancy and childbirth, including the release of prolactin and oxytocin, stimulate milk production and ejection.

The milk let-down reflex is triggered by the suckling stimulus, causing the contraction of myoepithelial cells surrounding the alveoli, resulting in the expulsion of milk from the mammary glands.

## LET US SEE, HOW MUCH YOU HAVE LEARNT?

### Review Questions

#### Long/Short Answer Questions

Q1. What is capacitation of sperm? How does it help in fertilization of ovum?
Q2. What will happen to corpus luteum, if the fertilization occurs?
Q3. What is the physiological role of hCG in pregnancy?
Q4. What is the physiological (Immunological) basis of pregnancy test?
Q5. Enumerate various Placental hormones. Describe their functions.
Q6. Describe the physiological changes, occurring in the pregnancy.
Q7. Define the parturition reflex. Describe it mechanism.
Q8. Describe the milk let down reflex.

#### Explain Why? (Reasoning Questions)

Q1. Only one sperm can fertilize an ovum.
Q2. Progesterone levels remain elevated throughout pregnancy.
Q3. Oxytocin plays a crucial role in the initiation and progression of labor during childbirth.
Q4. Process of lactogenesis occurs shortly after childbirth.

### Critical Thinking Case-Based Questions

Q1. A 30-year-old woman, presented to her obstetrician for her routine prenatal check-up. She was in her third trimester of pregnancy with her first child. Neha expressed concerns about the upcoming delivery and her ability to breastfeed successfully. She had a history of anxiety and wanted to understand the physiological processes of pregnancy, childbirth, and lactation to alleviate her worries. Based on this scenario, answer the following questions on behalf of doctor:
  a. What are the hormonal changes and physiological adaptations that occur during pregnancy?
  b. How does the process of parturition occur, including the stages of labor and delivery?
  c. What are the key hormones involved in lactation?

### Multiple Choice Questions

Q1. During which trimester of pregnancy does the fetus undergo rapid development of organs and structures?
  a. First trimester
  b. Second trimester
  c. Third trimester
  d. Preconception
Q2. Which hormone is primarily responsible for promoting uterine relaxation during pregnancy?
  a. Estrogen
  b. Progesterone
  c. Relaxin
  d. Oxytocin
Q3. What is the main function of oxytocin during pregnancy?
  a. Stimulate uterine contractions
  b. Maintain uterine relaxation
  c. Inhibit progesterone production
  d. Promote fetal growth
Q4. Which physiological change occurs in the maternal respiratory system during pregnancy to meet increased oxygen demands?
  a. Decreased tidal volume
  b. Increased respiratory rate
  c. Reduced lung capacity
  d. Constriction of airways
Q5. What is the primary role of human chorionic gonadotropin (hCG) during early pregnancy?
  a. Stimulate milk production
  b. Support the corpus luteum
  c. Regulate uterine contractions
  d. Promote fetal lung development
Q6. A pregnant woman experiences frequent urination and increased thirst. What physiological change during pregnancy is most likely responsible for these symptoms?
  a. Increased blood volume and renal blood flow
  b. Decreased blood volume and renal blood flow
  c. Reduced bladder capacity
  d. Constriction of blood vessels

Q7. A pregnant woman presents with mild, intermittent uterine contractions. What physiological process is most likely occurring?
   a. Braxton Hicks contractions
   b. Onset of labor
   c. Uterine rupture
   d. Placental abruption

Q8. A pregnant woman experiences occasional dizziness and lightheadedness upon standing. What physiological change during pregnancy is most likely responsible for these symptoms?
   a. Increased blood pressure
   b. Decreased blood volume
   c. Elevated heart rate
   d. Reduced cardiac output

Q9. A pregnant woman presents with leg cramps and swelling in her lower extremities. What physiological change during pregnancy is most likely contributing to these symptoms?
   a. Increased venous pressure and reduced venous return
   b. Decreased venous pressure and increased venous return
   c. Constriction of blood vessels
   d. Increased blood viscosity

Q10. A pregnant woman experiences increased appetite and weight gain during the second trimester. What physiological process is most likely occurring?
   a. Accelerated fetal growth
   b. Maternal fat storage
   c. Reduced metabolic rate
   d. Enhanced nutrient absorption

Q11. A pregnant woman complains of shortness of breath and difficulty breathing while lying flat. What physiological adaptation during pregnancy is most likely responsible for these symptoms?
   a. Elevated diaphragm
   b. Increased lung capacity
   c. Reduced lung compliance
   d. Constriction of airways

Q12. A pregnant woman experiences heartburn and regurgitation after meals. What physiological change during pregnancy is most likely contributing to these symptoms?
   a. Relaxation of the lower esophageal sphincter
   b. Increased gastric motility
   c. Reduced stomach acid production
   d. Enlargement of the stomach

Q13. A pregnant woman reports feeling fatigued and experiencing occasional fainting episodes. What physiological change during pregnancy is most likely responsible for these symptoms?
   a. Reduced blood pressure
   b. Increased blood volume
   c. Elevated heart rate
   d. Constriction of blood vessels

Q14. A pregnant woman presents with occasional headaches and visual disturbances. What physiological change during pregnancy is most likely contributing to these symptoms?
   a. Reduced blood pressure
   b. Elevated blood glucose levels
   c. Increased blood viscosity
   d. Constriction of blood vessels

Q15. A pregnant woman experiences an increase in vaginal discharge and urinary frequency. What physiological change during pregnancy is most likely responsible for these symptoms?
   a. Increased blood volume
   b. Enhanced renal blood flow
   c. Enlargement of the uterus
   d. Constriction of the bladder

## ANSWERS

1. b   2. c   3. a   4. b   5. b   6. a   7. a   8. b   9. a   10. a   11. a   12. a   13. b   14. d   15. c

# Contraception

CHAPTER 78

> **COMPETENCY ADDRESSED**
> PY9.6: Enumerate the contraceptive methods for male and female. Discuss their advantages and disadvantages.

**LEARNING OBJECTIVES**
**At the end of this chapter, the learner should be able to:**
- Enumerate various contraceptive methods for males and females.
- Describe the physiological basis of the use of the contraceptive methods.
- Describe the physiological basis of the use of contraceptive methods in various conditions.
- Discuss the advantages and disadvantages of commonly used contraceptive methods.

## DEFINITION

These are various methods to prevent conception/pregnancy along with a regular sexual contact.

### Methods Commonly used to Prevent Conception

See **Flowchart 78.1**.

## RHYTHM METHOD

It is to observe abstinence (no sexual activity) near ovulation **(Fig. 78.1)**.

### Physiological Basis

In a woman with a regular cycle of 28 days, *ovulation occurs 14 days prior to menstruation*. The cervical mucus

**Flowchart 78.1:** Different methods of contraception.

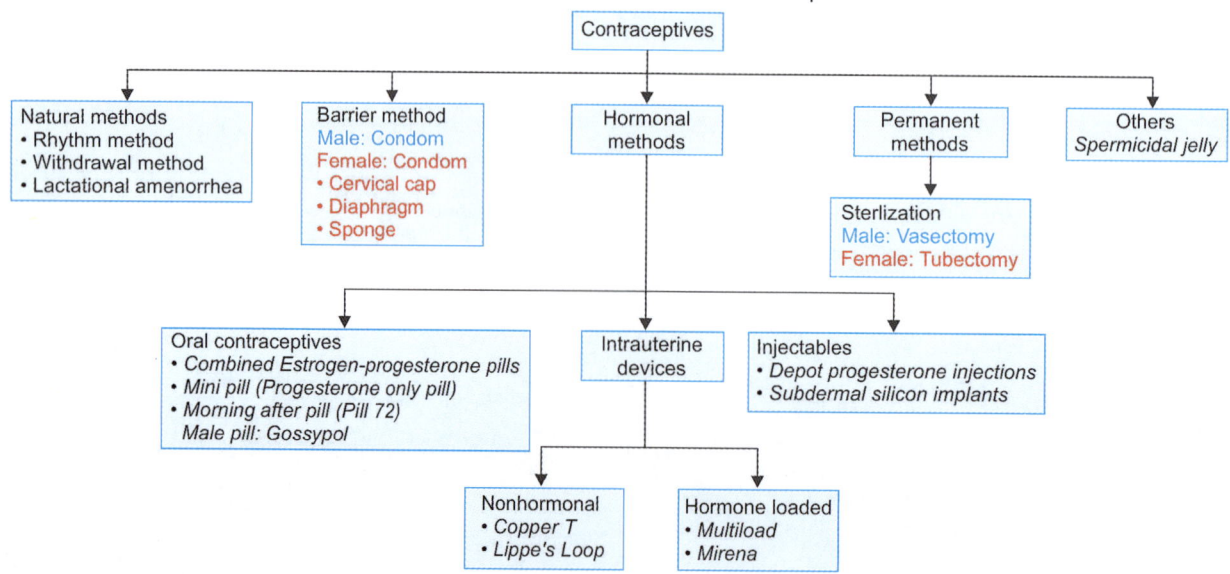

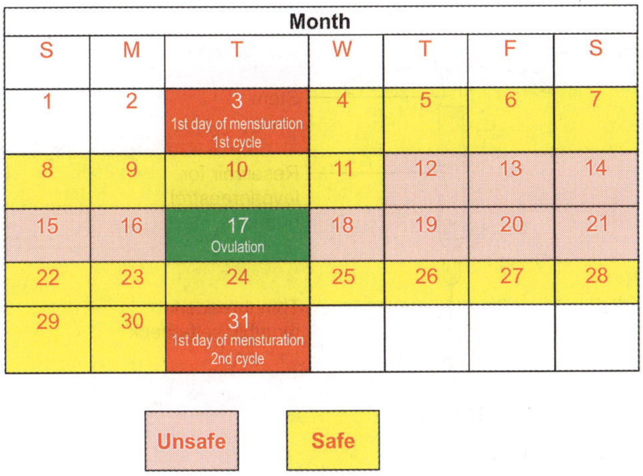

Fig. 78.1: Rhythm method based on menstrual cycle.

is viscous, elastic, and thick 3 to 4 days before ovulation. Sperm and ovaries have a vitality of 4 to 5 days and 24 hours, respectively. Because of this, each month, the female reproductive window is brief, only 4 to 5 days long. As a result, it is typically said that refraining from sexual activity for 4 days prior to and 3 days following the estimated day of ovulation inhibits conception. However, this method of birth control is only successful when the menstrual cycle is regular.

The ***formula*** used to calculate the safe period is by determining the shortest and longest cycle of the female.

The shortest cycle marks the ***onset of fertile (unsafe) period; subtract 18 from the length of shortest cycle.***

Example: If the shortest cycle of female is 26 days, then subtract 18 from 26, i.e., 8. Hence, the fertile period begins from 8th day of menstrual cycle, considering 1st day of the menstrual cycle being the day of onset of menstruation.

The longest cycle marks the ***end of fertile (unsafe) period; subtract 11 from the length of longest cycle.***

Example: If the shortest cycle of female is 30 days, then subtract 11 from 30, i.e., 19. Hence, the fertile period ends on 19th day of menstrual cycle, considering 1st day of menstrual cycle being the day of onset of menstruation.

Hence, for a woman with a menstrual cycle length of 26–30 days, the unsafe/fertile period ranges from day 8 to day 19, where the couple needs to use additional contraceptives.

**Advantage:** Safe, affordable, and does not need a prescription.

**Disadvantage:** Least effective.

> A 21-year-old woman and her husband are interested in natural family planning techniques. Her monthly cycle lasts for a normal 28 days. What is the longest period of fertility that should be avoided by abstinence? Explain why?

## LACTATIONAL AMENORRHEA METHOD

There is no ovulation and menstruation while breastfeeding. While nursing, the female ovarian cycle is inhibited.

**Physiological basis:** High prolactin prevents ovulation. When the baby is suckling occurs, it causes the inhibition of the release of dopamine from hypothalamus. Dopamine function is to inhibit the secretion of dopamine. The dopamine inhibitory effect on prolactin is removed and there increase level of prolactin inhibits the release of hypothalamic GnRH and Prolactin FSH, LH, which causes anovulation and amenorrhea.

**Advantage:** Natural method with no side effects.

**Disadvantage:** Not effective.

> A couple has come to the postpartum unit for family planning advice. The husband is 24-years-old and wife is 20-years-old. Their only child is a 4-months-old baby girl who is exclusively on breastfeeding. What are the contraceptive methods for the couple?

## BARRIER METHODS

Mechanical barriers are devices that provide a physical barrier between the sperm and the egg.

Examples: Male condom, female condom, diaphragm, cervical cap, and sponge.

**Physiological basis:** They acts by preventing the passage of sperms into the female genital tract.

**Advantage:** They are safe, no hormonal side effects, easy to use, and prevent sexually transmitted infections (STIs).

## INTRAUTERINE DEVICE

These are the devices which are inserted into the uterine cavity. The intrauterine devices (IUDs) are broadly classified as **(Fig. 78.2)**:
- **Non hormonal IUDs:**
  - Copper T
  - Lippe's loop
- **Hormonal IUDs:**
  - Hormone-loaded IUD
  - Mirena

**Physiological basis:** Implantation of a foreign body into the uterus (an intrauterine device) causes foreign body reaction in the endometrium, thus preventing fertilization and implantation. They cause phagocytosis of sperm by causing leucocyte infiltration. Prostaglandin releases uterine contractility, which prevents implantation. The copper IUD has a spermicidal action by releasing copper into the uterus. It also affects sperm motility. Progesterone is progressively released by hormonal IUDs, which thickens cervical mucus and prevents sperm from entering the uterus.

**Advantages:** Highly effective, long-term protection can be used during breastfeeding, no systemic side effects.

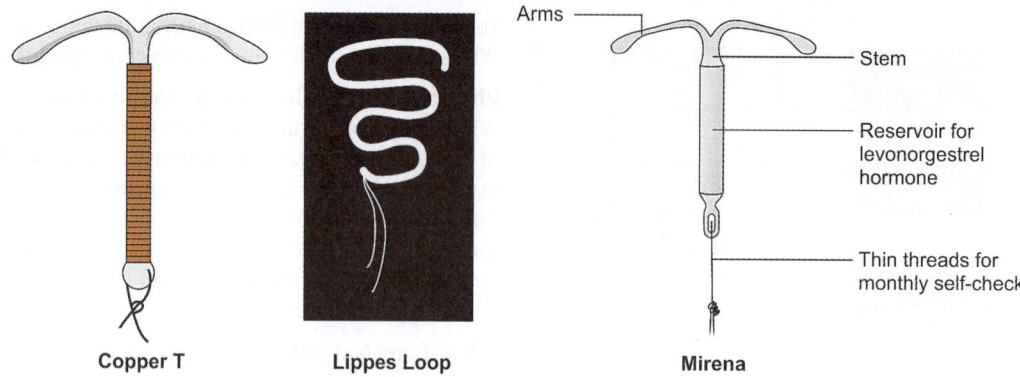

**Fig. 78.2:** Intrauterine devices (IUDs).

**Disadvantages:**
- They do not offer any protection from sexually transmitted disease.
- Insertion and removal need a trained heart care provider. It may cause pelvic infection. It is the second most common cause of ectopic pregnancy.

 *A 26-years-old woman presents for a health maintenance visit. The patient is sexually active and want to know about female contraceptive methods. Which contraceptive method would be avoided in this patient and why?*

## ORAL CONTRACEPTIVES PILLS

Oral contraceptives pills (OC pills) contain estrogen and progesterone. The different types of OC pills that are available are:
- **Combined estrogen-progesterone pill:** Estrogen inhibits pituitary FSH and hypothalamic GnRH secretion through a negative feedback mechanism **(Fig. 78.3)**. A low level of FSH inhibits the growth of ovarian follicles. Progesterone inhibits the secretion of pituitary LH and thus inhibits ovulation. Additionally, progesterone causes thinning of endometrium that prevents implantation also causes thickening of cervical mucus that prevents the penetration of sperms.
- **Progesterone-only pill/mini pill:** This pill has only progesterone. It is prescribed to women who do not tolerate estrogen in the combined pill.
- **Morning after pill (pill 72):** It is an emergency pill containing levonorgestrel. It is an emergency contraceptive, can be taken after unprotected sexual contact during fertile/unsafe period.

**Advantages:** Highly effective. Periods become regular.
**Disadvantages:**
- It must be taken regularly.
- The adverse effects include headaches, nausea, breast tenderness and weight gain.
- OC Pill is contraindicated in deep vein thrombosis and cardiovascular events. It should not be used by high-risk women who are older than 35, have diabetes or

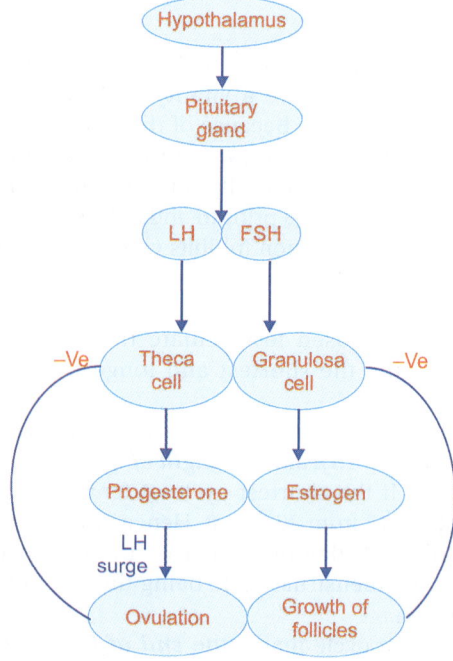

**Fig. 78.3:** Hypothalamic pituitary gonadal axis.

hypertension, smoke more than 20 cigarettes per day, have a history of heart disease, or have illnesses that cause an excess of estrogen.

## OTHER METHODS

**Spermicidal jelly:** It provide chemical barrier by destroying spermatozoa which is inserted into vagina before sexual contact.

**Permanent method:** In this method the surgical ligation is done.
- **Vasectomy:** It is a surgical procedure in which there is bilateral ligation of the vas deferens preventing mature sperm from being transported to the urethra.
- **Tubectomy/tubal ligation:** It is the method of sterilization in females.

These are the permanent methods of sterilization, hence preferred for couples who have completed their family.

## SUMMARY

- This chapter comprehensively covers various contraceptive methods available for both males and females, along with their physiological basis, application in different conditions, and associated advantages and disadvantages.
- The chapter begins by enumerating a wide range of contraceptive methods, including barrier methods (condoms, diaphragms), hormonal methods (oral contraceptives, patches, injections), intrauterine devices (IUDs), sterilization procedures (vasectomy, tubal ligation), and fertility awareness methods. Each method is described in terms of its mechanism of action, efficacy, and usage instructions.
- Furthermore, the physiological basis of contraceptive methods is discussed, focusing on how each method interferes with the process of conception or pregnancy. This includes inhibiting ovulation, altering cervical mucus consistency to prevent sperm penetration, and creating a hostile uterine environment for implantation.
- Moreover, the chapter explores the application of contraceptive methods in various conditions, such as polycystic ovary syndrome (PCOS), endometriosis, and irregular menstrual cycles. It discusses how specific contraceptive methods can address underlying hormonal imbalances or alleviate symptoms associated with these conditions.
- Additionally, the advantages and disadvantages of commonly used contraceptive methods are analyzed in detail. Factors such as efficacy, reversibility, side effects, convenience, and cost are considered when evaluating the suitability of each method for individual preferences and health needs.
- Overall, this chapter serves as a comprehensive guide to understanding contraceptive options, their physiological mechanisms, clinical applications, and considerations for informed decision-making regarding reproductive health and family planning.

## LET US SEE, HOW MUCH YOU HAVE LEARNT?

### Review Questions

Q1. Describe the physiological basis of mechanism of action oral contraceptive pills.

Q2. Describe the physiological basis of intrauterine devices.

Q3. Explain how the lactational amenorrhea act as contraceptive barrier?

### Critical Thinking Case-Based Questions

Q1. Riya and Aryan, a young couple in their late 20s, visited their healthcare provider to discuss contraception options. They wanted to prevent unintended pregnancies while considering their individual health needs and preferences. Riya had concerns about the potential side effects of hormonal contraceptives, while Aryan was interested in learning about male contraceptive methods. They seek guidance on effective and suitable contraceptive options for both of them.

Based on the concerns of couple, answer the following questions:
a. Explain the physiological mechanisms of contraception in males and females.
b. Enumerate the contraceptives methods for male and female in this case.
c. What are the potential benefits and limitations of hormonal contraceptives for females?
d. What are the emerging options for male contraception?

### Multiple Choice Questions

Q1. Which of the following is NOT a barrier method of contraception?
   a. Condoms           b. Diaphragm
   c. Oral contraceptives   d. Cervical cap

Q2. How do hormonal contraceptives primarily prevent pregnancy?
   a. By inhibiting ovulation
   b. By blocking sperm from entering the uterus
   c. By preventing implantation of the fertilized egg
   d. By thickening cervical mucus

Q3. Which contraceptive method involves the insertion of a small T-shaped device into the uterus?
   a. Condoms           b. Diaphragm
   c. Intrauterine device (IUD)   d. Cervical cap

Q4. What is the mechanism of action of condoms in preventing pregnancy?
   a. By blocking sperm from entering the uterus
   b. By inhibiting ovulation
   c. By preventing implantation of the fertilized egg
   d. By thickening cervical mucus

Q5. Which contraceptive method involves the surgical sealing or blocking of the fallopian tubes?
   a. Vasectomy         b. Tubal ligation
   c. Contraceptive implant   d. Oral contraceptives

Q6. What is the primary advantage of hormonal contraceptives?
   a. High efficacy         b. Reversible
   c. Long-lasting protection   d. No side effects

Q7. Which contraceptive method is NOT suitable for individuals with latex allergies?
   a. Condoms           b. Diaphragm
   c. Copper IUD        d. Hormonal implants

Q8. How does the contraceptive implant prevent pregnancy?
   a. By inhibiting ovulation
   b. By blocking sperm from entering the uterus

c. By thickening cervical mucus
d. By preventing implantation of the fertilized egg

Q9. Which contraceptive method is suitable for women who cannot use estrogen-based contraceptives?
a. Copper IUD
b. Combined oral contraceptives
c. Contraceptive patch
d. Progestin-only pill

Q10. What is the primary disadvantage of barrier methods of contraception?
a. Low efficacy
b. High cost
c. Require frequent healthcare provider visits
d. Interrupt spontaneity during sexual intercourse

Q11. Which contraceptive method is associated with the highest risk of ectopic pregnancy?
a. Copper IUD
b. Hormonal implants
c. Vasectomy
d. Tubal ligation

Q12. How do emergency contraceptive pills primarily prevent pregnancy?
a. By inhibiting ovulation
b. By blocking sperm from entering the uterus
c. By thickening cervical mucus
d. By preventing implantation of the fertilized egg

Q13. Which contraceptive method requires consistent daily use for maximum efficacy?
a. Copper IUD
b. Contraceptive patch
c. Hormonal implants
d. Condoms

Q14. Which contraceptive method is reversible and does not affect hormonal balance?
a. Tubal ligation
b. Vasectomy
c. Contraceptive implant
d. Intrauterine device (IUD)

Q15. What is the primary disadvantage of hormonal contraceptives?
a. Low efficacy
b. High cost
c. Increased risk of cardiovascular events
d. Require surgical procedure for insertion

## ANSWERS

1. c  2. a  3. c  4. a  5. b  6. a  7. a  8. a  9. d  10. d  11. a  12. a  13. b  14. d  15. c

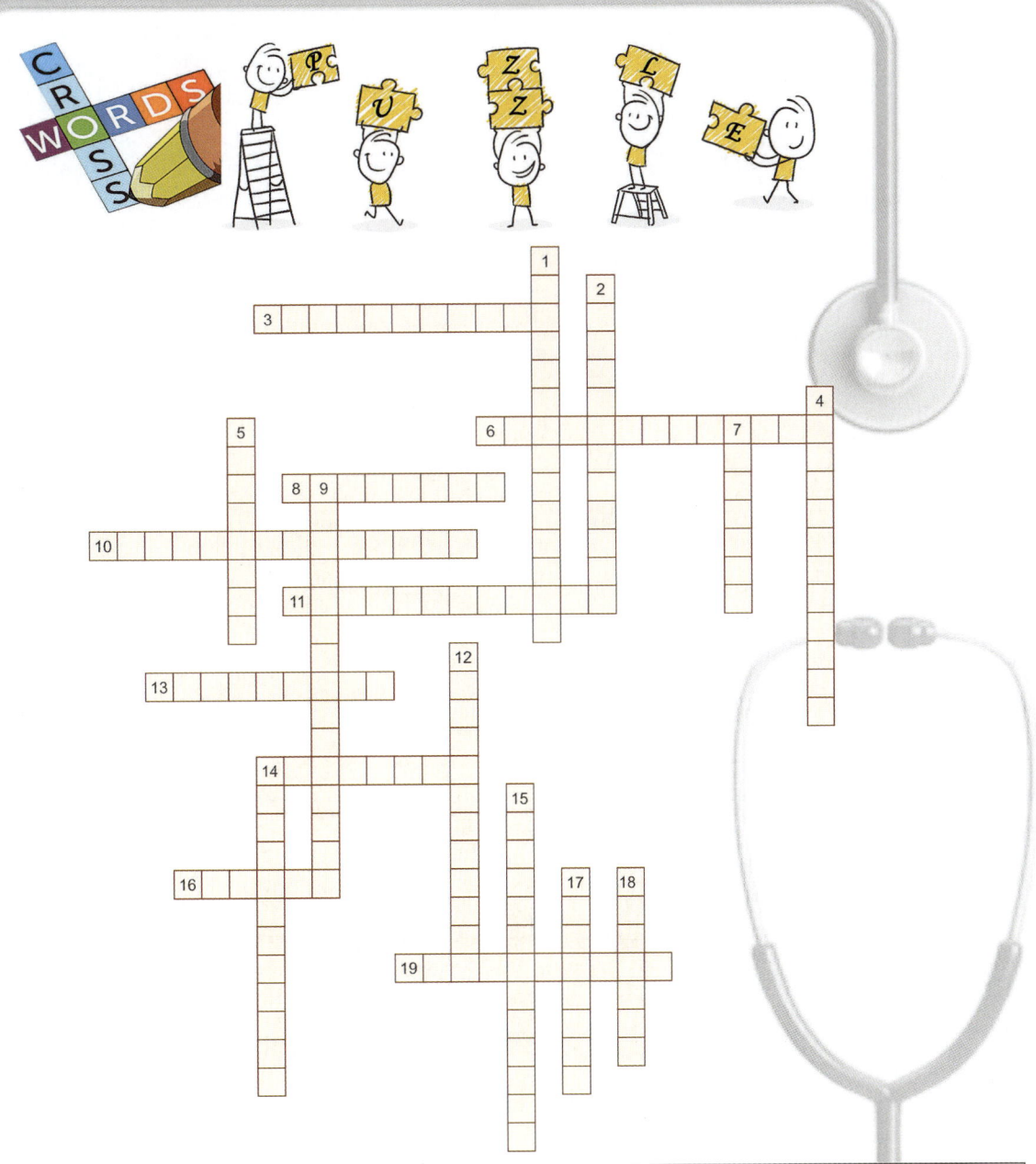

### Across

3. Enzyme involved in the breakdown of the ovarian follicle during ovulation
6. Phase of the menstrual cycle characterized by the thickening of the uterine lining
8. Hormone, primarily produced by the ovaries, peaks around the middle of the menstrual cycle
10. Compound present in emergency contraceptive pill
11. Process by which the fertilized egg implants into the uterine wall
13. Surgical procedure of bilateral ligation of the vas deferens for contraception
14. Onset of the first menstrual cycle at puberty
16. Gland responsible for producing testosterone in males
19. Condition characterized by the absence of menstruation

### Down

1. The process of sperm maturation that occurs in the epididymis
2. Changes occurring in spermatozoa in the female genital tract for fertilization
4. Male sex hormone responsible for development of secondary sexual characteristics
5. The hormone responsible for milk ejection during breastfeeding
7. Pair of chromosomes do not separate during meiotic division resulting in gamete having 24 chromosomes
9. Process by which spermatozoa are produced in the seminiferous tubules
12. The hormone responsible for maintaining the uterine lining during pregnancy
14. The phase of the menstrual cycle characterized by the shedding of the uterine lining
15. Enzyme present in acrosome of sperm responsible for acrosome reaction
17. Inactive X chromosome of each somatic cell forms a condensed mass
18. Period of life during which reproductive organs become functional

# SECTION 10

# NEUROPHYSIOLOGY AND SPECIAL SENSES

## Section Outline

- **Chapter 79:** Organization of Nervous System
- **Chapter 80:** Synapse
- **Chapter 81:** Neurotransmitters
- **Chapter 82:** Physiology of Sensory Receptors
- **Chapter 83:** Postural Reflexes and their Regulation
- **Chapter 84:** Cerebral Cortex
- **Chapter 85:** Thalamus
- **Chapter 86:** Role of Cerebellum and Basal Ganglia (Motor Planning, Programming and Execution)
- **Chapter 87:** Spinal Cord and the Pathways between Cerebrum and Peripheral Parts of Body
- **Chapter 88:** Reticular Activating System (RAS)
- **Chapter 89:** Physiology of Limbic System, Speech, Memory, EEG and Sleep
- **Chapter 90:** Vestibular System
- **Chapter 91:** Autonomic Nervous System
- **Chapter 92:** Cerebral Blood Flow
- **Chapter 93:** Physiology of Olfaction
- **Chapter 94:** Physiology of Taste Sensation (Gustatory Sensation)
- **Chapter 95:** Physiology of Vision
- **Chapter 96:** Physiology of Hearing

# Organization of Nervous System

**CHAPTER 79**

### COMPETENCY ADDRESSED
PY10.1: Describe and discuss the organization of nervous system.

### LEARNING OBJECTIVES
**At the end of this chapter, the learner should be able to:**
- Describe the basic divisions of the central nervous system.
- Describe the functional anatomy of the central nervous system.
- Describe the functional organization of CNS.
- Describe the principles of neuronal signal processing in CNS.

The nervous system, is the main controlling system of all the muscle, glands and organs of our body. The nervous system is broadly divided into:
1. **Central nervous system:** It is comprised of brain and spinal cord. These are the vital organs, which are protected in the bone covering. The brain is enclosed in the skull and the spinal cord is enclosed in the vertebral column.
2. **Peripheral nervous system:** The peripheral somatic nerves which emerge from the spinal cord and the cranium forms the PNS.
3. **Autonomic nervous system:** This division of nervous system which is not in our voluntary control is called autonomic nervous system (ANS). It is further subdivided to two divisions: sympathetic and parasympathetic nervous system. The ANS regulates the normal visceral functioning for proper functioning of various organ systems.

## CENTRAL NERVOUS SYSTEM

### BRAIN
The brain is further classified on the basis of embryological development (**Fig. 79.1** and **Table 79.1**).

### FUNCTIONAL ANATOMY OF BRAIN AND SPINAL CORD

#### Brain
From the **Table 79.1**, we have seen that the different parts of the brain with their function.

- The brain and spinal cord are organized into *gray matter* (consisting of cell bodies of neurons with their dendrites and proximal parts of neurons) and the *white matter* (made by axons). Both the gray and white matter contain neuroglial cells.
- **The brain is classified as:**
  - *Cerebral cortex:* There are two cerebral hemispheres, connected through the corpus callosum. The surface of cerebral cortex has many folds called sulci (the grooves) and gyri (the elevations). These folds increase the surface area of the cerebral cortex.

The deepest fissure is present on the superior surface between the two hemispheres **(Fig. 79.2)**.

The lateral view of cerebral cortex shows **(Fig. 79.3)**:
- **Four lobes:** Frontal, parietal, temporal and occipital lobes.
- **The lateral fissure:** It separates temporal lobe from frontal lobe.
- **The central sulcus:** It runs between the frontal and parietal lobe.
- **Specific areas:** The cerebral cortex has specific motor, premotor, primary somatosensory area, visual area, speech area, etc., discussed in detail in cerebrum.

The basal surface of cerebrum shows **(Fig. 79.4)**:
- The olfactory bulbs
- Two surfaces: The orbital and tentorial surfaces
- The optic nerves and optic chiasma are also visible.
- The cerebellum is located on both sides.
- The brainstem is also clearly appreciated in this view.

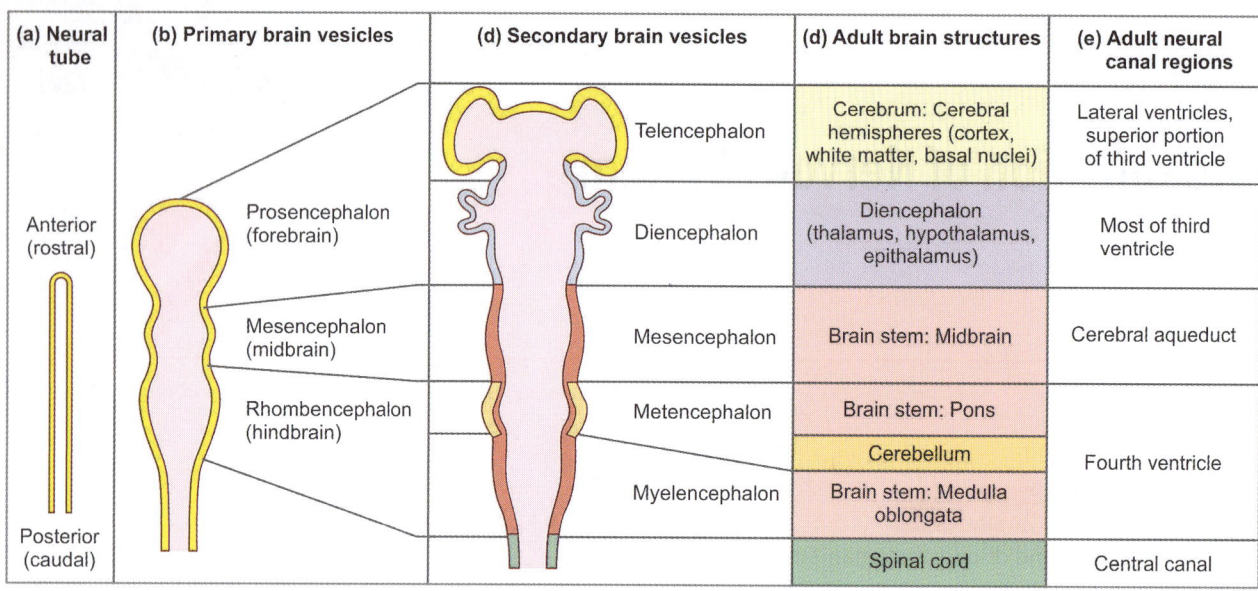

**Fig. 79.1:** Embryonic development of CNS.

**Table 79.1:** Parts of brain based on embryonic development.

| | Prosencephalon | | Mesencephalon | Rhombencephalon | |
|---|---|---|---|---|---|
| | **Telencephalon** | **Diencephalon** | | **Metaencephalon** | **Myelencephalon** |
| Parts of brain | Both cerebral hemispheres | Thalamus, hypothalamus, metathalamus, subthalamus | Corpora quadrigemina, cerebral peduncles, substantia nigra, tegmentum, midbrain nuclei | Pons, cerebellum | Medulla oblongata |
| Functions | Perception of sensations, cognition, learning, memory, planning, programming, etc. | • Relay of information to cortex<br>• Control of ANS and endocrines | | • Also called as brainstem<br>• CVS and Respiratory control<br>• Motor activity<br>• Sleep wakefulness cycle<br>• Visceral functions | |

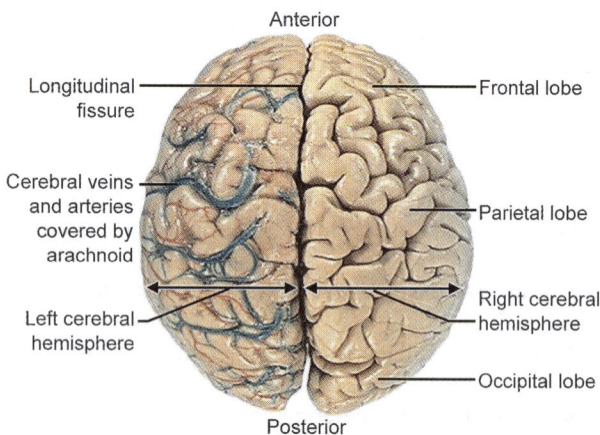

**Fig. 79.2:** Superior view of cerebral cortex.

The medial view shows the following structures (**Fig. 79.5**):
- The medial surface of the frontal, parietal, temporal and occipital lobes

- **The corpus callosum:** A structure which connects both the cerebral hemispheres. It has the fibers which cross from one hemisphere to another.
- Other structures seen here are thalamus, hypothalamus, pituitary gland, optic chiasma, mamillary body, fourth ventricle, cerebellum, pons and medulla oblongata.

Deep inside the brain, structures present are:
- Ventricular system, which contains the cerebrospinal fluid
- Basal ganglia
- Limbic system

All these anatomical structures have specific functions to play. The functional organization of CNS can be done as:
- **Somatosensory nervous axis:** This receives the inputs from the sensory organs/receptors which are processed in the cerebral cortex. The response to stimulus is then integrated with the motor cortex
- **Skeletal motor nervous axis:** The movements are planned and executed by the motor cortex of cerebrum which are controlled and coordinated to desired level by basal ganglia and cerebellum.

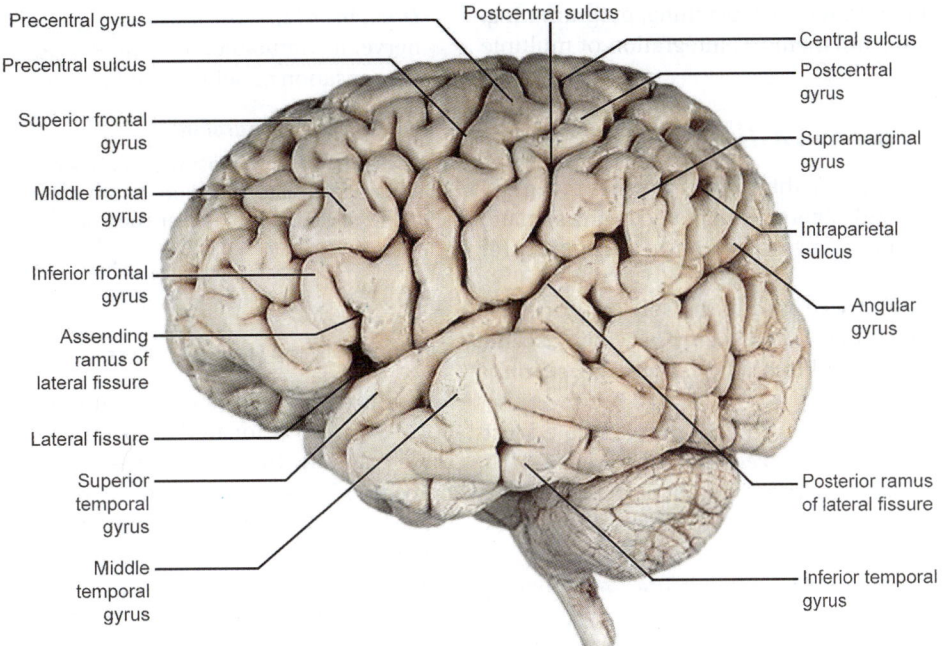

**Fig. 79.3:** Lateral view of left cerebrum.

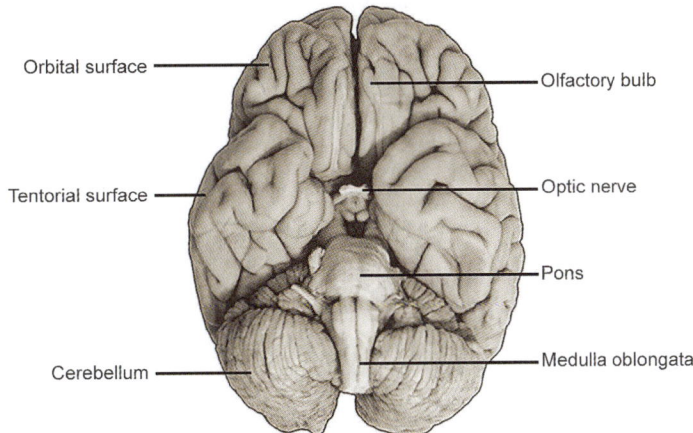

**Fig. 79.4:** Basal view of cerebrum.

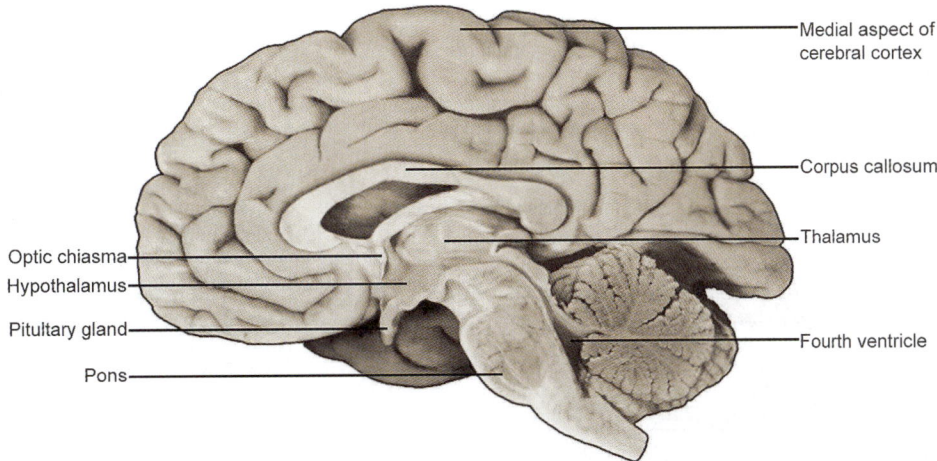

**Fig. 79.5:** Medial view of cerebrum after sectioning the corpus callosum.

- **Higher mental functions** like planning, programming, speech, learning and memory, integration of multiple inputs, etc.

### Somatosensory Nervous Axis

In **Figure 79.6**, we can see the various somatic receptors present in the skin and joints get stimulated by the somatic sensations like touch, pressure, pain, temperature, proprioception etc.

- These sensations are carried to the sensory cortex of the brain through the *sensory neurons* which ascend up from the spinal cord to brain (*ascending neurons/pathways*).
- The *somatosensory cortex* in the brain is located just behind the central sulcus (**Area 3,2,1 and Area 5,7**).
- The sensations received from different parts of the body are represented on specific parts of the cerebral cortex *'Sensory homunculus'*.
- All the somatic senses relay through *Thalamus,* before being relayed to sensory cortex.
- An input is also shared with *cerebellum* for **unconscious kinesthetic inputs.**
- All the nerve fibers are coded for a single sensation from receptor to cerebral cortex. It is explained by *'Muller's Doctrine of specific nerve energies.'* It explains that the nerve, if stimulated, anywhere in its course, produces the sensation of being stimulated at the receptor.

**Phantom Limb Syndrome**

In patients, who have lost their limb (amputated), still feel the pain/sensation in the nonexistent (phantom) limb due to Muller's doctrine of specific nerve energies/labeled line code.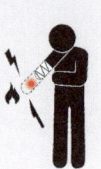

### Skeletal Motor Nervous Axis

The **Figure 79.7**, shows the motor area in the cerebral cortex, which is located in front of the central sulcus (area 4 and 6). The motor areas for different parts of the body are represented on specific parts of the motor area on cerebral cortex *'Motor homunculus'.* There is a close sensory motor coordination for the perfect execution of motor activities.

- The neurons arising from the motor cortex descend down to the spinal cord through the descending or motor tracts.
- Thes activity of these neurons is influenced by the activity of basal ganglia and cerebellum.

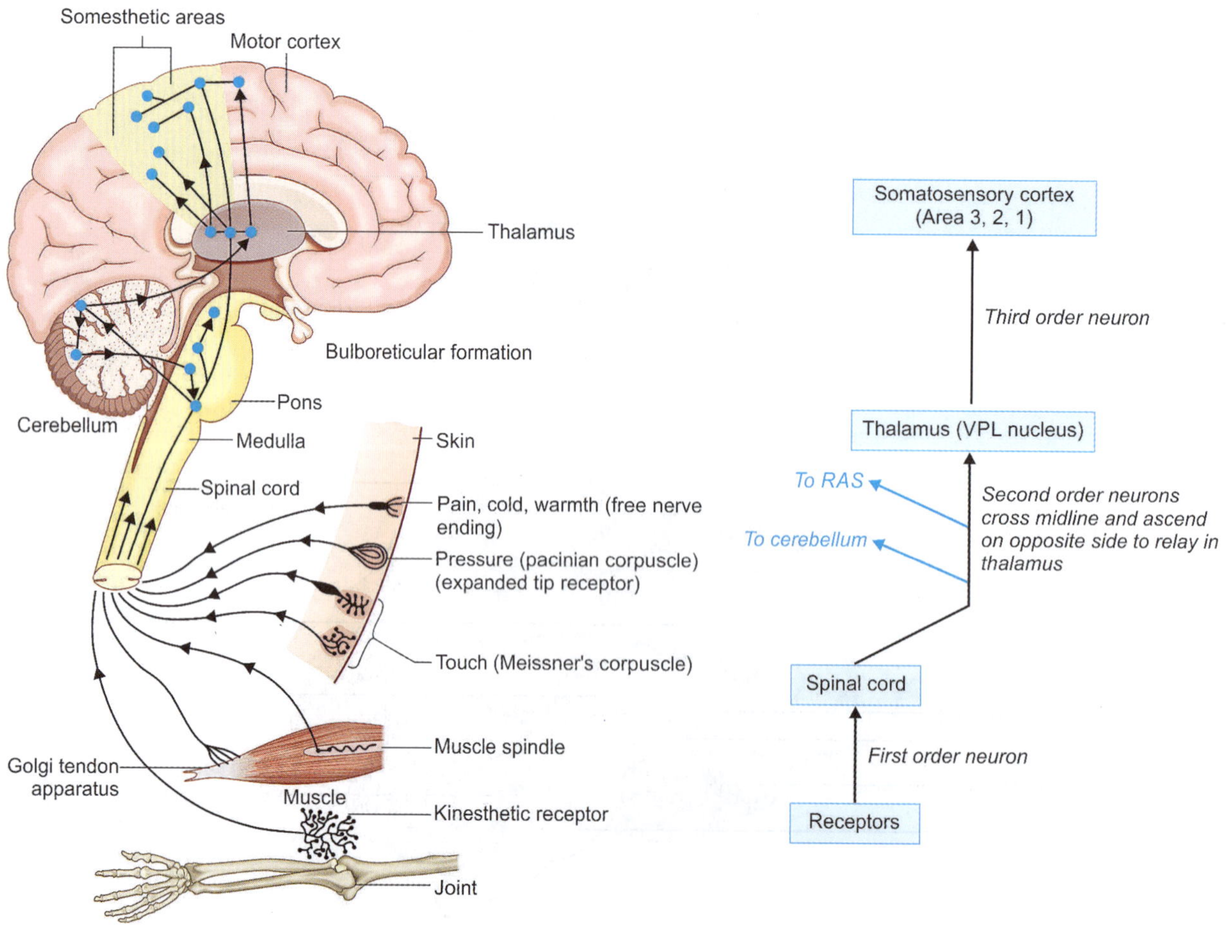

**Fig. 79.6:** Somatosensory nervous axis.

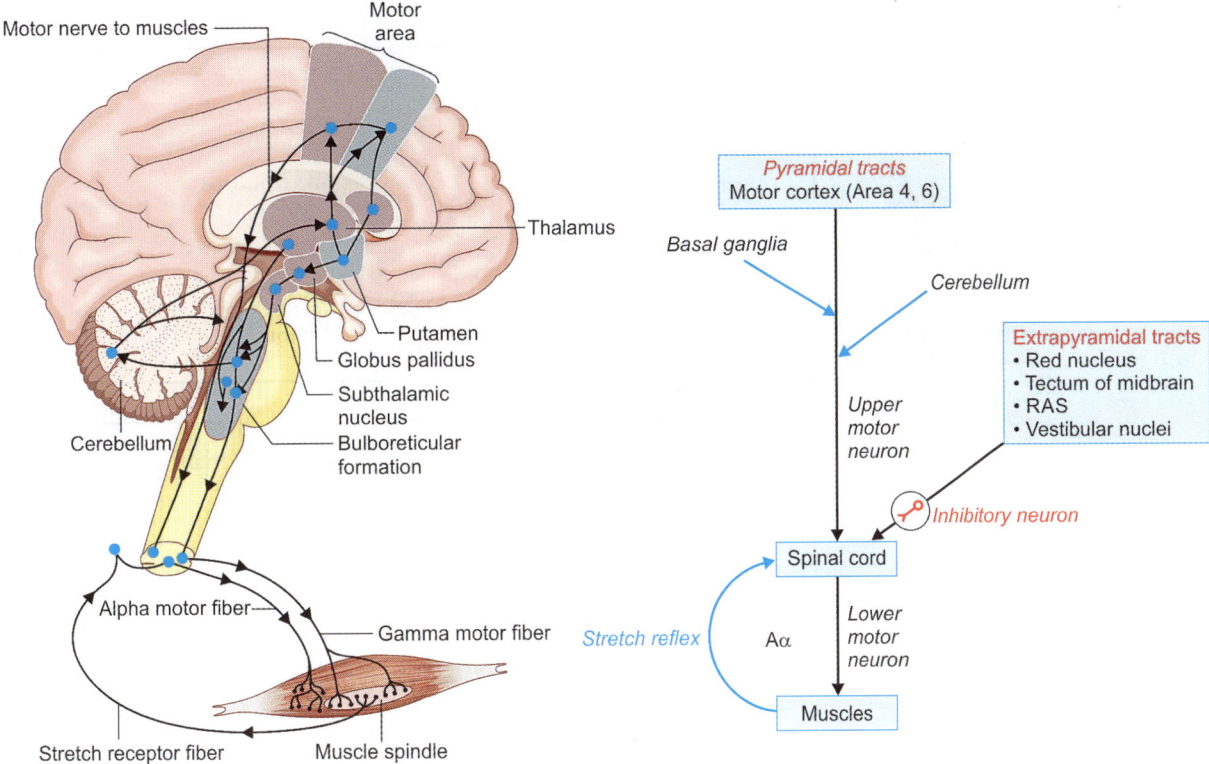

**Fig. 79.7:** Skeletal motor nervous axis.

- Some motor neurons, instead of arising from motor are of the cerebral cortex, arise from the other structures like red nucleus, reticular formation, etc., influences the motor activity.
- These tracts are called as motor, as the influence the activity of skeletal muscles.
- The neurons arising from CNS and terminating in the spinal cord on motor neurons of spinal cord are called the *Upper motor neurons*. Whereas the motor neurons arising from the anterior horn of spinal cord (***alpha and gamma***) are called the *Lower motor neurons*, as they innervate the skeletal muscle at motor end plates.

## Higher Mental Functions

The cerebral cortex along with the deeper structures is responsible for various higher mental functions like:
- Planning, programing and execution of the motor activity.
- Responsible for thinking, mentation and solving the problems.
- Makes the personality of an individual (docile/aggressive, etc.)
- The memorization of the learned activity by the temporal cortex.
- The synthesis of speech by the motor speech area. Ability to interpret heard/written or spoken form of speech.
- The understanding of reward and punishment, which alters the behavior of the person.
- Integration of many functions producing complex

## Spinal Cord (Fig. 79.8)

- Originates from base of skull and extends up to L1 vertebra. Below that, the spinal cord rise to many rootlets, resembling the horse tail, hence called the *cauda equina*.

> The spinal cord terminates at the level of L1 vertebrae in adults and the canal below this contains only cerebrospinal fluid. Hence, L3–L4 is the most common site used for lumbar puncture. Lumbar puncture is performed to:
> - Collect the sample of CSF for diagnostic purposes
> - Administration of spinal anesthesia
> - Administration of drug via intrathecal route.

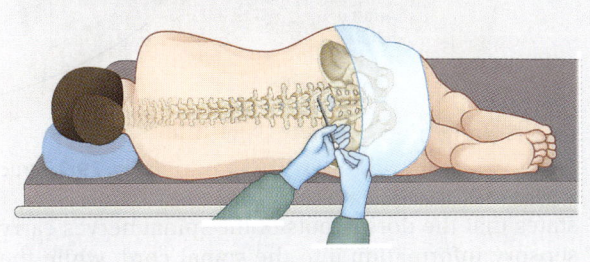

- The spinal cord has the outer white matter which consists of nerve fibers and inner H-shaped grey matter which has many cell bodies.
- There are 31 spinal nerves are named as 8 cervical, 12 thoracic, 5 lumbar, 5 sacral and 1 coccygeal nerves.
- The spinal segment has each having a motor and a sensory root/horn (**Fig. 79.9**). **Bell-Magendie Law**

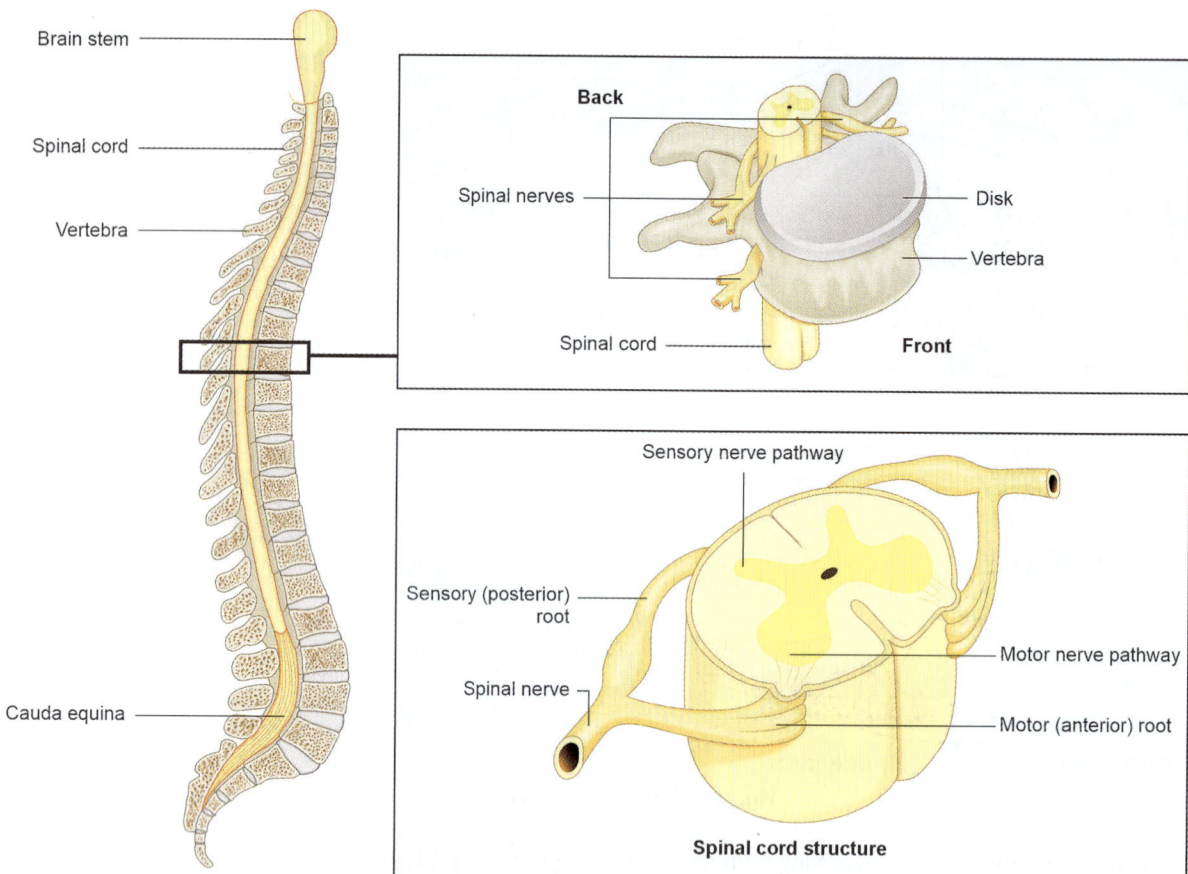

**Fig. 79.8:** The spinal cord: extent, location and structure.

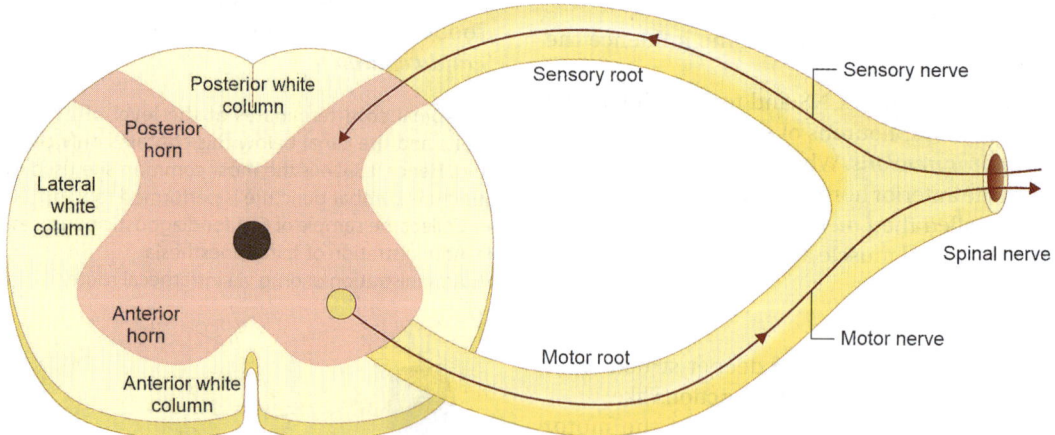

**Fig. 79.9:** Structure of spinal cord.

states that the dorsal roots of the spinal nerves carry sensory information into the spinal cord, while the ventral roots carry motor information out of the spinal cord.

- The *sensory root* is also called the *Posterior/Dorsal root/horn*. It brings the sensory fibers from the receptors to the spinal cord.
- The *motor root* is also called the *Anterior/Ventral root/horn*. The motor neurons (alpha and gamma) arise from this root.
- The thoracolumbar segment has an additional intermediate horn, which gives rise to the sympathetic neurons.
- There are two main type of neurons present in spinal cord:
  1. **Motor neurons:**
     - *Alpha (Aα) neurons:* They are the main motor neurons, innervating the muscle fibers
     - *Gamma (Aγ) neurons:* They are motor to the intrafusal fibers of muscle spindle.

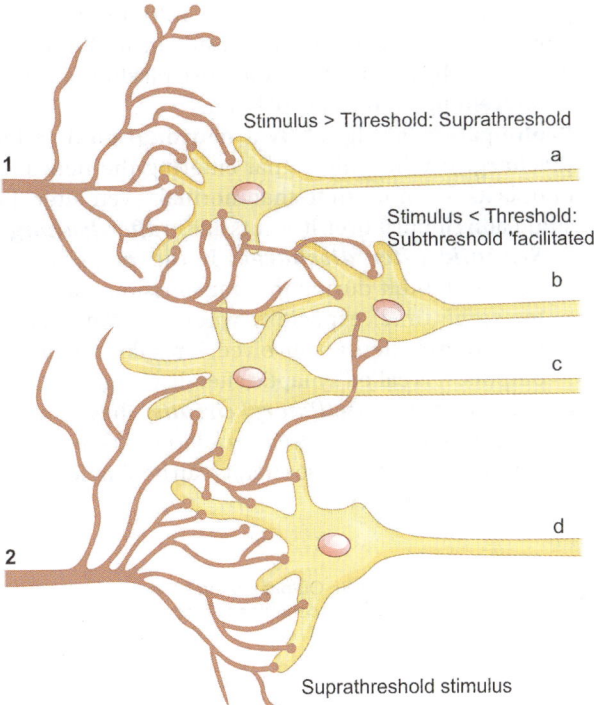

**Fig. 79.10:** Organization of neuronal pool.

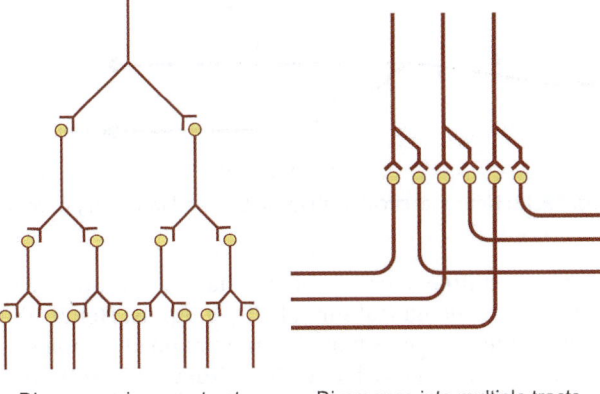

**Fig. 79.11:** Divergence of signal in neuronal pool.

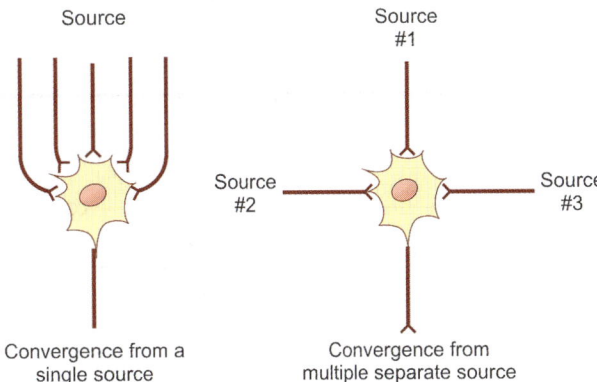

**Fig. 79.12:** Convergence of signal in neuronal pool results in summation of stimulus.

2. *Interneurons:* These are small neurons present in the spinal cord responsible for signal modulation at the level of spinal cord. These neurons can cause presynaptic inhibition (as seen in Renshaw cells) or facilitation, repetitive discharge, convergence, divergence, etc.
- **Function:** Convey sensory signals from periphery to brain and motor signals from brain to target organs.

**Processing of signal in neuronal pool:**
As we know that the brain and spinal cord are primarily formed by the neurons. There are millions of neurons in the neuronal pool. These neurons connect to each other through the synapse. Each input neuron divides into hundreds and thousands of terminal fibers which influence the other neurons in the neuronal pool **(Fig. 79.10)**. The neuronal area stimulated by each incoming nerve fiber is called the *stimulatory field*. The information is processed in many ways in the neuronal pool, which is described below:
- **Threshold stimulus:** Each neuron has to be stimulated to a *minimum potential*, so that it can get excited and result in the significant change in the voltage/potential of the neuron. *Change of potential in second neuron, occurring due to the activity of first (Input) neuron, is called the postsynaptic potential*.
  - In **Figure 79.10**, Neuron 1 synapses on neurons a, b and c. Stimulus from neuron 1 (excitatory stimulus) synapsing with neuron a, excites it. This stimulation is above the threshold of neuron a. Hence it is called *suprathreshold stimulus* and genesis of *excitatory postsynaptic potential (EPSP)*. For neuron 2, the neuron d is excited by suprathreshold stimulus.
  - Similarly, neuron 1 also stimulates b and c, but the stimulus is below the threshold stimulus *(subthreshold stimulus)*. These neurons b and c are said to be *facilitated*. Neuron 2 facilitates neuron c and d.
  - Some fibers inhibit the neuronal pool, instead of stimulating it. They result in *inhibitory postsynaptic potentials (IPSP)*.
- **Divergence:** The input neuron spread the impulse on thousands of other neurons. This is called divergence. The divergence is of two types:
  1. *Divergence into same tract (amplifying type)* **(Fig. 79.11):** The signal spreads to an increasing number of neurons as it passes from one neuron to another. It is seen in *corticospinal pathway*, supplying the skeletal muscles.
  2. *Divergence into multiple tracts* **(Fig. 79.11):** The impulse spreads from one neuronal pool to another structure of brain or neuronal impulse. For example, spread of impulse into cerebellum, thalamus, etc.
- **Convergence (Fig. 79.12):** When a neuron is excited by multiple stimuli, which may either arise from a single source or multiple sources. If the input is converging

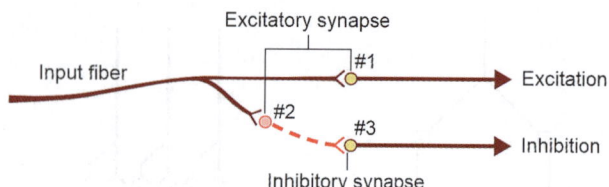

**Fig. 79.13:** Neuronal circuit with excitatory and inhibitory output.

from multiple sources, the resultant stimulation will be the mathematical sum of all the inputs. Hence, the convergence results from the summation of stimulus.

- **Neuron circuits with both inhibitory and excitatory output (Fig. 79.13):** Some neuronal circuits have both types of outputs, excitatory and inhibitory due to an inhibitory neuron in the second pathway converting the excitatory output to inhibitory. Such type of neuronal pathways are seen in reciprocal inhibition, where stimulation of flexor muscle result in inhibition of extensors. These types of circuits are typically important for preventing overactivity of brain.

- **Prolongation of signal by a neuronal pool (after discharge):** When the signal entering the neuronal pool lasts for more time than normal, even after the stimulating input is over. It occurs due to *after discharge*.
  - *Synaptic after discharge:* If the postsynaptic potential, built during the transmission continues for some time, especially when the long acting neurotransmitters are involved, it results in multiple outputs. It is called synaptic after discharge.
  - *Reverberatory (oscillatory) circuits:* These circuits are based on *positive feedback loops* created in the neuronal circuits. These circuits can be simple to very complex **(Fig. 79.14)**.

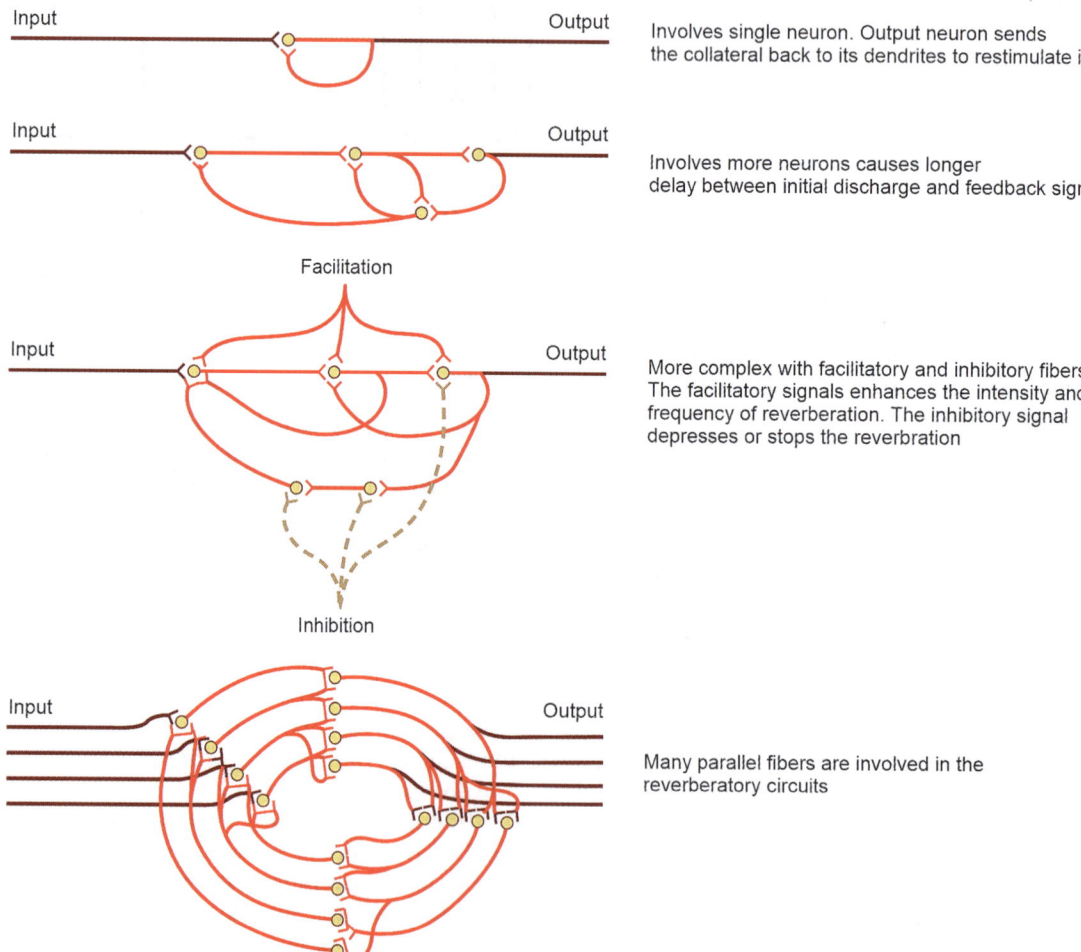

**Fig. 79.14:** Reverberatory circuits with increasing complexity.

The duration of output in a reverberatory circuit is dependent upon the exhaustion of neurotransmitter (synaptic fatigue). Hence the output ceases after some time.

- **Continuous signal output:** Some neuronal circuits exhibit continuous output signal, even after the cessation of the input. It occurs due to:
  - *Continuous discharge by intrinsic neuronal excitability:* Some neurons continuously emit the impulses and discharge repetitively as their threshold is not so high enough. Hence the increase in firing rate of these neurons give facilitatory output and decreased firing rate gives the inhibitory signal. These types of neurons are present in cerebellum and interneurons of spinal cord.
  - *Continuous signals emitted from reverberatory circuits:* The continuous discharge from reverberatory circuits, increases the intensity of output signal in excitatory input signal, whereas the inhibitory input reduces the output.

**Flowchart 79.1:** Rhythmical signal control of respiration during hypoxia.

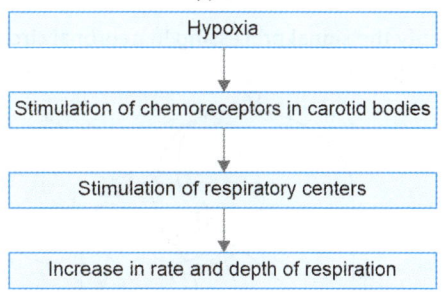

- **Rhythmical signal output:** Many neuronal circuits emit the rhythmical neuronal discharge. The rate of firing of these neuronal circuits determines whether the output is facilitatory or inhibitory. For example, the respiratory neurons discharge rhythmically and controls the respiratory rate (**Flowchart 79.1**).

## SUMMARY

- The embryonic development of various parts of brain as
  - Prosencephalon:
    - Telencephalon: cerebral hemispheres
    - Diencephalon: Thalamus, hypothalamus
  - Mesencephalon: Corpora quadrigemina, Cerebral peduncles, Substantia nigra, Tegmentum, Mid brain nuclei
  - Rhombencephalon:
    - Meta encephalon: Pons and cerebellum
    - Myelencephalon: Medulla oblongata
- The functional organization of CNS is done on the basis of:
  - **Somatosensory nervous axis:** This receives the inputs from the sensory organs/receptors which are processed in the cerebral cortex. The response to stimulus is then integrated with the motor cortex
  - **Skeletal motor nervous axis:** The movements are planned and executed by the motor cortex of cerebrum which are controlled and coordinated to desired level by basal ganglia and cerebellum.
  - **Higher mental functions** like planning, programing, speech, learning and memory, integration of multiple inputs, etc.
- The spinal cord is an extension of the medulla oblongata into the vertebral column, extending up to L1. It gives rise to 31 pairs of spinal nerves carrying the sensory, motor and autonomic fibers.
  - The spinal cord has H-shaped grey matter consisting of cell bodies of neurons, with anterior motor horn and posterior sensory root.
  - The white matter has nerve fibers which is divided into anterior, lateral and posterior white column.
- The signal processing in neuronal pool includes:
  - Threshold stimulation
  - Facilitation and inhibition
  - Divergence
  - Convergence
  - Neuronal circuits with excitatory and inhibitory output.
  - Prolonged signal output due to:
    - Synaptic after discharge
    - Reverberatory circuits
    - Continuous discharge of neurons
    - Rhythmic neuronal discharge

## LET US SEE, HOW MUCH YOU HAVE LEARNT?

 *Review Questions*

Q1. Describe the physiological basis of phantom limb.
Q2. Describe the principles of signal processing in neuronal pool.
Q3. What is Bell-Magendie's law?
Q4. What is threshold stimulus? What does it signify?

## Multiple Choice Questions

**Q1. Identify the signal processing in neuronal circuit in the given figure:**

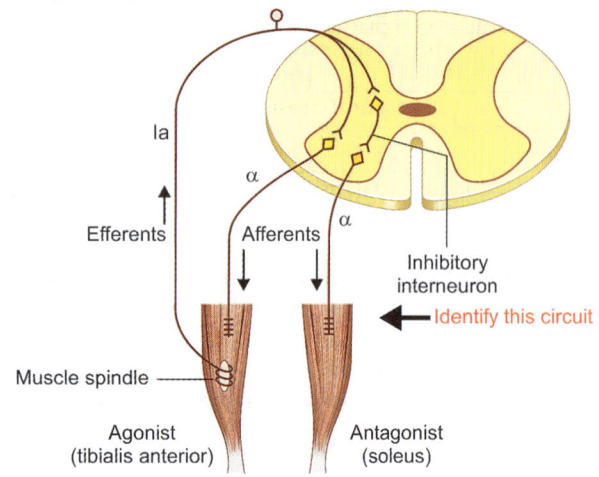

a. Convergence
b. Divergence
c. Reciprocal inhibition
d. Reverberatory circuit

**Q2. Which neuronal signal processing is seen in the figure given below?**

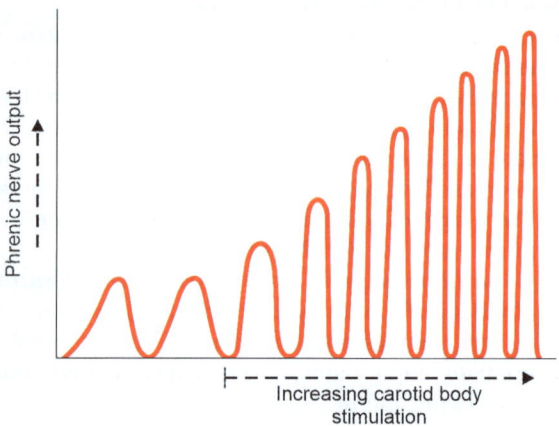

a. Increased stimulation of carotid body due to hypoxia
b. Increased stimulation of respiratory neurons due to carotid body stimulation
c. Increased output from reverberatory circuits due to convergence of neuronal signal
d. None of the above

### ANSWERS

1. c   2. b

# Synapse

**CHAPTER 80**

### COMPETENCY ADDRESSED
PY10.2: Describe and discuss the functions and properties of synapse, reflex, receptors.

### LEARNING OBJECTIVES

**At the end of this chapter, the learner should be able to:**
- Define the synapse.
- Enumerate different types of synapse, based on structural and functional characteristics.
- Describe the structure of synapse.
- Describe the transmission of impulse across the synapse.
- Describe the potential changes in the postsynaptic membrane.
- Describe the properties of synapse.

---

Synapse is defined as the junction between the neurons, which results in the transmission of impulse from one neuron to another.

## TYPES OF SYNAPSE

- **Depending on the type of transmission, the synapse is classified as:**
  - *Chemical synapse:* It is a type of synapse which involves a chemical (neurotransmitter) (*see* **Fig. 80.3**). It is the most common type of synapse present in neurons. The transmission of impulse in a chemical synapse is described below, in the next section. There are more than 50 types of neurotransmitters involved in the chemical synapse.
  - *Electrical synapse:* It is the transmission of impulse from one neuron to another through the gap junctions (**Fig. 80.1**). It is not a common form of synapse. However, a single neuron can have both types of synapses (chemical and electrical). The transmission of impulse across the electrical synapse have certain peculiarities, described below:
    ♦ The transmission across the electrical synapse is faster than the chemical synapse.
    ♦ Usually, the chemical synapse shows only one way conduction, but the electrical synapse allows the bidirectional transmission of impulse.

- **Depending on the location of synapse, it is classified as (Fig. 80.2):**
  - *Axo-dendritic synapse:* The axon of one neuron synapses on the dendrites of another neuron
  - *Axo-somatic synapse:* The axon of one neuron synapses on the soma/cell body of another neuron
  - *Axo-axonic synapse:* The axon of one neuron synapses on the axon of another neuron

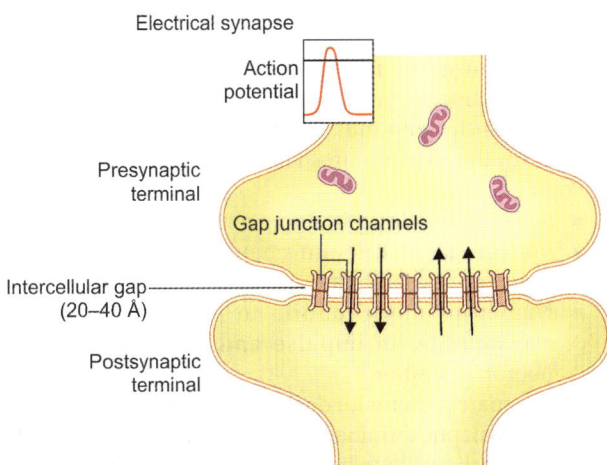

**Fig. 80.1:** Structure of electrical synapse.

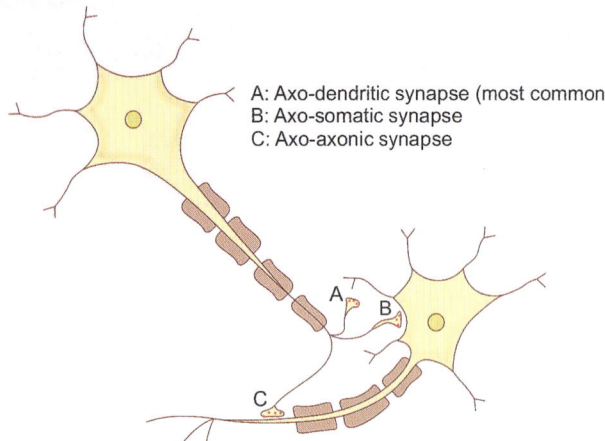

Fig. 80.2: Types of synapse, based on location of synapse.

- A: Axo-dendritic synapse (most common)
- B: Axo-somatic synapse
- C: Axo-axonic synapse

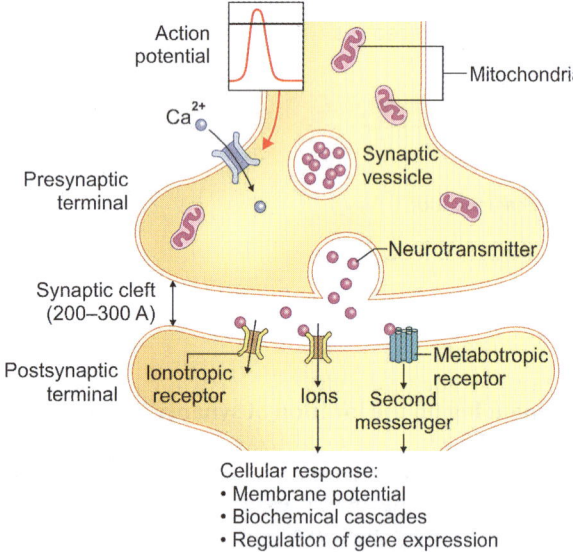

Fig. 80.3: Structure of synapse.

## STRUCTURE AND FUNCTIONING OF THE SYNAPSE

Synapse in the junction between the two neurons. We will discuss the most common type of synaptic structure. It has following components **(Fig. 80.3)**:

- **Presynaptic terminal:** The presynaptic terminal is made by the axon terminal knobs, which are dilated and contain:
  - Synaptic vesicles containing neurotransmitters
  - Voltage gated calcium channels located on the presynaptic membrane.
  - Numerous mitochondria to provide energy for transmission of impulse and replenishment of neurotransmitter
  - The snare proteins for docking of the synaptic vesicles. The presynaptic terminal of synapse and neuromuscular junction are structurally and functionally similar, which we read in Chapter 3, except the different types of neurotransmitters, being secreted in synapse.

**Flowchart 80.1:** Presynaptic release of neurotransmitter.

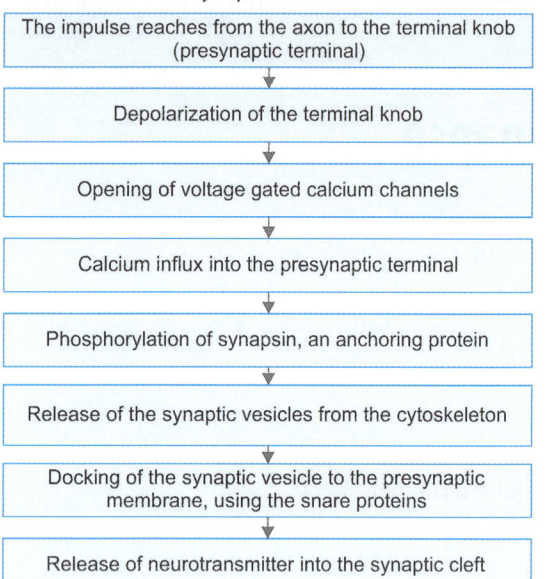

Release of neurotransmitter from presynaptic terminal shown in **Flowchart 80.1**.

- **Synaptic cleft:** It is the space between the pre and postsynaptic terminals, usually 200–300 Å wide. It has the extracellular fluid present here.
  - The neurotransmitters are released from the presynaptic terminal into the synaptic cleft.
  - The neurotransmitters bind to the specific receptors on postsynaptic membrane. These binding site of the receptors project into the synaptic cleft.
  - The neurotransmitters are quickly removed from the synaptic cleft to prevent the excessive/prolonged stimulation of postsynaptic receptors.
  - The neurotransmitter is taken back into the presynaptic terminal which is used for resynthesis of neurotransmitter.
- **Postsynaptic terminal:** Unlike the neuromuscular junction, the postsynaptic membrane is also a neuron. Depending upon the type of neurotransmitter released by the presynaptic terminal, the postsynaptic membrane may have either of the following receptors:
  - Ionotropic receptors: These receptors gate the ion channels
  - Ion channels: These channels transmit the ions and are classified as **(Fig. 80.4)**:
    - **Cation channel:** Allows positively charged ions through it. *The most commonly ion which is allowed to pass through it is sodium.* Other ions which are allowed to pass through cation channel is potassium and calcium. They repel the negatively charged ions ($Cl^-$ and other anions). These cation channels when activated result in *increased $Na^+$ influx/$Ca^{2+}$ influx/decreased $K^+$ efflux and hence depolarizes* the postsynaptic neuron. The neurotransmitter resulting in opening or closing of cation channels resulting in

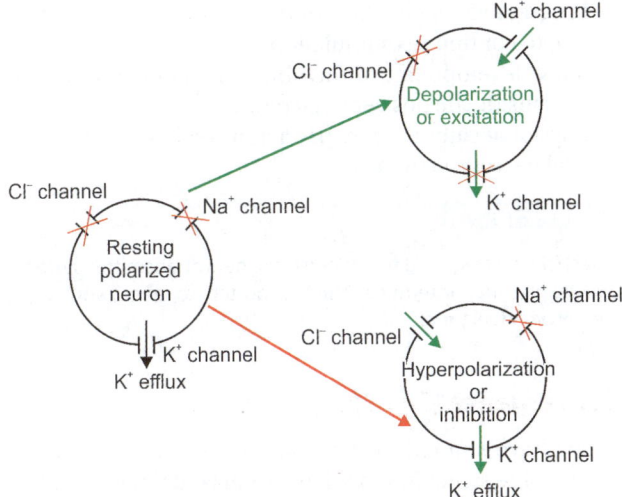

**Fig. 80.4:** Ionic channel activity during facilitation and inhibition.

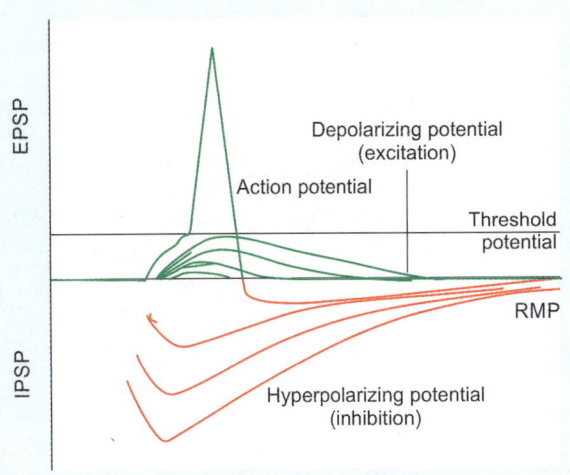

**Fig. 80.5:** The excitatory and inhibitory postsynaptic potentials.

excitation/depolarization of postsynaptic neuron is called the *excitatory neurotransmitter*.

- **Anion channel:** Allows negatively charged ion *(mostly chloride ion)* to pass through them resulting in Cl⁻ influx. The cations are repelled from these receptors and not allowed to pass through them. The neurotransmitters stimulating the anion channels are called the *inhibitory neurotransmitter*.
- *Metabotropic receptors:* These receptors are the G protein coupled receptors, which act through the second messenger. These receptors get activated and results in
    - Opening of specific ion channels resulting in change of the membrane potential (postsynaptic potentials).
    - Activation of cAMP/cGMP, which in turn activates the biochemical enzyme cascades.
    - Activation of one or more intracellular enzymes, modulating cellular function.
    - Activation of gene transcription and can modulate the gene expression of the cells.

## Postsynaptic Potentials

The potential developed in the postsynaptic terminal after the transmission of impulse from the presynaptic terminal are called the postsynaptic potentials (PSP). Depending on the type of neurotransmitter, the postsynaptic potentials can be excitatory or inhibitory (**Fig. 80.5**).

### Excitatory Postsynaptic Potential

The excitation of the postsynaptic terminal, resulting in the *depolarization of the neuron*, is called the excitatory postsynaptic potential (EPSP). This raises the intracellular potential towards the threshold potential for excitation. The excitation/depolarization hence occurs due to increased concentration of positive ion inside the postsynaptic neuron, which can occur due to:

- *Increased Na⁺ influx, raising Na⁺ levels in the cells*
- *Decreased K⁺ efflux from the cell. This raises the concentration of K⁺ inside the cell.*
- *Decreased Cl⁻ influx into the cell also depolarizes the cell.*
- *Increase in the number of receptors responsible for causing excitation.*

### Inhibitory Postsynaptic Potential (IPSP)

This leads to the inhibition/hyperpolarization of the postsynaptic membrane. Contrary to the EPSP, the membrane potential decreases below the resting membrane potential, becoming more negative. Hence, all the ionic movements, which increases the negativity inside the cell, will be activated like:

- *Decreased Na⁺ influx*
- *Increased K⁺ efflux from the cell. This decreases the concentration of K⁺ inside the cell.*
- *Increased Cl⁻ influx into the cell hyperpolarizes the cell.*
- *Activation of receptor enzymes, which increases the inhibitory receptors or decreases the excitatory receptors.*

## PROPERTIES OF SYNAPSE

The synapse is the basic junction between the two neurons required for transmission of impulse in the neuronal pool. Hence, most of the signal processing in the neuronal pool is influence by the synaptic transmission. Some of the common properties of synapse are described below:

### One Way Conduction

The chemical synapse has a unique property of transmission in one direction, i.e., *from the axon to terminal knobs and then to the other neuron through axo-dendritic/axo-somatic or axo-axonic synapses* (**Fig. 80.6**). There is no transmission from the dendrites to the axons in a chemical synapse. However, the electrical synapse can result in

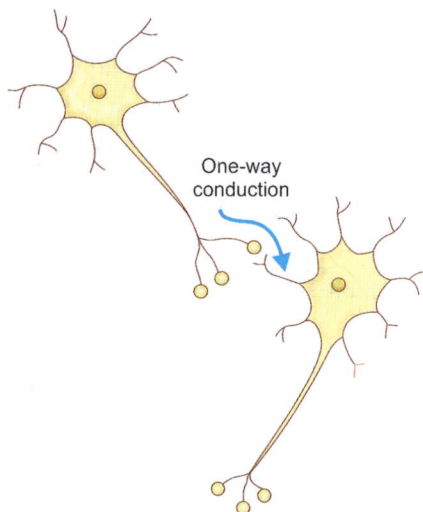

**Fig. 80.6:** Unidirectional transmission of impulse.

the two-way transmission of impulse between both the neurons.

## Synaptic Delay

The transmission of impulse across a single chemical synapse can take *around 0.5 milliseconds*. Hence, the total reaction time of a neural circuit can predict the number of neurons involved in it.

> *While testing the pain sensation of an individual, the time taken by the person to appreciate the sensation of pain, is around 1.0 milliseconds. How many neurons are involved in this pathway?*
>
> Since the synaptic delay for each synapse in 0.5 msec, the delay of 1.0 msec means that there are two synapses present in the pathway. Hence, it is a three-neuron pathway.

**Physiological basis of synaptic delay:** The various events taking place in the synapse, mentioned below are responsible for delay in a chemical synapse.
- Depolarization of presynaptic terminal
- Opening of voltage gated calcium channels resulting in calcium influx.
- Release of synaptic vesicle from cytoskeletal anchor
- Docking and release of the neurotransmitter from the presynaptic terminal
- Binding of the neurotransmitter to the postsynaptic receptor.
- Generation of appropriate postsynaptic potential
- Response in the postsynaptic neuron.

## Synaptic Fatigue

Repetitive stimulation of a neuron results in the setting of the synaptic fatigue. It occurs due to:
- Depletion of a neurotransmitter stored in the presynaptic terminal.
- Progressive inactivation of the postsynaptic receptors due to continuous stimulation.
- Slow development of the abnormal concentration of ions inside the postsynaptic neurons.

Physiologically, the synapse acts as seat of fatigue in the central nervous system.

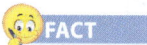 **FACT**

> Rest/sleep is required to replenish the neurotransmitter stores in the presynaptic terminal. This is important to refresh yourself, when you feel tired.

## Convergence (Fig. 80.7)

As we have studied in the Chapter 79, a single neuron receives the signal from various (thousands) neurons. It is required for the sharpening of the signal.

## Divergence (Fig. 80.8)

Each neuron synapses on thousands of the neurons and results in the propagation of the signal in the neuronal

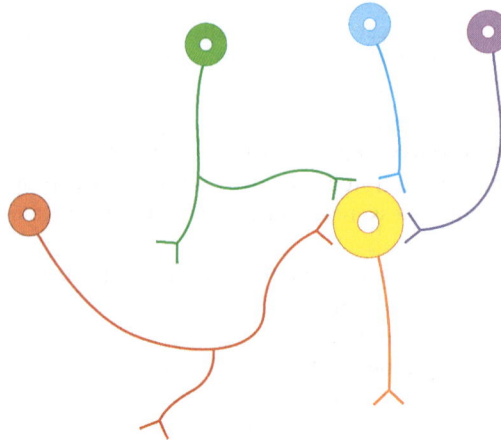

**Fig. 80.7:** Convergence of signal through synapse.

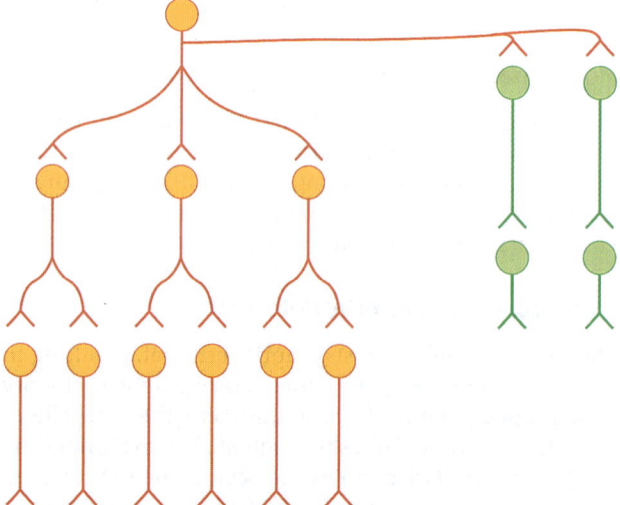

**Fig. 80.8:** Divergence of neuronal signal through synapse.

pool. In the Chapter 79, we had also discussed that the divergence can occur in the same tract/pathway as seen in corticospinal pathway. It results in *amplification of signal*. If the divergence occurs in multiple pathways, which can result in spread of signal into the associated circuits. Example: the sensory signal arising from spinal cord is also transmitted to cerebellum while its transmission to thalamus.

## Threshold Stimulus

A minimum threshold stimulus is required to excite the postsynaptic membrane. The neuronal zone process the signal in the following way:

- **Discharge zone:** Where the neurons are stimulated with suprathreshold stimulus. This result in excitation of postsynaptic membrane.
- **Occlusion (Fig. 80.9A):** It is a property of the neuronal pool, in which the presynaptic neurons facilitate less number of neurons, when stimulated together rather than when acting alone. This can be explained using the following example:
  - Neuron 1 when stimulated, further synapses on 3 neurons (a, b, c), resulting in their activation.
  - Neuron 2, also synapses of 4 neurons (b, c, d, e), resulting in activation of these 4 neurons.
  - But when Neurons 1 and 2 are co-stimulated, they should have stimulated 7 (a, b, b, c, c, d, e) neurons. Rather, only 5 (a, b, c, d, e) neurons are stimulated, as 2 neurons (b, c) were receiving the input from both Neurons 1 and 2.
  - Hence, these two neurons (b and c) are said to be occluded.
- **Subliminal fringe (Fig. 80.9B):** It is a property of the neuronal pool, in which the presynaptic neurons facilitate more number of neurons, when stimulated together rather when acting alone. This can be explained using the following example:
  - Neuron 1 when stimulated, further synapses on 3 neurons (a, b, c). But there is activation of only 2 neurons (a and b). The third neuron c is stimulated with subthreshold stimulus and hence not propagated.
  - Neuron 2, also synapses of 3 neurons (c, d, e), resulting in activation of 2 (d, e) neurons. The neuron c is still not propagated, as it is stimulated with subthreshold stimulus.
  - But when Neuron 1 and 2 are co-stimulated, they should have stimulated 4 (a, b, d, e) neurons. Rather, they stimulate 5 (a, b, c, d, e) neurons, as neuron c was receiving the input from both Neuron 1 and 2, and hence reached the threshold stimulation.
  - Hence, the neurons c is said to be in subliminal fringe.
- **Summation (Fig. 80.9C):** The stimulus received from the same or different input neurons is added up, so that the postsynaptic neuron reaches its threshold; and results in propagation of impulse. The summation can happen in two ways:

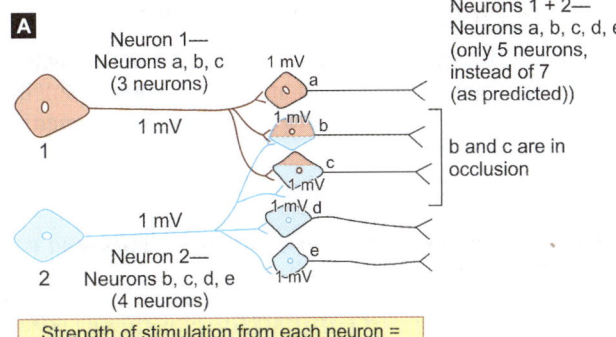

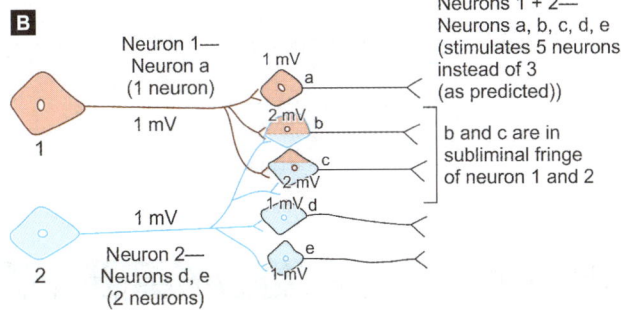

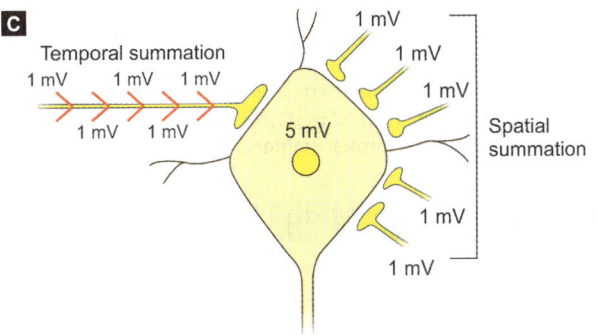

**Figs. 80.9A to C:** Synapse properties. (A) Occlusion; (B) Subliminal fringe; (C) Summation.

- *Spatial summation:* The multiple input neurons synapse on the postsynaptic neuron. This results in adding up of the stimuli to reach the threshold for postsynaptic neuron. Example: Neuron 1 has a threshold of 5 mV and receives the input of 1 mV from 5 neurons, adding up to 5mV of threshold stimulation.
- *Temporal summation:* The single input neuron sends the successive repetitive stimulations, resulting in attainment of the threshold of the postsynaptic neuron.

## Effect of Hypoxia

The synaptic transmission requires adequate supply of oxygen. Hence, even small fall in oxygen concentration adversely affects the synaptic transmission. Even 3–7 seconds of interruption of cerebral blood flow can result in unconsciousness. It can result in complete inexcitability of some neurons.

## Effect of pH on Synaptic Transmission

The change in pH greatly influences the neuronal activity.
- If the pH falls from 7.4 to 7.0 or below, it would result in depression of neuronal activity. *The patient appears comatose in acidosis.*

**Why does hyperventilation precipitates the seizure in a patient of epilepsy?**

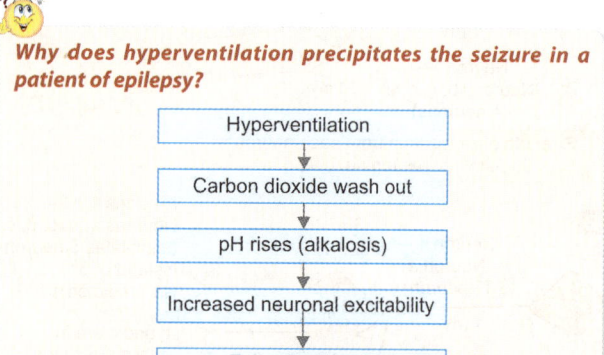

- On the contrary, if pH rises from 7.4 to 7.8 or above, it can greatly increase the neuronal excitability. For this reason, the epileptic patients are asked to avoid hyperventilation as it may precipitate an attack of epilepsy.

## Effect of Drugs on Synaptic Transmission

There are many drugs which affect the excitability of neurons:
- **Drugs increasing the neuronal excitability:**
    - Caffeine, theophylline, theobromine; found in tea and coffee increase the neuronal excitability by reducing the threshold for excitation of neurons.
    - Strychnine greatly increases the neuronal excitability. It inhibits the inhibitory neurotransmitter glycine in the spinal cord; resulting in severe tonic clonic muscle spasms.
- **Drugs decreasing the neuronal excitability:**
    - Anesthetics are lipid soluble which increases the threshold of the neuronal membrane, making them less responsive to excitatory agents.

---

### SUMMARY

- Synapse is the junction between two neurons.
- Based on the type of transmission, the synapse is classified as chemical and electrical synapse.
- Based on the location of the synapse, it is classified as axo-dendritic, axo-somatic and axo-axonic synapse.
- The synapse has a presynaptic terminal having the synaptic vesicles, synaptic cleft and postsynaptic membrane having the receptors for the neurotransmitter.
- The potential changes in postsynaptic potential is called the postsynaptic potentials. The excitatory potentials are called EPSP and inhibitory potentials are called IPSP.
- The various properties of synapse are same as the processing the signal in neuronal pool: one way conduction, synaptic delay, synaptic fatigue, threshold stimulation, occlusion, subliminal fringe, convergence, divergence, summation, effect of pH, oxygen levels and drugs on synaptic transmission.

---

### LET US SEE, HOW MUCH YOU HAVE LEARNT?

#### Review Questions

##### Long/Short Answer Questions

Q1. Define synapse. Describe the structure of synapse with the help of a well labeled diagram.
Q2. Differentiate between the chemical and electrical synapse.
Q3. Describe the properties of synapse.
Q4. Describe the role of postsynaptic receptors in transmission of impulse across the synapse.
Q5. Define postsynaptic potentials. Describe the different types of postsynaptic potential, and how can they be achieved?
Q6. What is the physiological significance of EPSPs and IPSPs?

##### Explain Why? (Reasoning Questions)

Q1. Synaptic delay is an important property of chemical synapses.
Q2. The balance between excitatory and inhibitory synapses is vital for neural network function.
Q3. The neurologists tell their epileptic patients to avoid hyperventilation.
Q4. Synaptic dysfunctions, can lead to psychiatric and neurodevelopmental disorders.

# Multiple Choice Questions

**Q1.** From the graph given below, identify the correct statement:

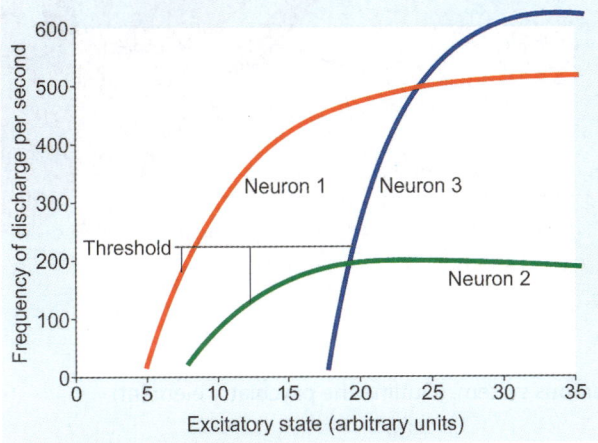

a. Neuron 3 can be stimulated easily
b. Neuron 2 shows a high discharge frequency
c. Neuron 1 has lowest threshold stimulus
d. Neuron 2 is inhibited while 1 and 3 are excited

**Q2.** A patient with diabetic ketoacidosis is brought to the medical ICU with blood sugar level of 460 mg/dL, pH of blood is 7.2. He appears comatose and drowsy. What do you think is the cause of his mental status?
a. The high blood sugar level causes dehydration of brain
b. pH of 7.2 shows acidosis, and hence depresses the synaptic transmission
c. The ketone bodies present in this condition, causes drowsiness
d. Hypovolemia causes decreased cerebral perfusion

**Q3.** Which of the following is NOT a type of synapse based on structural characteristics?
a. Axodendritic      b. Axosomatic
c. Axon-terminal     d. Chemical

**Q4.** What is the main function of a synapse?
a. Production of neurotransmitters
b. Transmission of electrical impulses between neurons
c. Protection of neurons
d. Maintenance of neuron's shape

**Q5.** What potential changes occur in the postsynaptic membrane during synaptic transmission?
a. Depolarization       b. Hyperpolarization
c. Both a and b         d. None of the above

**Q6.** Which of the following properties are NOT associated with synapses?
a. Plasticity                 b. Growth of neurons
c. Amplification of signal    d. Spreading of signal

**Q7.** Which type of synapse is characterized by direct electrical connections between neurons?
a. Electrical synapse       b. Chemical synapse
c. Axodendritic synapse     d. Axosomatic synapse

**Q8.** What is the space between the pre and postsynaptic neurons called?
a. Neurotransmitter     b. Synaptic cleft
c. Synaptic vesicle     d. Dendrite

**Q9.** Which of the following neurotransmitters is commonly associated with excitatory synapses?
a. GABA         b. Serotonin
c. Dopamine     d. Glutamate

**Q10.** The release of neurotransmitters into the synaptic cleft is triggered by:
a. An influx of calcium ions into the presynaptic neuron
b. An efflux of potassium ions from the postsynaptic neuron
c. An influx of sodium ions into the postsynaptic neuron
d. An efflux of chloride ions from the presynaptic neuron

**Q11.** Which of the following structures is responsible for reuptake of neurotransmitters in the synaptic cleft?
a. Synaptic vesicles
b. Axon terminal
c. Postsynaptic membrane
d. Transporter proteins

**Q12.** Inhibitory postsynaptic potentials (IPSPs) are typically associated with:
a. Hyperpolarization of the postsynaptic membrane
b. Depolarization of the postsynaptic membrane
c. No change in membrane potential
d. Generation of action potentials

**Q13.** Which of the following is NOT a structural component of a chemical synapse?
a. Neurotransmitter     b. Synaptic cleft
c. Myelin sheath        d. Postsynaptic density

**Q14.** Long-term potentiation (LTP) refers to:
a. The strengthening of synaptic connections over time
b. The weakening of synaptic connections over time
c. The release of neurotransmitters from presynaptic neurons
d. The reuptake of neurotransmitters into presynaptic neurons

**Q15.** Which of the following is a characteristic of neuromuscular junctions?
a. They are chemical synapses
b. They are found between neurons and muscle cells
c. They utilize acetylcholine as the neurotransmitter
d. All of the above

**Q16.** The process of synaptic pruning is associated with:
a. Strengthening synaptic connections
b. Weakening synaptic connections
c. Elimination of unnecessary synapses
d. Inhibition of neurotransmitter release

**Q17.** Which of the following is an example of a neuromodulator?
a. Acetylcholine    b. Serotonin
c. Glutamate        d. GABA

## ANSWERS

1. c  2. b  3. d  4. b  5. c  6. b  7. a  8. b  9. d  10. a  11. d  12. a  13. c  14. a
15. d  16. c  17. b

# Neurotransmitters

**CHAPTER 81**

> **COMPETENCY ADDRESSED**
> PY10.10: Describe and discuss chemical transmission in the nervous system. (Outline the psychiatry element).

>  **LEARNING OBJECTIVES**
> At the end of this chapter, the learner should be able to:
> - Classify various neurotransmitters.
> - Describe the functions and mechanism of actions of each of the neurotransmitters.
> - Describe the various clinical/applied aspect associated with neurotransmitters.

The chemical synapse requires certain chemicals which act as neurotransmitters. These neurotransmitters are broadly classified as *small and large molecule neurotransmitters*.

## SMALL MOLECULE NEUROTRANSMITTERS

The small molecule neurotransmitters are responsible for the acute responses in the neuron **(Table 81.1)**. Hence, they are *fast acting* biomolecules. They are synthesized in the cytoplasm of the presynaptic terminal and stored in the synaptic vesicles. Once the presynaptic neuron is stimulated, these vesicles fuse with the presynaptic terminal and release the neurotransmitter. The neurotransmitter and the vesicles are recycled to synthesize fresh synaptic vesicles.

The small molecule neurotransmitter results in the changes in conductance (increase or decrease) of the ion channels on the postsynaptic membrane.

**Table 81.1:** Types of small molecule neurotransmitters.

| Class I | Acetylcholine |
|---|---|
| Class II | **Amines:** Norepinephrine, epinephrine, dopamine, serotonin, histamine |
| Class III | **Amino acids:** γ-amino butyric acid (GABA), glycine, aspartate |
| Class IV | Nitric oxide |

Let us now discuss all the neurotransmitters, shown in **Table 81.1**.

## Class I

### Acetylcholine (ACh)

It is a small molecule neurotransmitter which is synthesized in synaptic terminals from *acetyl coenzyme A (CoA) and choline*, and, after release, is degraded in the synaptic cleft by acetylcholinesterase. Choline is taken up and recycled from the synaptic cleft. It is found in:
- Terminals of large pyramidal cells
- Neurons of basal ganglia in corpus striatum
- Motor neurons at neuromuscular junction
- Preganglionic autonomic neurons
- Postganglionic parasympathetic neurons
- Cholinergic postganglionic sympathetic neurons

**Actions:**
- Cholinergic neurons **initiate rapid eye movement (REM) sleep** and facilitate the activity of hippocampal neurons in memory consolidation

**Receptors:**
- The preganglionic autonomic neurons act on nicotinic ($N_N$ receptors)
- The postganglionic parasympathetic neurons act on muscarinic (M receptors)
- The lower motor neurons act on skeletal muscle through nicotinic $N_M$ receptors

### Disorders Associated with Cholinergic Neurons

- In the CNS, cholinergic neurons in the ventral forebrain (basal nucleus of Meynert) are a main type of neurons that degenerates in patients with **Alzheimer's disease**.
- In **organophosphorus poisoning**, such as mustard gas and insecticides, it binds irreversibly to acetylcholinesterase at the neuromuscular junction. ACh accumulates in the synaptic cleft and causes prolonged depolarization of skeletal muscle. This makes the muscle, less sensitive to additional ACh release. The excessive stimulation of nicotinic receptors results in increased GI secretions.
- **Tobacco smoke** contains nicotine which binds to the N_N receptors of autonomic ganglia and results in its effects.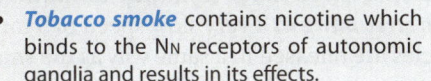

**Dopamine receptors:** G-protein coupled receptors
- D1 like (D1 and D5): Increase in cAMP
- D2 like (D2, D3 and D4): Reduces cAMP

### Dopaminergic Neurons, Parkinson's Disease, and Schizophrenia

- **Selective loss of the dopaminergic neurons** in the substantia nigra, pars compacta, results in **Parkinson's disease, a motor disorder of the basal ganglia.**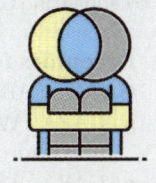
- Changes in the levels of dopamine in the mesolimbic and mesocortical circuits may result in the positive and negative symptoms of schizophrenia, respectively.
- **Cocaine and amphetamines** are addictive substances that act by *increasing dopamine levels*, particularly in the mesolimbic pathway.
- Overstimulation of D2 causes Schizophrenia

## Class II

### Norepinephrine (NE)

It is a catecholamine that is converted from dopamine and is the only small neurotransmitter synthesized inside synaptic vesicles at the synaptic terminal instead of in the cytoplasm of the terminal. It is present in some of the *neurons of brainstem and hypothalamus, postganglionic sympathetic neurons, and locus coeruleus in pons* secrete nor epinephrine. These neurons send signals all over the brain and control the overall activity of the brain, affect the mood, and increase the level of wakefulness. Nor epinephrine always *activates the nervous system* hence acts as the excitatory neurotransmitter.

**Receptors:** α and β receptors.

### Epinephrine

It is converted in small amounts from norepinephrine in the CNS. It is found in:
- Adrenergic neurons in the CNS are found mainly in the medulla oblongata.
- Most epinephrine is synthesized and released outside the CNS is from the adrenal medulla.
- After release, all catecholamines are taken up by axon terminals and degraded by either monoamine oxidase (MAO) or catechol-o-methyltransferase (COMT).

### Dopamine (DA)

It is a catecholamine synthesized from the amino acid *tyrosine*; tyrosine hydroxylase, the rate-limiting enzyme in catecholamine synthesis, catalyzes the conversion to dopamine. It is present in:
- Substantia nigra forming the *nigrostriatal pathway*. Dopamine acts as the inhibitory neuron in the basal ganglia.
- The *arcuate nuclei* of the hypothalamus use dopamine to regulate the release of prolactin from the anterior pituitary.

### Serotonin

It is an indolamine synthesized from *tryptophan*. Serotonin is an *excitatory neurotransmitter* that influences neuronal circuits, which function in *sleep, arousal, eating, and circadian rhythms*. It is secreted by the neurons arising in the *median raphe of the brain stem* which projects to brain and spinal cord areas.

### Depression

- **Changes in the synthesis, release, or activation of catecholamines and serotonin may cause depression,** the most common unipolar mood disorder, or **bipolar disorder,** during which patients experience both depression and manic episodes.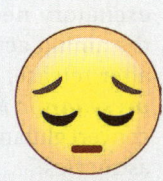
- **Antidepressant drugs include MAO inhibitors,** which limit the reuptake of catecholamines. Drugs such as fluoxetine for moderate depression, selectively block the uptake of serotonin without affecting the reuptake of other catecholamines, and tricyclic compounds, for severe depression, inhibit the uptake of both serotonin and norepinephrine.

### Histamine

It is an excitatory neurotransmitter used by neurons in the posterior hypothalamus. It has effects similar to acetylcholine and norepinephrine in facilitating arousal and an awake state. It is synthesized from *histidine* and, after its release, is transported back into axon terminals and metabolized by MAO. Histamine is also released from mast cells in allergic reactions and in response to tissue damage.

## Class III

- **GABA:** It is secreted at the nerve terminals in the *spinal cord, cerebellum, basal ganglia and cerebral cortex*. It is one of the main inhibitory neurotransmitters.

### Antianxiety Medications

Benzodiazepines, such as diazepam and chlordiazepoxide, are effective **antianxiety drugs that act by enhancing the effects of GABA neurons.** Benzodiazepines and barbiturates also act as antiepileptic drugs by enhancing GABA inhibition.

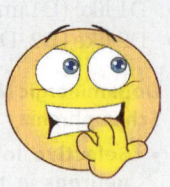

- **Receptors for GABA:** It has three types of receptors $GABA_A$, $GABA_B$ and $GABA_C$
    - $GABA_A$: Widely distributed in *CNS*. Allows *$Cl^-$ influx* into neuron
    - $GABA_B$: Widely distributed in *CNS*. GPCR *alters $K^+$ and $Ca^{2+}$ influx.*
    - $GABA_C$: Present in *retina*. Allows *$Cl^-$ influx* into neuron.
- **Glycine:** It is present in the synapses are the spinal cord it is an important inhibitory neurotransmitter.
    *GABA and glycine are major inhibitory* CNS transmitters; GABA is used by about 30% of all CNS neurons, and glycine is used mainly by neurons in the *brainstem and spinal cord*. Both GABA and glycine *prevent prolonged excitation* in many neuronal systems.
- **Glutamate:** It is a present in the presynaptic terminals in sensory pathways entering the CNS. It is an important *excitatory neurotransmitter*, secreted by 75% of the excitatory neurons. Glutamate is synthesized from the amino acid *glutamine* in the axon terminal and, after release, is rapidly taken up by *transporters in presynaptic terminals and in astrocytes*. Astrocytes convert glutamate to glutamine which is released by the astrocytes.
    **Receptors:** There are three subtypes of glutamate receptors:
    1. *AMPA* (α amino-3-hydroxy-5 methylisoxazole-4-propionate) with 4 subunits (GluR1 to GluR4). Present on *all neurons and glia*.
    2. *Kainite receptors* with 5 subunits (GluR5 to GluR7, KA1 and KA2). Present on *GABA secreting neurons and glia*.
    3. *NMDA receptors* with 6 subunits (NR1, NR2A-NR2D). Present on *all neurons*.

### Glutamate-Induced Excitotoxicity

The uptake process of glutamate from synaptic cleft is energy dependent which is slowed by oxygen deprivation results in **glutamate-induced excitotoxicity** in ischemic neurons in stroke patients.

The epilepsy, characterized by multiple seizures that arise from excessive neuronal activity in the cerebral cortex, may also cause glutamate-induced excitotoxicity.

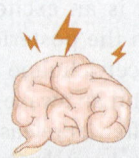

## Class IV

**Nitric oxide (NO):** It is secreted by the nerve terminals responsible for *long-term behavior and memory*. It is different from the neurotransmitters because it is not preformed and stored in the synaptic vesicles. It is *synthesized instantaneously* and diffuses out of the presynaptic terminal to diffuse into postsynaptic terminal. It brings changes in the intracellular metabolic functions modifying neuronal excitability.

## LARGE MOLECULE NEUROTRANSMITTERS

These are slow acting neuropeptides synthesized in the rough endoplasmic reticulum by the ribosomes. These are packed by Golgi apparatus into the vesicles. These vesicles are *transported to the presynaptic terminal by the axoplasmic streaming at* a very slow speed of 5 mm/day. These vesicles are released in a same way as the small molecule neurotransmitter. These vesicles once released are *not recycled*. The neuropeptides are slow to act and produce prolonged effects which can last for days to years. These actions occur due to prolonged:
- Closure of $Ca^{2+}$ channels
- Changes in metabolic mechanism
- Changes in activation/deactivation of genes
- Changes in alteration in number of excitatory or inhibitory receptors.

There is a large list of neuropeptides, which can act as the large molecule neurotransmitters.

### Hypothalamic-releasing Hormones

They are synthesized by neurons in the *arcuate and periventricular nuclei of the hypothalamus* and influence the release of anterior pituitary peptide hormones; dopamine acts as an inhibitory factor that regulates the release of prolactin.
- Thyrotropin-releasing hormone
- Luteinizing hormone–releasing hormone
- Somatostatin (growth hormone inhibitory factor)

### Pituitary Neuropeptides

These include the hormones *oxytocin and vasopressin*, which are produced by the neurons in the hypothalamus and released from axon terminals of those neurons into the posterior pituitary (neurohypophysis). Other peptides are:
- Adrenocorticotropic hormone
- β-endorphin
- α-melanocyte-stimulating hormone
- Prolactin
- Luteinizing hormone
- Thyrotropin
- Growth hormone

### Opioid Peptides

There are three classes of about 20 **opioid peptides,** including enkephalins, endorphins, and dynorphins, that act mainly as analgesics; their effects are mimicked by narcotic drugs. *Enkephalins are used by neurons in the dorsal horn of the spinal cord in the suppression* *of pain.* Opioid peptides are also used by neurons in the periaqueductal gray matter of the midbrain in the suppression of pain.

## Peptides Acting on Brain-gut

- Leucine enkephalin
- Methionine enkephalin
- **Substance P:** The best-known *brain-gut peptide*. It is found in neurons in the cerebral cortex, basal ganglia, hippocampus, and gastrointestinal tract. It is used by axons of neurons that respond to pain and project into the spinal cord in dorsal roots of spinal nerves.
- Gastrin
- Cholecystokinin
- Vasoactive intestinal polypeptide

- Nerve growth factor
- Brain-derived neurotropic factor
- Neurotensin
- Insulin
- Glucagon

## From Other Tissues

- Angiotensin II
- Bradykinin
- Carnosine
- Sleep peptides
- Calcitonin

The mechanism of action of all the neurotransmitters and neuropeptides have been discussed in detail in Chapter 3.

### SUMMARY

In this chapter, we have learnt about the two main types of neurotransmitters, small molecule and large molecule transmitter required for chemical transmission across the neuronal synapse.

The small molecule neurotransmitters are rapidly acting and promptly recycled whereas the neuropeptides are formed slowly and not recycled. They are required for prolonged actions.

### LET US SEE, HOW MUCH YOU HAVE LEARNT?

*Review Questions*

#### Long/Short Answer Question

Q1. Define and classify the neurotransmitters.

#### Explain Why? (Reasoning Questions)

Q1. An imbalance in serotonin levels is associated with mood disorders such as depression.
Q2. Blocking acetylcholine receptors can lead to muscle paralysis.
Q3. Excessive glutamate release can cause excitotoxicity and neuronal damage.
Q4. Dopamine dysregulation is a key factor in the development of Parkinson's disease.
Q5. GABAergic drugs are effective in treating anxiety disorders.
Q6. The reuptake of norepinephrine can improve symptoms of attention deficit hyperactivity disorder (ADHD).

*Answer in One Word*

Q1. An inhibitory neurotransmitter used by neurons found throughout the CNS.
Q2. Used by preganglionic autonomic axons.
Q3. Used by autonomic neurons derived from neural crest cells.
Q4. Released by lower motor neurons.
Q5. An excitatory neurotransmitter used by 50% of CNS neurons.
Q6. Used by neurons in the nucleus accumbens.
Q7. Produced by neurons in the locus coeruleus.
Q8. Used by neurons that promote memory consolidation.

#### ANSWERS

1. GABA
2. Acetylcholine
3. Acetylcholine and norepinephrine
4. Acetylcholine
5. Glutamate
6. Dopamine
7. Norepinephrine
8. Acetylcholine

*Critical Thinking Case-Based Questions*

Q1. Amit, a 30-year-old farmer, was brought to the emergency department with symptoms of muscle twitching, excessive salivation, sweating, difficulty breathing, and confusion. His family reported that Amit was spraying pesticides in the fields before the onset of symptoms. The attending physician suspected poisoning and began the treatment immediately. Based on the given history, answer the following questions:
  a. What is the probable diagnosis?

b. What is the role of acetylcholine and acetylcholinesterase in normal neurotransmitter function?

c. How does this condition affect the activity of acetylcholinesterase?

## Multiple Choice Questions

**Q1.** An anticancer drug acts by disrupting microtubules in cancer cells but also disrupts fast anterograde axonal transport. Movement of which of the following neurotransmitters or precursors of neurotransmitters will be most affected?
   a. Neuropeptides
   b. Glutamate
   c. Small molecule neurotransmitters
   d. Acetylcholine

**Q2.** A medical student is studying transmission through autonomic ganglia. She studied the effects of two drugs on the activity of a postganglionic neuron. Drug A induced an EPSP in the postganglionic neuron, and drug B blocked the EPSP produced by electrical stimulation of a preganglionic nerve. Drugs A and B might be the following drugs, respectively:
   a. Glutamate and glycine
   b. Nicotine and atropine
   c. Strychnine and atenolol
   d. Nicotine and trimethaphan

**Q3.** A 38-year-old woman was referred to a psychiatrist after telling her primary care physician that she had difficulty sleeping (awakening at 4 AM frequently for the past few months) and a lack of appetite causing a weight loss of over 20 lb. She also said she no longer enjoyed going out with her friends or doing volunteer service for underprivileged children. What type of drug is her doctor most likely to suggest as an initial step in her therapy?
   a. A serotonergic receptor antagonist
   b. A selective serotonin reuptake inhibitor
   c. An inhibitor of monoamine oxidase
   d. An amphetamine-like drug

**ANSWERS**

1. a   2. d   3. b

# Physiology of Sensory Receptors

**82 CHAPTER**

### COMPETENCY ADDRESSED
PY10.2: Describe and discuss the functions and properties of synapse, reflex, **receptors**.

### LEARNING OBJECTIVES
At the end of this chapter, the learner should be able to:
- Define a receptor.
- Classify the receptors based on stimulus and location.
- Describe the generation of receptor potential/generator potential.
- Describe the structure and functions of muscle spindle.

## HOW ARE SENSATIONS CARRIED AND RECOGNIZED?

Our body recognizes various stimuli applied on the skin called the *somatic senses*; whereas some senses require special organs called *special senses*.

The various sensations can be classified as:
- **Somatic sensations:**
  - Simple somatic sensation
    - Touch
      - Crude touch
      - Fine touch
    - Pressure
    - Temperature
    - Pain
    - Proprioception
    - Vibration
  - *Complex somatic sensation:*
    - Itch
    - Tickle
- **Visceral sensation:** Due to the receptors present in the walls of the viscera.
- **Special senses:**
  - Vision
  - Hearing
  - Olfaction (smell)
  - Gustation (taste)

## RECEPTORS

The receptors are the transducers which convert various types of environmental energies to action potentials (electrical signal) in sensory neurons.

### Classification of Somatic Receptors

Somatic receptors, crucial for sensory perception, are classified based on stimulus type, location, and function **(Table 82.1)**. Mechanoreceptors detect mechanical stimuli like touch and pressure; thermoreceptors sense temperature changes; nociceptors respond to painful stimuli, and proprioceptors monitor body position and movement. These receptors vary in their sensitivity thresholds, adaptation rates, and transmission speeds, tailored to their specific roles in sensory processing **(Table 82.2)**.

**Table 82.1:** Classification of receptors.

| Based on function | Based on stimulus | Based on location |
|---|---|---|
| 1. **Exteroreceptors:** Cutaneous sense organs | 1. **Mechanoreceptors:** For touch (Fig. 82.1) | 1. Superficial |
| 2. **Interoreceptors:** Present inside the body. Baroreceptors, osmoreceptors | 2. **Thermoreceptors:** For temperature (Fig. 82.1) | 2. Deep |
| 3. **Proprioceptors:** Joint position | 3. **Nociceptors:** For pain (Fig. 82.1) | 3. Visceral |
| 4. **Teleceptors:** Sense from a distance; auditory receptors | 4. Chemoreceptors | |
| | 5. Photoreceptors | |

**Table 82.2:** Difference in major somatic receptors.

| | Structure | | Type of fiber | Adaptability | Location | Sensation perceived |
|---|---|---|---|---|---|---|
| Pacinian corpuscle (Fig. 82.1) | | | Concentric lamellae, largest | Aβ fibers | | Skin and deep tissues | Pressure and vibration |
| Meissner's corpuscle (Fig. 82.1) | | | Encapsulated | Aβ fibers | Rapid | Dermal ridges of hairless skin | Touch, vibration |
| Merkel's Disc | | | Flattened | Aβ fibers | Slow | Superficial, epidermis | Touch, pressure |
| Ruffini's endings | | | Smallest | Aβ fibers | Slow | Both hairless and hairy skin | Crude touch |
| Krauze's end bulb | | | Encapsulated | Aβ fibers | Rapid | Dermis | Touch, pressure |

## Transduction of Sensory Stimuli: Generation of Action Potential (Generator Potential/Receptor Potential)

All the sensory receptors when stimulated. Results in the change in the membrane electrical potential of receptor called *receptor potential*. The receptors as discussed above are stimulated by the:

- By mechanical deformation of the receptor, which stretches the receptor membrane and opens ion channels
- By application of a chemical to the membrane, which also opens ion channels;
- By change of the temperature of the membrane, which alters the permeability of the membrane
- By the effects of electromagnetic radiation, such as light on a retinal visual receptor, which either directly or indirectly changes the receptor membrane characteristics and allows ions to flow through membrane channels.

## Physiological Basis of Receptor Potential

The change in membrane potential occurs due to the change in the permeability of the receptor allowing the diffusion of various ions across the membrane, hence changing the *transmembrane potential*.

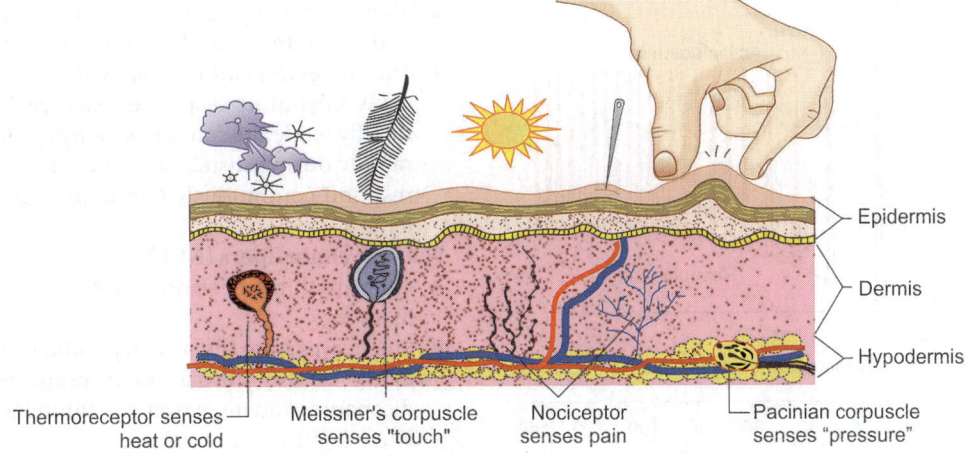

**Fig. 82.1:** Various sense receptors in the skin.

### Receptor Potential of the Pacinian Corpuscle— an Example of Receptor Function

The Pacinian corpuscle has a central nerve fiber extending through its core. There are multiple concentric capsule layers surrounding the nerve fiber core, so that compression anywhere on the outside of the corpuscle will elongate, indent, or otherwise deform the central fiber.

The tip of the central fiber inside the capsule is unmyelinated, but the fiber becomes myelinated before leaving the corpuscle to enter a peripheral sensory nerve.

The small area of the terminal fiber that has been deformed by compression of the corpuscle, opens, the ion channels, resulting in $Na^+$ influx. This creates increased positivity inside the fiber, which is the **"receptor potential."** The receptor potential in turn induces a *local circuit* of current flow, shown by the arrows, that spreads along the nerve fiber. At the first node of Ranvier, which itself lies inside the capsule of the Pacinian corpuscle, the local current flow depolarizes the fiber membrane at this node, which then sets off typical action potentials that are transmitted along the nerve fiber toward the central nervous system **(Fig. 82.2)**.

## PROPERTIES OF RECEPTORS

- **Specificity:** The receptors are specific for the specific modalities. Example touch receptors, pressure receptors etc. Each sensory receptor and its nerve transmit a single sensation (modality). This is called the *labelled line principle*.
- **Adequate stimulus:** Adequate stimulus in the form of type of stimulus and threshold is required for the stimulation of receptor.
- **Stimulus intensity:** if the intensity of the stimulation increases (due to progressive stronger compression, in case of Pacinian corpuscle).

  Once the receptor potential rises above the threshold level, the frequency of action potentials generated also increase as seen in the **Figure 82.3**.
- **Adaptation**
  - *Phasic receptors:* These are the **rapidly adapting receptors that detect change in strength of stimulus.** They are also called *"rate receptors, movement receptors or phasic receptors."*

    These rapidly adapting receptors cannot transmit a continuous signal because they are stimulated only

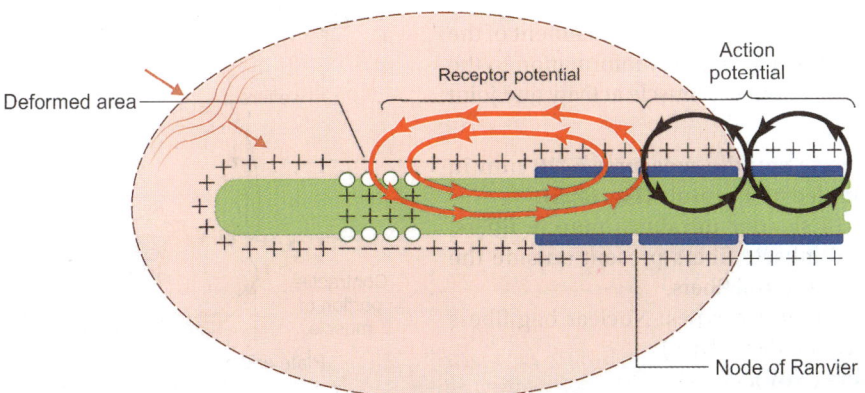

**Fig. 82.2:** Transduction of pressure into electrical nerve signal.

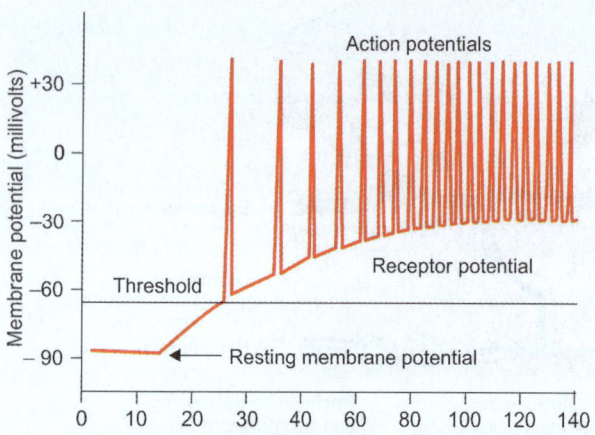

**Fig. 82.3:** Action potential frequency of a receptor stimulated above receptor potential.

when the strength of stimulus changes. For example, Pacinian corpuscle

- **Tonic receptors:** These receptors are *slowly adapting receptors which detect continuous stimulus.* They transmit impulses to the brain as long as the stimulus is present (or at least for many minutes or hours). Therefore, they keep the brain constantly appraised of the status of the body and its relation to its surroundings. These receptors are present in:
  - Receptors of the macula in the vestibular apparatus
  - Pain receptors
  - Baroreceptors of the arterial tree
  - Chemoreceptors of the carotid and aortic bodies
  - Muscle spindle and Golgi tendon organ

We have discussed briefly about all the receptors responsible for somatic sensations such as pain, temperature, touch, pressure. However, the muscle spindle and Golgi tendon organ; the receptors for proprioception, are described in detail in the section given below.

## Muscle Spindle

It is a *spindle shaped receptor*, found in skeletal muscle. It is mostly located towards the tendinous attachment of the muscle (**Fig. 82.4**). It provides sensory information to the central nervous system about the muscle activity and joint position sense.

**Structure:** The muscle spindle measures 5–10 mm in length and is surrounded by a capsule (**Fig. 82.5**).

It consists of 2–14 slender intrafusal muscle fibers, whereas the skeletal muscle fibers present outside the spindle are called as extrafusal fibers.

Intrafusal fibers are of two types: Nuclear bag fibers (NBF) and nuclear chain fibers (NCF)

- **Nuclear bag fibers (NBF):**
  - They are dilated in center and consists of numerous nuclei.
  - They are longer than NCF.
  - They extend beyond the capsule and attaches to the endomysium of extrafusal muscle fibers.
  - The nerves from the endings in the nuclear bag region show a **dynamic response**, i.e., they discharge most rapidly while the muscle is being stretched and less rapidly during sustained stretch. Hence these fibers respond continuously to rate pf change of stretch/length.
- **Nuclear chain fibers (NCF):**
  - They are thin and slender and have nuclei arranged in a row.
  - The nerves from the primary endings on the nuclear chain fibers show a **static response,** i.e., they discharge at an increased rate throughout the period when a muscle is stretched.

Both these fibers have the striations and the ends. The ends of these intrafusal fibers contracts and stretch the central portion of the spindle resulting in the stimulation of these fibers.

> **Spindle is stretched due to:**
> 1. Stretching of muscle
> 2. Contraction of ends of intrafusal fibers (due to gamma efferent).
>
> This results in stimulation of spindles and increased Ia and II discharge.

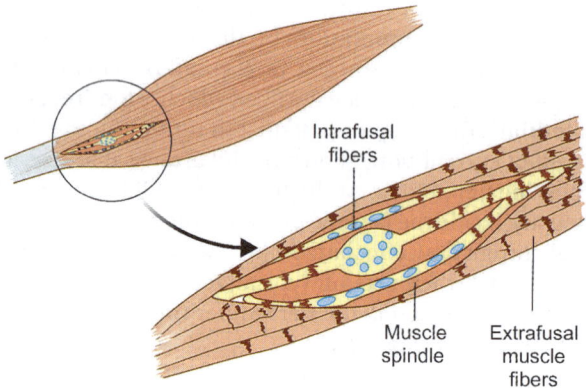

**Fig. 82.4:** Location and overview of muscle spindle.

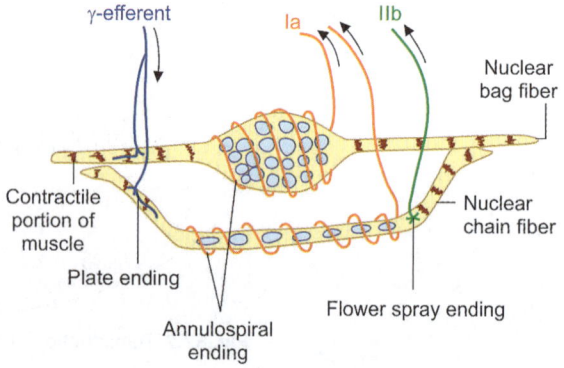

**Fig. 82.5:** Structure of muscle spindle.

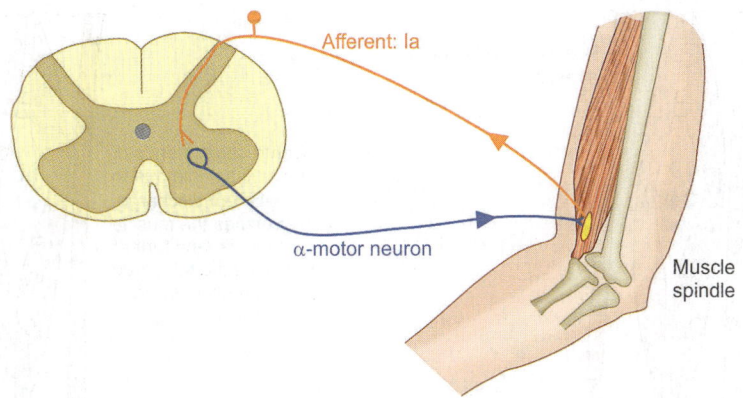

**Fig. 82.6:** Working of a muscle spindle.

## Innervation of Muscle Spindle

Muscle spindle have both afferent (sensory) and efferent (motor) innervation.
- **Afferent innervation:**
    - *Ia fibers:* Faster than Type II fibers. These fibers are coiled spirally around the center of both types of intrafusal fibers (NBF and NCF) and are called as *Annulospiral endings*.
    - *II Fibers:* Mostly innervate the nuclear chain fibers and are located in paracentral part of spindle. These fibers have *flower spray endings*, as they appear like flowers.
- **Efferent innervation:**
    - *γ-efferent:* They are small motor neurons arising from the anterior horn of the spinal cord and constitute only about 30% of fibers arising from anterior horn. They supply the peripheral part of intrafusal fibers. They have plate endings on NBF and trail endings on NCF.

## Working of a Muscle Spindle (Fig. 82.6)

- **Resting skeletal muscle and muscle spindle (Fig. 82.7):** The skeletal muscle, which is attached to the bones, is constantly stretched. This results in the stretching of the muscle spindle also (loading of spindle). Whenever the muscle spindle is stretched it sends the sensory signals to the spinal cord through Ia afferent fibers. The sensory fibers synapse on the motor neurons arising from the anterior horn cell of the spinal cord which in turn innervate the extrafusal skeletal muscle fibers and result in its contraction, relaxing the spindle (unloading of muscle spindle). Hence, the extrafusal skeletal muscle fibers remain partially contracted generating the muscle tone.

    Due to the constant stretching of the muscle spindle, there is a continuous discharge (action potentials) arising from the muscle spindle, hence the muscle spindle has the tonic discharge.
- **Passive stretching of muscle spindle (Fig. 82.8):** Whenever the muscle is stretched beyond its resting

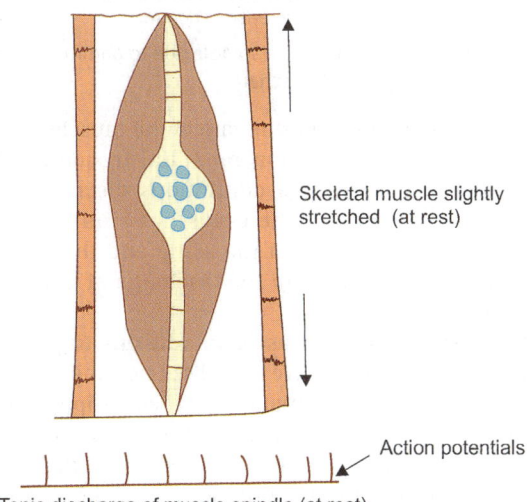

**Fig. 82.7:** Tonic discharge of muscle spindle at rest, with no external stimulation.

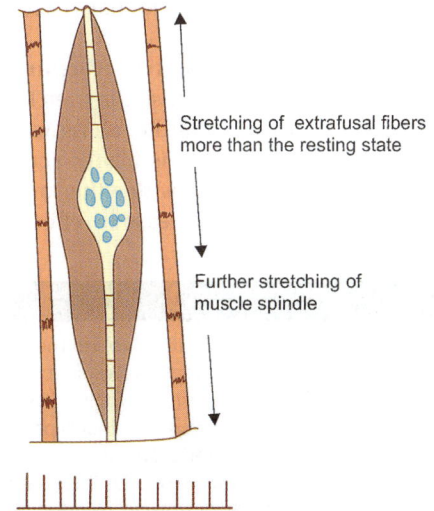

**Fig. 82.8:** Activation of muscle spindle due to passive stretching of extrafusal fibers.

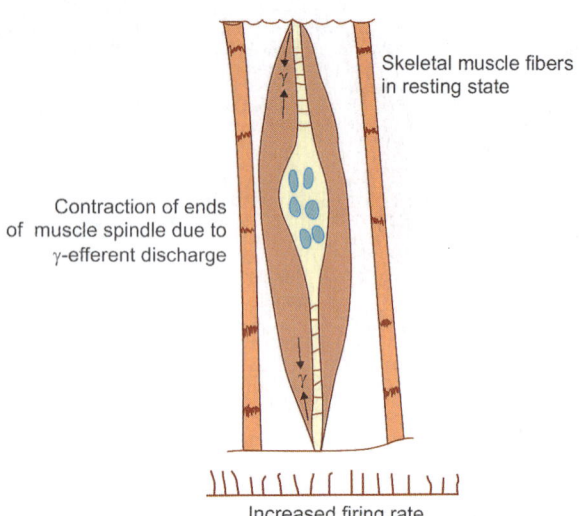

Fig. 82.9: Activation of muscle spindle due to gamma efferent discharge.

Fig. 82.10: Alpha gamma co-activation.

stage it increases the firing rate of the muscle spindle, i.e., increases the action potential frequency. The **Figure 82.7** shows the continuous discharge from the muscle spindle when it is not stimulated (b). However, stimulation of the static and the dynamic fibers shows increase in the discharge of the muscle spindle.

- **Active stretching of muscle spindle due to γ-efferent discharge (Fig. 82.9):** We have discussed above, that the intrafusal fibers have striations on their peripheral ends, hence they are contractile. This portion of the muscle spindle also receives the innervation from the gamma motor neurons. Contraction of the peripheral portion of the muscle spindle fibers results in the stretching of the central sensory part and increases the frequency of action potentials generated by the muscles spindle. This increase in firing rate is due to the activation of gamma neurons rising from the anterior horn cells of the spinal cord.
- **Combined passive and active stretching of muscle spindle (Fig. 82.10):** The muscle is stretched, passively stretching the muscle spindle, along with increased γ-efferent discharge; there is higher action potential frequency generated than with either of the active or passive stretching. The increased γ-efferent discharge along with the activation of Aα motor neurons is called **'α-γ co-activation'**

> **How do the γ-motor neurons monitor the muscle length and also the speed of change of length?**
>
> There are two types of γ-motor neurons: dynamic γ motor neurons, which terminate on the NBF and sense the dynamic muscle stretch, i.e., rate of change of muscle length and static γ-motor neuron, which terminates on NCF which sense the maintained stretch.
>
> Depending upon these two type of neurons, the afferent discharge also occurs as dynamic and static response.
>
> **β-efferent:** They have both dynamic and static β-efferents.

### Functions of Muscle Spindle

- Receptors sensitive to stretch
- Feedback device that controls the length of the muscle.
    - If the muscle is stretched, spindle discharge increases, and reflex shortening occurs in the muscle.
    - The contraction of the muscle stretches the antagonist muscle which stimulates its muscle spindle. The reciprocal innervation hence inhibits the further contraction of the skeletal muscle which was stimulated earlier.

## SUMMARY

- The perceives various sensations through the somatosensory system. There are specific receptors present for each sensation. In this chapter we had learnt about the various receptors present for the somatic sensation, i.e., touch, pain, temperature, pressure, vibration and proprioception.
- The receptor for the proprioception is important for the joint position sense, called the muscle spindle, located at the musculotendinous junction. It contains specialized muscle fibers called intrafusal fibers, which are of two types (nuclear bag fibers and nuclear chain fibers). The skeletal muscle fibers present in the belly of muscle, outside the spindle are called the extrafusal fibers.
- The muscle spindle responds to stretch of extrafusal fibers, which may occur due to passive or active stretching of muscle and results in contraction of the skeletal muscle. It forms the physiological basis of muscle tone.

# LET US SEE, HOW MUCH YOU HAVE LEARNT?

## Review Questions

Q1. Describe the structure of the muscle spindle with the help of a well labeled diagram.
Q2. Describe the functions of muscle spindle.
Q3. What is receptor potential? Describe the generation of receptor potential.

## Multiple Choice Questions

Q1. When dynamic γ-motor neurons are activated at the same time as α-motor neurons to muscle.
   a. Prompt inhibition of discharge in spindle Ia afferents takes place.
   b. Clonus is likely to occur.
   c. The number of impulses in spindle Ia afferents is smaller than when α discharge alone is increased.
   d. The number of impulses in spindle Ia afferents is greater than when α discharge alone is increased.

Q2. The multiple Merkel discs are connected to a large myelinated fiber in the Iggo dome receptor, shown in figure below; is responsible for:

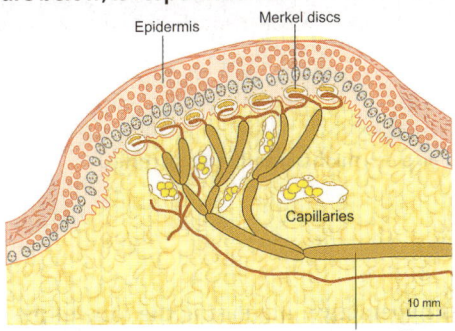

   a. Sensing the pressure sensation and carried by Aβ nerve fiber
   b. Sensing the touch sensation and carried by Aβ nerve fiber
   c. Sensing the temperature sensation and carried by Aβ nerve fiber
   d. Sensing the pain sensation and carried by Aβ nerve fiber

Q3. Identify the fastest adapting receptor from the figure given below:

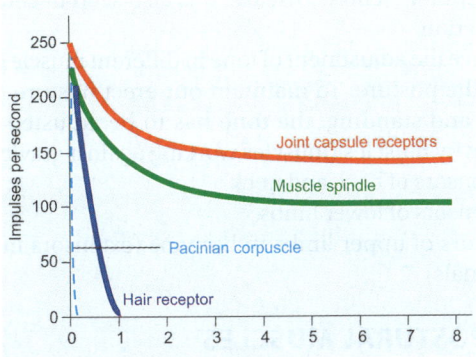

   a. Pacinian corpuscle      b. Muscle spindle
   c. Hair receptor           d. Joint capsule receptors

Q4. The property of accommodation of receptors occurs due to:
   a. Readjustment of receptor potential
   b. Inactivation of sodium channels
   c. Stimulus becomes weak over time
   d. Nerve becomes refractory to stimulus

Q5. The sensation of tickle, is a complex sensation, sent to spinal cord and lower brain through:
   a. Myelinated Aα fibers    b. Myelinated Aβ fibers
   c. Myelinated Aγ fibers    d. Unmyelinated C fibers

Q6. What is the primary function of alpha-gamma coactivation in the neuromuscular system?
   a. To regulate muscle tone
   b. To initiate muscle contraction
   c. To inhibit sensory input
   d. To synchronize motor neuron firing

Q7. Which of the following best describes the relationship between alpha and gamma motor neurons during alpha-gamma coactivation?
   a. Alpha motor neurons innervate extrafusal muscle fibers, while gamma motor neurons innervate intrafusal muscle fibers
   b. Alpha motor neurons innervate intrafusal muscle fibers, while gamma motor neurons innervate extrafusal muscle fibers
   c. Alpha and gamma motor neurons innervate the same type of muscle fibers but control different aspects of muscle function
   d. Alpha and gamma motor neurons work independently and do not interact during muscle contraction

Q8. What is the primary function of receptor potentials in sensory neurons?
   a. To propagate action potentials
   b. To amplify sensory signals
   c. To convert external stimuli into electrical signals
   d. To regulate neurotransmitter release

Q9. Which of the following best describes the relationship between receptor potentials and action potentials?
   a. Receptor potentials directly trigger action potentials in sensory neurons
   b. Receptor potentials are the same as action potentials
   c. Receptor potentials modulate the threshold for action potential generation
   d. Receptor potentials inhibit the generation of action

## ANSWERS

1. d    2. b    3. a    4. b    5. d    6. a    7. a    8. c    9. c

# Postural Reflexes and their Regulation

## 83 CHAPTER

> **COMPETENCY ADDRESSED**
> **PY10.2:** Describe and discuss the functions and properties of synapse, reflex, receptors.
> **PY10.4:** Describe and discuss motor tracts, mechanism of maintenance of tone, control of body movements, posture, and equilibrium and vestibular apparatus.

>  **LEARNING OBJECTIVES**
> **At the end of this chapter, the learner should be able to:**
> - Define a postural reflex.
> - Define the muscle tone.
> - Describe the physiological basis of the muscle tone.
> - Describe the various postural reflexes integrated at the level of spinal cord, brainstem, midbrain and cerebral cortex.
> - Describe the physiological significance of the postural reflexes.
> - Describe the clinical significance of the postural reflexes.

## WHAT IS A POSTURAL REFLEX?

It is defined as a sudden action mediated at the local level, without the involvement of higher centers, for sudden postural correction/maintenance.

The postural reflexes maintain the body posture due to the muscle tone. We had studied about muscle tone in Section 3, Nerve Muscle Physiology. To revise, the tone is defined as the state of partial contraction of the muscle. Since our muscle are attached to our skeleton, they remain slightly stretched at their resting state. This activates the stretch reflex (discussed below), resulting in the state of partial contraction of muscle. Hence, the continuous activation of stretch reflex forms the physiological basis of muscle tone.

Further, the skeletal muscles receive the motor control from the motor area of cerebral cortex (Chapter 79, Skeletal Motor Nervous Axis). The main motor tract controlling the motor activity is corticospinal tract ('*cortico*' means arising from cerebral cortex and *'spinal'* means it ends in spinal cord). There are some other motor tracts too, which we will learn about in later chapters. All these tracts influence the muscle tone and power.

An increase in the muscle tone is called *Hypertonia*, which is seen in diseases where there is loss of inhibitory influence of higher centers (corticospinal or other motor tracts) on the stretch reflex arc. Hence, the stretch reflex becomes hyperactive, increasing the tone of the muscle. This type of lesion is called as the upper motor neuron lesion. It can lead to:
- Clasp knife spasticity (due to pure corticospinal tract lesion)
- Cogwheel/Lead pipe rigidity (due to associated extrapyramidal tract lesion).

However, the decrease in muscle tone is called *hypotonia*. It occurs when the lower motor neurons (A$\alpha$ motor neurons) are damaged. The stretch reflex is lost resulting in hypotonia. This condition is called the Lower Motor Neuron Disease. It is also seen in cerebellar dysfunction.

Hence the adjustment of tone in different muscle groups affect the posture. To maintain our erect posture during sitting and standing, the tone has to be adjusted in the antigravity muscles (muscles working against gravity) like:
- Extensors of back and neck
- Extensors of lower limbs
- Flexors of upper limbs in humans (extensors in lower animals)

## THE POSTURAL MUSCLES

All these postural muscles are the red muscle, which can remain contracted for long durations.

There are many postural reflexes controlled by various levels of central nervous system. These are isometric and subtetanic contractions. The motor units discharge asynchronously and result in smooth sustained contractions. The tension generated in the muscles due to stretch reflex is not strong enough to hold the body weight and hence the support of higher centers is required through:
- Corticospinal tracts and other extrapyramidal motor tracts
- Impulses controlling the muscle tone from
  - Labyrinthine apparatus
  - Neck muscles
  - Eyes

## POSTURAL REFLEXES INTEGRATED AT DIFFERENT LEVELS OF CNS

**Postural reflexes integrated at the level of spinal cord**
- Stretch reflex
- Inverse stretch reflex
- Flexor reflex/withdrawal reflex
- Crossed extensor reflex
- Positive supporting reaction
- Walking movements

**Postural reflexes integrated by medulla oblongata**
- Upright posture
- Tonic neck reflexes
- Tonic labyrinthine reflex

**Postural reflexes integrated by midbrain**
- Righting reflexes
  - Optical righting reflex
  - Neck righting reflex
  - Labyrinthine righting reflex
  - Body righting reflex
    - Body on head righting reflex
    - Body on body righting reflex

**Postural reflexes integrated at the level of cerebral cortex**
- Hopping and placing reactions

### Postural Reflexes Integrated at the Level of Spinal Cord (Spinal Reflexes)

Spinal cord is an extension of the central nervous system into the back which can independently execute various commands and responses at its local level. However, it does send the information to the higher centers like medulla, pons, midbrain and cerebral cortex for appraisal except in stretch reflex.

The various reflexes integrated at the level of spinal cord are:
- Stretch reflex
- Inverse stretch reflex
- Flexor reflex/withdrawal reflex
- Crossed extensor reflex
- Positive supporting reaction
- Walking movements

In Chapter 82, we had studied about the structure and functions of muscle spindle which forms an important receptor for the initiation of proprioceptive/postural reflexes.

### Stretch Reflex (Fig. 83.1)

It can also be explained that if a muscle with intact nerve supply is stretched, it results in the contraction of the muscle. It is also called as the
- **Monosynaptic reflex:** Based on the number of synapses (only one) involved in this reflex, it is called monosynaptic reflex.
- **Myotatic reflex:** Since the continuous stretching of muscles is seen in normal conditions (the attachment of muscles to the bones, keeps them stretched), they always remain partly contracted. This is called tone of muscles. Hence this reflex is also called myotatic reflex.

**How it works?**
- **Stimulus:** That initiates the reflex is **stretch** of the muscle
- **The sense organ (Receptor):** Muscle spindle
- **Sensory fiber (Afferent):** Ia afferent fibers arising from muscle spindle
- **Center:** Spinal cord
- **Motor fiber (Efferent):** Alpha motor neurons to the extrafusal fibers
- **Effector:** Extrafusal/skeletal muscle fibers
- **Response:** Is contraction of the muscle being stretched.

**Physiological significance:** It is responsible for the generation of muscle tone.

**Clinical significance:** During the clinical examination of motor system, the testing of stretch reflex is called the deep tendon reflexes (DTR) or jerks. They are used to differentiate between the lower and upper motor neuron lesion, this reflex requires an intact lower motor neuron for eliciting it.

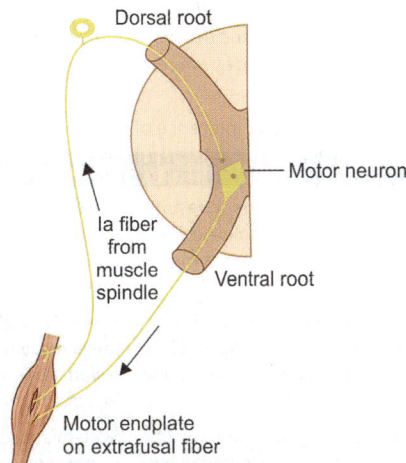

**Fig. 83.1:** Stretch reflex.

These reflexes are tested for the main muscles, i.e.:
- **Testing of triceps and biceps brachii:** Tapping on the tendon of the triceps muscle, for example, causes an extensor response at the elbow as a result of reflex contraction of the triceps (Triceps reflex). Tapping on the tendon of the biceps brachii muscle, causes a flexor response at the elbow as a result of reflex contraction of the biceps (Biceps reflex).
- **Testing the quadriceps femoris:** Tapping on the patellar tendon elicits the **knee jerk,** a stretch reflex of the quadriceps femoris muscle, because the tap on the tendon stretches the muscle. A similar contraction is observed if the quadriceps are stretched manually. Stretch reflexes can also be elicited from most of the large muscles of the body.
- **Testing of gastrocnemius and soleus:** Tapping on the Achilles tendon causes an ankle jerk due to reflex contraction of the gastrocnemius (Ankle reflex).

**What does these reflexes mean?**

The normal expected response to stretch, caused by tapping on the tendon of muscle, is the contraction of the muscle. There could be the observations and inferences drawn from the same as shown in **Table 83.1**.

> **Control of Gamma Efferent Discharge**
>
> The motor neurons of the γ efferent system are regulated to a large degree by descending tracts from a number of areas in the brain. These γ efferent neurons are coactivated along with the α- motor neurons from anterior horn cells.
> Factors influencing γ efferent discharge.
> - **Anxiety** causes an increased discharge, a fact that probably explains the hyperactive tendon reflexes sometimes seen in anxious patients.
> - Sometimes, the stretch reflex is not elicited, in that case, we perform the Jendrassik's maneuver. This maneuver results in increased gamma discharge and increases the sensitivity of muscle spindle, which is described below: *Stimulation of the skin, especially by noxious agents, increases γ efferent discharge to ipsilateral flexor muscle spindles while decreasing that to extensors and produces the opposite pattern in the opposite limb. It is well known that trying to pull the hands apart when the flexed fingers are hooked together facilitates the knee jerk reflex (Jendrassik's maneuver), and this may also be due to increased γ efferent discharge initiated by afferent impulses from the hands.*

**Table 83.1:** Observation and inference of reflexes.

|  | Observation | Inference |
|---|---|---|
| **Normal** | Tapping of tendon results in stretching followed by a brief contraction of muscle | Skeletal muscle has intact innervation and functional stretch reflex |
| **Absent** | Tapping of tendon results in stretching followed by a no response in the muscle | Skeletal muscle has **lower motor neuron lesion** (denervated) and loss of stretch reflex |
| **Exaggerated** | Tapping of tendon results in stretching followed by an exaggerated contractile response in the muscle | Skeletal muscle has **upper motor neuron lesion** and overactivity of stretch reflex |

## Inverse Stretch Reflex (Fig. 83.2)

When the muscle is overstretched, the stretch reflex produces a stronger reflex contraction. It leads to stretching of the tendons of the muscles, so much so that it can avulse the tendons from its insertion. Hence, the inverse stretch reflex involves an inhibitory neuron, which inhibits the α-motor neuron, inhibiting the contraction. Hence, there is relaxation of muscle. The relaxation in response to strong stretch is called the inverse stretch reflex or autogenic inhibition.

**Physiological significance:** The inverse stretch reflex prevents the rupture of tendon from its insertion; hence it is a *protective reflex*. Like every reflex, this reflex has the following components, specific to it:
- **Stimulus:** Muscle contraction and overstretching of tendon
- **Receptor:** Golgi tendon organ
- **Afferent:** Ib group of myelinated, rapidly conducting sensory nerve fibers
- **Center:** Spinal cord. (The Ib fibers end in the spinal cord on inhibitory interneurons that, in turn, terminate directly on the motor neurons.)
- **Efferent:** Alpha motor neurons
- **Effector:** Extrafusal muscle fiber
- **Effect:** Relaxation of muscle

### Golgi tendon organs (Fig. 83.3)

As, we have studied in Chapter 82, the Golgi tendon organs are proprioceptors which are located near musculo-tendinous junction; and consists of an encapsulated knobby nerve endings entwined in the collagen fibers of the tendon.

### How is it stimulated?

When muscle contraction pulls on the tendon, the collagen fibers come together like the two sides of a stretched rubber band and squeeze the nerve endings between them.

The nerve fiber then sends signals to the spinal cord that provide the CNS with feedback on the degree of muscle tension at the joint.

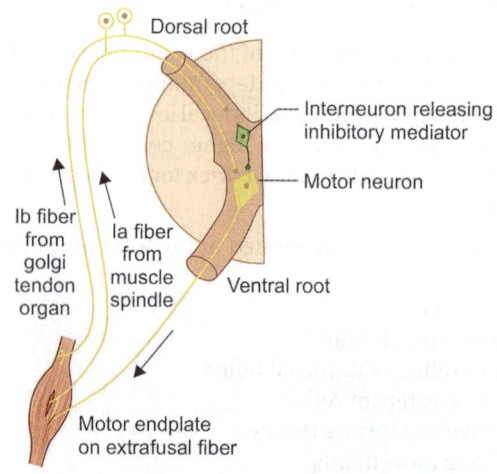

**Fig. 83.2:** Inverse stretch reflex.

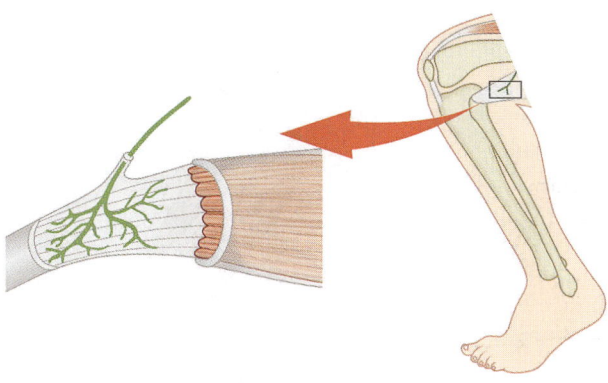

**Fig. 83.3:** Golgi tendon organ.

**Function**

The function of the inverse stretch reflex appears to be a *tension feedback system* that can *adjust the strength of contraction during sustained activity.*

## Flexor Reflex (The Withdrawal Reflex) (Fig. 83.4)

It is a *polysynaptic reflex,* as it involves *many synapses* which are required to provide information to motor neurons of *flexor and extensor muscles of same side and also to the higher centers.*

A flexor reflex is the quick contraction of flexor muscles resulting in the withdrawal of a limb from an injurious stimulus.
- Involves more complex neural pathways.

The reflex arc constitutes of:
- **Stimulus:** Exposure to noxious stimulus
- **Receptor:** Free nerve endings (pain receptors)
- **Afferent:** Sensory fibers carrying the sensation of fast pain
- **Center:** Spinal cord
- **Efferent:** Alpha motor neurons
- **Effector:** Extrafusal muscle fiber (flexors of same side)
- **Effect:** Contraction of flexor muscles of ipsilateral limb and inhibition of extensors of same limb.

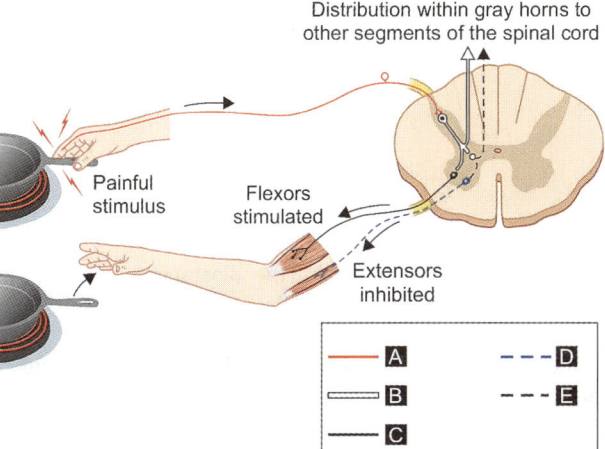

**Fig. 83.4:** Flexor reflex.

## Crossed Extensor Reflex (Fig. 83.5)

The **crossed extensor reflex** is the *contraction of extensor muscles* in the limb opposite from the one that is withdrawn. The crossed extensor reflex employs a **contralateral reflex arc,** in which the input and output are on opposite sides.

*Ipsilateral* extensors are inhibited; flexors contract resulting in removal of the effected limb from the noxious stimulus **(flexor reflex).**

*Contralateral* flexors are inhibited and extensors are stimulated. This results in extension of the opposite limb. It helps in maintaining balance and support weight, hence resulting in postural adjustment **(Fig. 83.6)**.

The reflex arc constitutes of:
- **Stimulus:** Exposure to noxious stimulus
- **Receptor:** Free nerve endings (pain receptors)
- **Afferent:** Sensory fibers carrying the sensation of fast pain
- **Center:** Spinal cord
- **Efferent:** Alpha motor neurons
- **Effector:** Extrafusal muscle fiber (extensors of opposite side)
- **Effect:** Contraction of extensor muscles and inhibition of flexion in contralateral limb.

## Positive Supporting Reaction (Magnet Reaction)

It is a primitive reflex that is present in infants and young children. It is the first postural reflex to develop and is present by 3 to 4 months of age. When a baby is placed in vertical suspension with the feet touching the mat, the baby will extend the legs and attempt to support their weight while being balanced by the examiner. This reflex is important for the development of standing and walking. Even in the adults, we make an attempt of get up from the bed only when our feet touch the ground. Hence, this reflex is important for our standing and posture maintenance. Since, the person extends his foot to the stimulus (hard surface below foot), it is also called the magnet reaction.

## Walking Movements (Fig. 83.7)

The walking movements which include the alternate coordinated flexion and extension of both the upper and lower limbs. This reflex is also integrated at the level of spinal cord due to the presence of neural circuits producing rhythmic outputs called central pattern generators (CPGs).

## Effect of Spinal Cord Transaction on Spinal Reflexes

*(The diseases of spinal cord are discussed in Chapter 80)*
The role of spinal cord in maintaining the spinal reflexes can be studied by removing the influence of higher centers on the spinal cord. This is done by making a complete transaction of spinal cord below the brainstem in lower

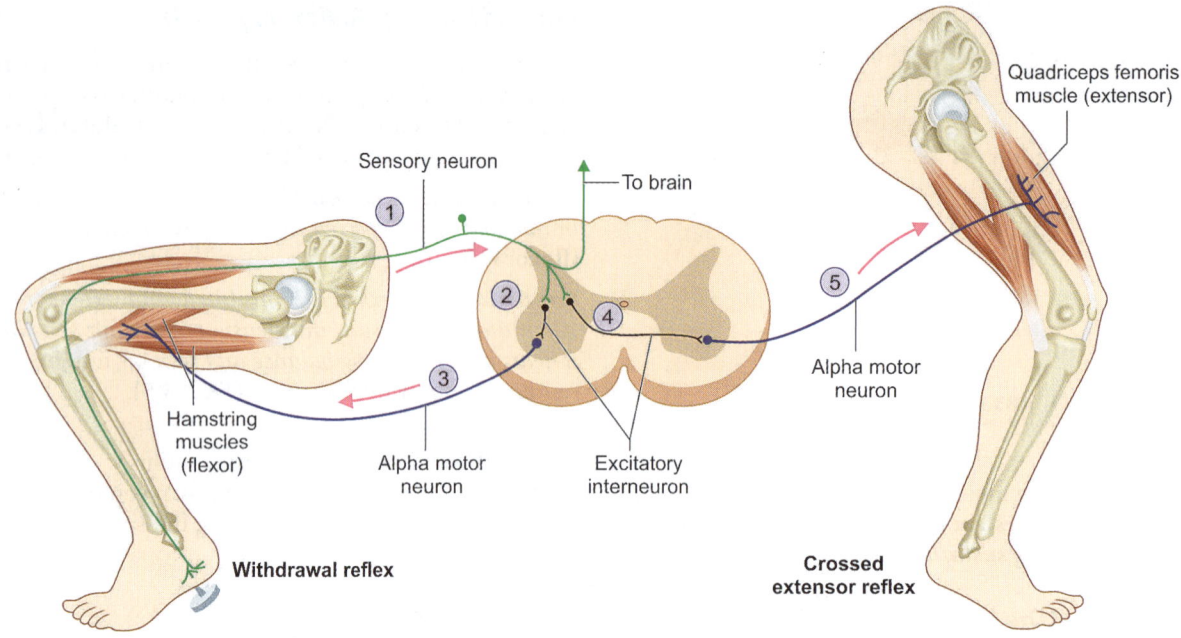

**Crossed extensor reflex:**
1. During the withdrawal reflex, sensory neurons from pain receptors conduct action potentials to the spinal cord.
2. Sensory neurons synapse with excitatory interneurons that are part of the withdrawal reflex.
3. The excitatory interneurons that are part of the withdrawal reflex stimulate alpha motor neurons that innervate flexor muscles, causing withdrawal of the limb from the painful stimulus.
4. Collateral branches of the sensory neurons also synapse with excitatory interneurons that cross to the opposite side of the spinal cord as part of the crossed extensor reflex.
5. The excitatory interneurons that cross the spinal cord stimulate alpha motor neurons supplying extensor muscles in the opposite limb, causing them to contract and support body weight during the withdrawal reflex.

**Fig. 83.5:** Crossed extensor reflex.

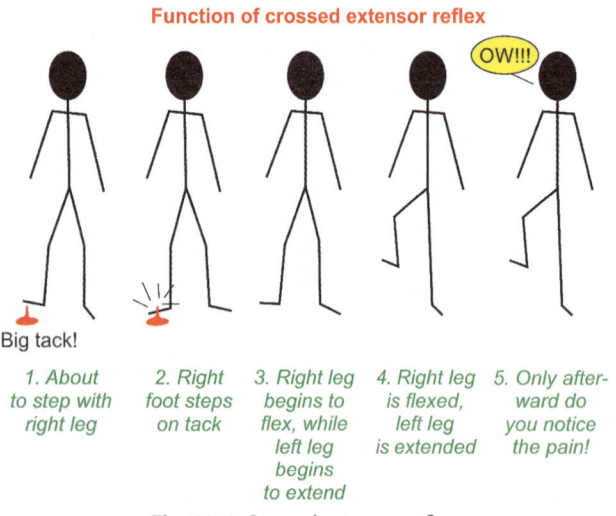

**Fig. 83.6:** Crossed extensor reflex.

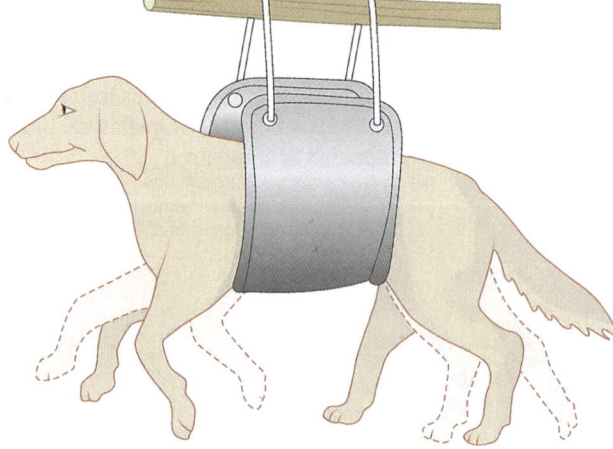

**Fig. 83.7:** Walking movements in the spinal animal suspended in a sling.

animals like cats, dogs and monkeys. Experimentally, we call such an animal as *spinal animal/spinal preparation*.

This is similar to the clinical condition, when a person suffers a spinal cord damage either due to injury or tumor, disconnecting it from the brainstem. The spinal cord works autonomously without any influence from higher centers.

Whenever there is sudden transection (transverse section/cut) of spinal cord, the animal/patient experiences the stage of spinal shock due to sudden loss of control of

higher centers. The stages of spinal injury and recovery are described below:
- **Stage of spinal shock:** Complete loss of sensory and motor functions
- **Stage of recovery:** We can study the spinal reflexes in this stage of experimental animals. Duration of stage of recovery Hence in such spinal preparation (in experimental animal)/patients, the following spinal reflexes are *present*:
  - Stretch reflex (exaggerated due to loss of higher inhibitory influence).
  - Inverse stretch reflex
  - Flexor reflex
  - Crossed extensor reflex
  - *Positive supporting reaction:* When the paw of the animal is touched, it moves the paw towards the stimulus.
  - *Walking movements:* Though the animal/human is not able to maintain the standing upright posture, but he can still exhibit the walking movements, when suspended in the sling. This is clear evidence that walking movements are produced at the level of spinal cord.

The reflexes integrated at the brainstem and above are *absent* in this animal (in experimental condition)/patients:
  - Upright posture
  - Righting reflexes
  - Hopping and placing reaction.

## Postural Reflexes Integrated at the Level of Medulla Oblongata and Pons (Brainstem)

The brainstem nuclei are responsible for maintaining the posture against gravity. The brainstem (except midbrain) receives the inputs from the following nuclei (**Fig. 83.8**):
- **The reticular activating system (RAS):** It is an important tract conveying signals to and from between the spinal cord and cerebral cortex. On its way to cortex, it also transmits the sensory and motor signals to various parts of brain. The main function of RAS is general consciousness/awareness about the senses and the motor signals. The RAS has two broad divisions:
  1. *Pontine/facilitatory neurons*: It facilitates the anterior horn cell motor neurons and increases the tone of the antigravity muscles. The muscle tone due to facilitation by the pontine RAS is strong enough to increase the tone in extensors to maintain the upright posture.
  2. *Medullary/inhibitory neurons*: It inhibits the pontine RAS neurons. They are facilitated by the corticospinal and extrapyramidal tracts. They balance the tone in the extensor muscles, due to the pontine RAS.
- **Vestibular nuclei:** The vestibular nuclei function in association with pontine RAS, it strongly facilitates the antigravity muscles. It selectively controls the excitatory

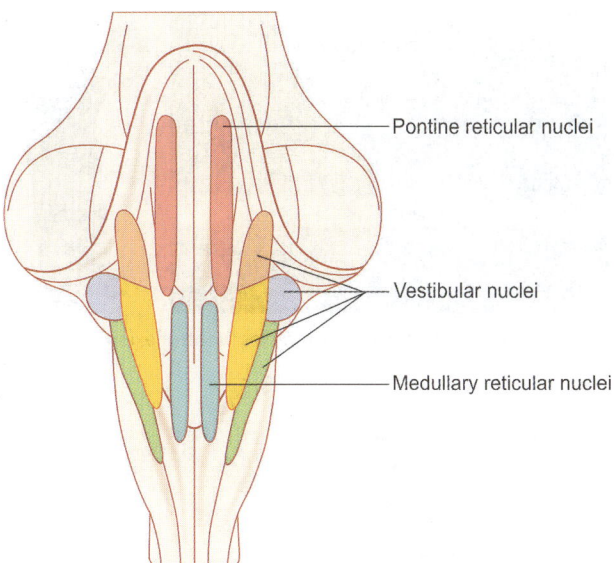

**Fig. 83.8:** Pons and medulla oblongata showing the pontine and medullary RAS and vestibular nuclei.

signals to different antigravity muscles, as required to maintain the posture.

The various inputs from RAS and vestibular nuclei are integrated to produce the following reflexes at the level of brainstem.

### Tonic Neck Reflexes

Impulses passing from neck muscles to spinal cord.

It refers to the postural adjustment, i.e., change in the position of the limbs in response to the neck movement.
- The movement of the neck to one side results in the flexion of vertex limb (towards back of head) and extension of jaw limb (towards chin), as seen in **Figure 83.9**.

*Physiological basis:* The **pathway** for the tonic neck reflex is mediated by two pathways:
1. An excitatory pathway from the lateral vestibular nucleus
2. An inhibitory pathway from the medial part of the medullary reticular formation.

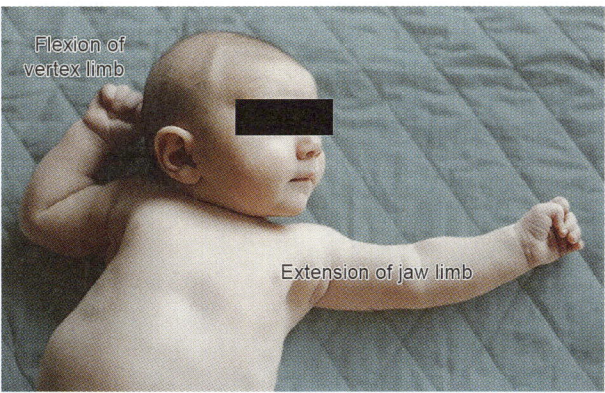

**Fig. 83.9:** Tonic neck reflex.

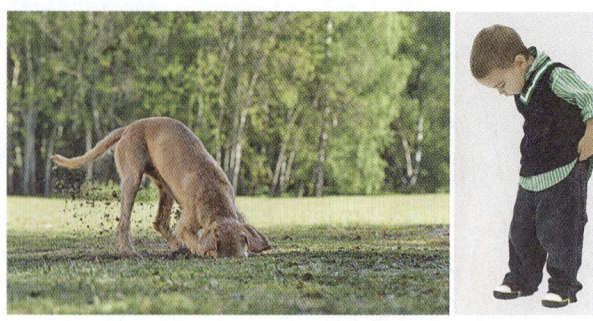

**Fig. 83.10:** Tonic neck reflexes (Ventroflexion).

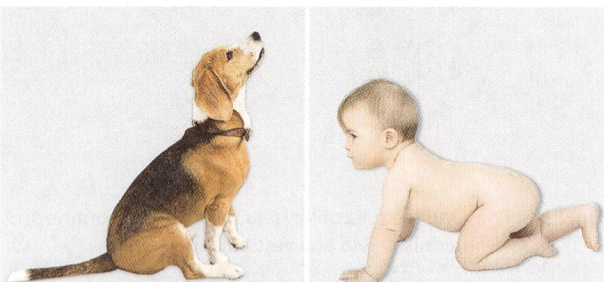

**Fig. 83.11:** Tonic neck reflexes (Dorsiflexion).

The activity of these pathways leads to the extension of the limb on the side to which the chin is pointed and flexion of the limb on the contralateral side.
- The ventroflexion of neck (as if the dog is looking into the hole/digging in the ground), the fore legs are in flexion and the hind legs are extended (**Fig. 83.10**).
- While the dorsiflexion of neck (as if the dog is looking towards the sky), the fore legs are extended and the hind legs are flexed (**Fig. 83.11**).

## Tonic Labyrinthine Reflexes

Impulses passing from vestibular apparatus to spinal cord. As mentioned above, the vestibular nucleus facilitates the pontine RAS. Hence, the tonic labyrinthine reflexes maintain the tone of extensors with respect to the position of the torso.
- When a person is lying on his back (supine position), the tone is increased in the back muscles/extensor muscles (**Fig. 83.12**).
- When the person is lying on the abdomen (prone position), the tone in the muscles of neck and the flexors increases (**Fig. 83.13**).

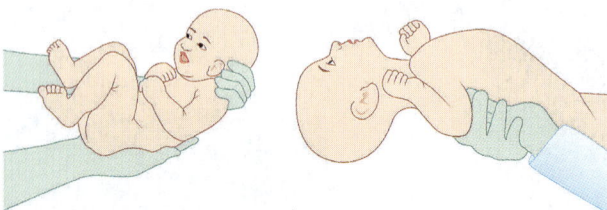

**Fig. 83.12:** Tonic labyrinthine reflexes (Supine).

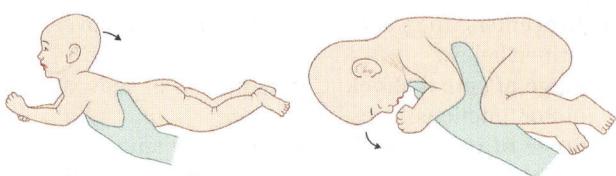

**Fig. 83.13:** Tonic labyrinthine reflexes (Prone).

## Effect of Transection above Brainstem

(Between the Superior and Inferior Colliculus/ Midcollicular Level).

In experimental lab, the midcollicular section is made in the lower animal to study the reflexes integrated at the level of brainstem. The influence of midbrain and cerebral cortex is abolished in the section. In that case, we call this animal as *Decerebrate preparation/midcollicular section*.

However, the patients with either **tumor/injury or hemorrhage** at the level of pons and medulla can present with the similar findings. The injury to brainstem is more dangerous and carries poor prognosis as the vital autonomic functions are located on the brainstem.

**The decerebrate animal shows the following features:**
- All the **spinal reflexes are preserved,** i.e., stretch reflex, inverse stretch reflex, flexor reflex, crossed extensor reflex, positive supporting reaction.
- The **upright posture is maintained,** i.e., the animal can stand upright due to hypertonia. There is increased tone in the extensors.
- There is **unopposed activation of pontine RAS** because the medullary RAS, which usually inhibits the pontine RAS is not facilitated due to loss of input from corticospinal tract and other inputs from higher centers. The patient attains the *decorticate posture: increased tone in extensors of neck, back, arms, legs and feet, the arms are pronated and hands and fingers are flexed*. The increased tone of the muscles is called the **decerebrate rigidity** (**Fig. 83.14**).

In animals, there is also the increased tone in limbs, neck, back muscles and tail resulting in hyperextension of back (***Opisthotonus/Caricature***) (**Fig. 83.15**).
- A decerebrate animal is not able to maintain its posture, if disturbed. Hence, the equilibrium is lost. The *righting reflexes are absent* in this animal. The righting reflexes are hence integrated above the brainstem.
- The tonic neck and labyrinthine reflexes integrated at the level of brainstem, without the influence of higher centers; can be studied in the experimental decerebrate preparation.
  - To demonstrate the tonic neck reflex, the animal is rotated very fast to destroy the vestibular apparatus, so that the pure tonic neck reflex is elicited. Once the vestibular apparatus is destroyed, the posture of the limbs with respect to the movement of neck is studies (as mentioned in the section above).

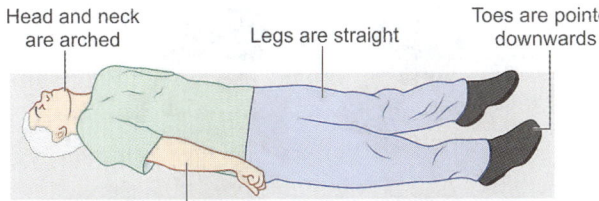

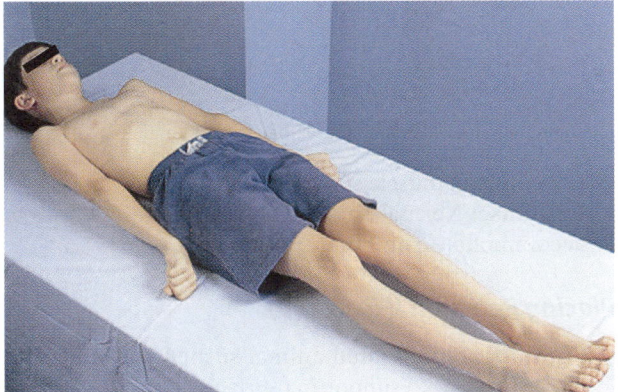

**Fig. 83.14:** Decerebrate rigidity.

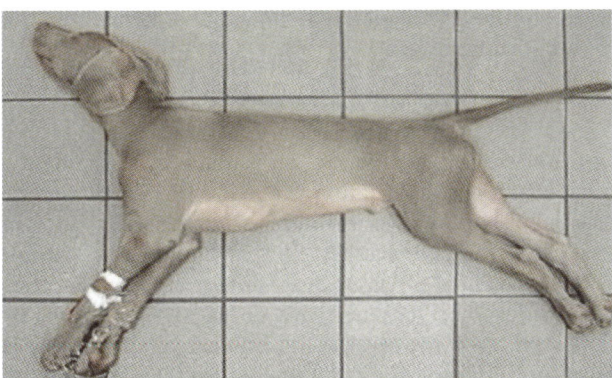

**Fig. 83.15:** Decerebrate rigidity in a dog (Opisthotonus).

- To demonstrate the tonic labyrinthine reflex, the nerves supplying the neck muscles (C1, C2 and C3) are cut to remove the effect of neck reflex. Then the labyrinthine reflex is demonstrated, as mentioned in tonic labyrinthine reflex.

## Postural Reflexes Integrated at the Level of Midbrain

The midbrain has red nucleus from where one of the main extrapyramidal tracts, rubrospinal tract (*arising from red nucleus and terminating in spinal cord*) originates. It primarily increases the tone of flexor muscles and inhibit the extensors. Various other inputs are integrated at the level of midbrain for maintenance and postural correction. Various reflexes involved in the correction of posture are called the **righting reflexes**.

### Righting Reflexes

Based on the neural circuit integrating the postural reflex, the righting reflexes are classified as:

- **Optical righting reflex:** Tectospinal, tectobulbar and spinotectal tracts. It is responsible for integration of *spinovisual reflex*. In this reflex, the posture maintenance is done by midbrain in response to sudden movement of head due to the visual stimulus. It is responsible for the postural correction in response to the visual stimuli, called the **Optical righting reflex.**
- **Labyrinthine righting reflex:** The impulses from the vestibular apparatus and cerebellum are integrated in the midbrain. The change in the position of head stimulates the labyrinthine and it sends the signals to midbrain. The cerebellum then compares the expected posture of body with the perceived posture and readjusts the tone in the muscles in such a way that it is corrected as per the expected posture. This is called the *Labyrinthine righting reflex*. It is different from the tonic labyrinthine reflex, since it involves the cerebellar comparison here.
- **Neck righting reflex:** Impulses from neck muscles pass and changes the tone resulting in the correction of posture of neck, thorax, abdomen and pelvis.
- **Body righting reflex:** When the person attempts to get up from the floor, the tone in the muscles readjusts in a way that helps the person to maintain his posture during the same. This is called the *Body righting reflex* (Table 83.2). The body righting reflex is further of two types:
  1. **Body on head righting reflex:** Raising the neck first to have upright posture. Further, the stretching of the neck muscles result in the correction of body posture.

**Table 83.2:** Types of body righting reflexes and their features.

| Reflex | Site | Stimulus | Receptor | Response |
|---|---|---|---|---|
| **Visual righting reflexes** | Center in cerebral cortex | Visual stimulus | Eye receptors | Adjustment of posture according to the visual image |
| **Labyrinthine righting reflexes** | Midbrain | Covered eyes and tilting the head | Otolith organs to stimulate neck muscles to correct the head level | Righting of head |
| **Body on head righting reflexes** | | Pressure on side of body | Trunk proprioceptors | Reflex correction of head |
| **Body on body** | | Pressure on side of the body and head is fixed | Trunk proprioceptors | Reflex correction of body |
| **Neck righting reflexes** | | Stretch of neck muscles (if head is corrected and body still tilted) righting of shoulders and body | Muscle spindles of neck muscles | Righting of body |

2. ***Body on body righting reflex:*** Body is raised first to have the upright posture. If the head is not allowed to right itself. The exteroceptors of the body can result in the correction of posture of the body.

## Effect of Transection above Superior Colliculus

In experimental lab, the section is made above the superior colliculus with intact brainstem in the lower animal to study the reflexes integrated at the level of midbrain. The influence of cerebral cortex is abolished in the section. However, the inputs from Vestibular apparatus, Cerebellum, RAS are integrated here. In that case, we call this animal as *Midbrain preparation*.

However, the patients with either *tumor/injury or hemorrhage* at the level of midbrain can present with the similar findings.

**The midbrain preparation shows the following features:**
- All the ***spinal reflexes are preserved,*** i.e., stretch reflex, inverse stretch reflex, flexor reflex, crossed extensor reflex, positive supporting reaction
- The ***upright posture is maintained***
- The rigidity is present. There is increased tone in the extensors as well as the flexors.
- The righting reflexes are present which are mainly due to the red nucleus present in the midbrain.

## Postural Reflexes Integrated at the Level of Cerebral Cortex

The cerebral cortex is the main motor control system of the body. It is mostly concerned with the initiation of the motor activity. But it is also responsible for the posture maintenance while hopping and placing reactions. This means the posture regulation during the movement is primarily controlled by the cerebral cortex. Below this level (up to midbrain) all the postural reflexes were static, i.e., the posture maintenance was done at rest.

### Hopping Reaction (Fig. 83.16)
- **Stimulus:** The animal is moved laterally (the majority of its weight is on one limb).

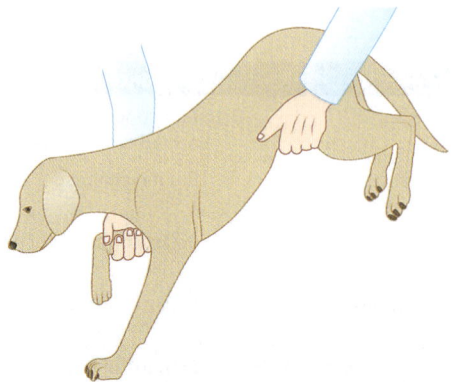

**Fig. 83.16:** Hopping reaction.

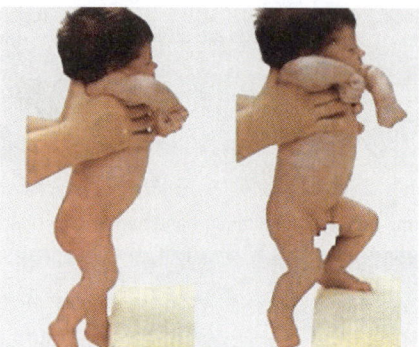

**Fig. 83.17:** Placing reaction.

- **Receptor:** In muscle spindles.
- **Response:** Normal animals hop on the tested limb to accommodate a new body position.

### Placing Reaction (Fig. 83.17)
- **Stimulus:** Blind folded animal suspended in air and moved towards a supporting surface.
- **Receptor:** Touch receptors and proprioceptors in soles of feet.
- **Response:** The feet will be placed firmly on the supporting surface.

## Effect of Damage to Cerebral Cortex

In experimental lab, the section is made by stripping the area 4s and corpus striatum in the lower animal to study the reflexes integrated at the level of cerebral cortex. In that case, we call this animal as *Decorticate preparation* **(Fig. 83.18)**.

However, the patients with either *tumor/injury or hemorrhage* at the level of internal capsule can present with the similar findings on the contralateral side of the body.

**The decorticate preparation shows the following features:**
- All the ***spinal reflexes are preserved,*** i.e., stretch reflex, inverse stretch reflex, flexor reflex, crossed extensor reflex, positive supporting reaction
- The ***upright posture is maintained***
- The rigidity is present. There is increased tone in the extensors as well as the flexors.
- The righting reflexes are present

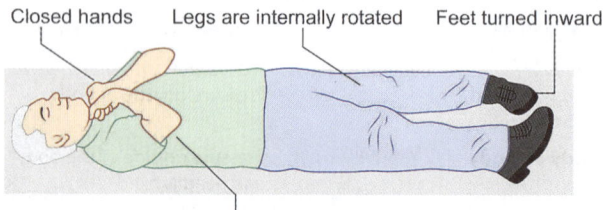

**Fig. 83.18:** Decorticate rigidity.

- Some rigidity is present. In case of pure corticospinal tract lesion there is spasticity of extensors of lower limbs and flexors of upper limbs. This results in flexion of upper limbs and extension of lower limbs. The spasticity is phasic i.e. it is more at rest and decreases with movement (Clasp knife spasticity) **(Fig. 83.19)**.
- Hoping and placing reaction is severely impaired.

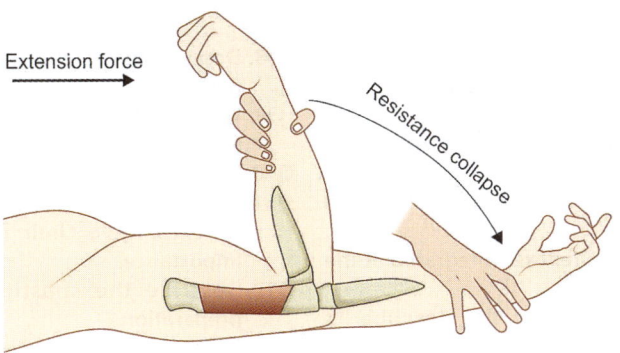

**Fig. 83.19:** Clasp knife spasticity.

## SUMMARY

| | Reflex | Receptor | Stimulus | Response | Center |
|---|---|---|---|---|---|
| **Static — Spinal** | Stretch | Muscle spindle | Stretch | Contraction of muscle | Spinal cord |
| | Negative supporting | Proprioceptors in extensors | | Release of positive supporting reaction | |
| | Positive supporting | Proprioceptors in distal flexor | Contact with sole or palm | Foot extended to support body | |
| | Segmental as: Crossed extensor | Pain receptors | Sharp painful | Flexion of stimulated limb and extension of other limb | |
| **Static — Medullary** | Labyrinthine | Otolithic organ | Gravity → Ventroflexion of head | Flexion of four limbs | Medulla |
| | | | Gravity → Dorsiflexion of head | Extension of four limbs | |
| | Neck | Neck proprioceptors | Head to side | Extension of limbs on that side and flexion of other side | |
| | | | Dorsiflexion of head | Arms extended and flexed hindlimb | |
| | | | Ventroflexion of head | Arms flexion and extend hindlimb | |
| **Righting** | Visual | Eye receptors | Visual cues | Adjustment of posture according to the visual cues | Cerebral cortex |
| | Labyrinthine | Otolith organ | Covered eyes and tilting the head | Righting of head | Midbrain |
| | Body on head | Trunk proprioceptors | Pressure on side of body | Reflex correction of head | |
| | Body on body | | Pressure on side of body | Reflex correction of body | |
| | Neck righting | Muscle spindles | Stretch of neck muscles | Righting of body | |
| **Phasic** | Hopping reaction | Muscle spindles | The animal is moved laterally | Normal animals hop on the tested limb to accommodate a new body position | Cerebral cortex |
| | Placing reaction | Touch receptors and proprioceptors in soles of feet | Blind folded animal suspended in air and moved towards a supporting surface | The feet will be placed firmly on the supporting surface | |

# LET US SEE, HOW MUCH YOU HAVE LEARNT?

## Review Questions

### Long/Short Answer Questions

Q1. Define the postural reflex.
Q2. Define the muscle tone. Describe the physiological basis of generation of muscle tone.
Q3. Describe stretch reflex. Also describe its physiological and functional importance.
Q4. Describe inverse stretch reflex. Give its physiological and functional importance.
Q5. Describe the various postural reflexes integrated at the level of spinal cord.
Q6. Describe flexor/withdrawal reflex. Also describe its physiological and functional importance.
Q7. Describe crossed extensor reflex. Also describe its physiological and functional importance.
Q8. Describe the postural reflexes integrated at the level of medulla and pons.
Q9. What is decerebrate rigidity? What are the salient features seen in decerebrate rigidity?
Q10. Describe the physiological basis of decerebrate rigidity.
Q11. Define righting reflexes. Describe the various righting reflexes. Give their physiological and functional importance.
Q12. Describe the spasticity seen in the decorticate preparation.
Q13. Differentiate between spasticity and rigidity.

### Explain Why? (Reasoning Questions)

Q1. The deep tendon reflexes become hyperactive in upper motor neuron lesion.
Q2. The deep tendon reflexes are lost in lower motor neuron lesion.
Q3. Postural reflexes involve both spinal cord and higher brain centers.
Q4. Impairment of postural reflexes can lead to gait abnormalities and falls.
Q5. Muscle tone is essential for maintaining posture and preventing joint instability.
Q6. Damage to upper motor neurons can lead to spasticity and hypertonia in muscles.

### Critical Thinking Case-Based Questions

Q1. Rajesh, a 65-year-old man, visited his physician with complaints of unsteadiness while walking and frequent falls, especially when getting up from a sitting position or changing directions. He reported no recent injuries but mentioned increasing difficulty with balance over the past few months. His physician suspected impairment in postural reflexes and wanted to explore the physiological basis and regulation of these reflexes to better understand Rajesh's symptoms. Based on the above scenario, answer the following questions:
a. What are postural reflexes, and how do they contribute to maintaining balance and stability during various movements such as standing, walking, and changing positions?
b. Discuss how impairment in these reflexes could contribute to Rajesh's symptoms.

### Multiple Choice Questions

Q1. A 63-year-old female is brought to the emergency with loss of consciousness and increased tone of all four limbs. She is hypertensive for 30 years. Physical examination shows BP 170/120 mm Hg, irregular respiration. Her legs and feet are extended, upper limbs are also extended. Her hands are pronated with flexed wrists and fingers. What do you think is the probable site of hemorrhage?
a. Internal capsule
b. Paramedian vertebrobasilar artery
c. Posterior cerebellar artery
d. Anterior cerebellar artery

Q2. A 6-month-old baby is placed in a prone position. When the baby's head is turned to one side, the arm and leg on that side extend while the opposite side flexes. What reflex is being exhibited by the baby in this situation?
a. Tonic labyrinthine reflex
b. Neck righting reflex
c. Tonic neck reflex
d. Labyrinthine reflex

Q3. Identify the postural reflex in the baby shown below:

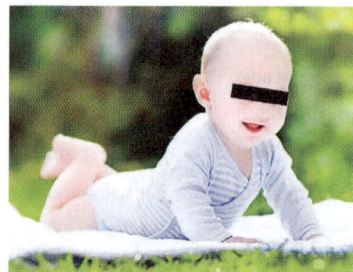

a. Tonic labyrinthine reflex
b. Neck righting reflex
c. Tonic neck reflex
d. Labyrinthine reflex

Q4. Esha, a 30-year-old woman, is brought to the emergency room after a car accident resulting in a head injury. Upon assessment, the medical team notices that Esha has flexed arms with clenched fists and extended legs. What type of spasticity is Esha exhibiting?
  a. Decorticate spasticity
  b. Decerebrate rigidity
  c. Flaccid paralysis
  d. Hyperreflexia

Q5. Sarah is driving her car on a bumpy road, and she notices that her friend sitting in the passenger seat is experiencing discomfort and difficulty maintaining an upright posture. Which postural reflex is likely to be engaged in Sarah's friend due to the motion of the moving vehicle?
  a. Tonic labyrinthine reflex
  b. Neck righting reflex
  c. Tonic neck reflex
  d. Labyrinthine reflex

## ANSWERS

**1.** b   **2.** c   **3.** a   **4.** a   **5.** a

# Cerebral Cortex

**CHAPTER 84**

> **COMPETENCY ADDRESSED**
>
> **PY10.7:** Describe and discuss functions of **cerebral cortex**, basal ganglia, thalamus, hypothalamus, cerebellum and limbic system and their abnormalities.

>  **LEARNING OBJECTIVES**
>
> **At the end of this chapter, the learner should be able to:**
> - Describe the functional divisions and histology of cerebral cortex.
> - Describe the functions of each lobe of cerebral cortex.
> - Name the important Broadman's areas and their functions.
> - Describe the physiological importance of sensory and motor homunculus.
> - Describe the concept of cerebral dominance.
> - Describe the role of cerebral cortex in higher functions.
> - Describe the clinical significance of lesions in different parts of the cerebral cortex.

The cerebral cortex is the most important part of the central nervous system which is protected inside the skull. In Chapter 79 we had discussed that it has 2 hemispheres, the right and the left which are connected with the help of corpus callosum. The cerebral cortex has an enormous area which is thrown into folds resulting in the formation of sulci and gyri. The cerebral cortex has an outer grey matter comprising of the cell bodies and inner white matter having the nerve fibers.

## FUNCTIONAL ANATOMY OF CEREBRAL CORTEX

The cerebral cortex has an outer thin layer (2–5 mm) made up of nearly 100 billion neurons with a total surface area of ¼ m². The cortical tissue in arranged in the vertical microcolumns of diameter 0.3 to 0.5 mm. In the sensory cortex, each column serves single sensory modality. These columns interact with each other through the association and projection fibers.

The cerebral cortex has six layers, as shown in **Figure 84.1** and their functions are tabulated in **Table 84.1**.

## LOBES OF CEREBRUM

Each hemisphere of the cerebral cortex has four lobes, the frontal, parietal, temporal and occipital lobes (**Fig. 84.2**). Let us now broadly discuss the functions of each lobe:

### Frontal Lobe

The frontal lobe is present at the front of the cerebral cortex, hence the name!

It is made up of very important areas, classified as (**Fig. 84.3**):
- **Motor cortex:** Primary motor cortex, premotor cortex, and supplementary motor cortex
- **Prefrontal cortex:** For planning and programming of complex motor movements, frontal eye field, etc.
- **Broca's area:** The motor area for speech/word formation.

> **Cerebral cortex has three types of neurons:**
> 1. Pyramidal cells
> 2. Granule/stellate cells: Excitatory (glutaminergic) and inhibitory (GABAergic)
> 3. Polymorphic/fusiform cells
>
> **Cerebral cortex has two types of fibers:**
> 1. Horizontal fibers: Association fibers
> 2. Vertical fibers: Projection fibers

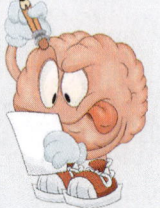

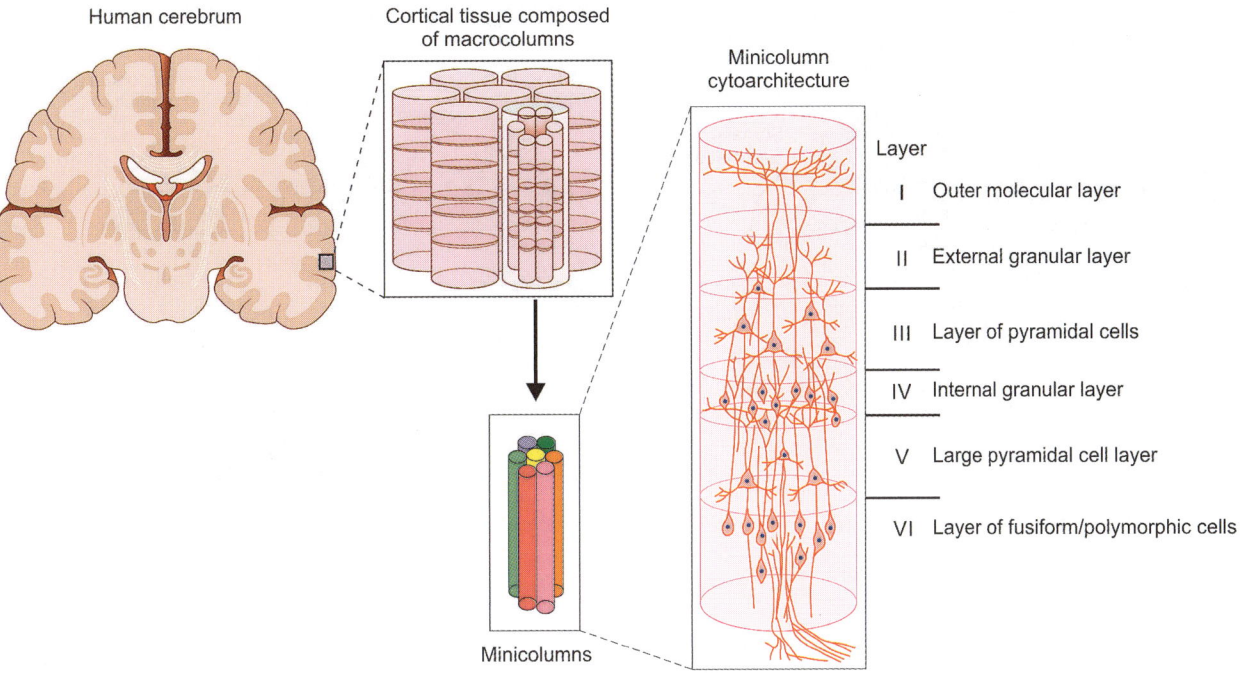

**Fig. 84.1:** The structural organization of cerebral cortex.

**Table 84.1:** The functions of each layer of the cerebral cortex.

| Layers | Name of layers | Functions |
|---|---|---|
| I | Outer molecular layer | It has the dendrites of the neurons (horizontal fibers) running in this layer, which connects the different parts of the cerebral cortex. They act as the association fibers |
| II | External granular layer | The granular layer consists of granular/stellate neurons, which are short neurons. These neurons transmit the signals only for short distances within the cortex. These neurons can be excitatory (neurotransmitter glutamate) or inhibitory (neurotransmitter GABA). These granular neurons process the sensory signals within the sensory areas and association areas. The vertical fibers extend to and from the cortex and to spinal cord |
| III | Layer of pyramidal cells | Intracortical association function through the short neurons |
| IV | Inner granular layer | Same as layer II. It receives most of the incoming specific sensory signals from body in cortical layer |
| V | Large pyramidal cell layer | It is the main output layer of the cerebral cortex. These neurons give rise to the major motor tract (corticospinal tract) which descend down to spinal cord |
| VI | Layer of fusiform/polymorphic cells | The fibers from this layer of cerebral cortex go to thalamus and other deeper structures of brain |

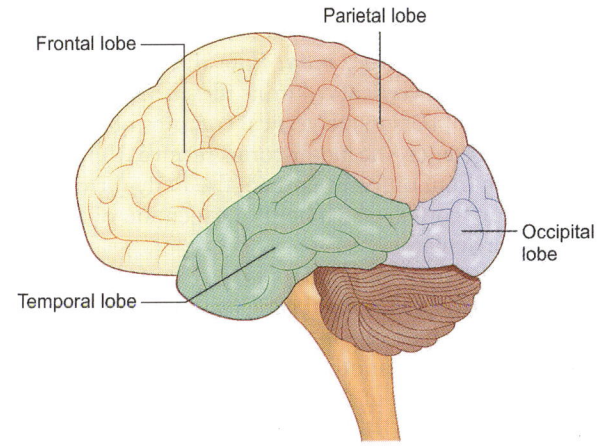

**Fig. 84.2:** The lobes of the cerebral cortex.

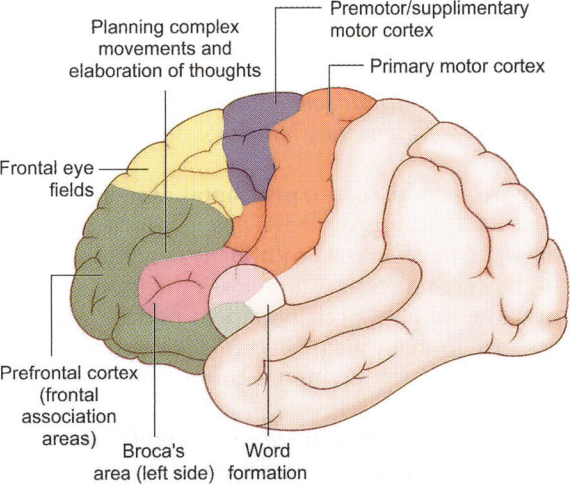

**Fig. 84.3:** Parts of frontal lobe.

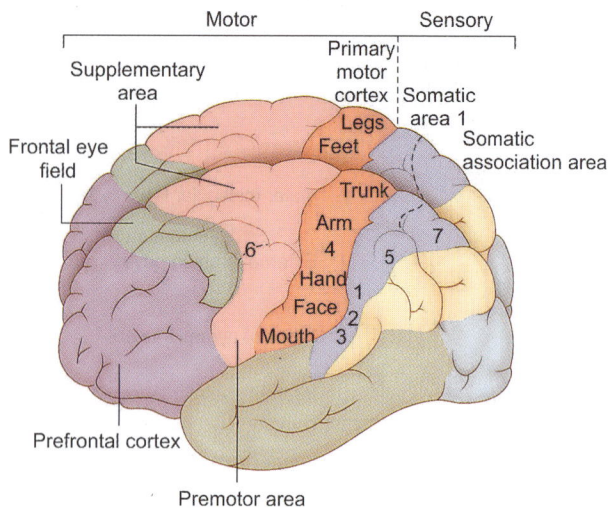

**Fig. 84.4:** The motor cortex.

## Functions of Frontal Lobe

- **The motor cortex** of the frontal lobe is further classified as primary motor area (Broadman Area 4), premotor and supplementary motor area (Area 6) **(Fig. 84.4)**. It lies anterior to central sulcus and constitutes posterior half of the frontal lobe. The main function of these areas is to:
  - *Receive the sensory input* from the somatosensory cortex. The vertical columns in the sensory cortex send the fibers to the vertical columns of the motor cortex. Hence, the motor cortex receives the sensory inputs from different parts of the body through the sensory cortex, which helps it execution of relevant motor activity.
  - *Relay the information to spinal cord* and other deeper nuclei (thalamus, basal ganglia and cerebellum) for the fine and precise motor activity.
  - The primary motor cortex has *topographical representation* of the entire body on the primary cortex **(Figs. 84.4 and 84.9)**. The topographic representation on the primary motor area is same as on the sensory cortex.
  - The *premotor area* has the same topographic arrangement as the motor area. However, the it is associated with *performing complex motor movements*.
  - The *supplementary motor area* is associated with the *bilateral rudimentary hand movements like grasping etc.*
- **The prefrontal cortex/prefrontal association area (Fig. 84.5):** It is also called as the prefrontal association area and in concerned with many complex functions of the cerebral cortex. It receives the inputs from all over the brain, especially parieto-occipito-temporal association area, which delivers the preanalyzed sensory information. The prefrontal cortex uses this sensory information for:
  - *Planning and programming of complex movements and sequences of movements.* This information is

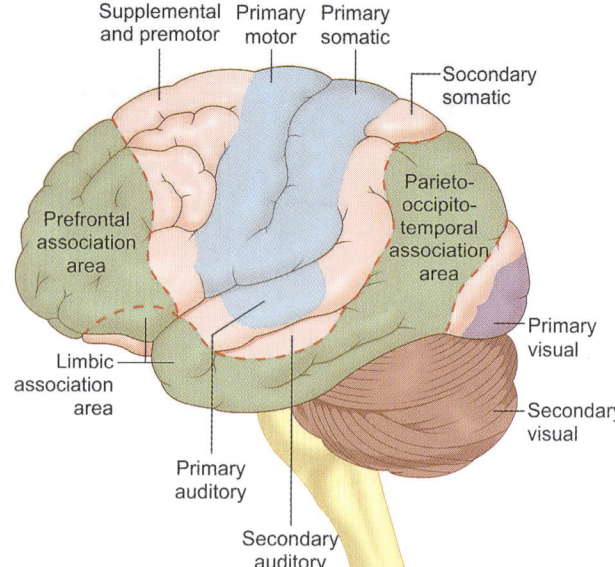

**Fig. 84.5:** The cerebral association areas (prefrontal association area, parieto-occipito-temporal association area and limbic association area).

sent back to the motor cortex for execution through the basal ganglia-thalamic feedback loop. Hence the motor cortex can execute the *sequential and parallel* components of the movement.
  - *Elaboration of thoughts* takes place in prefrontal cortex. The information from all parts of brain provides enough information to prefrontal cortex to *elaborate the thoughts in depth and abstractness*. The prefrontal cortex provides the working memory for this purpose, where the thoughts and information are stored for short term basis.
  - *Provides working memory* for prognostication, i.e., *prediction, planning for future, weighing the motor* actions before performing them, solve complex mathematical problems, analyses the available information, controls our social behavior according to moral laws.
- **Motor speech area (Broca's area):** This area is located partly in posterior lateral prefrontal cortex and partly in premotor area. The Broca's area plans the motor patterns for expressing words or short phrases.
- **Hand skill area:** It is located in the dominant hemisphere (left cerebral hemisphere) of the prefrontal cortex and supplementary motor area in 90% of individuals, hence responsible for right handedness of individuals.
- **Frontal eye fields:** The frontal eye field (FEF) is a region in the frontal lobe of the brain, specifically in Brodmann area 8 and 6. It plays a crucial role in the control of eye movements, particularly voluntary saccadic eye movements, which are rapid movements of the eyes between fixation points.

The FEF is involved in *directing visual attention and coordinating eye movements* with other sensory

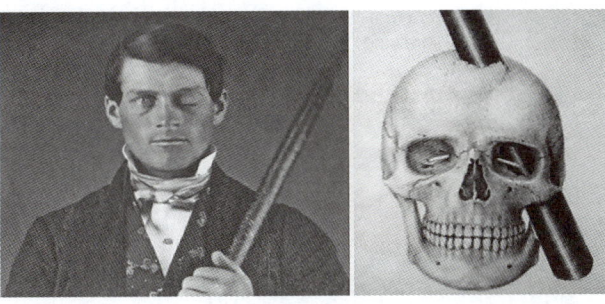

**Fig. 84.6:** Phineas Gage got injured with an iron rod, piercing through his frontal lobe resulting in major personality changes in him.

and motor systems. Damage to this area can lead to difficulties in focusing attention, following objects with the eyes, and making accurate saccades **(Fig. 84.6)**.

**Prefrontal lobotomy/lesion of prefrontal lobe/frontal lobe syndrome:**
In the lesions of prefrontal lobe, the patients show:
- Inability to solve complex problems
- Inability to comprehend the sequential tasks to reach complex goals
- Inability to learn parallel tasks at the same time
- Abulia: Lack of motivation/will or initiative
- Lack of regard for social rules resulting in inappropriate and immoral behavior
- Impulsive behavior
- Loss of organization of thought

## Parietal Lobe

The parietal lobe is present behind the central sulcus, between the primary motor cortex and the occipital cortex **(Fig. 84.2)**. It has three main areas located in it, mentioned below:

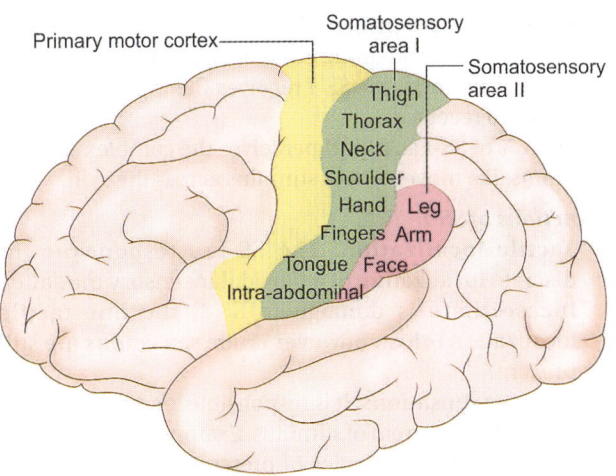

**Fig. 84.7:** Somatosensory areas I and II.

### Somatosensory Area I and II (SS-I and SS-II)

In **Figure 84.7**, the SS-I (Area 3, 1, 2) and II (Area 5, 7) are represented on the anterior part of parietal cortex. The topographical representation of the body is present on the SS-I **(Fig. 84.8)**, is similar for both the motor and sensory cortices.

SS-I is organized into the vertical columns of diameter 0.3 to 0.5 mm with around 10,000 neurons. Each column serves as a single sensory stimulus. The neuron of each column act separately, but send horizontal fibers for the analyzing the meaning of sensory inputs. SS-II is located behind the SS-I in the parietal cortex.

The sensory cortex (SS-I) is organized in a way that:
- The most anterior part of SS-I (deep in central fissure, area 3A) responds to muscle, tendon and joint stretch receptors. The signals from here spread anteriorly to the motor cortex, located anteriorly in frontal lobe (mentioned above).

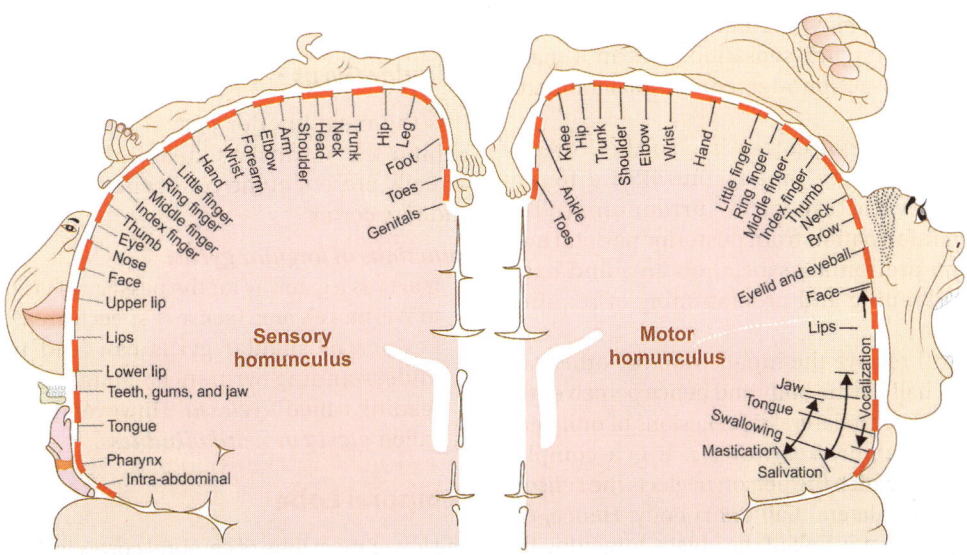

**Fig. 84.8:** Sensory and motor homunculus indication similar topographical representation, on sensory and motor cortex.

- Behind the proprioceptive sensory input, the SS-I receives slowly adapting cutaneous receptors.
- Most posteriorly, the SS-I receives the input from deep pressure receptors.
- Last 6% of SS-I and SS-II perceives the complex sensory inputs like movement of stimulus across the skin.

### Functions of SS-I:

- **Tactile localization:** The SS-I is responsible for discrete localization of a particular sensory modality. Incase there is damage to SS-I, the fine tactile localization is lost, however crude sensations are still present.
- **Epicritic sensations:** It is responsible for differentiating in the degree/extent of stimulus. Example differentiating between different grades of pressure. In the damage of SS-I, the person is unable to judge the difference in critical degree of pressure applied. Other epicritic sensations like difference in weight are also affected. *The sensation of pain and temperature are preserved in quality and intensity in the lesions of SS-I, however localization of these senses is affected.*
- **Texture of materials:** When the hand is moved across the surface of any object, we are able to appreciate the texture of that surface/cloth. This sensation is also perceived by SS-I. In case of damage of SS-I, this sensation is also lost.
- **Stereognosis:** It is the ability of the SS-I to synthesize the complex sensation from the simple somatic sensation. Example, we can judge the 3-dimensional shape and form of an object by holding it in our hand, with eyes closed. This phenomenon is called stereognosis. Damage to SS-I causes *astereognosis*, i.e., inability to judge the shape and form of the objects.

### Functions of SS-II (area 5, 7) and parietal association area:

- The SS-II receives sensory inputs from SS-I, visual cortex, auditory cortex, thalamus (VPL nucleus and other area), hence creates a complex sensation. It form a major part of the parieto-occipito-temporal association area **(Fig. 84.5)**.
- The posterior parietal cortex is also the locus of spatial coordinates for motor control of different parts of body with respect to surroundings. The preanalyzed information from posterior parietal area is sent to the prefrontal association area and basal ganglia for planning and programming of required motor activity.
- The SS-I and II receive the inputs from the other half (contralateral half) of the body and hence perceives the sensations from contralateral side. Lesions of unilateral SS-II results in *amorphosynthesis*. It is a complex sensory deficit in which the person neglects the sensory inputs from contralateral half of his body. Hence, the person recognizes only half of the object, forgetting the other half. It is also called the *Hemineglect syndrome*.

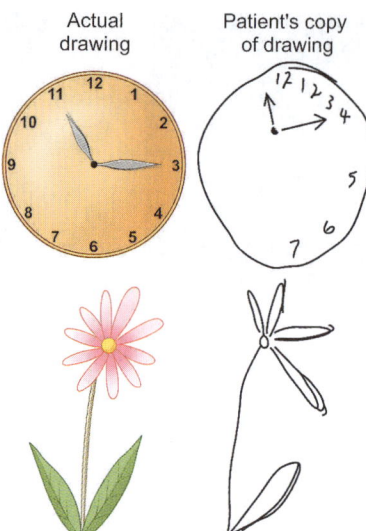

**Fig. 84.9:** Left side of the drawing is missing in a patient with right posterior parietal lobe lesion (hemineglect syndrome).

The lesions in the posterior parietal cortex are described below:

- There is inability to perceive parietal cortex though the sensory mechanisms are normal. This is called *agnosia*.
- **Lesion of right posterior parietal cortex:** The patient is not able to copy the drawings on the left side of drawing **(Fig. 84.9)**. He will avoid using his left arm, left hand and forgets to use left side of the body (personal neglect syndrome). In this case, the person forgets to shave half of his face.
- **Lesions of left posterior parietal cortex:** In most (95%) of the people, the left cerebrum is the dominant hemisphere where the Wernicke's area and angular gyrus are more developed as compared to the right parietal cortex. This results in loss the functions of angular gyrus (mentioned below) along with the above-mentioned lesions (agnosia and amorphosynthesis) of right posterior parietal lobe.

## Angular Gyrus

It is the most inferior part of the parietal cortex, lying behind the Wernicke's area of the temporal lobe. It is actually present at the confluence of parietal, visual and auditory cortex.

### Functions of angular gyrus:

- It acts as a gateway for the passage of visual information to Wernicke's area (sensory speech area).
- Lesions of angular gyrus can lead to difficulty in understanding written language, i.e., difficulty in reading called *dyslexia*. However, inability to read is called *alexia or word blindness*.

## Temporal Lobe

The lower most lobe of cerebral cortex is the temporal lobe. It has many important areas located on it like **(Fig. 84.10)**.

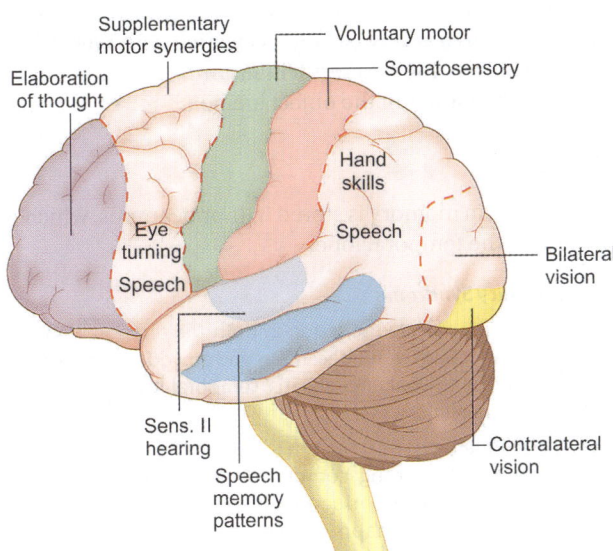

**Fig. 84.10:** Parts of temporal lobe.

## Primary Auditory Cortex (Fig. 84.11)

This area (Area 23) is located on *the supratemporal plane of superior temporal gyrus, extending to lateral side of temporal lobe.* It is divides into:
- **Primary auditory cortex:** It is directly excited by the auditory pathway.
- **Auditory association area/secondary auditory cortex:** It is excited by the impulses arising from the primary auditory cortex and thalamic association areas.

**Tonotopic maps:** There are six different tonotopic maps in primary auditory cortex and auditory association areas. As we can see in **Figure 84.11**, the low frequency sounds are located anteriorly, and high frequency sounds are located posteriorly. The utility of these tonotopic maps is described below:
- Each tonotopic map analysis the specific features of the sound. Example: pitch of this sound helps in analyzing the emotional sensation of that sound.
- It helps in judging the direction of the sound, onset of this sound, sound modulations etc.
- Lesions of both the auditory cortices reduce this sensitivity for hearing. However, the lesions on one side only slightly reduce the hearing in the opposite ear. In these patients the localization of sound is affected.
- Lesions of the auditory association area result in inability to interpret the meaning of the sounds heard by the patient.

## Wernicke's Area for Sensory Speech

Wernicke's area (Area 22) is located behind the primary auditory cortex in the posterior part of the superior gyrus of the temporal lobe **(Fig. 84.12)**. This area is very important and serves the following functions:
- **Higher intellectual (executive) functions:** Earlier it was thought that the higher intellectual functions are

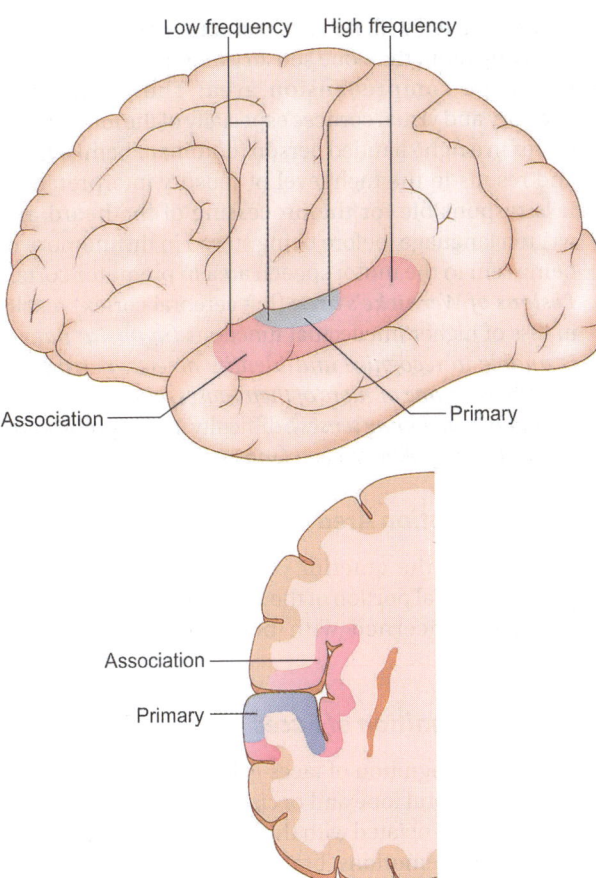

**Fig. 84.11:** The auditory cortex in the temporal lobe.

processed in the prefrontal cortex. But the scientists have studied that the Wernicke's area along with the angular gyrus, in the dominant hemisphere, has a major role to play in the intellectual functions. Hence, it is the seat of intelligence and also called *general interpretive area/ gnostic area/knowing area/tertiary association area.* It is responsible for the generation of complex thought process, especially associated with visual scenes. It is

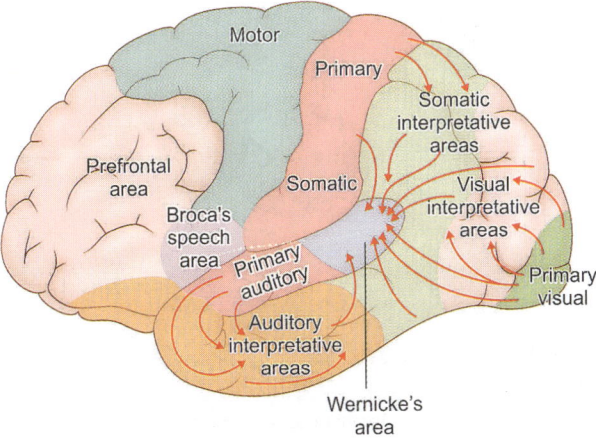

**Fig. 84.12:** The Wernicke's area showing the input of various inputs from auditory, visual and somatic sensation.

also associated with recall of complex memory patterns involving more than one sensory modality.
- **Language comprehension area:** The inputs from auditory and visual cortices especially of the left cerebral cortex in a right-handed person (dominant hemisphere) and results in the high level of sensory interpretation. It is responsible for the processing of the heard and written language, before being stored in the memory or being sent to the motor speech area in premotor cortex.
- **Lesions of Wernicke's area** (left cerebral cortex) results in loss of higher intellectual functions *(agnosia: patient is unable to recognize and identify objects, persons, or sounds using one or more of their senses despite otherwise normally functioning senses)*, difficulty in comprehension of written or spoken speech *(sensory aphasia)*.

### Limbic Association Area

It is present in the anterior pole of the temporal lobe (**Fig. 84.5**), ventral portion of the frontal lobe and cingulate gyrus. It is concerned with behavior, emotions and motivation.

### Area for Recognition of Faces

The area for recognition of faces is located on the inferior surface of temporal lobe and occipital lobes (**Fig. 84.13**).

It is closely associated with the limbic system and hence responds to the emotions, brain activation and control of behavioral responses. Lesions of this area result in inability to recognize the faces called *prosopagnosia*.

### Area for Naming Objects

The areas located in lateral portion of occipital lobe and posterior temporal lobe are concerned with naming of an object. The naming is learnt through auditory while physical attributes of objects are learnt though visual inputs. This area is very closely associated with Wernicke's area. Lesions of this area result in *anomia*, i.e., difficulty in recalling the names of the object/person.

### Memory

The long-term memory is stored in hippocampus, which is present in the temporal lobe.

> **Klüver–Bucy Syndrome**
>
> It is a rare disorder due to lesion in both the temporal lobes, especially affecting the hippocampus and amygdala. The lesion can occur due to viral encephalitis, temporal lobe infarction, traumatic brain injury, etc.
>
> *Clinical features:*
> - **Hyperorality:** Strong compulsion to put everything in mouth. Compulsive and socially inappropriate licking.
> - **Hypersexuality:** Inappropriate sexual activity. Patient attempts to copulate with inappropriate objects and species
> - **Hyperphagia:** The patient eats without any control
> - **Placidity:** Decreased response to emotional stimuli. No aggression.
> - **Visual agnosia (psychic blindness):** Inability to recognize familiar objects or faces presented visually.
> - Impaired memory resulting in anterograde amnesia

## Occipital Lobe

The posterior part of the cerebral cortex makes the occipital lobe. It is primarily concerned with the perception of visual sensation, hence also called the visual cortex (**Fig. 84.14**). It is further classified as:

### Primary Visual Cortex (Area 17)

It lies in the calcarine fissure of the medial surface of the occipital lobe, as seen in **Figure 84.14**. It is also called the visual area I/striate cortex because of its striated appearance. The retinal representation on primary visual cortex is summarized as:

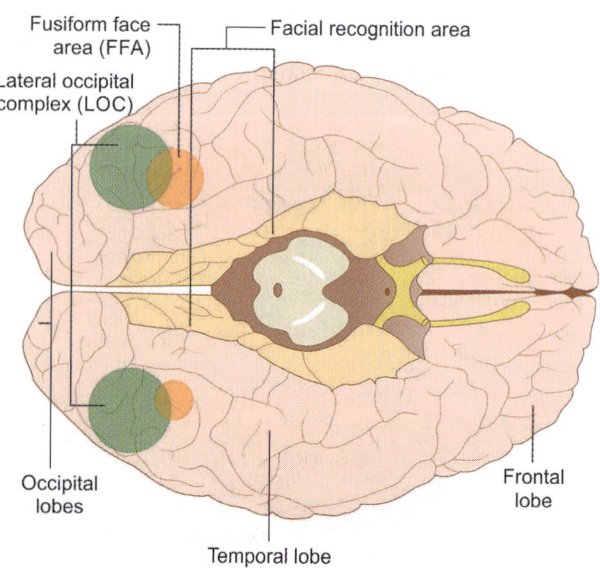

**Fig. 84.13:** The inferior surface of temporal and occipital lobes with area for recognition of faces.

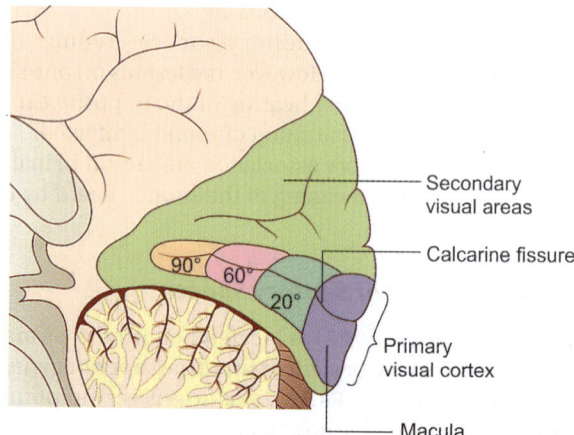

**Fig. 84.14:** The primary visual cortex located in calcarine fissure of medial occipital lobe.

- The macular area of retina is widely represented on the visual cortex, near occipital pole. It is responsible for the highest visual acuity of fovea centralis.
- The peripheral retina is represented in concentric half circles, along the calcarine fissure. Upper part of retina is represented superiorly while lower retina is represented inferiorly.

**Histology of primary visual cortex:** Like any other part of cerebral cortex, the primary visual cortex also has six layers (Fig. 84.15). But there are a few peculiarities, discussed below:
- Like other parts, the main input in visual cortex occurs in layer IV, from geniculocalcarine fibers.
- Rapidly conducting *retinal "M ganglion cells"*, carrying black and white visual information, terminate in layer *IVcα*, which relay vertically towards surface of cortex and deeper structures.
- Medium sized *"P ganglion cells"*, carrying color vision from retina, also terminate in layer IVa and IVcβ. These transmit an accurate point to point vision.
- Even the primary visual cortex, like other areas, is arranged in the vertical columns of diameter 0.3 to 0.5 mm. The vertical *'color blobs'* are interspersed in the primary and secondary visual areas, which decipher the color vision.
- The input received from both the eyes relay in layer IV and is fused to form a single image. This helps in judgement of the distance of object by the mechanism of *stereopsis*.
- Lesions of primary visual cortex result in *loss of vision/blindness.*

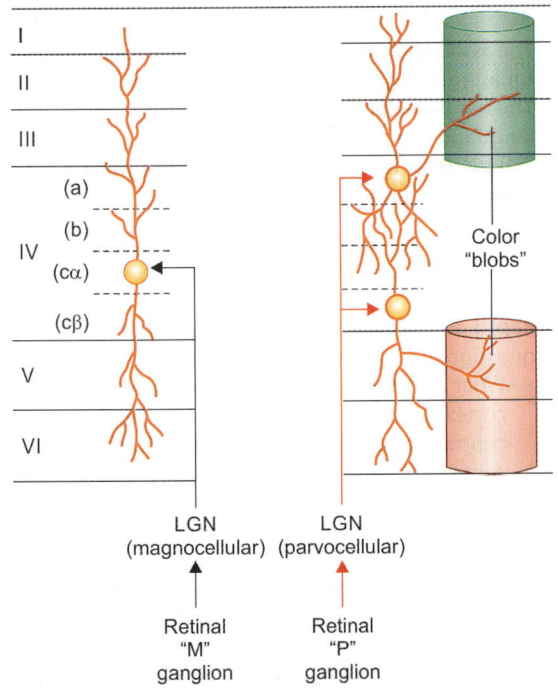

**Fig. 84.15:** Layers of primary visual cortex.

## Secondary Visual Cortex/Visual Association Area (Area 18, 19)

It lies around the primary visual cortex (laterally, anteriorly, superiorly and inferiorly). Signals from primary visual cortex are transmitted to the secondary area for processing of visual signals and analyzing their meaning. The area 18 is also called visual area II/V2 whereas, other distant areas are called the V3, V4 etc., which analyze various aspects of visual information. The information received from primary cortex is transmitted to secondary visual area for analysis of the following information:
- 3-dimensional position of the object
- Gross physical form of the object/visual scene
- The position-form-motion pathway, originating from M optic nerve fibers, transmitting black and white signals.
- Analysis of visual detail and color. The pathway for color vision is concerned with recognizing letters, reading, determining texture of surfaces, detailed colors of objects etc.
- Detects orientation of lines and borders by simple cells.
- Detects line orientation during displacement by complex cells.
- Detects lines of specific lengths, angles or other shapes.

### Other Functions

- The occipital lobe sends the visual information to Wernicke's area for written language.
- Along with temporal lobe, it participates in recognition of faces.

## COMMUNICATION BETWEEN BOTH THE CEREBRAL HEMISPHERES

Both the cerebral hemispheres are joined with the help of *corpus callosum*, which provides the bidirectional flow of information. The anterior portions of the temporal lobes especially the amygdala are connected through the *anterior commissure*.

### Functions of corpus callosum and anterior commissure:

- The intellectual functions of Wernicke's area is transferred to the nondominant hemisphere.
- Hence, damage to corpus callosum result in
  - Loss of control over right motor cortex that initiates voluntary movements in left side of body.
  - The failure of visual and somatic information from left side to reach the Wernicke's area
  - Both the hemispheres work separately. But the emotional stimulus is not compromised because the amygdala is connected through the anterior commissure, which incase is intact.

## CEREBRAL DOMINANCE

We have studied above that the left brain has a well-developed Wernicke's area and hand skill area in about 95% people. It results in majority of population with the right handedness. The left cerebral hemisphere is concerned with logic, calculation, reasoning whereas the right brain is concerned with art, music, abstract thinking, daydreaming.

## SUMMARY

In this chapter, we have studied that there are four main lobes of the cerebrum. Summarizing their functions as:
- **Frontal lobe:** It has the primary motor cortex, premotor cortex and supplementary motor cortex. There is a prefrontal association area which is responsible for planning and programming of complex sequential motor activity. It also has the motor speech area (Broca's area).
- **Parietal lobe:** It has a primary somatosensory cortex and somatosensory association area. The posterior parietal cortex forms the part of parieto-occipito-temporal association area. This area sends the information to prefrontal cortex and modulates the motor activity. The lowermost part of parietal cortex is formed by the angular gyrus.
- **Temporal lobe:** It has the primary and secondary auditory areas, Wernicke's area and limbic association area. Wernicke's area act as the general interpretive area and seat of intelligence; which integrates all the sensory inputs. It is also the language comprehension center.
- **Occipital lobe:** It receives the sensory information from the visual pathway and then analyses the complex patterns of visual input.
- The left brain is the dominant hemisphere in 95% of the population. It has a well-developed Wernicke's area.
- Both these hemispheres are connected by the corpus callosum and anterior commissure resulting in the communication between both the hemispheres.

## LET US SEE, HOW MUCH YOU HAVE LEARNT?

### Review Questions

**Long/Short Answer Questions**

Q1. Describe the functions of:
   a. Frontal lobe
   b. Parietal lobe
   c. Temporal lobe
   d. Occipital lobe

Q2. Describe the physiological significance of:
   a. Wernicke's area
   b. Association areas

Q3. Describe how the sensory-motor coordination occurs in the cerebral cortex.

**Explain Why (Reasoning Questions)**

Q1. The primary motor cortex is essential for voluntary movement control.

Q2. Damage to the prefrontal cortex can affect decision-making and personality.

Q3. The somatosensory cortex is critical for processing tactile information.

Q4. The occipital lobe is primarily responsible for visual processing.

Q5. The left hemisphere of the cerebral cortex is typically dominant for language in right-handed individuals.

Q6. The association areas of the cerebral cortex are important for integrating sensory and motor information.

Q7. The temporal lobe is crucial for auditory processing and language comprehension.

Q8. The parietal lobe is essential for integrating sensory information and spatial awareness.

### Critical Thinking Case-Based Questions

Q1. Anita, a 40-year-old woman, presented to a neurology clinic with complaints of difficulty speaking and understanding spoken language. She also experienced weakness on the right side of her body. MRI imaging revealed a lesion in the left hemisphere of her brain, specifically in the area corresponding to Broca's area and the motor cortex. The neurologist suspected a stroke affecting Anita's cerebral cortex and wanted to explain the functions, roles, and divisions of the cerebral cortex to better understand her symptoms.

Based on the given case history, answer the following questions:
   a. What are the main functions and roles of the cerebral cortex, and how do different areas within the cortex contribute to higher cognitive functions, motor control, sensory perception, and language processing?
   b. How does damage to Broca's area affect Anita's ability to produce speech and control movements on her right side?
   c. What are the underlying physiological mechanisms?

### Multiple Choice Questions

Q1. Which of the following somatosensory deficits is typically not seen with lesions that involve the postcentral gyrus?
   a. Inability to discretely localize touch sensation over the contralateral face and upper limb

b. Inability to recognize the position of the contralateral arm and leg
c. Inability to accurately assess the texture of common objects by touching them with the fingers
d. Inability to move the contralateral arm and leg

Q2. Within the primary somatosensory cortex, the various parts of the contralateral body surface are represented in areas of varying size that reflect which of the following?
a. Relative size of the body parts
b. Density of the specialized peripheral receptors
c. Size of the muscles in that body part
d. Conduction velocity of the primary afferent fibers

Q3. Which of the following statements regarding events in the primary visual cortex is correct?
a. "Color blobs" are interspersed among primary visual columns and are the primary areas for deciphering color
b. Primary visual columns contain signals from both eyes, with adjacent columns also receiving signals from both eyes
c. Rapidly changing black-and-white visual signals are transmitted by parvocellular neurons of the lateral geniculate nucleus to the primary visual cortex
d. Visual signals are transmitted by X ganglion cells, the majority of which form synapses in layer V of the primary visual cortex

Q4. Match the cortical functions described in the questions below with the correct region from the list below:
a. Parieto-occipital association cortex in nondominant hemisphere
b. Wernicke's area
c. Visual association cortex in dominant hemisphere
d. Broca's area
e. Ventral portion of medial occipitotemporal association cortex
  i. Lesions in this cortical region cause prosophenosia (or prosopagnosia), the inability to recognize faces ( )
  ii. A cortical region that provides the neural circuitry for word formation or the motor aspects of language ( )
  iii. A cortical region that provides the analysis of the spatial coordinates of the body in space as well as the environment surrounding the body ( )
  iv. A cortical region that provides the processing of information necessary for reading ( )

Q5. There is an area in the dominant hemisphere that, when damaged, might leave the sense of hearing intact but not allow words to be arranged into a comprehensive thought. Which of the following terms is used to identify this portion of the cortex?
a. Primary auditory cortex
b. Wernicke's area
c. Broca's area
d. Angular gyrus
e. Limbic association cortex

Q6. Evaluation of a patient reveals the following deficits: decreased aggressiveness and ambition, inappropriate social responses, inability to process sequential thoughts in order to solve a problem inability to process multiple bits of information could then be recalled instantaneously to complete a thought or solve a problem. Damage to which the following brain regions might be responsible for such deficits?
a. Premotor cortex
b. Parieto-occipital cortex in nondominant hemisphere
c. Limbic association cortex
d. Prefrontal association cortex

Q7. The phylogenetically new cerebral cortex, the neocortex, is composed of six layers tangential to the pial surface of the hemisphere. Which of the following statements concerning the organization of these six layers is correct?
a. The neurons in layers I, II, and III perform most of the thalamocortical connections within the same hemisphere
b. The neurons in layers II and III form connections with the basal ganglia
c. Specific incoming signals from the cerebellum terminate primarily in layer IV
d. The neurons in layer V have axons that extend beyond layer V to subcortical regions and the spinal cord

## ANSWERS

**1.** d  **2.** b  **3.** a  **4.** i. d  ii. c  iii. a  iv. b  **5.** b  **6.** d  **7.** a

# Thalamus

**CHAPTER 85**

### COMPETENCY ADDRESSED
**PY10.7:** Describe and discuss functions of cerebral cortex, basal ganglia, **thalamus**, hypothalamus, cerebellum and limbic system and their abnormalities.

### LEARNING OBJECTIVES
**At the end of this chapter, the learner should be able to:**
- Describe the structure and nuclei of thalamus.
- Describe the functions of the thalamus.
- Describe the connections of the themes with the cerebral cortex.
- Describe the applied aspects of the thalamic syndrome.

## STRUCTURE AND NUCLEI OF THALAMUS

Thalamus is an egg-shaped structure that is separated by the 3rd ventricle. It is located in each of the cerebral hemispheres which are connected by an inter-thalamic adhesion called **Massa intermedia.** The Y shaped internal medullary lamina divides each thalamus into anterior, medial and lateral regions.

### Thalamic Nuclei
- **Anterior region:** Anterior nucleus
- **Medial region:** Massa intermedia, Medial dorsal nuclei
- **Lateral region:**
  - *Dorsal tier:* Lateral Dorsal **(LDA)**, Lateral posterior **(LDP)**, Pulvinar
  - *Ventral tier:* Ventroanterior **(VA)**, Ventrolateral **(VL)**, Ventrobasal complex **(VPL, VPM)**, Caudal pole has the **LGB and MGB**

- **The anterior region:** it is situated between the fibers of internal medullary lamina and contains anterior nucleus
- **The medial region:** it is situated media to the internal medullary lamina and contains medial dorsal nuclei
- **The lateral region:** the lateral region can be divided into 2 tiers of the nuclei; dorsal tier Andy ventral tier.
  - **Dorsal tier** has 2 nuclei lateral dorsal anterior (LDA) nucleus and lateral dorsal posterior (LDP) nucleus.

  It also has the broad posterior end called as the Pulvinar.
  - **Ventral tier** has 3 main nuclei, ventroanterior nucleus (VA), ventrolateral nucleus (VL), ventrobasal complex having 2 subdivisions, ventral posterolateral (VPL) and winter postero medial nucleus (VPM ). The **Lateral and Medial Geniculate bodies (LGB, MGB)** are suspended from the ventral tier of the caudal pole of the thalamus.

## Functional Classification of the Nuclei

Based on the functions the thalamic nuclei are classified as specific or relay nuclei and nonspecific or generalized nuclei **(Fig. 85.1)**.

### Specific or Relay Nuclei

Nuclei relay the tracks (sensory information), received by it to the cerebral cortex.
- **Lateral geniculate body:** It is a 6th layered nucleus that receives the topographically organized inputs from the retina of each eye. Layers 1, 4, 6 receive the input from contralateral retina whereas layers 2, 3, 5 receive the input from the ipsilateral retina. LGN projects in the same topographically ordered manner to the primary visual cortex in the occipital lobe.

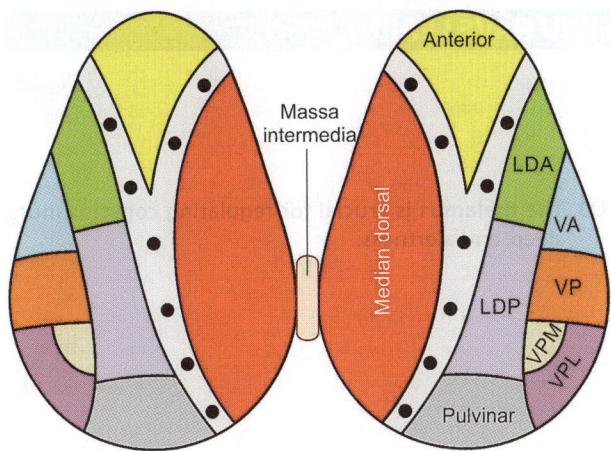

**Fig. 85.1:** Various thalamic nuclei showing in right thalamus. Note, the two thalami are connected with massa intermedia.

- **Medial geniculate body:** It receives the bilateral topically organized auditory input from the inferior colliculus and projects to the primary auditory cortex which is in the superior temporal gyrus of the temporal lobe.

**Ventrobasal Complex**
- **VPL:** This nucleus (especially VPL) receives the somatosensory information from the limbs, neck, trunk and the head. This information is projected to the primary somatosensory cortex.
- **VPM:** The dorsal trigemino-thalamic tract projects bilaterally to each VPM from the main sensory nuclei, whereas the ventral trigemino-thalamic tract arises exclusively from the contralateral spinal nucleus.

- **Anterior nucleus:** Anterior nucleus of the thalamus participates in the Papez circuit of the limbic system. It receives the afferents from mammillary nucleus of the hypothalamus and projects to the cingulate gyrus of the cerebral cortex.
- **Ventrolateral nucleus (VL):** This nucleus receives the afferents from the deep cerebellar nuclei and from the basal ganglia. The fibers from the cerebellum are projected to the primary motor cortex. Whereas the fibers from basal ganglia are projected to frontal lobe, supplementary motor area and premotor area.
- **Ventral anterior nucleus (VA):** This nucleus receives all its inputs from substantia nigra, pars reticularis and GPi (basal ganglia).

## Nonspecific or Generalized Nuclei of the Thalamus

(Mediodorsal nucleus, lateral dorsal nucleus, lateral posterior nucleus, intralaminar nuclei and reticular nucleus)
- **Mediodorsal nucleus:** It receives the inputs from amygdala, basal ganglia and projects to the frontal lobe.
- **Lateral dorsal nucleus:** It receives inputs from hypothalamus and projects to the singularity cyrus.
- **Lateral posterior nucleus and pulvinar** act as visual association nucleus. They received the input from superior colliculus, pretectal nuclei, and visual cortex. They project to visual association areas in the occipital parietal and temporal lobes.
- **Intralaminar nuclei:** They are present within the internal medullary lamina and include midline nuclei and centromedian nucleus. The midline nuclei receive inputs from reticular formation, pain and temperature from anterolateral system. The centromedian nucleus receives inputs from motor cortex and basal ganglia and projects back to the basal ganglia.
- **Reticular nucleus:** This is a sheath of cells on the outside of external medullary lamina. It receives the excitatory collaterals from thalamocortical and cortico thalamic axons. The reticular nucleus contains GABA neurons this provides inhibitory feedback to the nuclei of thalamus.

**Thalamic pain syndrome** commonly results from a lacunar stroke involving thalamoperforating branches of a posterior cerebral artery, which supply the ventrobasal complex. In these patients, there may be an **impairment of all forms of somatic sensations in the body and limbs** contralateral to the affected thalamus. Central pain may also occur if the lesion affects the anterolateral system part of the ventrobasal complex. Pain in thalamic pain syndrome does not respond to anti-inflammatory analgesics, which act to suppress pain at brainstem or spinal cord levels.

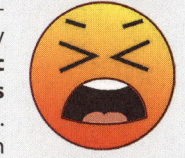

## SUMMARY

In this chapter we have learnt about the anatomical antifunctional nuclei of thalamus which are summarized as below:
- The anterior, mediodorsal, lateral dorsal nuclei participate in limbic system.
- Ventrobasal complex participate in the transmission of the somatic sensations.
- Lateral posterior nucleus and Pulvinar act as visual association nuclei.
- The ventral anterior and the ventrolateral nuclei receive their inputs from cerebellum and basal ganglia and projects to the cerebral cortex.
- The intralaminar nuclei received the inputs from the reticular formation for pain and temperature. It also receives the input from motor cortex and basal ganglia which projects back to basal ganglia.
- The reticular nuclei provide the inhibitory feedback to the other nuclei of thalamus.

# LET US SEE, HOW MUCH YOU HAVE LEARNT?

### Review Questions

#### Explain Why? (Reasoning Questions)

Q1. The thalamus is considered the relay center for sensory information in the brain.
Q2. Damage to the thalamus can result in sensory deficits or altered perception.
Q3. The thalamus is crucial for regulating consciousness, sleep, and alertness.

### Answer in One Word

#### Write in Reference to Which Nucleus

Q1. Projects to Brodmann areas 41 and 42.
Q2. Projects to prefrontal cortex.
Q3. Receives input from the dentate nucleus of the cerebellum.
Q4. Projects to cingulate gyrus.
Q5. Retinal ganglion cells synapse here.
Q6. Spinothalamic axons synapse here.
Q7. Projects to Brodmann area 17.
Q8. Projects to same cortical area as the lateral dorsal nucleus.
Q9. Receives input from both basal ganglia and cerebellum.
Q10. Receives input from the trigeminal nuclei.

**ANSWERS**

1. Medial geniculate nucleus
2. Medial dorsal nucleus
3. Ventral lateral nucleus
4. Anterior nucleus
5. Lateral geniculate nucleus
6. Ventral posterior lateral nucleus
7. Lateral geniculate nucleus
8. Anterior nucleus
9. Ventral lateral nucleus
10. Ventral posterior medial nucleus

# Role of Cerebellum and Basal Ganglia
## (Motor Planning, Programming and Execution)

**CHAPTER 86**

### COMPETENCY ADDRESSED

**PY10.4:** Describe and discuss motor tracts, mechanism of maintenance of tone, control of body movements, posture and equilibrium and vestibular apparatus.
**PY10.7:** Describe and discuss functions of cerebral cortex, **basal ganglia**, thalamus, hypothalamus, **cerebellum** and limbic system and their abnormalities.

### LEARNING OBJECTIVES

At the end of this chapter, the learner should be able to:
- Describe the functional anatomy, connections, physiological actions, and lesions of cerebellum.
- Describe the functional anatomy, connections, circuits, physiological actions, and lesions of basal ganglia.
- Describe the role of cerebellum and basal ganglia in planning and programming of motor activity for smooth execution of motor activity.

We have learnt in previous chapters 79, 83, 84 that the motor activity, i.e., muscular activity is initiated by the cerebral cortex from the motor area 4, premotor and supplementary motor area 6. To further add on to this, we will study that the motor activity (which is primarily transmitted through the corticospinal tract) is initiated in the motor areas but its planning and programming in also influenced by cerebellum and basal ganglia as per the need.

The **Figure 86.1** shows that the motor cortex gives out the following signals:
- The main motor tract (shown in red), the *corticospinal tract* arises from cortex and terminates in the spinal cord.
- The Betz cells also give out *short axons* which inhibit the adjacent areas of cerebral cortex and leads to the sharpening of signal.

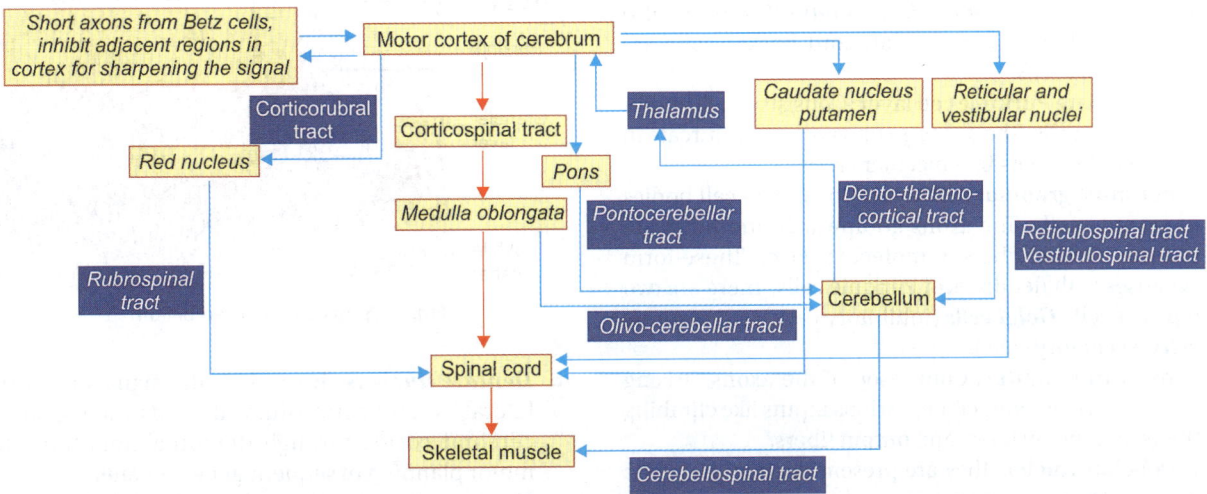

**Fig. 86.1:** The motor connections of cerebral cortex with other parts of cerebral cortex.

- The motor area sends *corticonuclear (corticorubral) fibers* to red nucleus in midbrain. The red nucleus then transmits the signal through *rubrospinal tract*, which is an alternative motor tract, influencing the activity of muscles.
- The cerebral cortex has no direct connections with *cerebellum*, but it sends the motor signals to it through the *cortico-reticular-cerebellar, cortico-vestibulo-cerebellar, cortico-ponto-cerebellar, cortico-olivo-cerebellar fibers*. The cerebellum then sends its signals to thalamus through *dento-thalamo-cortical fibers* and to spinal cord through the *cerebellospinal tract*. This result weighing the need of motor activity through sensory inputs and execution of appropriate motor activity.
- The fibers to *basal ganglia* (caudate nucleus and putamen) the *caudate and putamen circuits* helps in scaling, prediction of motor activity.
- The vestibular nuclei and reticular formation also influence the motor activity.

Let's now study the role of cerebellum and basal ganglia separately in detail.

## CEREBELLUM

The cerebellum is present attached to the brain stem, also called the hind brain. It has a size of 10% of cerebral cortex but area is 75% more area than the cerebral cortex. It is attached to brain stem by 3 cerebral peduncles; superior, middle, and inferior cerebellar peduncles **(Fig. 86.2A)**.

Anatomically, it has an outer gray and inner white matter. It has a vermis in center, 2 lateral lobes which are extensively folded on themselves. Each fold is called FOLIUM. The diagrammatic representation of the folia in midsagittal section is shown below in **Figure 86.2B**.

Histologically, the cerebellum has three layers **(Figs. 86.3 and 86.4)**:

- **Outer molecular layer:** It is a layer of parallel fibers and has very few nuclei.
  - *Parallel fibers* are the axons of granular cells and dendrites of Purkinje cells.
  - Nuclei of the **stellate cells** and **basket cells** are also present here. These stellate and basket cells are *inhibitory cells*.
- **Intermediate Purkinje cell layer:** Consists of cell bodies of Purkinje cells. The axons go upwards and bifurcate to form parallel fibers in molecular layer.
- **Inner most granular cell layer:** Consists of cell bodies of granule cells. The axons go upwards and bifurcate to form parallel fibers in molecular layer. These form synapses with dendrites of Purkinje cells. There are two types of cells *Golgi cells* (inhibitory cells) and *granule cells* (excitatory cells).
- **Inner white matter:** Composed of the axons, arising from within the cerebellum, various inputs like climbing fibers and mossy fibers and output fibers.
- **Cerebellar nuclei:** They are present deep in the white matter. There are primarily three sets of cerebellar nuclei:

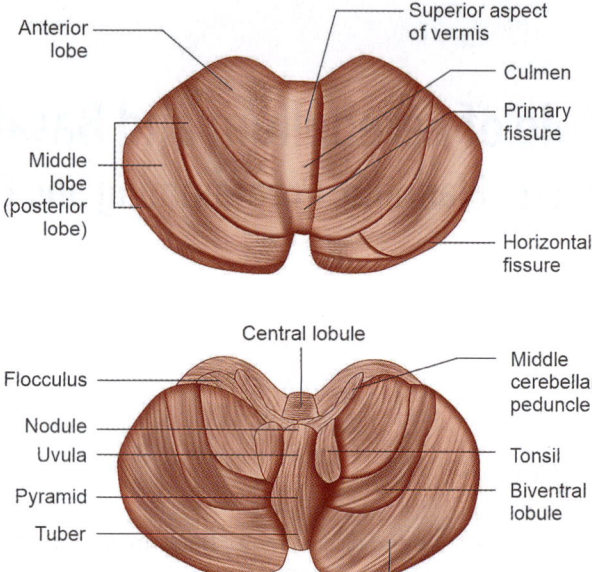

**Fig. 86.2A:** The superior and inferior surfaces of cerebellum.

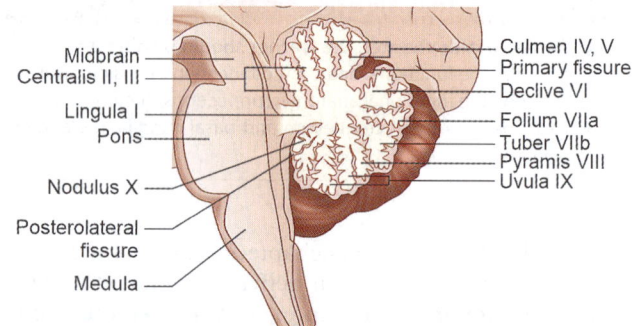

**Fig. 86.2B:** Midsagittal section of cerebellum showing all the folia.

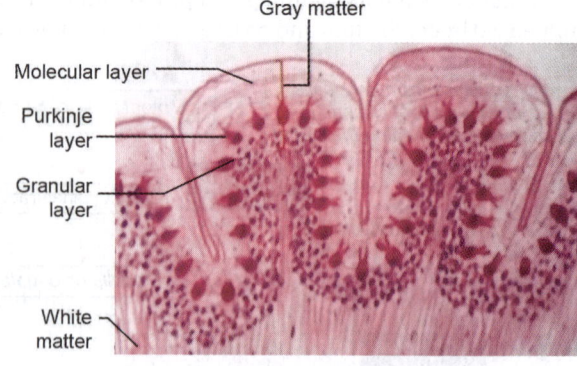

**Fig. 86.3:** Histology of cerebellum.

- **Dentate nucleus:** It receives the signals from the lateral/cerebrocerebellum. It sends the signals to cerebral cortex through dentothalamic tract, for motor planning of sequential movements.
- **Nucleus interpositus (nucleus globose and nucleus emboliform):** It receives the signals from

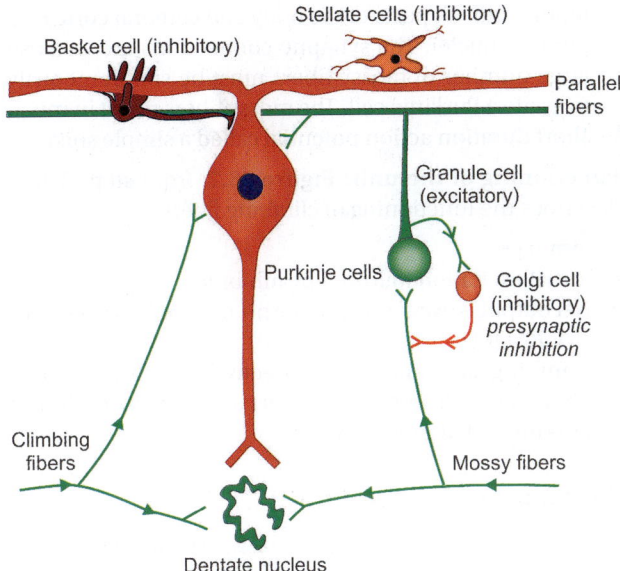

**Fig. 86.4:** Functional unit of cerebellum.

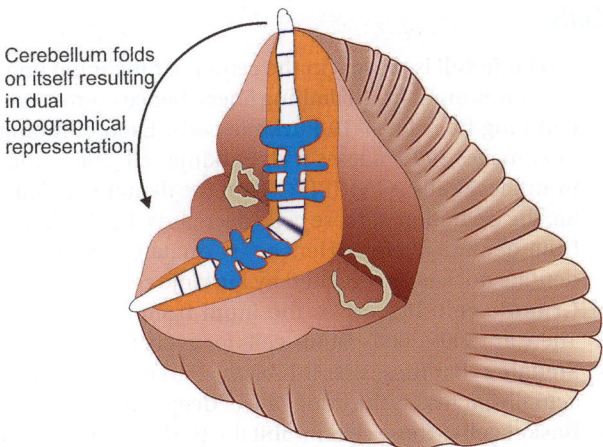

**Fig. 86.6:** Topographical representation of body on cerebellum.

the intermediate lobe. It sends the output signals to lateral descending pathways (lateral corticospinal tract) for motor execution. Hence, it is responsible for sequential of coordinated activity of limbs.

- *Fastigial nucleus:* It receives the signals from the vermis of the cerebellum. It sends the output signals to medial descending systems (anterior corticospinal pathway). Hence, it is responsible for maintaining the tone of neck and back muscles.

- **The physiological division of cerebellum:** As seen in **Figure 86.5**, phylogenetically, the cerebellum has three main functional divisions:
  - *Vestibulocerebellum/archicerebellum:* It is the oldest division of cerebellum, hence called archicerebellum. Since it projects to the vestibular nuclei, it is called as vestibulocerebellum. It is concerned with the equilibrium and balance of the body. Anatomically this region is also called the flocculonodular lobe.
  - *Spinocerebellum/paleocerebellum:* The vermis and intermediate lobe forms the spinocerebellum.

Topographically, *the body has dual representation on this region* (**Fig. 86.6**). The *trunk and axial parts of body are represented on the vermis, while the limbs are Ipsilaterally represented on the intermediate lobe*. As discussed earlier, the cerebellum is folded on itself, the dual representation of body is also overlapping. The intermediate lobe has nucleus interpositus and fastigial nucleus, as described above.

- *Cerebrocerebellum/neocerebellum:* It is the most lateral lobe of the cerebellar hemisphere. It is most advanced of all the lobes. There is no topographic representation of body in this lobe, but the input and output signals result in a close association with cerebrum. Hence, it participates in programming and planning of the motor activity. The most advanced dentate nucleus is present in the lateral lobe.

## Functional Unit of Cerebellum

Before we discuss the functions of cerebellum, we must understand the functional unit and its functioning. **Figure 86.4**, also shows the functional unit of cerebellum. There are around 30 million functional units in the cerebellum. Each functional unit is made of:

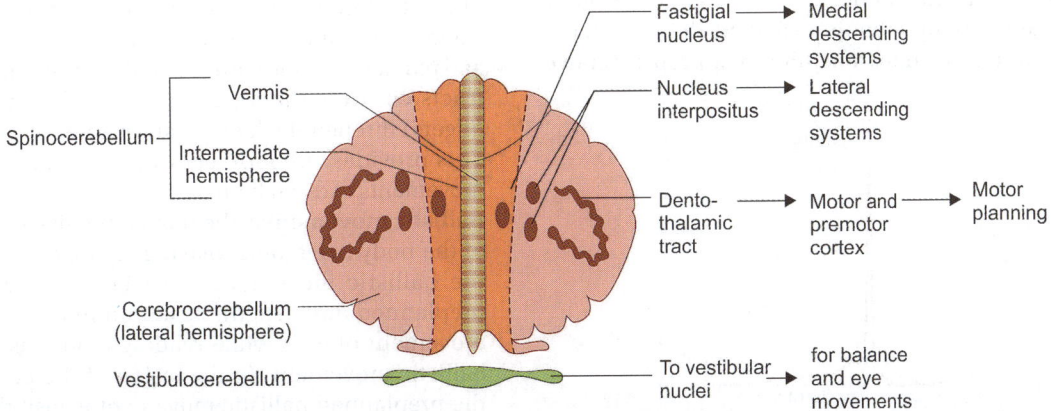

**Fig. 86.5:** Cerebellar nuclei.

## Cells

- **Purkinje cell** is present in the center of functional unit. It receives input from climbing fibers, hence there is one climbing fiber for 5-10 Purkinje cells. Each climbing fiber makes 300 synapses with Purkinje cell. The output from these cells is INHIBITORY to the dentate nucleus. So, the excitation of these cells decreases the discharge from dentate nucleus. Hence, the excitatory output of dentate nucleus is regulated by Purkinje cell.
- **Granule cell:** It receives the input from mossy fiber. There are 500–1,000 granule cells for every Purkinje cell.
- **Stellate cells:** These cells inhibit the Purkinje cell, which actually increases the firing rate of deep nucleus.
- **Basket cells:** These cells inhibit the Purkinje cell, which actually increases the firing rate of deep nucleus.
- **Golgi cell:** These cells are excited by granule cells but they in turn inhibit the granule cells by presynaptic inhibition.

## Fibers

- **Climbing fibers:** Provide input from Inferior Olivary Nucleus of medulla oblongata. They excite the deep nucleus and the Purkinje cells. They carry the sensory input from the proprioceptors and the cerebrum. A single impulse from climbing fiber causes a single, prolonged (up to 1 second) action potential in Purkinje cell which begins with a spike followed by a trail of weak impulses called *complex spike*.

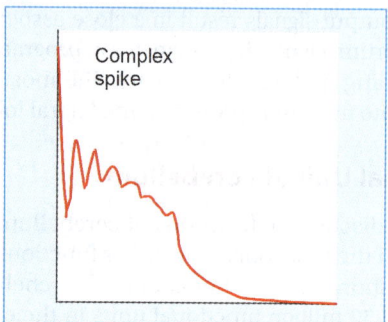

- **Mossy fibers:** All other inputs from cerebrum (reticulocerebellar, vestibulocerebellar tracts etc.) reach the cerebellum through these fibers. These mossy fibers excite many granule cells and deep nucleus/dentate nucleus. They transmit direct proprioceptive

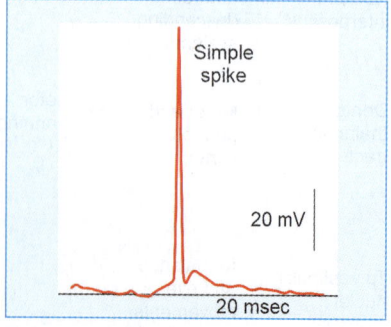

inputs from all parts of the body and cerebral cortex via pontine nuclei. The synaptic connections are weak so large number of mossy fibers must be simultaneously to excite a Purkinje cell. The mossy fibers result in much short duration action potential called a simple spike.

**Functioning of the unit: Figure 86.7**, from steps 1 to 6 describes the functioning of climbing fibers.

**Summary:**
- Initial excitation followed by inhibition
- Net output is excitatory but the no. of impulses decreases → GRADED
- Climbing fibers are more effective input than mossy fibers, coz climbing fiber exert a strong excitation of Purkinje cell than mossy fiber.

## Functions of Cerebellum

- The cerebellum *maintains the muscle tone* by facilitation the motor cortex and brainstem motor nuclei by tonic signals from deep cerebellar nuclei. The cerebellar lesions cause hypotonia due to loss of this facilitation.
- Along with the vestibular nuclei, spinal cord and other nuclei the vestibulocerebellum *maintains the equilibrium of body and the postural movements*. This part of cerebellum controls balance between agonist and antagonist muscle contraction of spine, hips and shoulders during rapid changes in posture. The change in body position is sensed by vestibular apparatus, which is transmitted to vestibular nuclei. The vestibulocerebellum predicts the change in position, which is going to happen in next few milliseconds. Hence, it sends the anticipatory correction signals to vestibular nuclei and spinal cord. This readjusts the tone in muscles, maintaining the equilibrium and body posture.
- **For precise smooth coordinated voluntary activity:** The cerebellum receives the information about
  - Intended sequential plan of movement from cerebral motor cortex and red nucleus of midbrain
  - Actual movement from skeletal muscles (through proprioceptors).

  Both the information are compared in intermediate zone of cerebellum in nucleus interpositus and corrective signals are send to cerebral cortex through thalamus and red nucleus. The corticospinal tract and rubrospinal tracts controls the distal part of limbs (hands and fingers) through the lateral part of anterior gray horns. This provides, smooth, coordinated and purposeful movements of distal limbs.
- **Ballistic movements:** The rapid repetitive movements of the body like typing, playing piano, etc., are called the ballistic movements. The entire movement is preplanned and sets the task into motion. Even the movement of eyes while reading a book is a type of ballistic movement. In the lesion of the cerebellum, the preplanned ballistic movement is lost, the motor

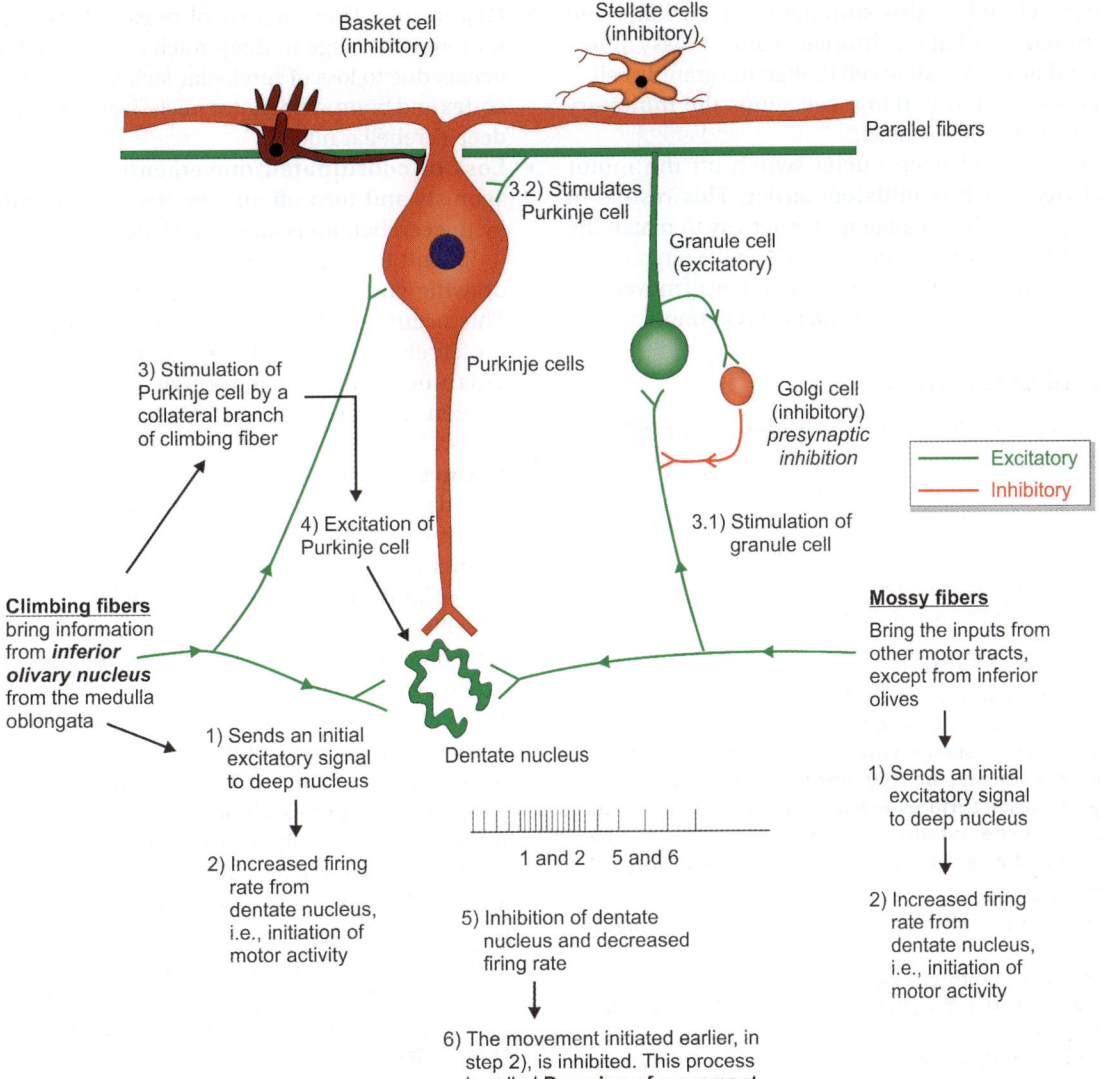

**Fig. 86.7:** Functional unit of cerebellum.

cortex takes more task to perform the activity in steps. If ballistic movements of eyes are disturbed, it results in nystagmus.

- **Planning and programming of sequential movements:** The cerebellum takes the input from sensory and premotor areas of cerebral cortex, which is transmitted to lateral hemispheres of cerebellum. The dentate nucleus is involved in the sequential movement of the limbs. Hence it enables the smooth progression from one movement to the another in a planned sequence. In the lesions of cerebellum, there is severe deficiency of planning of movements.

- **Predictive functions:** It provides the appropriate timing for each succeeding movement. In case of cerebellar lesions, the person is unable to smoothly progress the movements. It also integrates the visual and auditory inputs to time the motor activity. For example, the person can judge the speed of the approaching vehicle before crossing the road and can act accordingly. Hence, we can say that cerebellum helps in interpreting rapidly changing spatiotemporal relations.

- **Turn on and turn off activity of agonist and antagonist muscle:** The cerebellum provides rapid turn on signal for agonist muscle and turn off signal for antagonist muscle at the onset of movement. After the completion of intended activity, it sends turn off signals to agonist muscle and turn on to the antagonists muscles. Hence, it results in damping of motor activity, preventing the past pointing by damping the momentum.

*Mechanism of damping of movement:* As seen in **Figure 86.7**.

- The climbing fibers and mossy fibers directly stimulate the deep nucleus and initiates the movement by increasing the discharge of action potentials from deep nuclei. This results in the intended movement.

- These climbing also stimulate the Purkinje cell through a collateral branch, while mossy fibers stimulate the Purkinje cell though the granule cell.
- The stimulated Purkinje cell sends the inhibitory signal to the deep nuclei.
- The inhibited deep nuclei switch off the motor activity which is initiated earlier. This results in damping of the ongoing motor activity to match the intended activity. Cerebellar lesion result in damage to this circuitry and affects the damping of movement resulting in overshooting and past pointing.

## Lesions of Cerebellum

The lesions of cerebellum affect the *ipsilateral side of body*. Since the main functions of cerebellum are to maintain tone, posture, coordination of movement, planning of sequential movements as we have studied above, the patient presents with the loss of all the above-mentioned functions. For a clear understanding, let's see a clinical case study of cerebellar ataxia, mentioned in the box below.

> **CLINICAL CASE SCENARIO**
> 
> **Mrs Parul Sharma, a 55-year-old female, presents to the neurology clinic with complaints of progressively worsening coordination and balance issues over the past few months. She reports experiencing frequent falls, particularly when walking on uneven surfaces or in poorly lit areas. Mrs Sharma mentions that she has also noticed a deterioration in her handwriting, with her letters becoming increasingly illegible.**
> 
> *Presenting Complaints:*
> - Mrs Sharma reports frequent falls, especially on uneven surfaces.
> - Handwriting has become increasingly illegible.
> - She mentions slurring of speech and difficulty articulating words clearly.
> - Mrs Sharma notices tremors, particularly in her hands, when performing fine motor tasks.
> 
> *Physical Examination Findings:*
> - On examination, Mrs Sharma demonstrates a wide-based and unsteady drunken gait. She has difficulty with tandem walking and tends to sway from side to side.
> - Speech is dysarthric with slurring of words and irregular intonation.
> - There is intention tremor noted in both upper extremities, exacerbated with reaching for objects.
> 
> *Abnormal Cerebellar Function Tests:*
> a. **Finger-to-nose test:** Mrs Sharma demonstrates dysmetria with overshooting and undershooting when attempting to touch her nose with her index finger.
> b. **Knee heel test:** She has difficulty smoothly running her heel down the shin of the opposite leg, with irregular movements and overshooting.
> c. **Dysdiadochokinesia:** There is impaired rapid alternating movements of the hands, characterized by irregular and slow movements when performing tasks such as rapidly pronating and supinating the hands.

Physiological basis of all the clinical features of lesions of cerebellum:
- There is *no motor loss* in cerebellar lesion.
- **Hypotonia:** There is loss of muscle tone especially if there is damage to deep nuclei of cerebellum. This occurs due to loss of cerebellar facilitation of the motor cortex and brain stem motor nuclei by tonic signals from deep cerebellar nuclei.
- **Loss of coordinated movements:** The turn on of agonists and turn off antagonists, usually controlled by the cerebellum is affected. Hence, the person finds it difficult to execute the coordinated movements like drawing circles in the air with the extended hands. This occurs during the lesion of the lateral zone of the cerebellar hemisphere, along with deep nuclei. This uncoordinated movement is called ataxia. It is seen in patients with lesions of spinocerebellar tracts.
- **Dysmetria:** The inability of a person to predict the intended movement, which results in the overshooting. This is called as dysmetria. It is seen in patients with lesions of spinocerebellar tracts.
- **Loss of ballistic movements:** There is loss of automatism of ballistic movements. The motor cortex has to think extra hard to turn on the ballistic movements and then again think hard to turn it off.
- **Truncal ataxia:** The patients with lesions in the vermis, suffer from the truncal ataxia. Truncal ataxia is inability to maintain posture of the truncal muscles due to hypotonia of muscles of back and neck.
- **Intention tremor:** The patient experiences the tremor, whenever he intends to do an activity. It occurs due to loss of damping of the motor activity and overshooting the intended activity resulting in past pointing. In an attempt to correct the overshoot, there is reversal of activity again resulting in past pointing. The series of past pointing episodes result in the intention tremor (**Fig. 86.8**).
- **Dysdiadochokinesia (Fig. 86.9):** Rapid alternate movement of both the limbs. If we split the word 'dia' means both limbs, 'docho' means alternating and 'kinesia' means movement. Hence diadochokinesia means the alternating rapid movements of both limbs. If a person finds it difficult to perform, he is said to have dysdiadochokinesia, whereas inability to perform these movements is called adiadochokinesia. There is failure of progression of movement.
- **Dysarthria:** The patient finds it difficult to plan and progress the motor activity resulting in difficulty to speak. The speech becomes *slurry*, in which the person runs over the words making them difficult to understand. If you ask him to repeat 'What is your name", he would say that as "*whashyoname*". The person can even have a *scanning speech*, in which he takes a pause after each word. In this case the person would repeat as "*what....is....your.....name*"
- **Cerebellar nystagmus:** The person is not able to fixate the eyes on a scene to one side of head. This result in rapid tremulous movement of eyes rather than steady fixation because of loss of damping movement

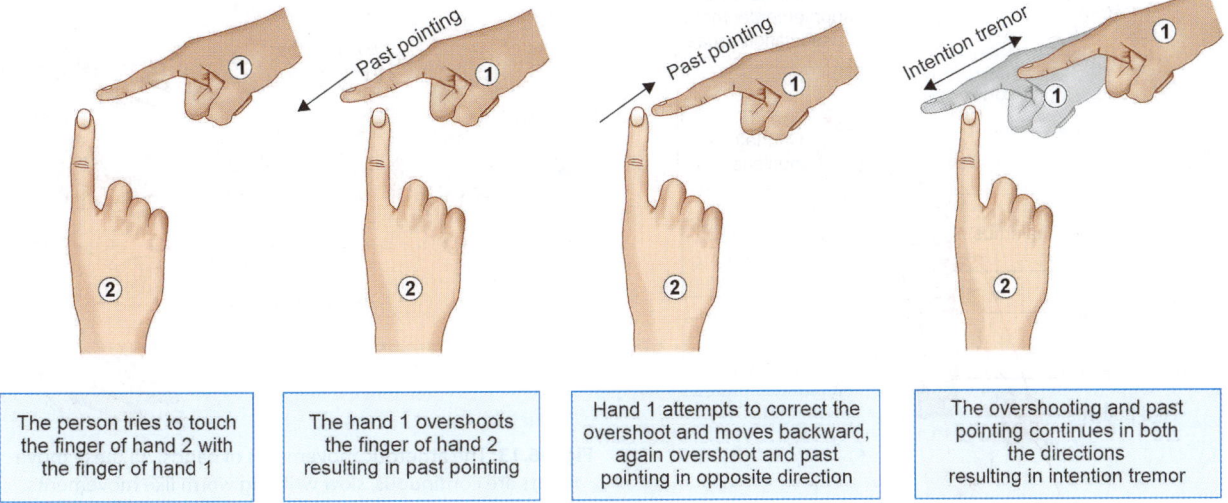

**Fig. 86.8:** The mechanism of past pointing.

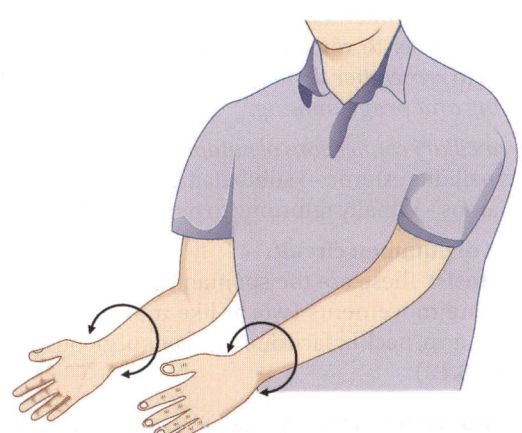

**Fig. 86.9:** Diadochokinesia: Rapid supination and pronation of forearms.

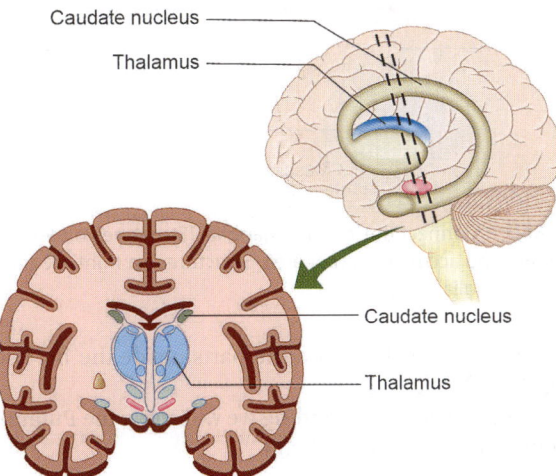

**Fig. 86.10:** Anatomical location of basal ganglia.

of eyes. It is seen in the lesions of flocculonodular lobe.
- **Drunken/reeling gait:** The person has a wide based staggered gait, as he is drunk. It occurs due to dysmetria, ataxia and loss of coordinated repetitive motor activity.
- The person with cerebellar ataxia cannot stand straight with his feet together (Rhomberg's test*) or cannot walk on a straight line (tandem walking) due to truncal hypotonia and difficulty in maintaining the posture.

## BASAL GANGLIA

It is group of nuclei present deep inside the cerebral cortex. It forms the accessory motor system like the cerebellum (Fig. 86.10). The basal ganglia (BG) extensively communicate with the cerebral cortex. Various nuclei of BG are:
- Corpus striatum
  - Caudate nucleus
  - Putamen
- Globus pallidus (externa and interna)
- Substantia nigra
- Subthalamic nuclei

All these nuclei surround the thalamus; arranged in the shape of a coma.

The area of the cerebral cortex between the caudate nucleus and putamen is the internal capsule, through which the corticospinal tract passes down to spinal cord. Hence, BG is closely associated with the corticospinal tract.

### Connections of BG

The basal ganglia is extensively connected with the other motor areas (motor cortex, thalamus, brain stem and

---

*__Rhomberg's test:__ It is test for identifying the sensory ataxia when a person is asked to stand with his feet close to each other. A person with sensory ataxia will be able to stand with his eyes open but will fall to one side on closing his eyes. But a patient with cerebellar lesion will not be able to stand with his feet put together, either with eyes open or closed. He will sway to the side of lesion.

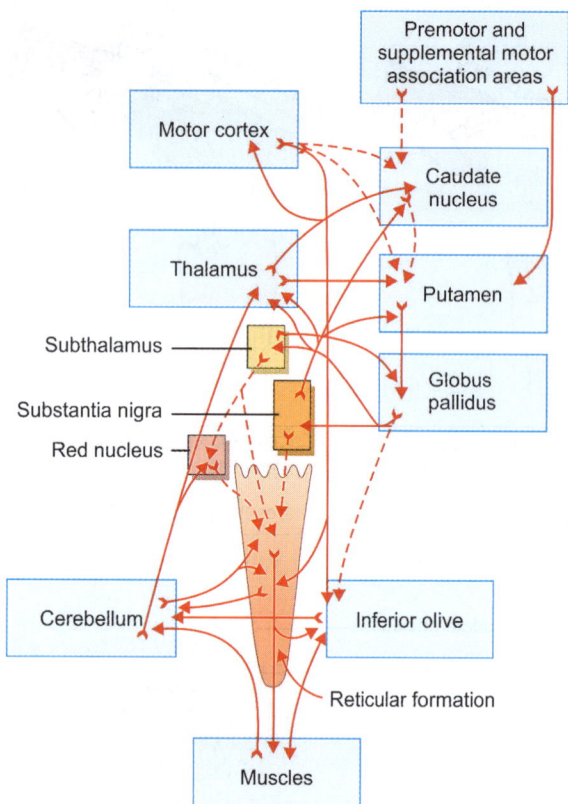

**Fig. 86.11:** Connections of basal ganglia. (Structures on left side are main and accessory motor area. Structures on right are nuclei of basal ganglia).

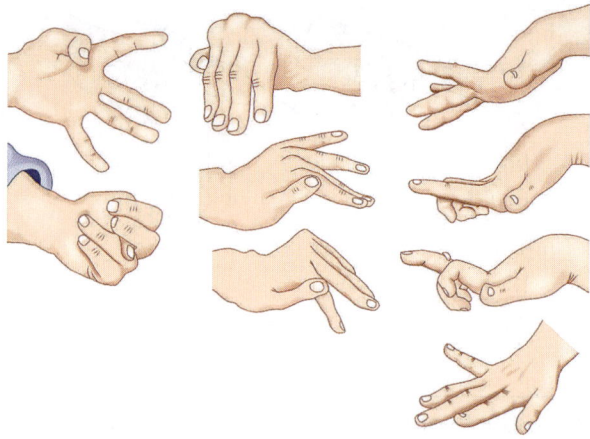

**Fig. 86.13:** The athetotic movements of hands. All these movements are continuous, slow writhing worm like movements.

cerebellum) as well as with the parts inside the BG itself **(Fig. 86.11)**.

For a simpler understanding we will study the Putamen Circuit and the Caudate Circuit.

## Putamen Circuit (Indirect Circuit)

This pathway is required for the ***execution of learned patterns of movements***. It doesn't receive the inputs from primary motor area but from the premotor, supplementary motor area and also from sensory cortex.

The primary putamen circuit is shown in **Figure 86.12**. The easiest way to remember the function of putamen circuit is to *remember 'P', where P for Putamen and P for Planning and programming.*

*Other ancillary connections of putamen circuit:* Putamen → globus pallidus externa → subthalamus → substantia nigra → thalamus → finally returning to motor cortex

**Lesions of putamen circuit:**
- **Athetosis:** These are the spontaneous and continuous writhing movements (worm-like movements) of the hands, arm, neck or face due to lesions of globus pallidus **(Fig. 86.13)**.

**Athetosis:** Lesion in globus pallidus
**Hemiballismus:** Lesions in subthalamus
**Chorea:** Lesions in Putamen
**Parkinsonism:** Lesions in substantia nigra
**Huntington's chorea:** Lesions of straitum due to mutant huntingtin protein

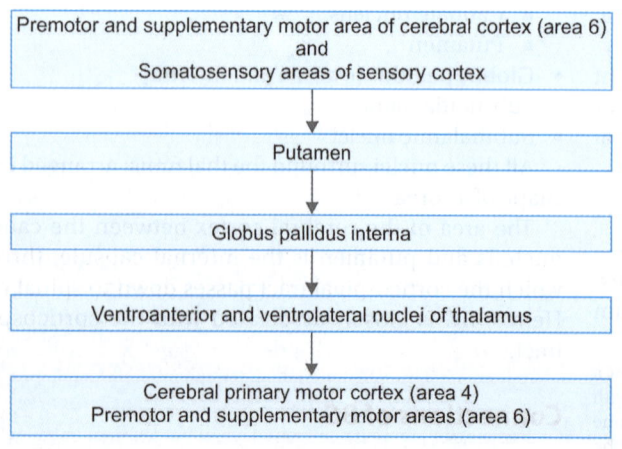
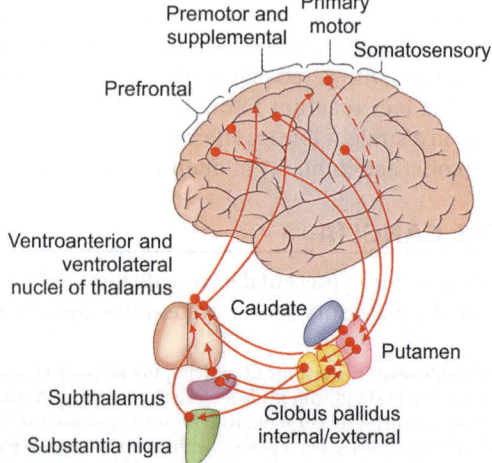

**Fig. 86.12:** Putamen circuit for planning and programming.

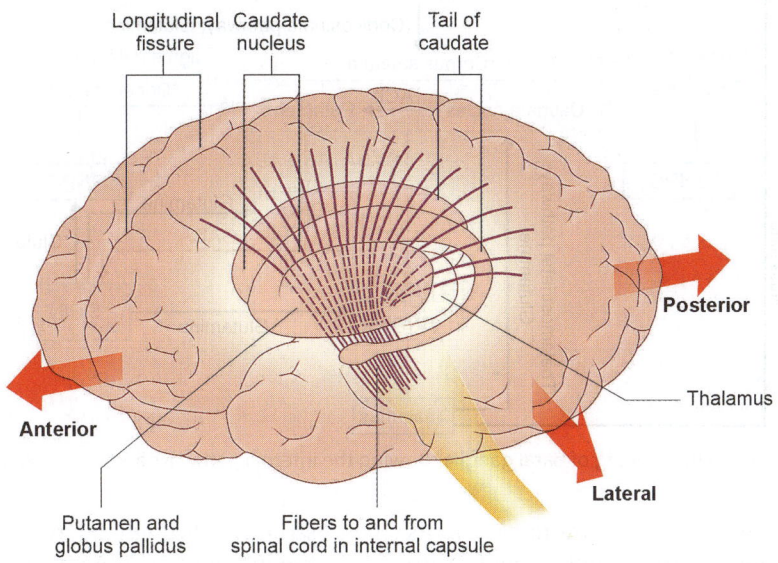

**Fig. 86.14:** Location of basal ganglia in the cerebrum and relationship of corticospinal tract.

- **Hemiballismus:** The sudden violent flailing movements (to wave something, esp. arms or legs, energetically but with little or no control) of an entire limb. These violent, jerky, high amplitude movements occur due to the lesions of subthalamus.
- **Chorea:** The dancing/flicking movements of hands, face and other parts of body due to the lesions of Putamen.
- **Parkinson's disease:** The lesions of substantia nigra causes a common and severe disease, characterized by rigidity, akinesia and tremors called Parkinson's disease.
- **Huntington's chorea:** Autosomal dominant disease on chromosome no. 4. There is degeneration of GABAergic and AChergic neurons in the striatum (head of caudate nucleus).

## Caudate Circuit (Direct Circuit)

The higher cognitive control of motor activity is regulated by the caudate circuit of the BG. (cognition: thinking process, hence the motor activity resulting as a consequence of thoughts generated in the mind are called cognitive control of motor activity).

### Neural connections of caudate circuit:

The caudate nucleus **(Fig. 86.14)** extends into all lobes of the cerebrum, which begins in frontal lobe, then passes posteriorly through parietal and occipital lobes and then finally curving into temporal lobes. Hence, the C-shaped caudate nucleus receives inputs from association areas overlying the caudate nucleus. The primary caudate circuit is shown in **Figure 86.15**.

### Lesions of caudate circuit/direct pathway:

- Pill rolling tremor is seen in the fingers at rest due to lesion in the direct pathway/caudate circuit

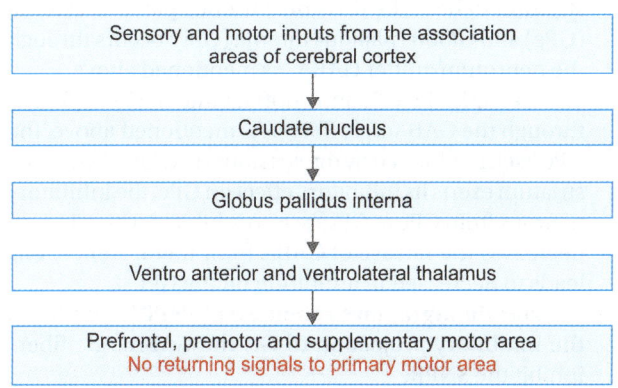

**Fig. 86.15:** Primary caudate circuit.

- Rigidity of muscles due to upper motor neuron type of lesion.
- Stooping posture
- Expressionless face
- Shuffling or accelerating gait

## Functioning of Basal Ganglia (Fig. 86.16)

The corpus striatum (caudate nucleus and Putamen) receives the inputs from

- **Cerebral cortex (corticostriate pathway):** From specific cortical areas to caudate nucleus and putamen (as mentioned in caudate and putamen circuit above). These fibers secrete **Glutamine**, which is an excitatory neurotransmitter.
- **Thalamus (thalamostriatal projection):** The intralaminar nuclei of thalamus, relay in the corpus striatum through the excitatory *glutaminergic* pathways. The thalamostriatal pathway acts as a feedback signal from the thalamus, which regulates the GABAergic discharge from striatum to GP and SNPR.

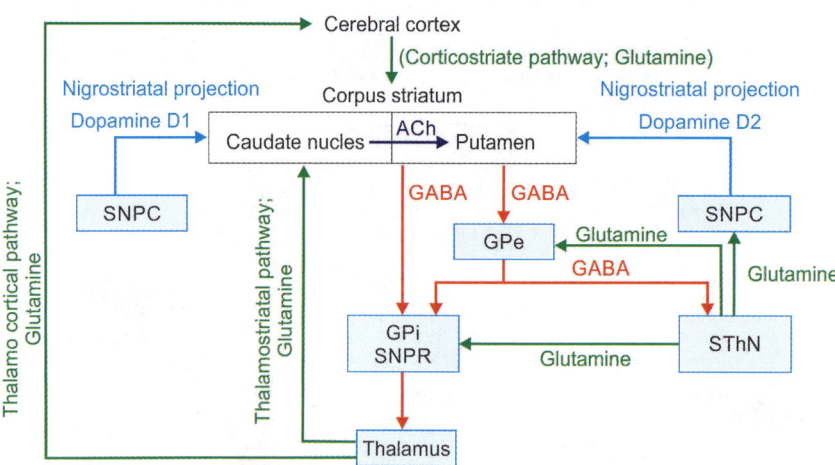

**Fig. 86.16:** The functioning of basal ganglia showing the internal pathways and neurotransmitters.

Both these inputs stimulate the striatum to secrete its inhibitory neurotransmitter, GABA (γ-amino butyric acid) which projects to:

- **Globus pallidus (GP):** The inhibitory projection from striatum to both the divisions; Globus pallidus externa (GPe) and Globus pallidus interna (GPi); occurs through the neurotransmitter GABA, as mentioned above.

  The GPe inhibits GPi and subthalamic nucleus (SThN) through the GABAergic fibers. As mentioned above, the GPe itself is inhibited by the striatum via GABA. When the striatum exerts its inhibitory effect on GPe, the inhibitory neurons from GPe to GPi are also inhibited which in turn decreases the release of GABA from them. Hence, this leads to decreased in inhibition on the GPi.

- **Substantia nigra pars reticularis (SNPR):** Similar to the inhibitory projection to GP, the GABAergic fibers inhibit the SNPR.

  Hence, with the stimulation of striatum, the GPi and SNPR gets inhibited through the GABAergic fibers. This decreases the GABAergic neuronal discharge from both, the GPi and SNPR. Thus, inhibition on thalamus is decreased, resulting in indirect stimulation by striatum. *Here again, the double inhibition results in the stimulation of thalamus.*

The other nuclei of basal ganglia also play an important role in direct and indirect circuitry:

- **Subthalamic nuclei:** The subthalamic nuclei are under the inhibitory GABAergic neurons but instead secrete excitatory glutamine. The excitatory output from SThN, stimulates, the GPe, GPi, SNPR and SNPC. The resultant effect of subthalamic inhibition by GPe is decreased stimulation of GPi, SNPR and SNPC and vice versa. Excitatory output to GPe acts as feedback loop for SThN.
- **Substantia nigra pars compacta (SNPC):** The nigrostriatal pathway, originating form substantia nigra secretes the neurotransmitter dopamine, which acts either through D1 receptors (stimulates the striatum) and D2 receptors (inhibits the striatum).
  - *Effect of stimulation of corpus striatum by SNPC through direct pathway* results in excitation of striatum through D1 receptors which increases the inhibitory GABAergic discharge from striatum. The inhibition of GPi and SNPR, decreases the inhibition of thalamus through the direct pathway. The decreased inhibition of thalamus increases the discharge in thalamocortical and thalamostriatal projections. During the initiation of movement, the thalamocortical oscillations initiate the movement and keeps it stable.
  - *Effect of stimulation of corpus striatum by SNPC through indirect pathway* results in inhibition of inhibitory GABAergic discharge through D2 receptors. This inturn increases the inhibition of the thalamus, decreasing the thalamic discharge. Hence the indirect pathway inhibits the thalamocortical and thalamostriatal discharge. At rest, the indirect pathway keeps the thalamic oscillations inhibited.

The **Figure 86.17**, simplifies the direct and indirect pathway and the neurotransmitters working in it.

Some neurotransmitters affecting the activity of BG, secreted from the brainstem are noradrenaline, enkephalins and serotonin.

## Functions of Basal Ganglia

- **Planning and programming of the motor activity** especially for the learned activities through the Putamen/indirect circuit.

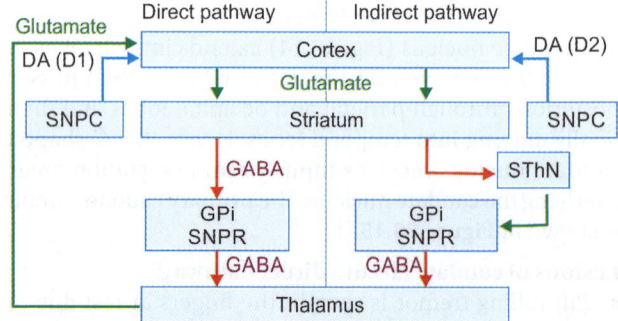

**Fig. 86.17:** The direct and indirect pathway of basal ganglia.

- **Cognitive control and learning the motor activity** and action selection through the direct/caudate circuit. It results in initiation of movement.
- **Timing and scaling of the movement** is maintained by basal ganglia. It determines the speed of the movement which allows many predictive functions. For example, passing the ball to other person, crossing the busy road etc.

  It also scales the movement according to the requirement. For example, the movement of hand is changed for writing the same alphabet of paper and blackboard. The timing of scaling of movement is processed along with the posterior parietal lobe (association area).
- **Behavioral control** due to its close association with the limbic system. The emotions associated with the movements are expressed here.

### Parkinson's Disease (Paralysis agitans)

**Definition:** It is a slowly progressing chronic degenerative disorder affecting the dopaminergic nigrostriatal neurons of basal ganglia

**Etiopathogenesis:** There is loss of dopamine secreting neurons in nigrostriatal pathway due to apoptosis occurring due to excessive free oxide radicals and oxidative stress which can occur due to:
- Old age/geriatric patients
- Familial predisposition
- Exposure to environmental toxins like a herbicide permethrin
- Other environmental factors

**Clinical Features (Fig. 86.18):**
- **Slow progression of disease:** Parkinsonism is a progressive disease, which appears around 50 years of age.
- **Mask like face** because of absence of emotional expression on the face.
- **Stooped posture:** There is flexion at hip and knee joint giving a stooped look.
- **Resting tremor:** The thalamocortical oscillation are usually kept inhibited by the indirect pathway. The absence of dopamine results in loss of inhibition on thalamus increasing the thalamocortical oscillations, even during the rest. This results in the resting tremor of the Parkinson's disease. *This tremor is however abolished, when a person attempts to work or hold something, which activates the direct pathway.* The tremor of Parkinson's disease begins as *'pill rolling tremor at rest'* but as the disease progresses, it becomes more severe resulting in **supination and pronation** of forearm and further progressing to add **the flexion and extension**. Hence a typical resting tremor of an advanced Parkinsons is having all three components.
- **Motor dysfunction:**
  - *Difficulty in initiating the movement (akinesia):* The loss of dopamine in direct pathway decreases the excitation of striatum. There is decrease in GABA secreted from striatum. There is less inhibition of GPi and SNPR which increases the thalamic inhibition. Hence, it becomes difficult to initiate the movement akinesia), the movements become slow (bradykinesia)
  - *Lead pipe/cogwheel rigidity:* The destruction of the dopaminergic neurons in substantia nigra of parkinsonian patient increases the activity of the striatum and indirectly affect the affects the corticospinal tracts. There is increased excitation of skeletal muscles resulting in muscle rigidity.
  - **Dysphagia:** Due to loss of planning and programming of tongue and pharyngeal muscle, the patient finds difficulty in swallowing resulting in dysphagia.
  - **Speech disorder:** Due to damage in motor activity, the person has speech problems. He may have slurred or stuttering speech. There is no change in the tone of the speech.
- **Postural instability** caused by impaired postural reflexes
- **Gait:** The patient with Parkinsons disease has the **festinating gait**, which is narrow based with short shuffling steps, with flat foot strike (entire foot strikes the floor), reduced arm swinging. The patient walks with flexion of hip and the knee joint. He walks in a way that he is trying to find the center of gravity. The phenomenon of **retropulsion** is seen in these patients, which means when a person is walking in one direction, say forwards, is suddenly stopped, we would walk a few steps backwards before stopping. This phenomenon seen in Parkinson's patients is due to inability to stop the ongoing movement.
- **Emotional disturbances:** The Parkinson's patient can undergo depression, sleeping disorder, etc.

**Treatment:** There is no definitive treatment of Parkinson's disease but however, its progressing can slowed down and symptomatic relief is given to the patient.
- **Administration of L-Dopa** to the patients give the symptomatic relief, because it gets converted to dopamine in brain.
- **Monoamine oxidase inhibitors:** Decreases the destruction of available dopamine and increases its half-life.
- **Surgical treatment:**
  - *Transplantation of dopamine secreting fetal cells* into striatum.

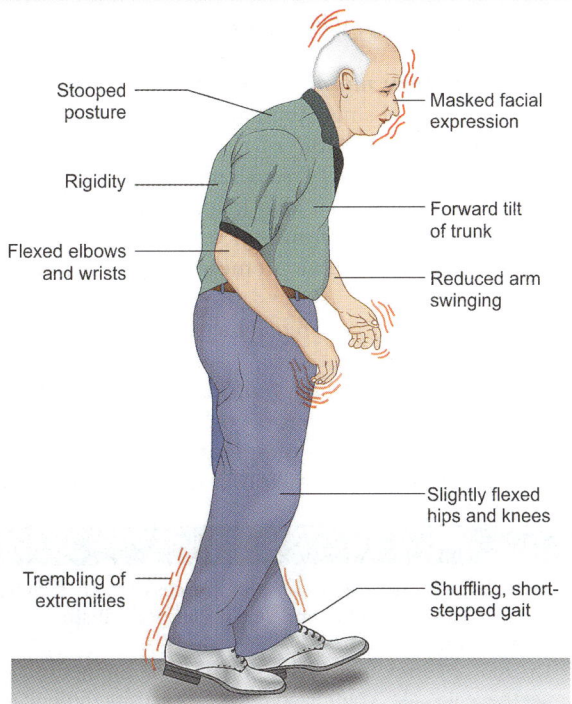

**Fig. 86.18:** Clinical presentation of Parkinson's disease.

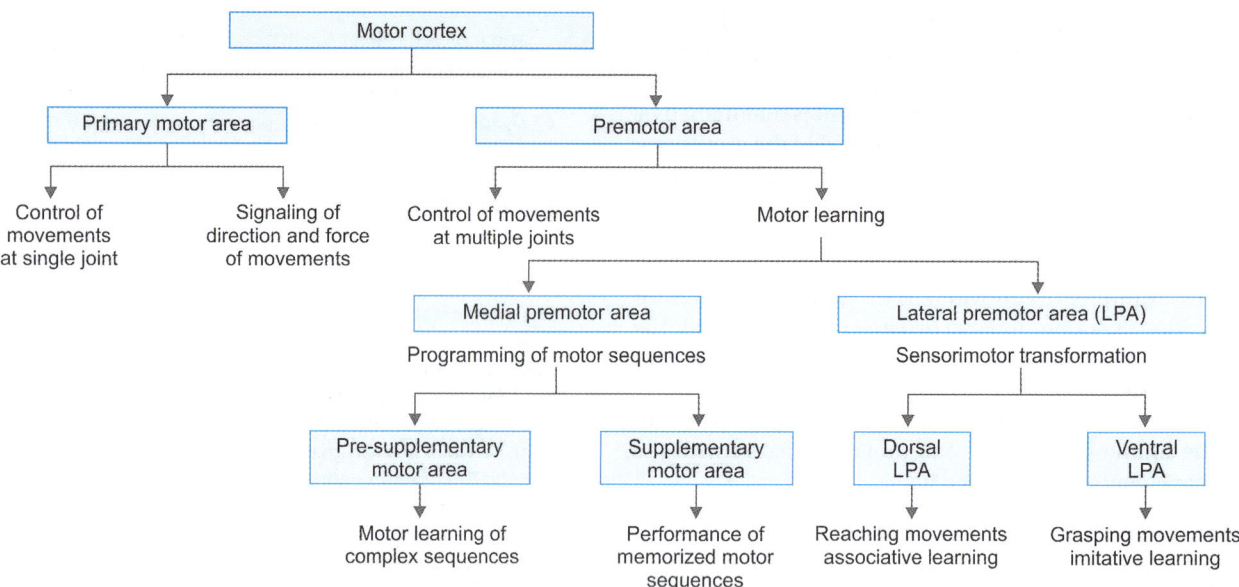

Fig. 86.19: The role of motor cortex, in execution of motor activity.

- **Ablation of feedback circuitry of basal ganglia** by creating the surgical lesions in ventrolateral and ventro anterior nuclei of thalamus.
- **Deep brain stimulation.** The electrodes are planted deep into the basal ganglia, which are connected to battery for stimulation of the basal ganglia nuclei.

## SUMMARY OF MOTOR PROGRAMMING AND PLANNING IN MOTOR EXECUTION

- **Role of motor cortex (Fig. 86.19):** The motor cortex has the most important role to play in the execution of the motor activity.
  - *The primary motor area (Area 4)* controls the movements of single joint and signals the direction of force of movement.
  - *The premotor area (Area 6)* controls the movements at multiple joints. It also helps in learning motor movements. The premotor area further has two subdivisions, medial premotor area, and lateral premotor area.
    - *Medial premotor area:* It helps in programming of motor sequences
      - *Presupplementary motor area:* It is the area for the motor learning of complex sequences
      - *Supplementary motor area:* This area is for performing the memorized motor sequences.
    - *Lateral premotor area (LPA):* It participates in sensory motor transformation
      - *Dorsal LPA:* This area results in the execution of movements, which aids to reach out for the object. It helps in associative learning.
      - *Ventral LPA:* It is responsible for grasping movements and initiative learning.
- **Role of cerebellum:**
  - Higher motor planning
  - *Dentato-rubro-olivo-cerebello-dentate loop:* Mental rehearsal of ballistic movements. Lesions in dentate nucleus delays initiation of movements
  - *Coordinates simultaneous performance of multiple motor subprograms.* Damage to cerebro-cerebellum leads to decomposition of complex motor programs into simple sequential sub routines.
- **Role of basal ganglia:**
  - *Through caudate loop: Motor sequencing,* i.e., transition from one motor program to another. It's damage needs to akinesia
  - *Through putamen loop: Scaling* the intensities of movement
- **Role of sensory feedback:** Proprioceptive/somatic/visual/vestibular sensory inputs provide the feedback for the intended activity, which is planned by the motor and accessory motor areas for execution.

## SUMMARY

- The motor activity is a complex process which requires programming, planning and sensory motor transformation before being executed.
- The motor cortex (primary motor area and premotor area) are the main areas controlling the motor activity through the corticospinal tract.
- The accessory motor areas (cerebellum and basal ganglia) are required for the smooth execution, coordination, ballistic movements, timing, scaling of the motor signal, initiated by motor cortex.

## LET US SEE, HOW MUCH YOU HAVE LEARNT?

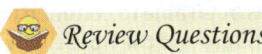
### Review Questions

#### Long/Short Answer Questions

Q1. Describe the working of functional unit of cerebellum.
Q2. Describe the physiological basis of the following, seen in cerebellar dysfunction
   a. Intention tremor
   b. Dysmetria and ataxia
Q3. Why does a person with cerebellar ataxia, not able to stand with his feet together?
Q4. Describe the functioning of caudate circuit and putamen circuit of basal ganglia.
Q5. What is the role of basal ganglia in planning and programming of motor activity?

Q6. Describe the physiological basis of the following, seen in Parkinsonism:
   a. Resting tremor
   b. Akinesia
   c. Rigidity
   d. Festinating gait
Q7. Describe the mechanism of motor execution of movements, required for picking up the pen from the table and putting a cap on it.
Q8. 'Parkinsons disease where hyperkinesia (tremor) and hypokinesia (akinesia), coexist'. Explain this statement.

#### Explain Why? (Reasoning Questions)

Q1. Damage to the cerebellum leads to ataxia and impaired coordination.
Q2. The basal ganglia are critical for initiating and regulating voluntary movements.
Q3. Lesions in the cerebellum can affect balance and posture.
Q4. Dysfunction in the basal ganglia can result in movement disorders such as Parkinson's disease.

Q5. The cerebellum is involved in motor learning and adapting movements based on feedback.
Q6. Disruptions in the basal ganglia circuitry can cause both hyperkinetic and hypokinetic movement disorders.
Q7. Parkinsons disease where hyperkinesia (tremor) and hypokinesia (akinesia), coexist.

### Critical Thinking Case-Based Questions

Q1. Mr Gupta, a 65-year-old man, presented to the OPD with complaints of tremors, difficulty initiating movements, and unsteady gait. He had noticed that his handwriting has become smaller and more illegible over the past year, and he struggles with tasks requiring fine motor skills. Upon examination, he exhibited a resting tremor in his hands, bradykinesia (slowness of movement), and a shuffling gait. The neurologist suspected a neurological disorder involving the cerebellum and basal ganglia and orders further diagnostic tests.

Based on the given case scenario, answer the following questions:
a. What is the probable diagnosis?
b. Explain the physiological roles of the cerebellum and basal ganglia in motor planning and execution.
c. Discuss how dysfunction in these areas can lead to Mr Gupta's symptoms.
d. What diagnostic tests and imaging techniques are useful in assessing the function and structure of the cerebellum and basal ganglia?

### Multiple Choice Questions

Q1. Both basal ganglia pathways use disinhibition to mediate their effects. Which of the following pairs of structures contain the 2 inhibitory neuron cell bodies that interact to create a disinhibition?
   a. Substantia nigra, pars compacta—putamen
   b. Globus pallidus external segment—subthalamic nucleus
   c. VA nucleus of the thalamus—motor cortex
   d. Putamen—globus pallidus internal segment

Q2. A 55-year-old male patient develops dancelike involuntary movements. You diagnose the patient as having a degenerative neurological disease that was also evident in the patient's father and uncle. Where is the most likely site of the degeneration?
   a. Globus pallidus, internal segment
   b. VL nucleus of the thalamus

   c. Head of caudate nucleus
   d. Substantia nigra, pars compacta

Q3. A hypertensive patient suffers a lacunar infarct and develops uncontrollable violent flinging movements of the left upper limb. Where is the lesion?
   a. Left globus pallidus internal segment
   b. Right subthalamic nucleus
   c. Left substantia nigra
   d. Right VL nucleus

Q4. Over a period of years, a construction worker begins to have difficulty hammering nails using his right arm and hand. When he walks, he seems to teeter to the right. Neurological exam reveals that muscle strength is 5/5 in both the upper and lower limbs, but the patient exhibits a tremor when attempting to touch his right

index finger to the tip of his nose. Cranial nerve testing and the rest of the neurological exam are normal. Where might a lesion be located that accounts for all of the patient's symptoms?
   a. Anterior part of the vermis bilaterally
   b. Lateral part of the hemisphere on the right
   c. The vermis and cerebellar hemisphere on the right
   d. Head of the caudate nucleus on the right

Q5. Which of the following describes a connection between components of the basal ganglia?
   a. The subthalamic nucleus releases glutamate to excite the globus pallidus, internal segment
   b. The substantia nigra pars reticulata releases dopamine to inhibit the striatum
   c. The substantia nigra pars compacta releases dopamine to excite the globus pallidus, external segment
   d. The striatum releases acetylcholine to excite the substantia nigra pars reticulata

Q6. A 60-year-old man with Parkinson disease, which was diagnosed 15 years ago, has been taking carbidopa and levodopa; until recently, he has been able to continue to work and help with routine jobs around the house. Now his tremor and rigidity interfere with these activities. His clinician has suggested that he undergo deep brain stimulation therapy. The therapeutic effect of L-dopa in patients with Parkinson disease eventually wears off because:
   a. Antibodies to dopamine receptors develop
   b. Inhibitory pathways grow into the basal ganglia from the frontal lobe
   c. The normal action of nerve growth factor (NGF) is disrupted
   d. The dopaminergic neurons in the substantia nigra continue to degenerate

## ANSWERS

**1.** d    **2.** c    **3.** b    **4.** c    **5.** a    **6.** d

# Spinal Cord and the Pathways between Cerebrum and Peripheral Parts of Body

**87 CHAPTER**

### COMPETENCY ADDRESSED

**PY10.3:** Describe and discuss somatic sensations and sensory tracts.
**PY10.4:** Describe and discuss motor tracts, mechanism of maintenance of tone, control of body movements, posture and equilibrium and vestibular apparatus.
**PY10.6:** Describe and discuss spinal cord, its functions, lesion and sensory disturbances.

### LEARNING OBJECTIVES

At the end of this chapter, the learner should be able to:
- Describe the basic functional anatomy of spinal cord.
- Enumerate various ascending (sensory) and descending (motor) tracts of spinal cord.
- Outline the course of various ascending (sensory) and descending (motor) tracts of spinal cord.
- Enumerate the functions of each sensory motor tract.
- Describe the mechanism of sensory motor coordination, i.e., processing of sensory signal to generate the motor commands.
- Describe the various lesions of spinal cord along with their clinical presentation and effect on the sensory motor function.

## FUNCTIONAL ANATOMY

As we have studied in Chapter 79, the spinal cord is the continuation of medulla oblongata, which extends through the vertebral column. It is 45–50 cm in length and extends up to L1 in adults. Below this level, the spinal roots are present which looks like the horse tail, hence the name cauda equina. The spinal cord is covered by three meninges: *Outer dura mater, arachnoid mater and innermost pia mater.* The spinal cord is cushioned by cerebrospinal fluid present in subarachnoid space present between arachnoid mater and pia mater. There are 31 pairs of spinal nerves, emerging from the spinal cord. These are 8 cervical, 12 thoracic, 5 lumbar and 5 sacral. Then there is cauda equina and filum terminale in the end.

## ORGANIZATION OF SPINAL CORD (FIG. 87.1)

As studied in Chapter 79, the spinal cord has an outer white matter and inner H shaped gray matter.
- **Inner gray matter:** The gray matter can be classified based on their anatomical organization and functional classification. We will learn about both these classifications, simultaneously for the ease of study. In the functional classificational, the entire gray matter is divided into ten (X) laminae, shown in **Figure 87.2**.

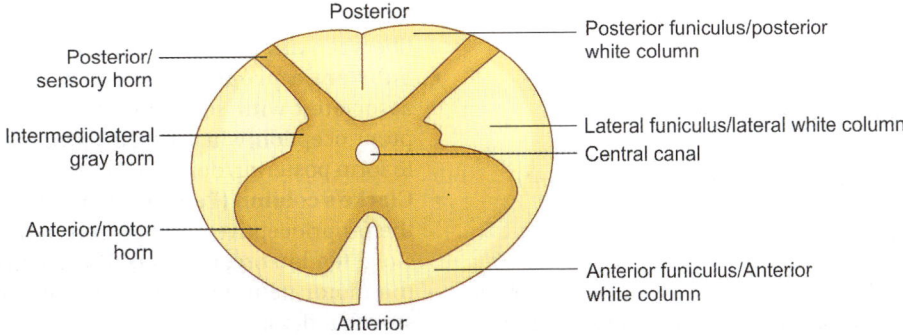

Fig. 87.1: Organization of spinal cord.

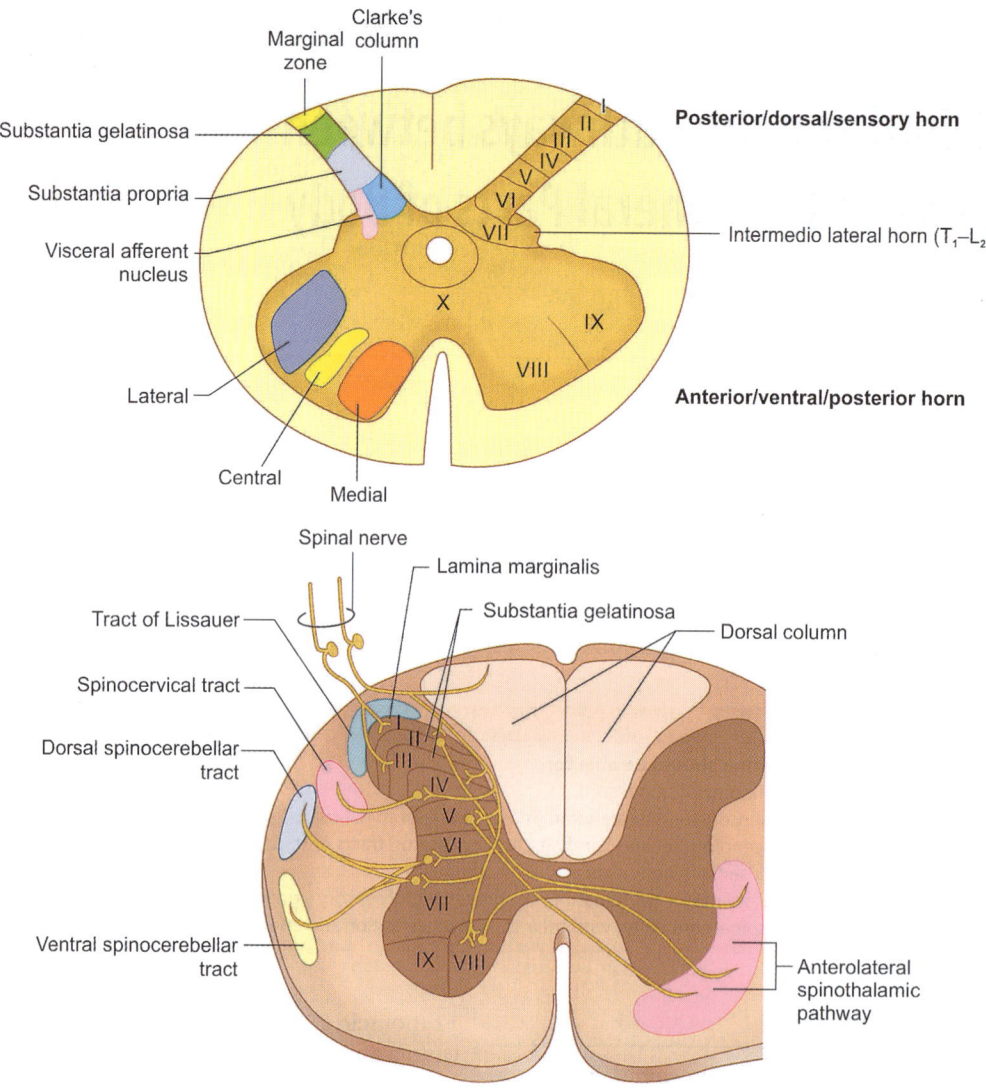

**Fig. 87.2:** Organization of gray matter in spinal cord.

According to the anatomical classification, the H shaped inner gray matter has two roots and two main horns. However, there is a third horn in thoracolumbar segments. All these details are discussed below.

## Spinal Roots

Anterior/motor root and posterior/sensory root. The **Bell Magendie law** states that the posterior root of spinal cord is sensory and the anterior root is motor.

## Horns

- *Posterior/dorsal/sensory horn*
- *Anterior/ventral/motor horn*
- *Intermediolateral horn (in thoracolumbar segment)*

## Posterior/Sensory Horn

This horn acts as the entry gate for the sensory nerves to enter into the spinal cord. The various sensory nerves entering through here either synapse here or just pass from posterior root to synapse on other neurons. The posterior horn has the following nuclei (collection of cell bodies, from where the second order neuron arise). These are:

- **Marginal zone (Lamina I):** The fibers entering the spinal cord sends the fibers to 2 segments above and below through the short Tracts of Lissauer.
- **Substantia gelatinosa (Laminae II and III):** Receives inputs of pain, temperature and touch from posterior root forming the spinothalamic pathways. Hence, the sensory fibers carrying these sensations first synapse here.
- **Substantia propria (Lamina IV):** It receives fibers associated with sensation of vibration, fine touch, proprioception; which pass from here without synapsing to form posterior/dorsal white column.
- **Clarke's column (Laminae V and VI):** (C8-L4) Receive the proprioceptive endings from muscle spindles and Golgi tendon organ (GTO). These neurons synapse on the motor neurons in anterior horn to complete the stretch reflex arc.

- **Visceral afferent nucleus (Lamina V):** (present in the thoracolumbar segments, T1-L3) It receives visceral afferent information.

## Anterior/Motor Horn

This horn contains:
- Large multipolar cells; **Aα type of fibers** {innervate the skeletal muscles (LMN)}
- Small multipolar cells; **Aγ type of fibers** (innervate the intrafusal muscle fibers of muscle spindle)

The anterior horn is divided into four regions based on its anatomical location:
1. **Medial part (Lamina VIII):** The lower motor neurons arising from this part innervate the neck, trunk and intercostal muscles (i.e., the medial/axial part of the body)
2. **Central part (Lamina VIII):** The lower motor neurons arising from this part innervate the diaphragm, sternocleidomastoids and trapezius
3. **Lateral part (Lamina IX):** The lower motor neurons arising from this part innervate the muscles of the limbs. Hence this area is larger in the cervical and lumbar region.
4. **Lamina X** is present around the central canal.

## Intermediolateral Gray Horn (Lamina VII)

This is the site of origin of the autonomic sympathetic fibers from the thoracolumbar segment.

## SENSORY TRACTS: ASCENDING TRACTS OF SPINAL CORD

These tracts (bundles of nerve fibers) carry the sensory information from sensory receptors to the somatosensory cortex of the brain and other parts of brain. Since, the information ascends upwards from lower body towards the CNS, they are named as ascending tracts. Before we further study the various ascending tracts, there are certain general rules followed by these tracts, mentioned below:
- All the ascending tracts begin with word *"spino"* and end with the area of destination

**Example:**
- Spinothalamic tracts (From spinal cord to ventro-postero-lateral nucleus of thalamus)
- Spinocerebellar tracts (From spinal cord to cerebellum)
- Spino-olivary tract (From spinal cord to olivary nucleus of medulla oblongata)
- Spinotectal tract [From spinal cord to superior colliculus in midbrain (tectum)]
- Each tract is a **system of three neurons:**
  1. *First order neuron* → enters the spinal cord; *from receptor to first synapse*
  2. *Second order neuron* → **cross to the other side of spinal cord**, and ends in thalamus; *from first synapse to 2nd synapse*
  3. *Third order neuron* → from thalamus to the sensory cortex; *from 2nd synapse to relay in post central gyrus*
- All the tracts (ascending and descending), are present in the white matter. Depending on the location of these tracts, they carry a prefix of anterior (ventral)/lateral/posterior (dorsal) tracts.
- There are two lemniscal systems: Medial and lateral. The medial lemniscus carries the medial tracts while the lateral lemniscus carries the lateral tracts. Various ascending and descending tracts are shown in the **Figure 87.3**.

After the basic structural rules, lets study the course and functions of various sensory tracts. Depending on the location in the white column, the ascending tracts are described below.

### The Ascending Tracts and the Sensations (Fig. 87.4 and Table 87.1)

- **Anterior spinothalamic tract:**
  - Crude touch
  - Pressure
- **Lateral spinothalamic tract:**
  - Pain
  - Temperature

Type of fibers in spinothalamic tracts:
- Aδ fibers and C fibers

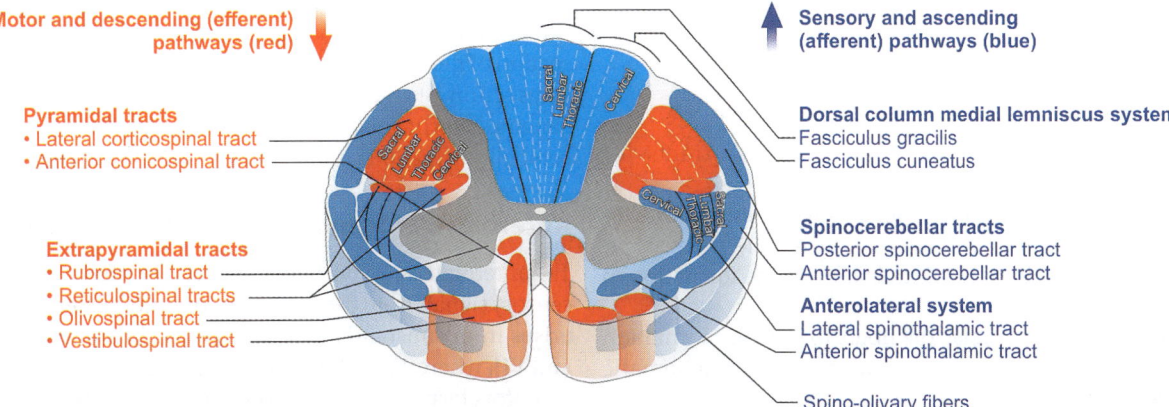

**Fig. 87.3:** Ascending and descending spinal tracts (blue tracts are ascending tracts, red tracts are descending tracts).

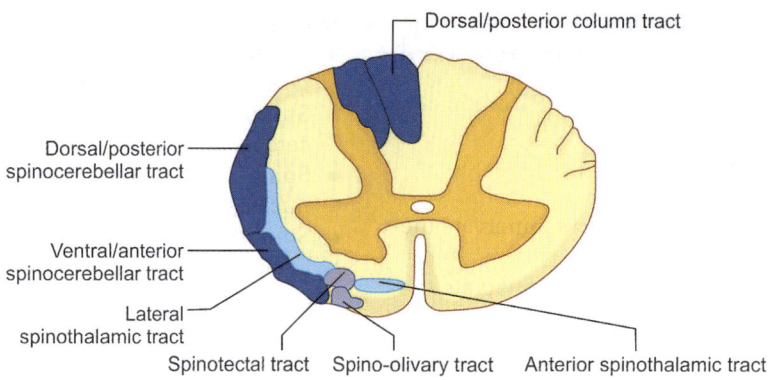

**Fig. 87.4:** Ascending tracts in the spinal cord.

**Table 87.1:** Summary of various ascending tracts.

| Name of tract | First order neuron | First synapse/ terminates in | Second order neuron | Second synapse/ terminates in | Third order neuron | Terminates in |
|---|---|---|---|---|---|---|
| Anterior spinothalamic tract | Arises from sensory receptor (touch and pressure) | Substantia gelatinosa | Arises from substantia gelatinosa and ascends upwards in anterior white column of opposite side | Ventral posterolateral (VPL) nucleus of thalamus | Arises from VPL nucleus of thalamus | Somatosensory cortex (Area 3, 1, 2) |
| Lateral spinothalamic tract | Arises from sensory receptor (pain and temperature) | Substantia gelatinosa | Arises from substantia gelatinosa and ascends upwards in lateral white column of opposite side | Ventral posterolateral (VPL) nucleus of thalamus | Arises from VPL nucleus of thalamus | Somatosensory cortex (Area 3, 1, 2) |
| Posterior column tract (Tract of Goll and Burdach) | Arises from sensory receptor (touch, proprioceptors). Enter the spinal cord and reach substantia propria. Ascends upwards without synapsing in spinal cord in the posterior white column | Nucleus cuneatus and nucleus gracilis in medulla oblongata of same side | Arises from nucleus cuneatus and nucleus gracilis and crosses midline to reach thalamus | Ventral posterolateral (VPL) nucleus of thalamus | Arises from VPL nucleus of thalamus | Somatosensory cortex (Area 3, 1, 2) |
| Anterior spino- cerebellar tract | Arises from sensory receptors | Substantia gelatinosa | Arises from substantia gelatinosa and ascends upwards in anteriorly in lateral white column of opposite side | Cerebellum | Arises from VPL nucleus of thalamus | Somatosensory cortex (Area 3, 1, 2) |

- **Posterior column tracts/dorsal column tracts**
  - Fine touch
  - Two point discrimination
  - Vibration
  - Joint positioning, proprioception
- Anterior and posterior spinocerebellar tracts for unconscious kinesthetic impulses
- Spino-olivary tracts for the sensory input to inferior olives of medulla oblongata. It forms the main input for the cerebellum by participating in the formation of climbing fibers.
- **Spinoreticular tracts:** The fibers to reticular formation are responsible for general awareness about somatic sensations.
- Spinotectal tracts for the spinovisual reflex

We will outline the course/pathway of various ascending tracts in a simple and reproducible way. The coronal section of the entire CNS pathway showing cerebrum with the section of thalamus (with lateral ventricles), basal ganglia, internal capsule is visible along with brainstem, cerebellum, medulla oblongata and spinal cord (**Fig. 87.5**).

## Anterolateral Spinothalamic Tracts (Fig. 87.6)

The anterolateral spinothalamic tracts are carry less critical sensory signals from the receptors. The anterolateral system arises from substantia gelatinosa (S.G.) (Laminae I, IV, V and VI), where 1st order neurons arising from the sensory receptors terminate. The second order neurons arise from here forming the anterolateral system and immediately

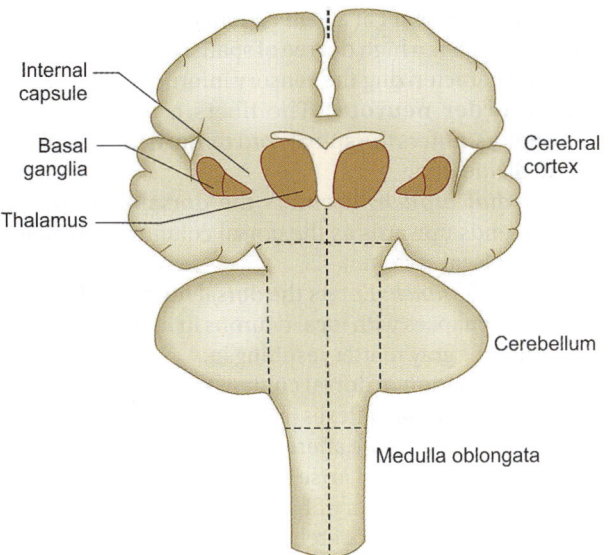

**Fig. 87.5:** A line diagram of coronal section of cerebrum, midbrain, medulla and spinal cord for showing the ascending and descending tracts.

activation system, thus forming the spinoreticular system. Even in the thalamus, it transmits the signals to medullary intralaminar reticular nuclei of thalamus. The 3rd order neurons from VPL nucleus relay in the somatosensory cortex (Area 3, 1, 2) of the cerebral cortex.

> ***Intramedullary spinal cord tumors/lesions*** (arising from within the spinal cord) will have present initial compressive symptoms in most medial fibers, depending on the site of lesion. For example, the intramedullary tumors in thoracic lesion will affect the anterolateral system, if present in its vicinity, in the sequence of thoracic followed by lumbar and then sacral.
> 
> Similarly, ***extramedullary lesions tumor/injury*** would present with the involvement of most lateral fibers (sacral to cervical, depending on extent of lesion).

The anterolateral spinothalamic tract is responsible from the crude transmission of senses as compared to dorsal column because:
- The conduction velocity of around 8 to 40 m/sec, which is much slower than the dorsal column tract.
- The degree of localization of signal is not well developed.
- Gradation of intensity is not very accurate, far more less than the dorsal column.
- The modalities transmitted by the anterolateral system only are pain, temperature, tickle, itch, pressure and sexual sensations. However, the touch sensation is crude here.

***Physiological significance of crude touch:*** Just hearing the word crude touch, it gives us a feeling that it is not important. But let me tell you the how we are actually using

cross to the anterior and lateral white columns of opposite side, hence forming anterior spinothalamic tract and lateral spinothalamic tract.

The fibers entering from the lower part of body are most lateral and the upper part of body are most medial, arranged from lateral to medial as sacral, lumbar, thoracic and cervical (S, L, T, C). On its way to the VPL nucleus of the thalamus, the anterolateral spinothalamic tract transmits the information to the lower brainstem and some parts of midbrain. This send the information to the reticular

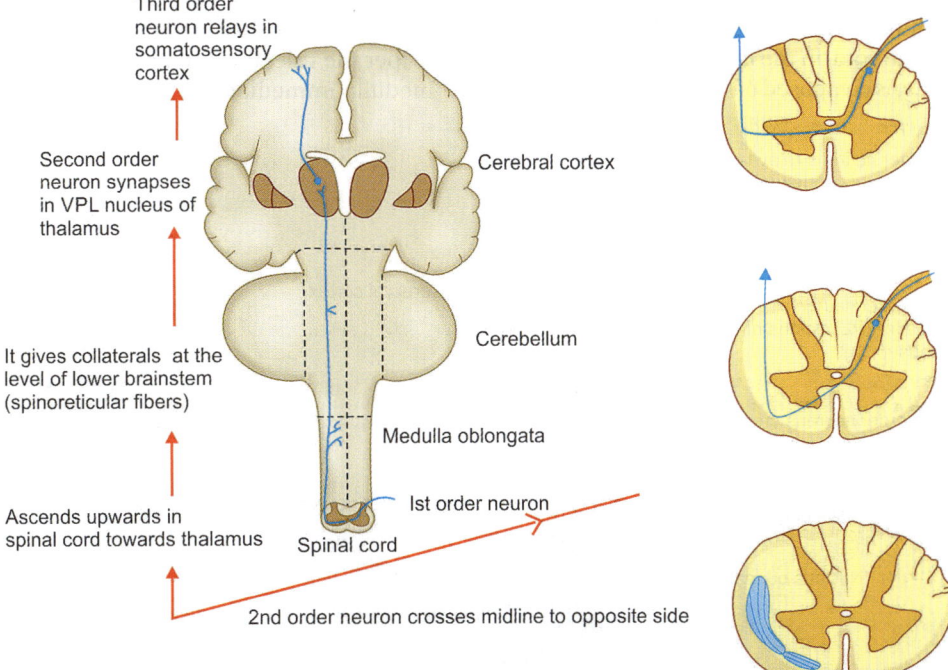

**Fig. 87.6:** The anterior and lateral spinothalamic tracts showing the course and topography of fibers in spinal cord.

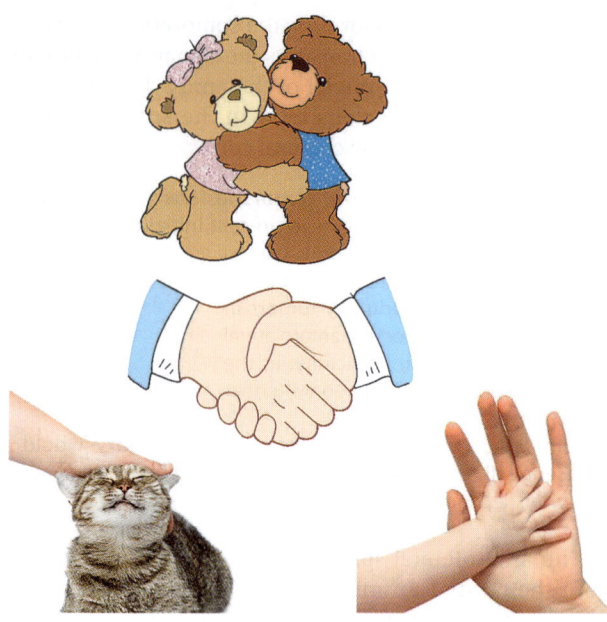

**Fig. 87.7:** Expressions of crude touch.

crude touch in our day to day life. The crude touch is used in everyday life to express our feelings, emotions through gestures and touch. Apart from these, whatever we do or tasks we perform are a result of crude touch **(Fig. 87.7)**.

### Dorsal Column–Medial Lemniscal System (Fig. 87.8)

*(Posterior column tract/fasciculus cuneatus and fasciculus gracilis/tract of Goll and Burdach)*
Dorsal column tract carries the sensations of fine touch, proprioception, two point discrimination, vibration. It carries the fibers from the body to the brain in dorsal column of the spinal cord, in the medial lemniscus, hence the name. This tract is composed of large myelinated nerve fibers which transmit at a high conduction velocity of 30 to 110 m/sec. It has a high degree of spatial orientation which helps in characterizing the sensory information.

- **First order neurons:** The fibers arising from the receptors, enters the spinal cord through the dorsal root and divide into:
  - *Medial branch:* It enters the dorsal column and ascends upwards as the dorsal column tract/medial lemniscal system.
  - *Lateral branch:* Enters the dorsal horn of spinal cord and synapses with local neurons in intermediate and anterior gray matter resulting in:
    ♦ Formation of dorsal column tract.
    ♦ Local spinal reflexes (stretch reflex, inverse stretch reflex, etc.): The afferents for these reflexes and the dorsal column arise from proprioceptors, hence common sensory fibers.
    ♦ Origin of spinocerebellar tracts, which transmits unconscious kinesthetic impulses to the cerebellum.
- Fibers from lower part of body enter first and form F. gracilis and the fibers from upper part of body enter later and form F. cuneatus. Hence, the fibers from the lower part of the body are present most medially and the upper part are located most laterally. (Tip: The Fasciculus '**G**'racilis has fibers from lower body (which is near '**G**'round), it is more medial. Similarly, the Fasciculus '**C**'uneatus has fibers from upper body (which is near '**C**'rown), it is more lateral.
- The first order neurons ascend upwards towards the medulla in medial lemniscus, without synapsing in spinal cord. These neurons synapse in nucleus cuneatus and nucleus gracilis located in the medulla oblongata. After these nuclei, this tract is also named as the fasciculus cuneatus and gracilis.
- As per the rule, the 2nd order neuron arising from the medulla immediately crosses the midline to synapse

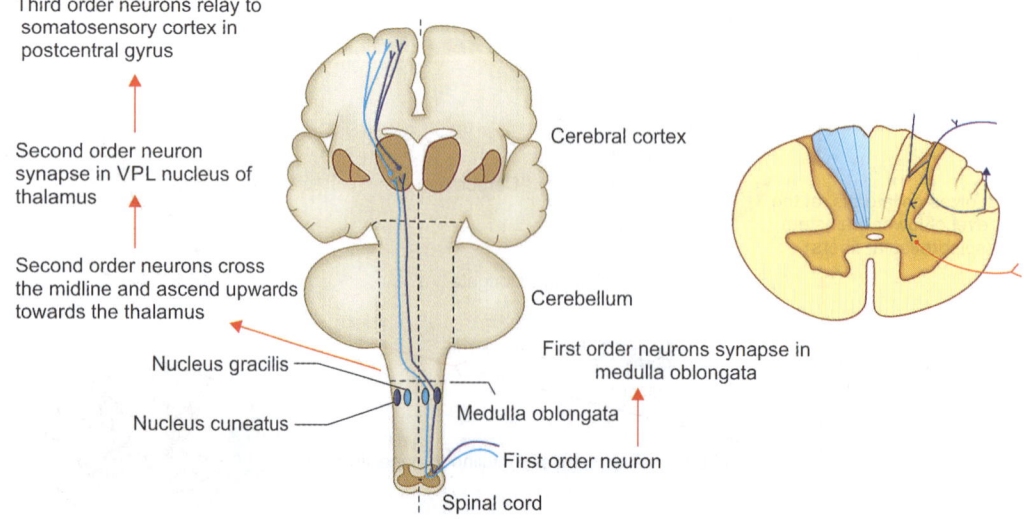

**Fig. 87.8:** Dorsal column tract.

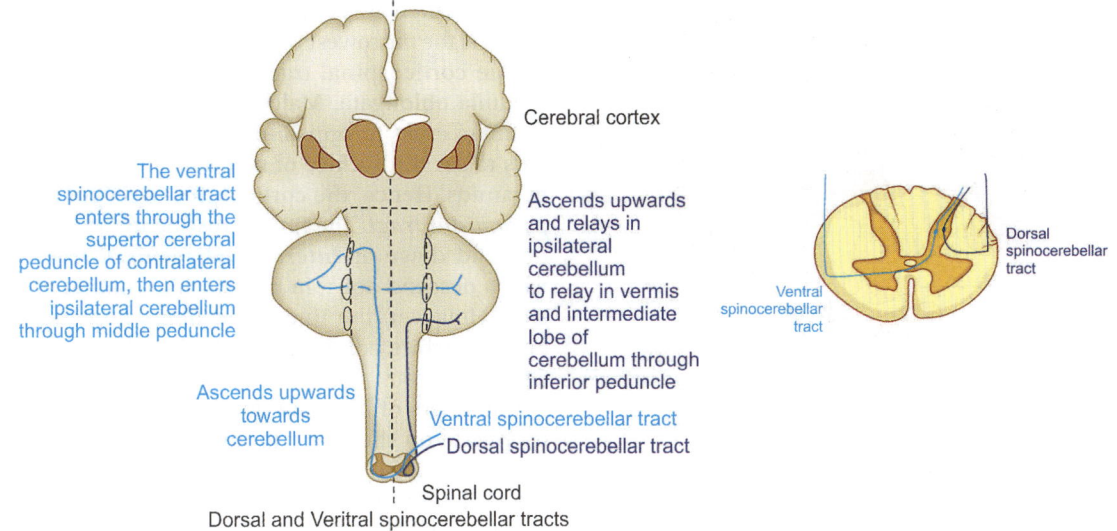

**Fig. 87.9:** Dorsal and ventral spinocerebellar tracts.

in VPL nucleus of thalamus. During this course to thalamus, the sensory nucleus of trigeminal nucleus also joins the dorsal column.
- In the thalamus, the 2nd order neurons synapse in VPL nucleus and the 3rd order neurons arise.
- The 3rd order neurons project to the postcentral gyrus (SS-I).

The dorsal column tract has some special features mentioned below:
- Spatial orientation of nerve fibers from individual parts of the body. This spatial organization is maintained in thalamus and cerebral cortex.
- The conduction velocity is higher.

Hence, this sensory pathway is more advanced than anterolateral system.

## SPINOCEREBELLAR TRACTS (FIG. 87.9)

The spinocerebellar tract originates in the spinal cord and terminates in the cerebellum. It *receives its impulses from the proprioceptors* and is responsible for sensory feed to cerebellum regarding muscle tone, joint position and posture. Hence, it is concerned with unconscious kinesthetic impulses. Since, sensory fibers are large myelinated fibers, their conduction velocity is very fast. They transmit the *impulses to same side (ipsilateral)* cerebellum, unlike the rest of the tracts. There are main two tracts transmitting the information to cerebellum, the *dorsal/posterior spinocerebellar tract* and the *ventral/anterior spinocerebellar tract*.

## Spino-olivary Tract

This tract conveys information to cerebellum from cutaneous and proprioceptive organs from the inferior olives of medulla oblongata. The fibers arising from olivary nucleus than participate in the formation of climbing fibers from the main input of cerebellar circuits.

## Spinotectal Tract

This tract provides afferent information for spinovisual reflex and brings about the *movements of eyes and head towards the source of stimulus*. The second order neuron relays in tectum of the midbrain.

## MOTOR TRACTS: THE DESCENDING TRACTS OF SPINAL CORD

As we had studied in Chapter 84, the sensory signals perceived by the somatosensory areas I and II are analyzed in posterior parietal cortex. Further, the somatosensory, auditory and visual inputs are processed in parieto-occipitotemporal association area and then projected to the prefrontal cortex in association with basal ganglia and cerebellum. This information is processed in prefrontal cortex, programs and plans the complex sequential motor activity. The primary motor cortex and premotor area then receives the complex input from somatosensory area and prefrontal cortex, which then initiates the motor activity through the motor tracts, which innervate the skeletal muscles. The motor activity initiated by motor cortex is fine tuned and scaled by basal ganglia and cerebellum. The main motor/descending tracts required for execution of motor activity are described below.

### Various Descending Tracts (Fig. 87.10)

- Pyramidal tract or corticospinal tract (main motor tract)
- Extrapyramidal tracts
    - Rubrospinal tract
    - Vestibulospinal tract
    - Reticulospinal tract
    - Tectospinal tract
    - Olivospinal tract

*Some important concepts*:
- *All the motor tracts are mainly two neuron system; the upper and lower motor neurons.*

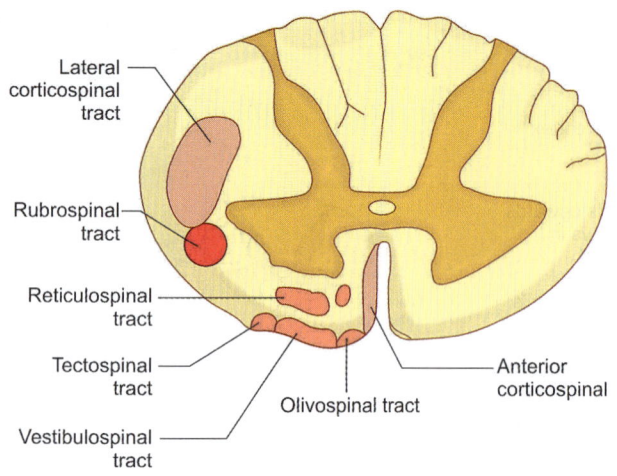

**Fig. 87.10:** Descending (motor) tracts.

- *Pyramidal tracts end directly and indirectly on lower motor neurons.*
- *Extrapyramidal tracts first end on internuncial cells and then on α and γ-neurons (lower motor neurons).*

## Corticospinal Tract/Pyramidal Tract (Fig. 87.11)

It is the main motor tract originating from motor area terminating in spinal cord. It has two divisions:
- Anterior corticospinal tract
- Lateral corticospinal tract.

> The hemorrhage or ischemia of internal capsule results in contralateral hemiplegia, i.e., complete paralysis of opposite side of the body.

The tract originates from area 4,6 of cerebrum and also from area 3,2,1, layer V, neurons called as **BETZ CELLS**.

The fibers then descend down through the internal capsule, which is the narrowest part of the entire tract.

The corticospinal tract then descends down till the medulla oblongata. Majority of fibers (around 90–95%) of fibers cross to opposite side at the level of medulla. This raises the surface of medulla, giving it the shape of pyramids. Hence, the corticospinal tract got its name as *pyramidal tract*. The fibers crossing to the opposite side descend down as *lateral corticospinal tract (LCST)*, which descend down in lateral white column of opposite side. However, the uncrossed fibers descend down in anterior white column as *anterior corticospinal tract (ACST)*.

The fibers of both the divisions of corticospinal tract terminate on the lower motor neurons of contralateral side. The LCST terminates on the neurons supplying the skeletal muscle of limbs whereas ACST terminates on the neurons supplying the axial muscles of neck and trunk.

### Functions of Pyramidal/Corticospinal Tract

- **Lateral CS tract:** Control of voluntary movements esp. the *fine, precise movements of fingers and hands* to carry out *skilled movements*.
- **Anterior CS tract:** Control of *muscles of trunk* and *proximal portions of the limbs* to carry out postural adjustments and gross movements.
- Forms a part of *superficial reflexes*
- *Sensory motor coordination*

### Extrapyramidal Tracts

All the other motor tract originating from CNS and terminating in the spinal cord are grouped under the

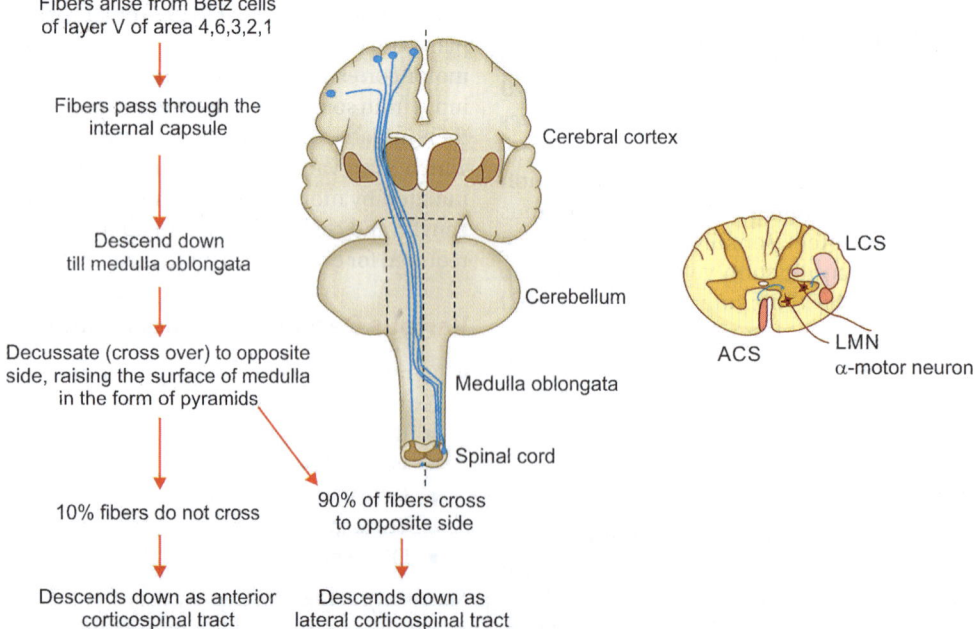

**Fig. 87.11:** Origin, course and termination of lateral and anterior corticospinal tracts.

extrapyramidal tracts. All these tracts are primarily concerned with the maintenance of tone and posture by affecting the antigravity muscles. **Table 87.2** summarizes the origin, course and functions of all the extrapyramidal tracts.

### Rubrospinal Tract (Fig. 87.12)

It is an alternate route of pyramidal system to influence the lower motor neuron. The fibers originate from the red nucleus of the midbrain. It is primarily concerned with maintenance of *muscle tone and posture*. It *increases the tone in flexors and inhibits the extensors*.

The lesions of rubrospinal tract result in increased tone of extensors resulting the rigidity of antigravity muscles.

### Functions of Extrapyramidal Tracts

- They are responsible for *control of tone, posture and equilibrium*.
- Control of *movement of body and limbs* such as co-ordinated movements of arms and legs during walking.
- Exert *tonic inhibitory control* over the lower centers. Their damage increases rigidity of the muscles.

**Table 87.2:** Origin, course and functions of extrapyramidal tracts.

| Tract | Origin and course | Functions |
|---|---|---|
| **Rubrospinal tract (Fig. 86.12)** (alternate route of pyramidal system to influence LMN) | • Red nucleus in the midbrain<br>• Descends down in the lateral white column<br>• End on α and γ neurons in anterior horn cells | • Facilitates the activity of flexor muscles<br>• Inhibits the activity of extensors or antigravity muscles |
| **Tectospinal tract** | • From superior colliculi<br>• Cross to opposite side and descend in anterior white matter (tectospinal tract)<br>• Most of fibers terminate in anterior gray column in Upper Cervical Segments of spinal cord by synapsing on internuncial neurons | • Concerned with reflex postural movements of head and neck with visual stimuli<br>• Corticonuclear fibers of control the movements of the eye balls |
| **Reticulospinal tract** | • Reticular nuclei present in brain stem (pontine and medullary)<br>• Crossed fibers and uncrossed fibers end on α and γ neurons | • Influence voluntary movements and reflex activity<br>• Facilitatory and inhibitory to the muscles |
| **Vestibulospinal tract** | • From vestibular nuclei at the junction of pons and medulla<br>• Axons descend in vestibulospinal tract<br>• End on α and γ neurons<br>• No crossing of fibers | • Effects mainly extensor muscles of the body<br>• Concerned with posture regulation of the body |

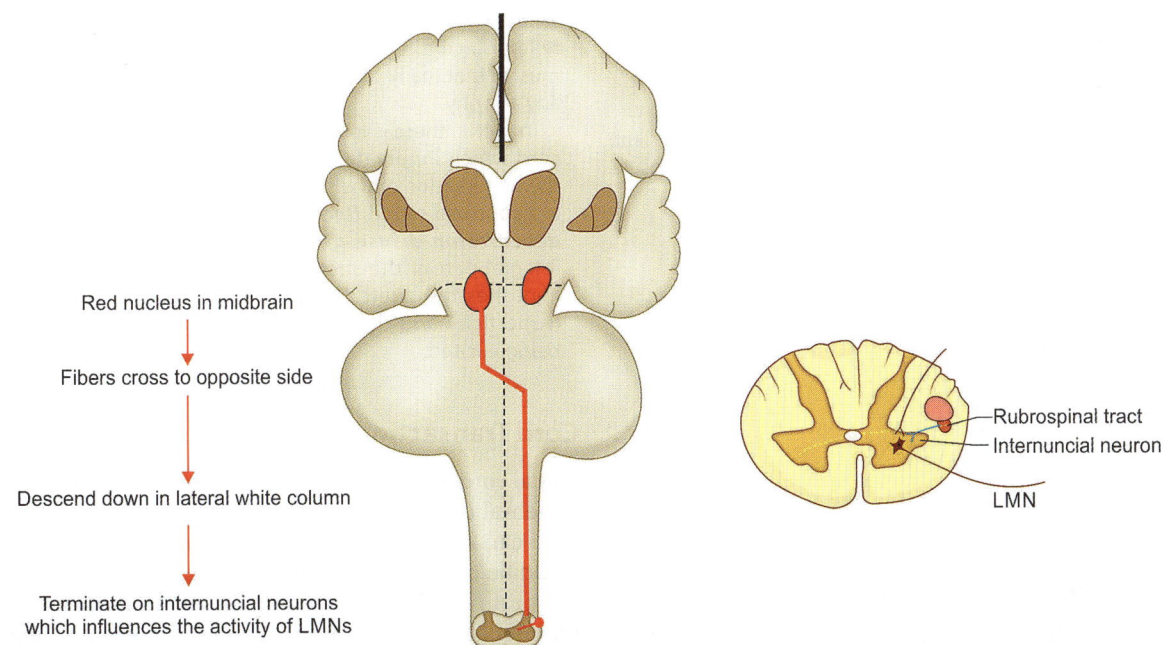

**Fig. 87.12:** Rubrospinal tract.

## SOME COMMON LESIONS OF SPINAL CORD

The spinal cord lesions in the form of trauma, tumor, compression, ischemia or hemorrhage result in functional loss in spinal cord. The specific clinical presentation helps in diagnosis and management of spinal lesions. Let's start with the specific lesion of the tracts and then the generalized lesion.

### Lesions of Pyramidal Tracts (Fig. 87.13)

The most common site of pyramidal tract lesion is internal capsule, which is the narrowest part in the entire tract. The lesion most commonly occurs due to hemorrhage or ischemia. In common language, it is called as *'Brain Attack or Stroke.'*

It results in contralateral hemiplegia, i.e., paralysis of opposite half of the body. There is muscle weakness and the patient has spasticity.

There is upper motor neuron type of lesion. The patient has hemiplegic or spastic gait **(Fig. 87.14)**. In this, the patient is not able to flex the spastic limb, hence drags his paralyzed foot on the ground, making a semicircle and supports his body weight on the other side of the body.

The hemorrhage in left internal capsule, the dominant hemisphere, there is hemiplegia of the right half of the body along with the damage to the Wernick's area resulting in aphasia and agnosia. The patient may not be able to communicate with his family members in this case.

Post stroke spasticity of left lower extremity

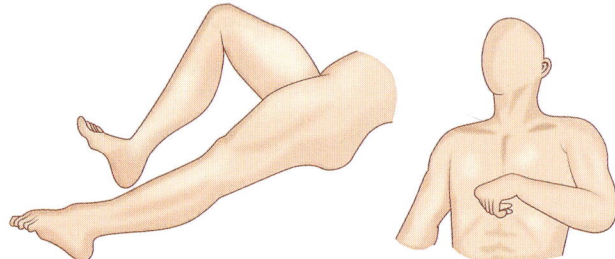

**Fig. 87.13:** The spasticity of the left upper and lower limb (contralateral hemiplegia) after the stroke in right internal capsule.

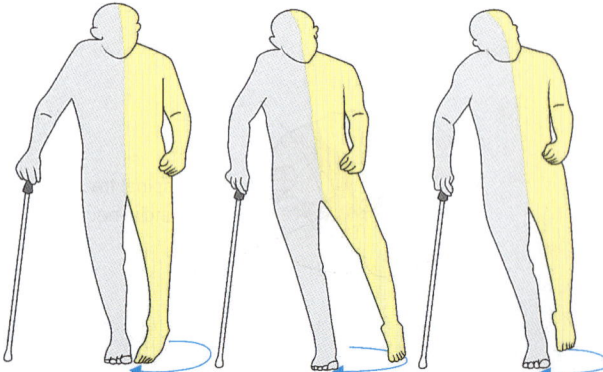

**Fig. 87.14:** Spastic gait in the patient with left sided contralateral hemiplegia.

### Upper Motor Neuron and Lower Motor Neuron Lesion

The upper motor neuron lesion (UMNL) refers to damage/ *lesion of the pyramidal or extrapyramidal tract or both resulting in loss of inhibitory influence of upper motor neurons* on the lower motor neurons.

The lower motor neuron lesion (LMNL) occurs when there is a *lesion of alpha motor neuron, arising from anterior horn cells*. **Table 87.3** tabulates the differences between upper and lower motor neuron lesions.

> *Explain the physiological basis of:*
> - *Hyperactive deep tendon reflexes in upper motor neuron lesion*
> - *Absent deep and superficial reflexes in LMNL*
> - *Spastic paralysis in UMNL and flaccid paralysis in LMNL*
> - *Why there is not so significant muscle atrophy in UMNL?*
>
> The answers to all the questions mentioned above lies in the fact that UMNs influence (inhibit) the locally active stretch reflex operational between the skeletal muscle and the spinal cord.
>
> In a normal person, the stretch reflex is always active due to the anatomical stretching of muscle. The UMNs keep the stretch reflex under control by controlling the discharge from the UMNs (pyramidal and extrapyramidal tracts).
>
> **In UMNL,** there is loss of the inhibitory influence of the UMNs, which leaves the stretch reflex unchecked. Hence, there is increased contraction of skeletal muscle in response to the stretch. This results in **hypertonia** in skeletal muscle. When this hypertonia occurs in only one group of muscles (due to pure corticospinal tract lesion), it results in **spasticity**. However, if both the flexors and extensors are involved (mixed lesion involving damage to pyramidal and extrapyramidal tracts), there is **rigidity** of the muscles. When the deep reflexes are examined in these patients, they show an **exaggerated** response due to the hyperactive stretch reflex. Since, the LMNs are intact in this type of lesion, the muscle is actually NOT denervated and hence doesn't show any atrophy.
>
> In LMNL, there is loss of the LMNs arising from the spinal cord which innervate the skeletal muscles. This results in the denervation of the skeletal muscles and hence resulting in hypotonia called **flaccid paralysis**. The muscle undergo **denervation disuse atrophy**. Further, the LMNs are an integral part of the stretch reflex, making its efferent arm, abolishes the stretch reflex. Hence, NONE of the reflexes (superficial and deep), mediated through the LMNs are being elicited.

### Cord Transaction

Spinal cord is a very delicate structure, housed in the bony vertebral column. But still in some situations, the spinal cord can be damaged/cut (transacted). This transaction could be complete in which it is completely severed from the brain stem or there could be a partial injury. It can happen at any level, depending on the site and type of injury.

**Table 87.3:** Differences between upper and lower motor neuron lesion.

| | Upper motor neuron | Lower motor neuron |
|---|---|---|
| Definition | The motor fibers arising from higher centers and influencing the activity of α and γ neurons | The motor fibers arising from higher centers and influencing the activity of α and γ neurons |
| Diagram | *Stretch reflex showing upper and lower motor neurons* | |
| Muscle involvement | Involves a group of muscles | Involves single muscle |
| Paralysis | Spastic paralysis | Flaccid paralysis |
| Muscle atrophy | Not severe | Severe disuse atrophy |
| Deep reflexes | Hyperactive | Absent |
| Superficial reflexes | Lost | Absent |
| Babinski sign | Positive | Not elicited |

## Complete Cord Transaction

Here are a few causes complete cord transaction:
- Fracture dislocation of vertebrae
- Gunshot injuries
- Experimental section of cord in animals

There are three stages of events occurring after complete cord transaction:
- **Stage of spinal shock**
  - Here the person is conscious
  - All the sensations below the cord are absent on both the sides
  - All reflexes (superficial and deep) are absent at the level of lesion, indicating the lower motor neuron lesion
  - If the spinal cord transaction occurs between the levels of T1 to L2, the sympathetic fibers are damages. This is followed by the fall in blood pressure due to lack of sympathetic supply and sympathetic tone.
  - The damage to cervical region results in diaphragmatic paralysis but the blood pressure is normal because the sympathetic nerves are not damaged.
  - There is loss of tone of smooth muscles of bladder and rectum resulting in retention of urine and feces.
  - The duration of spinal shock depends on degree of encephalization of the animal. More the encephalization more is the duration of spinal shock.

  In a cat, spinal shock last from few minutes–few hours, in a monkey, spinal shock last for few days. However in humans, spinal shock last from days–weeks.

- **Stage of recovery:**
  - *At the level of injury:* The muscles show a typical LMN lesion showing:
    - Flaccid paralysis
    - Hypotonia
    - Absent reflexes
    - Reaction of degeneration is present
  - *Below the level of injury:* The muscles show features of UMN damage:
    - Hypertonia in present (spasticity or rigidity) **(Table 87.4)**

**Table 87.4:** Lesions of pure corticospinal and extrapyramidal tract lesion.

| Pure corticospinal tract lesion | Extrapyramidal tract lesion |
|---|---|
| Loss of fine skilled movements | Gross movements lost |
| Hypotonia | • Hypertonia (CS and Ex Pyr: Spasticity; Only Pyr Tracts: Rigidity)<br>• Clasp knife spasticity |
| • Absent superficial reflexes<br>• Exaggerated deep reflexes<br>• Babinski's positive<br>• Clonus present | |

During the recovery process:

> TIP: is **SaFE**
> **S**- Smooth muscle
> **F**- Flexor muscles
> **E**- Extensor muscles

- The tone in *smooth muscles* appear first in which the:
    - Urinary bladder becomes autonomous
    - Blood vessels regain tone → improvement in BP
- Then the tone appears in *flexor muscles* resulting in:
    - **Paraplegia in flexion:** The tone in the flexor muscles increases. There is spastic paralysis, which is overlapped by the sudden flexor spasms
    - **Flexor reflex develops:** Painful stimulus results in sudden flexor contraction.
    - **Mass reflex appears:** There is mass evacuation of bowel and bladder on stimulation.
- In the end, the tone appears in *extensor muscles*: There is increase in the tone of extensor muscles called paraplegia in extension.
- **Fatal outcome**: If the patient shows any improvement, as described above due to infection or low nutrition, the patient can go into fatal outcome. The patient may go into stage of degeneration. In this condition,
    - Extensor muscles lose their tone first
    - Flexor muscles lose their tone next
    - Smooth muscles lose their tone in the end resulting in dribbling urine and fall in BP.

### Hemisection of Spinal Cord (Brown-Sequard Syndrome)

There is a lesion in one half of the spinal cord (hemisection of spinal cord). This shows a typical response, shown in **Figure 87.15**. A patient with hemisection of spinal cord would present with the complaints loss of sensations carried by spinothalamic tracts (touch, pain, temperature and pressure) on one half of the body and sensations carried by dorsal column tract (fine touch, vibration and proprioception) in the other half of body below the level of injury. The physical examination of this patient suggests that the *spinothalamic tract is affected on the contralateral side, while dorsal column is affected on the same side below the level of lesion*. To find out the level of lesion, the patient will have *lower motor neuron type of flaccid paralysis* along with hyperalgesia (increased pain sensation, touch feels like pain). As we can see the **Figure 87.15**, the ipsilateral muscles *below the lesion have UMNL* while the *contralateral side has no motor deficit*.

### Syringomyelia (Fig. 87.16)

Syringomyelia is a developmental abnormality, where there is *dilation of central canal*. It is mostly present just below medulla oblongata which leads to *compression of lateral spinothalamic tracts* of both sides. Hence, the patient presents with loss of pain, touch, temp, pressure in neck, shoulder and upper limbs *'SHAWL LIKE distribution of clinical presentation'.*

### Poliomyelitis

Poliomyelitis is an acute *ascending viral infection* of neurons of *anterior gray column of spinal cord and the motor nuclei of cranial nerves* (**Fig. 87.17**). There is flaccid paralysis; wasting of muscles due to the involvement of lower motor neurons. The lower limbs are more affected than upper limbs.

### Multiple Sclerosis

There is *demyelination of ascending and descending tracts*. It has the autoimmune/hereditary/infective pathology. There is invasion of brain and spinal cord by some

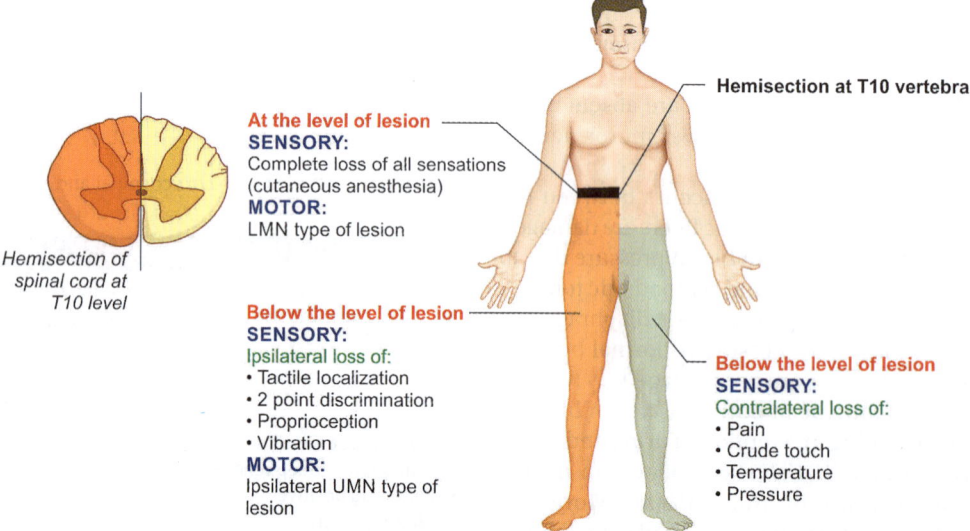

**Fig. 87.15:** Brown-Sequard syndrome.

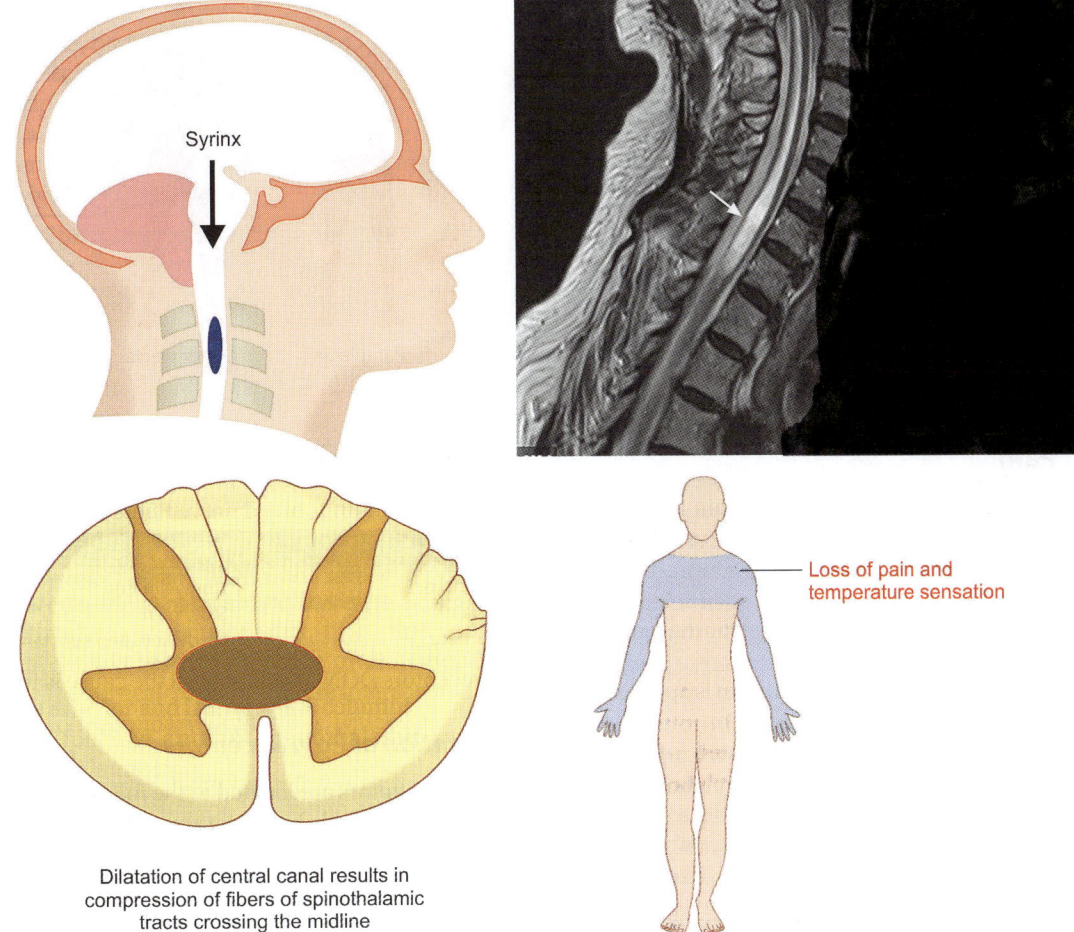

Fig. 87.16: Syringomyelia.

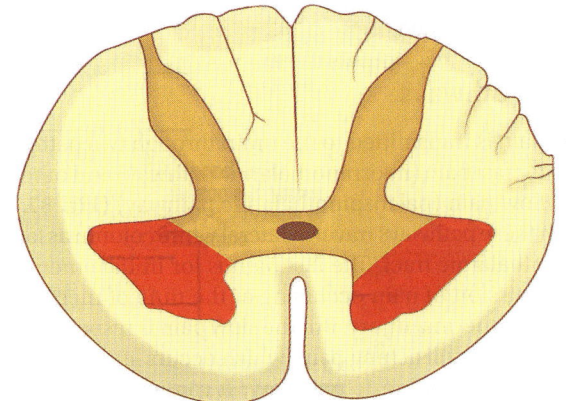

Fig. 87.17: Viral infection of anterior gray horns of spinal cord resulting in lower motor neuron damage.

infection allowing leukocytes to enter immunologically protected CNS, resulting in weakness of muscles, ataxia and spastic paralysis.

## Types of Paralysis (Fig. 87.18)

- Hemiplegia—paralysis of one side of body
- Monoplegia—paralysis of one limb only
- Diplegia—paralysis of two corresponding limbs
- Paraplegia—paralysis of two lower limbs
- Quadriplegia—paralysis of all four limbs

# PAIN AND ANALGESIA SYSTEM

## PAIN

Pain is defined as an unpleasant sensory and emotional experience associated with actual or potential tissue damage.

### Causes of Pain

- **Mechanical deformity/stimuli:** Too much distortion, injury or cut
- **Thermal stimuli:** Any temperature >45°C and < 10°C
- **Chemical stimuli:** Histamine, bradykinin, serotonin, excess $K^+$, excess Ach, prostaglandins, lactic acid
- **Biological stimuli:** Bacterial/viral/parasitic infections, etc.

### Physiological Responses to Pain

Change in blood pressure, heart rate, respiration and vasomotor tone, sweating and other protective responses primarily mediated by the sympathetic nervous system.

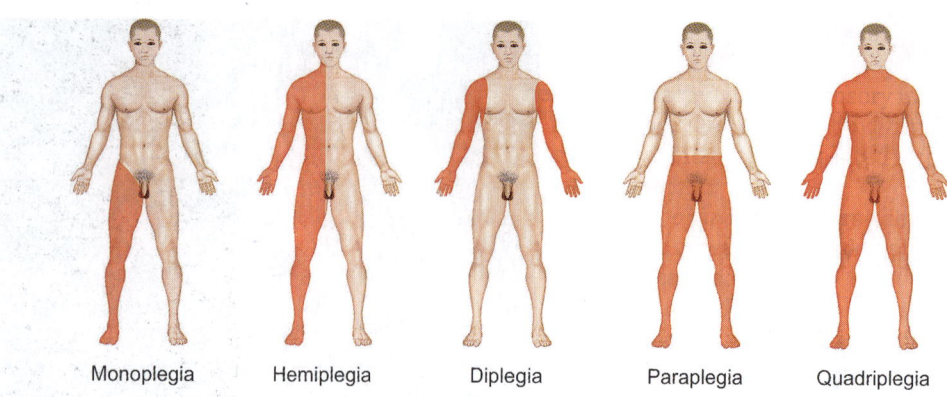

Fig. 87.18: Types of paralysis.

## Types of Pain

Depending on the duration of onset, the pain is classified as:
- **Acute pain:**
  - Sudden onset
  - Sharp pain/fast pain/pricking pain/cutting pain/first pain
  - Against a painful stimulus the first pain is appreciated as sharp, bright and localized sensation
  - The fast pain travels through myelinated A-fibers
- **Chronic pain:**
  - Present for considerable time
  - Slow pain/ache/dull pain/throbbing pain/second pain
  - Inflammatory pain or neuropathic pain
  - It follows first pain and is dull, aching and more diffuse.
  - The slow pain travels through unmyelinated C-fibers.

Differences between fast and slow pain are summarized in **Table 87.5**.

**Table 87.5:** Differences between fast and slow pain.

| First pain/acute pain/fast pain | Second pain/chronic pain/slow pain |
|---|---|
| The first pain is appreciated as sharp, bright, localized sensation | The second pain is follows the first pain as dull, aching, more diffuse |
| Felt within 0.1 second | Felt after 1 second or more |
| Acute in nature | Chronic in nature |
| Person react immediately | Person react—trying to relieve the cause of pain |
| Myelinated fibers A delta type | Nonmyelinated C type of fibers |
| Rate of conduction of impulse 6–10 meters/second | Rate of conduction of impulse 0.5–2 meter/second |
| Pricking type (needle) | Burning, aching, throbbing, nauseous |
| Superficial tissue damage | Deep tissue damage |
| Pricking pain pathway | Tissue destruction too; made burning pain pathway |

## Receptors for Pain

Naked nerve endings of A d nerve fibers

| A d fibers | C fibers |
|---|---|
| Myelinated | Unmyelinated |
| Fast pain | Slow pain |
| Glutamate | Bradykinin and substance P |

Pain receptors DONOT adapt until the cause is REMOVED

### Localization of Pain Receptors

The pain receptors are located at the following sites:
- Cutaneous (in skin) → most abundant
- In periosteum
- In joints
- In deeper tissues (muscle, viscera) → less
- Walls of arteries/blood vessels
- *Brain has no pain receptors*, but they are present in Falx tentorium and crus cerebri which produces pain when stretched.

## Pain Pathways

The pain is transmitted to the brain through two pathways, one for fast pain (neospinothalamic pathway) and other for the slow pain (paleospinothalamic pathway) **(Fig. 87.19)**. Both these pathways travel in lateral white column as lateral spinothalamic tract. The fast pain is for initial emergency transmission of pain occurring at the time of mechanical injury or thermal injury. But the slow pain is responsible for the chronic dull aching pain, which occurs later.

- **Neospinothalamic pathway:** It carries the *sensation of fast pain* through *A$\delta$ glutaminergic* fibers. It transmits *mechanical and acute thermal pain*. Some fibers terminate in the reticular areas of the brain stem while most of them relay in VPL nucleus of thalamus. From here the third order neurons send the signals to somatosensory cortex and basal portions of cerebrum. This pathway can help the exact localization of pain provided the touch receptors are also stimulated along with it. The tactile stimulation is mediated by dorsal column, hence resulting in better localization.

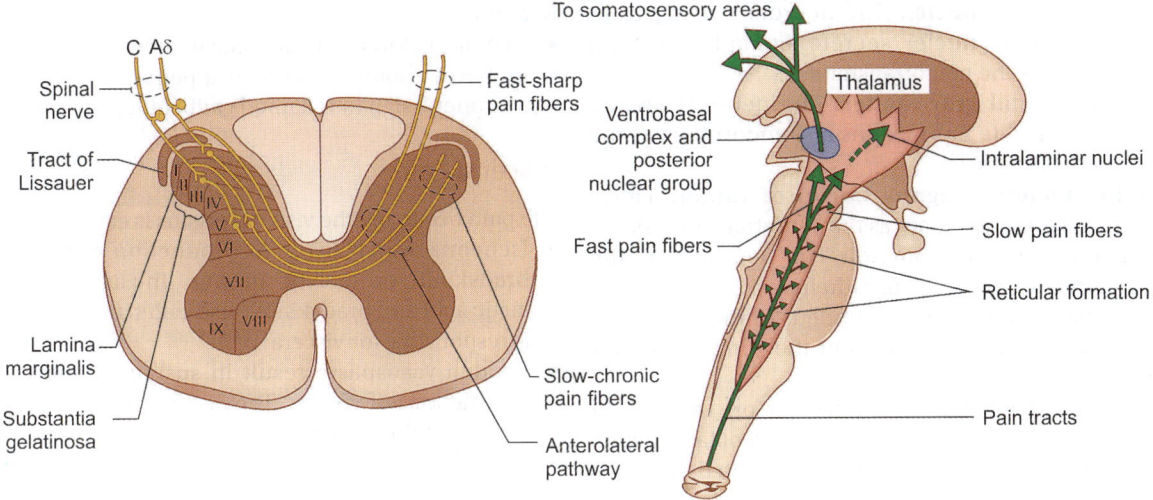

**Fig. 87.19:** Origin, course and termination of neospinothalamic and paleospinothalamic pathways

- **Paleospinothalamic pathway:** It is a much older system, which transmits pain sensation received from slow *chronic C type of pain fibers*. The fibers synapse multiple times in dorsal horn of spinal cord before giving the neuron with long axon which ascend upwards carrying the pain sensation. The type C fibers secrete the neurotransmitter *substance P and glutamate*. This pathway terminates widely in brainstem, while some fibers pass to thalamus terminating in any of these areas:
  - *Reticular nuclei of medulla, pons and mesencephalon*
  - *The tectal area of mesencephalon*
  - *The periaqueductal gray matter*.

The localization of pain in this pathway is very poor.

**Management of intractable cancer patients—a palliative treatment:** The patients with intractable cancer pain are often advised palliative pain management by cutting the pain pathway or cauterizing the specific pain area in intralaminar nuclei in thalamus.

## ANALGESIA SYSTEM

Our body has an inherent mechanism to cope up with pain, called the analgesia system of the body. It originates from the nuclei present in third ventricle as shown in **Figure 87.20**.

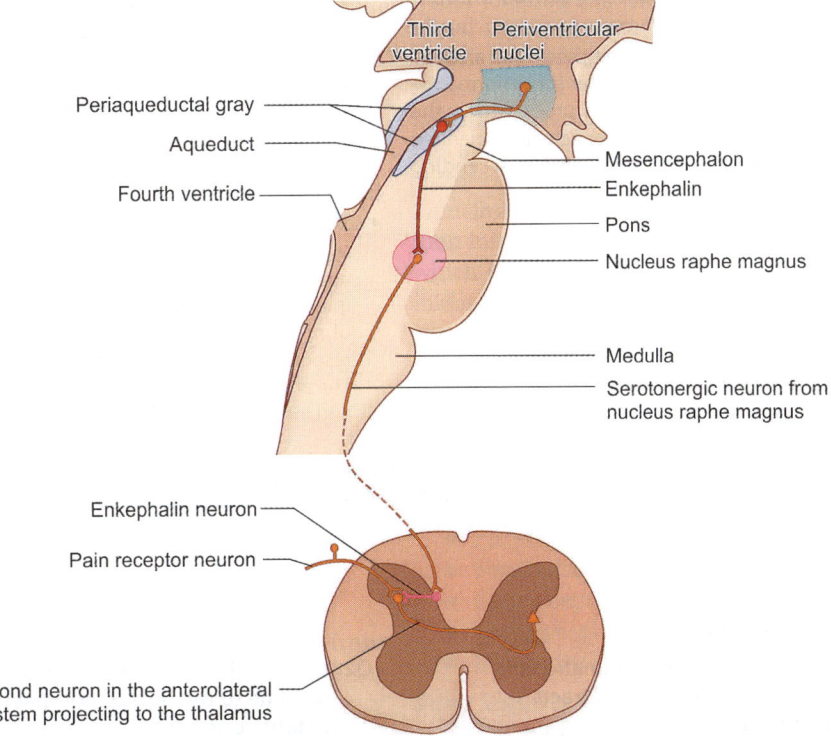

**Fig. 87.20:** Analgesia pathway.

- **Periventricular nuclei:** The neurons arising from periventricular nuclei secrete Enkephalins and endorphins as the neurotransmitters.
- **Periaqueductal gray matter:** The neurons arising from here secrete Enkephalins and endorphins as the neurotransmitters.
- **Raphe nucleus/magnus nuclei of raphe:** These neurons secrete serotonin as the neurotransmitters.
- **Paragigantocellular nuclei:** The neurons arising from here are part of the noradrenergic system, which originates from the locus coeruleus in the brainstem and projects widely throughout the central nervous system.

Since, these neurotransmitters act on the opioid receptors, they are called the opioid system/opiate system. The exogenous morphine, when administered, attaches to periventricular and PAG, hypothalamus, pituitary and relieves pain. Similarly, endogenous opioids (Enkephalins and endorphins) act on these opioid receptors. Hence, they are also called as mood elevators.

## Referred Pain

Referred pain is the pain produced in viscera, due to some reason, but felt at some other point on the surface of the body due to the same dermatomal innervation of somatic part and viscera. Further, there is poor localization of viscera on brain.

**Example:**
- Angina pectoris in myocardial infarction
- McBurney point in inflamed appendix
- Murphey's sign in inflamed gallbladder

## Visceral Pain

The pain occurring the visceral organs is caused due to:
- Ischemia which leads to production of lactic acid, bradykinin, proteolytic enzyme. The accumulation of lactic acid and bradykinin (also called the substance P) is responsible for visceral pain.
- Sudden vasospasm result in sustained and forceful contractions of viscera. The occlusion of blood vessels result in ischemic pain.
- Whenever there is over distension of viscera, it result in occlusion of blood vessel and result in ischemic pain.
- Various chemicals like hydrochloric acid in stomach during peptic ulcer stimulate nerve endings (peptic ulcer).
- Pain fibers from above thoracic pain line and below the pelvic pain line are carried by parasympathetic pathways.
- Between these two lines are carried by sympathetic pathways.

**Anesthesia:** No sensation of pain
**Hyperalgesia:** Increased pain sensation
**Analgesia:** Relief of pain
**Allodynia:** Touch causing pain

## SUMMARY

- Spinal cord is located in the vertebral column have 31 spinal segments. The anterior root is motor and posterior root is sensory (Bell Magendie Law).
- The spinal cord is a conduit between the peripheral and the central nervous system, which carries the sensory information from the receptors to the CNS, which is processed in the cerebral cortex and the appropriate motor activity is planned in the motor cortex, which is executed. Various ascending tracts are:
    - Anterolateral spinothalamic tracts
    - Dorsal column tracts
    - Anterior and posterior spinocerebellar tracts
    - Spinotectal, spinoreticular and spino-olivary tracts
  
  The descending tracts are:
    - Corticospinal tract/pyramidal tracts
    - Extrapyramidal tracts like rubrospinal tract, olivospinal, tectospinal, reticulospinal tract
- The spinal cord lesions result in the loss of spinal cord function.
    - Motor loss: Lower motor neuron lesion occurs at the level of lesion and upper motor neuron lesion below the level of lesion.
    - Sensory loss: Complete transaction results in complete sensory loss. But hemisection results loss of sensations carried by spinothalamic tract on the contralateral side and sensations carried by dorsal column on the same side, below the lesion (Brown-Sequard syndrome).
- The pain pathway, lateral corticospinal pathway, is composed of two types of fibers, neospinothalamic tract for fast pain and paleospinothalamic tract for slow pain. The fast pain is for initial emergency transmission of pain occurring at the time of mechanical injury or thermal injury. But the slow pain is responsible for the chronic dull aching pain, which occurs later. The analgesia system in the body acts on the opiate receptors and inhibits the pain fibers by the gate control theory of pain.

### LET US SEE, HOW MUCH YOU HAVE LEARNT?

 *Review Questions*

### Long/Short Answer Questions

Q1. Describe the origin, course and termination of:
   a. Anterior and lateral spinothalamic tracts
   b. Dorsal column tract
   c. Corticospinal tract

Q2. What will happen to the sensory system if there is damage to the dorsal root ganglia, as seen in a patient of tabes dorsalis?

Q3. Describe the Brown-Sequard syndrome in terms of cause, and physiological basis of clinical presentation.
Q4. Differentiate between upper and lower motor neuron disease.
Q5. Differentiate between fast and slow pain.
Q6. What will happen, if there is hemorrhage in the right internal capsule?
Q7. Describe the analgesia system.

## Explain Why? (Give Reasons)

Q1. Damage to the dorsal columns of the spinal cord affects proprioception and fine touch sensation.
Q2. Lesions in the lateral spinothalamic tract result in loss of pain and temperature sensation.
Q3. A complete spinal cord injury at the cervical level can lead to quadriplegia.
Q4. Damage to the corticospinal tract results in muscle weakness and spasticity.
Q5. Lesions of the pyramidal tract cause hyperreflexia and a positive Babinski sign.
Q6. The spinocerebellar tracts are essential for coordinating muscle movements.
Q7. The anterolateral system is involved in transmitting pain and temperature sensations to the brain.
Q8. Hemisection of the spinal cord (Brown-Séquard syndrome) results in ipsilateral loss of motor function and contralateral loss of pain and temperature sensation.
Q9. Central cord syndrome typically affects upper limb function more than lower limb function.
Q10. The descending tracts are crucial for voluntary motor control and the modulation of reflexes.

## Multiple Choice Questions

Q1. A ventrolateral cordotomy is performed that produces relief of pain in the right leg. It is effective because it interrupts the:
 a. Left dorsal column
 b. Left ventrolateral spinothalamic tract
 c. Right ventrolateral spinothalamic tract
 d. Right medial lemniscal pathway

Q2. A 32-year-old woman experienced the sudden onset of a severe cramping pain in the abdominal region. She also became nauseated. List some of the common features of visceral pain.
 a. It results from activation of nociceptors in the viscera that are innervated by the same fibers as innervate skin, induces rapid sharp pain, causes spasms of the visceral muscle, and shows relatively rapid adaptation
 b. It is mediated by Aδ and C fibers in the ventral roots of spinal nerves, radiates to a nearby or distant somatic structure, is accompanied by sweating, and is relayed to the cortex by the spinothalamic tract
 c. It is poorly localized, is accompanied by sweating, radiates to a somatic structure that may be some distance away, and is relayed to the somatosensory cortex via the spinothalamic tract
 d. It requires simultaneous activation of nociceptors within and outside of the viscera, causes spasms of the visceral and skeletal muscle, and is relayed to the cortex by the dorsal column pathway

Q3. Your patient complains that he burned his hand on his portable heater but did not feel the stimulus. The patient also notes that he has difficulty using either hand. You note that the patient has no response to pinprick in skin of either hand, arm, or shoulder and a bilateral wasting of intrinsic hand muscles. You suspect that the patient has:
 a. Syringomyelia
 b. Multiple sclerosis
 c. Poliomyelitis
 d. Brown-Sequard syndrome

Q4. A construction worker falls off a ladder and fractures a vertebra. A neurological exam conducted 2 weeks after the accident reveals that the individual has a complete hemisection of the right side of the spinal cord at T5. In this patient, you might expect a pain and temperature loss:
 a. In the upper and lower limbs on the left
 b. In all dermatomes below T7 on the left
 c. In the T3 dermatome on the right
 d. Below the T5 dermatome on the right

Q5. A tumor is beginning to compress the right side of the spinal cord at the C3 spinal cord segment and is impinging on the corticospinal and spinothalamic tracts. What might you expect to observe first in the patient?
 a. Alteration of pain and temperature sensations from the left upper limb
 b. Alteration of pain and temperature sensations from the left lower limb
 c. Spastic weakness of the left upper limb
 d. Spastic weakness of the left lower limb

Q6. Your patient has suffered trauma to the spinal cord. During a period of spinal shock, what might you expect to observe in the patient?
 a. Hyperactive reflexes below the lesion
 b. Flaccid weakness below the lesion
 c. A spastic bladder
 d. A clasp knife reflex

Q7. Cutting a dorsal root of a spinal nerve may result in:
 a. Hypotonia in skeletal muscles innervated by the cut root
 b. Fasciculations in skeletal muscles innervated by the cut root
 c. Reversed cutaneous reflexes in skin over the denervated muscle
 d. Anterograde degeneration of axons in the spinothalamic tract

Q8. A neurological exam of your patient reveals a loss of vibratory sense in the lower limb on the right, weakness and hyperactive reflexes in the lower limb on the right, and a loss of pain and temperature that begins below the T8 dermatome on the left. Where is the lesion?

a. T6 spinal cord segment on the right
b. T8 spinal cord segment on the right
c. T10 spinal cord segment on the right
d. T8 spinal cord segment on the left

## ANSWERS

**1.** b    **2.** c    **3.** b    **4.** b    **5.** b    **6.** b    **7.** a    **8.** a

# Reticular Activating System (RAS)

**CHAPTER 88**

**COMPETENCY ADDRESSED**

PY10.5: Describe and discuss structure and functions of **reticular activating system**, autonomic nervous system (ANS).

**LEARNING OBJECTIVE**

At the end of this chapter, the learner should be able to:
- Describe the structure and the functions of the reticular activating system.

## ANATOMY AND STRUCTURE OF RAS

The reticular formation is a complex group of nuclei located in the brainstem. Based on their location they are classified as medullary reticular formation, pontine reticular formation and mid brain reticular formation. The neurons pass from these nuclei and end in nonspecific nuclei of thalamus. From the thalamus, neurons project to all the parts of cerebral cortex. All the sensations give collateral to reticular nuclei in pons and medulla. The ascending fibers, hence, activates the brain.

These nuclei received the inputs from the somato-sensory projections in the spinal cord; which further project to all parts of the cerebral cortex and results in diffuse cortical excitation.

Physiologically, the afferent connections of the reticular formation send collaterals to ascending reticular formation and involves slow pain.

The *gigantocellular neurons of reticular excitatory area*, located in pons and midbrain, secrete *acetyl choline* which is an excitatory neurotransmitter. The fibers arising from pons and midbrain divide into two branches, ascending and descending reticular formations. Hence, the efferent connections, based on direction of neurons, are classified as:

1. **Ascending reticular formation (Fig. 88.1):** The neurons arising from the brainstem reticular nuclei ascending towards the cerebral cortex via thalamus. Example, spinoreticular tract and thalamocortical fibers.
2. **Descending reticular formation:** The neurons descending into the spinal cord. Example reticulospinal tract. It affects the extensor tone, as it forms the part of the extrapyramidal system.

- It gives collaterals to cerebellum and basal ganglia for maintain the tone of muscle and body posture.
- It also gives collaterals to substantia gelatinosa and forms the analgesia system.
- The collateral to respiratory, vagal, sympathetic preganglionic neurons are given out to control respiratory, cardiac and vasomotor tone.

## FUNCTIONS OF RAS

- Awakeness, alertness, awareness, consciousness is a function of RAS
- Perception of other sensations also depends on RAS which is more when RAS is activated
- It is responsible for maintaining the conscious

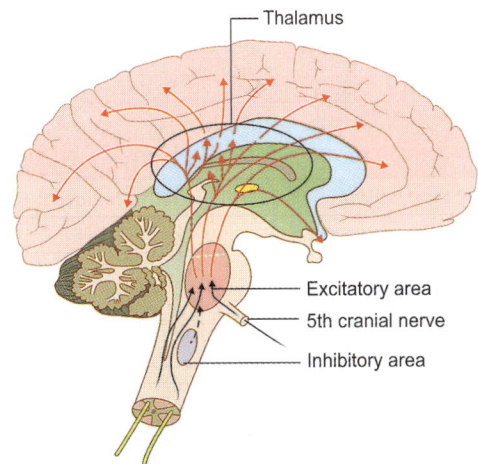

**Fig. 88.1:** Reticular ascending system showing the pontine and medullary reticular formation.

- Along with the extrapyramidal tracts, it is responsible for maintenance of tone and posture.
- It modulates pain by analgesia system.
- It maintains sleep wakefulness cycles through:
  - Serotonin (5-HT) secreting neurons induce slow wave sleep
  - Noradrenergic and acetylcholinergic neurons influence REM sleep
  - RAS through the intralaminar nuclei of the thalamus is responsible for wakefulness
- Autonomic function through its connections with limbic system.

## SUMMARY

The reticular activating system is group of interconnected nuclei, scattered in the brainstem, responsible for the generalized overall awareness about the sensations in the brain. In return, it also maintains the tone and posture of the body. It plays an important role in sleep, emotions and analgesia system.

## LET US SEE, HOW MUCH YOU HAVE LEARNT?

### Review Questions

Q1. Explain the physiological anatomy of reticular activating system.

Q2. Discuss the role of reticular activating system in sleep wake cycle.

Q3. What are the various functions of RAS?

### Multiple Choice Questions

Q1. The reticular formation plays a crucial role in regulating the sleep-wake cycle. During which phase of sleep is the reticular formation most active?
   a. Rapid eye movement (REM) sleep
   b. Nonrapid eye movement (NREM) sleep
   c. Deep sleep
   d. Transition from wakefulness to sleep

Q2. Imagine a person is involved in a car accident, and emergency responders are trying to assess their level of consciousness. Which part of the reticular formation is likely to be involved in maintaining arousal and attention in this situation?
   a. Raphe nuclei
   b. Locus coeruleus
   c. Medial geniculate nucleus
   d. Pontine reticular formation

Q3. In a noisy classroom, a teacher is able to focus on the student's question and ignore the background noise. Which function of the reticular formation is demonstrated in this scenario?
   a. Motor coordination
   b. Sensory filtering
   c. Autonomic control
   d. Emotional processing

Q4. A patient presents with difficulties in maintaining consciousness and shows signs of impaired arousal. After a brain injury, which part of the reticular formation might be affected?
   a. Mesencephalic reticular formation
   b. Pontine reticular formation
   c. Medullary reticular formation
   d. Lateral reticular nucleus

Q5. During a medical examination, a doctor taps the knee of a patient, and the leg jerks involuntarily. Which aspect of the reticular formation is involved in this reflex activity?
   a. Sensory filtering
   b. Autonomic control
   c. Descending motor pathways
   d. Ascending sensory pathways

**ANSWERS**

1. b   2. b   3. b   4. a   5. c

# Physiology of Limbic System, Speech, Memory, EEG and Sleep

**89 CHAPTER**

## COMPETENCY ADDRESSED

**PY10.7:** Describe and discuss functions of cerebral cortex, basal ganglia, thalamus, hypothalamus, cerebellum and limbic system and their abnormalities.
**PY10.8:** Describe and discuss behavioral and EEG characteristics during sleep and mechanism responsible for its production.
**PY10.9:** Describe and discuss the physiological basis of memory, learning and speech.
**PY10.12:** Identify normal EEG forms.

## LEARNING OBJECTIVES

**At the end of this chapter, the learner should be able to:**
- Describe the physiology of emotions through the limbic system.
- Describe the disorders related to the limbic system.
- Describe the physiology of speech and the disorders of speech.
- Describe the physiology of learning and memory and the related disorders.
- Describe the physiology of normal electroencephalography.
- Describe the stages and types of sleep and the physiology of sleep.
- Describe the EEG changes in each stage of sleep.
- Describe the disorders of sleep.

In the previous chapters we had studied the highly specialized sensory and motor functions of the cerebral cortex. But the cerebrum is not just pure sensory and motor system, it is actually a whole central processing unit which handles many other functions like speech, emotion, sleep learning and memory. All these functions are carried out through a wide variety of neuronal connections and neurotransmitters. Let us study these functions one by one in detail.

## PHYSIOLOGY OF EMOTIONS—THE LIMBIC SYSTEM

The limbic system derives its name from the border, as it is made of the bordering structures around the basal regions of cerebrum. But now, the studies have shown that these basal structures also participate in the limbic system. **Figure 89.1** shows the parts of the limbic system, which are interconnected with diencephalon and basal ganglia.

The overall functioning of limbic system can be consolidated into a single pneumonic: HOME, which means homeostasis, Olfaction, Memory processing and Emotions. Talking about each of the parts separately; we can see that the hypothalamus is an important part of the

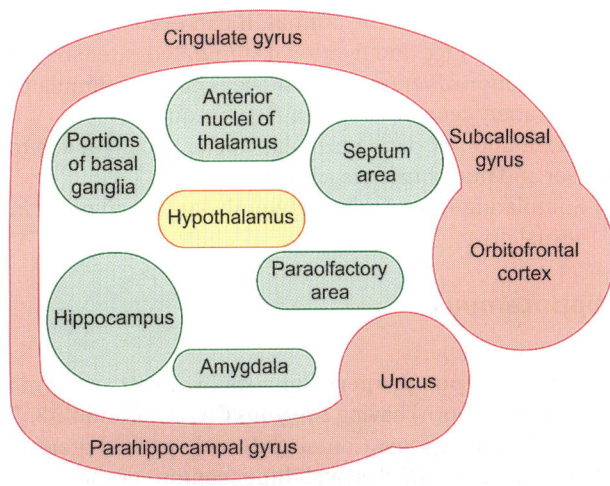

**Fig. 89.1:** The limbic system.

limbic system and occupies the central place in the limbic system. Now, we will discuss the functions of each of the important parts of limbic system.

**Parts of limbic system:**
- Hypothalamus
- Septum
- Paraolfactory area
- Anterior nucleus of thalamus
- Portions of basal ganglia
- Hippocampus
- Amygdala

## Hypothalamus

The hypothalamus forms the major part of the limbic system controlling the vegetative functions of the body like regulation of body temperature, maintaining osmolality of body fluids, feeding and satiety, control of body weight. Box below shows the various vegetative functions of the hypothalamus.

**Endocrine functions:**
- Regulation of anterior pituitary hormones by Hypothalamo-pituitary gland axis
- Synthesis of hormones secreted from posterior pituitary

**Autonomic functions:**
- Regulation of cardiovascular functions

**Behavioral effects:**
- Effect of stimulation of hypothalamic nuclei
- Effect of hypothalamic lesions
- Reward and Punishment function

**Other vegetative functions:**
- Regulation of feeding
- Body temperature regulation
- Body water regulation
- Regulation of circadian rhythm

Hypothalamus and associated structures of limbic system controls the following behavioral functions:
- Stimulation of lateral hypothalamus stimulates the thirst and feeding behavior. It also increases the general level of activity of the animal. It can even sometimes lead to the rage and fighting if stimulated extensively.
- Stimulation of ventromedial nucleus not only stimulates the satiety center but also causes tranquility.
- Stimulation of periventricular nuclei usually leads to fear and punishment reactions.
- Stimulating several areas of hypothalamus can result in sexual drive of the animal.

## Hippocampus

It has three subparts:
1. **Hippocampus proper:** Consists of cornu ammonis (Ammon's horn) having 3 regions CA1, CA2 and CA3.
2. **The dentate gyrus:** Contains densely packed granule cells and is interlocked with hippocampus proper.
3. **Subiculum:** It is a 3 layered cortex containing pyramidal cells.

### Functions of Hippocampus

- All type of sensory inputs cause the activation of some part of the hippocampus. It generates the *behavioral reactions to the sensory inputs* like pleasure, rage, passivity or excessive sexual drive.
- The hippocampus can become *hyper excitable* even with the week electrical stimuli resulting in focal epileptic seizures in small areas of hippocampi. This suggests that hippocampus can give prolonged output signals even under normal functioning conditions. The hippocampus seizures can result in the various psychomotor experiences to the patient like olfactory visual auditory and other type of hallucinations.
- Hippocampus has an important role in *learning and memory* hence the damage to the hippocampus can result in the anterograde amnesia. It *consolidates* short term declarative *memory* (retained from minutes to hours) to long term declarative memories (stored for days to years).

We will learn more about the learning and memory in the subsequent sections of this chapter.

## Amygdala

It is a complex of multiple small nuclei located beneath the cerebral cortex of the medial anterior pole of each temporal lobe. It receives the neuronal signals from all portions of limbic cortex, neocortex of temporal, parietal, occipital lobes. Because of these multiple connections India is also called as the *window through which the limbic system sees the place of the person in the world*.

When the amygdala is stimulated can result in the:
- Effects which are *mediated through hypothalamus* example changes in blood pressure, heart rate, gastrointestinal motility and secretion, defecation, micturition, secretion of various anterior pituitary hormones like gonadotrophins, ACTH
- Increases *several type of involuntary movements* like tonic movements, circling movements, occasionally clonic rhythmical movements, ejaculation, ovulation and premature labor.

### Bilateral Ablation of Amygdala Results in Kluver-Bucy syndrome

Damage to the anterior parts of both temporal lobes also damages the amygdala, that lie inside this part of the temporal lobe. It changes behavior of the animal/patient which is demonstrated by the following characters:
- Not afraid of anything
- Extreme curiosity about everything
- Forgets rapidly

- Increased oral tendencies. the animal/patient tries to put everything in the mouth and even tries to eat the solid inedible object.
- Hypersexuality. The animal/patient has a strong sexual drive that it attempts to copulate with immature animals or animals of different species.

### Reward and Punishment Function of Limbic System

The limbic structures are concerned with the motivational function which is carried out through the reward and punishment centres.

#### The Reward Centers

Experimentally the scientists have identified the major reward centers along the course of the medial forebrain bundle specially in the lateral and ventromedial nucleus of hypothalamus. They have identified these centers by implanting the electrical stimulators deep into the brain of the experimental animals. The less potent reward centers are found in hypothalamus, septum, amygdala, certain areas of thalamus and basal ganglia.

#### The Punishment Centers

The similar experiments have helped the scientists to identify the punishment centers which has been found in the central grey area surrounding the aqueduct of Sylvius in mesencephalon, which extends outwards into the ventricular zones of hypothalamus and thalamus. Less potent punishment areas are found in some locations in amygdala and hippocampus. The stimulation of punishment centers can completely inhibit the reward center demonstrating that punishment and fear can take precedence over pleasure and reward.

#### Rage

Strong stimulation of the punishment centers of brain especially the periventricular zone of hypothalamus and the lateral hypothalamus causes the animal to show the emotions of rage, which are characterized by developing a defensive posture, extending the claws lifting its tail by the animal. The animal hisses, spits, growls develop piloerection, his eyes are wide open and dilated pupils. The slightest provocation can cause an immediate savage attack.

In normal animals the rage is inhibited by the ventromedial nucleus of the hypothalamus along with the help of portions of hippocampi, anterior limbic cortex (interior single gyri and subcallosal gyrus).

#### Placidity and Tameness

When the reward centers are over stimulated the animal shows the behavior of placidity and tameness.

## PHYSIOLOGY OF SPEECH

In the Chapter 85, we had learnt about various cerebral lobes and their functions. Let's quickly do a recap of the speech areas in the cerebral cortex (**Fig. 89.2**) and their functions.

### The Sensory Speech Area (Wernicke's Area, Broadman Area 22)

It is located behind the primary auditory cortex in the posterior part of the superior gyrus of the temporal lobe. It is concerned with the comprehension of auditory and visual inputs received through the angular gyrus. It is present in the dominant hemisphere of the cerebral cortex, i.e., left hemisphere for 95% of people, who are right-handed.

> It is recommended that the reader should read the functions of Wernicke's area in Chapter 85.

### The Motor Speech Area (Broca's Area, Broadman Area 44)

It is present in the posterior lateral prefrontal cortex and premotor area in the frontal lobe. It processes information received from Wernicke's area into a detailed coordinated pattern of vocalization. It then projects to speech articulation area in insula to motor cortex. The movements of the lips, tongue and larynx to produce speech.

### Arcuate Fasciculus

It is the tract of nerve fibers which projects from the Wernicke's area to the Broca's area to transmit the processed visual and auditory input for the further motor processing there (**Fig. 89.3**).

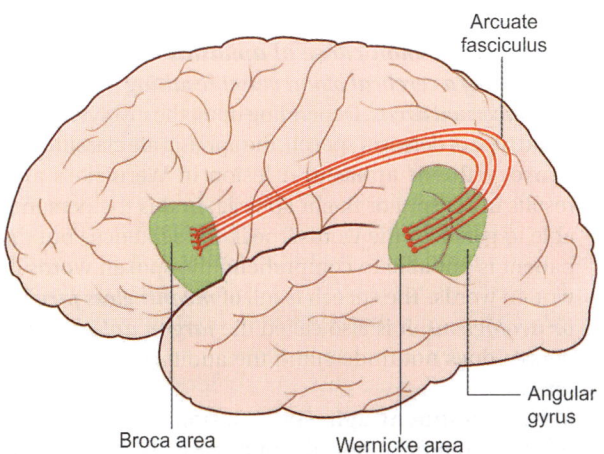

**Fig. 89.2:** The speech area.

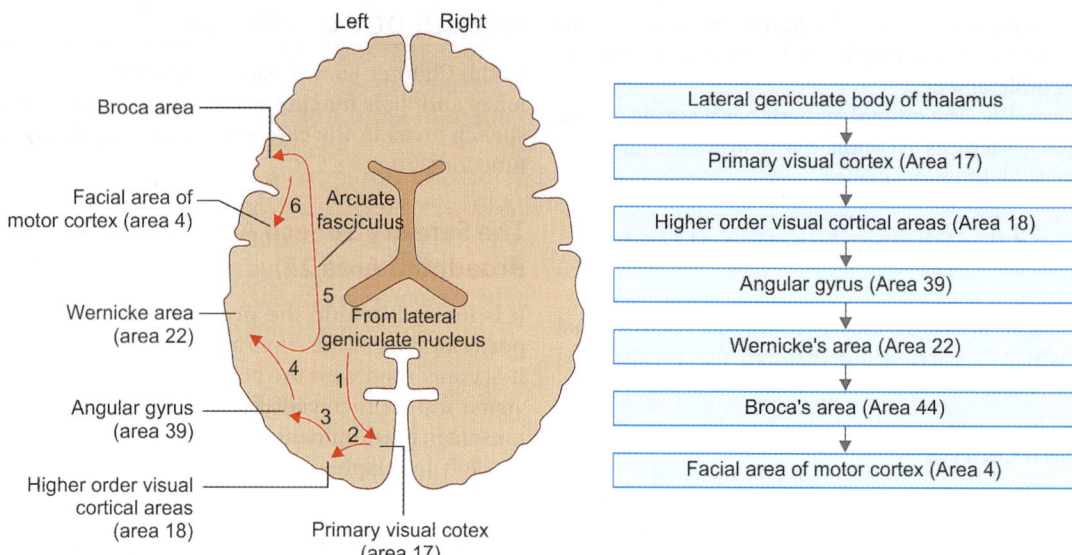

Fig. 89.3: The projection of impulses from visual area for language production.

**Processing of auditory signal for language production:**

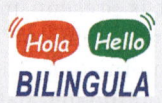
**Learning two languages**

When we try to learn a second language in adulthood, a portion of Broca's area is formed which is distinct from the area concerned with the native language.

But, if the children are taught two languages, in early life, they have only a single Broca's area for both the languages.

## Disorders of Speech (APHASIA)

Aphasias are the abnormalities of language function due to involvement of either sensory or motor speech areas, or arcuate fasciculus or all the areas involved in language processing in the dominant hemisphere. However, the patients with aphasias have a normal vision, hearing and motor functioning involving the facial muscles and tongue.

The most *common cause of aphasias is embolism or thrombosis of a cerebral blood vessel resulting in ischemia of the concerned areas*. Depending upon the involvement of area and type of defect in speech, the aphasia are classified as:

- **Sensory/fluent aphasia:** A lesion in Wernicke's area results in sensory or fluent aphasia. In this the person is able to generate the words/speak the sentences but the patient is not able to comprehend the spoken words or written words. The speech is full of *meaningless jargons or neologisms*. It is also called the *jargon aphasia*. The person does not understand the auditory or the visual input.
- **Motor/nonfluent aphasia:** A lesion in Broca's area results in motor or non-fluent aphasia. It is also called as *expressive aphasia*. The patient with motor aphasia has slow speech and difficulty in generating verbal or written words.
- **Anomic aphasia:** It occurs due to the *lesion of angular gyrus of dominant cerebral hemisphere*. The Wernicke's area and the Broca's area are normal in this case. The auditory information is interpreted without any problem, but the visual information is not processed. This results in *difficulty is interpretation of written language*. This is called *word blindness or anomic aphasia*.
- **Global aphasia:** The lesion involving the *Wernicke's area, Broca's area and arcuate fasciculus* result in loss of interpretation of all types of visual and auditory form of language and affecting the motor component of speech. The patient has both the sensory and motor aphasia.

## PHYSIOLOGY OF LEARNING AND MEMORY

A memory is a result of formation of new pathway called *memory trace*. It is formed by changing the basic sensitivity to the synaptic transmission between the neurons by the following changes:

- **Habituation:** It is the property of synapse where repetitive stimulus fails to produce an action potential across synapse. Similarly, the brain has capability of *ignoring the redundant and continuous information* (like background noises). This property of habituation results from the inhibition of synaptic pathways. This results in the formation of *negative memory*. Hence, *most* of our memories are made up of negative memories.
- **Sensitization:** If the information is *associated with pain or pleasure*, the brain stores these memory traces in the form of positive memory. It occurs because of facilitation of synaptic pathways. It is called the *memory sensitization*.

## Classification of Memory

Classification of memory is shown in **Figure 89.4**.

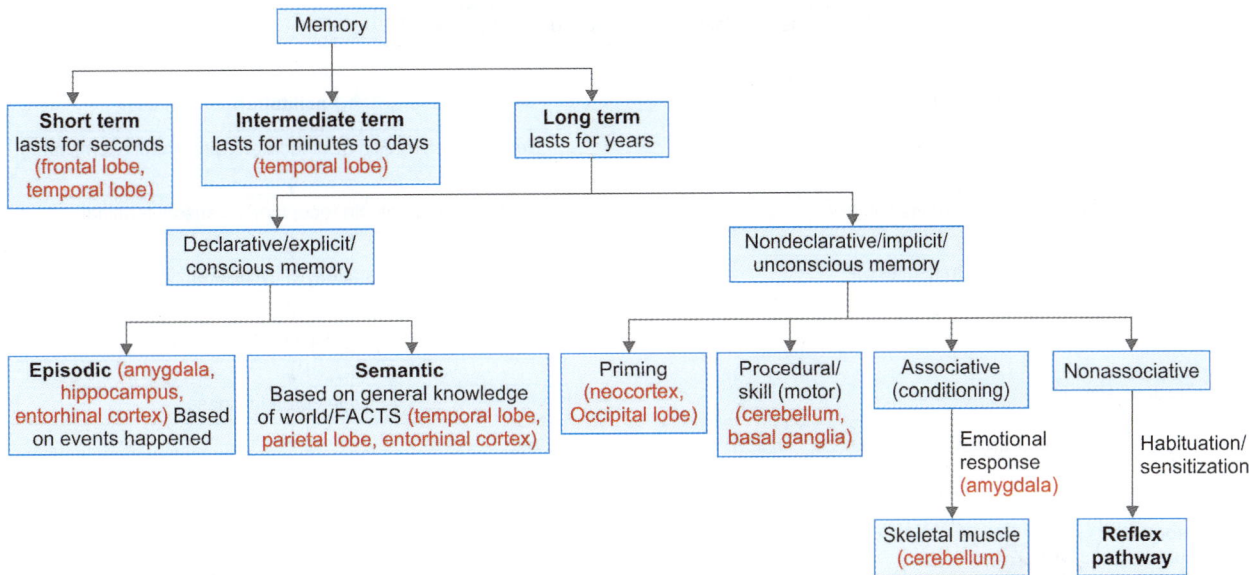

**Fig. 89.4:** Classification of memory.

## Short-term Memory

The short-term memory lasts for only *few seconds to minutes*, i.e., till the time he continues to think about the task he is performing. It is also called as the *working memory*. For example you may remember a phone number while dialing it but will forget soon after the job is done.

**Physiological basis of short-term memory:**
- It occurs due to the *continuous neuronal discharge in the reverberatory circuits*.

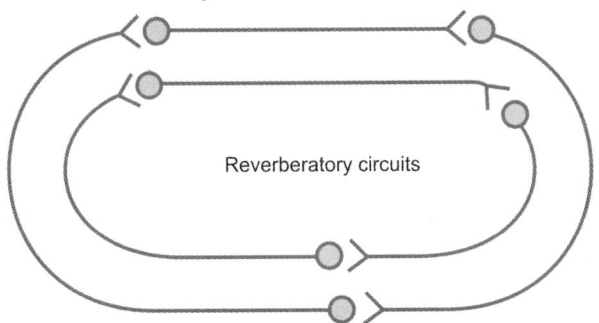

- It can also occur due to *presynaptic inhibition or facilitation*.

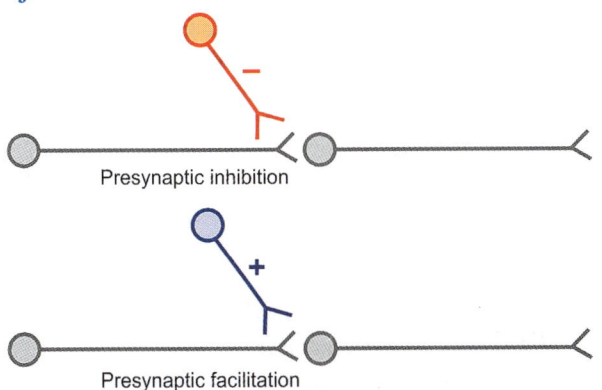

## Intermediate Long-term Memory

This memory may last for minutes to weeks, but eventually gets lost and doesn't get consolidated to become a permanent memory. The intermediate memories are formed by certain chemical changes in the pre and post synaptic membranes shown in **Figure 89.5**.

The habituation or facilitation affects the presynaptic sensory neuron, as shown in the **Figure 89.5**.

## Long-term Memory

Long-term memory is formed due to actual structural changes instead of chemical changes at the synapses, mentioned above. Various structural changes occurring in long term memory are summarized below:
- Increased number of available *synaptic vesicles* in presynaptic terminals
- Increased in the number of *docking sites* for the release of neurotransmitter
- Increased number of *presynaptic terminals and dendritic spines*. In a nutshell, there is increase in number of *synapses* (demonstrating the property of synaptic plasticity).

## Consolidation of Memory

The short-term memory gets converted into the long-term memory through a series of changes involving the *chemical and structural (physical and anatomical)* in the synapses due to active repetitions of the event **(Fig. 89.6)**. The process and duration of consolidation, is mentioned below:
- **Rehearsal/repetition enhances the transference of short-term memory into long term memory.** The rehearsals fix the sensory experiences in the

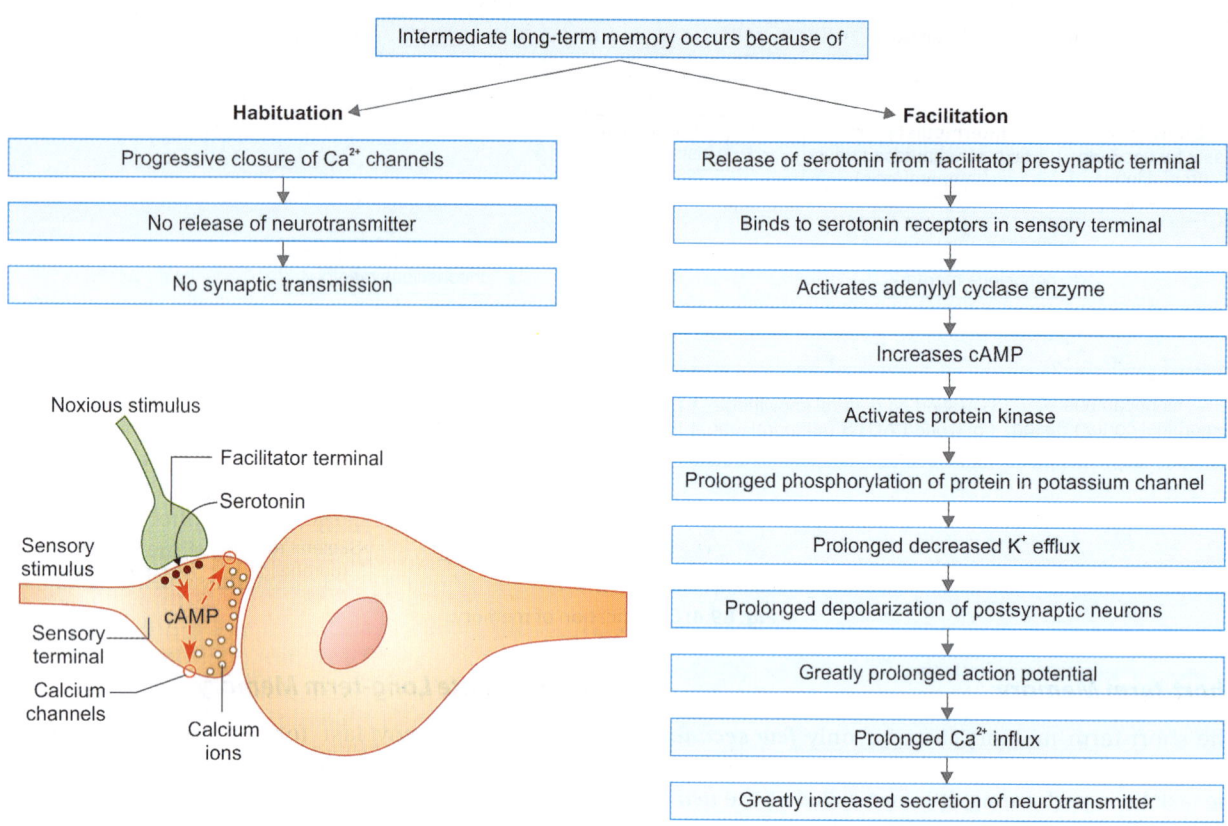

**Fig. 89.5:** The physiological basis of Intermediate Long-term memory.

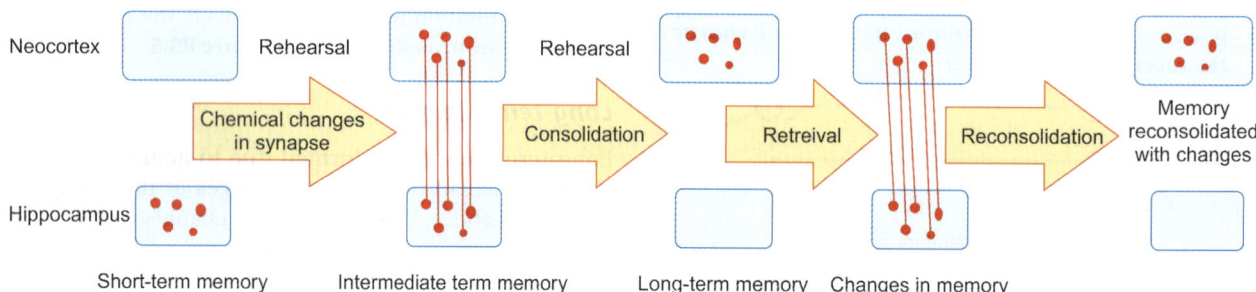

**Fig. 89.6:** Flow diagram to show consolidation of memory.

memory stores. A memory is consolidated in a better way, if a person is wide awake than a state of mental fatigue.

- **Coding of new memories:** Similar memories are stored together hence they are compared and coded. It allows the easy retrieval of memories.

The short-term memories are formed in the hippocampus of the temporal lobe. The hippocampus receives all the inputs through its dentate gyrus which are then projected into the CA3 and then to CA1 portions of hippocampus. From CA1, some fibers in fornix enters septum. The post commissural fibers of septum, cholinergic fibers and Basal nucleus of Meynert from amygdala project to hippocampus. This circuit is responsible for consolidation of memory **(Fig. 89.7)**.

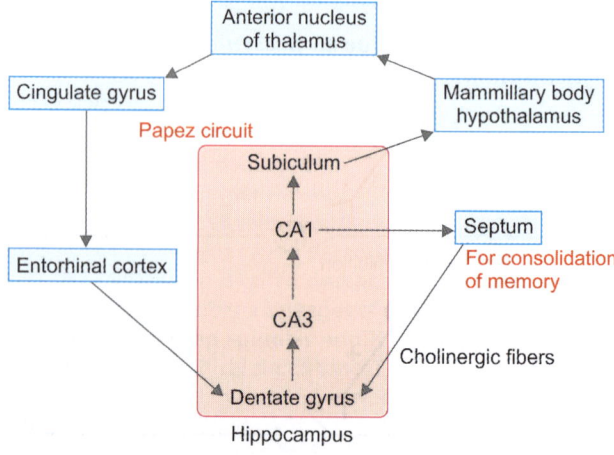

**Fig. 89.7:** Consolidation of memory.

Once the memory is consolidated, it is stored in the neocortex, in a way that it could be easily retrieved. During the process of retrieval, if a memory is modified, the reconsolidated memory will also be modified. It is very interesting to learn that *when we recall our memory with words our left frontal lobe and left parahippocampal gyrus are activated* as seen on fMRI. But when we try to *recall images or scenes, our right frontal lobe and both the parahippocampal gyri show activity*.

We have often observed that the chronic alcoholics have some impairment of memory. It happens because of damage to the mammillary bodies and the mammillothalamic tract due to associated thiamine deficiency, called *Korsakoff psychosis*. The recent memory is particularly affected in them.

## Lesions of Hippocampus

### Anterograde Amnesia

Bilateral removal of temporal lobes to treat the patient of temporal lobe epilepsy, result in removal of hippocampi. The patient is not able to form new long term memories. This is called *anterograde amnesia*. The patient can perform adequately till the time he is focusing on the task. The moment he is distracted, even by a trivial stimulus, he forgets what he was doing. He cannot form intermediate or long term memories.

The hippocampal lesion can result in some amount of *retrograde amnesia* (inability to recall the already consolidated memory). Pure retrograde amnesia occurs in the lesions of thalamus. Hence, we can deduce from this, that the thalamus is required for searching and retrieving the memories.

The patients with hippocampal lesions, retain the reflexes he had already learnt before the lesion like driving etc. The patient can actually learn a few motor skills after the lesion as it involves the reflexive learning.

### Temporal Lobe Epilepsy

The hyperexcitability of hippocampus is responsible for temporal lobe epilepsy, which is associated with psychomotor effects including olfactory, visual, auditory, tactile and other hallucinations. Stimulation of some parts of temporal lobe can result in the feeling of similarity in unknown surroundings. This phenomenon is called *'deja vu'* in French, which means *already seen*. This can occur in healthy persons or during the aura preceding the temporal lobe epilepsy.

The hyperexcitability of hippocampus can be explained on the basis of its histology, that it is 3 layered cortex as compared to 6 layered in other places.

### Alzheimer's Disease

It is an age-related progressive neurodegenerative disorder characterized by short term memory loss, followed by general loss of cognitive brain functions, agitation and depression.

**Etiopathogenesis:**
- It is seen in middle aged people (old, aged people, usually have senile dementia). The risk of developing Alzheimer's disease increases with increase in age.
- It is more prevalent in women.
- The etiology of this disease could be genetic (autosomal dominant) due to mutations in the genes for
  - *Amyloid* precursor protein on chromosome *21*
  - *Presenilin 1* protein on chromosome *14*
  - *Presenilin 2* protein on chromosome *1*
- The mutations can lead to the overproduction of β-amyloid protein, which is found in neuritic plaques.

**Cytopathological changes (Fig. 89.8):**
- Intracellular *neurofibrillary tangles* (made up of tau proteins that normally binds to microtubules and extracellular amyloid plaques, having a core of *β-amyloid protein* surrounded by altered nerve fiber and reactive glial cells.
- The polypeptides formed after the hydrolyses of *amyloid precursor proteins (APP)* are toxic and initiate the inflammatory response with production of intracellular tangles. These cells eventually die leading to neurodegenerative disease associated with *narrowing of the gyri, widening of sulci, enlargement of ventricles and reduction in brain weight.*

## PHYSIOLOGY OF ELECTROENCEPHALOGRAPHY

The electroencephalography (EEG) is the surface recording of the neural activity from the scalp by using the electrodes. The electrical activity is recorded as the waves of different frequency and amplitudes indicating the neuronal activity. *Hans Berger* was the first to describe these EEG waves, hence they are also named after him and called Berger waves.

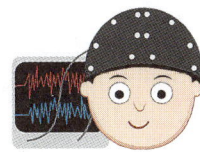

### Types of EEG Waves (Fig. 89.9)

The intensity of brain waves range from *0 to 200 μV* and frequency range from once a few seconds to *50/sec*. Depending on the frequency of these waves, they are classified as:

### Alpha Waves

These waves are recorded in awake state with eyes closed. The frequency of waves is *8–13/sec*, with amplitude of *50 μV*. This wave is generated in healthy adults during *awake, quiet and resting state of mind*. They are best present in *occipital region, parietal and frontal regions*.

**Origin of alpha waves:** Alpha waves result from the spontaneous feedback oscillations in diffuse

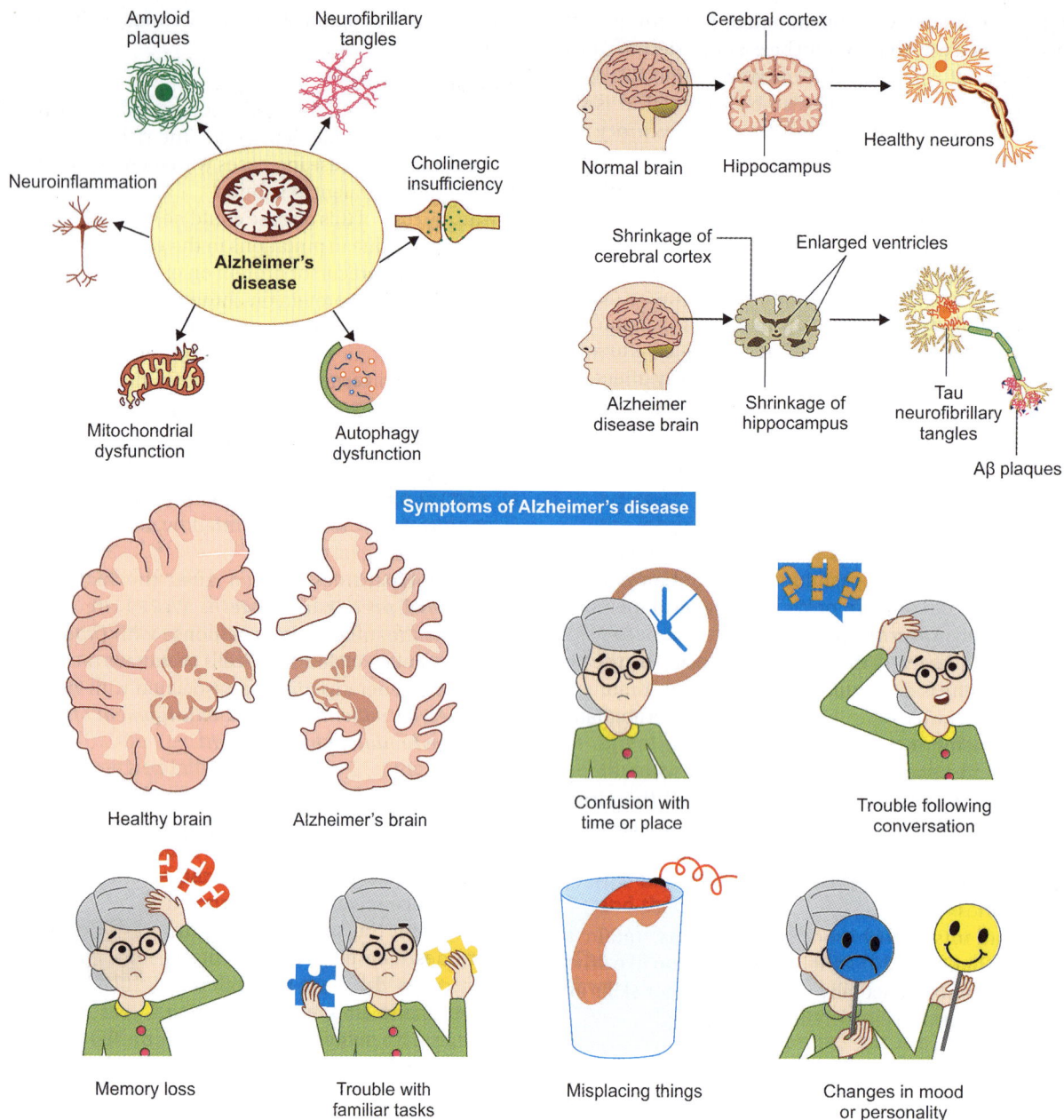

**Fig. 89.8:** Alzheimer's disease.

*thalamocortical system*, including reticular activating system and brainstem.

### Beta Waves

These are asynchronous waves with *high frequency 14–80/sec and low amplitude/voltage.* These waves are recorded in awake state with eyes open, indicating the activity of brain. They are mainly recorded from *parietal and frontal regions of brain*.

**Origin of beta waves:** The millions of neurons fire synchronously to allow the pick-up of electrical signal from the scalp. Hence the wave with larger amplitude has the synchronous neuronal discharge; whereas the asynchronous discharge nullify one another because of opposite polarities, resulting in lower amplitudes. 'During periods of mental activity, the waves usually become *asynchronous* rather than synchronous, so the voltage falls considerably despite markedly increased cortical activity'.

### Theta Waves

They are low frequency waves *4–7/sec*. They are generated during *emotional stress in adults* especially during stress and frustration. They are normally seen in *parietal and temporal regions in children*. These waves are also seen in *degenerative brain disease*.

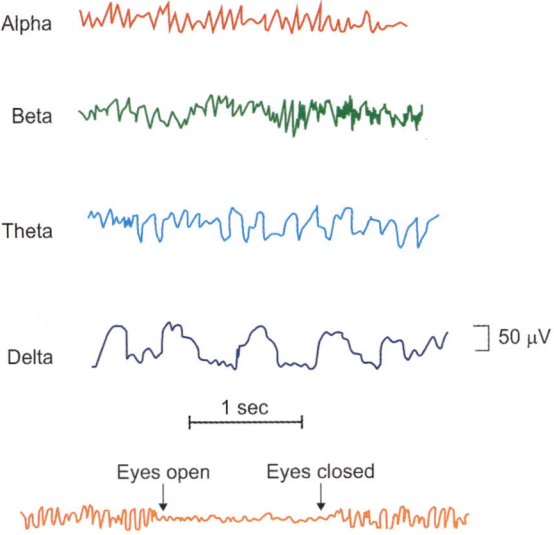

Fig. 89.9: Normal EEG waves.

## Physio-clinical Significance of EEG Waves

- The EEG waves are recorded during the sleep studies to identify the EEG changes during the sleep (**Fig. 89.10**). Various EEG changes during sleep are discussed in the next section.
- To study the abnormal brain activity during epilepsy/seizures.

> **Epilepsy:** Epilepsy is a chronic condition which is a collection of clinical symptoms that are heterogeneous and can occur due to multiple underlying causes like:
> - Cerebral dysfunction
> - Injury occurring due to trauma, malignancy infection or degenerative diseases.
> - It can also have the genetic predisposition.
> - Any factor which leads to the increased neuronal excitation or impaired inhibition.
> Example: the drugs which predispose a person to epilepsy (epileptogenic drugs). Where has the antiepileptic drugs decrease the excitation and facilitate the inhibition.

### Delta Waves

They are slowest of all waves with a *frequency of 3.5/sec* with the highest voltage of all the brain waves. It is generated by the neurons *during deep sleep, in infancy and in persons with serious brain disease*.

**Origin of delta waves:** The synchronizing mechanism occurring in the cortical neuron system itself causes the delta waves. The delta waves during *deep sleep* indicate that the cortex is released from the activating influence of *thalamus and lower centers*.

## Types of Epileptic Seizures

- *Focal/partial seizures:* They are limited to one area (focal area) of one cerebral hemisphere.
- *Generalized seizures:* Result in diffuse activity of both the hemispheres of cerebral cortex.

### Focal/Partial Seizures

The epileptic future begins in the small, localized region of the cerebral cortex reflect as the function of the

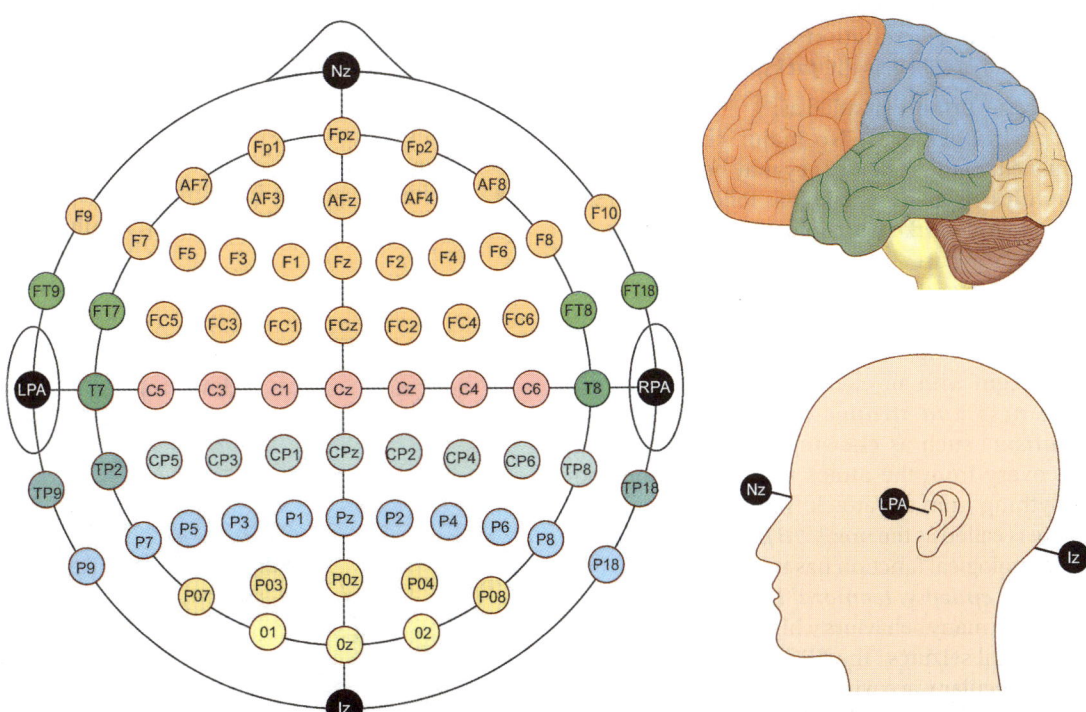

Fig. 89.10: Electrode placement in EEG.

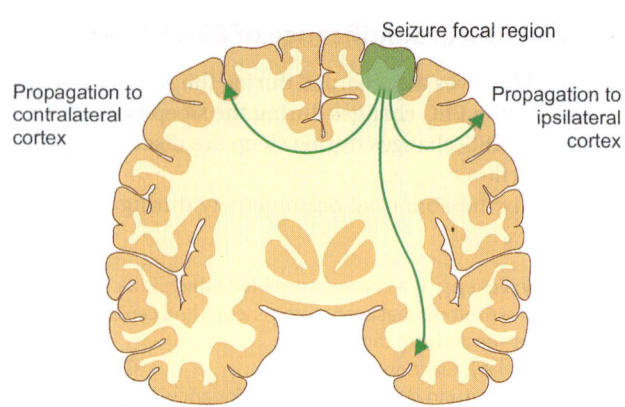

**Fig. 89.11:** Propagation of focal seizures.

effected brain area **(Fig. 89.11)**. the focal seizures occur due to:
- Scar tissue in the brain
- Malignancy, that compresses an area of the brain
- Abnormal neuronal circuits.

**How it happens?**

Extremely rapid discharges the local neurons occur due to the lesions, mentioned above. When these discharges occur at a very high rate, they send the synchronous waves to the adjacent cortical regions. This sets up the local reverberating circuits which further spread over the adjacent cortex. *The focal seizures can spread locally from a focus to the contralateral cortex and subcortical areas of the brain through the thalamic projections.*

When the wave of excitation spreads over the motor cortex it causes the excitation of the muscles as represented on the motor homunculus. The muscular contractions appear *'marching'* from a mouth region the legs below. This phenomenon of excitation of the muscles in a particular manner is called as the *Jacksonian March*.

Focal seizures are further classified as:
- **Simple partial seizures:** No major change in the consciousness of the patient. They may be preceded by an *aura* with sensations such as fear, followed by motor signs like rhythmic jerking or tonic stiffening movement of a single body part. The focal epileptic attack most commonly involves the *temporal lobe*.
- **Complex partial seizures:** When the patient has loss of consciousness or impaired consciousness. This seizure may also begin with an *aura* followed by *impaired consciousness and strange repetitive movement (automatism)* such as chewing our lips smacking. After recovery from the attack the person does not recall anything from the attack. The time period after the seizure is called as the *postictal period* in which the normal neurological function has not yet returned.

*Psychomotor epilepsy, temporal lobe epilepsy limbic seizures* describe many behaviors which are now classified as complex partial seizures. The EEG tracing shows a low frequency rectangular wave with the frequency between 2 to 4 per second with the locational superimposed 14 per second waves as shown in **Figure 89.12**.

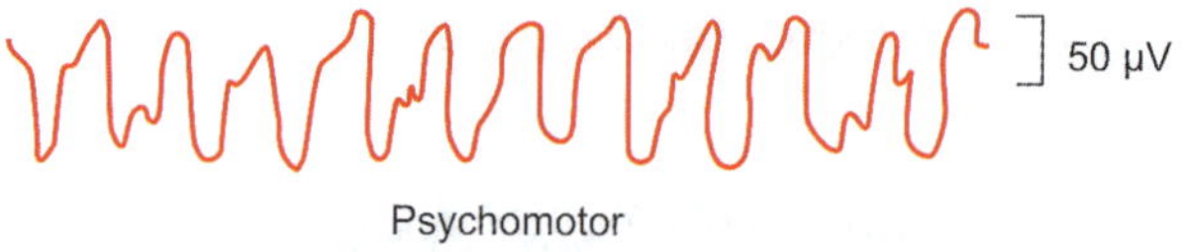

**Fig. 89.12:** EEG in psychomotor epilepsy.

### Generalized Epileptic Seizures

These seizures are diffuse, excessive and uncontrolled neuronal discharges that spread rapidly and simultaneously to both cerebral hemispheres to interconnections between the thalamus and cortex. They are further classified as:
- Generalized tonic clonic seizures/Grand Mal epilepsy
- Absence seizures/Petit Mal epilepsy
- **Generalized tonic clonic (GTC) seizures/Grand Mal epilepsy:** They are characterized by sudden loss of consciousness and extreme neuronal discharge in all the areas of cerebral cortex, deeper parts of the brain and even the brain stem **(Fig. 89.13)**.
  - There is generalized tonic seizure of the entire body followed by the alternating tonic spasmodic muscle contractions called tonic clonic seizures.
  - The person may bite or swallow his or her tongue which may cause difficulty in breathing or cyanosis.
  - The person can have urination or defecation during the seizure.
  - GTC seizure can last for few seconds to 3 to 4 minutes.
  - After the seizure is over, the person can remain in super for several minutes. This is called as *post seizure depression.* During this period, the person remains severely fatigued and may sleep for hours.
  - The EEG recording during the GTC show high voltage activity from thalamus, reticular formation and cerebral cortex **(Fig. 89.14)**.

GTC seizures may occur due to any of the following reasons:
- Abnormal or epileptogenic circuitry
- Strong emotional stimuli
- Alkalosis occurring due to hyperventilation: when the person hyperventilates, the carbon dioxide washout

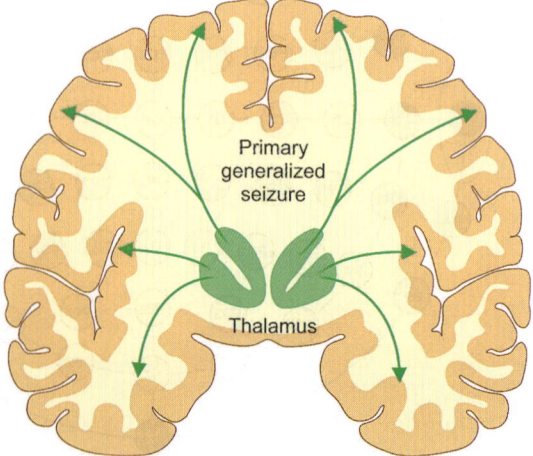

**Fig. 89.13:** Propagation of GTC seizure.

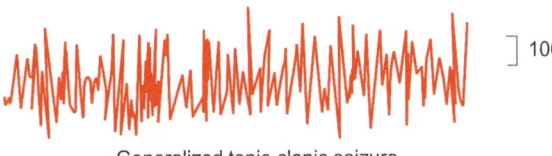

**Fig. 89.14:** EEG tracing in GTC Seizure.

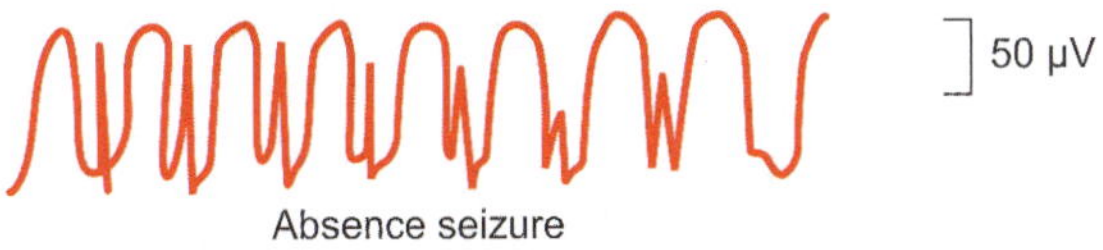

**Fig. 89.15:** EEG tracing in Absence seizure, a typical spike and dome pattern.

results in the alkalosis of the blood which increases when you run excitability and hence precipitates the epilepsy.
- Drugs increasing neuronal excitability
- High grade fever
- Loud noises or flashing lights
- Traumatic religions of the brain

- **Absence seizures (Petit Mal epilepsy):** It begins in childhood or early adolescence. It is characterized by a brief period of unconsciousness or diminished consciousness, during which the person often stars and has twitch like contractions of muscles of the facial region especially blinking of eyes, this phase is followed by rapid return of consciousness and that resumption of previous activity.
EEG shows a typical *Spike and Dome pattern* which is recorded from the thalamocortical activating system of brain and associated with 3/s doublets **(Fig. 89.15)**. This activity lasts for about 10 seconds. This suggest that it results from the oscillations of inhibitory thalamic reticular GABAergic neurons and excitatory thalamocortical and thalamocortical neurons. It occurs due to low threshold T-type $Ca^{2+}$ channels in thalamic neurons.

## Physiological Basis of Treatment of Epilepsy

The mainstay to treat the epilepsy is to block the initiation or spread of the seizures with the help of anti-epileptic drugs which can act on the following mechanisms:
- Blockage of voltage gated sodium channels (Carbamazepine and phenytoin)
- Altered calcium currents (Ethosuximide)
- Increased GABA activity (Phenobarbital and benzodiazepines)
- Inhibition of receptors for glutamate (Perampanel)
- Multiple mechanisms, voltage gated sodium channel blocker and increases GABA in brain (Valproate and topiramate).

## PHYSIOLOGY OF SLEEP

Sleep is defined as the state of unconsciousness from which a person can be aroused by the sensory stimulus.

## Types of Sleep

Based on the eye movement and brain activity, the sleep is divided into two main stages, the Rapid eye movement (REM) sleep and nonrapid eye movement (NREM) or slow wave sleep.

### Rapid Eye Movement (REM) Sleep

This type of sleep is characterized by rapid movements of eyes, increased brain activity and dreaming. The characteristics of REM sleep are described below:
- It is also called the *desynchronized or paradoxical sleep*.
- REM sleep has the characteristic *rapid movements of the eyes*.
- It *lasts for 5–30 minutes* and occurs after every 90 minutes.
- It constitutes about **25%** of the total sleep.
- It is *not restful* sleep.
- The *duration of REM sleep increases towards the end of the night* when the person becomes more rested.
- It is *difficult to arouse the person* during REM sleep. But the person usually wakes up spontaneously during the REM sleep in the morning.
- REM sleep is associated with the *dreaming and bodily movements*. The dreams during this stage can be recalled.
- The *heart rate* and *respiratory rate* becomes *irregular* in this phase.
- The *brain activity increases* in this type of sleep, resulting in the *low voltage high frequency waves* on EEG. These waves resemble the β waves when a person is wide awake, which is a paradox that the person is actually asleep. Hence this sleep is called as the *'paradoxical sleep'*. Further, the synchronized high voltage slow wave sleep becomes desynchronized to yield low voltage waves. Hence it is called as the *'desynchronized sleep'*.
- The muscle tone decreases due to inhibition of spinal muscle control areas.
- When a person takes an afternoon nap/powernap, he usually gets the REM sleep.

### Nonrapid Eye Movement (NREM) or Slow Wave Sleep

This type of sleep is characterized by extremely restful sleep with slow movements of eyes, decreased brain activity resulting in high voltage low frequency brain waves. The characteristics of NREM sleep are described below:
- 75–80% of the total sleep is the slow wave sleep.
- There is *decreased vegetative functions* of body. The body repairs itself during this phase, replenishment of neurotransmitters occurs during this phase.
- The *blood pressure, respiratory rate decreases*. The vasomotor tone also decreases.
- The *basal metabolic rate decreases* during slow wave sleep.

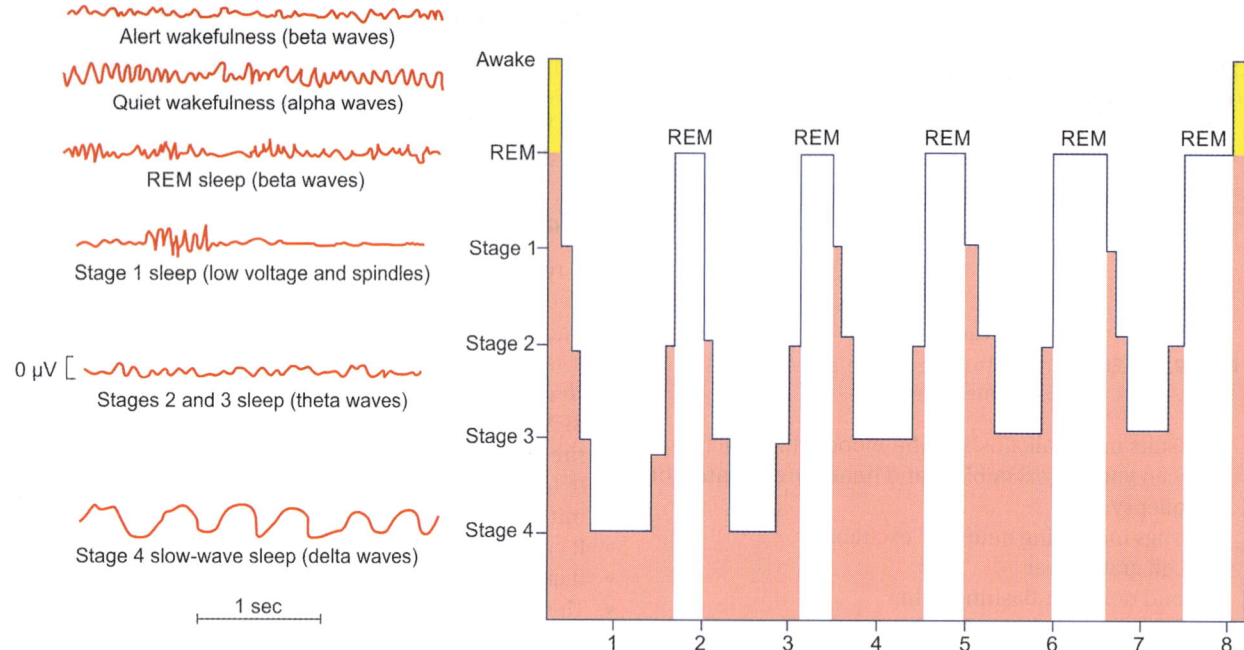

**Fig. 89.16:** Hypnogram showing EEG waves during different stages of sleep.

- The people in slow wave sleep is *don't get dreams*. Actually, the dreams can't be remembered as the consolidation doesn't occur.
- The EEG during slow wave sleep shows high voltage low frequency waves with Sleep spindles and K complexes.
- The muscle tone decreases in some postural muscles.
- The body movements are very low during this phase.
- A person usually gets 5 sleep cycles, where each cycle has all the four stages. The graphical representation of this 8 hours of sleep is called as the *'hypnogram'* **(Fig. 89.16)**.

The hypnogram shows the following stages of the sleep **(Fig. 89.17)**:
- During first sleep cycle, the Slow wave sleep/NREM sleep is predominant. But in fifth sleep cycle, the REM sleep becomes predominant.
- If we study the first sleep cycle:
  - We see that when a person is *awake* and his *eyes are open*, the brain waves show the *beta waves* indicating the alert awake state.
  - On the *closure of the eyes*, the brain waves become *synchronized*, increasing the voltage of the EEG waves resulting in the *alpha waves*. This indicated the *quiet wakefulness*.
  - **NREM stage 1:** During *first 5 minutes*, there is *decrease in the tone of the muscles* and the person gets a feeling as if he is going to fall. Sometimes, it might result in a jerk which can awaken the person, this is the NREM stage 1. The person is falling asleep, he can be easily awakened in this stage. The *heart beat and respiration slows down and muscles begin to relax*. The EEG shows *alpha rhythm*.
  - **NREM Stage 2:** In *next 20–25 minutes*, the person is in light sleep, where the heart rate and respiratory rate drops further. There is *no eye movement*. The EEG shows *high voltage very low frequency theta waves with sleep spindles and K complexes* **(Fig. 89.18)**.

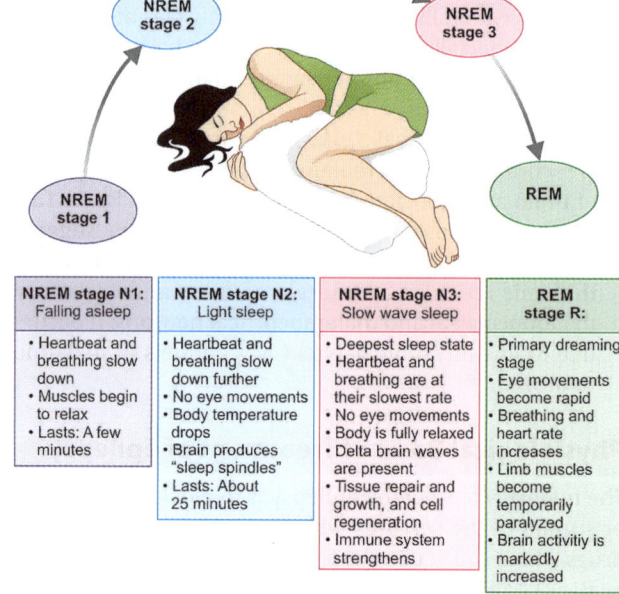

**Fig. 89.17:** Stages of sleep.

**Sleep spindles:** They are the sinusoidal waves with a frequency of 7–15 Hz produced by the thalamo-reticular nuclei. They are thought to reduce the sensory input during the sleep.
**K-complexes:** Are the *high voltage biphasic waves* seen along with sleep spindles. These waves are important for the consolidation of memory. Also they suppress the cortical arousal in response to non-threatening sensory stimulus.

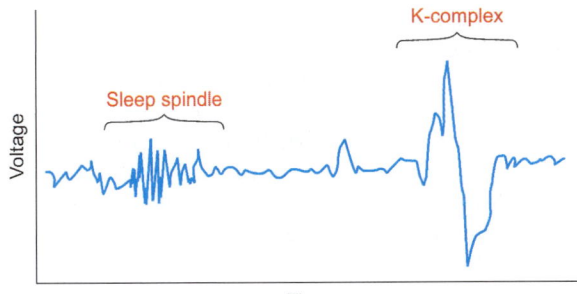

**Fig. 89.18:** Sleep spindles and K-complexes.

- **NREM stage 3:** This stage is the stage of *deep sleep* where the body carries out its repair work. The *immune system is strengthened*. The muscles are completely relaxed and heart rate and respiratory rate slows down further. There is *no eye movement*. The EEG shows the *delta waves*.
- **REM stage:** It is followed by the rapid eye movement sleep, where there is rapid movement of the eyeballs. The *muscles lose their tone*. The *heart rate and respiratory rate becomes irregular*. The *brain activity increases* and the EEG shows *low voltage high frequency beta waves*. The *dreams* are present in this stage. These cycles repeat themselves resulting in increase in the duration of REM sleep. In the morning the person wakes up spontaneously in the REM stage of sleep.

> *Differentiate between REM and NREM sleep.*
> *Why REM sleep is called 'paradoxical sleep'?*
> *Why REM sleep is called 'desynchronized sleep'?*
> *What are the different stages of sleep?*
> *What are sleep spindles and K complexes? What are their physiological significance?*
> *What are the different EEG waves recorded in the sleep?*
> *What will happen if a person is deprived of NREM sleep?*

## Functions of Sleep

The sleep is an important physiological process which is required for the restoration of the natural balances of the neuronal homeostasis, repair and restoration of the physical structures of the body. The functions of the sleep can be enumerated as

- It is required for the *neural maturation*
- The sleep helps in *consolidation of memory* and helps in formation of *long-term memories*.
- The sleep *replenishes the neurotransmitters* and restores the neural functioning. It takes care of the synaptic fatigue. Hence, increases the cognitive ability of brain.
- It *reduces the basal metabolic rate* and hence conserves the metabolic energy.
- The sleep wakefulness cycles help in *maintenance of the circadian rhythm*, which act as the biological clock for the release of hormones required for maintaining the normal functioning of body.
- It leads to the *clearance of the metabolic waste products* generated by the neural activity.

If a person is sleep deprived all the above functions will be affected. The *total/selective deprivation* results in the *'catch-up'* or *'rebound sleep'*. However **prolonged deprivation of slow wave sleep can affect the:**

- **Memory and cognitive function:** Sleep deprivation affects the consolidation of memory, hence affects the memory retention, and decreased ability to learns new information.
- **Inadequate repair and restoration of the body:** This affects the repair of the skin, muscles, bones etc. Hence it hinders the vital restoration process.
- **Hormonal imbalance:** The decreased secretion of growth hormone occurs due to the disruption of the circadian rhythm, which affects the metabolism, bone and muscle growth. Prolonged sleep deprivation and hormonal imbalance predisposes to the insulin resistance and diabetes mellitus.
- **Appetite and body weight:** Sleep deprivation causes the food craving for the high calorie foods resulting in the weight gain. This also predisposes to the insulin resistance and diabetes mellitus.
- **Chronic fatigue**

Hence, proper sleep at the night is important for the adequate functioning of the body.

## Neurohormonal Control of Sleep (Fig. 89.19)

The neurohormonal control of sleep involves the regulation of sleep-wake cycles by neurotransmitters and hormones,

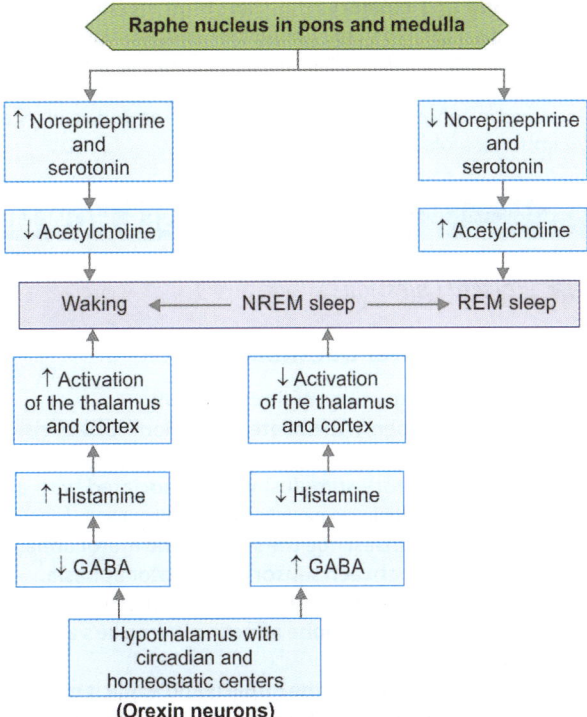

**Fig. 89.19:** Neurohormonal control of sleep.

such as **melatonin**, which promotes sleep, and cortisol, which supports wakefulness. The **hypothalamus** plays a key role in this process, mediating the release of these chemicals in response to the circadian rhythm.

## Sleep Disorders

- **Obstructive sleep apnea (OSA):** It is the most common cause of day time sleepiness due to fragmented sleep at night. There is cessation of breathing for more than 10 seconds due to frequent upper airway obstruction due to reduced muscle tone. This causes brief period of arousal in order to re-establish the muscle tone. The patient with OSA snores after falling asleep, which gets progressively louder until interrupted by an episode of apnea. It is followed by loud snort and gasp as the patient tries to breathe. There is an *increase in stage 1 NREM sleep and reduction in stage 3 and 4 of NREM*.
- **Narcolepsy:** It is a chronic condition where the person has a difficulty in maintaining the normal sleep and wake cycles. He *sleeps at any time*, even during the day. It is characterized by sudden onset of REM sleep. The patients with narcolepsy have a *fewer hypocretin (orexin) producing neurons in the hypothalamus*.
- **Cataplexy:** Sudden loss of muscle tone
- **Somnambulism:** Sleep walking
- **Insomnia:** Inability to sleep at night
- **Periodic limb movement disorders:** There is rhythmic extension of big toe and dorsiflexion of ankle and knee during sleep. The movement could be shallow but can be wild and strenuous kicking and flailing of legs and arms. *Stage 1 of NREM may be increased while stage 3 and 4 may be decreased*. A similar condition, restless leg syndrome or Willis-Ekbom disease presents with an irresistible urge to move their legs while at rest all day long.
- **Nocturnal enuresis:** Bed wetting.

---

### SUMMARY

- **Physiology of emotions:** The limbic system plays an important part in the physiology of emotions, memory consolidation and olfaction. The reward, punishment, rage and placidity are processed in the limbic system. Hence, it controls the behavior of an individual.
- **Speech:** The Wernicke's area receives the sensory inputs from the auditory cortex and the occipital cortex for the heard and written language. This enables us to hear and read and also understand their meaning. This information is sent to the motor speech area through arcuate fasciculus, which generated the speech through the motor cortex. Any lesion in these areas result in speech disorder called aphasias.
- **Learning and memory:** The short term memory/working memory is created in the frontal lobe and the hippocampus. The rehearsals consolidate this short term memory into the intermediate term memory and long term memory, which is stored in neocortex. The hippocampus and amygdala plays an important role in consolidation of memory.
- **EEG:** The electrical activity of the brain is picked up by the surface electrodes. This recording is called the electro-encephalogram (EEG). The main EEG waves are
  - Alpha waves, recorded with quiet wakefulness with eyes closed.
  - Beta waves, recorded with eyes open and the person is awake.
  - Theta waves, recorded during NREM stage 2 and during emotional rage.
  - Delta waves are recorded during deep sleep and organic brain disease.
- **Physiology of sleep:** The sleep is classified as NREM (Slow wave sleep) and REM sleep. Typically a person falls asleep in the stage 1 of NREM sleep, then progresses to stage 2, 3 and REM sleep. In the 8 hour sleep, the duration of NREM is more in the beginning and duration of REM sleep is more near the morning. The sleep is important to restore and repair the normal physiological wear and tear of the body.

---

### LET US SEE, HOW MUCH YOU HAVE LEARNT?

 *Review Questions*

### Long/Short Answer Questions

Q1. Describe the functions of limbic system.
Q2. What will happen, if the bilateral temporal lobe excision is done in a patient of temporal lobe epilepsy?
Q3. Why the olfactory stimulus, when associated with any memory, results in an easy retrieval of memory?
Q4. Define aphasia. Describe the sensory and motor aphasia.
Q5. Differentiate between sensory and motor aphasia.
Q6. What will happen to a person with hemorrhage in the left posterior parietal lobe affecting Wernicke's area and angular gyrus?
Q7. Differentiate between the implicit and explicit memory.
Q8. Describe the mechanism of consolidation of memory.
Q9. What will happen to the memory, if both the hippocampi of a person are damaged?
Q10. Describe the Berger waves.
Q11. Differentiate between NREM and REM sleep.
Q12. Why REM sleep is called 'paradoxical sleep'?
Q13. Why REM sleep is called 'desynchronized sleep'?
Q14. What are the different stages of sleep?
Q15. What are sleep spindles and K complexes? What are their physiological significance?
Q16. What are the different EEG waves recorded in the sleep?
Q17. What will happen if a person is deprived of NREM sleep?

## Explain Why? (Reasoning Questions)

Q1. Damage to the hippocampus can result in severe anterograde amnesia.
Q2. The limbic system is crucial for emotional regulation and behavior.
Q3. Broca's area is essential for speech production and its damage leads to expressive aphasia.
Q4. Wernicke's area is critical for language comprehension and its lesions result in receptive aphasia.
Q5. EEG patterns change across different stages of sleep.
Q6. REM sleep is important for memory consolidation.
Q7. Disorders of the limbic system can lead to changes in mood and behavior, such as in depression and anxiety.
Q8. Damage to the amygdala can affect emotional responses, such as fear and aggression.
Q9. Disruptions in sleep architecture can impair cognitive function and memory.
Q10. The thalamus plays a key role in regulating sleep-wake cycles and consciousness as evidenced by EEG patterns.

## Critical Thinking Case-Based Questions

Q1. Mrs Sharma, a 58-year-old woman, presented with complaints of recent memory loss, difficulty finding words, and disturbed sleep patterns. Her family reported that she had become increasingly forgetful, often misplacing items and struggling to recall recent conversations. Additionally, she had started waking up frequently at night and feels fatigued during the day. A neurological exam revealed mild cognitive impairment. The neurologist suspected a disorder involving the limbic system and related brain areas and recommends further evaluation, including EEG and sleep studies. Based on the given scenario, answer the following questions:
   a. What are the primary functions of the limbic system in regulating emotions and memory?
   b. How might dysfunction in this system lead to the cognitive and memory issues observed in Mrs Sharma?
   c. What can EEG and sleep studies reveal about the underlying causes of Mrs Sharma's?

## Multiple Choice Questions

Q1. Which part of the limbic system is responsible for processing and storing emotional memories?
   a. Amygdala  b. Hippocampus
   c. Thalamus  d. Hypothalamus

Q2. Which part of the limbic system regulates the autonomic nervous system and the endocrine system, and controls body temperature, hunger, thirst, and circadian rhythms?
   a. Amygdala  b. Hippocampus
   c. Thalamus  d. Hypothalamus

Q3. Which part of the limbic system acts as a relay station for sensory information, and filters out irrelevant stimuli before sending them to the cerebral cortex?
   a. Amygdala  b. Hippocampus
   c. Thalamus  d. Hypothalamus

Q4. Which part of the limbic system is essential for forming new declarative memories, such as facts and events, and consolidating them from short-term to long-term memory?
   a. Amygdala  b. Hippocampus
   c. Thalamus  d. Hypothalamus

Q5. Which part of the limbic system is involved in spatial navigation, spatial memory, and spatial reasoning?
   a. Amygdala  b. Hippocampus
   c. Thalamus  d. Hypothalamus

Q6. Which of the following is the main area of the cerebrum that controls speech comprehension?
   a. Broca's area  b. Wernicke's area
   c. Heschl's gyrus  d. Angular gyrus

Q7. Which of the following is the main area of the cerebrum that processes auditory information, including speech sounds?
   a. Broca's area  b. Wernicke's area
   c. Heschl's gyrus  d. Angular gyrus

Q8. Which of the following is the main area of the cerebrum that integrates visual and linguistic information, such as reading and writing?
   a. Broca's area  b. Wernicke's area
   c. Heschl's gyrus  d. Angular gyrus

Q9. Which of the following is the main pathway that connects Broca's area and Wernicke's area, allowing for fluent and meaningful speech?
   a. Arcuate fasciculus  b. Corpus callosum
   c. Corticospinal tract  d. Pyramidal tract

Q10. Which of the following brain structures is most involved in the formation of long-term declarative memories?
   a. Amygdala  b. Cerebellum
   c. Hippocampus  d. Hypothalamus

Q11. Which of the following types of memory is characterized by unconscious, implicit, and procedural learning?
   a. Semantic memory  b. Episodic memory
   c. Working memory  d. Nondeclarative memory

Q12. Which of the following is a neurotransmitter that plays a key role in memory consolidation and synaptic plasticity?
   a. Dopamine  b. Serotonin
   c. Glutamate  d. GABA

Q13. Which of the following is a phenomenon in which prior exposure to a stimulus enhances the subsequent recognition or recall of that stimulus?
   a. Priming  b. Rehearsal
   c. Chunking  d. Spacing

Q14. Which of the following is a memory improvement technique that involves repeating information over and over to keep it active in short-term memory?
   a. Elaboration  b. Mnemonics
   c. Maintenance rehearsal  d. Retrieval practice

Q15. A 7-year-old girl is brought to the pediatrician by her mother, who is concerned about her daughter's school performance. She says that her daughter often seems to "zone out" during class and misses important instructions. She also notices that her daughter sometimes blinks rapidly or twitches her eyelids. The episodes last for a few seconds and then she resumes her normal activity. The mother denies any history of fever, trauma, infection, or drug exposure. What is the most likely diagnosis for this girl?
   a. Absence seizures
   b. Attention deficit hyperactivity disorder (ADHD)
   c. Complex partial seizures
   d. Narcolepsy

Q16. A 45-year-old man with a body mass index of 32 kg/m2 complains of snoring, morning headaches, and excessive daytime sleepiness. He has a history of hypertension and type 2 diabetes. His wife reports that he often stops breathing for a few seconds during sleep and then gasps for air. What is the most likely type of sleep apnea affecting this man?
   a. Obstructive sleep apnea (OSA)
   b. Central sleep apnea (CSA)
   c. Mixed sleep apnea (MSA)
   d. Cheyne-Stokes breathing (CSB)

Q17. A 72-year-old woman suffers a stroke that damages the left parietal lobe of her brain. She has fluent and grammatical speech, but she often has trouble finding the right words to express herself. She uses circumlocutions, vague terms, and gestures to compensate for her word-finding difficulties. She can understand and repeat speech well, but she has some problems with naming objects and reading aloud. What type of aphasia does she have?
   a. Broca's aphasia        b. Wernicke's aphasia
   c. Conduction aphasia     d. Anomic aphasia

## ANSWERS

1. a   2. d   3. c   4. b   5. b   6. b   7. c   8. d   9. a   10. c   11. d   12. c   13. a   14. c
15. a   16. a   17. d

# Vestibular System

**CHAPTER 90**

### COMPETENCY ADDRESSED
PY10.4: Describe and discuss motor tracts, mechanism of maintenance of tone, control of body movements, posture and equilibrium and **vestibular apparatus**.

### LEARNING OBJECTIVES
**At the end of this chapter, the learner should be able to:**
- Describe the relevant functional anatomy of vestibular apparatus, vestibular nuclei, and the neuronal pathways associated with equilibrium.
- Describe the functions of vestibular system.
- Describe the vestibular pathways, vestibular nuclei, and its connections.
- Describe the applied physiology associated with vestibular apparatus.

The Vestibular system is formed from the vestibular apparatus and central vestibular nuclei, that forms an intricate system that allowing organisms to sense and respond to changes in head position, motion, and orientation in space, facilitating activities such as maintaining balance, stabilizing gaze, and coordinating movements.

## VESTIBULAR APPARATUS

The vestibular apparatus, situated within the petrous portion of the temporal bone, is crucial for maintaining equilibrium. It comprises the bony labyrinth, which houses the functional part known as the membranous labyrinth (**Fig. 90.1**). This membranous structure consists primarily of the cochlea for hearing and three semicircular canals, along with the utricle and saccule, all essential for equilibrium.

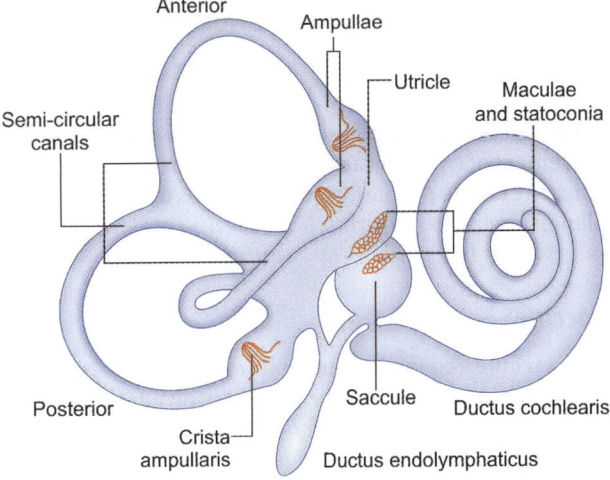

**Fig. 90.1:** Membranous labyrinth.

### Utricle and Saccule

The utricle and saccule are two key components of the membranous labyrinth within the vestibular apparatus, responsible for detecting *linear acceleration and the orientation of the head with respect to gravity* (**Fig. 90.2**).

### Utricle

The utricle is *larger* than the saccule and is *positioned horizontally* within the vestibular apparatus. It *detects linear movements in the horizontal plane, such as forward/backward or side-to-side motions.* The macula of the utricle, located on its inferior surface, contains hair cells embedded in a gelatinous layer. These hair cells

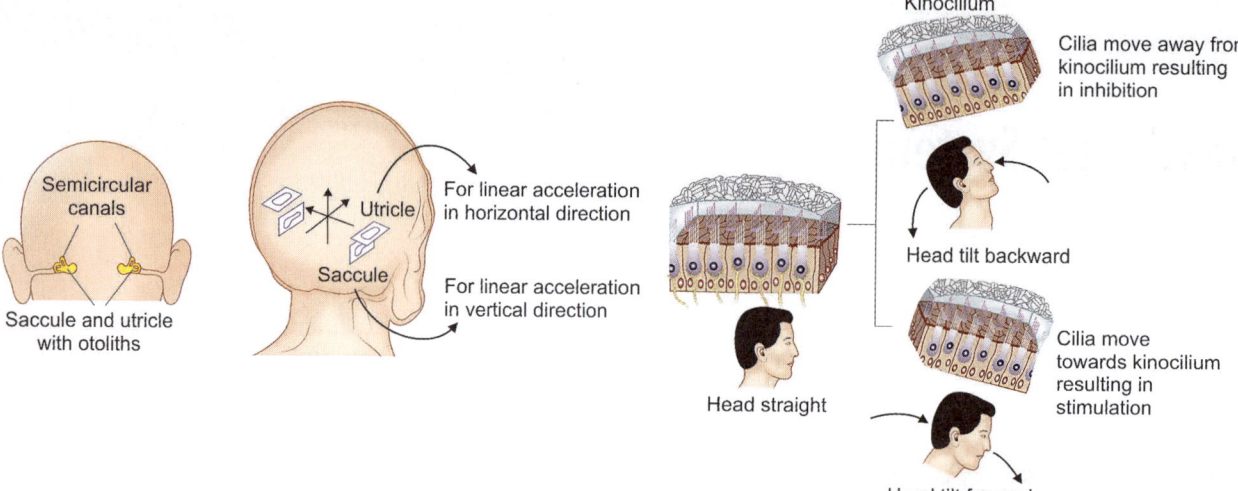

**Fig. 90.2:** Role of utricle and saccule in linear movements.

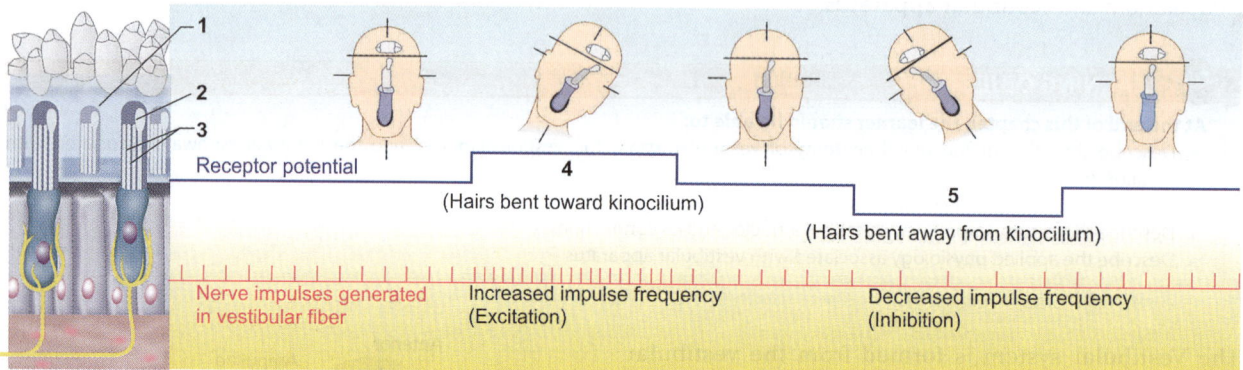

**Fig. 90.3:** Maintenance of balance and spatial orientation.

have stereocilia and a kinocilium, which respond to the movement of calcium carbonate crystals called statoconia. Since the utricle primarily senses changes in the horizontal plane, it helps to *maintain balance and stability during movements like walking or running.*

### Saccule

The saccule is *smaller* and *situated vertically* in the vestibular apparatus. It is primarily involved in *detecting linear movements in the vertical plane*, such as changes in head position *when lying down or standing up.* Similar to the utricle, the saccule contains a macula with hair cells that respond to the movement of statoconia. The macula of the saccule is mainly oriented in a vertical plane, *allowing it to sense changes in head orientation relative to gravity* (like movement in an elevator).

Within the utricle and saccule, small sensory areas called *maculae* detect the head's orientation concerning gravity. These maculae contain hair cells embedded in a gelatinous layer with calcium carbonate crystals called *statoconia*. When the head moves, the weight of these crystals bends the hair cells, initiating nerve impulses through the vestibular nerve **(Figs. 90.3 and 90.4).**

- When the *stereocilia bend towards the largest kinocilium*, it results in the *depolarization* of the cell, thus stimulating it. When the stereocilia and

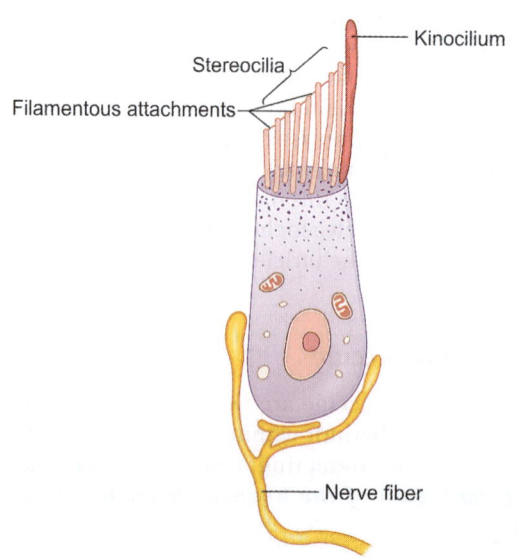

**Fig. 90.4:** Structure of hair cell.

kinocilium are bent in the direction of the kinocilium, the filamentous attachments between them tug on the stereocilia, pulling them outward from the cell body. This action opens several fluid channels in the neuronal cell membrane surrounding the bases of the stereocilia. These channels allow positive ions to flow into the cell from the surrounding endolymphatic fluid. This influx of positive ions leads to depolarization of the receptor membrane, which means the inside of the cell becomes less negative compared to the outside.

- When the *stereocilia bend away from the largest kinocilium*, it results in the *hyperpolarization* of the cell. When the pile of stereocilia is bent in the opposite direction, away from the kinocilium, the tension on the attachments is reduced. This movement results in the closure of the ion channels, causing receptor hyperpolarization. Hyperpolarization makes the inside of the cell more negative relative to the outside.

These signals are then transmitted to the brain via the vestibular nerve, providing information about the direction and intensity of mechanical stimuli, such as changes in head position or movement, to help maintain balance and spatial orientation.

## Semicircular Canals

The semicircular canals are another vital component of the vestibular system, responsible for detecting rotational movements of the head in three-dimensional space. There are three semicircular canals in each vestibular apparatus, oriented at right angles to each other to cover all three planes of motion.

### Anterior Semicircular Canal

This canal is *oriented vertically* and detects *rotational movements of the head in the sagittal plane*, such as nodding the head up and down (Nodding to say YES)

### Posterior Semicircular Canal

The posterior canal is also *oriented vertically* but in a different plane than the anterior canal. It detects *rotational movements of the head in the transverse plane*, such as tilting the head from side to side (Nodding to AGREE).

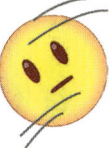

### Lateral (Horizontal) Semicircular Canal

This canal is *oriented horizontally* and detects **rotational movements of the head in the frontal plane**, such as turning the head from side to side.

Each semicircular canal has an enlargement at one end called the ampulla. Inside the ampulla is a sensory organ called the *crista ampullaris*, which contains hair cells.

When the head rotates, the inertia of the fluid within the semicircular canals causes the fluid to remain stationary while the canal itself moves. This movement of the canal causes the fluid to flow within the ampulla, deflecting a gelatinous structure called the cupula. The cupula deflects in the direction opposite to the head movement, bending the hair cells within the crista ampullaris **(Fig. 90.5)**.

Similar to the mechanism described for the utricle and saccule, the bending of the hair cells in the semicircular canals results in changes in membrane potential, which generate electrical signals. These signals are then transmitted via the vestibular nerve to the brain, providing information about the direction, speed, and intensity of head movements, allowing for the maintenance of balance and coordination.

Overall, the vestibular apparatus, with its intricate structures and mechanisms, plays a vital role in maintaining balance and spatial orientation.

## FUNCTIONS OF VESTIBULAR APPARATUS

### Maintenance of Static Equilibrium

The utricle and saccule play crucial roles in the maintenance of static equilibrium, primarily by detecting the orientation of the head with respect to the pull of gravity.

#### Orientation Detection

The hair cells within the maculae of the utricles and saccules are oriented in different directions, allowing them to be stimulated differently based on the position of the head. This pattern of stimulation provides the brain with information about the head's orientation relative to gravity. The brain then uses this information to activate appropriate postural muscles via the vestibular, cerebellar, and reticular motor nerve systems, ensuring proper equilibrium is maintained **(Fig. 90.6)**.

#### Detection of Linear Acceleration

When the body experiences sudden linear acceleration, such as being thrust forward, the statoconia within the utricles and saccules, due to their greater mass inertia, fall backward on the hair cell cilia. This triggers the sensation of disequilibrium, making the person feel as though they are falling backward. In response, the nervous system automatically causes the person to lean forward until the anterior shift of the statoconia equals the tendency for them to fall backward due to acceleration. Once equilibrium is achieved, the nervous system stops further forward leaning. Essentially, the maculae help maintain equilibrium during linear acceleration by adjusting the body's position to counteract the perceived imbalance.

**Note:** That's exactly the reason, why you don't fall, when the driver hits the sudden brakes, when you are standing in a moving bus.

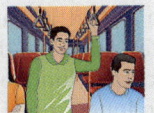

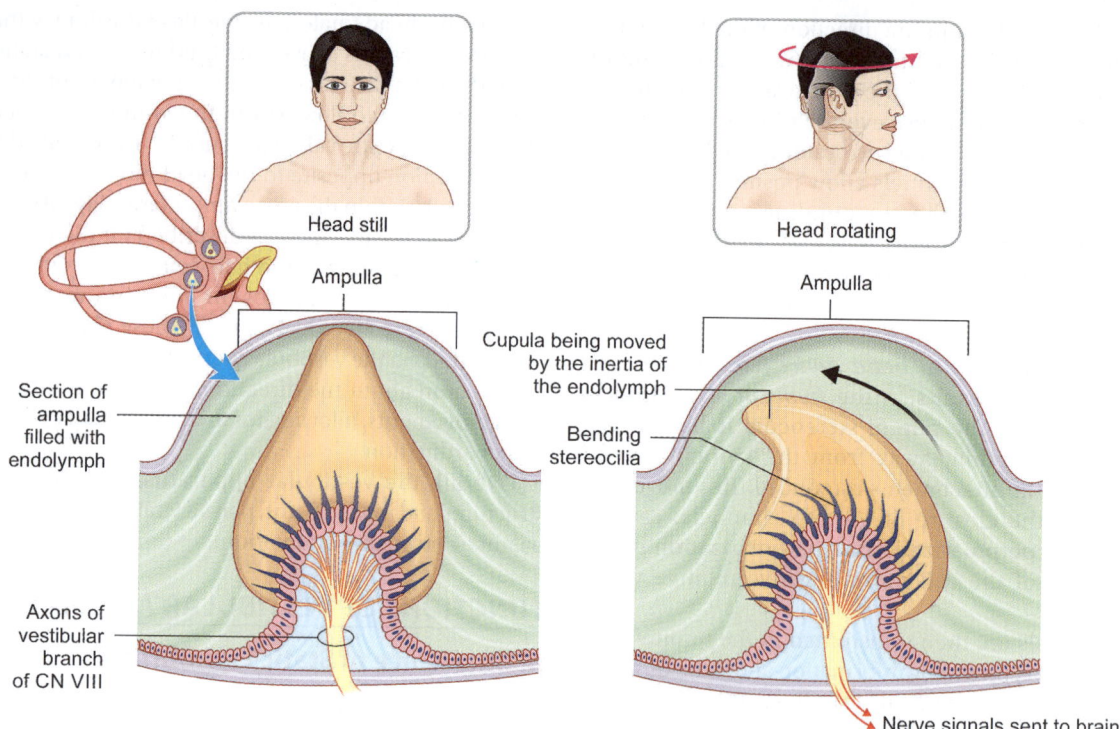

**Fig. 90.5:** Movement of cupula with head movement.

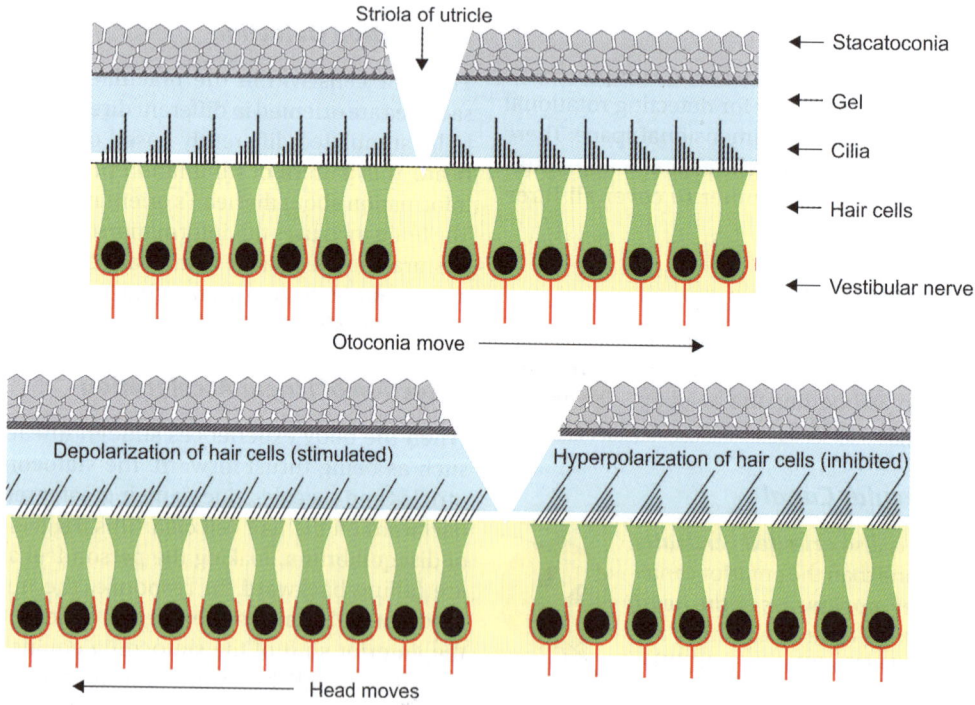

**Fig. 90.6:** Orientation detection of hair cell.

### Linear Velocity Detection

Unlike linear acceleration, the maculae do not operate to detect linear velocity. For instance, when runners start running, they lean forward to counteract the initial acceleration. However, once they reach running speed, they no longer need to lean forward to maintain equilibrium unless there is air resistance. In such cases, it's the pressure end-organs in the skin, not the maculae, that initiate equilibrium adjustments to prevent falling.

Hence, the utricle and saccule contribute significantly to maintaining static equilibrium by detecting head orientation, responding to linear acceleration, and ensuring appropriate adjustments are made to keep the body balanced and stable.

## Predictive Function of the Semicircular Canals for Maintaining the Equilibrium

The semicircular duct system serves a "predictive" function in the maintenance of equilibrium by detecting rotational movements of the head and providing anticipatory signals to the central nervous system. While the maculae of the utricle and saccule detect static orientations and linear accelerations, the semicircular canals detect beginning or stopping rotation in one direction or another.

### Anticipatory Corrections

When a person initiates a rapid, intricate movement involving rotation, such as suddenly turning while running, there is a brief delay before the maculae of the utricle and saccule can detect the change in balance. However, the semicircular ducts detect the rotational movement almost instantly. This early detection allows the central nervous system to anticipate the loss of balance that may occur in the next fraction of a second.

### Predictive Adjustments

Armed with information from the semicircular ducts, the central nervous system can make anticipatory adjustments to prevent the person from falling off balance. These adjustments may involve activating appropriate postural muscles or adjusting the position of the body to maintain equilibrium before the imbalance occurs.

The cerebellum plays a crucial role in processing signals from the semicircular ducts and coordinating anticipatory adjustments to maintain balance. Removal of the flocculonodular lobes of the cerebellum affects the normal detection of semicircular duct signals but has less impact on detecting signals from the maculae. This highlights the cerebellum's role as a "predictive" organ for rapid body movements and equilibrium maintenance.

## VESTIBULAR PATHWAYS AND CONNECTIONS (FIG. 90.7)

The nerves from the semicircular canals and the otolithic organs project to the Scarpa's ganglion in internal acoustic meatus. Axons of the Scarpa's ganglion form the vestibular nerve (CN VIII).

## VESTIBULAR NUCLEI

The vestibular nuclei are clusters of neurons located in the brainstem, specifically in the medulla and pons. These nuclei receive input from the vestibular nerve and are involved in processing and integrating vestibular signals. They play a crucial role in maintaining balance, spatial orientation, and stabilizing gaze. The vestibular nuclei are also responsible for relaying vestibular information to other parts of the brain, such as the cerebellum, thalamus, and cerebral cortex. Additionally, the vestibular nuclei are involved in generating motor responses to maintain the position of the head in space. Tracts descending from these nuclei, such as the vestibulospinal tract, mediate adjustments of the head relative to the neck and body.

There are around 19,000 neurons supplying the cristae and maculae on each side. Each vestibular nerve

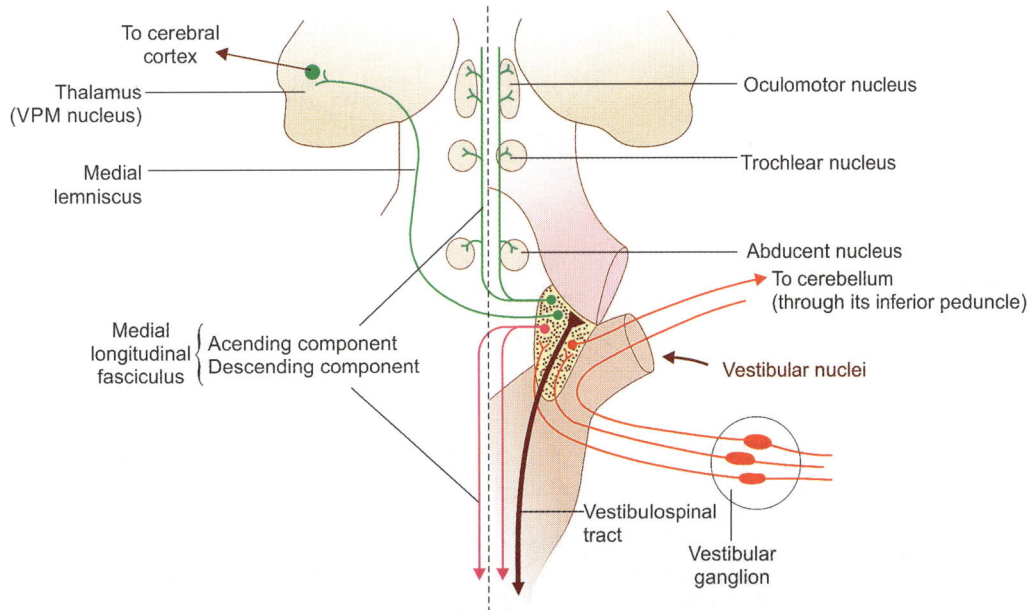

**Fig. 90.7:** Central connections of the vestibular system.

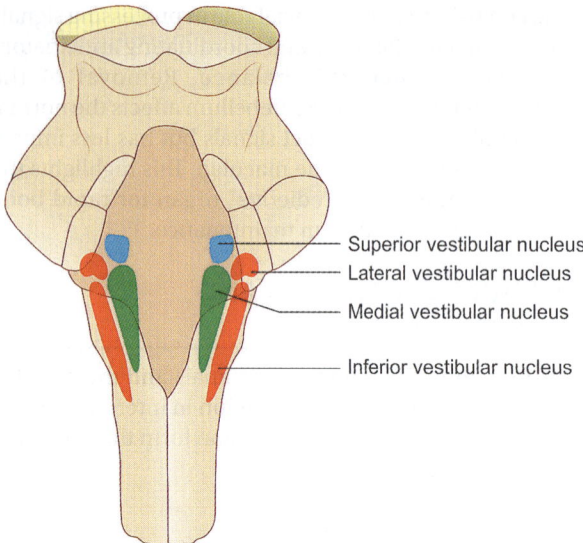

**Fig. 90.8:** Parts of vestibular nucleus.

terminates in flocculonodular lobe of cerebellum and ipsilateral vestibular nucleus having four parts **(Fig. 90.8)**, mentioned below:

- **Superior vestibular nucleus** (also called as angular or Bechterew's). This nucleus contributes particularly to the medial longitudinal fasciculus (MLF). It receives the inputs from horizontal semicircular canals. It supplies the muscles of eyes for the vestibulo-occular reflex.
- **Lateral (deiters) vestibular nucleus:** It receives the inputs from utricle and saccule. From here the fibers project to the contralateral spinal cord.
- **Medial (triangular nucleus of Schwalbe) vestibular nucleus:** It receives the inputs from anterior and posterior semicircular canals.
- **Descending (inferior or spinal) vestibular nuclei.** It receives the inputs from otolith organs and projects to cerebellum, reticular formation, and spinal cord. The major output of this nucleus are the vestibulospinal tracts.

## Connections of Vestibular Nucleus

*See* **Figure 90.9**.

### VESTIBULAR REFLEXES

Vestibular reflexes are a set of automatic responses mediated by the vestibular system. These reflexes help maintain balance, stabilize gaze, and adjust posture in response to changes in head position or movement.

- **Vestibulo-ocular reflex (VOR):** This reflex helps stabilize gaze during head movements by generating eye movements in the opposite direction of head movements. For example, when you turn your head to the right, your eyes move to the left to maintain fixation on a target.

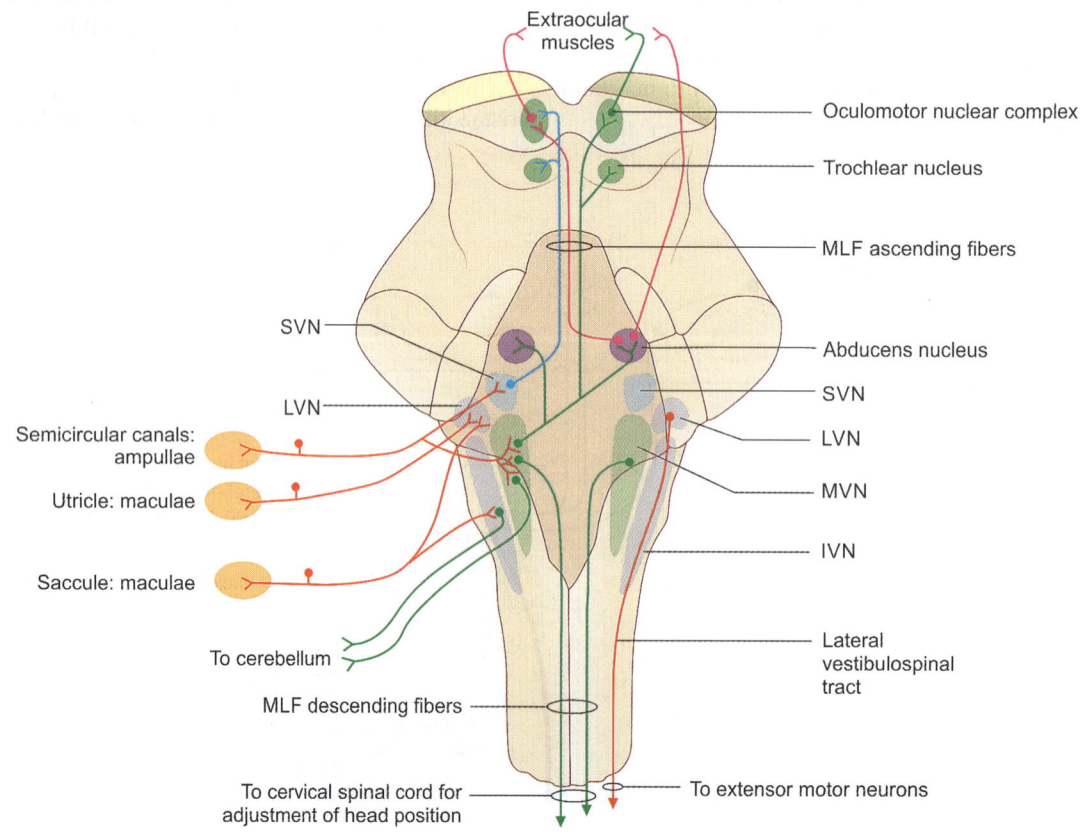

**Fig. 90.9:** Connections of vestibular nucleus.

- **Vestibulospinal reflex (VSR):** The VSR helps maintain posture and balance by adjusting muscle tone and activity in response to signals from the vestibular system. It plays a crucial role in coordinating movements to prevent falls.
- **Vestibulocollic reflex (VCR):** This reflex adjusts neck muscle activity to stabilize the head during head movements, helping to maintain visual stability and balance.
- **Otolith reflexes:** These reflexes involve the utricle and saccule, which are structures in the inner ear that detect linear acceleration and gravity. Otolith reflexes contribute to postural control and stabilization during activities such as walking and standing.
- **Vestibulo-autonomic reflexes:** These reflexes involve connections between the vestibular system and the autonomic nervous system, influencing functions such as blood pressure, heart rate, and sweating in response to changes in posture or motion.

These reflexes are essential for everyday activities such as walking, running, and maintaining balance while standing or sitting upright. Dysfunction of the vestibular system can lead to symptoms such as dizziness, vertigo, and imbalance, affecting a person's quality of life and ability to perform daily tasks.

## DISORDERS ASSOCIATED WITH VESTIBULAR APPARATUS

### Nystagmus

Nystagmus is a rhythmic, involuntary movement of the eyes characterized by alternating smooth pursuit in one direction followed by a fast, jerky movement in the opposite direction. This eye movement can occur horizontally, vertically, or even in a rotary pattern. It can be congenital (present at birth) or acquired later in life due to various causes. This reflex serves to maintain visual fixation on stationary points while the body is in motion, particularly during rotation (vestibulo-ocular reflex).

There are two main types of nystagmus.

### Peripheral Nystagmus

This type is often associated with dysfunction or abnormalities in the vestibular system or the peripheral parts of the inner ear. Conditions such as vestibular neuritis, Meniere's disease, and benign paroxysmal positional vertigo (BPPV) can lead to peripheral nystagmus. These conditions disrupt the normal balance of signals sent from the inner ear to the brain, resulting in abnormal eye movements.

### Central Nystagmus

Central nystagmus originates from abnormalities in the central nervous system, particularly in regions responsible for controlling eye movements and gaze stability. It can be a sign of underlying neurological disorders such as multiple sclerosis, brainstem strokes, or brain tumors affecting the cerebellum or brainstem.

Nystagmus is a characteristic eye movement observed during rotation, characterized by a slow drift in one direction followed by a quick return movement in the opposite direction. The slow component of nystagmus is initiated by impulses from the vestibular labyrinths, while the quick component is triggered by a center in the brainstem.

Caloric stimulation, a test used to assess vestibular labyrinth function, involves irrigating the external auditory meats with warm or cold water. In healthy individuals, warm water induces nystagmus towards the stimulated side, while cold water induces nystagmus towards the opposite side (COWS mnemonic). However, in cases of unilateral vestibular pathway lesions, nystagmus may be reduced or absent on the affected side.

When performing ear irrigations for the treatment of ear infections to avoid inducing nystagmus, vertigo, and nausea, it's essential to use fluid at body temperature. This helps maintain equilibrium within the inner ear and minimizes adverse effects.

### Benign Paroxysmal Positional Vertigo

Benign paroxysmal positional vertigo (BPPV) is characterized by episodic vertigo triggered by specific changes in body position, such as rolling over in bed or bending over. In BPPV, 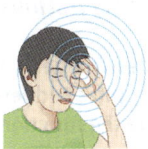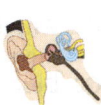 tiny calcium carbonate crystals called otoconia dislodge from the utricle and can become lodged within the semicircular canal or cupula. This displacement disrupts the normal fluid dynamics within the inner ear, resulting in abnormal deflections of the hair cells in response to head movements relative to gravity.

Effective treatment for BPPV typically involves otolith repositioning maneuvers, which aim to guide the displaced otoconia back into the utricle, alleviating symptoms. These maneuvers, such as the Epley maneuver, are often performed by healthcare professionals and can provide significant relief for individuals experiencing BPPV episodes.

### Ménière Disease

Ménière's disease is a chronic inner ear disorder characterized by episodes of vertigo or severe dizziness, tinnitus (ringing in the ears), fluctuating hearing loss, and a sensation of pressure or fullness in the affected ear. These symptoms can vary in intensity and duration, with episodes lasting several hours and occurring sporadically. Initially, hearing loss in Ménière's disease may be temporary, but it can progress to permanent hearing loss over time. The exact cause of Ménière's disease is not fully understood, but it is believed to involve a combination of factors, including abnormal fluid buildup in the inner ear and possibly immune system dysfunction. Inflammation and increased fluid volume within the membranous labyrinth of the inner ear can lead to rupture, resulting in the mixing of endolymph and perilymph fluids.

## Motion Sickness

Motion sickness is a transient condition characterized by nausea, vomiting, sweating, pallor, and changes in blood pressure, often triggered by conflicting sensory information received by the vestibular and other sensory systems.

Space motion sickness, experienced by astronauts during spaceflight, occurs due to mismatches in neural input caused by changes in gravity and spatial orientation cues. It typically resolves after a few days in microgravity but can recur upon reentry to Earth's gravity.

### SUMMARY

- Vestibular system is comprised of the vestibular apparatus and the vestibular nuclei.
- The vestibular system is primarily concerned with maintenance of the body equilibrium and various participate in various postural reflexes.
- The membranous labyrinth of vestibular apparatus is present along with the inner ear, housed in the bony labyrinth. It has the receptors present in utricle, saccule and ampullae of semicircular canals.
- The utricle and saccule have maculae containing the hair cells, whose stereocilia are embedded in the gelatinous material containing otoliths. They are responsible for maintaining the posture during linear acceleration (horizontal and vertical).
- The semicircular canals, have cristae ampullaris, which is cup like receptors having numerous hair cells. It detects the beginning and stoppage of the rotational movement.
- The vestibular nerve originates from these hair cells and projects to the ipsilateral vestibular nuclei, which has four parts, the superior, medial, lateral, and inferior vestibular nuclei.
- The fibers arising from vestibular nuclei project into cerebellum, cerebrum, spinal cord for maintaining the posture and equilibrium of the body.

### LET US SEE, HOW MUCH YOU HAVE LEARNT?

#### Review Questions

**Q1.** Why doesn't a person standing in the bus fall when the driver applies sudden brakes?

**Q2.** Describe the functions of vestibular apparatus.

**Q3.** How does the vestibular apparatus detect the head rotation?

**Q4.** Why don't one fall when he suddenly looks back while running?

#### Critical Thinking Case-Based Questions

**Q1.** A 50-year-old man, presented to OPD with complaints of dizziness, vertigo, and a sensation of spinning, especially when moving his head quickly or standing up from a seated position. He also reported occasional nausea and imbalance, causing him to feel unsteady while walking. These symptoms began a few weeks ago without any apparent trigger. On physical examination, he showed signs of nystagmus (involuntary eye movements). His physician suspected a disorder of the vestibular system and recommends further evaluation. Based on the given case scenario, answer the following questions:
   a. What are the main components of the vestibular system?
   b. How do they work together to maintain balance, posture, and spatial orientation?
   c. How can disorders of the vestibular system cause symptoms in this case?

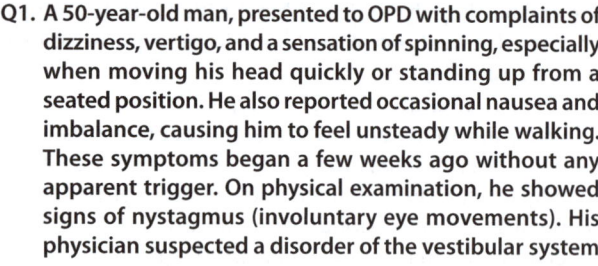
#### Multiple Choice Questions

**Q1.** Geeta is on a boat trip and suddenly experiences a sensation of spinning and loss of balance. Which of the following vestibular structures is likely responsible for her symptoms?
   a. Utricle
   b. Saccule
   c. Ampulla
   d. Cochlea

**Q2.** During a roller coaster ride, John feels his eyes automatically move in the opposite direction of his head movements to maintain focus on the horizon. Which vestibular reflex is responsible for this phenomenon?
   a. Vestibulo-ocular reflex (VOR)
   b. Vestibulospinal reflex (VSR)
   c. Vestibulocollic reflex (VCR)
   d. Otolith reflex

**Q3.** After spinning around several times, Michael feels dizzy and unsteady on his feet. Which part of the vestibular system is primarily responsible for detecting rotational movements?
   a. Semicircular canals
   b. Utricle
   c. Saccule
   d. Cochlea

Q4. Seema is standing on a moving train and notices that she can maintain her balance even when the train suddenly accelerates. Which vestibular reflex is primarily responsible for her ability to adjust her posture in response to changes in velocity?
   a. Vestibulo-ocular reflex (VOR)
   b. Vestibulospinal reflex (VSR)
   c. Vestibulocollic reflex (VCR)
   d. Otolith reflex

Q5. During a medical examination, the doctor observes involuntary eye movements in a patient when the head is rapidly rotated from side to side. Which vestibular reflex is likely impaired in this patient?
   a. Vestibulo-ocular reflex (VOR)
   b. Vestibulospinal reflex (VSR)
   c. Vestibulocollic reflex (VCR)
   d. Otolith reflex

Q6. The utricle and saccule are responsible for detecting which type of movement?
   a. Linear acceleration and gravity
   b. Angular acceleration
   c. Sound vibrations
   d. Visual stimuli

Q7. Which vestibular reflex adjusts neck muscle activity to stabilize the head during head movements?
   a. Vestibulospinal reflex (VSR)
   b. Vestibulo-ocular reflex (VOR)
   c. Vestibulocollic reflex (VCR)
   d. Otolith reflex

Q8. Which part of the brainstem plays a crucial role in integrating vestibular signals and coordinating balance and posture?
   a. Cerebellum
   b. Thalamus
   c. Medulla oblongata
   d. Hypothalamus

**ANSWERS**

1. a   2. a   3. a   4. b   5. a   6. a   7. c   8. c

# Autonomic Nervous System

**CHAPTER 91**

> **COMPETENCY ADDRESSED**
> 
> **PY10.5:** Describe and discuss structure and functions of reticular activating system and autonomic nervous system.

>  **LEARNING OBJECTIVES**
> 
> **At the end of this chapter, the learner should be able to:**
> - Describe the structural details of the autonomic nervous system
> - Describe the functions of autonomic nervous system
> - Describe the regulatory mechanisms under the influence of autonomic nervous system
> - Describe the applied aspects related to autonomic nervous system

Autonomic means self-control, hence the nervous system which controls its functioning is called an autonomic nervous system (ANS). The ANS is not under voluntary control; rather it takes care of the self-regulated homeostatic mechanisms and various visceral regulations.

The ANS serves following *functions* in our body:
- Maintenance of homeostasis
- Regulation of visceral activities
- Coordination of body responses towards exercise and stress
- Assists endocrine for various functions
- Controls circulation, respiration, digestion, excretion and reproduction.

## ORGANIZATION OF AUTONOMIC NERVOUS SYSTEM (FIG. 91.1)

Basic functional unit of the ANS comprises two neurons—the preganglionic and the postganglionic neurons.

1. **Preganglionic neurons:** These neurons arise from the central nervous system (cranial nerve nuclei) or from the spinal cord. They are *type B myelinated cholinergic fibers,* which end in the autonomic ganglia.
2. **Autonomic ganglia:** The autonomic ganglia is the collection of neurons where the preganglionic neurons terminate on the postganglionic neurons. The *neurotransmitter* secreted by the preganglionic neurons is *acetylcholine* and the *receptors* on the postganglionic neurons are *nicotinic ($N_N$) type*.
3. **Postganglionic neurons:** These neurons (mostly *type C, unmyelinated fibers*) arise from the autonomic ganglia and terminate on the target organs. The neurotransmitter secreted from the neurons and the receptors on the target organs depends on division of the autonomic nervous system.

Both anatomically and physiologically, the autonomic nervous system is classified into two broad divisions:
1. Parasympathetic nervous system
2. Sympathetic nervous system

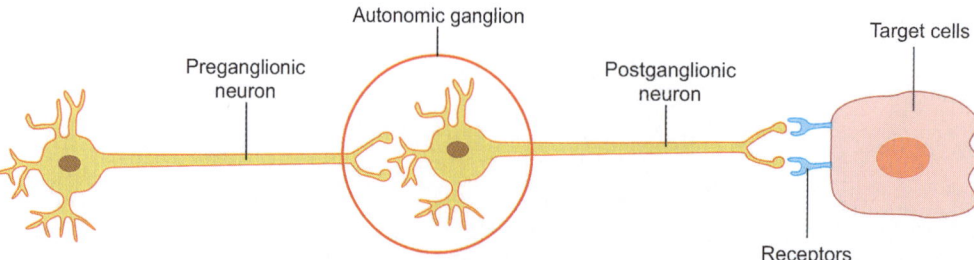

**Fig. 91.1:** Organization of autonomic nervous system.

However, the *enteric nervous system is also considered as the third division of the autonomic nervous system.*

## PARASYMPATHETIC NERVOUS SYSTEM (FIG. 91.2)

The parasympathetic division of the autonomic nervous system is primarily responsible for regulating the *basal homeostatic and visceral functions*. Hence, it is also called the nervous system for *'rest and digest'.*

## SYMPATHETIC NERVOUS SYSTEM (FIG. 91.2)

Sympathetic division of ANS is primarily responsible for the *emergency situations*. However, some basal functions such as *sympathetic vasoconstrictor tone are maintained even at rest*.

The various differences and similarities in sympathetic and parasympathetic nervous system are shown in the **Table 91.1**.

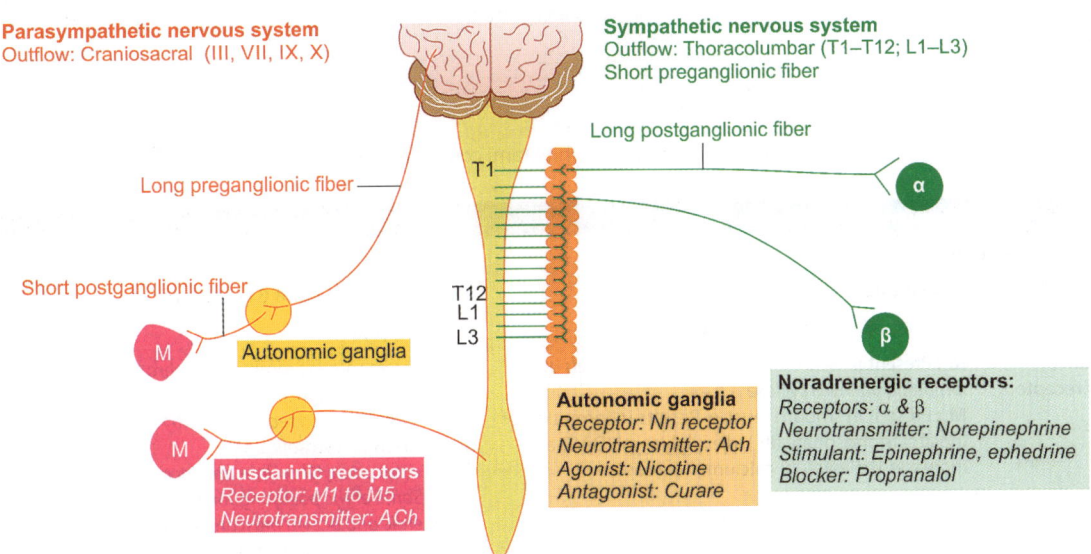

**Fig. 91.2:** Organization of parasympathetic and sympathetic nervous system.

**Table 91.1:** Similarities and differences between parasympathetic and sympathetic nervous system.

|  | Parasympathetic nervous system | Sympathetic nervous system |
|---|---|---|
| Origin | Craniosacral outflow<br>• Cranial nerve nuclei for III, VII, IX, X nerves<br>• Sacral (S2-4 or segments) | Thoracolumbar outflow **(Fig. 91.3)**<br>T1 to T12, L1 to L3 |
| Preganglionic (connector) fibers | Type B, myelinated, long, cholinergic nerve fibers | Type B, myelinated, short, cholinergic nerve fibers, exits the thoracolumbar segments of the spinal cord and enters the *white rami communicantes*, to reach chain of autonomic ganglia (paravertebral sympathetic chain) |
| **Applied Physiology** | Damage to preganglionic fibers results in *autonomic failure called Shy-Drager syndrome*. This condition when accompanied with parkinsonism and cerebellar ataxia is called *multiple system atrophy (MSA)*. It is a neurodegenerative disorder seen in elderly people. The most common presenting symptom in these patients is erectile dysfunction. | |
| **Autonomic ganglion** | | |
| Neurotransmitter | Acetylcholine | Acetylcholine |
| Receptor | **Nicotinic ($N_N$) type** | **Nicotinic ($N_N$) type** |
| Agonist | Nicotine | Nicotine |
| Blocker | Curare | Curare |
| Postganglionic (effector) fibers | Type C, unmyelinated, short-cholinergic nerve fibers | Type C, unmyelinated, long, noradrenergic nerve fibers. These fibers enter the *gray rami communicantes*, and travel to the effector organs. |
| **Applied Physiology** | Blockage of nicotinic receptors due to arrow poison containing d-tubocurarine results in blockage of $N_M$ receptors (other nicotinic receptors) present in the neuromuscular junction. This causes *transient paralysis of the skeletal muscles*. | |

*Contd...*

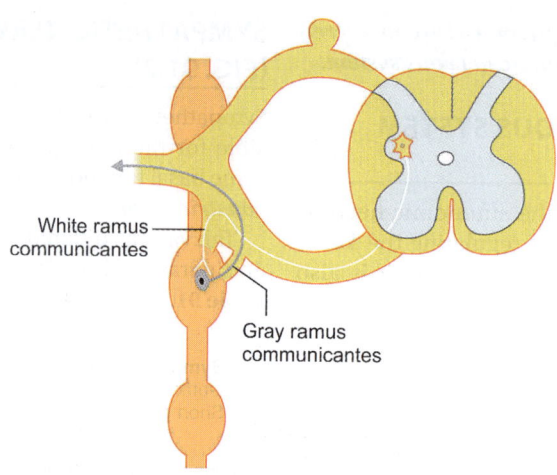

**Fig. 91.3:** Gray and white rami communicantes.

*Contd...*

| | Parasympathetic nervous system | Sympathetic nervous system |
|---|---|---|
| **Target organ receptors** | | |
| Type of receptor | Muscarinic | Noradrenergic (α and β receptors) |
| Subtypes | $M_1$ to $M_5$ ($M_2$ and $M_3$ are most abundant) | $α_1, α_2, β_1, β_2, β_3$ |
| Mechanism of action of receptors | $M_2$: Present in heart muscle. *Opens $K^+$ channels by inhibiting adenylyl cyclase*<br>$M_3$: Present in smooth muscle. Results in formation of inositol triphosphate ($IP_3$), diacylglycerol (DAG) and increases the levels of calcium in sarcoplasm | $α_1$: G protein coupled receptor acts through $IP_3$/DAG. It increases cytosolic calcium concentration<br>$α_2$: G protein coupled receptor acts by inhibiting adenylyl cyclase and decreasing cytosolic cAMP<br>β: Activates adenylyl cyclase and increases cAMP<br>*Note: Some of the postganglionic sympathetic fibers are cholinergic and act via muscarinic receptors. These fibers supply sweat glands (sudomotor fibers), for skeletal muscles (sympathetic vasodilator fibers)* |
| Agonist | Carbachol | Ephedrine, pseudoephedrine |
| Blocker | Atropine | α blocker: pentazocine, phentolamine<br>β blocker: propranolol |
| **Organization of parasympathetic and sympathetic fibers** | | |
| | **III nerve (oculomotor nerve)**<br>• *Origin:* Edinger-Westphal nucleus<br>• *Autonomic ganglia:* Ciliary ganglion<br>• *Innervate:* Sphincter pupillae, ciliary muscle<br>**VII nerve**<br>• *Origin:* Superior salivary nucleus<br>• *Autonomic ganglia:* Pterygopalatine ganglion and submandibular ganglion<br>• *Innervate:* Lacrimal gland, nasal and palatal glands. Submandibular and sublingual salivary glands<br>**IX nerve (glossopharyngeal nerve)**<br>• *Origin:* Inferior salivary nucleus<br>• *Autonomic ganglia:* Otic ganglion<br>• *Innervate:* Parotid gland, carotid and aortic sinus and bodies<br>**X nerve**<br>• *Origin:* Nucleus ambiguus, dorsal motor nuclei of vagus<br>• *Autonomic ganglia:* Intrinsic visceral plexus (vagosympathetic trunk)<br>• *Innervate:* All visceral organs of thorax and abdomen<br>**Sacral (pudendal nerve S2-4)**<br>• *Origin:* Intermediolateral nucleus gray matter of spinal cord<br>• *Autonomic ganglia:* Visceral ganglion<br>• *Innervate:* Pelvic organs | **I) Paravertebral sympathetic chain**<br>• *Cervical ganglia*<br>  ▪ Superior cervical ganglia: Head<br>  ▪ Middle cervical ganglia: Stellate ganglia<br>  ▪ Inferior cervical ganglia: Chest<br>• *Thoracic ganglia*<br>  ▪ T1, T2: Supplies head, neck<br>  ▪ T3, T4: Supplies thoracic viscera<br>  ▪ T5-9: Supplies upper limb<br>  ▪ T10-12: Supplies upper abdominal viscera<br>• *Lumbar ganglia*<br>  ▪ T10-L2: Supplies lower limb<br>  ▪ L1-2: Supplies lower abdominal viscera<br>**II) Collateral ganglia**<br>• *Celiac ganglia:* Supplies stomach, small intestine, liver, gallbladder, pancreas, spleen and kidneys<br>• *Superior mesenteric ganglia:* Supplies small and large intestines<br>• *Inferior mesenteric ganglia:* Supplies colon, rectum, urinary bladder, reproductive organs (pelvic organs)<br>**III) Terminal Ganglia**<br>• Adrenal Medulla<br>• Intrinsic cardiac adrenergic rec.<br>• Pancreas<br>• Urinary bladder |

*Contd...*

Contd...

| | Parasympathetic nervous system | Sympathetic nervous system |
|---|---|---|
| **Systemic effects/actions** | | |
| Eyes<br>• Pupil<br><br>• Lacrimal glands | Constriction of pupil (miosis) due to stimulation of sphincter pupillae muscle<br>Increased secretion of lacrimal glands | Dilation of pupil (mydriasis) due to stimulation of radial muscles of iris ($α_1$) |
| Heart<br>• SA node<br><br><br><br><br><br><br><br>• AV node<br><br><br>• Ventricular muscles<br><br><br>• Blood vessels | It is supplied by the right vagus nerve. It decreases the activity of the SA node by increasing the conductance of potassium channels ($K^+$ efflux). It exerts a—<br>• negative chronotropic effect (decreased heart rate)<br>• negative bathmotropic effect (decreased excitability)<br>• negative dromotropic effect (decreased conductivity)<br>It is supplied by the left vagus nerve. It also exerts a negative bathmotropic and dromotropic effects.<br><br>There is no parasympathetic supply to the ventricular muscles. Hence, the force of contraction is not affected by the parasympathetic stimulation. There is no parasympathetic supply to the blood vessels. | It is supplied by the right cardiac sympathetic nerves (C6-7 and T1-5). It stimulates the SA node and exerts a positive chronotropic, bathmotropic and dromotropic effects.<br><br><br><br><br><br>It is supplied by the left cardiac sympathetic nerves (C6-7 and T1-5). It stimulates the AV node and exerts a positive chronotropic, bathmotropic and dromotropic effects.<br>The sympathetic supply to the ventricular muscle increases the force of contraction, hence increasing the cardiac output on sympathetic stimulation.<br><br>The blood vessels maintained their diameter due to the sympathetic vasoconstrictor tone.<br>$α_1$ and $α_2$ receptors result in vasoconstriction, whereas some sympathetic vasodilator nerves act through M receptors resulting in vasodilation in some skeletal muscles. |
| Respiratory system | Bronchoconstriction resulting in increased airway resistance | Bronchodilation resulting in decreased airway resistance |
| Excretory system<br>• Urinary bladder | Contraction of detrusor muscle<br>Relaxation of sphincters<br>'Results in voiding of urine' | Relaxation of detrusor muscle ($β_2$)<br>Contraction of sphincters ($α_1$)<br>'Results in holding of urine' |
| Gastrointestinal system<br>• GI secretions<br>• GI motility | <br>Increases<br>Increases | <br>Decreases<br>Decreases |
| Sweat glands | No parasympathetic supply | Sympathetic fibers acts through the muscarinic receptors by secreting the neurotransmitter acetylcholine and increases the activity of sweat glands<br>*Note:* There are sweaty hands during anxiety, which occurs due to sympathetic overstimulation |
| Piloerector muscles | No parasympathetic supply | Contraction ($α_1$) |
| Reproduction<br>• Males<br>• Pregnant uterus in females | <br>Erection<br>No effect | <br>Ejaculation ($α_1$)<br>Contraction ($α_1$)/relaxation ($β_2$) |
| **Applied Physiology** | **1. Mushroom poisoning:**<br>Ingestion of wild mushrooms results in overstimulation of muscarinic receptors causing nausea, vomiting, diarrhea, urinary urgency, vasodilation, sweating and salivation. This can be treated by administering cholinesterase inhibitors like physostigmine.<br><br>**2. Organophosphorus compound (OPC) poisoning (Fig. 91.4):**<br>*Clinical features:* Miosis, salivation, sweating, bronchial constriction, vomiting and diarrhea | **1. Horner's syndrome:**<br>This syndrome occurs when the cervical sympathetic chain is disrupted. it is characterized by the presence of:<br>a. Ptosis (drooping of eyelid)<br>b. Miosis (constriction of pupil)<br>c. Anhidrosis (inability to sweat)<br>d. Hyperemia (flushed skin)<br>e. Loss of ciliospinal reflex<br>f. Enophthalmos.<br>**2. Pheochromocytoma:**<br>It is the tumor of the adrenal medulla resulting in excessive secretion of adrenaline. The clinical features are due to high levels of circulating adrenaline resulting in nausea, abdominal pain, weakness, headache, sweating attacks, hypertension, |

Contd...

| Parasympathetic nervous system | Sympathetic nervous system |
|---|---|
| *CNS toxicity:* Cognitive disturbances, convulsions, seizures, coma<br>*Other nicotinic effects:* Depolarizing NM blockade<br>*Pathogenesis:* Overstimulation of nicotinic and muscarinic receptors<br>*Diagnosis:* Mostly clinically, RBC and plasma cholinesterase level can be done for diagnosis<br>*Treatment:*<br>• Muscarinic receptor antagonist: IV Atropine is the treatment of choice<br>• Pralidoxime: To break the bond between OPC and acetylcholinesterase *'cholinesterase regenerator'*<br>• Sedatives: To abort seizures | anxiety and panic attacks, weight loss, elevated blood sugar levels, etc.<br>A 24-hour urine sample shows elevated levels of vanillylmandelic acid (VMA), which is the metabolite of adrenaline.<br>Treatment is the removal of the tumor. |

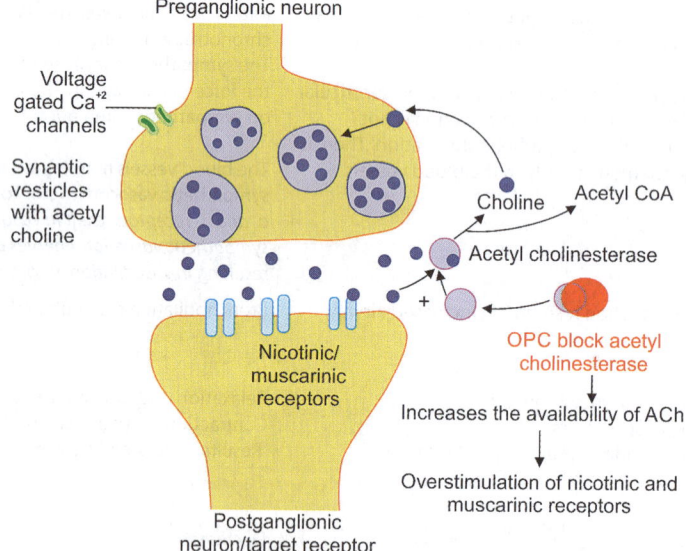

**Fig. 91.4:** Release of acetylcholine from the nerve endings acting of nicotinic receptors (in autonomic ganglia) and muscarinic receptors at postganglionic parasympathetic fibers.

## FIGHT OR FLIGHT RESPONSE (FIG. 91.5)

This term is used to represent the *mass activation of the sympathetic nervous system* in emergency situations, in which the body prepares itself for fight or flight.

There is overactivation of the sympathetic nervous system, resulting in
- *Mydriasis/pupillary dilation:* Which allows more light to enter eyes
- *Increased heart rate, cardiac output and blood pressure:* This permits more blood flow to the peripheral tissues
- *Increased respiratory rate:* Increasing the oxygen delivery to the peripheral tissues
- *Vasodilation in the muscles:* Allowing increased muscular performance
- *Inhibition of gastrointestinal secretions and motility*
- *Inhibition of micturition reflex*

## LEVELS OF CONTROL OF THE AUTONOMIC NERVOUS SYSTEM

Higher autonomic nervous centers (limbic system, forebrain structures) are further divided into the anterior hypothalamus and the posterior hypothalamus. The anterior hypothalamus further includes cranial nerve nuclei for IIIrd, VIIth, and IX nerves; nucleus ambiguus, sacral outflow from S2-4 sacral segments, and pontine nuclei. The posterior hypothalamus includes pontine nuclei, rostral medulla, and raphe nuclei **(Fig. 91.6)**.

## WORKING OF AUTONOMIC NERVOUS SYSTEM

The autonomic nervous system is concerned with regulation of various visceral reflexes and homeostatic mechanism like:
- Temperature regulation
- Regulation of blood volume

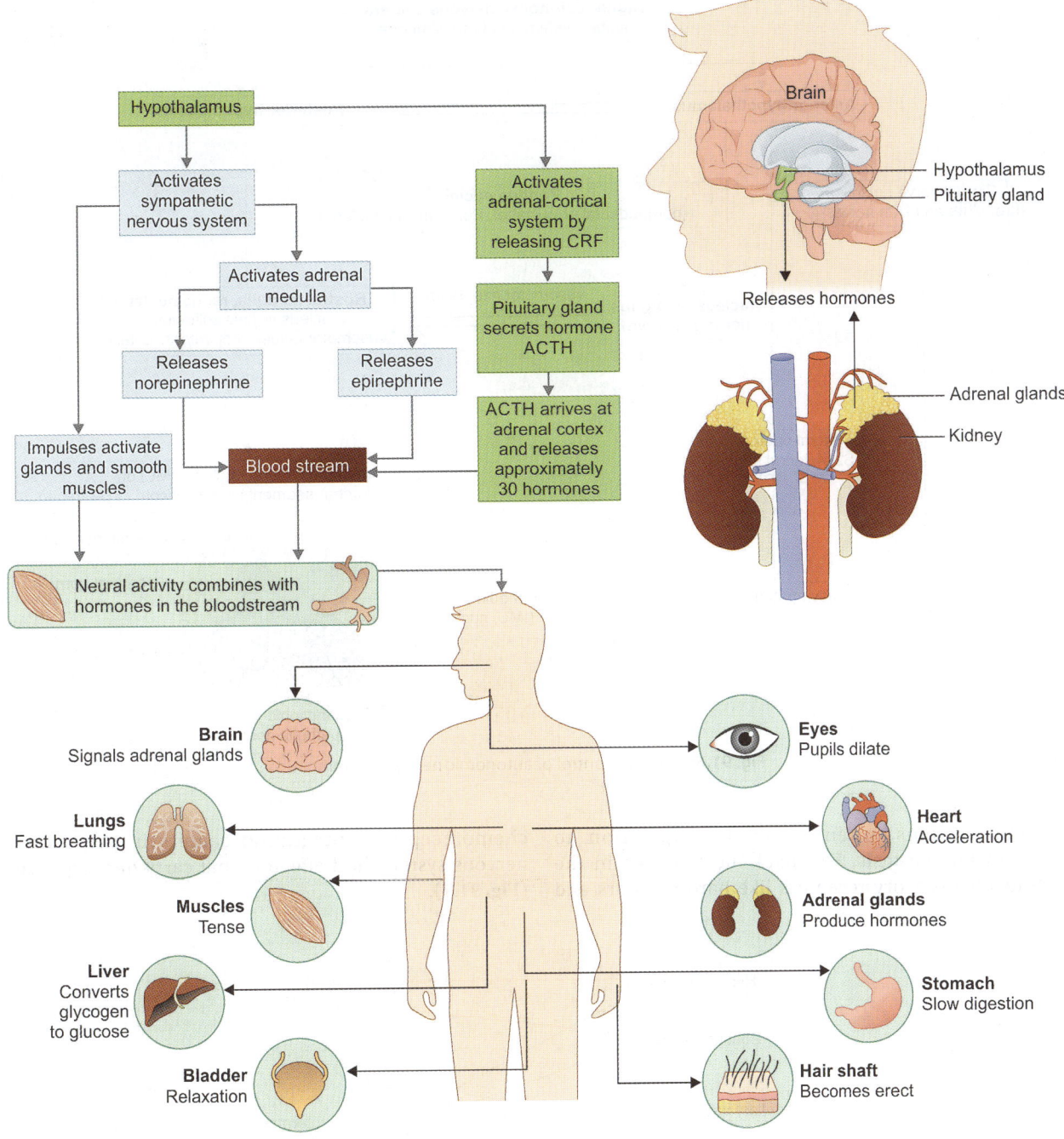

**Fig. 91.5:** Fight or flight response.

- Regulation of blood pressure
- Pupillary light reflex
- Accommodation reflex
- Vomiting reflex
- Deglutition reflex
- Defecation reflex
- Micturition reflex
- Erection and ejaculation

ANS is able to function efficiently due to the feedback and feedforward control mechanisms.

## FEEDBACK MECHANISM IN THE AUTONOMIC NERVOUS SYSTEM

The autonomic nervous system (ANS) operates largely unconsciously and regulates involuntary bodily functions, such as heart rate, digestion, and respiratory rate. A crucial aspect of its functionality is the feedback mechanism, which ensures dynamic adjustments in response to changing internal and external conditions. The ANS consists of two main branches: the sympathetic and parasympathetic

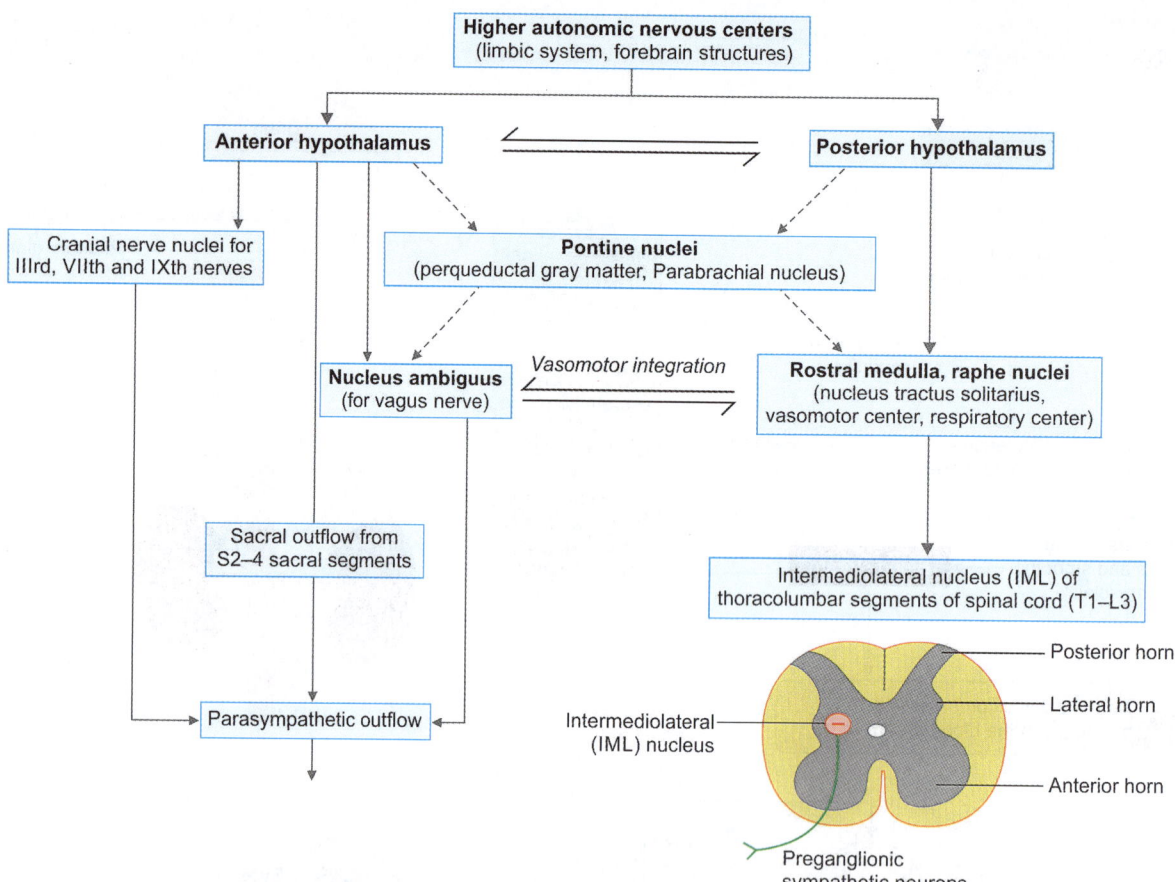

**Fig. 91.6:** Levels of control of autonomic nervous system.

nervous systems, often acting in opposition to maintain homeostasis. Feedback mechanisms in the ANS involve sensory receptors like baroreceptors and chemoreceptors, integrating centers in the central nervous system, and effectors that carry out responses **(Fig. 91.7)**.

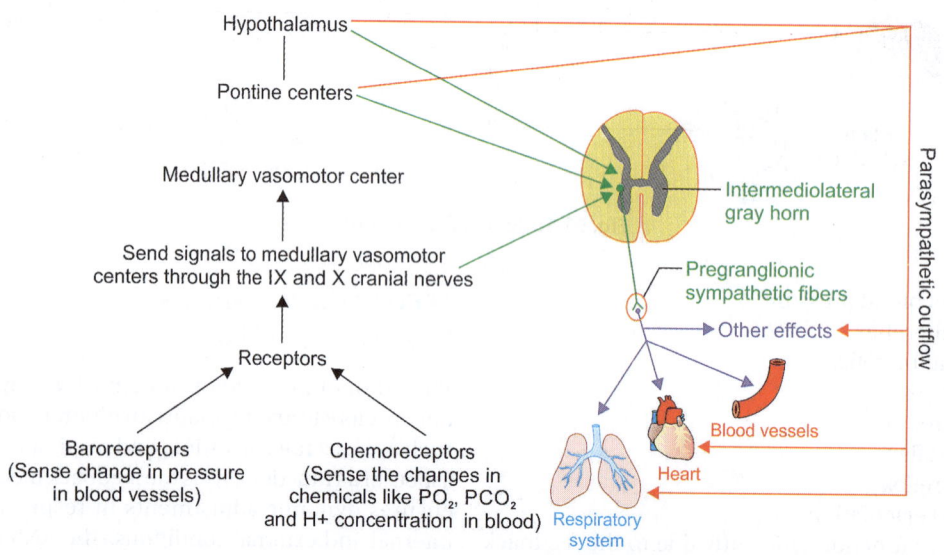

**Fig. 91.7:** Feedback control of autonomic nervous system.

## SUMMARY

- In this chapter we studied the autonomic nervous system (ANS), covering its structure, functions, regulatory mechanisms, and applied aspects.
- It delves into the control of homeostatic mechanisms and visceral regulations, as well as the coordination of bodily responses to stress and exercise.
- The autonomic nervous system is concerned with regulation of various visceral reflexes and homeostatic mechanisms like temperature regulation, regulation of blood volume, blood pressure, pupillary light reflex, accommodation reflex, vomiting reflex, and deglutition reflex.
- The ANS is divided into the parasympathetic and sympathetic nervous systems, each with distinct functions and effects on target organs. The parasympathetic system regulates basal homeostatic and visceral functions, while the sympathetic system is primarily responsible for emergency situations.
- The parasympathetic division of the autonomic nervous system is primarily responsible for regulating the basal homeostatic and visceral functions. Hence, it is also called the nervous system for 'rest and digest'.
- The sympathetic division of ANS is primarily responsible for emergency situations. However, some basal functions such as sympathetic vasoconstrictor tone are maintained even at rest.
- The feedback control and levels of control of the autonomic nervous system, including the role of higher autonomic nervous centers and the feedback mechanisms involving baroreceptors and chemoreceptors.

## LET US SEE, HOW MUCH YOU HAVE LEARNT?

### Review Questions

#### Long/Short Answer Questions

Q1. Differentiate between the sympathetic and parasympathetic nervous system.
Q2. Describe the effect of ANS on:
   a. Cardiovascular system
   b. Gastrointestinal system
Q3. Define vagal tone. What is its physiological significance?
Q4. Describe the physiological significance of sympathetic vasoconstrictor tone.
Q5. Describe the fight or flight response.
Q6. Describe the Horner's syndrome.
Q7. Why does a person with sympathetic overactivity has cold and sweaty hands?

#### Explain Why? (Reasoning Questions)

Q1. Activation of the sympathetic nervous system results in increased heart rate and blood pressure.
Q2. Parasympathetic stimulation causes constriction of the pupil (miosis).
Q3. The autonomic nervous system plays a crucial role in maintaining homeostasis.
Q4. Sympathetic activation leads to the release of adrenaline (epinephrine) from the adrenal medulla.
Q5. The autonomic nervous system is involved in regulating visceral functions such as digestion and urination.
Q6. Autonomic dysregulation can contribute to disorders like hypertension and gastrointestinal motility issues.

 *Critical Thinking Case-Based Questions*

Q1. A 35-year-old female presented to the emergency department with complaints of excessive salivation, sweating, vomiting, diarrhea, breathing difficulty, and seizure. Her attendant reported a history of consumption of toxic pesticides. On examination, the patient exhibited reduced air entry on both sides, miosis (constricted pupils), and altered sensorium. Based on the given scenario answer the following questions:
   a. What is the diagnosis?
   b. What is the physiological mechanism of action of organophosphates on the nervous system?

Q2. A 23-year-old male presented in emergency with complaints of nausea, vomiting, diarrhea, urinary urgency, sweating and excess salivation. The patient's attender gave a history of traveling to Manali for trekking and ingestion of wild mushrooms. On examination, there was vasodilation and signs of dehydration with reduced blood-pressure. Based on the case history, answer the following questions:
   a. What is the diagnosis?
   b. Explain the physiological reason behind this condition.

Q3. A 59-year-old woman with a history of hypertension without any treatment for 5 years presented in emergency with chest tightness, headache, sweating attacks, anxiety, panic attacks, nausea, abdominal pain, weakness, vital signs on arrival indicated a blood pressure of 78/50 mmHg. Twelve-lead electrocardiogram indicated ST-segment depression in leads II, III, aVF, and V3–V6 and QT prolongation. The coronary angiogram revealed no evidence of coronary artery disease. Contrast-enhanced computed tomography demonstrated an inhomogeneous right adrenal mass (2.5 × 3.0 cm). Based on the case history, answer the following questions:
   a. What is the diagnosis?
   b. Explain the physiological reason behind this condition.

## Multiple Choice Questions

**Q1.** The autonomic nervous system:
a. Controls smooth muscle, skeletal muscle and cardiac muscle
b. Controls smooth muscle, cardiac muscle and glandular activity
c. Mainly provides the afferent pathways for involuntary control of organs
d. Is subdivided into parasympathetic and sympathetic systems that mostly work antagonistically on blood vessels

**Q2.** The physiological effect in unacclimatised person suddenly exposed to cold is:
a. Tachycardia
b. Shift of blood from shell to core
c. Nonshivering thermogenesis
d. Hypertension

**Q3.** An injection of atropine causes all the following effects, *except*:
a. An increase in the heart rate.
b. Pupillo-dilatation.
c. Difficult micturition.
d. Constriction of the bronchi.

**Q4.** Nonshivering thermogenesis in adults is due to:
a. Thyroid hormone
b. Brown fat between the shoulders
c. Noradrenaline
d. Muscle metabolism

**Q5.** Activation of the sympathetic nervous system leads to the 'fight and flight' response. Which of these is *NOT* part of that process?
a. Vasodilatation in skeletal muscle
b. Sweating
c. Bladder relaxation
d. Increased gut motility

**Q6.** True about visceral pain:
a. It is poorly localized
b. Resembles 'fast pain' produced by noxious stimulation of the skin
c. Mediated by B fibers in the dorsal roots of the spinal nerves
d. Causes relaxation of nearby skeletal muscles
e. Shows relatively rapid adaptation

**Q7.** Sympathetic neurons:
a. Originate in the ventral horn of the spinal cord
b. Release nor-adrenaline at their target receptors
c. Release acetylcholine at their terminals
d. Have peripheral ganglia found close to or in the target organ

**Q8.** Damage to preganglionic fibers result in autonomic failure called:
a. Shy-Drager syndrome
b. Multiple atrophy syndrome
c. Horner's syndrome
d. Pheochromocytoma

**Q9.** Which part of the paravertebral sympathetic chain supplies the lower abdominal viscera?
a. Lumbar ganglia    b. Cervical ganglia
c. Thoracic ganglia    d. Celiac ganglia

**Q10.** An individual presented in emergency after an alleged history of consumption of toxic pesticides with miosis, salivation, sweating, bronchial constriction, vomiting and diarrhea; CNS toxicity: cognitive disturbances, convulsions and seizures. What is the most probable diagnosis?
a. Mushroom poisoning
b. Organophosphorus poisoning
c. Snake bite
d. Pheochromocytoma

## ANSWERS

**1.** a    **2.** b    **3.** d    **4.** b    **5.** d    **6.** a    **7.** b    **8.** a    **9.** d    **10.** b

# Cerebral Blood Flow

**CHAPTER 92**

### COMPETENCY ADDRESSED
**PY5.10:** Describe and discuss regional circulation including microcirculation, lymphatic circulation, coronary, **cerebral**, capillary, skin, fetal, pulmonary and splanchnic circulation.

### LEARNING OBJECTIVES
**At the end of this chapter, the learner should be able to:**
- Describe the functional anatomy of cerebral blood flow.
- Describe the physiology of cerebral blood flow.
- Describe the regulation of cerebral blood flow.
- Describe the applied aspects of the cerebral blood flow.

## FUNCTIONAL ANATOMY OF CEREBRAL BLOOD FLOW

The brain is supplied by two sets of arteries viz, internal carotid arteries (main blood supply) and vertebrobasilar arteries (lesser contribution). The internal carotid arteries form the anterior and middle cerebral arteries (ACA, MCA) forming the anterior circulation. The vertebrobasilar arteries form the posterior circulation through the posterior cerebral arteries (PCA) **(Figs. 92.1 and 92.2)**.

The anterior cerebral artery supplies the medial aspect of the cerebral hemisphere of its side, up to the parietal lobe, while the middle cerebral artery supplies the lateral aspect of the cerebral hemisphere except superior frontal

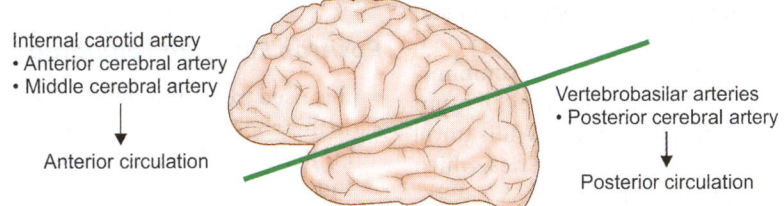

**Fig. 92.1:** The anterior and posterior circulation showing the main arteries participating in it.

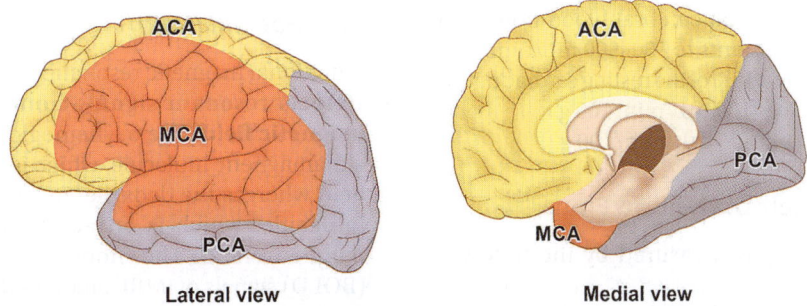

**Fig. 92.2:** The areas of cerebral cortex supplied by ACA (in yellow), MCA (in red) and PCA (in blue).

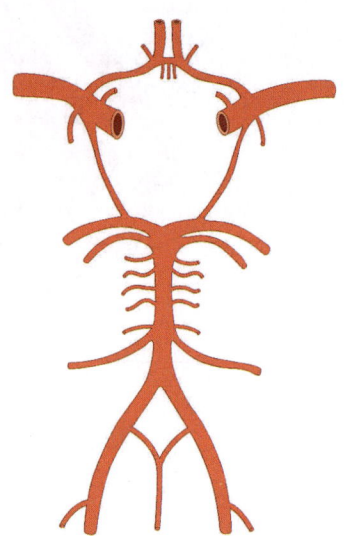

**Fig. 92.3:** Circle of Willis.

**Flowchart 92.1:** Flow of cerebral blood.

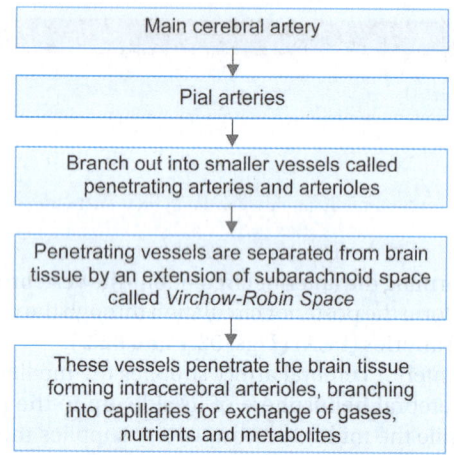

and inferior temporal cortex. The posterior cerebral artery supplies occipital lobe, temporal lobe (posterior, medial and inferior lobe).

The major arteries merge to form the intercommunicating circle of Willis along the basal surface of the cerebrum **(Fig. 92.3)**. The arteries arising from circle of Willis travel along the brain surface and give rise to pial arteries, which further branch as shown in the **Flowchart 92.1**.

## PHYSIOLOGY OF CEREBRAL CIRCULATION

In a healthy adult, the normal cerebral blood flow is 50–65 mL/100/min which amounts to 750–900 mL/min.
- The brain receives about 15% of the resting cardiac output.
- The gray mater receives 100 mL/min/100 g.
- White mater receives 20–25 mL/min/100 g.

## Measurement of Cerebral Blood Flow

The cerebral blood flow is measured by the following methods:
- Kety's method is based on the Fick's principle.
- $^{133}$Xe clearance curve technique
- Transcranial doppler sonography
- Positron emission tomography (PET)
- Functional MRI (fMRI)

### Kety's Method using Fick's Principle

This method uses the nitrous oxide ($N_2O$) to find out the arterio venous difference. The Fick's principle is described in detail with cardiac output.
- The person is asked to inhale 15% $N_2O$ in an $O_2$-$N_2O$ mixture for 10 minutes.
- The cerebral blood flow is calculated by finding out the total consumption of $N_2O$, arterial concentration of $N_2O$ from any artery and the venous concentration of $N_2O$ from internal jugular vein.
- These values are then substituted in the formula

$$\text{Blood flow} = \frac{\text{Total consumption of } N_2O}{\text{Arterial concentration of } N_2O - \text{Venous concentration of } N_2O}$$

- It gives the average value for perfused areas of the brain. It fails to provide information about the regional flow differences or the variations in blood flow with functioning of different brain areas.
- It is effective only when the cerebral blood flow remains unchanged/compensated.

### $^{133}$Xe Clearance Curve Technique

- It is used for studying regional distribution of cerebral blood flow during different activities.
- $^{133}$Xe dissolved in 2 mL saline, injected within 1–2 sec via thin catheter in internal carotid artery.
- Scintillation counters used to detect radioactivity in the brain.
- It is used for the diagnosis of various lesions in brain depending on blood flow.

### Positron Emission Tomography (PET)

- It is used to monitor regional blood flow.
- In this short-lived radio isotope of $^{18}$F, $^{11}$O or $^{15}$O positron emitter tagged to 2-deoxy-d-glucose is used. It is a good index of blood flow.
- Its concentration in various parts of brain can be monitored.

### Functional MRI (fMRI)

- Functional magnetic resonance imaging
- **Detects resonant signals from different tissues in magnetic field:** The oxyhemoglobin molecules act as a diamagnetic molecule, which is repelled by magnetic field whereas the deoxyhemoglobin is a paramagnetic molecule, which is attracted to externally applied magnetic field. The blood oxygen level dependent (BOLD) signals of fMRI, analyses the deoxyhemoglobin for blood flow, volume of blood and rate of oxygen

consumption of brain. Hence, it provides the indirect estimate of regional blood flow of brain.

## Regulation of Cerebral Blood Flow

The cerebral blood flow is primarily regulated by the tissue metabolism. The main metabolic factors affecting the cerebral blood flow are:

- **Concentration of oxygen in arterial blood [PaO$_2$]:** The brain is very sensitive to hypoxia and utilizes the O$_2$ at the rate of around 3.5 mL/100 g/min. If the cerebral blood flow decreases, it results in hypoxia causing vasodilation. This restores the cerebral blood flow. It is important to learn about the effect of hypoxia on the brain. A decrease in PaO$_2$ level 30 mm Hg (normal PaO$_2$ is 35–40 mm Hg), immediately increases the blood flow. However, the PaO$_2$ of 20 mmHg can result in the derangement of brain function, even leading to coma. Hence, even a little decrease in PaO$_2$ tightly controls the cerebral blood flow preventing the neuronal damage.
- **Concentration of carbon dioxide in arterial blood [PaCO$_2$]:** Increased [PaCO$_2$], greatly increases the cerebral blood flow. The CO$_2$ can easily cross the blood brain barrier, which readily binds with the water of CSF and forms the carbonic acid (H$_2$CO$_3$). The carbonic acid dissociates to form H$^+$, which increases the cerebral blood flow.
- **Concentration of H$^+$ [H$^+$]:** The increased concentration of H$^+$ in arterial blood, as well as in CSF (due to raised CO$_2$ levels), results in an increase in the cerebral blood flow. It happens to wash out the excessive metabolites and restore the pH of brain. The low pH/acidosis causes neuronal depression, hence, increase in cerebral blood flow acts as the protective measure. Various acids which cause acidosis are lactic acid, pyruvic acid and other metabolic acids.
- **Substances released by astrocytes:** The astrocytes form the part of astroglial system and surround the blood vessels of brain. They act as conduits between blood vessels and neurons; hence they secrete various substances influencing the neuronal activity providing neurovascular communication. They are non-neuronal cells which protect the neurons and provide the nutrition to brain. Studies have shown that vasoactive metabolites released by astrocytes result in vasodilation. These vasoactive metabolites are thought to be *nitric oxide (NO), metabolites of arachidonic acid, potassium ions, adenosine, etc*.
- **Sympathetic nervous system:** The cerebral blood vessels have a strong sympathetic tone, innervated by superior cervical sympathetic ganglia. This sympathetic tone protects the brain from vascular accidents in acute increase in arterial pressure during exercise or other similar states.
- **Autoregulation of blood flow:** Like any other vital circulation, the cerebral blood flow is autoregulated, which prevents the fluctuations in cerebral blood flow with changes in arterial pressure. The cerebral blood flow is tightly regulated between the mean arterial blood pressure (MAP) of 60–140 mm Hg (normal mean arterial pressure is calculated as DBP+ ⅓ pulse pressure). If the MAP falls below 60 mm Hg, the cerebral blood flow would decrease proportionately whereas the rise of MAP above 140 mmHg would result in increase in cerebral blood flow. However, the cerebral blood flow remains constant between 60–140 mm Hg. In the patients who have persistent hypertension, the range of autoregulation also rises accordingly, may be up to 160 or 180 mm Hg.

## CEREBROVASCULAR ACCIDENTS (CVA)/ STROKE

The terminal/feeder cerebral blood vessels are prone to CVAs resulting in loss of blood supply to the brain. The loss of blood supply results in loss of function of the respective region of the brain called *'stroke'.* Depending on the cause, the stroke is classified as ischemic stroke and hemorrhagic stroke.

- **Ischemic stroke:** The cerebral arteries develop some degree of *atherosclerotic blockage* resulting in the *decrease in lumen of the small arteries*. If this blockage become severe, then it can lead to the ischemia of the brain tissue resulting in *ischemic stroke*. The plaques can activate the *platelet aggregation* and formation of *thrombus*, which results in complete cutting of blood supply in that area (cerebral ischemia).
- **Hemorrhagic stroke:** High blood pressure in some patients may result in sudden bursting of a small blood vessel resulting in local hemorrhage. The collected blood compresses the local brain tissue and compromises its function.

The involvement of the artery determines the site and effects of the stroke, which can be studied as under:

- *Middle cerebral artery:* The blockage of MCA (which supplies midportion of brain hemisphere) results in the functional loss due to ischemia of that area. The loss of blood supply to motor area can result in contralateral spastic paralysis. However, blockage of left MCA, which supplies the Wernicke's area and Broca's area. Hence, the person becomes totally demented and or unable to speak.
- *Posterior cerebral artery:* The blockage of PCA results in infarction of occipital cortex on the same side as blockage. It causes loss of vision in both eyes in half of retina on the same side as the stroke lesion.
- *Ischemia involving the arteries of midbrain:* It can block the conduction in major pathways between brain and spinal cord, causing sensory and motor abnormalities.

## METABOLISM IN BRAIN

Under normal resting conditions, the brain has a basal metabolic rate of 15% of total BMR, which is 7.5 times the average BMR of non-nervous tissue.

The high metabolism of neuronal tissue occurs due to:
- Transport of ions across the neuronal membrane: Sodium and calcium influx, potassium efflux.
- Utilization of ATP for ionic transport.

High utilization of oxygen, as the brain is not able to carry out anaerobic metabolism. But in case of hypoxia, brain switches to anaerobic metabolism and utilizes more amount of glucose and glycogen for adequate production of ATP. *The entry of glucose in the neurons does not require insulin hence, the glucose utilization by the neurons is not affected in diabetics.*

**What will happen to neuronal function if a diabetic person is overtreated with insulin?**

When a diabetic person is overtreated with insulin, the entry of glucose into the insulin dependent tissues (skeletal muscle, adipose tissue and liver) increases, decreasing the blood glucose levels. It doesn't leave enough glucose in the blood for neurons causing derangement of the mental functions.

## SUMMARY

- The brain is primarily supplied by two internal carotid arteries and two vertebrobasilar arteries. The internal carotid arteries give rise to anterior and middle cerebral arteries, which supplies the forebrain. The vertebrobasilar arteries give rise to posterior cerebral artery, cerebellar arteries, basilar artery supplying the pons and midbrain and spinal arteries.
- In a healthy adult, the normal cerebral blood flow is 50–65 mL/100/min which amounts to 750–900 mL/min.
- The blood flow to brain is regulated by the arterial concentration of $CO_2$, $H^+$, $O_2$ and also various substances released by astrocytes.
- The cerebral blood flow remains unchanged between the mean arterial pressure of 60 to 140 mm Hg, called as autoregulation of blood flow.
- The blockage of blood flow to any part of brain result in cerebral stroke.

## LET US SEE, HOW MUCH YOU HAVE LEARNT?

 *Review Questions*

### Long/Short Answer Questions

Q1. Describe the various factors affecting the cerebral circulation.
Q2. Describe the physiological significance of autoregulation of cerebral blood flow.
Q3. What will happen, if the diabetic patient is overtreated with insulin?

### Explain Why? (Reasoning Questions)

Q1. Disruption of cerebral blood flow can lead to ischemic stroke.
Q2. Increased intracranial pressure can reduce cerebral perfusion and cause brain damage.
Q3. An aneurysm in the circle of Willis is a common cause of subarachnoid hemorrhage.

 *Multiple Choice Questions*

Q1. A 62-year-old male is brought to the neurology ICU with spastic paralysis of right half of body. He is having difficulty in understanding the simple commands. Which artery is most likely to be affected, in this patient.
  a. Anterior cerebral artery
  b. Middle cerebral artery
  c. Posterior cerebral artery
  d. Anterior superior cerebellar artery
Q2. The above patient is facing difficulty in understanding simple commands because:
  a. Broca's area is affected
  b. Occipital lobe is affected
  c. Wernicke's area is affected
  d. Angular gyrus is affected
Q3. An athlete finishes a 200 m race in 1 minute, his arterial pressure rises to 140/90 mm Hg. What will happen to his cerebral flow?
  a. Increases
  b. Decreases
  c. Will remain same
  d. Can't say

**ANSWERS**
  1. b    2. c    3. c

# Physiology of Olfaction

**93 CHAPTER**

### COMPETENCY ADDRESSED
PY10.13: Describe and discuss the perception of smell and taste sensation.
PY10.14: Describe and discuss pathophysiology of altered smell and taste sensation.

### LEARNING OBJECTIVES
**At the end of this chapter, the learner should be able to:**
- Describe the site of olfaction and the structure of olfactory cells.
- Explain the physiological basis of olfaction.
- Enumerate and explain the olfactory disorders.

## SMELL OR OLFACTION

A sense of smell or olfaction is well developed in animals like dog and rabbits to give warning of environmental dangers. Such animals are known as *macrosomatics*. In humans, apes, and monkeys this sense of smell is less developed but is important for pleasure and enjoying the taste of food. Therefore, these animals are known as *microsomatics*.

The receptors for taste and smell are *chemoreceptors* that are stimulated by molecules in solution in mucus in the nose and saliva in mouth. The smell receptors are distance receptors, i.e., *Telereceptors*.

## Site of Olfaction

Smell is detected by specialized receptors located on the free nerve endings of the olfactory nerves which are located in the **(Fig. 93.1)**:
- Olfactory mucosa of nose in human beings
- Vomeronasal organ in reptiles and certain animals

## Olfactory Mucosa

- The olfactory neuroepithelium, is crucial for our sense of smell, occupies a specific region within the nasal cavity. It is located in the *upper one-third of the nasal cavity*, forming the areas such as the roof of the nasal

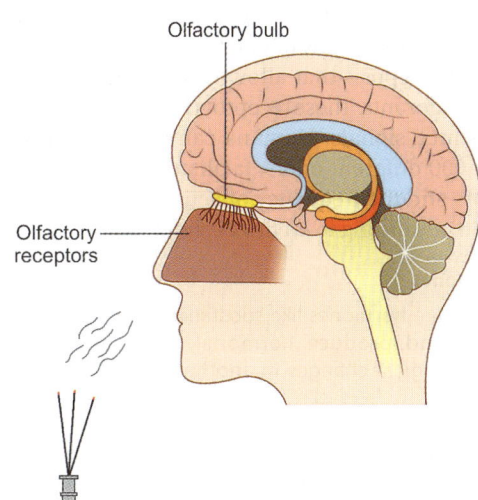

**Fig. 93.1:** Site of olfaction.

cavity, sections along the medial wall (septum), and the superior nasal concha on the lateral wall.
- This neuroepithelium is characterized by its appearance as a patch of *thin, dull yellow mucosa, covering approximately 5.0 cm² of surface area*. A layer of mucosa coats the entire epithelium, providing support and protection to the specialized receptor cells responsible for detecting various odors. These cells play a vital role in transmitting olfactory information to the brain, contributing significantly to our ability to perceive and distinguish different smells.

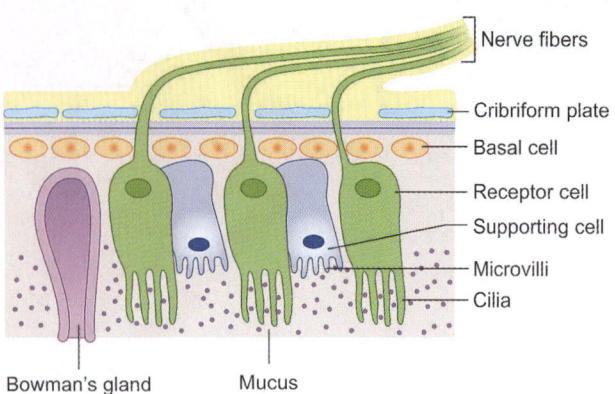

**Fig. 93.2:** Schematic histology of olfactory mucosa.

## Histology of Olfactory Mucosa (Fig. 93.2)

### Receptor Cells

These are bipolar neurons located between sustentacular cells. They possess short, thick dendrites with expanded ends called *olfactory rods*. Each neuron has *unmyelinated cilia* projecting to the mucosal surface, approximately *2 μm long and 0.1 μm in diameter, with 10–20 cilia per neuron*. These cilia are specialized for *odor detection*, equipped with specific receptors for odorants and transduction machinery to amplify sensory signals, generating action potentials. Receptor cells have a short lifespan of about 60 days and are continually replenished by basal cells, highlighting a unique turnover process for sensory neurons.

There's a large family of odorant receptors—potentially up to 1,000 types—that allow discrimination of a wide variety of odorants. These receptors interact with G-proteins to transduce signals. Humans can distinguish between 2,000–4,000 different odors, facilitated by the diversity of receptors and the frequency of action potentials reaching the brain, according to Weber Fechner Law.

---

**Pheromones**

- These are hormones like substances which emit specific odor and produce hormonal, behavioral or other physiological changes in another animals of the same species.
- These are secreted by animals during mating season only.
- Smell of pheromones often is the cause of sex and allow animals to find out its mating partners waiting at a distance.
- It is being assumed that these substances also exist in humans and that there is close relationship between smell and sexual functions.

---

### Vomeronasal Organ

It is found in animals like rodents and is a pouch-like structure along the nasal septum. It detects pheromones and specific odors related to food and sexual behavior. Nerve fibers from the vomeronasal organ project to the accessory olfactory bulb, which then sends signals to brain areas like the *amygdala and hypothalamus*, crucial for reproductive and eating behaviors. However, *in humans, the vomeronasal organ is vestigial*, appearing as a pit in the anterior nasal septum, suggesting evolutionary remnants of a structure once essential for odor-based communication.

### Sustentacular Cells

These are the columnar cells which provide structural support and maintenance to the olfactory epithelium. They have microvilli extending into the mucous layer and are involved in secreting mucus, which helps in trapping and processing odor molecules. *Bowman's glands*, located near the basement membrane, secrete mucus to aid in olfactory function.

### Basal Cells

They serve as stem cells from which new receptor cells (olfactory sensory neurons) are continuously generated. Unlike receptor cells, sensory neurons do not exhibit the same turnover rate. The turnover of basal cells is regulated by factors like *bone morphogenic protein (BMP), which promotes tissue growth and maintenance*.

## Nerve Supply of Olfactory Mucosa

The olfactory mucosa has a *dual innervation* from the cranial nerve I *(The olfactory nerve)* and V *(The trigeminal nerve)* through the general sensory nerve.

- Olfactory nerve is responsible for the transmission of sense of smell.
- The general sensory nerve is a branch of the trigeminal nerve which is stimulated by irritative odorants, activating the free nerve endings of the V Cranial Nerve. It leads to nasal irritation and excess mucus secretion, such as when inhaling ammonia vapors.

## MECHANISM OF OLFACTION

Mechanism of olfaction is shown in **Flowchart 93.1**.

### Olfactory Pathway

It is the only sensory pathway which does not relay in the thalamus. The various structures involved in olfactory pathway are discussed below:

### Olfactory Nerves

The olfactory pathway begins with *10–20 nerve filaments*, composed of the axons of bipolar olfactory neurons. These filaments pierce the *cribriform plate of the ethmoid bone* on either side to reach the olfactory bulb.

### Olfactory Bulb (Fig. 93.3)

The olfactory bulb is an oval, flattened strip of grey matter lying on the cribriform plate. It receives the olfactory nerve filaments. There is a point-to-point representation of the olfactory mucosa on the bulb: the upper part of the mucosa is represented on the anterior bulb, and the lower part on the posterior bulb. The olfactory bulb contains three types of cells: *mitral cells, tufted cells, and interneurons (granule and periglomerular cells)*.

**Flowchart 93.1:** Mechanism of olfaction.

```
Water soluble odoriferous substances dissolve in thin layer of mucus covering olfactory epithelium
and lipid soluble odorants binds to odorant binding proteins and reach the receptors
                                    ↓
        Odorants bind to receptors and results in G protein activation
                                    ↓
                • Calcium influx
                • Activation of adenylyl cyclase (Inc. cAMP)
                • Activation of PIP₂ pathway (IP₃ and DAG)
                                    ↓
        Depolarization of olfactory epithelium → generation of action potential
                                    ↓
    Dendrites of periglomerular cells and granule cells inhibit the olfactory
    glomeruli on which they synapse, sharpening and focusing AP in mitral and tufted cells
```

**Fig. 93.3:** Olfactory bulb and related structures.

- **Mitral cells:** They are named for their resemblance to a "mitre," an ancient headdress worn by bishops. Dendrites of mitral and tufted cells form synapses with axons of olfactory neurons (first-order neurons), creating olfactory glomeruli. Each glomerulus receives input from approximately *26,000 receptors* and transmits information to *24 mitral cells and 68 tufted cells*. The axons of mitral and tufted cells then leave the bulb and run in the olfactory tract.

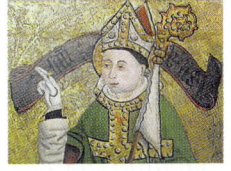

- **Tufted cells:** Function similarly to mitral cells, forming second-order neurons within the olfactory pathway.
- **Interneurons:** Granule and periglomerular cells are inhibitory neurons that form dendro-dendritic reciprocal synapses with mitral cells, modulating the output of the mitral cells.

## Olfactory Tract (Fig. 93.4)

The olfactory tract lies in the *olfactory sulcus on the orbital surface of the frontal lobe*. It proceeds backward from each olfactory bulb to the region of the anterior perforated substance at the base of the brain. The tract divides into *three olfactory striae: lateral, intermediate, and medial*.

## Anterior Olfactory Nucleus

It is scattered within the olfactory tract and receives synaptic connections from neurons of the olfactory bulb. It sends axons through the anterior commissure to inhibit neurons in the contralateral olfactory bulb.

## Olfactory Stria

There are three different striae, described below:
- **Lateral stria:** Axons synapse in the primary olfactory receiving area, which includes the prepiriform cortex/piriform cortex, activating it bilaterally. It also activates the orbitofrontal cortex, but only on the right side.
- **Medial stria:** Projections are sent to the amygdaloid nucleus and parts of the cortex of the basal forebrain.
- **Intermediate stria:** Terminates in the olfactory tubercle, an area of the cortex rostral to the anterior perforated substance.

## Olfactory Cortex

The olfactory cortex includes the anterior olfactory nucleus, piriform cortex, olfactory tubercle, and amygdala. It also influences other parts of the limbic system, such as the hypothalamus and hippocampus, aiding in the storage of smell in long-term memory.

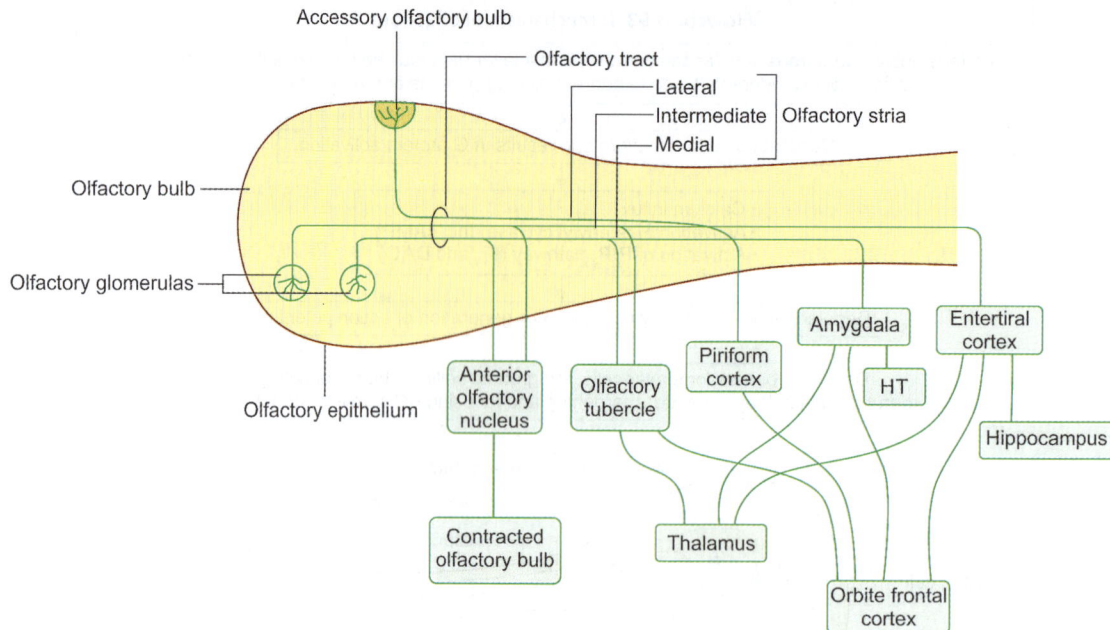

**Fig. 93.4:** Olfactory tract.

**Key Functions of Olfactory Pathway Components**
- **Amygdala:** Triggers emotional responses to different smells, linking scents to emotions and memories.
- **Entorhinal cortex:** Encodes and retrieves olfactory memories, helping to recall past experiences associated with particular scents.
- **Orbitofrontal cortex:** Facilitates the conscious perception and differentiation of odors, allowing us to identify and distinguish various smells.
- **Olfactory fibers and DMN of the vagus:** Project to the dorsal motor nucleus of the vagus, triggering parasympathetic responses to certain smells, such as the secretion of digestive juices.

## Odoriferous Stimuli

Odoriferous (smell-producing) stimuli enter the nasal cavity during breathing. These odorant molecules dissolve in the mucosa layer before coming into contact with the olfactory receptors. The process of detecting and distinguishing various smells involves several key features and mechanisms.

### Features of Odorant Molecules

- **Volatile:** Odorant molecules need to be volatile because olfactory receptors respond to airborne chemicals.
- **Water soluble:** To reach the olfactory receptor cell membranes, odorant molecules must be somewhat water-soluble to penetrate the watery nasal mucosa layer.
- **Lipid soluble:** To stimulate the olfactory receptor cells, odorant molecules should also be partially lipid-soluble to cross the cell membrane.

### Types of Odorant Stimuli

Humans can perceive more than 10,000 different odorous molecules, despite there being around 50 primary smell sensations. The concentration of an odoriferous substance must change by about 30% for a difference to be detected, compared to a 1% change required for visual discrimination.

The sensitivity of olfactory receptors varies depending on the substance. For example, methyl mercaptan, which emits a garlic odor, has an extremely low threshold and can be detected at a concentration of <500 pg/L of air. Typically, odoriferous molecules are small, containing 3 to 20 carbon atoms. Notably, molecules with the same number of carbon atoms but different structural configurations can produce different odors.

### Common Odors

- **Aromatic/Resinous:** Camphor, lavender, and cloves
- **Fragrant:** Perfume and flowers
- **Ethereal:** Ether and chloroform
- **Garlic:** Garlic, onion, and sulfur compounds
- **Burning:** Tobacco, burning feathers, meat, and bones
- **Nauseating:** Excreta, decomposed meat, and vegetables
- **Goat:** Sweat and ripe cheese
- **Repulsive:** Odors of bed bugs
- **Musky:** Musk

### Olfactory Transduction (Conversion of Olfactory Sensation to Electrical Signals)

When olfactory molecules attach to the mucous membrane, they generate a potential lasting 4–6 seconds. This triggers action potentials in the olfactory receptors, which are then conducted along the axons to the olfactory bulb.

## Steps in Transduction in Olfactory Receptor Neurons

### Binding of an odorant molecule to receptor:
- Odorant molecules enter the nasal cavity and dissolve in the mucous layer.
- The cilia of olfactory neurons project into this mucous layer.

### Odorant Binding Protein
- The mucous layer covering the olfactory mucosa contains one or more odorant binding proteins (OBP) that concentrate and transfer the molecule to the receptor on the cilia of the olfactory neurons.
- OBP is an 18 kDa protein in the nasal cavity, homologous to other proteins in the body that carry *small lipophilic molecules*.

### Activations of Receptors
When an odorant molecule binds to its receptor, it induces an interaction between the receptor and a heteromeric G-protein. This interaction releases the G-protein *GTP-coupled α-subunit*, which then stimulates adenylyl cyclase to produce *cyclic adenosine monophosphate (cAMP)*.

### Depolarization Receptor Potential (Fig. 93.5)
The increase in intracellular cAMP opens cyclic-nucleotide-gated (CNG) cation channels, leading to the influx of cations and a change in membrane potential in the cilium membrane, producing a depolarizing receptor potential. Specifically, there is an inward flow of $Na^+$ and $Ca^{2+}$ ions. This receptor potential lasts for 4–6 seconds and is converted to an action potential, which is then conducted to the olfactory bulb.

### Action Potential in Olfactory Receptors
The receptor potential depolarizes the initial segment of the axon to the threshold, generating an action potential in the sensory axon and transmitting the signal to the olfactory bulb. Each receptor responds to multiple odors, and no two receptor cells have identical responses to a series of stimuli. Sensory perception is thus based on the pattern of receptors activated by the stimulus.

### Membrane Potential and Action Potential in Olfactory Cells
The resting membrane potential of olfactory cells is around –55 mV. At this potential, most cells generate continuous action potentials (AP) at a rate varying from once every 20 seconds to two or three times per second. Most odorants cause depolarization of the olfactory membrane, decreasing the negative potential in the olfactory cells from –55 mV to as low as –30 mV or less. This increases the number of action potentials to about 20 per second. Some odorants, however, hyperpolarize the olfactory cell membrane, reducing the nerve firing rate. Over a wide range, the rate of olfactory nerve impulses is approximately proportional to the logarithm of the stimulus strength, indicating that olfactory receptors follow transduction principles similar to other sensory receptors.

## Processing of Olfactory Sensation
Information is spatially encoded in the olfactory bulb, where lateral inhibition is mediated by periglomerular and granule cells in the olfactory glomeruli. Additional signal refinement and adjustment occur due to multiple inputs to the olfactory bulb from the olfactory area of the cortex as well as the basal forebrain and midbrain. Thus, sensory information is extensively processed and refined in the bulb before being sent to the olfactory cortex.

### Transmission of Impulse to Olfactory Cortex and Neocortex
Information is first transmitted to the olfactory cortex, which includes the piriform cortex, part of the amygdala,

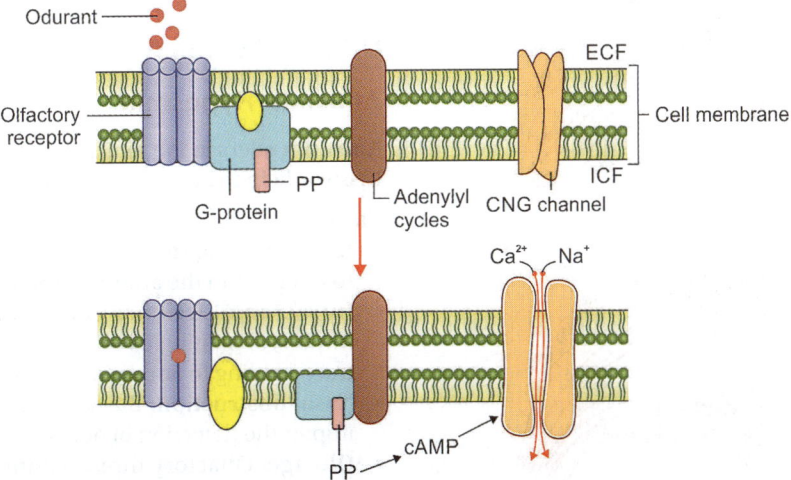

**Fig. 93.5:** Olfactory transduction (depolarization of receptor cell).

the olfactory tubercle, and part of the entorhinal cortex.

From the olfactory cortex, information is relayed to the frontal cortex directly and to the orbitofrontal cortex via the thalamus. Unlike other sensations, the olfactory tract projects directly to the cortex without relaying through the thalamus, reflecting the phylogenetic primitiveness of the olfactory system.

### Roles of Various Brain Regions in Olfactory Processing

- **Piriform cortex:** Activated by sniffing in humans.
- **Amygdala and hypothalamus:** Involved in the emotional and motivational responses to olfactory stimuli, as well as the behavioral and physiological effects of odors.
- **Entorhinal cortex:** Concerned with olfactory memory.
- **Neocortex (frontal and orbitofrontal cortex):** Involved in the conscious discrimination of odors. People with lesions in the orbitofrontal cortex are unable to discriminate odors.

## SNIFFING (FIG. 93.6)

The portion of the nasal cavity containing the olfactory receptors is poorly ventilated. During normal breathing, most of the air flows smoothly over the turbinates, although some eddy currents pass air over the olfactory mucous membrane. These eddy currents are likely created by convection as cool air strikes the warm mucosal surfaces.

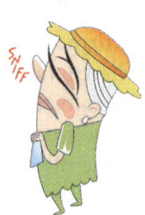

Sniffing significantly increases the amount of air reaching the olfactory region. This action involves contractions of the lower part of the nares on the septum, which helps deflect the airstream upward. Sniffing is a semi-reflex response that typically occurs when a new odor captures attention.

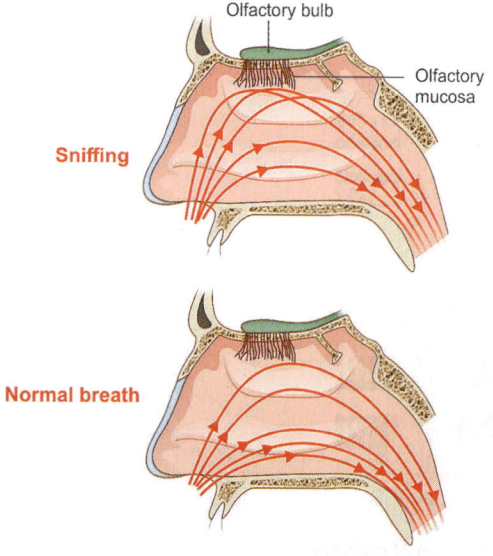

**Fig. 93.6:** Sniffing and normal breath.

## ADAPTATION OF OLFACTORY RECEPTORS

Olfactory receptors exhibit a phenomenon known as adaptation, where their response to a continuous or repeated stimulus decreases over time. This process allows the olfactory system to remain sensitive to new odors even in the presence of persistent smells.

### Mechanisms of Adaptation

1. **Receptor-level adaptation:**
   - When exposed to an odorant continuously, the olfactory receptors on the sensory neurons become less responsive.
   - This decreased responsiveness is due to the temporary desensitization of the receptors or a reduction in the number of active receptors available to bind new odorant molecules.
2. **Signal transduction pathways:**
   - Upon odorant binding, the initial cascade involving G-protein activation and cAMP production diminishes with prolonged exposure.
   - The continuous presence of cAMP can lead to the activation of phosphodiesterases, which break down cAMP, thereby reducing the receptor's sensitivity.
3. **Neuronal adaptation:**
   - The olfactory bulb and higher brain regions also play a role in adaptation.
   - Inhibitory interneurons within the olfactory bulb, such as granule and periglomerular cells, help modulate the signal by lateral inhibition, contributing to the decreased perception of persistent odors.
4. **CNG ion channel sensitivity:**
   - Adaptation also involves adjustments in the sensitivity of cyclic nucleotide-gated (CNG) ion channels to cAMP, which vary with different concentrations of the odorant.
   - Research indicates that knocking out NGA4 (a gene associated with this process) slows down adaptation, suggesting its crucial role in regulating this mechanism.

## DISORDERS RELATED TO OLFACTION

### Anosmia/Hyposmia

**Anosmia** refers to the total loss of the sense of smell, while **hyposmia** indicates diminished olfactory sensitivity.

#### Causes
- **Injury:** Damage to the olfactory bulb or nerve, often due to fractures in the anterior cranial fossa.
- **Intracranial lesions:** Conditions such as abscesses, tumors, or meningitis can exert pressure on the olfactory tract, leading to anosmia or hyposmia.
- **Nasal obstruction:** Blockage in the nasal passages can impair the detection of odors.
- **Old age:** Olfactory threshold increases with age, with >25% of individuals over 80 years experiencing some degree of olfactory loss.

- **Atrophic rhinitis:** Chronic inflammation and wasting away of nasal tissues can affect olfactory function.
- **Kallmann's syndrome:** Anosmia associated with hypogonadism, often due to abnormal development of the olfactory system.

## Parasomia/Dysosmia

**Parosmia** refers to the distortion or perversion of the sense of smell, where individuals interpret odors incorrectly and may perceive them as unpleasant or disgusting.

### Causes

- **Recovery phase of postinfluenza anosmia:** During the healing process following influenza, misdirected regeneration of nerves can lead to abnormal sensory perceptions.
- **Intracranial tumors:** Presence of tumors within the brain can disrupt the normal functioning of olfactory pathways, resulting in dysosmia or parosmia.

## METHOD OF QUANTITATIVE ESTIMATION OF THE SENSE OF SMELL USING AN OLFACTOMETER (FIG. 93.7)

The olfactometer is an instrument used to quantitatively measure the sense of smell. It consists of two glass tubes, an outer tube, and an inner sliding tube, which work together to determine an individual's olfactory threshold.

### Components

- **Outer tube:** Contains the smelling substance on its inner surface.
- **Inner tube:** Graduated for precise measurement and can slide within the outer tube.
- **Curved end:** The curved end of the inner tube is introduced into the nostril.

### Procedure

- The curved end of the inner tube is gently inserted into the nostril of the subject.
- The subject is asked to breathe quietly to avoid any turbulence that could affect the test.
- The distal end of the outer tube is initially closed and then gradually withdrawn.
- As soon as the subject first perceives the odor, they indicate this to the tester.
- The highest figure noted on the graduated inner tube at the point of odor detection is recorded. This reading represents the subject's threshold for smell in terms of olfactories.

This method provides a standardized approach to assess the olfactory sensitivity and can help in diagnosing olfactory disorders or evaluating the effectiveness of treatments for such conditions.

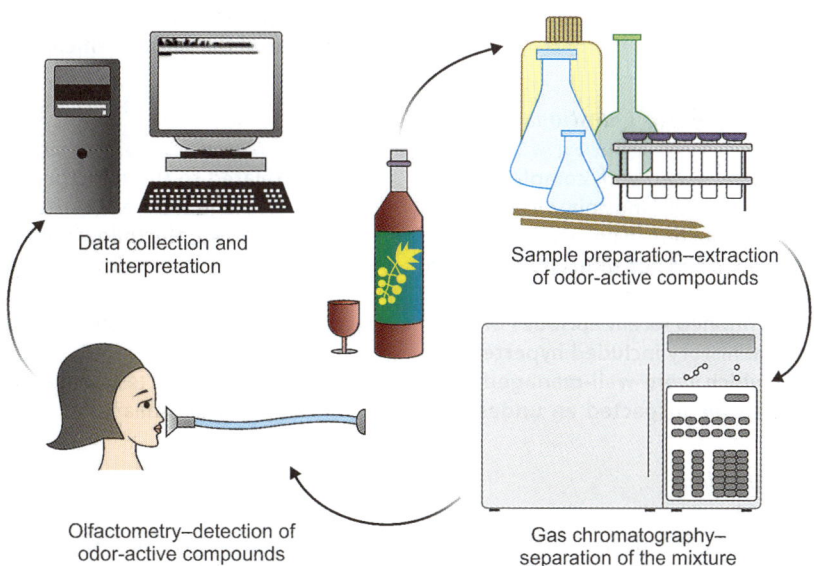

**Fig. 93.7:** Olfactometer.

## SUMMARY

- **Site of olfaction and structure of olfactory cells:** Olfaction, the sense of smell, occurs in the olfactory epithelium located in the upper part of the nasal cavity. The olfactory epithelium contains specialized sensory neurons called olfactory receptor cells. These cells have hair-like extensions called cilia that project into the mucus lining the nasal cavity. The cilia contain olfactory receptors, which are proteins that bind to odor molecules. When odor molecules enter the nasal cavity and bind to the receptors, they trigger electrical signals that are transmitted to the brain for processing.

- **Physiological basis of olfaction:** The physiological basis of olfaction involves a complex process that begins with the detection of odor molecules by olfactory receptor cells. When odor molecules bind to specific receptors on the cilia of olfactory receptor cells, they activate a signal transduction pathway, leading to the generation of electrical signals called action potentials. These action potentials are transmitted along the olfactory nerve fibers to the olfactory bulb, which is a structure located at the base of the brain. In the olfactory bulb, the electrical signals are processed and relayed to higher brain regions, including the olfactory cortex, where they are interpreted as specific odors.
- **Olfactory disorders:**
  - *Anosmia:* Anosmia refers to the partial or complete loss of the sense of smell. It can result from various causes, including viral infections (such as the common cold), nasal polyps, head trauma, neurodegenerative diseases (such as Alzheimer's disease), or congenital conditions. Anosmia can significantly impact quality of life, as it affects the ability to detect and enjoy food, detect danger (such as spoiled food or gas leaks), and experience pleasurable scents.
  - *Hyposmia:* Hyposmia refers to a reduced sense of smell. It can be temporary, such as during a cold or sinus infection, or it may be chronic due to conditions like nasal congestion, allergies, or aging.
  - *Dysosmia:* Dysosmia refers to a distorted sense of smell, where odors may be perceived differently than they actually are. Dysosmia can result from various factors, including head trauma, sinus infections, or exposure to certain chemicals or medications.
  - *Parosmia:* Parosmia is a specific type of dysosmia where familiar odors are perceived as unpleasant or offensive. It can occur following viral infections, head injuries, or as a side effect of certain medications.
  - *Phantosmia:* Phantosmia refers to the perception of phantom odors that aren't actually present. It can occur in conditions such as epilepsy, migraines, or as a result of olfactory hallucinations.

## LET US SEE, HOW MUCH YOU HAVE LEARNT?

### Review Questions

#### Long/Short Answer Questions

Q1. Describe the transmission of olfactory stimulus to brain.

Q2. What is the role of odorant binding proteins in the sense of smell?

#### Explain Why? (Reasoning Questions)

Q1. Offensive smells stop bothering us after some time/days.

Q2. Damage to the olfactory nerve can result in anosmia, the loss of the sense of smell.

### Critical Thinking Case-Based Questions

Q1. Kiran, a 60-year-old man, visited with complaints of a gradual loss of his sense of smell (anosmia) over the past few months. He reported that he can no longer enjoy the aroma of his favorite foods and had difficulty detecting smells that others around him can easily identify. Additionally, Kiran mentioned recent episodes of sinus infections. His medical history included hypertension and mild diabetes, which were well-managed with medication. The physician suspected an underlying issue related to the olfactory system and considered further diagnostic evaluation. Based on the above history, answer the following questions:
  a. What are the primary structures and pathways involved in the sense of olfaction?
  b. How do they function together to detect and process different odors?
  c. What diagnostic tests are available for evaluating and managing anosmia?

### Multiple Choice Questions

Q1. What is the primary site of olfaction in humans?
  a. Tongue
  b. Nasal cavity
  c. Eyes
  d. Ears

Q2. What are the specialized sensory neurons responsible for detecting odor molecules?
  a. Taste buds
  b. Auditory hair cells
  c. Olfactory receptor cells
  d. Photoreceptor cells

Q3. Which structure in the brain processes olfactory information?
  a. Hippocampus       b. Cerebellum
  c. Olfactory bulb    d. Medulla oblongata

Q4. What type of molecules bind to olfactory receptors to trigger the sense of smell?
  a. Sound waves       b. Light waves
  c. Odor molecules    d. Taste molecules

Q5. Anosmia refers to:
  a. Enhanced sense of smell
  b. Partial loss of taste

c. Loss of the sense of smell
d. Increased sensitivity to odors

Q6. What is the term for a distorted sense of smell?
   a. Hyposmia
   b. Parosmia
   c. Dysosmia
   d. Hyperosmia

Q7. Which of the following conditions results in the perception of phantom odors?
   a. Hyposmia
   b. Parosmia
   c. Dysosmia
   d. Phantosmia

Q8. What is the primary cause of temporary hyposmia?
   a. Aging
   b. Sinus infection
   c. Head trauma
   d. Exposure to chemicals

Q9. Which neurotransmitter is involved in transmitting olfactory signals to the brain?
   a. Dopamine
   b. Serotonin
   c. Acetylcholine
   d. Glutamate

Q10. Which part of the brain is responsible for interpreting olfactory information?
   a. Prefrontal cortex
   b. Olfactory cortex
   c. Temporal lobe
   d. Occipital lobe

Q11. What is the primary function of olfactory receptor cells?
   a. Transmitting sound signals
   b. Detecting light waves
   c. Sensing changes in temperature
   d. Detecting odor molecules

Q12. Which of the following is NOT an olfactory disorder?
   a. Anosmia
   b. Hyposmia
   c. Tinnitus
   d. Phantosmia

Q13. What is the term for the ability to detect and distinguish between different odors?
   a. Olfactory acuity
   b. Olfactory sensitivity
   c. Olfactory discrimination
   d. Olfactory adaptation

Q14. Which of the following is NOT a primary taste sensation?
   a. Sweet
   b. Sour
   c. Salty
   d. Bitter

Q15. Which nerve carries olfactory signals from the olfactory epithelium to the brain?
   a. Trigeminal nerve
   b. Olfactory nerve
   c. Optic nerve
   d. Facial nerve

Q16. What is the term for the tiny hair-like projections on olfactory receptor cells?
   a. Cilia
   b. Villi
   c. Microvilli
   d. Stereocilia

Q17. What is the role of the olfactory bulb in olfaction?
   a. Detecting odor molecules
   b. Transmitting olfactory signals to the brain
   c. Processing olfactory information
   d. Producing olfactory receptor cells

Q18. Which of the following is a common cause of parosmia?
   a. Aging
   b. Viral infection
   c. Head trauma
   d. Sinus congestion

Q19. What is the term for the loss of the sense of smell due to aging?
   a. Hyposmia
   b. Presbyopia
   c. Anosmia
   d. Ageusia

Q20. What is the primary sensory modality associated with the olfactory system?
   a. Taste
   b. Hearing
   c. Vision
   d. Smell

## ANSWERS

1. b   2. c   3. c   4. c   5. c   6. c   7. d   8. b   9. d   10. b   11. d   12. c   13. c   14. d
15. b   16. a   17. c   18. b   19. a   20. d

# Physiology of Taste Sensation
## (Gustatory Sensation)

**CHAPTER 94**

> **COMPETENCY ADDRESSED**
>
> PY10.13: Describe and discuss the perception of smell and taste sensation.
> PY10.14: Describe and discuss pathophysiology of altered smell and taste sensation.

> **LEARNING OBJECTIVES**
>
> At the end of this chapter, the learner should be able to:
> - Describe the taste sensation mechanism.
> - Explain the disorder of taste sensation.
> - Demonstrate clinical examination of taste sensations.

Why do we have different taste perceptions for different items we eat?

Sense of taste (gustation) is a chemical sense that is stimulated by food and drink. It contributes to the quality of life and is important for digestion. Taste must be distinguished from flavor, including the olfactory, tactile, and thermal attributes of food and taste.

## FUNCTIONAL ANATOMY OF TONGUE

**Site for taste sensation:** Detected by specialized chemoreceptors known as taste receptors/taste cells. They are clustered in the taste buds located on the tongue, palate, pharynx, epiglottis, and upper ⅓rd of the esophagus.

### Papillae Distributed Over the Tongue

Main taste detector, containing numerous taste buds on its dorsal surface. As it exhibits numerous papillae, which increases the surface area of the mucosa available for taste receptors. The taste buds are located in the walls of these papillae.

### Types of Papillae (Fig. 94.1)

**Four different types** of papillae are found all over the tongue.

1. **Circumvallate papillae:** Large (2-4 mm in diameter) about 10-20 in number forming a single row in front of Sulcus terminalis. Sulcus terminalis is a V-shaped

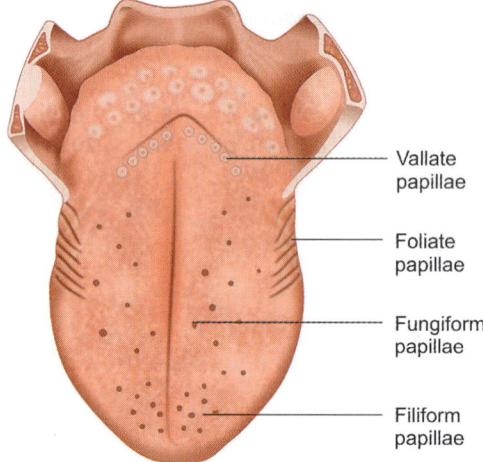

**Fig. 94.1:** Distribution of papillae on tongue.

groove that separates the tongue in the anterior ⅔rd and posterior ⅓rd part. About 200 taste buds are located along the side of each circumvallate papillae.

2. **Fungiform papillae:** Bright red, flat dot-like structure (each about 1 mm in diameter) located in the anterior ⅔ rd of the tongue along the edge, dorsum, and tip part. There are 8–10 taste buds on each papilla.

3. **Foliate papillae** are transverse mucosal folds found on the posterior-lateral surface of the tongue and anterior to the circumvallate papillae. Each folate papillae has numerous taste buds.

4. **Filiform papillae:** Small conical projections, covering the entire remaining surface of the dorsum of the anterior ⅔rd of the tongue, giving it a velvety appearance. They are arranged in rows parallel to the sulcus terminalis. They are not gustatory structures, i.e., do not contain taste buds. But plays a role in breaking up food particles and is called *mechanical papillae* in contrast to the other three forms which are known as gustatory papillae.

## Taste Buds

There are around *10,000 in number* in total having a *barrel-shaped structure*. The cluster of cells with a small opening (taste pore) on the surface allows the substance to reach the interior of the taste buds. Each taste bud measures about 50–70 μm diameter and 60–80 μm length and consists of different types of cells.

### Structure of Taste Bud (Fig. 94.2)

**Receptor/taste cells:** Each taste bud has around 100 receptor cells which are modified epithelial cells. They are elongated, bipolar structures and extend from the epithelial opening of the taste bud to its base. They have a short life span of about 10 days and are replaced continuously by new cells differentiating from basal cells. Through the taste pore, all the taste cells' microvilli (cilia) protrude into the oral cavity and encounter the saliva. Taste cells are innervated by sensory neurons (primary gustatory afferent fibers) at the basal pole. Although taste cells are non-neural epithelial cells, the contrast between these cells with sensory cells has more physiological characteristics of a chemical synapse. Each nerve innervates taste cells in several taste buds i.e., each taste bud is innervated by at least 50 nerve fibers.

**Basal cells:** Small round cells present at the bottom of the taste buds. They are thought to be stem cells that are continuously being differentiated into taste cells.

**Supporting cells:** They are the support of receptor cells and are also known as sustentacular cells.

### Innervation of Taste Buds

Special sensory nerve fibers innervating the taste cells come from the branches of the facial, glossopharyngeal, and vagus nerves. Tactile and temperature receptors of the mouth, tongue, and pharynx are innervated by the trigeminal nerve (V CN). The anterior ⅔rd of the tongue is by the facial nerve and the posterior ⅓rd of the tongue is by the glossopharyngeal nerve. The palate, larynx, etc., is by the vagus nerve. Sensory sensation by trigeminal nerve.

**Types of stimuli:** Five basic types of taste sensations. Sweet, salt, sour, bitter, and umami which has been recently listed. They are known as primary/basic taste sensations and all others are assumed to result from various combinations of these five. In addition to the above, associated sensations of olfaction, temperature, and texture contribute to different flavors.

### Location (Fig. 94.3)

- Sweet: Tip of tongue
- Salty and sour: Sides of tongue
- Bitter: At the base
- Umami: Center

However, it is now clear that all tastes are sensed from all parts of the tongue and adjacent structures containing taste buds.

1. **Sweet sensation:** Produced by the number of organic molecules including *sugars, glycols, alcohols, aldehydes, esters* etc. Saccharin is a chemical 600 times as sweet as sucrose and it is non-calorigenic and is often used as a sweetening agent for Diabetic patients. The tip was considered the most sensitive area to sweet stimuli.
2. **Salty sensation:** Produced by the *anion of ionizable salts, especially NaCl*. The front half of each side of the tongue was considered the area most sensitive to salty sensation. The threshold Sensitivity is *0.01M*.
3. **Sour sensation:** Produced by *acid*, and the intensity of this sensation relates to some degree to the pH of the stimulus solution. The lateral sides of the tongue is most sensitive area to sour stimuli.

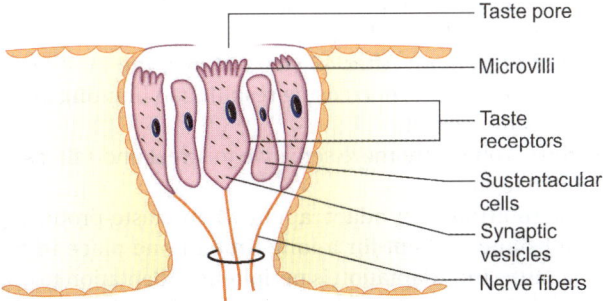

**Fig. 94.2:** Structure of taste bud.

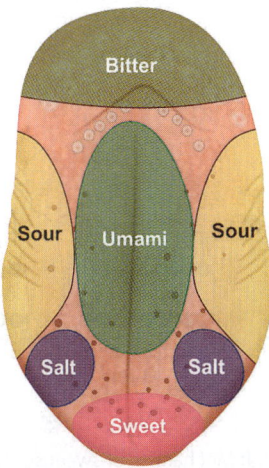

**Fig. 94.3:** Distribution of taste sensation on tongue.

4. **Bitter sensation:** Produced by *alkaloids*, e.g., quinine, caffeine, nicotine, and strychnine. Many alkaloids are harmful when swallowed so this prevents the individual to ingest it i.e., *Protective Mechanism*. The threshold Sensitivity is *0.000008M*.
5. **Umami sensation:** Recently been added. Produced by *glutamate*, particularly monosodium glutamate (MSG) used extensively in Asian cooking. This taste is pleasant and sweet but differs from the standard sweet taste.

## TRANSDUCTION OF GUSTATORY STIMULI

A gustatory stimulus transduced into the electrical signal is initiated at the level of receptors. Taste receptors are *chemoreceptors* that are stimulated by substances dissolved in the mouth by saliva. These dissolved substances act on the microvilli of taste receptors exposed in the pore of taste buds. **Proteins** that bind to taste-producing molecules have been cloned. It is *produced by Ebner's gland* and has probably concentrating and transport functions like olfactory binding protein (OBP). Then these proteins *bind to taste molecules* which in turn bind to the receptor on the microvilli of taste cells. This causes depolarization of cells either directly or via the action of the second messenger. This causes the development of **receptor potential** in the receptor cells which in turn **generates the action potential** in the sensory nerves.

## Mechanism

### Sweet Tastants: By Two Different Mechanisms (Fig. 94.4)

- **By activating adenylate cyclase:** Some sweet receptors couple to G-protein which interacts with adenylyl cyclase to increase cAMP which leads to the closing of K⁺ selective channels which in turn leads to depolarization of taste cell. Since they are normally open at RMP.
- **By stimulating inositol triphosphate (IP$_3$) production:** Some sweet receptors couple to *gustducin or G-protein* that stimulate IP$_3$ production. Thus, increased IP$_3$ is likely to cause the release of Ca$^{2+}$ from intracellular stores.

### Bitter Tastants: Depolarize by Three Mechanisms (Fig. 94.5)

- **By stimulating IP$_3$ production:** Receptors activate G-protein which in turn increases the production of IP$_3$ which then increases intracellular calcium level which leads to the release of synaptic transmitters and activation of gustatory nerve fibers.
- **By lowering intramolecular levels of cAMP and cGMP:** receptors for bitter tastants couple to specific taste cell G-protein gustducin. The G-protein gustducin activates a phosphodiesterase (PDE) that may reduce intracellular levels of cAMP and cGMP.
- **By blocking apical potassium channel:** At least one bitter stimulus the quinine may depolarize the taste cells by blocking the apical K⁺ channel.

### Salty Tastants (Fig. 94.6)

Depolarize taste cells by activating an *amiloride-sensitive Na⁺ channel*. No specific Na⁺ receptor has been identified. This allows the entry of sodium ions and causes the depolarization of cells.

### Sour Tastants (Fig. 94.7)

Depolarize the cell by permeation or blockage of the apical ion channel by proteins either causing the passage of *hydrogen ions through amiloride sensitive Na⁺ channels or blocking K⁺ channels* (which normally are open during RMP).

### Umami Taste

Transduction by a specific type of truncated metabotropic *glutamate receptor (mGluR4)* and the agonists are purine 5-ribonucleotide such as AMP/GMP in the food. The way this produces depolarization is still unsettled.

## FACTORS AFFECTING TASTE SENSATION

- **Area of stimulation:** Perception of sense of taste is directly proportional to the area of taste buds stimulated. Therefore, stimulation of a small area of the tongue by one drop of solution produces a weaker sensation than the same solution by the whole mouth.
- **Temperature of tastant:** Optimal response to taste-producing substance is obtained when their temperature is between 30 and 40°C.
- **Age of person:** After 45 years of age, the number of taste buds starts decreasing resulting in blunting of the sensation of taste.
- **Sex:** Women are more sensitive to sweet and salt tastes than to sour.
- **Adaptation:** They adapt rapidly when a taste-producing substance is kept for a long time in one place in the mouth. The adaptation is peripheral. Adaptation to one acid produces adaptation to other acids too because the H⁺ ion is the basic stimulus in all cases.

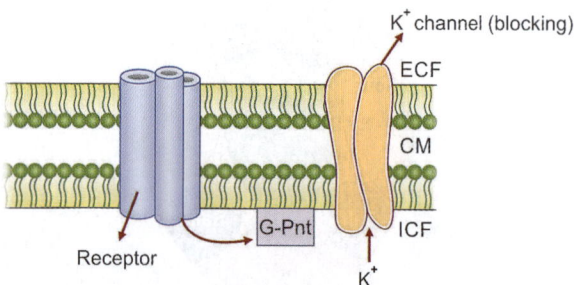

**Fig. 94.4:** Mechanism of sweet sensation.
(ECF: extracellular fluid; CM: cell membrane; ICF: intracellular fluid)

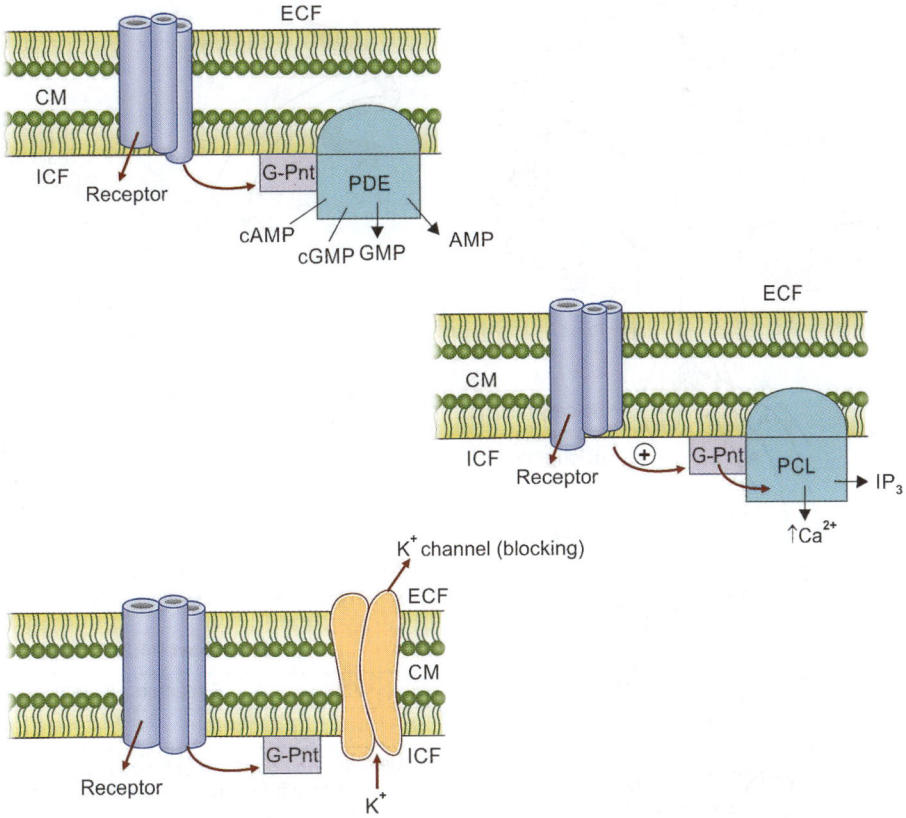

**Fig. 94.5:** Mechanism of bitter sensation.

(CM: cell membrane; ICF: intracellular fluid; cAMP: cyclic adenosine monophosphate; cGMP: cyclic guanosine monophosphate; GMP: guanosine monophosphate; AMP: adenosine monophosphate; ECF: extracellular fluid; IP: inositol trisphosphate; PDE: phosphodiesterase; PLC: phospholipase C)

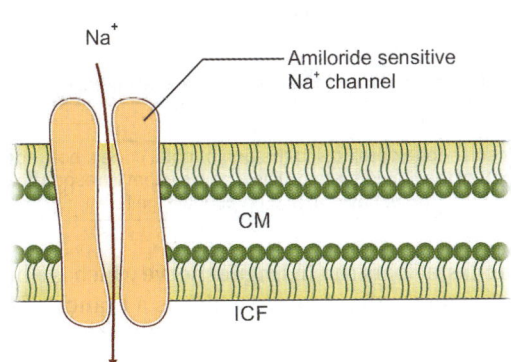

**Fig. 94.6:** Mechanism of salty sensation.
(CM: cell membrane; ICF: intracellular fluid)

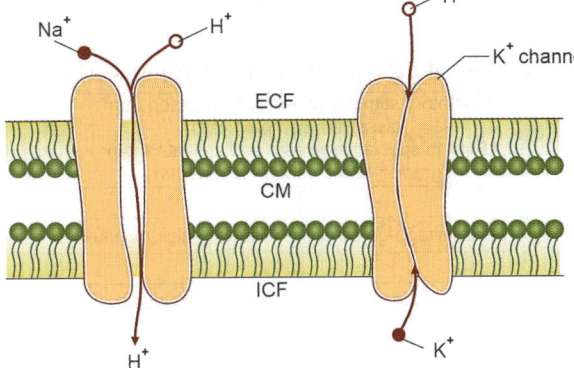

**Fig. 94.7:** Mechanism of sour sensation.
(ECF: extracellular fluid; CM: cell membrane; ICF: intracellular fluid)

- **Interaction between taste-producing substances:** It also affects taste sensation, e.g., the reduction of the sour taste of fruits by sucrose is a well-known phenomenon.
- **Effect of taste modifying proteins:** A taste-modifying protein known as miraculin has been discovered in plants of West Africa. When it is applied over the tongue, this protein makes acid taste sweet.
- **Gymnemic acid**—abolishes the sensation of sweetness, but does not affect other taste sensations.
- **Drugs**—captopril, penicillamine—temporary loss of taste
- **Nutrient deficiencies**—preference for salt arises due to salt deficiency while calorie deficiency produces the preference for sweet food.

## MECHANISM OF GUSTATORY TRANSDUCTION

See **Flowchart 94.1** and **Fig. 94.8**.

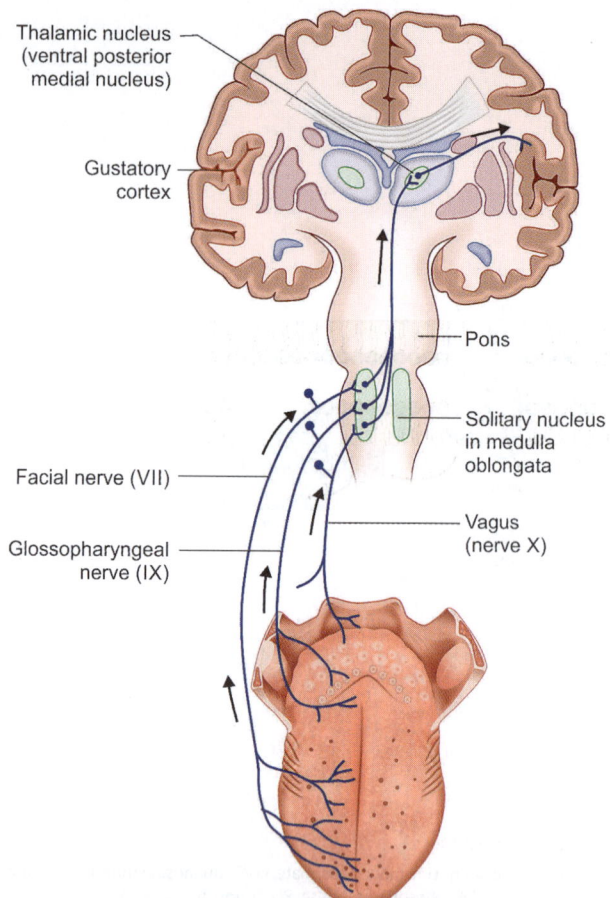

**Fig. 94.8:** Diagrammatic representation of gustatory transduction.

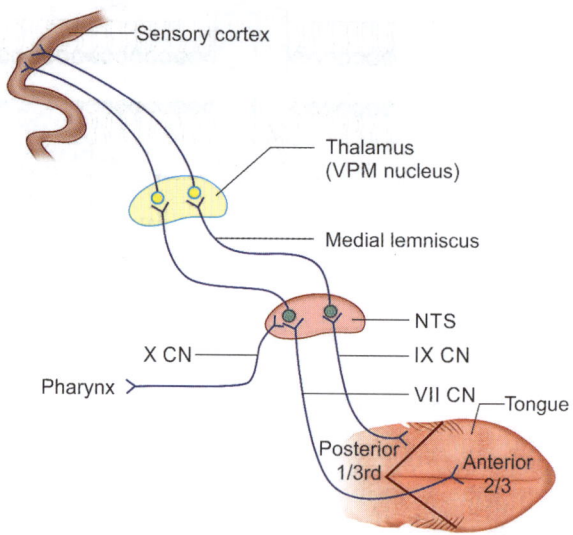

**Fig. 94.9:** Diagrammatic representation of taste pathway.
(VPM: ventral posteromedial; NTS: nucleus tractus solitarius)

**Flowchart 94.1:** Mechanism of gustatory transduction.

```
Gustatory stimulus (chemicals released from
dissolved food particles)
Bind to specific receptors and activate them
(graded depolarization of receptor)
            ↓
Opens voltage-gated Ca++ channels (calcium influx)
            ↓
Increased intracytoplasmic calcium levels
            ↓
Release of neurotransmitter (glutamate) from nerve
endings of taste cells
            ↓
Action potential in sensory nerve
```

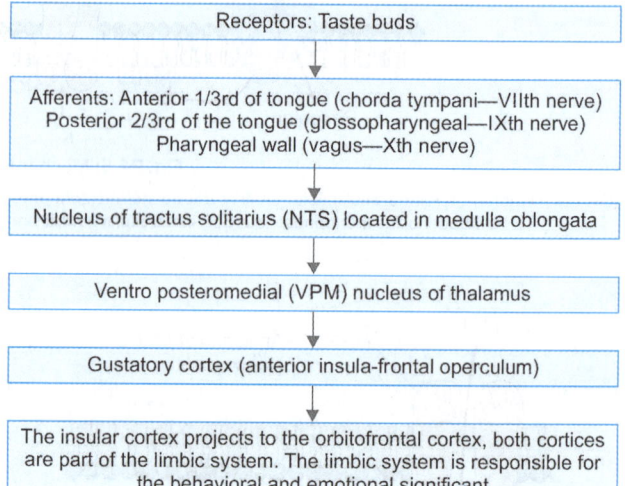

## TASTE PATHWAYS

See **Flowchart 94.2** and **Fig. 94.9**.

### Three-order Neurons of Taste Pathway

#### First Order Neuron

Cell bodies of the 1st order neuron are innervating the taste cells in taste buds are located in three different ganglia of VII, IX and X cranial nerve as; from anterior ⅔rd of the tongue: Taste fibers run in **lingual nerve** which is a branch from **chorda tympani nerve** which is a branch of **facial nerve** (VII CN) whose cell bodies are located in *geniculate ganglion*.

**From posterior ⅓rd of the tongue:** Taste fibers run in the Glossopharyngeal nerve. Cell bodies lie in the superior and inferior ganglia of this nerve.

**From pharynx, epiglottis, hard and soft palate:** Taste fibers run in the vagus nerve. Cell bodies are located in the superior and inferior ganglions of the vagus nerve. Ultimately all the taste fibers from different ganglions join the **tractus solitaries** to terminate in the *nucleus of tractus solitarius*.

#### Second Order Neuron

Cell bodies are located in the nucleus of tractus solitarius (NTS) in the medulla. Axon of 2nd order neurons joins the medial lemniscus and terminates with Vth CN fiber which carries pain, touch, and temperature sensation in the ventroposterior medial nucleus of the thalamus.

### Third Order Neuron

Cell bodies are in the **ventral posterior medial nucleus** of the thalamus. Axons proceed to terminate in the inferior part of the *post central gyrus*, i.e., part of the sensory cortex known as *taste cortex*. Perception of taste involves a complex mechanism extending from the tongue to the brain. In the brain, there is a pathway terminating in the cortex and another in the limbic system.

Brain, i.e., the former is possibly concerned with conscious perception while the latter, i.e., limbic system is responsible for the emotional reaction to taste. To the overall influence of civilization is to dissociate the two aspects, so that awareness of taste is possible without the accompanying emotional response, specifically if the taste is unpleasant. Thus, it can be said that "Real seat of taste is not the tongue but mind/brain" as well said by Mahatma Gandhi.

## APPLIED ASPECT

### Ageusia

Absence of taste sensation

**Causes:**
- Lesion of the mandibular division of Vth CN of which the chorda tympani nerve reaches the tongue.
- **Lesion of facial nerve:** Causes loss of taste sensation in the anterior ⅔rd part of the tongue.
- **Lesion of IXth CN:** Loss of taste sensation in posterior ⅓rd part of the tongue.
- Drugs like captopril, penicillamine which contain sulphydryl group cause temporary loss of taste sensation.
- **Familial dysautonomia:** Congenital widespread sensory disorder characterized by the absence of taste sensation associated with other abnormalities, e.g., postural hypotension, lacrimation, hyporeflexia, and insensitivity to temperature and noxious stimuli.

### Hypogeusia

Diminished taste sensation.

In them, there is an increase in the threshold for different taste sensations. Many different diseases can produce hypogeusia.

### Dysgeusia

Disturbed sensation of taste.

It is a feature of temporal lobe syndrome particularly when the anterior region of the temporal lobe is affected. The patient usually experiences paroxysmal hallucinations of taste and smell which are usually unpleasant.

### Selective Taste Blindness

It is an inherited autosomal recessive trait characterized by the markedly elevated threshold for phenyl thiocarbamide, i.e., PTC (a chemical substance with a very bitter taste). Such individuals are known as non-taster for PTC. The defect is highly selective since there is no taste blindness to other substances producing bitter taste and to the substance producing salty, sour, or sweet taste. Probably, there is a particular receptor protein that is not synthesized in these individuals.

**What is the life span of your taste receptor cell?**
10 days. New cells arise from the basal cells.

**What is taste-salivary reflex?**
Reflex stimulation of salivary secretion once taste bud receives tastant molecule. Afferent for reflex: 7th, 9th, and 10th cranial nerve to nucleus tractus solitarius—sends impulse to inferior and superior salivary nucleus of the facial and glossopharyngeal nerves.

Efferent from VII and IX cranial nerve innervates salivary gland for secretion.

---

## SUMMARY

Taste sensation, also known as gustation, is the sensory perception of flavor that arises from the stimulation of taste buds located on the tongue and other parts of the oral cavity.
- Taste buds are specialized sensory organs composed of clusters of taste receptor cells that detect different taste stimuli.
- There are five primary taste sensations: sweet, sour, salty, bitter, and umami (savory).
- Taste receptor cells are activated when specific molecules from food or beverages bind to receptors on their surface.
- Once activated, taste receptor cells generate electrical signals that are transmitted via nerve fibers to the brainstem and then to higher brain centers, where the taste perception is processed and interpreted.
- The process of taste sensation involves complex interactions between taste receptor cells, nerve pathways, and brain regions responsible for processing sensory information.

Disorders of taste sensation:
- Disorders of taste sensation, known as dysgeusia or ageusia, involve alterations or loss of the ability to perceive taste stimuli.
- Dysgeusia refers to distorted or abnormal taste perception, where tastes may be perceived as unpleasant, metallic, or altered in intensity.
- Ageusia refers to the complete loss of taste sensation, where individuals are unable to detect any taste stimuli.

Causes of taste disorders include:
- Infections of the oral cavity or upper respiratory tract.

- Medications that interfere with taste perception.
- Damage to taste buds or nerves, such as from head trauma, oral surgery, or neurological conditions.
- Systemic diseases, including diabetes, autoimmune disorders, and nutritional deficiencies.
- Aging, which can lead to a natural decline in taste sensitivity.
- Taste disorders can have a significant impact on quality of life, affecting appetite, nutritional status, and enjoyment of food.

## LET US SEE, HOW MUCH YOU HAVE LEARNT?

### Review Questions

#### Long/Short Answer Questions

Q1. Draw a well labeled diagram of taste bud.
Q2. Describe the gustatory pathway.
Q3. What is the physiological significance of dual nerve supply of tongue?

#### Explain Why? (Review Questions)

Q1. You feel the bitter taste at the time of swallowing.
Q2. You do not feel the taste, when your nose is blocked.
Q3. Gustatory dysfunction can be associated with conditions such as zinc deficiency or chemotherapy treatment.

### Multiple Choice Questions

Q1. Which of the following is NOT a primary taste sensation?
   a. Sweet        b. Spicy
   c. Sour         d. Bitter

Q2. Taste buds are primarily located on which of the following?
   a. Tongue       b. Esophagus
   c. Stomach      d. Liver

Q3. Dysgeusia refers to:
   a. Complete loss of taste sensation
   b. Normal taste perception
   c. Altered or distorted taste perception
   d. Inability to distinguish between taste sensations

Q4. Which cranial nerve is primarily responsible for transmitting taste sensations from the anterior two-thirds of the tongue?
   a. Olfactory nerve (CN I)
   b. Facial nerve (CN VII)
   c. Glossopharyngeal nerve (CN IX)
   d. Vagus nerve (CN X)

Q5. What is the fifth primary taste sensation, in addition to sweet, sour, salty, and bitter?
   a. Umami        b. Spicy
   c. Metallic       d. Astringent

Q6. Ageusia refers to:
   a. Complete loss of taste sensation
   b. Altered taste perception
   c. Normal taste perception
   d. Heightened taste sensitivity

Q7. Which of the following is NOT a common cause of taste disorders?
   a. Head trauma        b. Medications
   c. Nutritional supplements      d. Visual impairment

Q8. Which nerve is primarily responsible for transmitting taste sensations from the posterior one-third of the tongue?
   a. Facial nerve (CN VII)
   b. Glossopharyngeal nerve (CN IX)
   c. Trigeminal nerve (CN V)
   d. Vagus nerve (CN X)

Q9. Which of the following is NOT a method used for taste testing?
   a. Taste strips
   b. Applying taste stimuli to the skin
   c. Using taste solutions
   d. Identifying different foods with blindfolded participants

Q10. Gymnemic acid, found in Gymnema sylvestre, is known for its:
   a. Antidiabetic properties
   b. Antibacterial properties
   c. Antiviral properties
   d. Antifungal properties

Q11. Taste buds contain specialized cells known as:
   a. Sensory neurons
   b. Olfactory cells
   c. Taste receptor cells
   d. Epithelial cells

Q12. Which taste sensation is associated with the perception of acidic substances?
   a. Sweet        b. Sour
   c. Salty         d. Bitter

Q13. Which of the following is NOT a factor contributing to taste disorders?
   a. Aging
   b. Smoking
   c. Improved oral hygiene
   d. Medications

Q14. Taste receptor cells are primarily activated by:
   a. Light         b. Sound
   c. Chemicals     d. Temperature

Q15. Which taste sensation is associated with the perception of savory or meaty flavors?
   a. Sweet        b. Sour
   c. Salty         d. Umami

Q16. The taste sensation mechanism primarily involves interactions between taste receptor cells and:
   a. Skeletal muscles
   b. Blood vessels
   c. Nerve fibers
   d. Endocrine glands

Q17. Dysgeusia can be caused by:
   a. Headache
   b. Nasal congestion
   c. Allergic reactions
   d. Exposure to loud noises

Q18. Which of the following is NOT a method of clinical examination of taste sensations?
   a. Taste strips
   b. Snellen chart
   c. Taste solutions
   d. Identifying foods blindfolded

## ANSWERS

1. b   2. a   3. c   4. b   5. a   6. a   7. d   8. b   9. b   10. a   11. c   12. b   13. c   14. c
15. d   16. c   17. c   18. b

# Physiology of Vision

## CHAPTER 95

### COMPETENCY ADDRESSED

**PY10.17:** Describe and discuss the functional anatomy of eye, physiology of image formation, physiology of vision including color vision, refractive errors, color blindness, physiology of pupil and light reflex.
**PY10.18:** Describe and discuss the physiological basis of the lesion in the visual pathway.
**PY10.19:** Describe and discuss the visual evoked potential.

### LEARNING OBJECTIVES

**At the end of this chapter, the learner should be able to:**
- Describe the physio-anatomical basis of the eyeball and eye.
- Explain the composition, secretion and flow of the aqueous humor in eye.
- Describe the intraocular pressure and disorders associated with it.
- Describe the functional anatomy of layers of retina.
- Describe the photochemistry of vision, including color vision.
- Describe the neural circuitry of the retinal cells.
- Describe the visual pathway and the disorders associated due to lesions in it.
- Describe the physiological basis of different types of refractory errors.

Have you ever thought how do we see this beautiful, colorful world around us? As a first-year undergraduate medical student you need to have a good understanding about the anatomical background of the vision and its physiological action in terms of its function and mechanism of action.

## ANATOMY OF EYE

Basic structure by with we can our surrounding is eye. It is a *hollow globe structure* located in the orbital cavity with 24 mm in diameter, having *1/6th part of its visible outside* rest being protected inside the orbital cavity **(Fig. 95.1)**. It has three layers with two different fluids with ocular muscle leading to eyeball movements and areolar/fatty tissue leading to protective cushion to the eyeball.

It is made up of three layers **(Fig. 95.2)**:
A. *Outer layer OR Tunica externa/fibrosa: cornea and sclera*
B. *Middle layer OR Tunica media/vasculosa: choroid, ciliary body and iris*
C. *Inner layer OR Tunica intima/nervosa: retina*

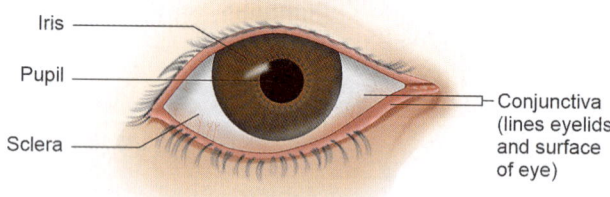

**Fig. 95.1:** External anatomy of the eye.

### Outer Layer or Tunica Externa/Fibrosa
#### Sclera

- Sclera is the tough, white avascular, fibrous structure-collagen fibers, covers posterior 5/6th of the eyeball.
- Extraocular muscles are inserted on it.
- Anteriorly, it is continuous with cornea.
- Posterior-most part of sclera is pierced by the optic nerve, in the form of thin perforations called lamina cribrosa.

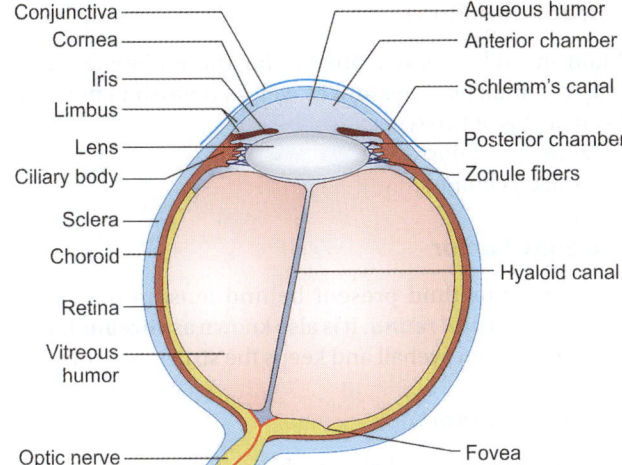

**Fig. 95.2:** Internal structure of the eyeball.

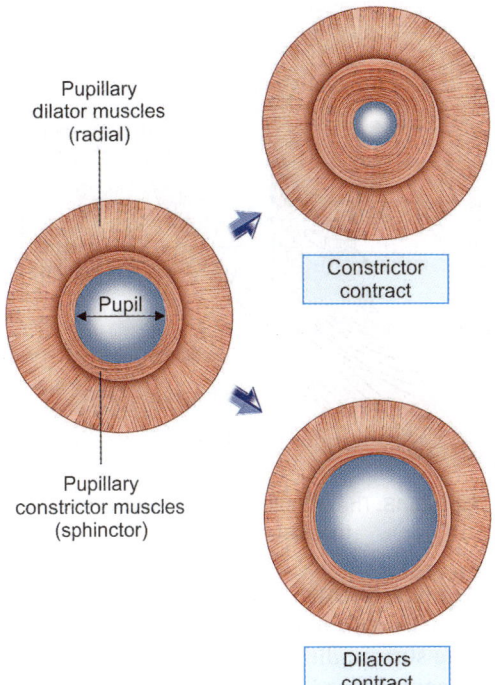

**Fig. 95.3:** Constriction and dilatation of pupil.

## Cornea

It is the transparent, avascular, convex, anterior portion of the outer layer of eyeball, covers the iris and pupil, forms the anterior 1/6th of eyeball. It is supplied by sensory nerve ending of V cranial nerve. The curvature of the cornea contributes to most of refractive power of eye.

The diameter of cornea is *12 mm horizontally and 11 mm vertically*. It is very sensitive to pain, touch, pressure and cold, because of rich supply of free nerve endings. Cornea is not vascularized but it derives its nourishment mainly from aqueous humor.

## Middle Layer or Tunica Media/Vasculosa

Middle layer surrounds the eyeball completely, except for a small opening in front known as pupil. This layer comprises of choroid, ciliary body, iris and crystalline lens.

## Choroid

A thin vascular layer situated between sclera and retina. *Membrane of Bruch* lines the inner side of the choroid and separates it from the retina. Its blood vessels are bound together by connective tissue containing pigmented cells called *chromatophores*.

## Ciliary Body

It is made up of two sets of *ciliary muscles*, namely outer longitudinal and inner circular muscles, both innervated by the parasympathetic III CN.

**The ciliary muscle**—made of circular and radial multiunit smooth muscle—supplied by the ciliary ganglion—gets activated by the Edinger-Westphal nucleus of oculomotor nerve.

## Iris

Iris is a thin circular diaphragm with a circular opening in the center called **pupil**. Iris is formed by muscles **(Fig. 95.3):**
- **Constrictor pupillae**
- **Dilator pupillae** or pupillary dilator muscle.

*It regulates the amount of light entering the eyeball.*

The intraocular muscles of iris are supplied by parasympathetic fibers of III CN which results in pupillary constriction (miosis). This cuts more diffracted rays and decreases spherical and chromatic aberrations. It sharpens image on the retina. Sympathetic fibers from cervical sympathetic chain supplies the dilator pupillae causing (mydriasis), letting more light into the retina.

## Crystalline Lens (Figs. 95.4A and B)

It is transparent, biconvex; developed from the **ectoderm**. It is 9–10 mm diameter and the thickness varies with age

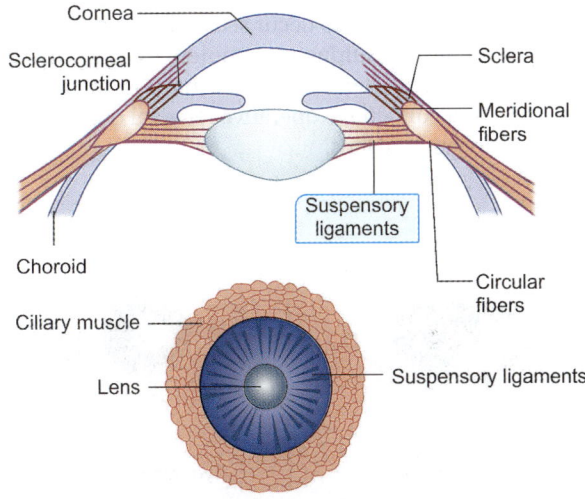

**Fig. 95.4A:** The crystalline lens is held in place by suspensory ligaments, just behind the posterior chamber.

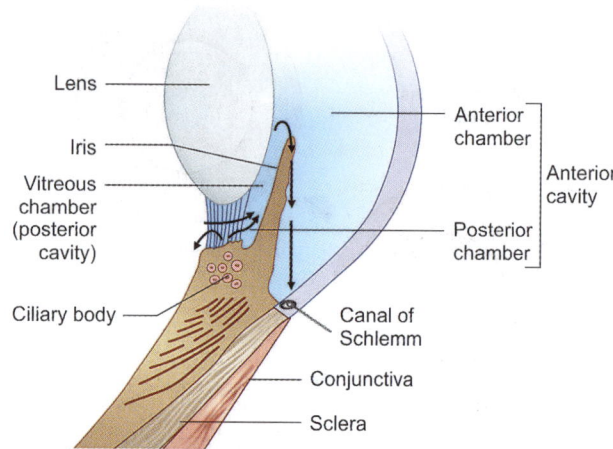

**Fig. 95.4B:** The crystalline lens located just behind the posterior chamber.

from 3.5 mm (at birth) to 5 mm (old age). It is enclosed in a capsule which is thin, tough, transparent, elastic and hyaline membrane surrounding the lens. It is semipermeable in nature. It contributes 17 diopters to total refractive power of the eye (discussed later).

**Lens transparency:** The transparency of the lens is maintained by the:
- Avascularity of the lens
- Arrangement of lens proteins
- Auto-oxidation
- High concentration of reduced glutathione (GSH) in the lens maintains the lens proteins in a reduced state and ensures transparency.

**Age-related changes:** With advanced age lens starts to lose its high-water content and becomes tougher and less elastic. Results in decreased convexity of the lens following relaxation of the suspensory ligament. Hence the lens becomes less transparent with age.

**Cataract:** It is defined as opacity in the lens or its capsule (Fig. 95.5). It occurs with aging due to degenerative/senile cataract. It can also occur secondary to disease like diabetes mellitus resulting in complete opacity (mature cataract). Absence of lens from its normal position is called *aphakia*. It occurs due to operative removal of the lens or due to dislocation of lens.

## Intraocular Fluid

Fluid in eyeball is responsible for the maintenance of shape, intraocular pressure as well as nourishment of the eyeball. It is of two types:
1. Vitreous humor
2. Aqueous humor

### Vitreous Humor

It is a viscous fluid present behind lens, in the *space between lens and retina*. It is also known as **vitreous body**. It gives shape to eyeball and keeps the structure in place.

### Aqueous Humor

It is a thin, **watery** fluid filled in the space between lens and cornea. This space is divided into *anterior and posterior chambers* by iris. Both the chambers communicate with each other through **pupil**.

**Composition:**
- pH 7.1–7.3, specific gravity 1.002–1.004
- Rich in vitamin C, hyaluronic acid
- High NaCl concentration and lactic acid
- Low glucose and protein

**Formation (Fig. 95.6):**
- Secreted almost entirely by ciliary processes.
- Sodium ions are actively transported first. $Cl^-$, $HCO_3^-$ and water follow this. Rate of formation—2 to 3 µL/min
- It is formed by the **ciliary processes** from plasma by diffusion, ultrafiltration and active transport through the epithelial cells linings. After formation, aqueous humor reaches the **posterior chamber** by passing through the suspensory ligaments. From here, it reaches the **anterior chamber** via pupil.

**Drainage of aqueous humor:** From anterior chamber, the aqueous humor passes into the angle between cornea and

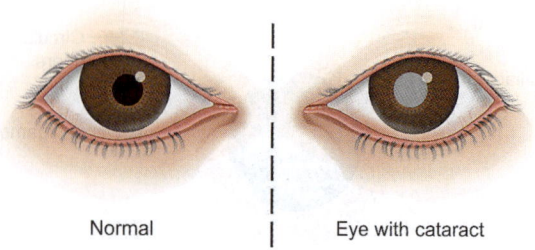

**Fig. 95.5:** Opacity of lens showing cataract.

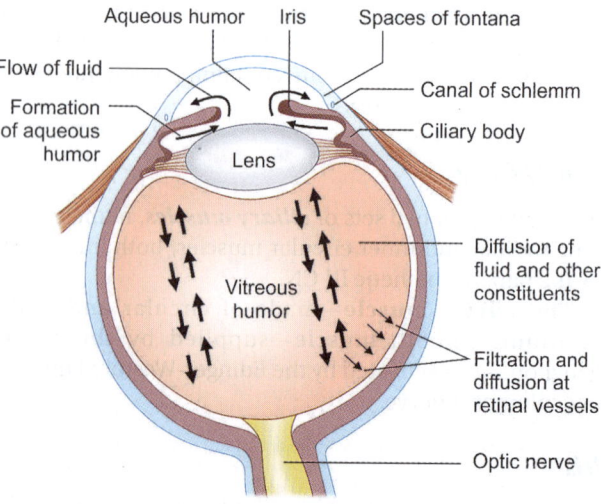

**Fig. 95.6:** Formation of aqueous humor.

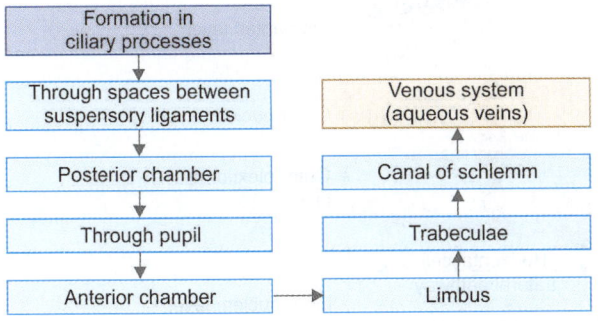

Flowchart 95.1: Aqueous flow and drainage.

iris. From here, it passes through meshwork of **trabeculae situated** here. Then it flows through **canal of Schlemm** and reaches the venous system via **anterior ciliary vein**.

**Aqueous flow:** *See* **Flowchart 95.1.**

**Intraocular pressure:**
- Intraocular pressure is the measure of fluid pressure in eye, exerted by aqueous humor.
- Normal intraocular pressure varies between 12 and 20 mm Hg.
- It is measured by **tonometer.**
- **When intraocular pressure increases**, it leads to the compression of the intraocular structures resulting in **glaucoma.**

**Glaucoma:** Most common cause of blindness:
- A group of diseases characterized by increased intraocular pressure, which causes damage of optic nerve, resulting in blindness.
- In glaucoma, the drainage of aqueous humor through trabeculae is blocked, resulting in increased intraocular pressure.
- Increasing intraocular pressure compresses retina, optic nerve and blood vessels.
- Late symptoms include blurred vision and halos around bright objects.

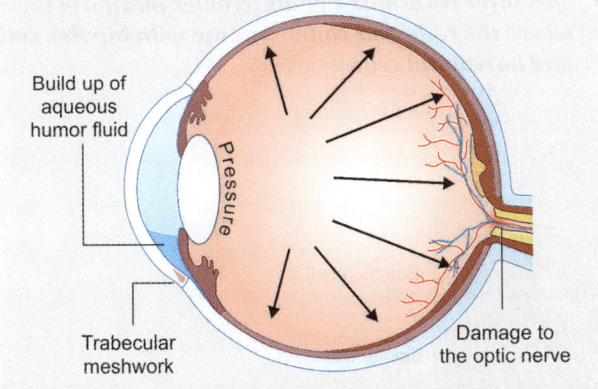

## Inner Layer or Tunica Intima/Nervosa

### Retina

The innermost neural layer is called retina. It has 10 layers, enumerated below (from outside to inside) **(Fig. 95.7)**:
1. Layer of pigment epithelium
2. Layer of rods and cones (photoreceptors)
3. External limiting membrane
4. Outer nuclear layer
5. Outer plexiform layer
6. Inner nuclear layer
7. Inner plexiform layer
8. Ganglion cell layer
9. Layer of nerve fibers
10. Internal limiting membrane.

*(These layers are described below)*

- **Fundus oculi:** Fundus oculi is the posterior part of interior eyeball, which can be seen through an **ophthalmoscope.** It has two important structures: Optic disc and Macula lutea with fovea centralis.
  - *Optic Disc:* It is also called a *blind spot*. It is a pale disc, situated near the center of the posterior wall of eyeball. It contains all the layers of retina, **except rods and cones**. It is situated 3mm medial to and slightly above posterior pole.
  - *Macula lutea (the yellow spot):* It is a small yellowish area, situated a little lateral to the optic disc. Macula lutea has **fovea centralis in its center (Fig. 95.8).**
  - Most acute vision because it contains *only cones* (**Note:** The rods are absent here).
- **Fovea centralis:** It is a small area with a diameter of 0.3 mm. It contains large number of tightly packed small-sized slender cones only **(Fig. 95.9).**
  - Other neural layers are displaced laterally to the side of the fovea—making light reach to photoreceptors.
  - **Cone cell to ganglion cell ratio is 1:1**—making receptive field of a ganglion cell smaller while it increases towards periphery of the retina.
  - Central artery and vein of retina pass at the side of macula, not over it.
  - **Nutrition of macula:** Choroidal blood vessels by diffusion.

As mentioned above, the various layers of retina are described below:

**Layer 1: Pigmented epithelium**
- Continues with epithelium of iris
- It is rich in melanocytes
- It contains melanin pigment which along with pigmented choroid and absorbs extra amount of light, thus preventing the reflection of rays back through the retina.

**Albinos** lack the melanin pigment hence the dark pigment layer is absent in them. On entering the bright room, the light gets reflected inside the retina in all directions that it excites many photoreceptors. Hence, the visual acuity be up to 20/100 to 20/200 instead of 20/20)

- If this light gets refracted back, it would result in blurring of vision.
- It also has phagocytic function.
- It acts as a storage site for vitamin A, which readily gets exchanged with the outer segment of photoreceptors.

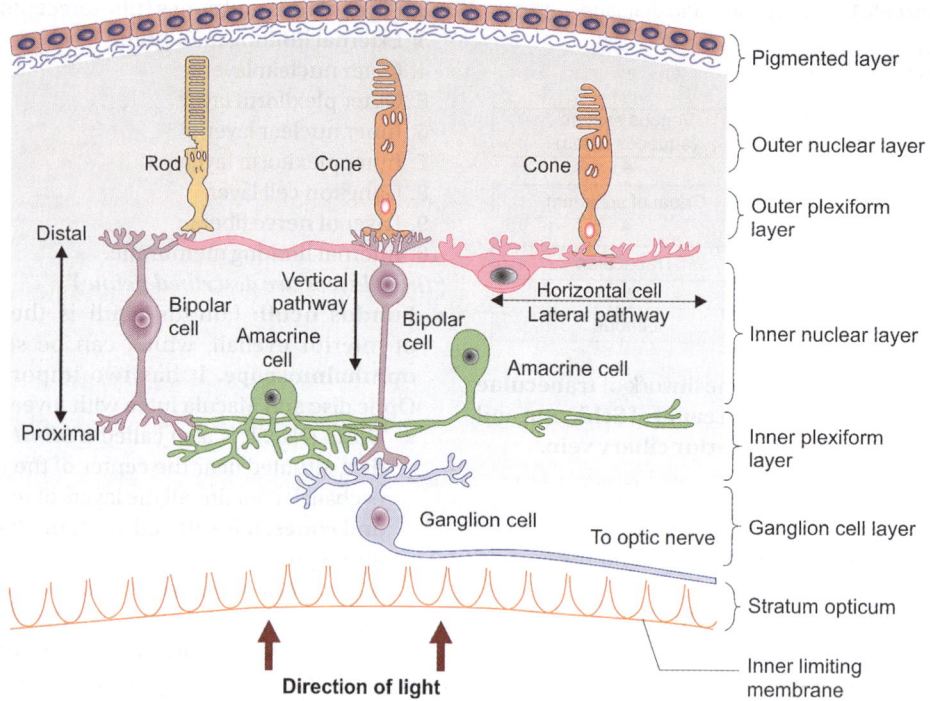

**Fig. 95.7:** The layers of retina.

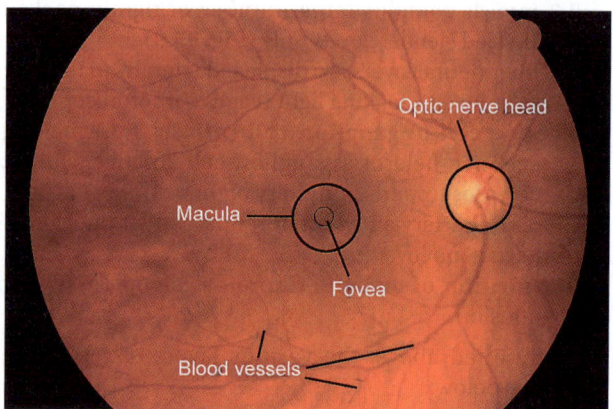

**Fig. 95.8:** The fundus of the eye showing the optic cup and the fovea.

- This layer is adherent to choroid. The layer of photoreceptors receives its nutrition from choroidal vessels by diffusion.

### Layer 2: Rods and cones layer—photoreceptors (Table 95.1)

- Also known as visual receptors; 120 million rods, 6 million cones only 1 million ganglion cells.
- Each photoreceptor (rod and cone) is divided into outer segment, inner segment and a synaptic zone.
- The outer and inner segment form the layers of rods and cones.
- *This layer transmits signals to outer plexiform layer, where the rods and cones synapse with bipolar cells and horizontal cells.*

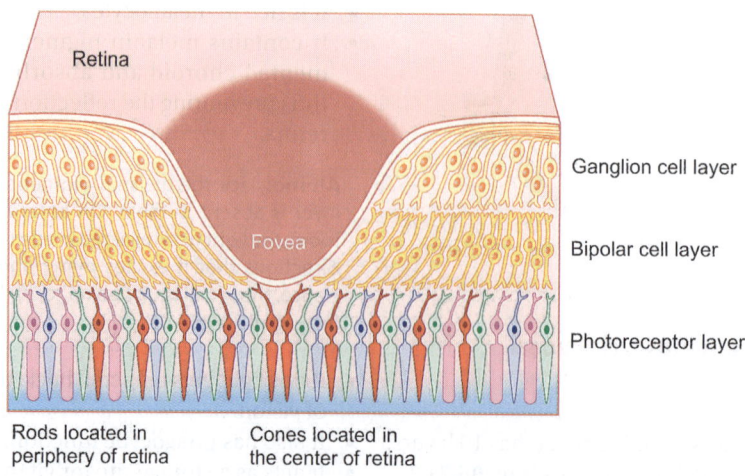

**Fig. 95.9:** The fovea centralis.

**Table 95.1:** Characteristics of rods and cones (similarities and differences).

| | Rods | Cones |
|---|---|---|
| Shape | Cylindrical/rod shaped. Narrower and longer than cones | Conical shaped |
| Number | Around 120 million | Around 6 million |
| Distribution | Present in the peripheral retina. Absent in fovea centralis | Most abundantly present in fovea centralis. The cones are thin and slender in fovea whereas fatter in peripheral retina |
| **Outer segment of photoreceptors** | | |
| Structure (Fig. 95.10) | There are around 1,000 folded shelves in both rods and cones, which contain the visual pigment. These pigments are conjugated G-proteins. They are responsible for 40% of entire mass of outer segment | |
| Pigment | Rhodopsin (visual purple) | Iodopsin. One of the three color pigments (red, green or blue) |
| Peak spectral sensitivity | 500 nm | Red-sensitive—560 nm<br>Green-sensitive—530 nm<br>Blue-sensitive—420 nm |
| Renewal of outer segments | Formation of new discs at the inner edge of the segments and **phagocytosis of old discs from the outer tip by cells of the pigment epithelium** | It is more diffused process and appears to occur at multiple sites in the outer segment |
| Clinical correlate | In **Retinitis Pigmentosa** the phagocytic process is defective and a layer of debris accumulates between the receptor and the pigment epithelium finally producing blindness | |
| **Inner segment of photoreceptors** | | |
| Mitochondria | Abundant | |
| Shape | Large and oval | |
| The inner segment pierce the outer limiting membrane, forming layer 3 of retina | | |
| **Nucleus (forms Layer 4, the outer nuclear layer)** | | |
| Both rods and cones pierces the external limiting membrane, then enlarge to form rod and cones nucleus respectively | | |
| **Synaptic body (forms Layer 5)** | | |
| Towards the inner side both rods and cones and finally enlarge into rod end bulb (knob-like fashion) and cone plate respectively | | |

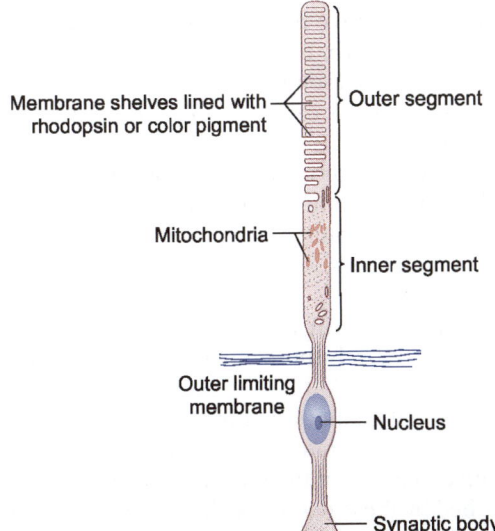

**Fig. 95.10:** Detailed structure of a photoreceptor (rods and cones)

**Different types of cells in retina:**
- Rods and cones (Layer 2)
- Horizontal cells (Layers 5 and 6)
- Bipolar cells (Layers 5 and 6)
- Amacrine cells (Layers 5 and 6)
- Ganglion cells (Layers 7 and 8)
- Interplexiform cells (Layers 7 to 6)
- Muller cells

**Layer 3: Outer limiting membrane**—it is formed by the glial tissues; it is the continuation of internal limiting membrane and is pierced by the rods and cones.

**Layer 4: Outer nuclear layer**—it is formed by the nucleus of rods and cones (as mentioned above).

**Layer 5: Outer plexiform/synaptic layer**—it is formed by synapse between the ends of rods and cones with dendrites of bipolar neuron cells and horizontal cells.

**Layer 6: Inner nuclear layer (Fig. 95.11)**—it is formed by the nuclei of bipolar cells, horizontal cells (which connect

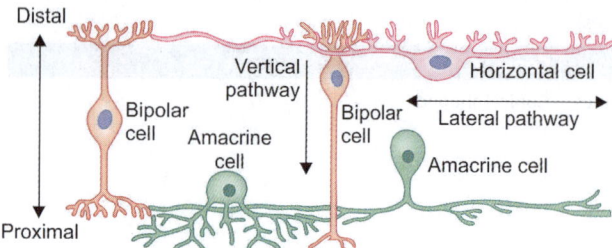

**Fig. 95.11:** Various cells present in outer nuclear layer.

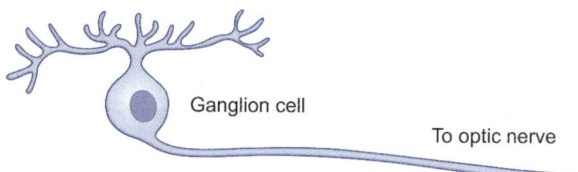

**Fig. 95.12:** Ganglion cells are present in the inner nuclear layer.

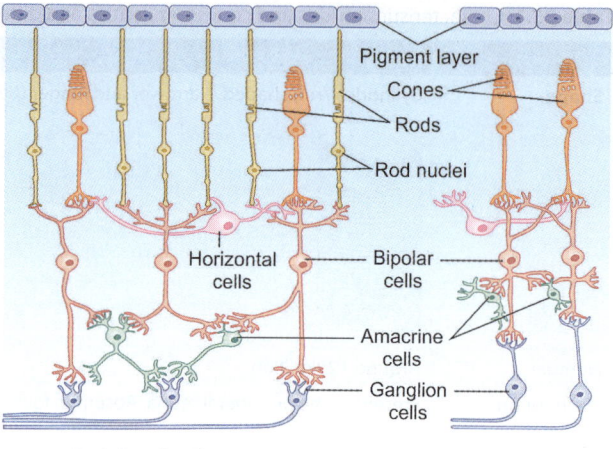

**Fig. 95.13:** The ratio of synapse between photoreceptors and ganglion cells in the peripheral retina and fovea centralis. It is responsible for the high visual acuity in the fovea.

one receptor cell to other receptor cell) and amacrine cells. The processes of amacrine cells make synaptic contacts with dendrites of both ganglion and bipolar cells and connect ganglion cells to one another.

- *Horizontal cells: Transmit signals horizontally in outer plexiform layer from rods and cones to bipolar cells.*
- *Bipolar cells: Transmit signal vertically from rods, cones and horizontal cells to inner plexiform layer, where they synapse with ganglion cells and amacrine cells.*
- *Amacrine cells: Transmit signals in two directions (directly from bipolar cells to ganglion cells; horizontally from bipolar cells to other cells in this layer).*

### Layer 7: Inner plexiform/synaptic layer

- The synapse between the axons of bipolar cells with the dendrites of ganglion cells occur in this layer.
- It is the site of major processing of the visual image.
  *Ganglion cells (Fig. 95.12): Transmit the output signals from the retina through the optic nerve into brain. Interplexiform cells: These cells are not prominent and they transmit signal in retrograde direction from inner plexiform layer to outer plexiform layer. These signals are inhibitory and controls the lateral speed of visual signals by the horizontal cells. They probably provide contrast to the visual image.*

### Layer 8: Ganglion cell layer

- It is a single layer of cell containing round cells.
- Functional convergence in peripheral is more than 100:1 from bipolar cells to ganglion cells, whereas the foveal cones have 1:1 synaptic ratio **(Fig. 95.13)**.

Various supporting glial cells are present interspersed between the neural elements called the *Muller cells*. They lie between bipolar and ganglion cell layer and send their process to inner part of photoreceptor and fixing these cells making the *outer limiting membrane*. They prevent the escape of the Intercellular photoreceptor matrix to other half of retina. Their other end extends to form foot plates as inner limiting membrane.

### Layer 9: Optic nerve
—it is formed by joining the axons of ganglion cells: All the *axons run parallel*.

### Layer 10: Internal limiting membrane
- It separates the retina from the vitreous humor.
- It is formed by the **glial tissues**.

## GENESIS OF ELECTRICAL ACTIVITY IN RETINA

The electrical activity in the retina is primarily generated in the layer of photoreceptors. But the other cells also participate in the electrical activity. Various changes are discussed below such as the photochemistry of vision and the transmission of visual signals to the occipital cortex.

- Photoreceptor potentials
- Responses of bipolar, amacrine and horizontal cells
- Response pattern of ganglion cells
- Responses of neurons in the lateral geniculate bodies and visual cortex

1. Visual images have different characteristics, such as color, form, depth, movement and texture and each image is processed simultaneously by a separate channel in the visual system, called *parallel processing of visual information.*
2. The processing of visual information in the retina involves the generation of electrical activity at 3 places:
   a. The photoreceptors
   b. The bipolar cells
   c. The ganglion cells
3. The electrical activity in the bipolar cells and ganglion cells is altered by the horizontal cells and amacrine cells respectively.
4. The potential changes that initiate action potential in the retina are generated by the action of light on photosensitive pigment in the rods and cones. When light is absorbed by these pigments, they trigger a sequence of events that initiates neural activity (photo-transduction).

5. **Sequence of events in photo-transduction in photo-receptors (Fig. 95.14):** When the light fall on the photoreceptor membrane, light absorbing pigment (rhodopsin) gets activated. This stimulates transducin (G-protein), which activates cGMP phosphodiesterase. This enzyme catalyzes the degradation of cGMP into 5'-GMP, which result in closure of sodium channels. This causes hyperpolarization of the photoreceptor.

## PHOTORECEPTOR POTENTIALS

See figure below for receptors potentials in dark and in light.

**In dark:**
- $Na^+$ channels in the outer segments are kept **open** by cGMP
- Steady current flow from the inner to the outer segment of the rods and cones
- Membrane potential is –40 mV

**In light:**
- Decreased cGMP and increased formation of 5'-GMP
- **Closure** of $Na^+$ channels; stoppage of $Na^+$ influx
- **Hyperpolarization** and generates local graded potentials (generator potentials).
- Membrane potential is –70 to –80 mV

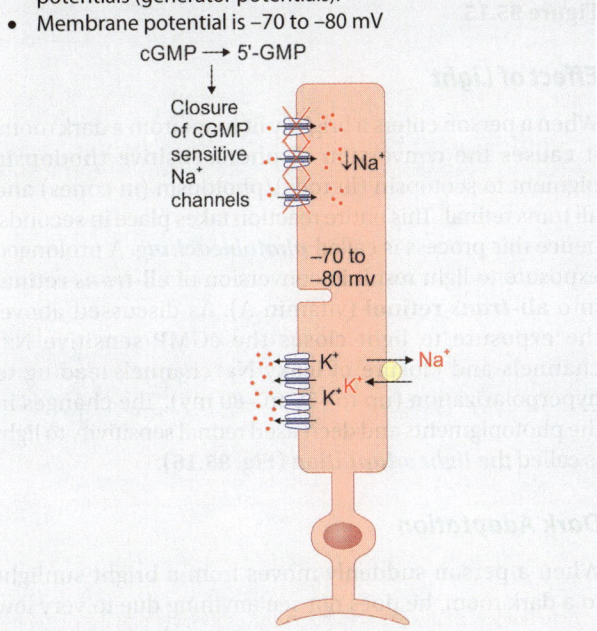

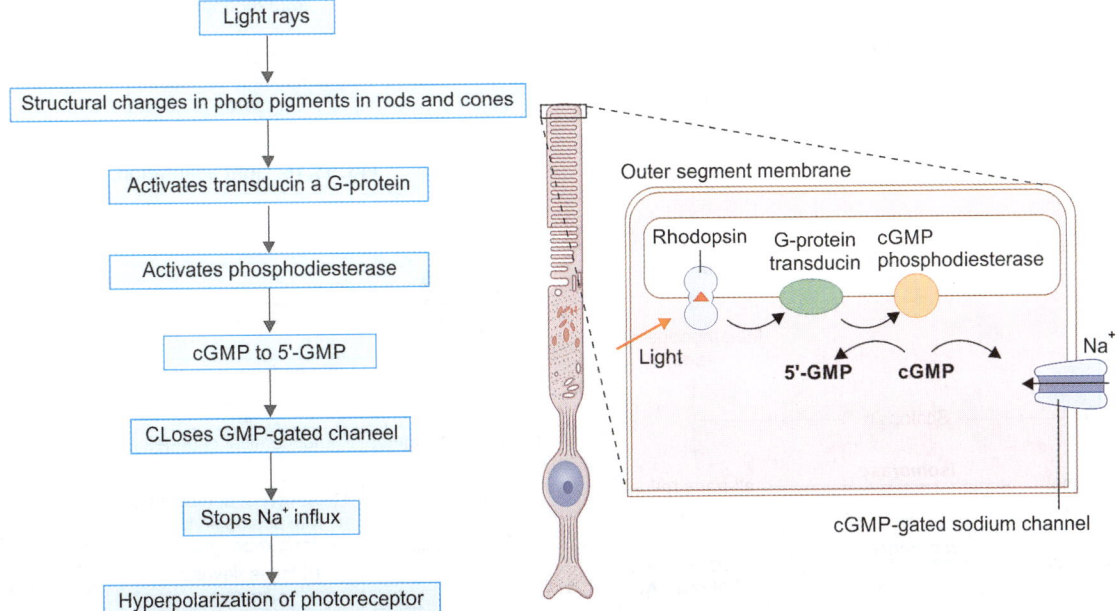

**Fig. 95.14:** Photo transduction in outer segment of photoreceptor membrane.

Receptor potential reaches peak in 0.3 s and lasts for more than a second in rods. These potentials are attained four times faster in cones.

Rods respond proportionately to stimulus intensity at levels of illumination that are below the threshold for cones, while cones respond proportionately to stimulus intensity at high levels of illumination.

## Photochemistry of Vision in Rods and Cones

**Rhodopsin:** Visual purple is made of protein scotopsin, conjugated with 11-*cis* retinal (a derivative of vitamin A). Metarhodopsin II: Activated rhodopsin—brings about electrical changes in rods. The visual cycle is shown in **Figure 95.15**.

### *Effect of Light*

When a person enters a brightly lit room from a dark room, it causes the conversion of photosensitive rhodopsin pigment to scotopsin (in rods)/photopsin (in cones) and all trans retinal. This entire reaction takes place in seconds, hence this process is called *photobleaching*. A prolonged exposure to light result in conversion of **all-*trans* retinal** into **all-*trans* retinol** (vitamin A). As discussed above, the exposure to light closes the cGMP sensitive $Na^+$ channels and closure of leaky $Na^+$ channels leading to hyperpolarization (up to −70 to −80 mv). The changes in the photopigments and decreased retinal sensitivity to light is called the *light adaptation* (Fig. 95.16).

### *Dark Adaptation*

When a person suddenly moves from a bright sunlight to a dark room, he does not see anything due to very low retinal sensitivity (as a result of light adaptation). When he stays there for a few minutes, the retinal sensitivity increases due to regeneration of Rhodopsin, as seen in **Figure 95.17**.

- All-*trans* retinol is enzymatically isomerized to 11-*cis* retinol
- Then enzymatically oxidized to 11-*cis* retinal then spontaneously combines with scotopsin, reforming rhodopsin

The reformation of rhodopsin takes a few minutes. Let's see the various changes in the eye occurring during dark adaptation.

The retinal sensitivity increases with an increase in concentration of rhodopsin formed in the photoreceptors.

- **Figure 95.18** shows the increase in retinal sensitivity with increase in duration of stay in dark. When a person enters the dark room, the retinal sensitivity is minimum. Initially the sensitivity of retinal increases by 10 folds in 1 minute but then increases exponentially by increasing to 6,000 times by the end of 20 minutes and 25,000 times by the end of 40,000 times.
- The pupils dilate to allow the entry of more amount of light.
- The bipolar cells and the ganglion cells also bring the necessary changes in transmission (discussed later).

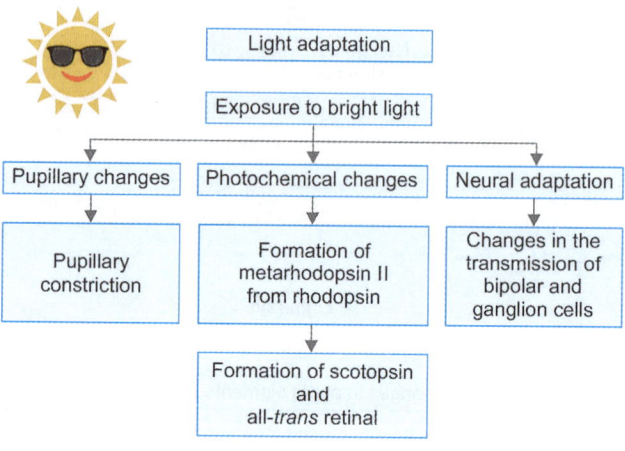

**Fig. 95.16:** Light adaptation.

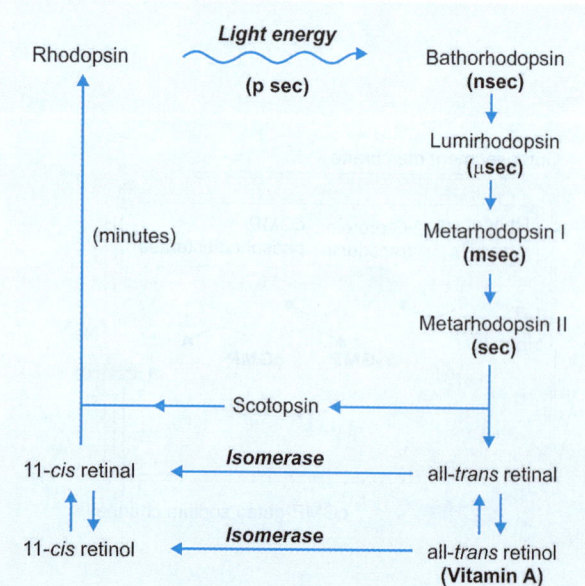

**Fig. 95.15:** The visual cycle.

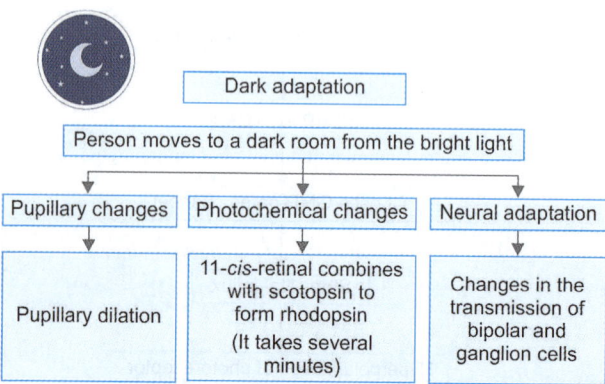

**Fig. 95.17:** Dark adaptation.

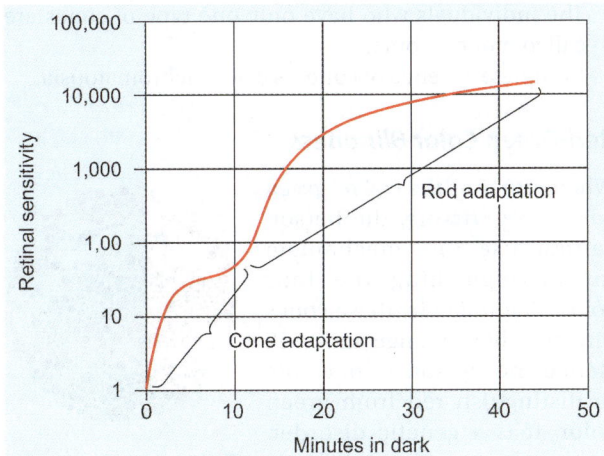

**Fig. 95.18:** The recovery of retinal sensitivity with duration in dark (minutes).

- The conversion of retinol to retinal is dependent on the pigment epithelium
- Deficiency of vitamin A prevents the regeneration of rhodopsin.

For this reason, lack of vitamin A leads to *night blindness*.

## Color Vision

The ability to discriminate between colors' excited by light of different wavelengths. The color vision has three main attributes: hue, intensity and saturation. The electromagnetic energy is wavelength between **380–760 nm.**

### Types of Color Vision

- **Achromatic:** Sensation of white vision with no color vision
- **Chromatic:**
  - Spectral color vision
  - Extra spectral color vision

If a person sees black, it is a positive sensation because black color is produced by absence of light. A blind eye *"sees nothing"*, not even black color.

### Type of Colors

- **Primary colors:** Blue, green, red and mixing of these colors.
- **Complementary colors (Fig. 95.19):** When two colors are mixed in appropriate amount it cancels the colors and produces while sensation. If a color is mixed with its complementary color, it leads to perception of white color.

### Theories of Color Vision

**Young-Helmholtz theory of color vision (Trichromatic color theory) (Fig. 95.20).**

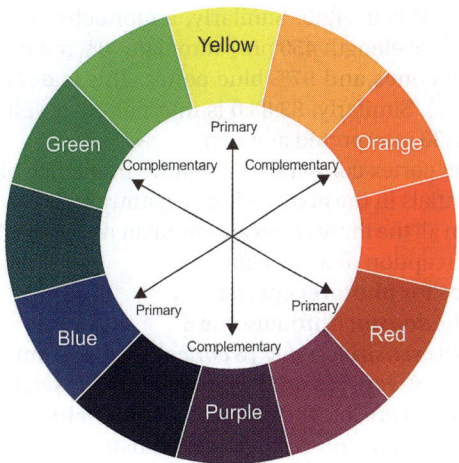

**Fig. 95.19:** The Newtons color wheel of complementary colors.

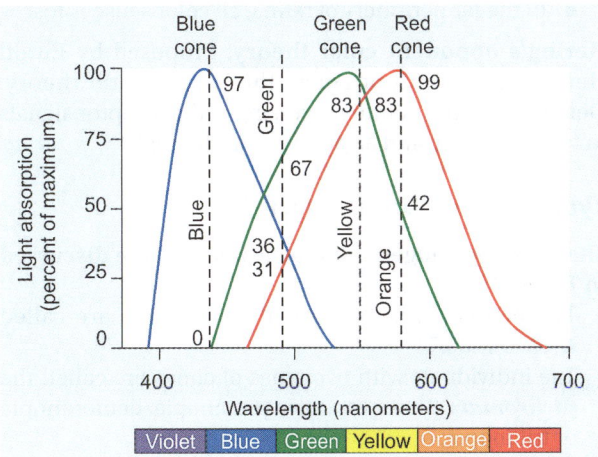

**Fig. 95.20:** The different spectral sensitivity of red, green and blue cones.

Operates at the receptor level. It was postulated by Young after color matching experiment by Helmholtz. It is based on three types of cones receptors which are responsible for color vision. **"Color match in the visible spectrum is possible by appropriate mixing of three primary colors."**

**Photochemistry of color vision:** Similar to the rods, cones have a photopigment called photopsin which combines to the retinal to form the visual pigment iodopsin. Depending on the sensitivity to the color spectrum, the cones are classified as:
- Red sensitive cones (570 nm)
- Green sensitive cones (535 nm)
- Blue sensitive cones (445 nm)

**Spectral sensitivity of cones:**
- Cone pigment can absorb a wide range of wavelengths
- Even, particular color produces different levels of stimulation in various cones. This means if an orange

light (wavelength of 580 nm) falls on the retina, it will stimulate the red cones (99%), green cones (42%) with no stimulation of blue cones. Thus the ratio of stimulation of R:G:B is 99:42:0. Similarly, a monochromatic blue light (wavelength 450 nm) stimulates 0% red cones, 0% green cones and 97% blue cones. This is depicted as (0:0:97). Similarly, 83:83:0 is interpreted as yellow and 31:67:36 interpreted as green.
- Visual cortex compares the relative frequency of action potentials in the activated cone pathway
- When all the three cones are stimulated equally, the lead to perception of white light.

    **Genes for photoreceptors:**
    - *Rhodopsin:* Chromosome 3
    - *Blue sensitive cones (S cones):* Chromosome 7
    - **Green sensitive (M cones)** and **red sensitive (L cones)** are located on the **q arm of X-chromosomes**

    Trichromatic color vision mechanism extends 20–30° from the point of fixation
    - Peripheral to this red and green become indistinguishable
    - In the far periphery of retina, all color sense is lost

**Hering's opponent color theory:** Proposed by Ewald Hering in 1878. Contradicts the trichromatic theory. Derived from the neural processing of the receptor signals in two chromatic and an achromatic channel.

### Types of Color Vision Defect

**These can be congenital or acquired and are discussed in Table 95.2.**
- The people with the normal color vision are called *trichromats*.
- The individuals with two types of cones are called the *dichromats*. These can have protanopia/deuteranopia or tritanopia.

> **Some terms:**
> - **Anomaly:** Weakness
> - **Anopia:** Absence or loss
> - **Prot:** Red color
> - **Deuter:** Green color
> - **Trit:** Blue color
>
> Hence,
> **Protanopia:** Absence of red color
> **Deuteranopia:** Absence of green color
> **Tritanopia:** Absence of blue color

**Table 95.2:** Color vision defects.

| Congenital | Acquired |
| --- | --- |
| Other visual functions like visual acuity, ERG are normal | Other visual functions like visual acuity, ERG are normal |
| The defect is stable | The defect may progress or regress |
| Symmetrical in both eyes | Often asymmetrical |
| Prevalent more in males than females | Equal predisposition people |

- The individuals who have only one type of cones are called monochromats.
- Complete absence of cones is called achromatopsia.

### Red-Green Color Blindness

When *either of the red or green cones are missing*, the person cannot use this mechanism for distinguishing the four colors, identified by these cones (green, yellow, orange and red). Hence the person is not able to distinguish red from green color. It is a genetic disorder, that occurs in males. It is having *X linked inheritance* (mentioned above), hence never occurs in females as other X chromosome is always normal.

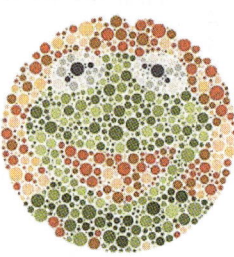

### Tests for Color Vision

- **Pseudo-isochromatic chart test (Ishihara's color plates) (Fig. 95.21A):** The two basic Ishihara's color plates can easily differentiate between a red-green color blind person from the person with normal vision. A person with normal color vision would read these plates as '74' and '42', whereas, the person with red-green color blindness will read the upper plate as 21, instead of 74. However, in the lower plate with '42'; a red blind person (protanope) will read 2; green blind (deuteranope) will read as 4. However, the Ishihara plates are the collection of other numbers and patterns for diagnosing the color blindness.
- **Edridge green lantern (Fig. 95.21B):** This is used to test the color vision especially in drivers and pilots.
- **Holmgren's wool test (Fig. 95.21C):** In this the patient is asked to match the skeins of the wool of same color from a cluster of wool skeins.

## RESPONSES TO BIPOLAR, AMACRINE AND HORIZONTAL CELLS (SEE FIGURE 95.22)

- The *bipolar cells do not generate action potentials,* instead they generate relatively steady hyperpolarizing or depolarizing potential (electrotonic/generator potential) up to 10 mV.
    - In some cells, hyperpolarizing potential are produced by a spot light, whereas depolarizing potentials by an annulus of light around the center. Hyperpolarizing bipolar cells are inhibited due by the horizontal cells, producing the inhibitory output. This helps in sharpening the signal and enhancing the contrast.
    - The receptive fields of the bipolar cells are organized into central and peripheral portions which generate opposite reactions.
    - If the periphery and the center are stimulated at the same time, the activities tend to cancel each other.

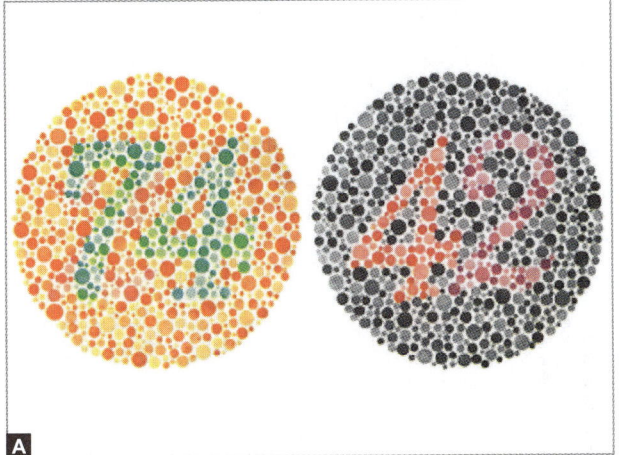

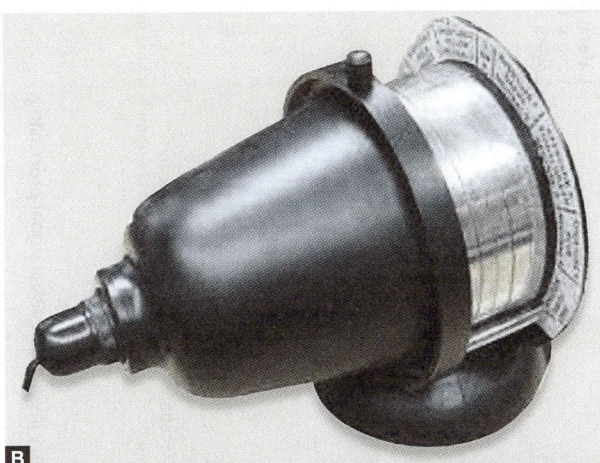

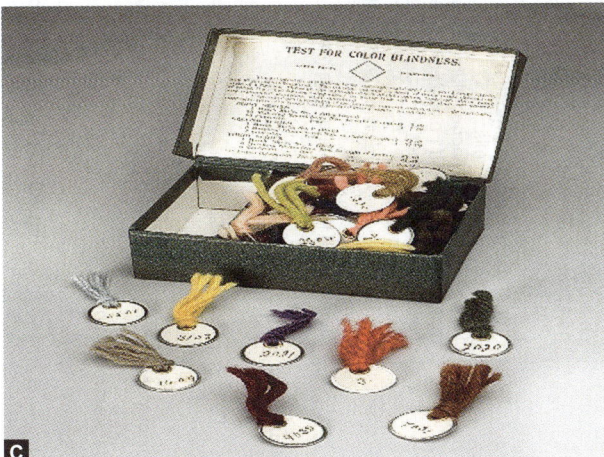

**Figs. 95.21A to C:** (A) Ishihara's color plates; (B) Edridge Green lantern; (C) Holmgren's wool test kit.

- The horizontal cells produce only graded hyperpolarizing and depolarizing responses.
  - Their neurotransmitters are **GABA, glycine, dopamine and indolamine.**
  - They appear to **play a role in color coding** and also **increase retinal sensitivity** by improving contrast.

- The amacrine cells **produce transient depolarizing potentials** and spikes at the onset and offset of visual stimulus.
  - These are the first cells in the visual pathway capable of generating impulses which are initiated during depolarizing.
  - The amacrine cells are responsible for directional sensitivity, i.e., they detect the motion of an object across the retina.

## RESPONSE PATTERN OF GANGLION CELLS

- These cells generate action potential which is transmitted along their axons in optic nerve to the lateral geniculate bodies.
- They discharge steadily at slow rate even in the absence of input from the rods and cones called *'Resting discharge'.*

### Types of Ganglion Cells

#### Large Ganglion Cells (α/M-cells/Parvo Cells)

- In the resting state discharge rate is of 20–50 spikes/sec
- Concentrated in the peripheral retina
- Mediate functions of rod system
- Conveys information regarding movements and stereopsis to LGB
- They are responsible for fast and black and white stimulus
- Also responsible for crude rod vision

#### Small Ganglion Cells (β-cells/P-cells/Midget Cells)

- Concentrated in the central retina
- Exhibits lateral inhibition
- Mediate function of cone system (color vision)
- Analyze and subtract response from one type of cone from response from another
- They send information regarding color, texture and shape of an object to LGB and finer details of the vision.

### Neurotransmitters within Retina

- Cones releases glutamic acid
  - It has inhibitory effect on hyperpolarizing bipolar cells produced by **opening $K^+$ channels and closing $Na^+$ channels**; both being operated via G-protein.
  - It has excitatory effect on depolarizing bipolar cells produced by opening $k^+$ channels and or $Na^+$ channels; both being operated via G-protein.
- Horizontal cells release GABA. It produces both its inhibitory effect and its excitatory effect by depolarizing cones.
- Amacrine cells release GABA, glycine, acetylcholine, dopamine to produce the effect.

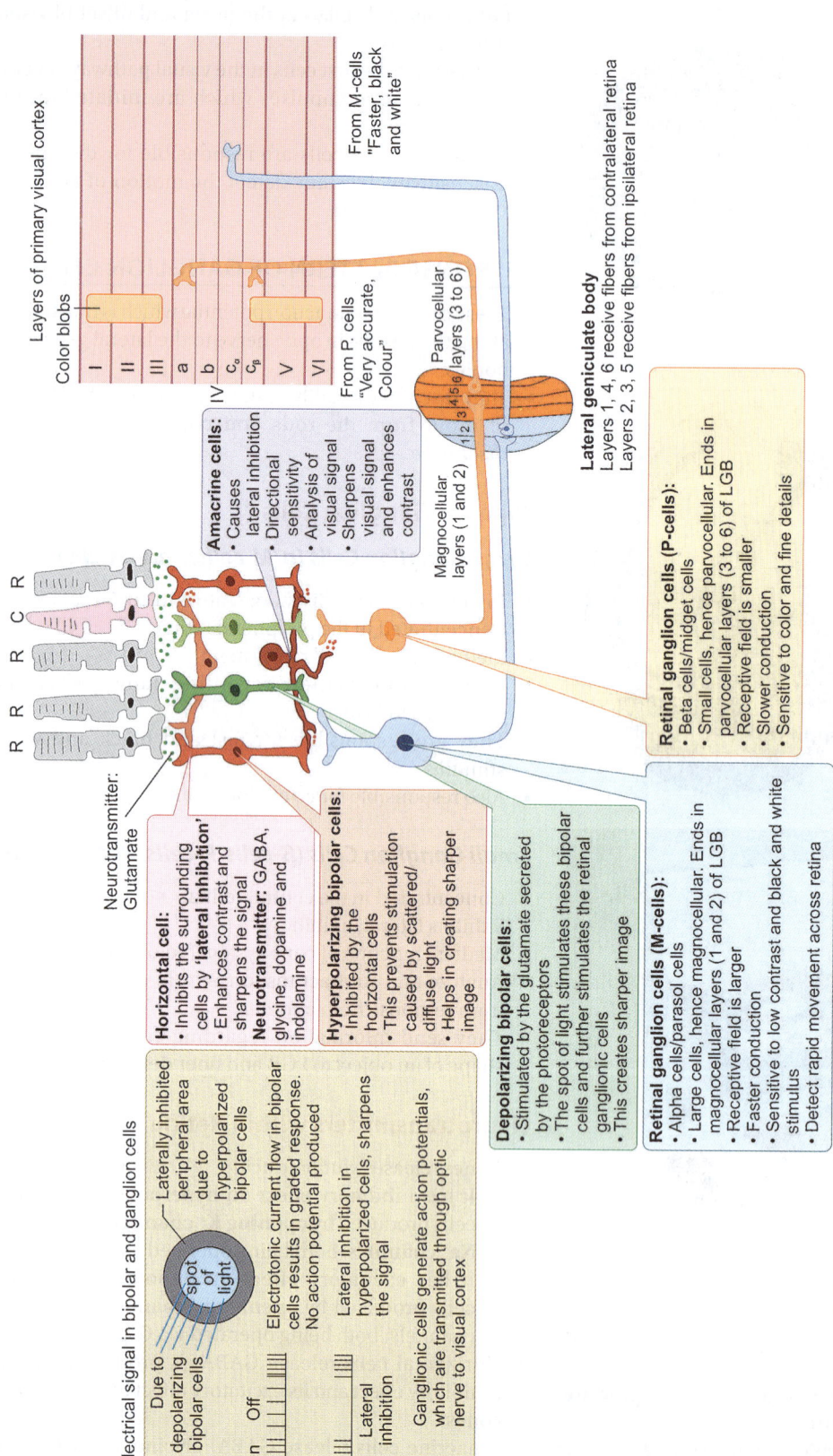

Fig. 95.22: The neural circuitry involved in visual signal processing.

## RESPONSES OF NEURONS IN LATERAL GENICULATE BODIES AND VISUAL CORTEX

- The optic nerve carries signals for detection of movements and flickers, and signals for color vision, texture, shape, and fine depth vision.
- Its function is to separate and relay these different kinds of information's from the retina to different cortical zones.
- In the visual cortex there are many neurons associated with each fiber projected from the LGB of thalamus.
  - Most neurons in one subdivision of the visual cortex are responsive only to stimuli oriented in a particular direction in the visual field. This is important in the detailed description of the form of an object.
  - Some neurons in another subdivision are most responsive to movements of an object across the visual field.
  - Some neurons respond best to color and some to depth perception.
- Layer 1 and 2 of the LGB are the magnocellular layer and layers 3 to 6 are parvocellular. Hence the M retinal ganglionic cells (RGC) terminate in layer 1 and 2 whereas P cells terminate in layers 3 to 6.
- The fibers from M cells and magnocellular layer of LGB relay in layer IVcα of the primary visual cortex. Whereas the fibers from P cells and parvocellular layer of the LGB relay in the layers IVa and IVcβ of primary visual cortex.

### Electroretinogram (ERG)

At rest, the potential difference between the front and back of the eye is 6 mV. When light falls on the eye it produces a series of potential changes which can be recorded by placing one electrode on the cornea and another indifferent electrode on in the mouth or forehead.

The record of this sequence is known as electroretinogram.

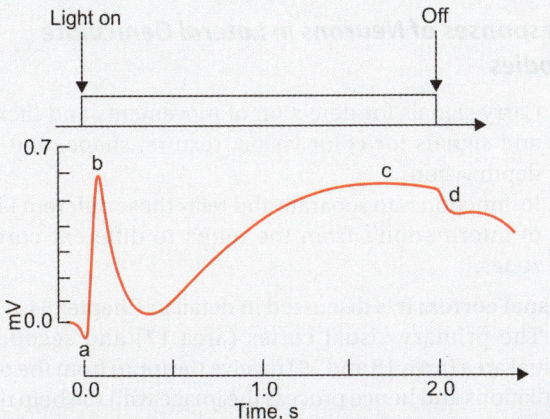

The sequence of potential changes which occur are:
- When the light stimulus is turned 'on' it produces, 'a', 'b', 'c' waves; while when the stimulus is turned 'off', a small negative 'off' deflection is produced (off response)
  - 'a' wave is the first sharp negative deflection due to rods and cones potential.
  - 'b' wave is a positive wave which follows the 'a' wave and results from activity in the bipolar cells or glial cells.
  - 'c' wave is due to activity in the pigmented epithelium of the retina.
- When the light stimulus is turned 'off', a small negative 'd' deflection is produced, called 'off' response.
  - They appear as a 'slow' decay in predominant rod retinae, called Remnant Negativity; and appear as a 'faster' decay from retinae containing only cones.

**Uses of ERG:**
- It is helpful in the diagnosis of diseases in which visualization of the retina is difficult because the ocular fluids are cloudy.
- It is helpful in congenital retinal dystrophies in which the retina appears normal by ophthalmoscopy.

## VISUAL PATHWAY

The visual pathway is the neural pathway beginning from the retina to occipital cortex. Like any other sensory pathway, it also has three neuron system.
1. **First-order neuron:** Bipolar cells
2. **Second-order neuron:** Ganglion cells to LGB. (The lateral geniculate body receives fibers from both the retinae)
3. **Third-order neurons:** From lateral geniculate body to visual cortex

### Optic Nerve

- The optic nerve is formed by the axons of the ganglion cells.
- It represents the **second order neurons** of the visual pathway.
- **80%** of the fibers originate from the macular region which represents 90% of retinal ganglion cells.
- There are **2.2 to 2.4 million fibers** in the two optic nerves representing 42% of all fibers entering and leaving the CNS.

### Formation of Image on the Retina (Fig. 95.23)

The light rays from the temporal field fall off the nasal half of the retina and from nasal field fall on the temporal half of the retina. This leads to the inversion of the image. It occurs due to the formation of real and inverted images on retina due to passage of light through the biconvex ocular lens. This image is not only vertically inverted but also horizontally flipped.

> David H Hubel and Torsten N Wiesel **The Nobel Prize in Physiology and Medicine (1981)** "For their discoveries concerning information processing in the visual system".

- Optic nerves carry information from nasal and temporal halves and upper and lower quadrants of retina.
- Due to the arrangement of fibers in the optic nerve, optic tract and radiations, the image interpreted by the brain is erect, as present in the visual field.

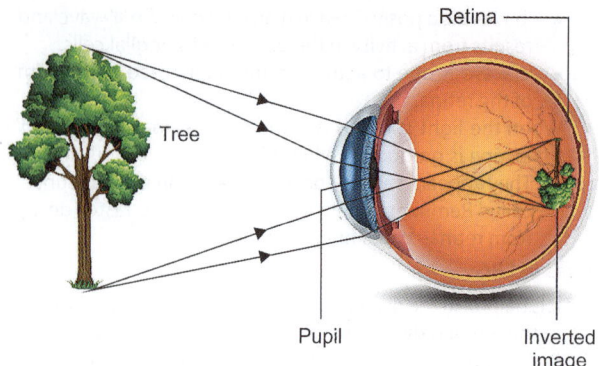

**Fig. 95.23:** Formation of horizontally and vertically inverted image on the retina.

## Optic Tract and Lateral Geniculate Body

Only the nasal fibers of the optic nerve (carrying the temporal field) cross to the opposite side in the optic chiasma
- The optic tracts end in LGB of thalamus. Few fibers from here move to suprachiasmatic nuclei and pretectal nuclei in brainstem for circadian rhythm and pupillary reflex **(Fig. 95.24)**.
- Fibers from **medial part** of LGB represent **superior** or upper quadrant of both retinas.
- Fibers from **lateral** part of LGB represent **inferior** or lower quadrant of both retinas.
- Vertically placed *layers 1 and 2 receive* input from **M ganglion cell**.
- Layers *3, 4, 5 and 6 receive input* from **P ganglion cell**.
- Further the layers 1, 4, 6 receives the input fibers from *contralateral retina (Tip: 146CL) while layers 2, 3, 5 receives input from ipsilateral retina (Tip: 235IL)* **(Fig. 95.25)**.
- Each LGB receives **half of the input from both** retina through the optic tract and the input from each eye project distinctly to specific layer of LGB.
- Right optic tract carries signals from right half of retina, i.e., left half of visual fields.
- **Some fibers from optic tract end in:**
  - *Pretectal area and are responsible for the pupillary light reflex*

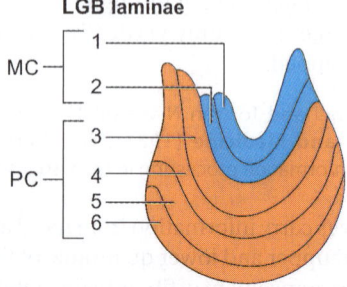

**Fig. 95.24:** The layers of LGB showing the magnocellular and parvocellular layers.

(MC: magnocellular layers; PC: parvocellular layer; LGB: lateral geniculate body)

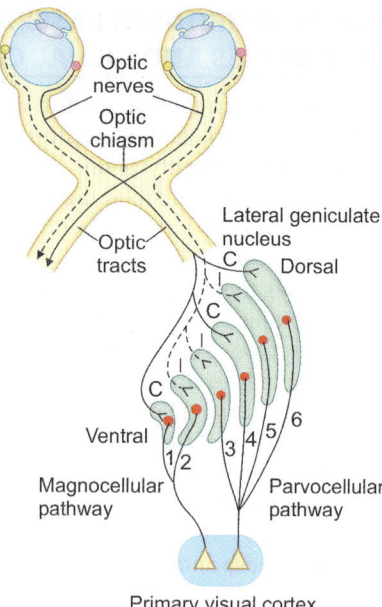

**Fig. 95.25:** The layers of LGB showing the ipsilateral and contralateral projection.

- *Suprachiasmatic nuclei and are responsible for the circadian rhythm*
- *Superior colliculus which are responsible for movement of eyeball.*
- *Inferior retina fibers/Meyer's loop* move fibers to occipital lobe through temporal lobe.
- *Superior retina fibers/Baram's loop* moves fibers from LGB to occipital lobe through parietal lobe which reaches to striate cortex known as *primary visual cortex,* where perception of images is seen.

The visual pathway is summarized in Figure 95.26.

## Responses of Neurons in Lateral Geniculate Bodies

- Carry signals for detection of movements and flickers, and signals for color vision, texture, shape, and fine depth vision.
- Its function is to separate and relay these different kinds of information's from the retina to different cortical zones.

**Visual cortex:** It is discussed in detail in Chapter 84.

The primary visual cortex (area 17) and secondary visual area (area 18 and 19) receive the input from the optic radiations and hence process the image with the help three main type of cells:

1. **Simple cells:** They respond best to *linear stimulus such as bars of light, lines, or edges,* but only when they have particular position. When the stimulus is rotated as little as 10° from the precise position, the response decreases.
2. **Complex cells:** They also require a particular position of a linear stimulus but are less dependent upon the

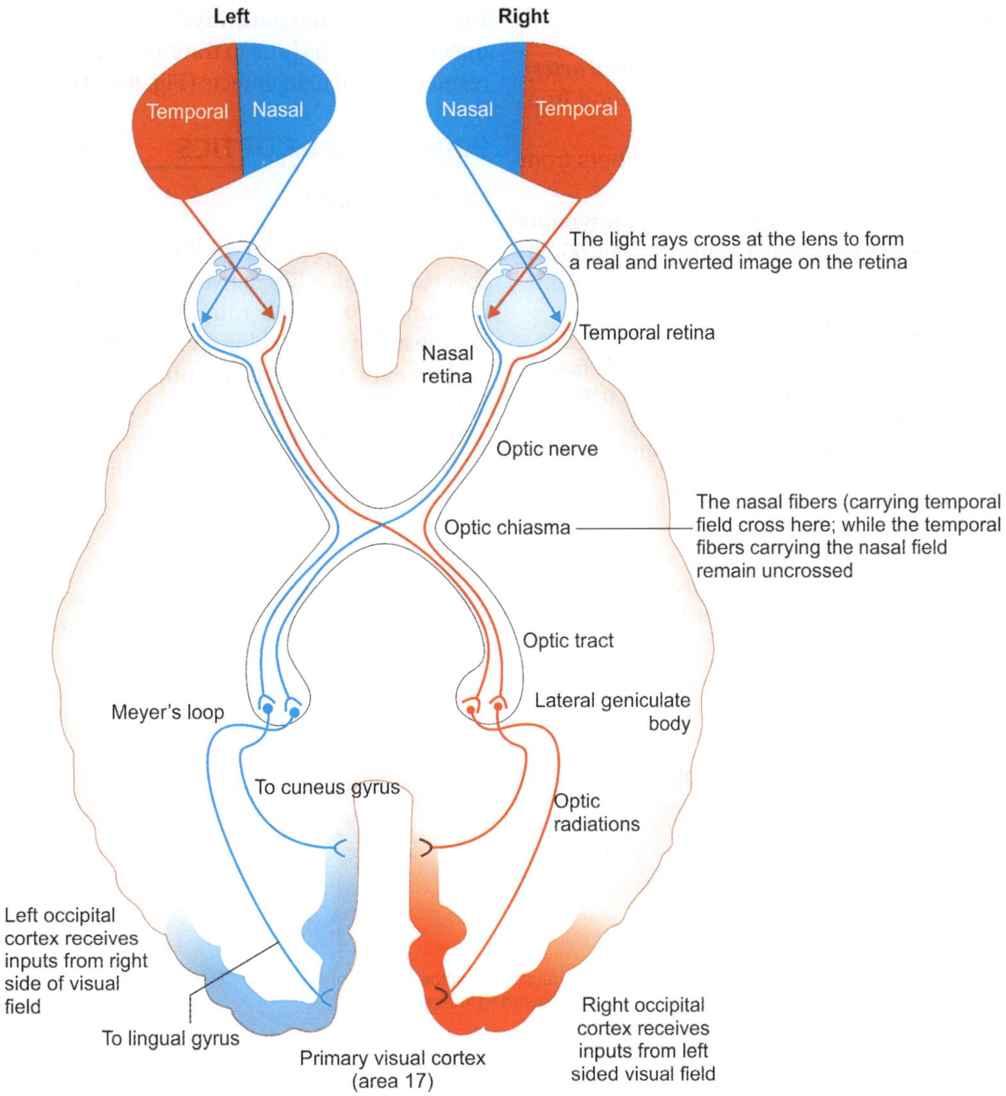

**Fig. 95.26:** Visual pathway.

location of a stimulus in the visual field than the simple cells.

They are concerned with *movement and velocity of the stimulus* and less with its central location.

3. **Hypercomplex cells:** Respond best to a moving bar with a precise orientation but also with a defined length.

There are two major pathways for the processing of visual signal **(Fig. 95.27)**:

1. *The fast "Position and Motion" pathway (magnocellular pathway):* Originate from layers I and II of LGB, the rapidly conducting fibers arise. These fibers bring the information from M type ganglion cells. They project into layer IVcα of primary visual cortex. This pathway is responsible for the analysis of 3-dimensional position, gross form and motion of objects.

2. *The accurate color pathway (Parvocellular pathway):* from layers III to VI of LGB, the fibers arising from P type ganglion cells. They project into layer IV and IVcβ of

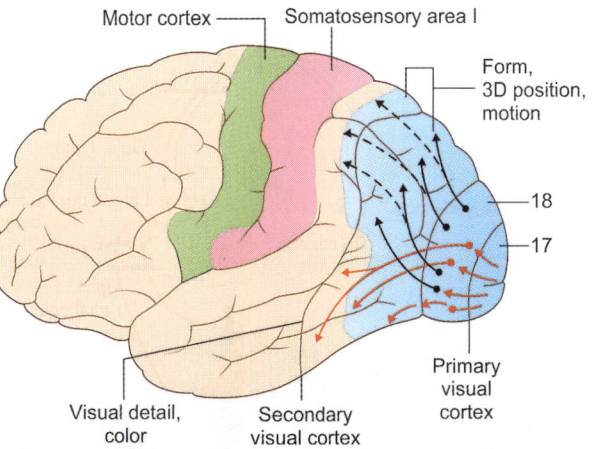

**Fig. 95.27:** Processing of visual signal in occipital lobe.

primary visual cortex. These are responsible for point-to-point spatial information and color vision.

### Macular Area in Visual Cortex

- This receives blood supply from *posterior cerebral artery*
- In case of its occlusion, it still will receive blood from *middle cerebral artery*
- So, this prevents the damage of the visual fibers from retinal macula.
- In this case the patient will have **right or left homonymous hemianopia but with sparing of macula** (*See* **Fig. 95.28**)

#### What is a visual field?

The total area in which objects can be seen in the **side (peripheral) vision** while you focus your eyes on a central point.
**Visual field/field of vision:** As discussed above,
- **Right temporal hemiretina:** Receives light from nasal field of right eye
- **Right nasal hemiretina:** Receives light from temporal field of right eye
- **At optic chiasma:** Crossing over fibers receiving light information from temporal visual field via nasal hemiretina
- **Uncrossed fibers** receive light information from nasal visual field via temporal hemiretina

**Disorder of visual pathway:** The defects in the visual field due to the lesions (due to trauma, tumor, or infection) may result in visual field defects (**Fig. 95.28**).

## PRINCIPLES OF OPTICS

### What is Light?

It is the visible portion of the electromagnetic radiation spectrum, which lies between the Ultraviolet and Infrared portion (400 to 700 nm). The white light is primary composed of seven colors (**VIBGYOR**).

The eyes perceive the objects due to reflection of light from the surface of object into the eye. The eye is composed of an optical system, which is quite similar to the photographic camera. It has a small adjustable aperture called the pupil, which controls the amount of light entering the eye.

The light rays travel in the following the principles of refraction (**Fig. 95.29**). In this, the incident light, when enters the medium with higher refractive index, will bend towards the normal and vice versa.

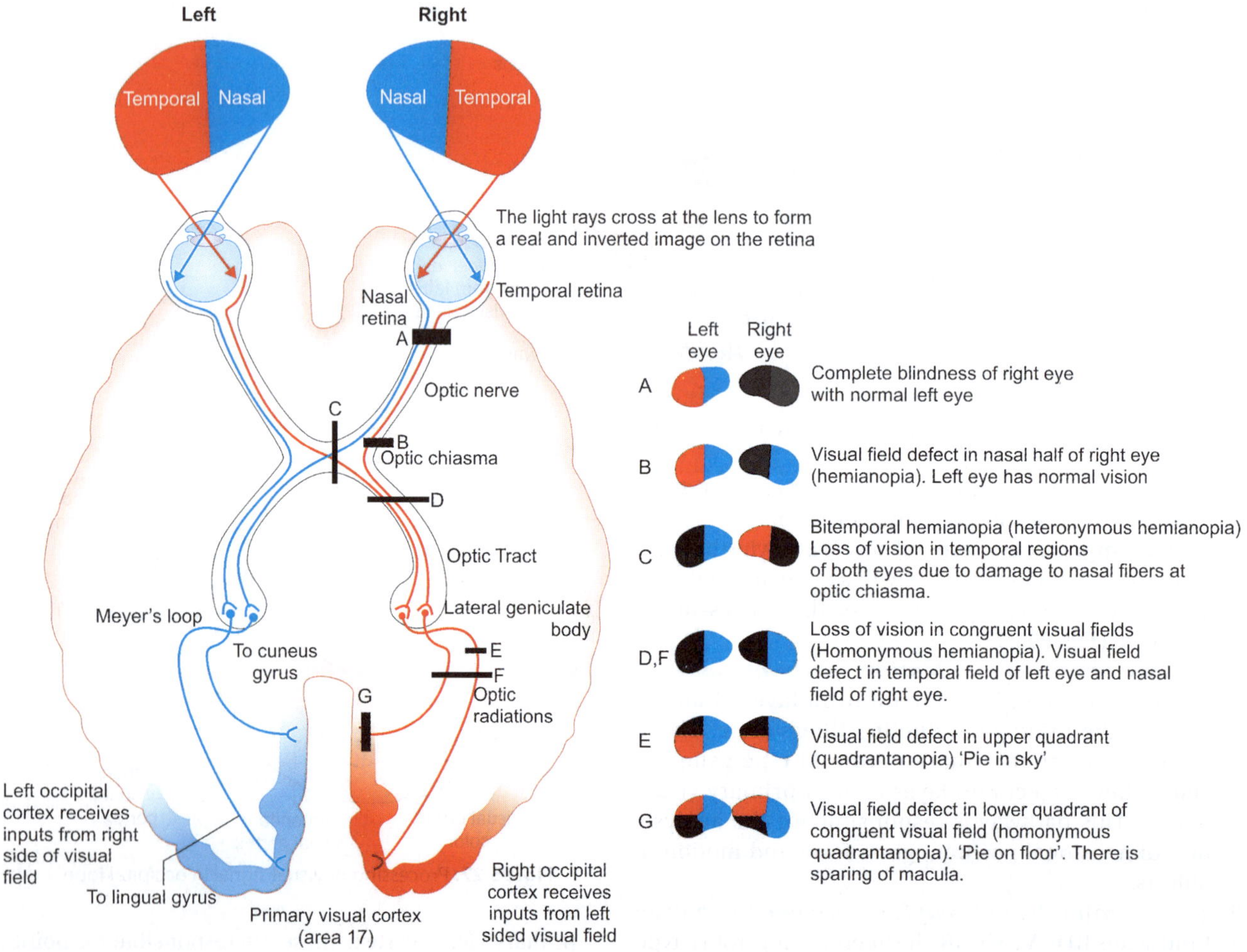

**Fig. 95.28:** The visual field defects.

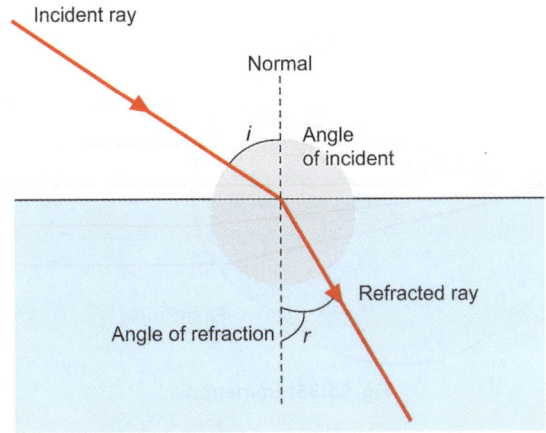

**Fig. 95.29:** Principle of refraction.

Refractive power is diopter (D), if the focal length of a spherical lens is 1m, its refractive power is one diopter (D)
$$D = 1/f$$
Corneal refractive system: 40 D
Lens refractive system: 20 D
Total refractive power of **globe: 59 D**

The eye is made up of four refractive surfaces (**Fig. 95.30**):
1. An interface between air ($\mu = 1.00$) and anterior surface of cornea ($\mu = 1.38$). This will bend the light rays inwards, towards the normal.
2. An interface between posterior surface of cornea ($\mu = 1.38$) and aqueous humor ($\mu = 1.33$). This will slightly bend the light rays outwards, away from normal.
3. An interface between aqueous humor ($\mu = 1.33$) and anterior surface of lens ($\mu = 1.40$). This will bend the light rays inwards, towards the normal.
4. An interface between posterior surface of lens ($\mu = 1.40$) and vitreous humor ($\mu = 1.3$).

In order to avoid the confusion of four refractive surfaces, a concept of reduced eye is introduced, in which it is believed to have a single refractive surface (**Fig. 95.31**). The reduced eye has a length of 22.6 mm and the nodal point (N), 17 mm in front of the fovea centralis (F'), where the image is formed. The object is placed at F, which is also 17 mm from the point N. The point on cornea, located on the line joining F, N and F', is called P (principal plane). The distance between P and N is

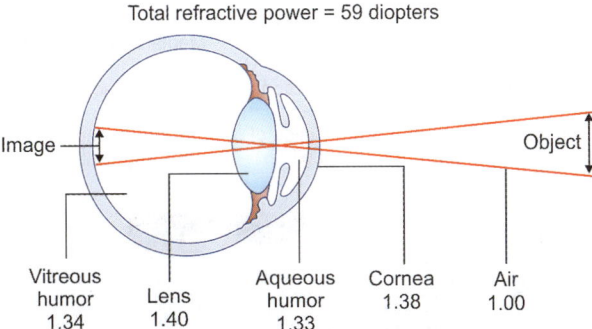

**Fig. 95.30:** Refractive indexes of various eye surfaces.

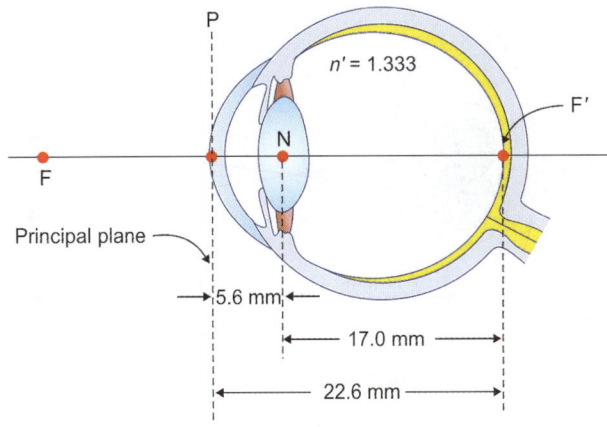

**Fig. 95.31:** Concept of reduced eye.

5.6 mm. The reduced eye has a single refractive surface (N) and is used to study and understand the physiological basis of the refractive errors. The ophthalmologists use the reduced eye to correcting the refractive errors and prescribing the suitable glasses.

## Ocular Optics-Focusing the Image on Retina

From our knowledge of physics, we know that when a parallel beam of light passes through the biconvex lens, it converges at the point to focus that beam of light at a point F (focus). The distance between the midpoint of lens and focus is called the focal length (f) (**Fig. 95.32**).

Considering the light is coming from a point sources a and b, as shown below, the light rays converge at different points on the retina, a' and b' resulting in the formation of a real and inverted image on retina (**Fig. 95.33**).

## Visual Acuity (Fig. 95.34)

It is the degree to which details and contours of the object are perceived.

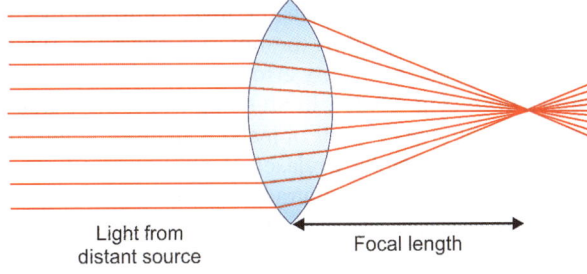

**Fig. 95.32:** Focal length.

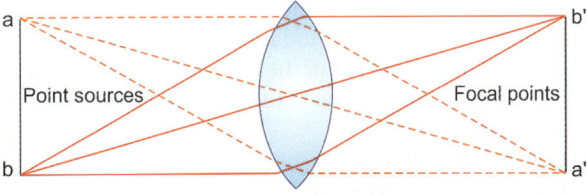

**Fig. 95.33:** Formation of image.

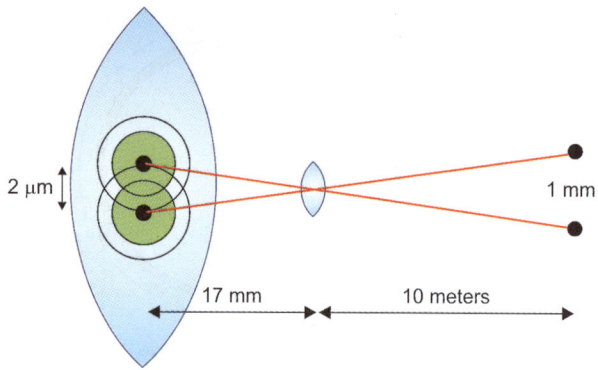

Fig. 95.34: Visual acuity.

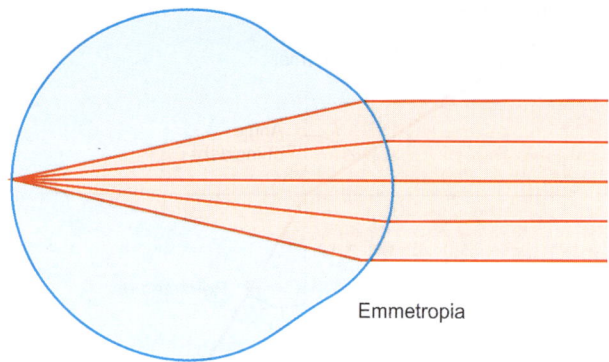

Fig. 95.35: Emmetropia.

- It is expressed in terms of visual angle.
- Normal visual acuity for discriminating between two-point sources is 1 minute of an arc.
- **Diameter of fovea is 0.5 mm.**
- The visual acuity of peripheral retina is poor.

Methods to assess the visual acuity:
- **For distant vision:** Snellen's chart (read from a distance of 6 m; for viewing distant objects) and
- **For near vision:** Jaeger's chart (read from a distance of 25 cm; for viewing near objects)

### Factors Affecting Visual Acuity

- **Optical factors:** State of image forming mechanisms of eye.
- **Retinal factors:** Fovea has better acuity as compared to peripheral retina due to presence of cones.
- **Stimulus factors:**
  - Size of the object
  - Color of the object
  - Illumination of the object and surrounding
  - Contrast of the object with its surrounding
  - Brightness
  - Duration of exposure

In our eye, the parallel beam of light/originating from a point source is focused on the fovea centralis by the crystalline lens located in the anterior chamber. When the person has no refractory error, the condition is called *emmetropia* (Fig. 95.35). In an emmetrope, the parallel beam of light (sees distant objects) is focused when the ciliary muscle is completed relaxed. However, to see the near objects, the ciliary muscle contracts to increase the curvature of lens due to accommodation for a clearer near vision.

### Accommodation

From this we learn that the ciliary muscles play an important role in accommodation to focus the same on distant and near objects. For the eye to accommodate from a distant object to near object the following changes occur in the eye: (Tip: 3 C)
- **C**onstriction of pupil
- **C**onvergence of eyeballs
- **C**urvature of lens increases

### Pathway of Accommodation (Fig. 95.36)

The accommodation of the eyes is controlled by the parasympathetic nervous system through the 3rd cranial nerve (oculomotor nerve), which originates from the Edinger Westphal nucleus (EW nucleus) in midbrain. The preganglionic fibers of 3rd nerve relay in autonomic ciliary ganglion, from where postganglionic short ciliary nerves arise which innervate the sphincter pupillae (resulting in

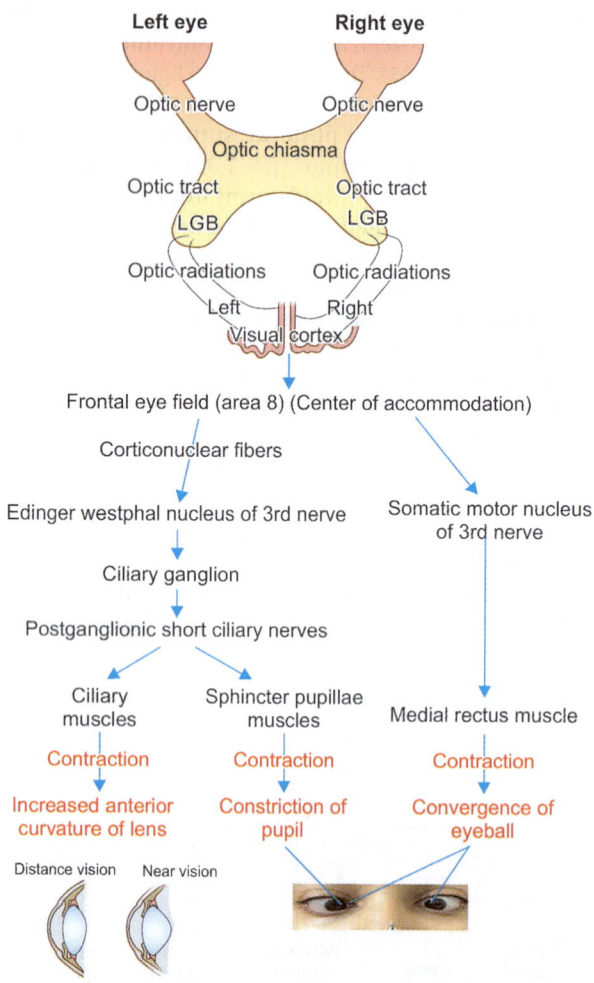

Fig. 95.36: Pathway of accommodation.
(LGB: lateral geniculate body)

miosis) and ciliary muscle (resulting in increased curvature of lens). The somatic nucleus of 3rd nerve supply the extraocular medial rectus muscle resulting in convergence of eyeballs.

## Physiological Significance of Accommodation

The refractive power of lens in 20 D, which can be increased voluntarily by accommodation to 34 D. This additional power of 14 D occurs due to accommodation.

In old age, the eyes lose its power to accommodate due to weakness of the ciliary muscles resulting in presbyopia and results in some loss of power due to weakness of accommodation. Presbyopia is discussed below in errors of refraction.

## Errors of Refraction

When a person is having trouble to see the objects clearly, he is said to have an error of refraction. Depending on the type of loss of visual acuity the errors of refraction are classified as:

## Myopia (Nearsightedness: Nearby Objects are Clear)

In this the children usually complain of headache and difficulty in seeing the black board clearly from their seat. Sometimes, they may often present with recurrent eye infections due to frequent rubbing of eyes. On examination, it is observed they have difficulty in seeing the distant objects but have clear near vision.

### Physiological basis of Myopia (Fig. 95.37)

When the person is not accommodating (ciliary muscles are relaxed), the parallel light rays refracted by the ocular refractive system come to focus *in front of the retina*. Hence, the image formed on retina is blurred (out of focus).

### Causes

- The cornea that is steeper, or an eye that is longer, than a normal eye.
- Axial length of the eye is quite more, but the refractive power is normal.
- The axis is normal but the refractive power increases.

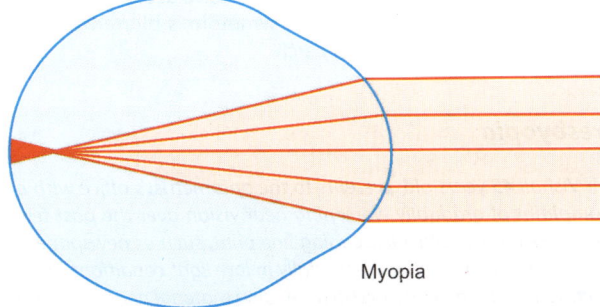

**Fig. 95.37:** Physiology of myopia.

### Classification

- **Mild:** Below -3D
- **Moderate:** From -3D to -6D
- **High myopia:** More than -6D

### Correction

- **Spectacles:** Concave lens **(Fig. 95.38)**.
  The concave lens neutralizes the excessive refractive power of the lens by diverging the rays falling on the cornea. The resultant beam of light focuses on the retina. The power of concave lens is determined by testing the visual acuity by Snellen's chart and correcting the error with the set of lenses on a trial frame.
- Laser surgery to slightly flattens the cornea and correct the refractive power of cornea.

## Hypermetropia (Fig. 95.39): (Farsightedness: Ability to See the Distant Objects Clearly)

The patients with hypermetropia/hyperopia have a problem is seeing the near vision, while reading. Young people with mild to moderate hyperopia are often able to see clearly because their natural lens can adjust or *accommodate* to increase the eye's focusing ability. However, as the eye gradually *loses the ability to accommodate* (beginning at about 40 years of age), *blurred vision* from hyperopia often becomes more apparent.

### Physiological basis of Hypermetropia

It is a state in which the unaccommodated eye would *focus the image behind the retina*. Parallel light rays refracted by the ocular refractive system focus behind the retina, forming a blurred image.

### Etiology

- Axial hyperopia is indicated that the ocular axis is short but refractive power is normal.

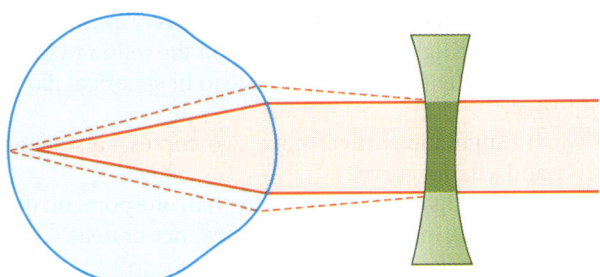

**Fig. 95.38:** Correction of myopia using concave lens.

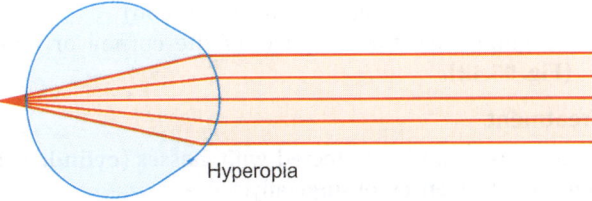

**Fig. 95.39:** Hyperopia.

- Refractive hyperopia is indicated that the ocular axis is normal, but refractive power is weak.

### Signs and Symptoms
- Difficulty seeing near objects clearly
- Blurred distance vision (occurs with higher amounts of hyperopia)
- Eye fatigue when reading
- Eye strain (headaches, pulling sensation, burning)
- Frequent infections of eyelids due to frequent rubbing

### Classification
- **Mild:** less than +3D
- **Moderate:** +5D or less than +5D
- **High:** More than +5D

### Correction
Spectacles with Convex lens (**Fig. 95.40**)

The convex lens adds up the refractive power to the weak refractory lens system, hence converging the light on the retina. Thus, correcting the refractory error.

## Astigmatism

> Geeta presents to the ophthalmologist's office with a complaint of blurred vision, particularly noticing difficulty focusing on objects both near and far. She describes her vision as "distorted" or "wavy" at times. These symptoms have been progressively worsening over the past few months, and she has noticed increased eye strain, especially during prolonged periods of reading or computer use. She denies any recent trauma to the eye or changes in her medications.

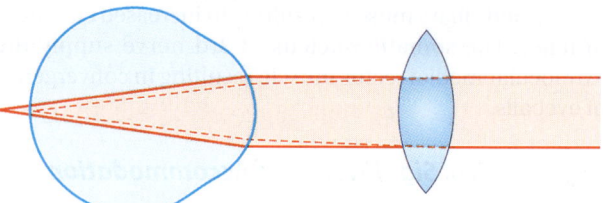

Fig. 95.40: Correction of hyperopia.

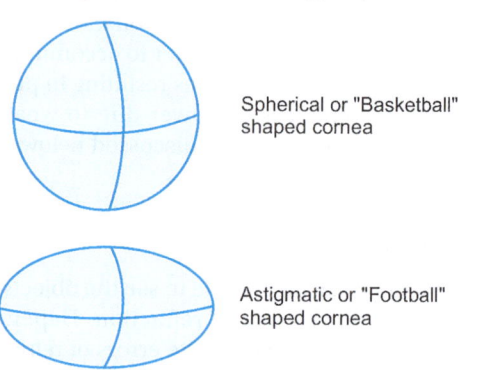

Fig. 95.41: Physiological basis of astigmatism.

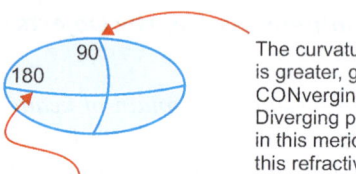

This meridian is flatter, giving it less (+) power than the meridian at 90 degrees. It will take less (−) power to neutralize the refractive error in this meridian in comparison to 90 degrees.

The curvature in this meridian is greater, giving it more CONverging (+) power. More Diverging power will be needed in this meridian to correct this refractive error.

Fig. 95.42: Irregular curvature.

Hence, the astigmatism is defined as the inability of the refractive apparatus of eye to focus on the retina resulting in the formation of distorted image for both the near and far vision.

### Physiological basis of Astigmatism (Fig. 95.41)
There is difference of refractive power in every meridian of eye, so outside light rays can't focus on the retina to form clear image. The cornea is oval instead of spherical like a basketball.

Most astigmatic corneas have two curves—a steeper curve and a flatter curve.

This causes light to focus on more than one point on the retina, resulting in blurred vision at distance or near.

### Causes
- The radii of curvature of cornea and lens are different in each meridian, generally, their difference between two main meridians is biggest. (most common)
- Irregular curvature in parts of the cornea or lens (**Fig. 95.42**).

### Treatment
Astigmatism can be corrected with glasses (**cylindrical lens**), contact lenses, or surgically.
- **Spectacles:** This may be corrected by specially ground lenses which compensate for the irregularity. Spherical correction, using concave/convex lens, if required, is done first for one of the two planes of astigmatism. Additional cylindrical correction is done in the perpendicular plane. The power and axis of lenses are prescribed by trial-and-error method.
- **Surgical correction:** The most common surgeries used to correct astigmatism are *astigmatic keratotomy* (procedures that involve placing a microscopic incision on the eye) and *LASIK*. The objective of these procedures is to reshape the cornea so it becomes more spherical or uniformly curved.

> **Asthenopia:** Long-term near work, excessive accommodation often may induce asthenopia, its symptom is blurred vision, distending pain in superciliary arch.

## Presbyopia

> Mr Vishal, 45 years old, presents to the optometrist's office with a complaint of gradually worsening near vision over the past few years. He reports difficulty reading fine print, such as newspapers, menus, or his smartphone, especially in low-light conditions. John mentions that he frequently holds reading material at arm's length to see it more clearly. He denies any recent changes in his distance vision or eye discomfort.

Presbyopia is defined as loss of accommodation with old age resulting in the difficulty in reading or focusing on the near objects.

### Physiological Basis of Presbyopia

With age, the lens becomes less elastic resulting in decreased accommodation power by 1D at 40 years, 2D by 50 years. It is also called as the "short arm syndrome," is a term used to describe an eye in which the natural lens can no longer accommodate.

### Clinical Features

- Most people first notice difficulty reading very fine print such as the phone book, a medicine bottle, or the stock market page. Print seems to have less contrast and the eyes become easily fatigued when reading a book or computer screen.
- The symptom of presbyopia is difficult to see near thing.
- Brighter, more direct light required for reading.
- Reading material must be held further away to see (for some)
- Fatigue and eyestrain when reading

### Correction

Spectacles with Convex lens/bifocal lens.

The convex lens adds up the loss of refractive power to the weak accommodation power, hence converging the light on the retina. However, if the person already has a pre-existing myopia, he will need both concave lens for distant vision and convex lens for reading. In that case, he is prescribed bifocal spectacles/progressive spectacles.

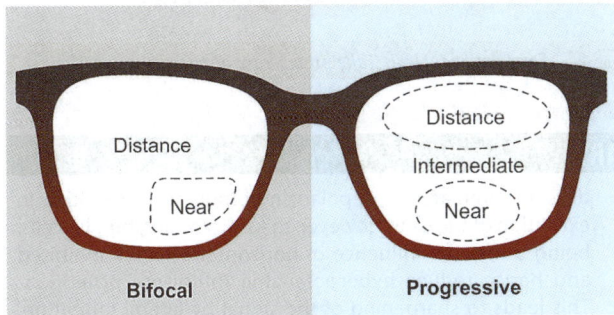

## EYE MOVEMENTS

Ocular muscles and their movements **(Fig. 95.43)**:
- **Superior rectus**—moves eye up (3rd nerve)
- **Inferior rectus**—moves eye down (3rd nerve)
- **Medial rectus**—moves eye in (adduction) (3rd nerve)
- **Lateral rectus**—moves eye out (abduction) (6th nerve)
- **Inferior oblique**—moves eye up when it is in an adducted position; also extorts the eye. (3rd nerve)
- **Superior oblique**—moves eye down when it is adducted; also, intorts the eye. (4th nerve)

### Targeting Eye Movements

- **Saccades:** Quick, darting conjugate movements which direct the eyes to a new target.

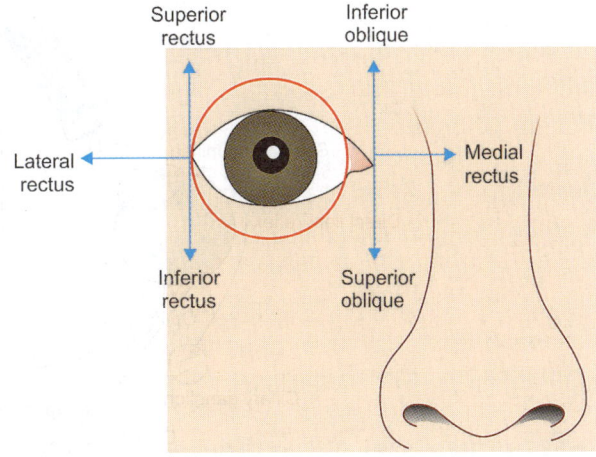

**Fig. 95.43:** Ocular muscles and their direction of movement.

- **Smooth pursuit:** A slower conjugate movement which allows for tracking of a moving object, or of a stationary object while we are moving.
- **Convergence:** A deconjugate movement of both eyes toward the midline to allow for focusing on a near object by adjusting the angle between the eyes.

## Pupillary Reflexes (To determine the integrity of visual pathway)

### Pupillary Light Reflex (Fig. 95.44)

- **Direct light reflex:** When light is thrown into one eye, it leads to constriction of pupil on the same side.
- **Consensual light reflex:** When light is thrown into one eye, it leads to constriction of pupil on the other side. It occurs due to crossing of fibers at the Edinger Westphal nucleus (Nucleus of 3rd nerve), supplying the sphincter pupillae.
  - The optic nerve fibers that carry the impulses initiating these pupillary responses leave the optic nerves near the lateral geniculate bodies.
  - On each side, they enter the midbrain via the brachium of the superior colliculus and terminate in the pretectal nucleus.
  - From this nucleus, the second-order neurons project to the ipsilateral and contralateral Edinger–Westphal nucleus.
  - The third-order neurons pass from this nucleus to the ciliary ganglion in the oculomotor nerve, and the fourth-order neurons pass from this ganglion to the ciliary body.
  - This pathway is dorsal to the pathway for the near response.

### Accommodation Reflex

When the object moves close to the eyes (distant vision to near vision), there is constriction of pupil, convergence of eyeball and increased anterior curvature of lens. It is already discussed above.

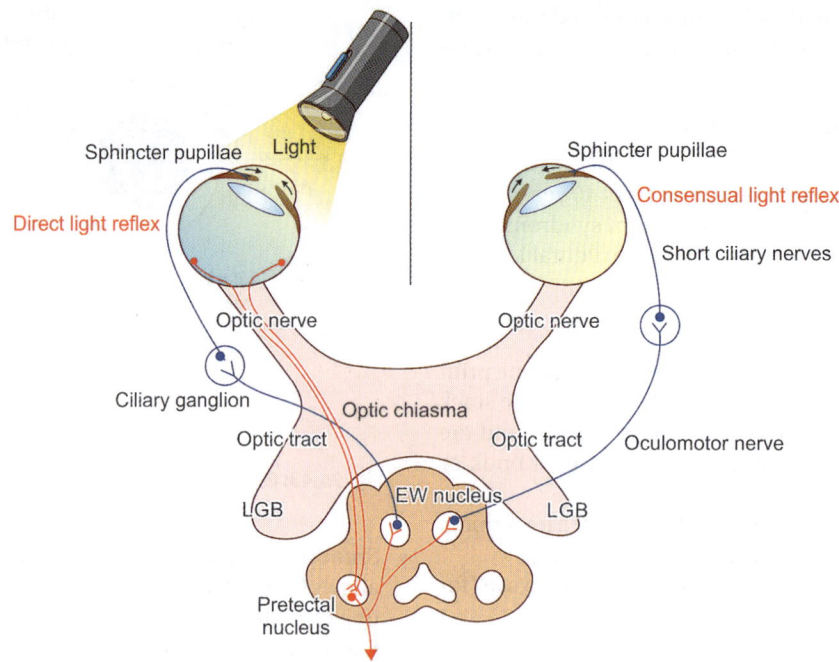

**Fig. 95.44:** Direct and consensual light reflex.
(LGB: lateral geniculate body)

**Abnormal pupillary response:**
- The pupillary reflexes are lost due to damage to afferent optic or efferent oculomotor nerve.
- **Argyll Robertson pupil (ARP):** The light reflex is lost, while the response to accommodation remains intact (**ARP: accommodation reflex present**). It is seen in neurosyphilis. It is also seen in other diseases producing selective lesions in the midbrain.

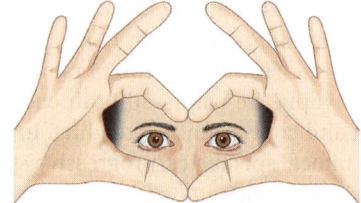

*"Eyes are beautiful, Take proper care of those beauties!!"*

## SUMMARY

In this chapter we had learnt about:
- The functional anatomy of the eye. The eyeball is a spherical organ housed in the orbit of the skull. The visible portion of the eyeball is protected by the eyelids. Externally we can see only the sclera (white portion) and iris (The pigmented ring) surrounding the pupil. The eyeball has three layers, sclera, vascular pigmented choroid, and inner most neural layer retina. The retina is made up of 10 layers: the pigmented layer, layer of photoreceptors (rods and cones), outer limiting membrane, outer nuclear layer, outer plexiform layer, inner nuclear layer, inner plexiform layer, layer of ganglion cells, layer have nerve fibers, inner limiting membrane.
- The retina has an optic cup which is also called a blind spot as it does not have any photoreceptors. This is where the optic nerve leaves the eyeball, and the central retinal blood vessels are present in the eyeball. Another point on retina is the macula lutea which has fovea centralis. This point has maximum number of cones and no rods. It is responsible for the accurate color vision.
- The rods and the cones synapse with the bipolar cells and the horizontal cells in the outer plexiform layer. The photoreceptors directly stimulate the depolarizing bipolar cells resulting in excitation of the cells. However, the surrounding bipolar cells, being under the influence of horizontal cells are inhibited and hence reduce hyperpolarizing inhibitory potentials. This leads to sharpening of the signal by lateral inhibition. The signal is then transmitted to the ganglion cells. The inner plexiform layer has another layer of amacrine cells which also participates in the lateral inhibition and further sharpens the signal. It leads to the initial signal processing at the level of retina itself.
- There are two types of ganglion cells. The larger ones are the magnocellular (M cells) and the smaller powerhouse cellular (P cells). The fibers arising from the M cells are faster and carry the direct rod vision (high contrast black and white stimulus) to the layer one and two of the lateral geniculate body. From here the fibers are projected into layer IVcβ of the primary visual cortex. On the other hand, the fibers arising from the P cells are slower but carry accurate color vision from the cones. They terminate in layer 3, 4, 5, 6 of the lateral geniculate body. From here the fibers project into layer IV and IVcα of the primary visual cortex.

- The projection of the fibers from the retina through the optic nerve, optic chiasma, optic tract, lateral geniculate body, optic radiation to the primary visual cortex is called the visual pathway. Any lesion in the visual pathway results in visual field defects.
- The eyes having the normal vision are called emmetropic eyes. However, if there is any error of refraction present in the eyes resulting in the inability to see clearly, it's called as an ametropia. Inability to see distant objects clearly is called myopia. it is corrected by the concave lenses. Whereas the inability to see the near objects is called hypermetropia and it is corrected by the convex lens. The irregular surface of the cornea or the lens results in inability to focus early on the retina and hence resulting in astigmatism. It is corrected by the use of cylindrical lenses.
- Our eyes ever refractive power of around 59D out of which 40D is because of the cornea and 20D is because of the crystalline lens. The power of the crystalline lens can be increased to 34D by the accommodation due to contraction of the ciliary muscles. In old age when the ciliary muscles lose their strength the individuals tend to find it difficult to read the final print and this condition is called presbyopia.

## LET US SEE, HOW MUCH YOU HAVE LEARNT?

### Review Questions

#### Long/Short Answer Questions

Q1. Describe the process of phototransduction in the rods with the help of a diagram.
Q2. Describe the visual cycle showing the role of vitamin A in vision.
Q3. What happens to the eyes when a person enters a dark room from a well-lit area?
Q4. Describe the various physiological events occurring when a person suddenly steps out of a dark room into bright light.
Q5. Why is it said that a person should not focus on the object, in the dark to see it clearly?
Q6. Draw a well labeled self-explanatory diagram of the visual pathway.
Q7. Describe the visual field defects seen when there is compression/lesion of:
   a. Right optic nerve
   b. Pituitary tumor pressing on the optic chiasma
   c. Aneurysm of the left internal carotid artery passing close to the optic chiasma
Q8. Describe the pathway for the accommodation reflex.
Q9. Describe the pathway for the pupillary light (direct and consensual) reflex.
Q10. Enumerate the various errors of refraction and describe under the following headings:
   a. Physiological basis of the error
   b. Correction along with its physiological basis

#### Explain Why? (Reasoning Questions)

Q1. Damage to the optic nerve can lead to unilateral vision loss.
Q2. The lens needs to change shape (accommodate) to focus on objects at different distances.
Q3. The retina's rod cells are essential for low-light (night) vision.
Q4. Lesions in the optic chiasm cause bitemporal hemianopia, the loss of peripheral vision in both eyes.
Q5. The fovea is crucial for sharp central vision and high acuity.
Q6. The pupillary light reflex involves both direct and consensual responses.
Q7. The occipital lobe is essential for processing visual information.
Q8. Damage to the visual cortex can result in cortical blindness despite intact eyes and optic nerves.
Q9. Macular degeneration primarily affects central vision.
Q10. Lesions in the parietal lobe can lead to difficulties in spatial awareness and visual perception.

### Critical Thinking Case-Based Questions

Q1. Chetna, a 55-year-old woman, visited her ophthalmologist with complaints of progressive vision loss in her right eye and occasional blurry vision in her left eye. She also reported experiencing frequent headaches and sometimes seeing flashes of light. On examination, the ophthalmologist found evidence of a visual field defect in her right eye and suspects a lesion in her visual pathway. An MRI was ordered to further investigate the cause of her symptoms. Based on the given clinical scenario, answer the following questions:

   a. What are the key structures and processes involved in the physiology of vision?
   b. How can lesions in different parts of the visual pathway result in specific types of visual field defects?
   c. What are the typical presentations associated with these lesions?
   d. What diagnostic tools and imaging techniques can be used to identify and locate lesions in the visual pathway?

## Multiple Choice Questions

**Q1.** If your patient has a visual field deficit caused by a complete lesion of an optic tract. Which of the following terms may be used to characterize the deficit?
a. Homonymous
b. Bitemporal
c. Ipsilateral
d. Monocular

**Q2.** Your patient has a complete lesion of the right optic nerve. Where might there be anterograde degeneration of the affected axon terminals?
a. In laminae 2, 3, and 5 of the left lateral geniculate nucleus
b. In the ganglion cell layer of the retina
c. In the supraoptic nucleus of the hypothalamus
d. In laminae 1, 4, and 6 of the left lateral geniculate nucleus

**Q3.** A 59-year-old retired autoworker complains of walking into things on his right. He trips over chair legs with his right foot and has trouble driving because he has difficulty seeing cars entering an intersection from the right. A neurological exam reveals a corrected vision of 6/6, normal ocular mobility, and no motor sensory or cranial nerve deficits. Both pupils react briskly to light, and the near response is normal. Visual field testing reveals a right homonymous hemianopsia. Where might the site of the lesion be located?
a. Optic tract on the left
b. Meyer's loop on the left
c. Primary visual cortex in the left occipital lobe
d. Visual radiations on the left

**Q4.** A 36-year-old woman who is prematurely amenorrheic is referred to an ophthalmologist because she is having headaches and trouble with her eyes. She could not see objects off to the side but could see them when they were directly in front of her. A magnetic resonance image reveals that a calcified craniopharyngioma is apparently the cause of the patient's visual problems and amenorrhea. How would you classify her visual field deficit?
a. Binasal hemianopsia
b. Contralateral superior quadrantanopia
c. Bitemporal inferior quadrantanopia
d. Bitemporal heteronymous hemianopsia

**5.** An 11-year-old boy was having difficulty reading the graphs that his teacher was showing at the front of the classroom. His teacher recommended he be seen by an ophthalmologist. Not only was he asked to look at a Snellen letter chart for visual acuity, but he was also asked to identify numbers in an Ishihara chart. He responded that he merely saw a bunch of dots. Abnormal color vision is 20 times more common in males than females because most cases are caused by an abnormal:
a. Dominant gene on the Y chromosome
b. Recessive gene on the Y chromosome
c. Dominant gene on the X chromosome
d. Recessive gene on the X chromosome

**Q6.** The correct sequence of events involved in photo-transduction in rods and cones in response to light is:
a. Activation of transducing, decreased release of glutamate, structural changes in rhodopsin, closure of cGMP-gated cation channels, and decrease in intracellular cGMP
b. Activation of transducing, structural changes in rhodopsin, closure of cGMP-gated cation channels, decrease in intracellular cGMP, and decreased release of glutamate
c. Structural changes in rhodopsin, decrease in intracellular cGMP, decreased release of glutamate, closure of cGMP-gated cation channels, and activation of transducing
d. Structural changes in rhodopsin, activation of transducing, decrease in intracellular cGMP, closure of cGMP-gated cation channels, and decreased release of glutamate

**Q7.** Which of the following parts of the eye has the greatest concentration of rods?
a. Ciliary body
b. Parafoveal region
c. Optic disk
d. Fovea

**Q8.** A 65-year-old woman was diagnosed with dry age-related macular degeneration with a foveal-sparing scotoma. The fovea of the eye
a. Has the lowest light threshold
b. Contains only red and green cones
c. Is the region of highest visual acuity
d. Contains only rods

**ANSWERS**
1. a    2. d    3. d    4. c    5. d    6. b    7. b    8. c

## Choose the Appropriate Visual Field Defect for the Conditions Given Below

| Clinical condition | | Visual field defect | |
|---|---|---|---|
| 1 | Caused by an aneurysm of the right internal carotid artery | A | |
| 2 | Caused by a right temporal lobe tumor | B | |
| 3 | Caused by complete compression of the optic chiasm | C | |
| 4 | Caused by a lesion of the right optic tract | D | |
| 5 | Caused by occlusion of the branches of the posterior cerebral artery to the right cuneus gyrus | E | |
| 6 | Caused by lesion to left lingual gyrus | F | |
| 7 | Caused by a lesion in the posterior limb of the internal capsule on the right | G | |
| 8 | Early manifestation of a pituitary adenoma | H | |
| 9 | Caused by a berry aneurysm at the juncture between the anterior cerebral and anterior communicating arteries | I | |

**ANSWERS**

**1.** I  **2.** D  **3.** B  **4.** C  **5.** E  **6.** F  **7.** C  **8.** G  **9.** H

# Physiology of Hearing

## 96 CHAPTER

### COMPETENCY ADDRESSED
**PY10.15:** Describe and discuss the functional anatomy of the ear and auditory pathways and physiology of hearing.
**PY10.16:** Describe and discuss the pathophysiology of deafness. Describe hearing tests.
**PY10.19:** Describe and discuss the auditory potential.

###  LEARNING OBJECTIVES
**At the end of this chapter, the learner should be able to:**
- Describe the physical properties of the sound waves with respect to hearing.
- Describe the functional anatomy of external, middle and inner ear.
- Describe the transmission of sound from external ear to inner ear.
- Describe the mechanism of mechanotransduction of sound wave into electrical impulses.
- Describe the physiology of endocochlear potentials.
- Describe the auditory pathway.
- Describe the different types of hearing disorders/deafness.
- Describe the role of hearing tests: tuning fork tests and audiometry in identifying the hearing loss.

Why do we assess students for physics during admission to the undergraduate medical program? Every student has this question in mind. Our body's functioning mechanism is based on the physics laws and principles and the biochemical mechanism works as per chemistry learned in our higher secondary course.

You might have known from childhood stories that a blind man had a sharp sense of hearing and smell. So, the increase in the functioning activity of special senses depends on how well we are training our body to utilize those senses.

Before we understand how we hear with our ear, let us explore the physics behind this mechanism.

## SOUND WAVES

### What is Sound?

Sound is pressure waves generated by vibrating air molecules (**Fig. 96.1**). It is a perception.

Sound travels as waves through the medium, we are not able to hear in space since it lacks the medium.

The molecules in the atmospheric air act as a medium causing alternating compression (dense molecules) and

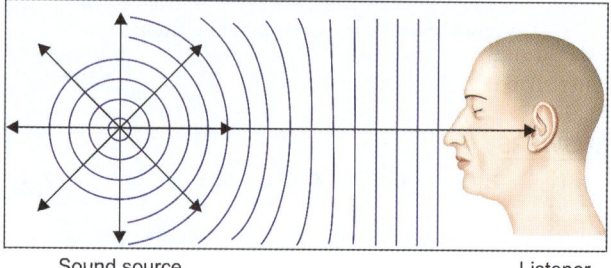

**Fig. 96.1:** The sound waves are the waves of compression and rarefaction.

rarefaction (loose molecules) waves as the sound travels through it. The simple sound is a sinusoidal wave or pure tone.

### Physiology of Hearing

- Transmission of sound depends on elastic medium.
- Sound waves travels more slowly than light (light travels at $3 \times 10^8$ m/s while the sound travels at 330 m/s at 20°C at sea level). This increases with temperature and altitude.

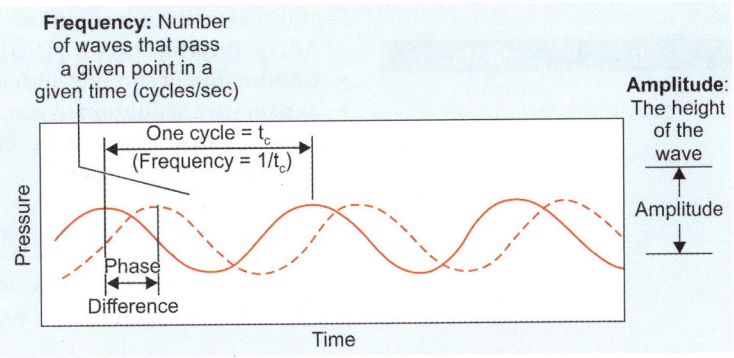

**Fig. 96.2:** Frequency and amplitude of sound waves.

- Speed of sound is more in the dense material. Hence, it is maximum in solids followed by liquid and then air. (solid > liquid > air).

The sound travels in the wave form, which are best described by its **(Fig. 96.2)**:
- Intensity (dB): Also called as loudness
- Frequency (Hz): Also called as pitch
- Complexity: Depends on many factors like pure tone/harmonics/noise

The properties of sound are tabulated in **Table 96.1**.

## How Sensitive is Your Ear?

- The human ear is sensitive to sound over a wide range:
- **Frequency:** 20–20,000 Hz
- **Amplitudes:** 0.0002–200 dynes/cm$^2$
- The human ear can detect the difference between two sounds occurring 10 μsec apart in time
- The wide sensitivity range of human hearing necessitates the use of **Logarithmic** (ratio) scales rather than **Linear** (numerical) scales.

**Table 96.1:** Properties of sound.

| Physical dimension | Perceptual dimension | |
|---|---|---|
| Intensity (dB) | **Loudness:**<br>It is correlated with amplitude of the sound waves<br>It is measured in decibels (dB)<br>1 dB = 0.01 bel<br>The intensity of sound at 0 dB at 1000 Hz (threshold of hearing) is represented as log of 0 dB = 10. It is considered as standard sound intensity<br>• 30 dB is faint sound<br>• 40–50 dB moderate sound<br>• 60–80 dB very loud sound<br>• 120–160 dB (painful) intensity of sound | Loud / Soft |
| Frequency (cycle/sec; Hertz) | **Pitch:**<br>• It is defined as the frequency range audible to the human ear. It is 20–20,000 cycles/sec (Hertz)<br>• The human ear is most sensitive to 1,000–4,000 cycles/sec best pitch discrimination occurs at 1,000–3,000 cycles/sec | Low frequency / High frequency |
| Complexity | **Timbre:**<br>Based on the complexity of the tone thus can be categorized as:<br>• **Pure tone:** Simple periodical regular sound of single frequency<br>• **Music tone:** A fundamental frequency with many harmonics<br>• **Noise:** Nonperiodical sound of no characteristic frequency<br>• i: Intensity p: Period t: Time | Music tone / Noise / Simple sound wave / Complex sound wave |

**Table 96.2:** Intensity of sound.

| Sound | dB SPL |
|---|---|
| Rocket launching pad | 180 |
| Jet plane | 140 |
| Gunshot blast | 130 |
| Car horn | 120 |
| Pneumatic drill | 110 |
| Power tools | 100 |
| Subway | 90 |
| Noisy restaurant | 80 |
| Busy traffic | 75 |
| Conversational speech | 66 |
| Average home | 55 |
| Library | 40 |
| Soft whisper | 30 |

(SPL: sound pressure level)

**Logarithmic scales** are used for the expressing the properties of sound:
- **Decibel (dB)** to represent sound pressure levels where 0 dB = 0.0002 dynes/cm$^2$ (threshold) and 120 dB: 200 dynes/cm$^2$ (maximum limit) **(Table 96.2).**
- **Octave scale for sound frequency in Hz:** The frequency range is measured in octave bands, i.e., each frequency is double the previous one, e.g., 250, 500, 1000, 2000, 4000 Hz, etc.

## What is the Importance of Hearing?

- We require hearing as it is an important mode of communication and it is essential for language.
- It helps us in localization of sound and helps us in determining the location of unseen sound sources.

For normal hearing we required:
- **Adequate stimulus** (SOUND)
- **Conduction** of stimulus to sensory organs of hearing
- **Sensory transduction** of stimulus at organs of hearing
- **Neural transmission** of the signal
- **Central auditory processing** of the signal at the brain

## FUNCTIONAL ANATOMY OF EAR

Based on the structure, the ear is divided into three parts: External, Middle, and Internal ear **(Fig. 96.3)**.

### External Ear (From Pinna Till Tympanic Membrane)

- **Pinna:** Helps to collect sound waves and to localize the source of the sound.
  - In lower animals pinna can be moved by muscular actions in the direction of a sound sour to collect sound in humans these muscles have little action.
- **External auditory canal—2.5 cm long**
  - Helps in transporting the sound waves to the middle ear.
  - Secrete wax and oil and trap the foreign bodies.

External ear is innervated mostly by **Vth** Cranial Nerve and **VIIth** cranial nerve; while tympanic membrane has add-on supply from **XI and Xth** cranial nerve.

### Functions of External Ear

- They collect the sound waves
- Amplification of frequencies 2000–4000 Hz (resonant frequency of EAC).
- Prevents mechanical injury to the tympanic membrane (TM).

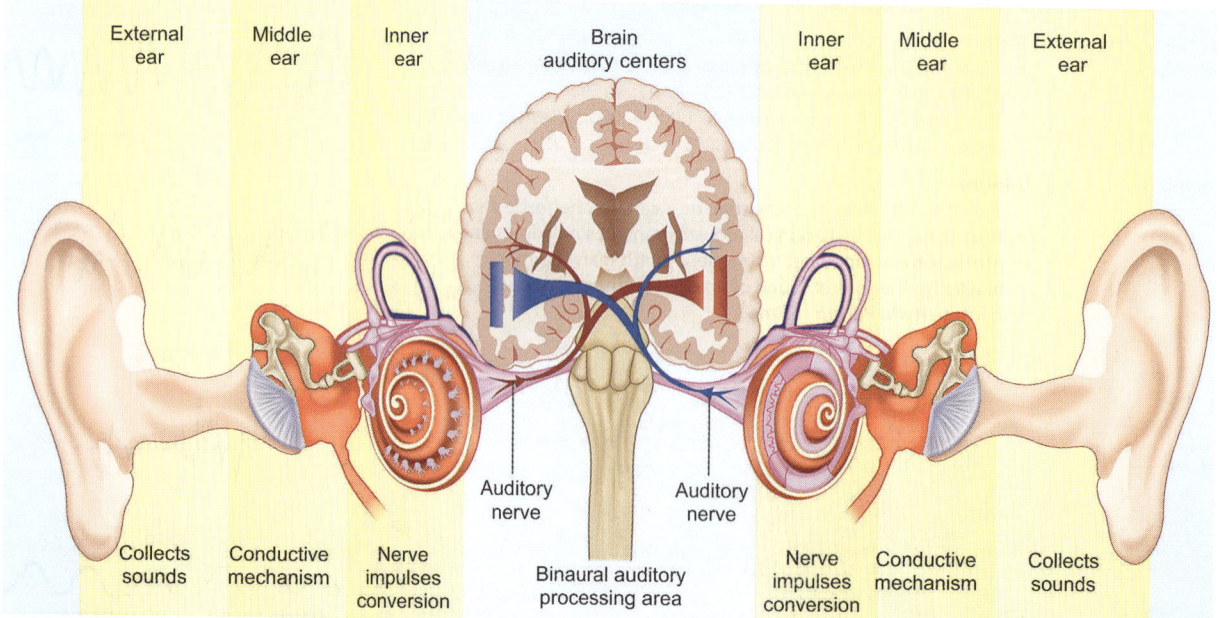

**Fig. 96.3:** The location of external, middle and inner ear inside the skull.

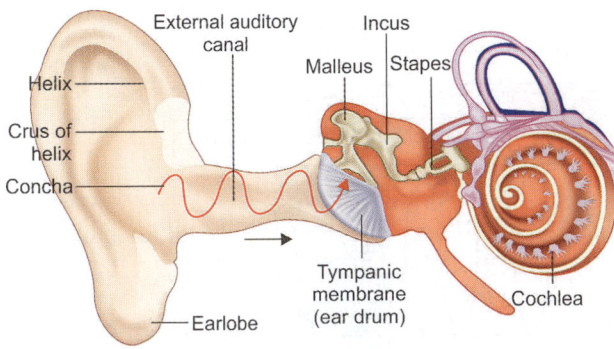

**Fig. 96.4:** Transmission of sound in external ear.

- Helps in maintaining favorable temperature and humidity for normal functioning of the TM.
- Providing cues about the vertical localization of a sound source (by the degree of sound reflection over the pinna).

### Sound Conduction in the Ear (Fig. 96.4)

- Sound waves are collected by the **pinna** and focused into the **EAC**.
- The vibration passes down the EAC and strikes the **TM**.

## Middle Ear

It is an air-filled cavity within the temporal bone that consists of:
- Tympanic membrane (Eardrum)
- **Ear ossicles:** Malleus, incus and stapes
- **Muscles:** Tensor tympani and stapedius
- Eustachian tube
- Mastoid antrum
- Facial nerve

### Tympanic Membrane (TM) (Fig. 96.5)

- Oval, thin, semi-transparent, pearly grey trilaminar membrane.
- **Diameter:** Max. 9–10 mm and Min. 8–9 mm
- **Position:** Placed obliquely at acute angle 55° with floor

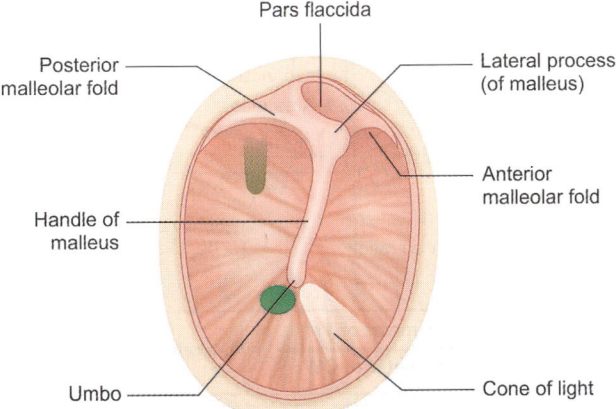

**Fig. 96.5:** Tympanic membrane.

- Facing downwards, forwards and laterally (children horizontal–can withstand even loud noisy sound).
- Anterior wall and floor are longer

It has two parts:
1. **Pars flaccida:** Areolar connective tissue
2. **Pars tensa:** Dense (irregular) connective tissue

### Ear Ossicles (Fig. 96.6)

- **Malleus–resembles a hammer:** The handle of the malleus is connected to the inner surface of TM.
- **Incus:** It is an anvil shaped bone which articulates with head of malleus.
- **Stapes looks like stirrup:** The head of the stapes articulates with the incus and the oval foot plate contacts the oval window of the cochlea.
- **Function:** To amplify the intensity of the sound by 1.2 to 1.3 times by lever action.

### Middle Ear Muscles (Fig. 96.6)

- **Tensor tympani:** It is attached to the neck of the malleus. Its contraction causes tension in the tympanic membrane.
- **Stapedius:** It is attached to the neck of the stapes and on contraction, it pulls the footplate of the stapes out from the oval window. This muscles tightens the ossicular chain and dampens its oscillations.

### Middle Ear Mechanics

- Effective transfer of sound energy from the air to the fluid medium is difficult because most of the sound is reflected as a result of the different mechanical properties of the two media.
- The middle ear thus acts as an **impedance-matching device** by amplifying the sound pressure.
- Amplification of sound intensity is greatest between **1000–3000 Hz** sounds below 16 Hz or above 20000 Hz are not amplified at all.

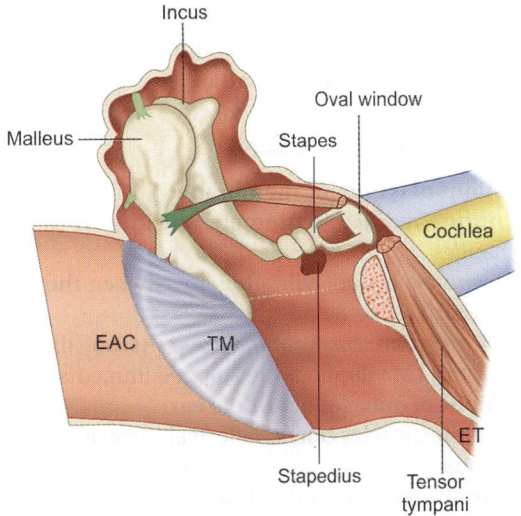

**Fig. 96.6:** Structures in middle ear.

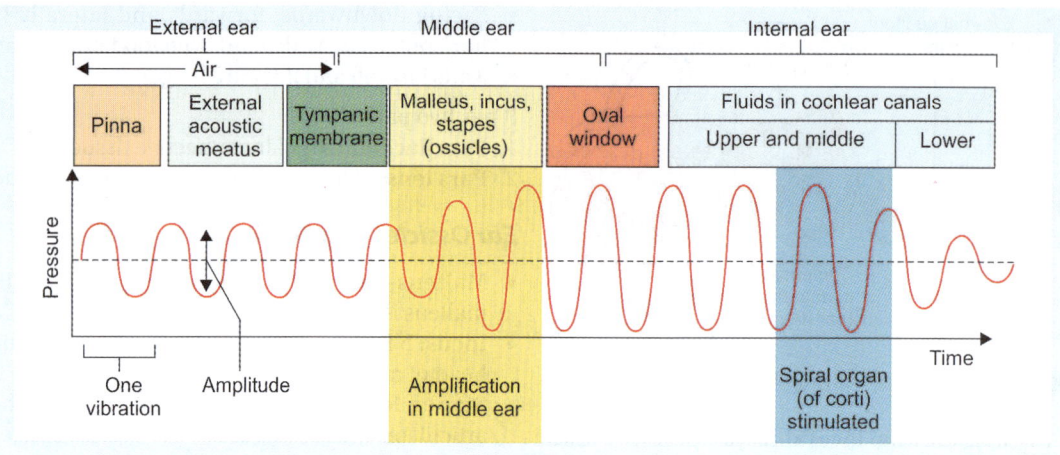

**Fig. 96.7:** Sound wave transmission through external ear to inner ear.

## Route of Sound Waves Through the Ear

See **Figure 96.7**.

### Tympanic/Attenuation Reflex

- It is a **protective reflex** caused by the **sudden contraction of the ear muscles** resulting is stiffening of ear ossicles. This dampens the ossicular oscillations and prevents the damage to tympanic membrane and ear ossicles.
- **Functions:**
  - It protects the cochlea from damaging vibrations caused by excessively loud sounds
  - It masks low frequency sounds in loud environments
  - It decreases a person's sensitivity to his or her own speech (muscles)
- It has a latency of 40 to 160 milliseconds, i.e., develops in 40 msec and completes in 160 msec. Hence, it may not be effective in sudden loud sounds like bomb explosions.
- **Mechanism:**
  - Contraction of tensor tympani and stapedius dampens the movement and ossicles and decreases the sensitivity of acoustic apparatus.
  - Reduce the intensity of sound transmission by 30–40 dB (↓ 1000 cycles/second).

### Functions of the Middle Ear

- **Functions of tympanic membrane:**
  - *Pressure receiver:* Extremely sensitive to pressure changes
  - *Resonator:* It starts vibrating freely when the sound wave strikes
  - *Critically dampens the sound waves:* As soon the sound will stop TM vibrations are stopped immediately
- **Functions of muscles of middle ear:**
  - Both the muscles can be reflexively activated by loud sounds
  - Amplitude of sound vibration of the tympanic membrane
  - Protection of the inner ear from the loud sound
  - *Tympanic reflex:* It has a reaction time 40 to 160 sec
- **Functions of ear ossicles:**
  - The ear ossicles result in amplification of sound intensity by 1.2–1.3 times, since the handle of the malleus is 1.3 times longer than the long process of incus—this provides a mechanical leverage advantage.
  - *Impedance matching:* They transmit the vibratory motion of the tympanic membrane to the oval window. The effective vibratory area of the tympanic membrane (about 45 mm$^2$) is much greater than the stapes—oval window surface area (about 3.2 mm$^2$) the difference in the size amplifies the pressure exerted on the oval window (14 folds). Movements of the TM are more at the periphery than at the center where the malleus handle is attached. This too provides some leverage. **Total amplification is 18 times (14 × 1.3).**
  - Hence, it matches the relatively low impedance of airborne sounds to the higher impedance of inner ear fluids. Focusing the forces at the larger diameter TM onto the much smaller diameter OW. Mechanical advantage gained by the **ossicular lever action (Fig. 96.8).**

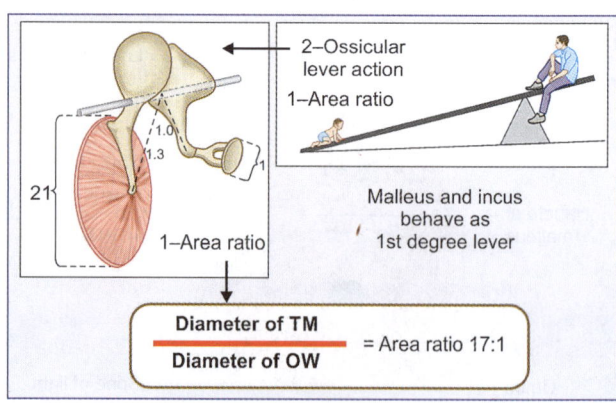

**Fig. 96.8:** Ossicular lever action.

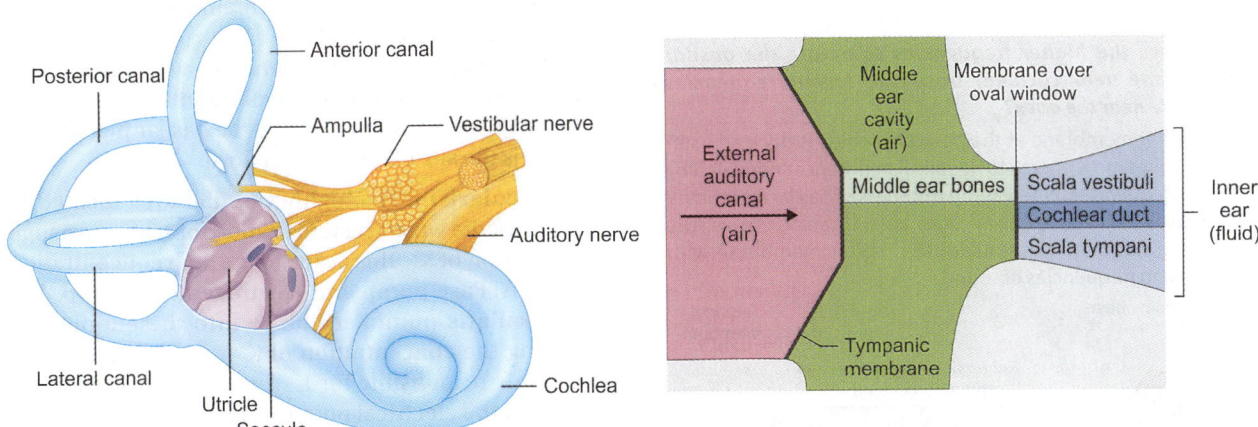

Fig. 96.9: Structure of inner ear and relation to external and middle ear.

### Auditory Tube

It was formerly called the eustachian tube. It serves as the link the middle ear with the pharynx and its opening equalizes pressure in the middle ear cavity with external air pressure.

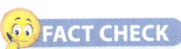 **FACT CHECK**

30–40% of sound energy is lost as sound travels from the middle to the inner ear.

### Inner Ear

#### Structure (Fig. 96.9)

The inner ear has a complex structure forming two important structures of the inner ear, the vestibular apparatus and the coiled structure for hearing, the cochlea. Together, the inner is call the labyrinth because of its complex structure. It has two parts, the bony and membranous labyrinth.

The membranous labyrinth is placed inside the bony labyrinth and comprises of one vestibule containing *saccule, utricle and three semicircular canals*. It also has a coiled structure *Cochlea*.

**STRUCTURES IN INNER EAR**
**Structures associated with equilibrium**
- **Utricle:** Detects linear acceleration in horizontal direction
- **Saccule:** Detects linear acceleration in vertical direction
- **Semicircular canal:** Detects the rotational acceleration

**Structures associated with hearing**
- **Cochlea**: For perception of sound

### Mechanism of Transmission of Sound Vibrations (Fig. 96.10)

- The tympanic membrane vibrates in response to sound perceived and moves the ear ossicles in middle ear.
- The vibration of the ossicles propagates the sound waves to the oval window.

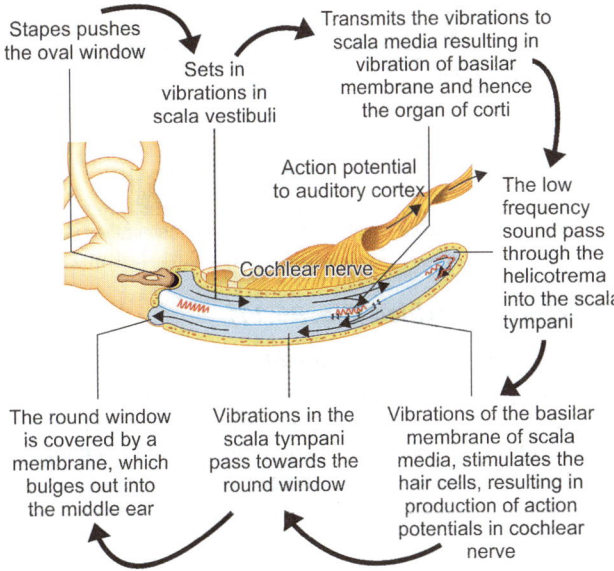

Fig. 96.10: Pathway of sound vibrations.

- Stapes push the perilymph fluid in the scala vestibuli at the oval window and transmits the vibrations from ear ossicles to the perilymph.
- The higher frequencies stimulate the basilar membrane near the base of cochlea whereas the lower frequencies travel to the apex, to stimulate the basilar membrane at appropriate place for that frequency. The lowest frequencies do not stimulate the basilar membrane, pass as such to scala tympani through helicotrema.
- These vibrations, when stimulate the basilar membrane, sets in the vibration in the basilar membrane, stimulating the hair cells in the scala media.
- At helicotrema, the low frequency vibration moves into the scala tympani.
- Fluid vibration dissipated at the round window which bulges into the middle ear.

> **Why does the higher frequencies stimulate the basilar membrane near cochlear base and lower frequencies stimulate near the apex?**
>
> The basilar membrane at the base of cochlea is thick and stiff and requires more energy to be stimulated, hence stimulated by higher frequencies. Whereas the thickness of basilar membrane decreases as it moves away from base to apex. Hence, the lowering frequencies stimulate the basilar membrane with decreasing frequencies of sound.
>
>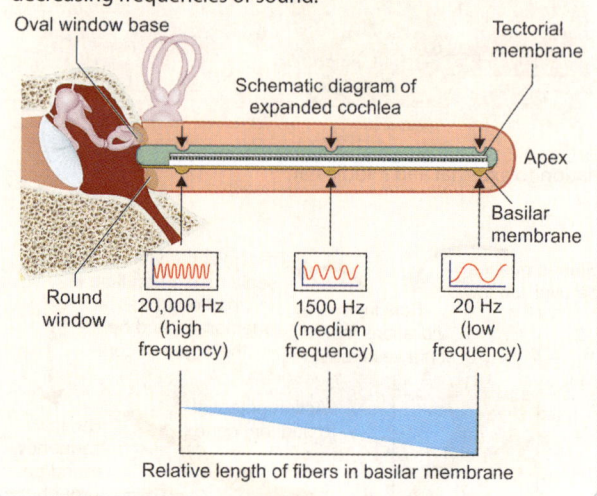

## Structure of Cochlea (Fig. 96.11)

Cochlea is a coiled blind tube of 39 mm which is coiled 2¾ turns on the base/modiolus. It contains three tubular canals, the scala vestibuli, scala media and scala tympani.

- The scala vestibuli and scala tympani contain *perilymph*, which has a *high Na+ concentration*. It communicates with the subarachnoid space of brain. Its composition is similar to cerebrospinal fluid.
- The scala media contain *endolymph*, which has a *high K+ concentration* which resembles intracellular fluid. The scala media is bordered by the basilar membrane, which is the site of the organ of Corti.

**Stria vascularis:** It is a highly vascular area located in the scala media which secretes endolymph having a high concentration of $K^+$. This is due to the high concentration of $Na^+ K^+$ ATPase pump and electrogenic $K^+$ pump. The stria vascularis pumps in the $K^+$ into the endolymph increasing the concentration of $K^+$ from the perilymph. Hence, it is responsible for $K^+$ recycling. This results in increase in the electrical potential inside the endolymph of +80mV, called the *endolymphatic/endocochlear potential*.

### Organ of Corti

Organ of Corti is located in the scala media on the basilar membrane, which separates it from scala tympani. The scala media is separated from scala vestibuli by Reissner's membrane. The basilar membrane is made up of elastic fibers.

- The vibration of fluid from scala vestibuli will move to scala tympani via helicotrema and vibrate different portions of the basilar membrane.
- **Tectorial membrane** in the scala media is stiff, thin gelatinous elastic structure, made of glycoproteins. The cilia from the inner and outer hair cells are embedded in the tectorial membrane **(Fig. 96.12)**. So, when the basilar membrane vibrates up and down, the hair cells bend to and for resulting in the mechanotransduction and generation of action potential.

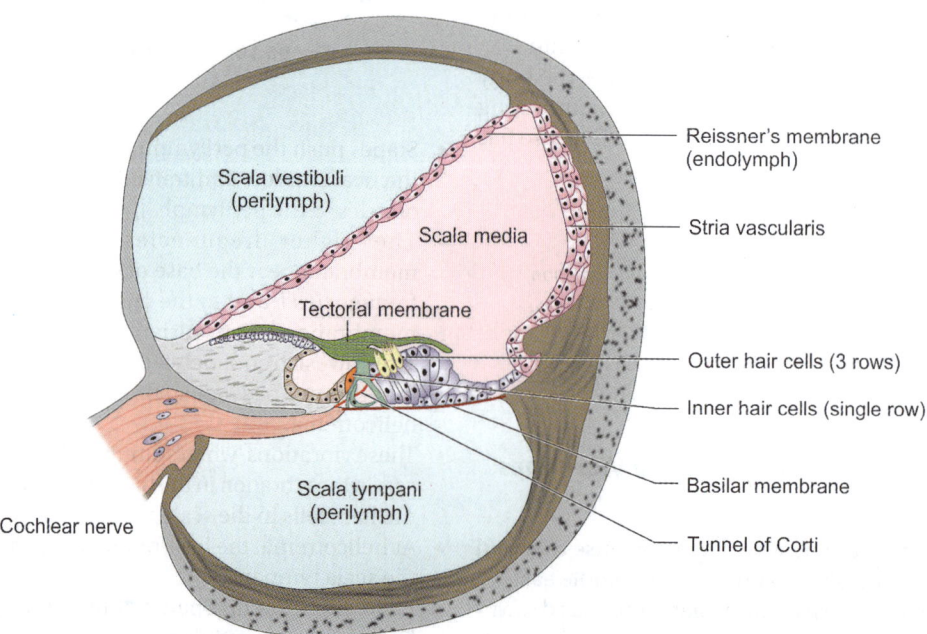

**Fig. 96.11:** Structure of cochlea.

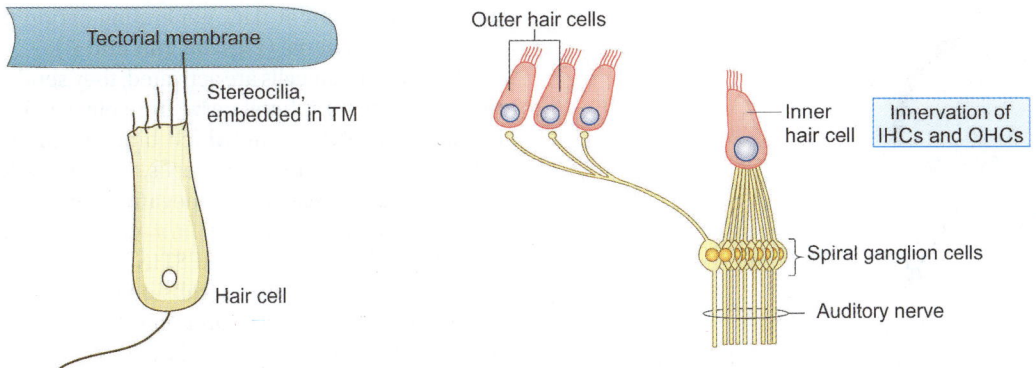

**Fig. 96.12:** Tectorial membrane and hair cell innervations.

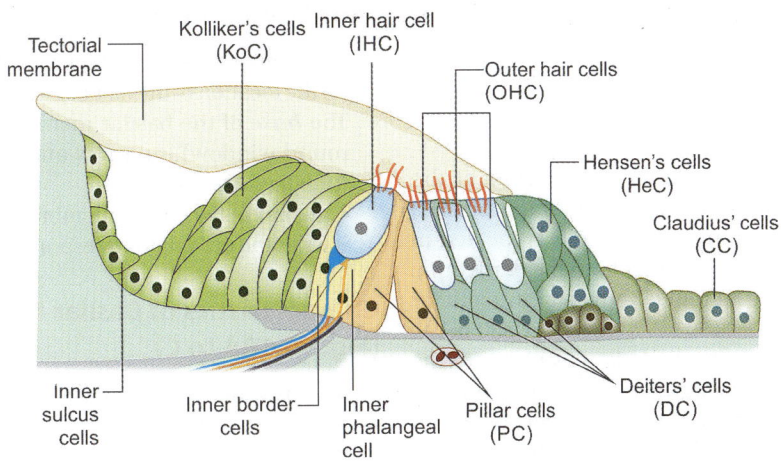

**Fig. 96.13:** Supporting cells of inner ear.

- **Hair cells:** They form the sensory part (receptor) of the inner ear, which converts the mechanical sound waves into electrical signals (mechanotransduction). These hair cells are present on the basilar membrane. Each hair cell has many cilia protruding from their upper end called stereocilia which are embedded in the tectorial membrane. These cilia are arranged in the ascending order. The hair cells are of two types:
  - *Inner hair cells* are flask-shaped, arranged in a single row, and are few in number (3000–5000). They are required for the transmission of auditory impulses especially for fine auditory transmission. IHC are richly innervated and are responsible for electrical transmission of sound signals **(Fig. 96.12)**.
  - *Outer hair cells* are cylindrical, arranged in parallel rows, and are greater in number (approx. 12000). They are responsible for detecting the presence of sound and receive efferent innervation from the olivary complex through the olivocochlear fibers. They are concerned with modulation and fine tuning of sound transmitted by inner hair cells in terms of amplitude and clarity of sound.
- **Rods of Corti:** Two projections (inner and outer rods) from the Basilar membrane into the SM—the tunnel of Corti is between the two rods containing cortilymph fluid (function unknown).
- **Supporting cells (Fig. 96.13):** There are mainly three types of the supporting cells, which support the hair cells and the organ of Corti.
  - Inner phalangeal cells—supports inner hair cells
  - Deiter's cells—supports the outer hair cells
  - Hensen's cells and Claudius cells: They are situated outside Deiter's cells and the Claudius cells are present further outside the Hensen cells. All these cells provide support to each other and hair cells. These cells have the gap junctions, which allows the $K^+$ ions to flow from the hair cells to the stria vascularis for the $K^+$ recycling.

## ELECTRICAL RESPONSES IN THE HAIR CELLS

As discussed earlier, the gap junctions between the hair cells and the support cells prevent the endolymph from reaching the base of the hair cells. However, the base of hair cells is permeable to the perilymph. This results in the generation of electrical gradient inside the hair cells called the resting membrane potential (discussed below). The electrical changes in the perilymph and endolymph are responsible for the generation of the impulse in the auditory nerve. Two type of potential changes are seen in inner ear:

- **Resting potential of the hair cells:** The hair cells are located in the endolymph but the base of the hair cells are bathed in perilymph of scala tympani. Hence,

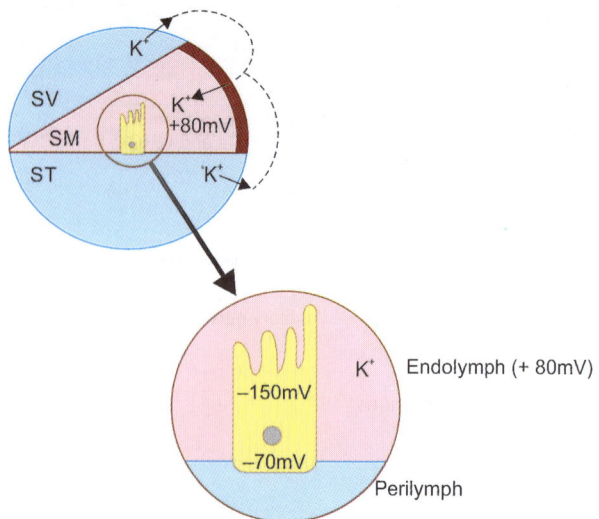

**Fig. 96.14:** Resting potential of hair cells.

the resting membrane potential of hair cells at the base is –70 mV with respect to the perilymph of scala tympani. But the upper end of hair cells is located in endolymph, which is 80 mV higher than the perilymph. Hence, the potential difference between intracellular fluid and endolymph is –150 mV [–70 mV – (+80 mV)]. The excessive potassium in the hair cells pause to the adjoining supporting cells through the gap junctions. It then reaches stria vascularis, from there the potassium is secreted back into the endolymph **(Fig. 96.14)**.

- **Endocochlear potential:** The endolymph contains a high concentration of $K^+$ (135 mEq/L) and is electrically positive with respect to perilymph and the potential of +80 mV higher than the perilymph. The high concentration of $K^+$ occurs due to its secretion from the stria vascularis (mentioned above). These potentials are called the endolymphatic/endocochlear potential.

## Transduction of Sounds

*'The conversion of the sound waves into the electrical signal is called as the mechanotransduction of the sound. The inner hair cells are responsible for the transmission of the sound signal to the cochlear nerve but the outer layer cells fine tune this signal.'*

The motion of the basilar membrane causes movement of the organ of Corti to vibrate up and down. This causes the back-and-forth movement of the cilia on hair cells, which is embedded in tectorial membrane. The tips of the stereocilia have the $K^+$ channels connected to each other by tip links. When the cilia move towards the stereocilia, the $K^+$ channels open resulting in $K^+$ influx causing depolarization **(Figs. 96.15A and B)**.

This causes opening of voltage-gated $Ca^{2+}$ to open on the lateral border of inner hair cells (IHC). This pushes the vesicles containing neurotransmitters to move toward the basal border of the hair cell, releasing Glutamate neurotransmitters from the vesicles. This stimulates the peripheral neuron at IHC, generating action potential in spiral ganglion nerve **(Figs. 96.16A and B)**.

Once inner hair cells are activated, they send the impulse to the efferent peripheral nerve from olivocochlear bundle. It releases acetylcholine which binds to the receptor on the basal level of outer hair cells. It releases $K^+$ ion from the cell, thus decreasing the negativity of the cell, causing *hyperpolarization* of the hair cell. This also causes relaxation of the protein "PRESTIN" which is a contractile protein, present on the lateral side of the outer hair cell, which lengthens the OHC and pulls the basilar membrane downward. This decreases the vibration of basilar membrane and activation of IHC, finetuning its output **(Fig. 96.17)**.

## How Sound is Encoded?

- The frequency that activates a particular hair cell depends on the location of the hair cell along the basilar membrane
- The *base* of the basilar membrane (near the oval and round window) is narrow and stiff. It responds best to *high frequencies*.
- The *apex* of the basilar membrane (near the helicotrema) is wide and complaint. It responds best to *low frequencies*.

## Characteristics of Basilar Membrane (Fig. 96.18A to C)

- Apex is wider than the base
- Tension is higher at the base than at the apex
- Base vibrates at a higher frequency than the apex (hence acts as a frequency analyzer)
- Length of the fibers is greater at the apex than at the base
- Fiber diameter is greater at the base than at the apex. The base is shorter and wider while apex is taller and slender
- High–frequency resonance (base), low-frequency resonance (apex)

The sound is discriminated based on two important attributes of sound:
1. Pitch
2. Loudness

### Pitch Discrimination

The pitch of frequency of sound is discriminated by the two principles/theories:
- **Place theory of hearing:**
  - The basilar membrane vibrations create the traveling waves which peak at the characteristic place on the basilar membrane according to the frequency of stimulating sound.
  - The high-frequency sound waves produce waves of maximum height near the oval window while low-frequency sounds produce waves of maximum height near the helicotrema.
  - The auditory nerve fiber activated by a particular sound frequency is similarly dependent on the location of the hair cell it innervates.

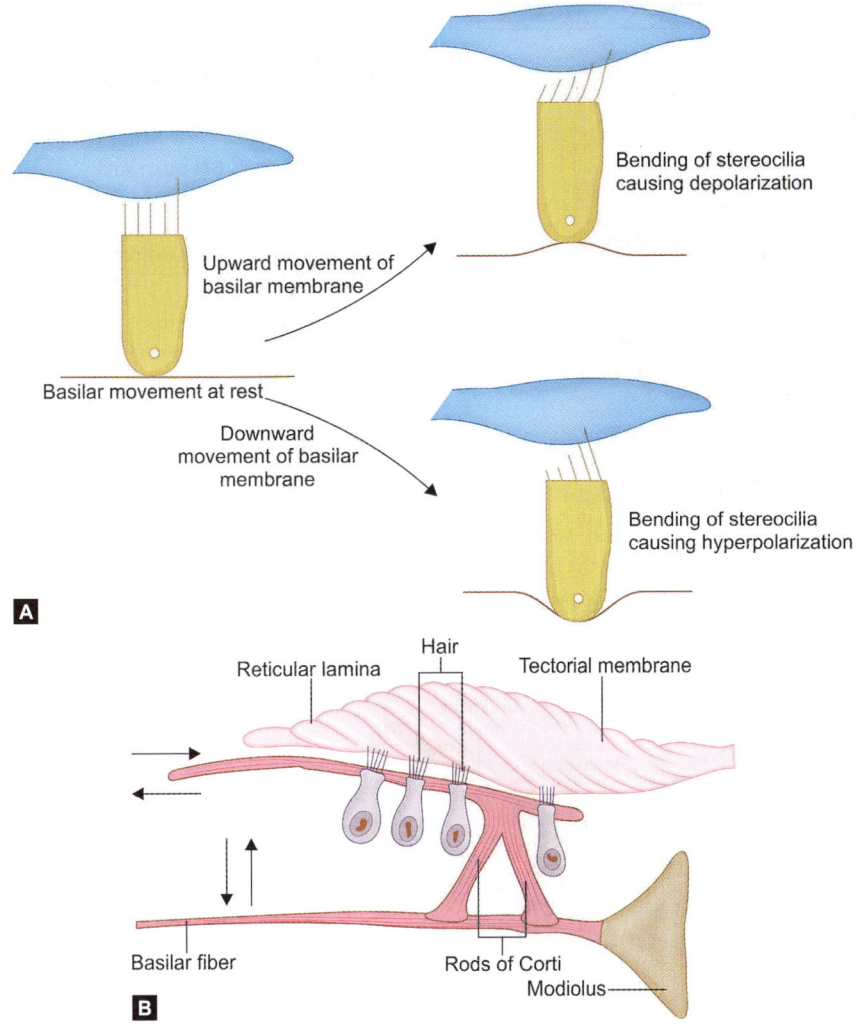

**Figs. 96.15A and B:** Transduction of sound.

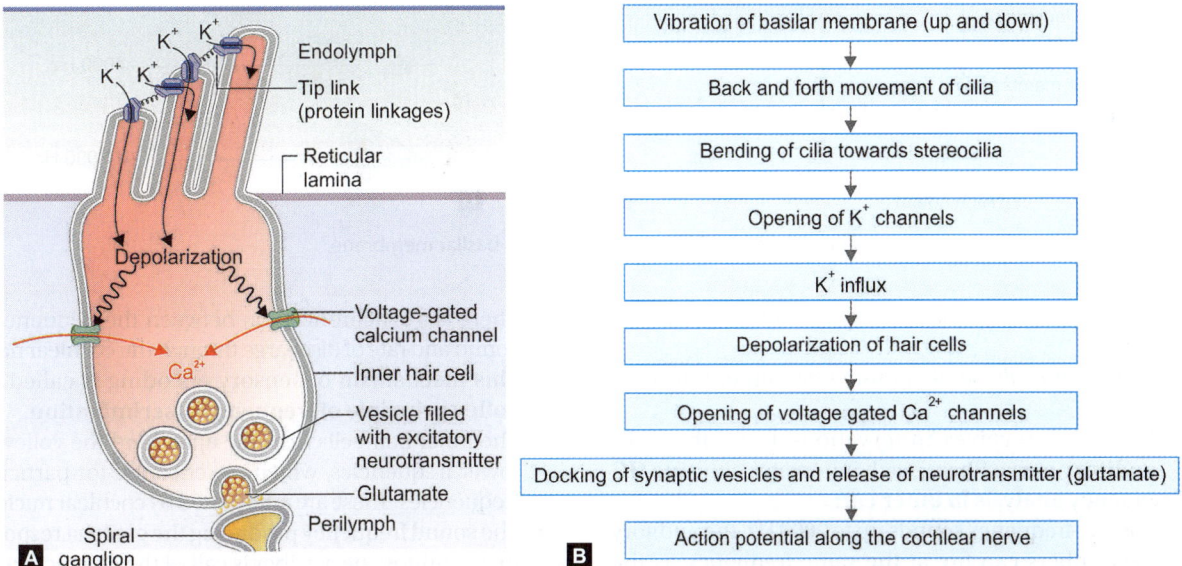

**Figs. 96.16A and B:** Generation of action potential in spiral ganglion nerve and cochlear nerve.

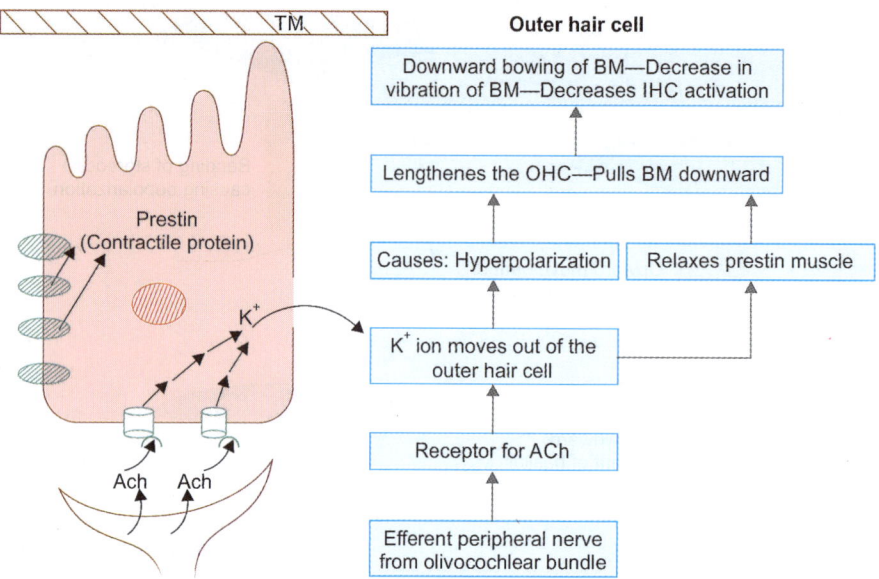

**Fig. 96.17:** Role of prestin in hyperpolarization.

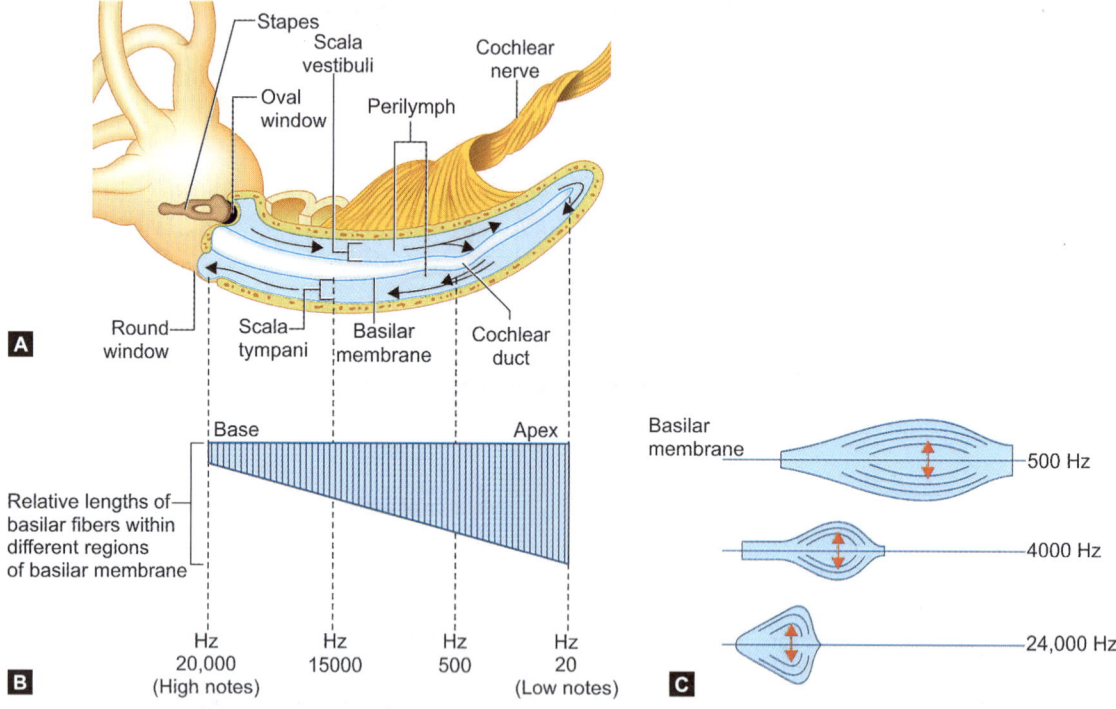

**Figs. 96.18A to C:** Frequency range of basilar membrane.

- There are about 30,000 nerve fibers in each auditory nerve.
- Over 90% of these fibers innervate inner hair cells (IHC).
- Each IHC receives innervations from about **10 auditory nerve fibers**; each innervates only **one HC**
• Frequency analysis in inner ear:
  - For low-frequency sounds up to 2000 Hz, the auditory nerve fibers can fire at the same frequency as the sound wave.
- There is a synchronization between the frequency of sound and rate of discharge through the cochlear nerve
- This mechanism of sensory encoding is called the **volley principle of frequency discrimination**.
- The inner hair cells near the apex send the volleys of lower frequencies, which are encoded for particular frequencies. These are interpreted by cochlear nucleus.
- The sound frequency producing the greatest response in an auditory nerve fiber is called the **characteristic frequency** of that nerve fiber.

## Loudness of the Sound

It refers to the intensity of the sound, which is measured in the bels.
- The frequency of firing in an auditory nerve fiber increase as the intensity of the sound wave increases.
- In addition, a **large portion of the basilar membrane** is vibrated as the sound intensity increases so that more auditory nerve fibers are activated.
- Thus, sound intensity is encoded by the **frequency of the auditory nerve discharge and by the number of auditory nerve fibers** that are active.

**What is the duplex theory of pitch discrimination?**
Place theory and the volley principle together are known as the duplex theory.

## Location of Sound in Space

- A human ear distinguishes sound originating from the sources separated by as little as $1^0$.
- Binaural receptive fields contribute to the sound localization.
- The time lag between the entry of sound in two ears—the detectable interaural time differences even 20 µs, especially for relatively low-frequency sounds (below 3000 Hz).
- Lesions of the auditory cortex disrupt sound localization.

## CENTRAL AUDITORY PATHWAY (TABLE 96.3)

As we have discussed above, the sound signals are converted to electrical signals, which are converted to the electrical signals by the IHCs. These are further transmitted

**Table 96.3:** Nuclei and ganglion of auditory pathway and their characteristics.

| Levels of brain | Part in auditory pathway | Characteristics and functions |
|---|---|---|
| | Spiral ganglion | • Pseudounipolar neuron<br>• Peripheral end stimulates hair cells |
| Medulla oblongata | Cochlear nuclei | • Has three groups of nuclei<br>• 2 Ventral (ventroanterior and ventroposterior)<br>• 1 Dorsal |
| Pons | Superior olivary nucleus | • Located at the lower part of the **Pons**<br>• Fibers move upward while some at the **Nucleus of the Lateral lemniscus**<br>• They move up together as Lateral Lemniscus (LL) ends at **Inferior Colliculus** (IC) at the midbrain<br>• There can be a **crossing over** of some fibers between two Nuclei of the Lateral Lemniscus<br>**Function:**<br>• Play a major role in the **Localization** of sound<br>• Has Medial and Lateral Halves<br>  ▪ Medial SON: Plays role in the relative **timing** of the sound<br>  ▪ Lateral SON: Plays a role in determining the relative **intensity** of sound stimuli<br>• It activates the **Olivocochlear bundle** in case of high sound stimuli thus activating the **Outer Hair cells** to relax the Prestin molecule and dampening the stimulation of Inner HC<br>**Sound localization:**<br>• Time lag between the entry of sound into one ear and its entry into the opposite ear<br>  ▪ Functions best at frequencies below 3,000 cycles/sec<br>  ▪ Neural analysis—**medial superior olivary nucleus**<br>• Difference between the intensities of the sounds in the two ears<br>  ▪ Functions best at frequencies above 3,000 cycles per second<br>  ▪ Neural analysis—**lateral superior olivary nucleus** |
| Midbrain | Inferior colliculus | • IC is a part of the downward tract known as **Tectospinal tract** which controls "**Auditory Reflexes**"<br>• This involves head movement on hearing the sound<br>• Most of the fibers move upwards from IC as Brachius of IC to the **Medial Geniculate Nucleus of Thalamus (MGB)** |
| Cerebral cortex | Auditory areas | • From there the fibers move to the superficial part of the **temporal cortex** (Superior Temporal cortex/Transverse Gyrus of Heschl/Primary Auditory Cortex) as **Auditory Radiation**<br>• Fibers may be **crossed or uncrossed**. As a result, a mixture of ascending auditory fibers represents both ears at all higher levels<br>• Therefore, lesions of the cochlea of one ear cause unilateral deafness, but most central unilateral lesions do not<br>• There are Associate Auditory Cortex for the interpretation of received sound<br>• **Wernicke's area**: Comprehend sound and send information to Broca's area (Controls muscles of speech) via fasciculus known as "**Arcuate fasciculus**"<br>• **Broca's area** sends information to the premotor, primary motor, and sensory area of the cortex—stimulating speech of other components via descending pathway |

*Contd...*

*Contd...*

| Levels of brain | Part in auditory pathway | Characteristics and functions |
|---|---|---|
| | | • There is a **Tonotopic Representation** of frequencies at all the levels of the central auditory pathways 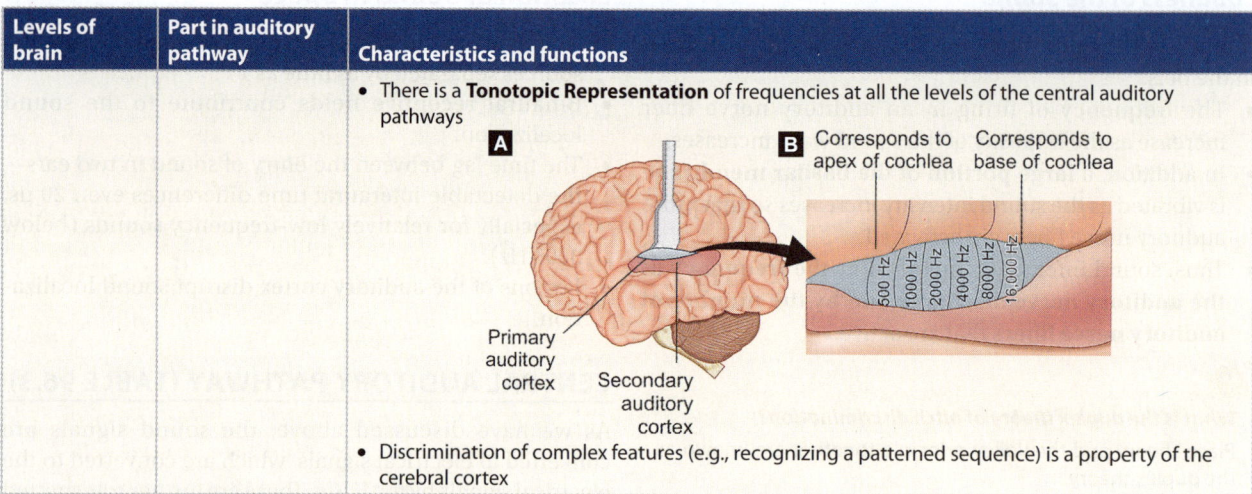 |
| | | • Discrimination of complex features (e.g., recognizing a patterned sequence) is a property of the cerebral cortex |

to the auditory area in the brain by the central auditory pathway, as shown in **Figure 96.19**. The inner ear sends its signals though the nerve fibers which pass through the spiral ganglion and terminates in the dorsal and ventral cochlear nucleus located in the medulla oblongata. The fibers from both the cochlear nuclei relay into ipsilateral and contralateral superior olivary nucleus. The fibers then ascend upward till the midbrain to relay in the inferior colliculus. From here the fibers relay in the medial geniculate body of thalamus.

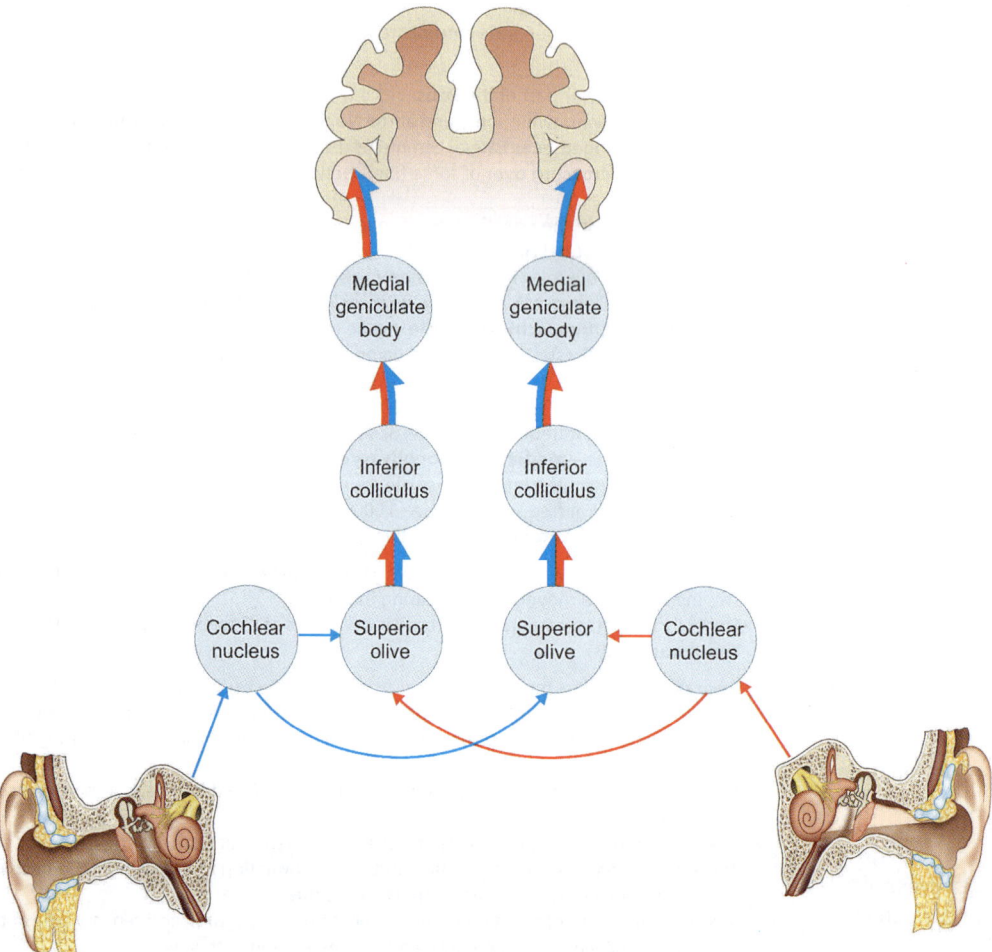

**Fig. 96.19:** Central auditory pathway.

Tip: Thalamus has two geniculate bodies; **M**edial for **M**usic (Auditory) and **L**ateral for **L**ight (Visual) pathways.

The fibers arising from MGB, end in the auditory cortex located in the temporal lobe.

*How does our body defend its hearing system due to very loud sounds?*
- Information from the auditory pathway to **Reticular Formation** nuclei present throughout the brain stem
- At the level of pons, it activates two nerves
- **Vth Cranial nerve**—Contracts tensor tympani—dampness sound conduction from tympanic membrane to middle ear
- **VIIth Cranial Nerve**—Contracts stapedius—dampness sound conduction from stapes to Inner ear via oval window

## PHYSIOLOGY OF HEARING DEFECTS/DEAFNESS

Before we study the different types of deafness, we must understand the difference between masking and noise.
- **Masking:** It is defined as the inability to process one type of sound in the presence of other sound. For example, the loud traffic sounds may provide the masking effect for a person and doesn't allow him to hear the conversation being carried with him clearly. Hence, the presence of one type of sound decreases the ability of the ear to hear another type of sound.

  It happens because the auditory mechanism is unable to process separate but simultaneous stimulation into separate components.
- **Noise:** It is a periodic complex sound which is composed of different frequencies. It is classified into three types:
  1. *White noise:* It is broadband noise which contains all frequencies in an audible spectrum. It is analogous to the white light that contains all the colors of the visible spectrum. It is used for masking.
  2. *Narrow-band noise:* White noise minus above and below the given noise when filtered out gives the narrow band noise. It is a frequency range that is smaller than the broadband white noise. Used to mask the tested frequency in pure tone audiometry.
  3. *Speed noise:* This noise has frequencies in the speech range (300–3000 Hz). All other frequencies are filtered out.

**Hearing defects:** When the person finds it difficult to hear, we call it as deafness or hearing defects. Based on the etiology, the deafness is classified as:
- Conductive deafness
- Sensorineural deafness

## Conductive Deafness

Conductive deafness occurs due to impaired sound transmission in the external and middle ear. It Impacts all sound frequencies.

### Causes
- Plugging of the EAC with cerumen (wax)/foreign bodies
- Otitis externa and otitis media
- Perforation of the eardrum
- Otosclerosis (immobility of ossicles)
- Disruption of auditory ossicles

## Sensorineural Deafness (SNHL)

Sensorineural deafness occurs due to loss of transmission of sound signal from the hair cells to the auditory cortex. The most common site of SNHL is cochlear hair cells, eighth cranial nerves or central auditory pathways (nerve deafness). There is impaired ability to hear certain frequencies. This type of hearing loss is permanent.

### Causes
- Exposure to sudden large-intensity noise
- Exposure to prolonged noise
- Tumors and vascular damage
- Ototoxic drugs (toxic drugs for hair cells) like aminoglycoside antibiotics, quinine, frusemide, tobramycin, kanamycin, gentamycin, etc.

## Presbycusis

There is gradual hearing loss associated with aging. It affects people in old age especially over 75 and is due to gradual loss of hair cells and neurons. There is loss of high frequency sounds but the lower frequencies are retained.

**Some syndromes associated with deafness:**
- **Pendred syndrome:** Mutation of an anion exchanger and goiter
- **Long QT syndrome:** Mutation of $K^+$ channel (KVLQT1) in stria vascularis and heart.
- **Bartter syndrome:** Mutation of protein barttin and kidney disease.

## Hearing Tests

These tests are done to differentiate the type of hearing loss:
- **Human voice:**
  - A conversation voice (60 dB) should be heard at 3.5 mts (12 feet) in each ear separately.
  - Lists of spondee (phonetically balanced) words are used for this test, which is repeated using whispered voice.
- **Tuning fork test:**
  - Tuning forks of 256 Hz or 512 Hz are used for this test.
  - Hearing threshold is lower at some frequencies than others thus low tones (<500 Hz) sound lowers and high tones (>4000 Hz) sound higher as their loudness increases.

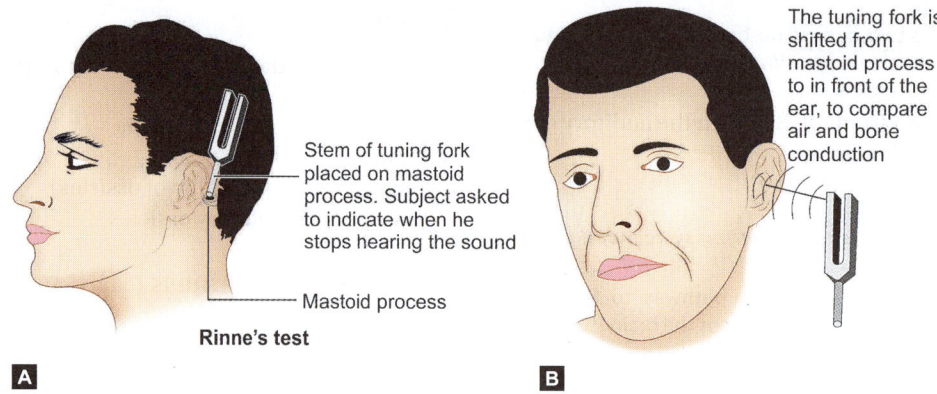

**Figs. 96.20A and B:** (A) Tuning fork placed on mastoid process to test bone conduction; (B) Tuning fork is placed in front of the ear to test air conduction.

### Rinne's Test

#### Procedure

This test compares air conduction (AC) and bone conduction (BC).
- Give proper instructions to the subject.
- The tuning fork is struck and kept at the mastoid process of the subject **(Fig. 96.20A)**.
- Subject indicates by raising hand when he stops hearing the sound through the bone. This part of the test examines the bone conduction of sound.
- In order to check the bone conduction, the tuning fork is then placed in front of the ear canal **(Fig. 96.20B)**.
- Subject responds (by saying yes or no) whether he is hearing the sound or not. In normal case, subject is able to hear the sound as the air conduction is better than the bone conduction (AC>BC).

### Weber's Test

#### Procedure

This test compares the bone conduction of both ears.
- Give proper instructions to the subject.
- The tuning fork is struck and kept at the vertex of the subject **(Fig. 96.21)**.
- He is instructed to indicate the side in which he hears well.

### Schwabach's Test

#### Procedure

This test compares the bone conduction of both the subject and examiner. We presume that examiner has normal bone conduction.
- Give proper instructions to the subject.
- The tuning fork is struck and placed on the mastoid process of the subject **(Fig. 96.22)**.
- Subject indicates when he stops hearing the sound.
- The tuning fork is then quickly shifted to the mastoid process of the examiner.

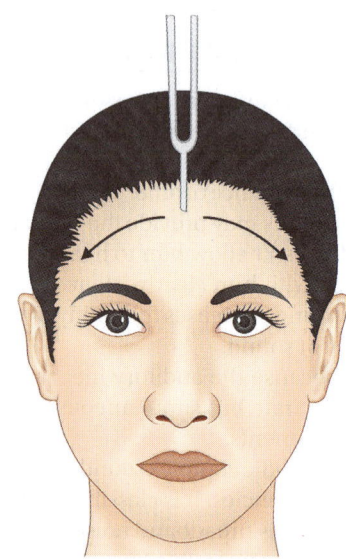

**Fig. 96.21:** Weber's test.

- Examiner observes whether he is able to hear any sound or not.

### Absolute Bone Conduction Test

#### Procedure

This test compares the absolute bone conduction of both the subject and examiner. We presume that examiner has normal bone conduction.
- Give proper instructions to the subject.
- The tuning fork is struck and placed on the mastoid process of the subject, with the tragus closed **(Fig. 96.23)**.
- Subject indicates when he stops hearing the sound.
- The tuning fork is then quickly shifted to the mastoid process of the examiner, with his tragus closed.
- Examiner observes whether he is able to hear any sound or not.

Summary of routinely done hearing tests and their findings are tabulated in **Table 96.4**.

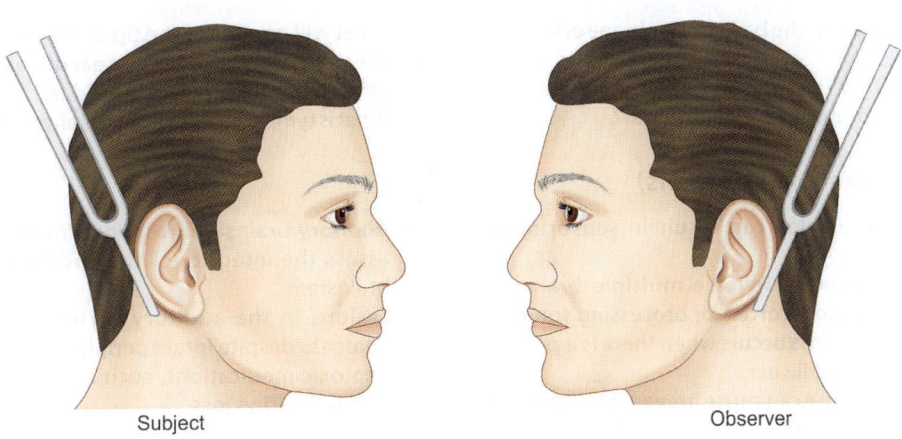

Fig. 96.22: Schwabach's test.

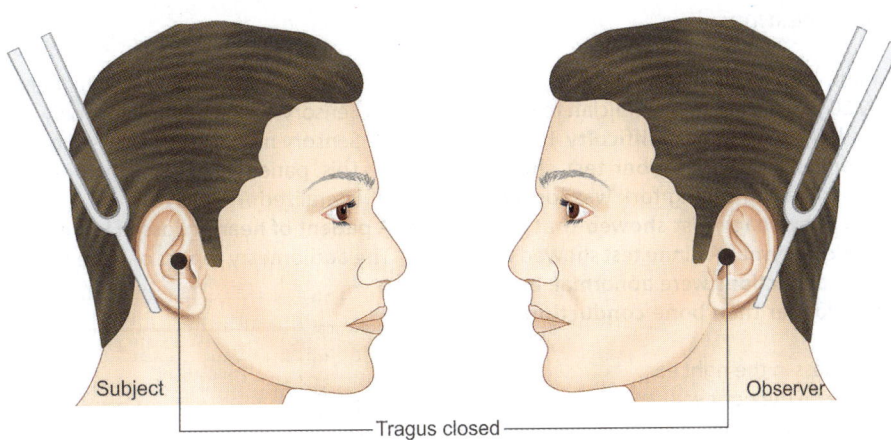

Fig. 96.23: Absolute bone conduction test.

**Table 96.4:** Different hearing tests and their findings in various conditions.

| Hearing test | Normal hearing | Conductive deafness | Nerve deafness |
| --- | --- | --- | --- |
| Rinne's test | Positive (AC>BC) | Negative (AC<BC) | Positive (AC>BC)<br>Though AC is less than normal |
| Weber's test | Equally heard in both ears | Lateralized to deaf ear | Lateralized to normal ear |
| Schwabach's test | Equal in subject and examiner | Subject's BC is better than the examiner's BC | Examiner's BC is better than the subject's BC |
| ABC test | Equal in subject and examiner | Equal in subject and examiner | Examiner's BC is better than the subject's BC |

## LET US SEE, HOW MUCH YOU HAVE LEARNT?

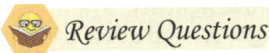 *Review Questions*

### Long Answer Questions

Q1. Describe the transmission of sound in the human ear.
Q2. Describe the functions of middle ear.
Q3. Draw a well labelled diagram of auditory pathway.
Q4. Differentiate between conductive hearing loss and sensorineural hearing loss.

### Short Answer Questions

Q1. Draw a well labelled diagram of organ of Corti.
Q2. Describe the functions of outer and inner hair cells.
Q3. Define the endocochlear potentials. What is its physiological basis?
Q4. Describe the process of mechanotransduction in the hair cell.
Q5. In space astronauts use sign language for communication. Justify your response.

Q6. How the movement of the basilar membrane affects hair cells?
Q7. What will happen in a person hearing if there is the complete absorption of air in middle ear?
Q8. What will happen, if the tip of cochlea is damaged?
Q9. How can prolonged used of ear dopes at a high volume, affect the hearing of an individual?
Q10. What is tympanic reflex? Give its physiological significance.

## Explain Why? (Reasoning Questions)

Q1. Damage to the cochlea can result in sensorineural hearing loss.
Q2. The auditory pathways involve multiple brainstem nuclei and the auditory cortex for processing sound.
Q3. Conductive hearing loss occurs when there is a problem with the outer or middle ear.
Q4. Exposure to loud noise can cause irreversible damage to hair cells in the inner ear.
Q5. Auditory brainstem response (ABR) testing is used to assess the integrity of the auditory pathways in the brainstem.
Q6. Lesions in the auditory cortex can lead to cortical deafness despite intact peripheral auditory structures.
Q7. Ototoxic medications, such as certain antibiotics, can lead to hearing loss.

## Multiple Choice Questions

Q1. A 40-year-old man, employed as a road construction worker for nearly 20 years, went to his clinician to report that he recently began to notice difficulty hearing during normal conversations. A Weber test showed that sound from a vibrating tuning fork was localized to the right ear. A Schwabach test showed that bone conduction was below normal. A Rinne test showed that both air and bone conductions were abnormal, but air conduction lasted longer than bone conduction. The diagnosis was:
  a. Conduction deafness in the right ear
  b. Sensorial deafness in the right ear
  c. Conduction deafness in the left ear
  d. Sensorineural deafness in the left ear

Q2. How does the brain determine the direction of a sound?
  a. By analyzing the intensity of the sound wave
  b. By comparing the time it takes for the sound to reach each ear
  c. By detecting the frequency of the sound wave
  d. By amplifying the sound vibrations in the cochlea

Q3. A 60-year-old female is having a some hearing loss. The audiometrist performs the pure tone audiometry and plots the audiogram shown below. What type of hearing loss is seen in this patient?

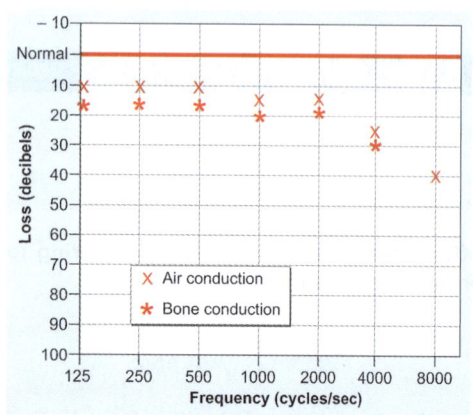

  a. Conductive hearing loss at higher frequencies
  b. Sensory neural hearing loss only at higher frequencies
  c. Sensory neural hearing loss suggestive of presbycusis
  d. This patient will show a positive Rinne's test and lateralized Weber's test

Q4. A patient of hearing loss in left ear, visits the ENT clinic. The audiometry report of left ear is shown below:

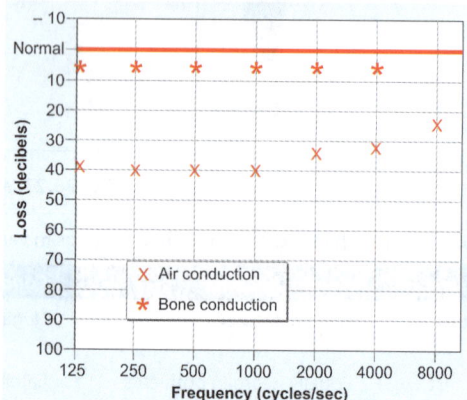

The tuning fork test for this test should show:
  a. Rinne's test is positive in both the ears and Weber's in lateralized to left ear
  b. Rinne's test is positive in right ear and negative in left ear and Weber's in lateralized to left ear
  c. Rinne's test is positive in right ear and negative in left ear and Weber's in lateralized to right ear
  d. Rinne's test is negative in right ear and positive in left ear and Weber's in lateralized to right ear

## ANSWERS

1. d   2. b   3. c   4. b

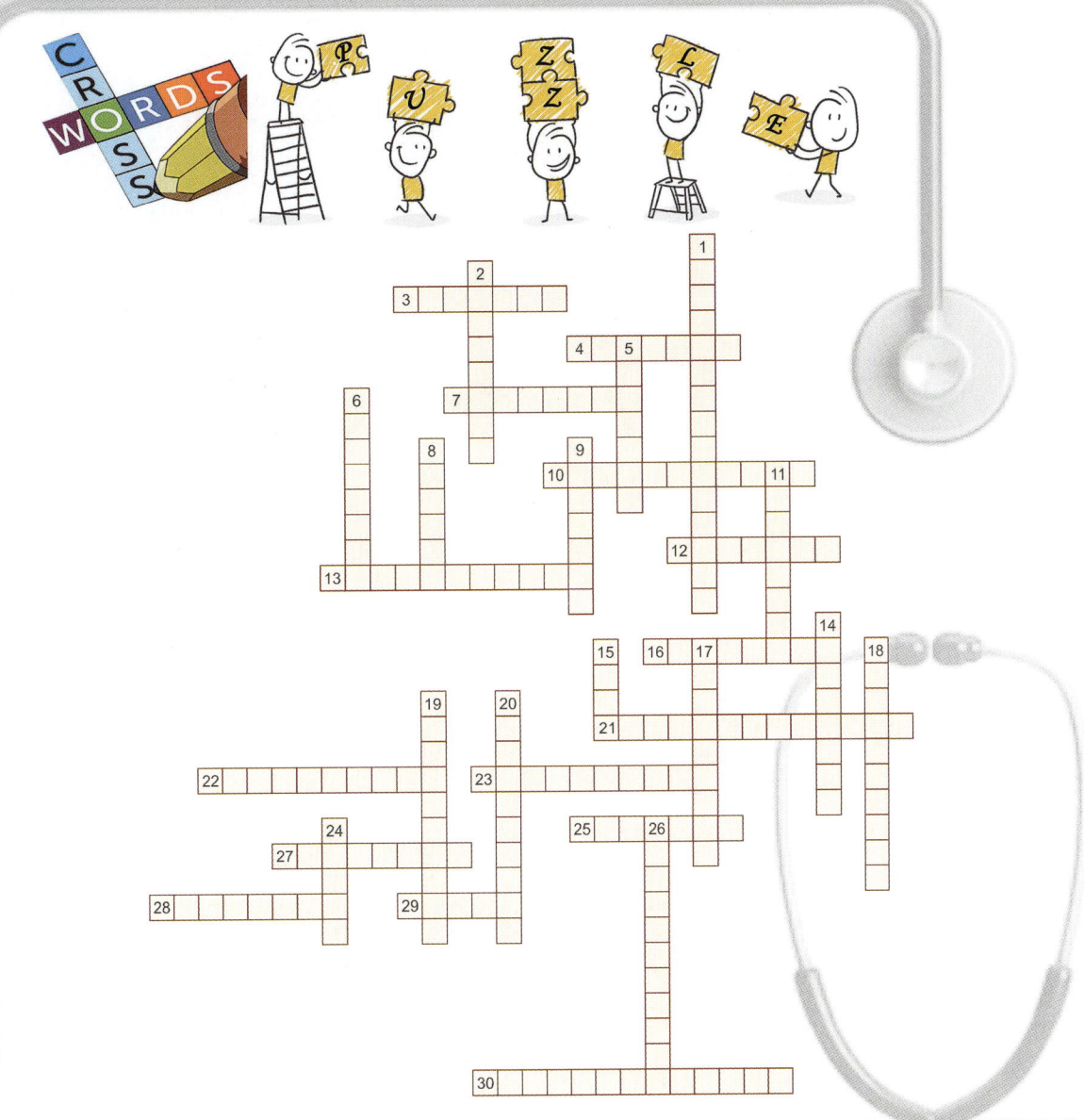

### Across

3. Lesion of Wernicke's area resulting in inability to recognize and identify objects
4. Frequency-detecting membrane in the cochlea
7. Brainstem structure that is involved in consciousness and alertness
10. Age-related hearing loss that presents bilaterally
12. Sensory structure providing information about head position
13. Division of spinal cord below L1 into many rootlets that resembles horse tail
16. Opacity in the lens or its capsule that occurs with aging
21. Pathway responsible for transmitting pain and temperature
22. Type of receptor for target organ in parasympathetic nervous system
23. Drug that inhibits the inhibitory neurotransmitter glycine in the spinal cord
25. Inner ear structure converting sound into neural signals
27. Primary motor area 4 located in motor cortex of frontal lobe
28. Area located behind the primary auditory cortex in the posterior part of the superior gyrus of the temporal lobe responsible for higher intellectual functions
29. Type of brain wave seen on EEG which is associated with deep sleep
30. Descending pathway for voluntary motor control

### Down

1. Type of receptors that are involved in detecting changes in pressure
2. Neurotransmitter linked to reward and pleasure pathways
5. Junction between the neurons, which results in the transmission of impulse from one neuron to another
6. Lesion of the angular gyrus resulting in difficulty in reading
8. Part of the retina that is responsible for sharp central vision
9. RAS role in sleep-wake cycle regulation
11. Test used to diagnose color blindness
14. Basal ganglia component involved in movement initiation
15. Retinal cell type detecting light intensity
17. Instrument used to measure the intraocular pressure
18. Type of receptor that is involved in pain perception
19. Cerebral cortex area involved in speech production
20. Reflex that helps maintain upright posture
24. Region of the retina with the highest visual acuity
26. Limbic system structure involved in long term memory

# SECTION 11

# INTEGRATED PHYSIOLOGY

## Section Outline

- **Chapter 97:** Temperature Regulation and Adaptation
- **Chapter 98:** Physiology of Physical Activity (Sedentary Lifestyle and Exercise)
- **Chapter 99:** Physiology of Infancy
- **Chapter 100:** Physiology of Aging, Free Radicals and Antioxidants
- **Chapter 101:** Physiology of Yoga and Meditation
- **Chapter 102:** Brain Death

# Temperature Regulation and Adaptation

## CHAPTER 97

> **COMPETENCY ADDRESSED**
> PY11.1: Describe and discuss mechanism of temperature regulation.
> PY11.2: Describe and discuss adaptation to altered temperature (heat and cold).
> PY11.3: Describe and discuss mechanism of fever, cold injuries and heat stroke.

> **LEARNING OBJECTIVES**
> At the end of this chapter, the learner should be able to:
> - Describe normal human body temperature, factors affecting it and why its regulation is needed?.
> - Describe heat producing and heat dissipating mechanisms of the body.
> - Describe regulation of temperature (adaptation to heat and cold).
> - Describe mechanisms of fever, cold injury and heat strokes.

## NORMAL HUMAN BODY TEMPERATURE

Human beings are homoeothermic with a very well-developed temperature maintaining mechanism in the body situated in the hypothalamus. The normal human body temperature ranges from 97°F to 99.5°F (36°C–37.5°C) and can be measured with a clinical thermometer. Extremities are generally cooler than rest of the body. The scrotal temperature is carefully regulated at 32°C (89.6°F) **(Fig. 97.1)**.

**Core temperature:** It is temperature of deeper body structures (e.g., temperature of intra-abdominal, intrathoracic and intracranial structures) and is maintained strictly constant.

- The core temperature **is always slightly more** than the oral temperature (about 37.8°C or 100°F).
- Rectal, vaginal and esophageal temperatures represent the core temperature.

### Factors Affecting Body Temperature

#### Physiological Variations

- **Diurnal variation:** Body temperature is highest in the evening (after day's labor—between 5 and 7 PM) and lowest in early hour of morning (after night's rest between 2 and 4 PM). There is difference between the two values may be 1°C. In the night workers, the rhythm is reversed. This diurnal variation is related to exercise and specific dynamic action of food. However, fasting and absolute bed rest abolish this variation.
- **Age:** Infants have an imperfect regulation of temperature. Hence, a fit of crying may raise and a cold bath may lower the body temperature. In old age, the body temperature tends to be subnormal due to decreased activity and decreased BMR. In addition, due to compromised circulatory system, older individuals cannot tolerate extremes of environmental temperature.
- **Sex:** *Females* have a slightly low body temperature due relatively low BMR and thick layer of subcutaneous fat (nonconductor). Due to thermogenic effect of

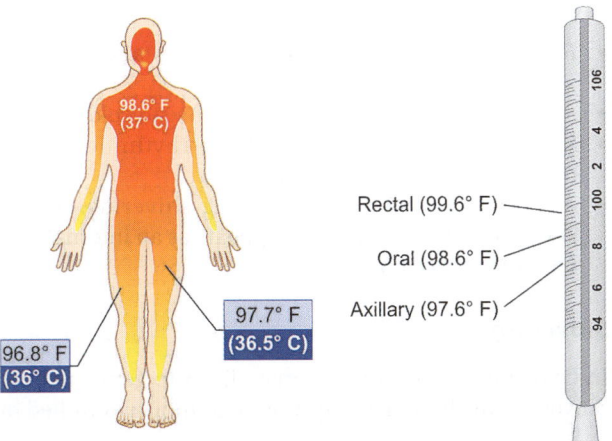

**Fig. 97.1:** Various body temperatures.

progesterone, the body temperature is higher in the secretory phase of menstrual cycle than in proliferative phase.
- **Size:** Heat production and heat loss depends upon the ratio of mass to body surface area.
- **Food:** Protein food, due to high specific dynamic action may raise body temperature. The ingestion of food may also raise BT
- **Exercise** increases temperature. Only 25% of muscular energy is converted into mechanical work, the rest comes out as heat.
- **Sleep:** Because of muscular inactivity, sleep results in a slight fall of body temperature.
- **Emotions:** Body temperature may rise due to emotional disturbances. The rise of temperature may be as high as 2°C due to tensing of muscles.

## Pathological Variations

- Hyperthermia or fever
- Hypothermia refers to the lowered body temperature (below normal) due to some pathological causes, such as:
  - Hypothyroidism
  - Hypopituitarism
  - Lesions in hypothalamus
  - Hemorrhage in certain parts of the brain, particularly pons.

Maintaining a constant body temperature is crucial for normal biochemical reactions because enzyme activities vary significantly with temperature. High body temperature can lead to nerve problems and protein damage. Severe cases may cause convulsions at temperatures of 41°C (106°F) or higher.

## HEAT PRODUCING AND HEAT DISSIPATING MECHANISMS OF THE BODY

Various mechanisms are involved in controlling the heat production or dissipation in human body. They are tabulated in **Table 97.1**.

## Heat Production Mechanisms (Fig. 97.2)

The body has various mechanisms for generating heat:

**Table 97.1:** Heat production and dissipation mechanisms.

| Heat producing mechanisms | Heat loss mechanisms |
| --- | --- |
| • BMR<br>• Muscular activity<br>• Shivering by sympathetic nerves<br>• Nonshivering thermogenesis (epinephrine, T3, T4)<br>• Skin and fat insulation | • Radiation, conduction convection<br>• Evaporation of water. (insensible perspiration–skin and RS membrane, sweating)<br>• Skin radiator system (blood flow 3 to 30 %) vaso (constriction/dilation) |

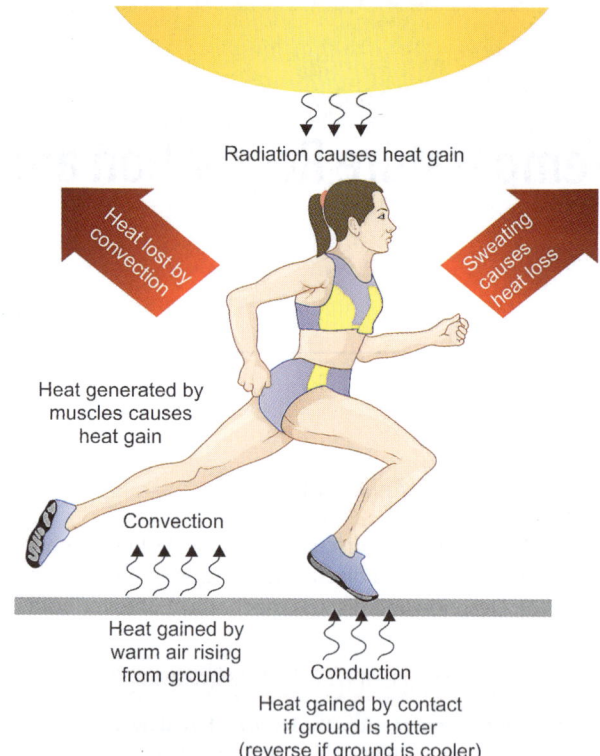

**Fig. 97.2:** Heat production.

## Basal Metabolic Rate (BMR)

All cells in the body constantly produce heat as part of their basic metabolic functions. Physiological oxidation of food materials, i.e., combustion of carbohydrates, proteins and fats. 1 g of each yields about 4, 4, and 9 calories, respectively. This is called *heat of metabolism*. Of all the organs, the liver contributes the highest amount of heat of metabolism. Heat produced by the liver and heart is relatively constant.

## Muscular Activity

Even at rest, muscles produce heat, with about 25% of their energy efficiency converting into heat. The heat produced during muscular activity is called *heat of activity*.
- *During exercise,* a great deal of heat is produced by the skeletal muscles.
- *Respiratory muscles activity* produces about 38% of activity heat.
- *Shivering* refers to the muscle response to cold.
- It is characterized by oscillating rhythmic muscle tremors occurring at a rate of 10–20/s.
- As no work is performed during shivering, all the energy liberated by muscles appears as an internal heat *(shivering thermogenesis)*.

## Shivering

In cold conditions, the body may shiver to generate heat. Shivering involves rhythmic muscle tremors controlled by the hypothalamus, increasing heat production significantly within seconds.

### Nonshivering Thermogenesis

Prolonged exposure to cold can increase metabolic rate due to hormonal changes, but this mechanism is minimal in adults.

### Heat Gain from Environment

*Ingestion* of hot fluids and food can add a small amount of heat to the body.

## Heat Dissipation Mechanisms (Fig. 97.3)

The body loses heat to the surroundings by radiation, conduction, convection and evaporation.
- Evaporation includes loss of water by sweating, respiration, etc.
- Vasodilatation leading to dissipation of heat from the surface of the skin to the environment
- Through the urine and feces by excretion

**Radiation:** Objects emit heat in the form of electromagnetic waves. Heat loss depends on the temperature difference between the skin and the environment.

**Conduction:** Heat transfer occurs through direct contact with cooler or warmer objects.

**Convection:** Heat loss is aided by the movement of air or water next to the body, carrying away heat and replacing it with cooler air.

**Evaporation:** Water evaporates from the skin and respiratory tract, cooling the body. Evaporation of sweat is a controlled process, crucial for heat dissipation.

## Heat Production and Distribution

Most heat is generated by deep organs like the liver, brain, muscles, and heart. Blood carries this heat to the skin, where it is dispersed to the surroundings through various mechanisms.

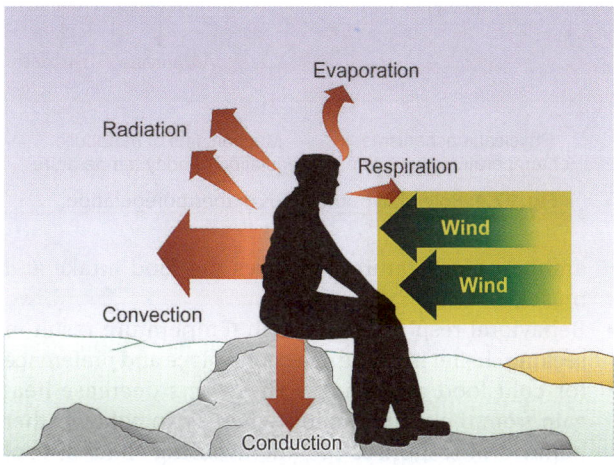

**Fig. 97.3:** Heat dissipation from body.

## REGULATION OF TEMPERATURE (OR ADAPTATION TO HEAT AND COLD)

The regulation of body temperature, known as *thermoregulation*, is maintained through a balance of heat production and heat loss, involving mechanisms like sweating, shivering, and blood flow adjustments. The hypothalamus in the brain acts as the body's thermostat, ensuring temperatures remain within a narrow, healthy range. They are tabulated in **Table 97.2**.

### Exposure to Heat

See **Flowchart 97.1**

### Exposure to Cold

See **Flowchart 97.2**.

### Temperature Control Mechanisms

- **Thermoreceptors:** Thermoreceptors or temperature receptors, which sense change in the body temperature and send information to the temperature control center in the hypothalamus. They are classified as peripheral

**Table 97.2:** Various regulatory mechanism for temperature adaptation.

| Center-hypothalamus | Anterior preoptic (heat loss, sweating) posterior nucleus (heat gain—shivering) |
|---|---|
| Input | • Peripheral thermoreceptors<br>• Central thermoreceptors<br>• Temperature of skin blood |
| Effects:<br>• Nervous<br>• Hormonal<br>• Metabolic<br>• Behavioral | • Readjust heat (gain/loss) mechanism)<br>• Vaso (constriction—sympathetic, dilation)<br>• Shivering—sympathetic, sweating<br>• Epinephrine and thyroid hormones<br>• Behavioral—clothes, body surface area, diet, activity, habits |

**Flowchart 97.1:** Regulation of body temperature on exposure to heat.

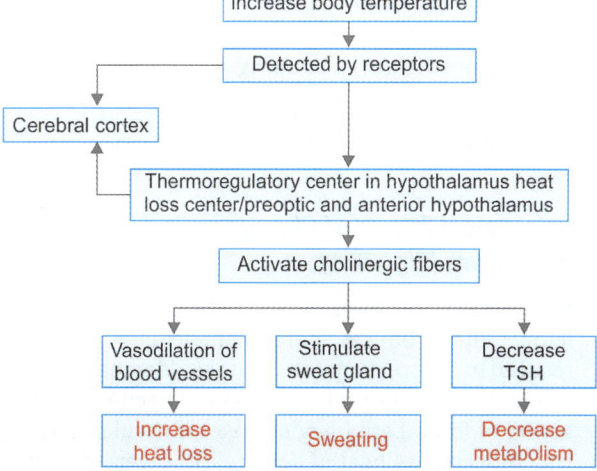

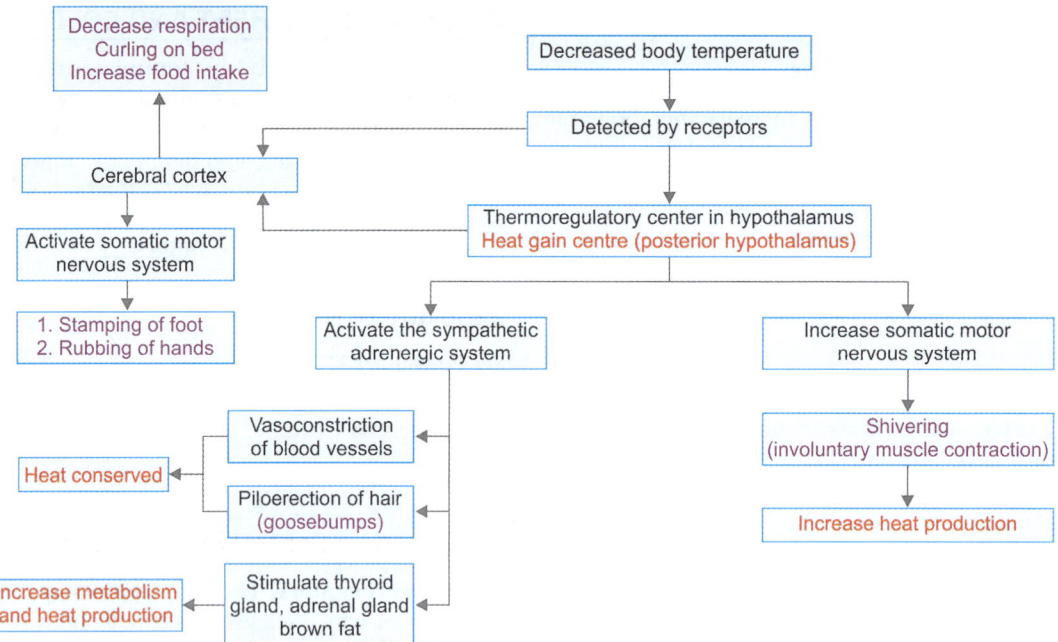

**Flowchart 97.2:** Regulation of body temperature on exposure to cold.

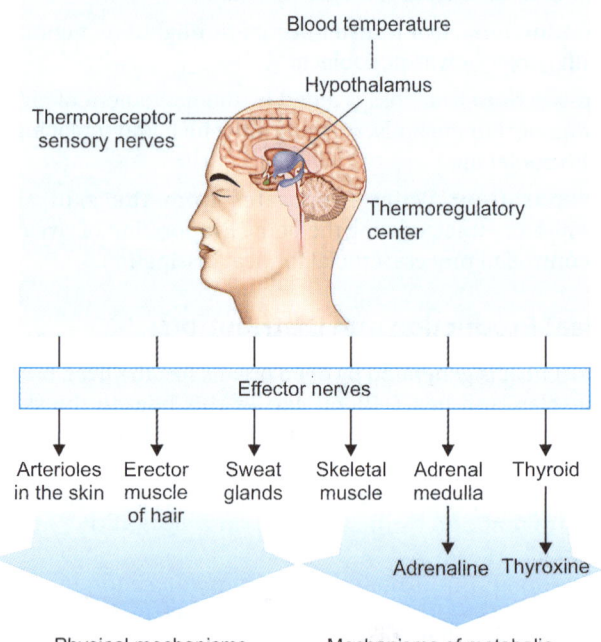

Fig. 97.4: Role of hypothalamus in thermoregulation.

**Thermoneutral zone:** It is **a range of temperatures of the immediate environment in which a standard healthy adult can maintain normal body temperature** without needing to use energy above and beyond normal basal metabolic rate. The values of thermoneutral zone in naked humans are:
- Adults: 26–28°C
- Newborn infants: 32–34°C and
- Premature infants: 35°C.

**Critical temperature:**
- It is the lower limit of thermoneutral zone.
- Below it the metabolic heat production of a resting thermoregulating animal increases to maintain thermal balance.

(present in skin, mucous membrane and viscera) and central (hypothalamus).
- Hypothalamus, the thermostat and integrator of temperature control system **(Fig. 97.4)**.

**Heat gain center:** Posterior hypothalamus
**Heat loss center:** Preoptic nuclei and anterior hypothalamus

### Physiological Effects of Change in Body Temperature (Fig. 97.5)

- **Food intake and muscle activity:** A rise in ambient temperature produces anorexia and lethargy. Anorexia results in decreased food intake, decreases heat production because of decrease in specific dynamic action of food. Lethargy decreases muscular activity, which decreases heat of activity. However, the fall in ambient temperature, increases the food intake and muscle activity.
- Behavioral responses to rise in temperature result in seeking shelter in shade or a cooler place and preference for cold food and drinks. These acts decrease heat gain from the environment. Whereas, in cold weather behavioral responses include avoiding shaded, cool places and preference for hot food and drinks.

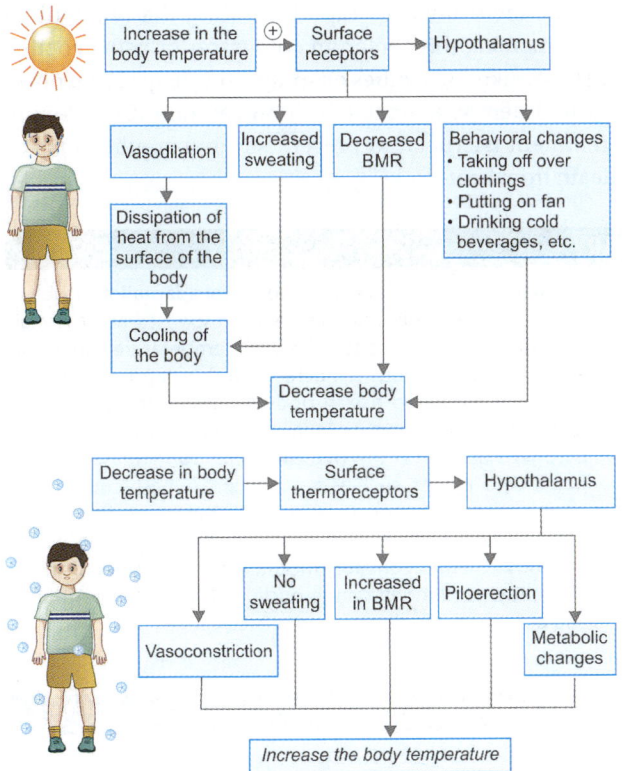

**Fig. 97.5:** Effects of increase and decrease in body temperatures.

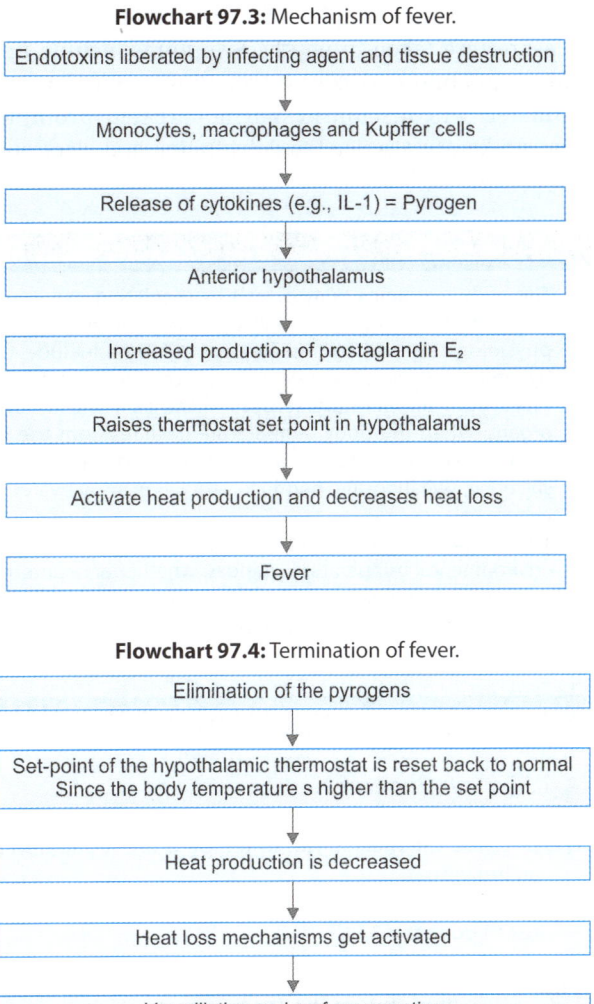

## Mechanisms of Fever, Cold Injury and Heat Strokes

### Fever Mechanism (Flowchart 97.3)

When the body's internal temperature controller, the hypothalamic thermostat, gets turned up due to invaders like bacteria or viruses, various processes kick into raise the body temperature back to its normal setting. This includes producing more heat and reducing heat loss. Initially, the body might shiver to generate extra heat, and the blood vessels under the skin tighten up to keep heat from escaping.

This rapid increase in temperature leads to flushed skin once it reaches its peak. During this time, sweat glands are inactive as the body tries to maintain its elevated temperature by boosting metabolism. If the trigger causing the high temperature is removed suddenly, the hypothalamic thermostat resets to normal, and the body starts cooling down through mechanisms like vasodilation (widening of blood vessels in the skin) and sweating. This sudden cooling phase is called *a "crisis" or "flush,"* where the skin becomes red and warm due to increased blood flow.

Antipyretic medications, such as aspirin, are thought to reset the hypothalamic thermostat back to normal, bringing down the body temperature.

### Termination of Fever

See **Flowchart 97.4**.

### Cold Injuries: Frostbite

When the body is exposed to extremely cold temperatures, certain areas like the ear lobes, fingers, and toes can freeze, leading to what's known as frostbite. If the freezing causes ice crystals to form within cells, it can result in permanent damage like impaired blood circulation, which can lead to tissue death (gangrene). Frostbitten areas often require surgical removal.

### Heat Stroke

Heat stroke is a serious condition commonly seen in hot climates or as a complication of conditions causing very high fever. It results from the body's inability to regulate its temperature. The body's tolerance to extreme heat depends on factors like humidity. Dry heat allows for more efficient cooling through sweat evaporation, while high humidity can make it harder for the body to cool down even at lower temperatures.

During heat stroke, the hypothalamic thermostat malfunctions, causing the body temperature to rise dangerously high (above 105–106°F). Sweating may stop, leading to further temperature increase unless cooling measures are taken promptly. Symptoms include high body temperature, dizziness, vomiting, confusion, and ultimately unconsciousness if not treated promptly. Heat stroke can also lead to dehydration and electrolyte imbalances.

Treatment involves rapidly cooling the body, often by immersing the person in cold water or using cooling methods like wet clothes or sprays. This helps bring down the body temperature to safer levels, around 101°F. Prompt treatment is crucial to prevent severe complications or death from heat stroke.

## SUMMARY

- The body maintains homeostasis by regulating its internal temperature through a complex process involving various physiological mechanisms. Key components include the hypothalamus, which acts as the body's thermostat, receiving input from temperature sensors in the skin and internal organs. When the body temperature deviates from the set point, mechanisms such as vasoconstriction or vasodilation, shivering, sweating, and hormonal regulation are activated to restore balance.
- The human body exhibits remarkable adaptability to environmental temperature changes, whether encountering extreme heat or cold. Adaptations include behavioral responses such as seeking shade or shelter, adjusting clothing layers, and altering activity levels. Physiological adaptations involve changes in metabolic rate, vasomotor responses, and thermal insulation mechanisms to cope with temperature variations and maintain core body temperature within narrow limits.
- Fever is a regulated rise in body temperature, typically in response to infection or inflammation. It is mediated by pyrogens acting on the hypothalamus to increase the set point. Cold injuries, such as frostbite and hypothermia, result from prolonged exposure to cold temperatures, leading to tissue damage and systemic effects. Heat stroke occurs when the body's thermoregulatory mechanisms fail to dissipate heat efficiently, resulting in dangerously high body temperatures and potentially life-threatening consequences.

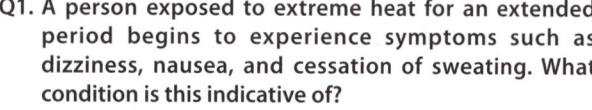

### Review Questions

Q1. Describe the mechanism of temperature regulation in an individual.
Q2. What will happen in a person, if his core temperature rises above the 37°C?
Q3. How the body temperature of a person is regulated, when he is exposed to 4°C of environmental temperature?

### Multiple Choice Questions

Q1. A person exposed to extreme heat for an extended period begins to experience symptoms such as dizziness, nausea, and cessation of sweating. What condition is this indicative of?
 a. Hypothermia b. Frostbite
 c. Heat stroke d. Chilblains
Q2. Which physiological response is activated by the body to conserve heat during cold exposure?
 a. Vasodilation b. Sweating
 c. Vasoconstriction d. Shivering
Q3. A hiker trekking in a snowy mountain region starts to notice numbness and discoloration of the fingers and toes. What cold-related injury is the hiker likely experiencing?
 a. Heat exhaustion
 b. Heat stroke
 c. Frostbite
 d. Hypothermia
Q4. What role does the hypothalamus play in temperature regulation?
 a. It synthesizes sweat glands
 b. It serves as the body's thermostat
 c. It promotes shivering responses
 d. It regulates blood pressure

Q5. A patient presents with symptoms of fever, including elevated body temperature, chills, and malaise. What mechanism underlies the development of fever?
 a. Increased production of sweat
 b. Vasodilation of blood vessels
 c. Activation of pyrogens acting on the hypothalamus
 d. Enhanced heat loss through radiation
Q6. How does the body respond to excessive heat to prevent overheating?
 a. By increasing shivering responses
 b. By promoting vasoconstriction
 c. By decreasing metabolic rate
 d. By initiating sweating and vasodilation
Q7. A person working outdoors in hot weather collapses and exhibits signs of confusion, rapid heart rate, and high body temperature. What condition is this indicative of?
 a. Hypothermia b. Heat stroke
 c. Frostbite d. Chilblains
Q8. What behavioral adaptation helps the body conserve heat in response to cold temperatures?
 a. Wearing light clothing
 b. Seeking shade
 c. Curling up to reduce surface area
 d. Sitting in direct sunlight

Q9. A person exposed to extreme cold develops symptoms such as slurred speech, confusion, and slowed heart rate. What condition is this indicative of?
   a. Frostbite
   b. Heat stroke
   c. Hypothermia
   d. Heat exhaustion

Q10. What physiological response helps the body dissipate heat during periods of elevated environmental temperature?
   a. Vasoconstriction
   b. Shivering
   c. Sweating
   d. Decreased metabolic rate

Q11. A person living in a tropical climate experiences persistent high body temperatures, dehydration, and confusion. What heat-related disorder might this person be at risk for?
   a. Frostbite
   b. Hypothermia
   c. Heat stroke
   d. Chilblains

Q12. What is the primary purpose of vasoconstriction during cold exposure?
   a. To conserve heat by reducing blood flow to the skin
   b. To increase heat loss through radiation
   c. To decrease metabolic rate
   d. To promote sweating

Q13. A person experiences prolonged exposure to cold temperatures and develops pale, numb skin accompanied by a tingling sensation. What cold-related injury is this indicative of?
   a. Frostbite
   b. Heat stroke
   c. Hypothermia
   d. Chilblains

Q14. What is the primary role of shivering during cold exposure?
   a. To increase metabolic rate
   b. To promote sweating
   c. To conserve heat through muscle contraction
   d. To enhance vasodilation

Q15. A person hiking in the desert starts to experience weakness, headache, and nausea due to prolonged exposure to high temperatures. What condition is this indicative of?
   a. Hypothermia
   b. Heat stroke
   c. Frostbite
   d. Chilblains

Q16. How does the body regulate core temperature during periods of elevated environmental temperature?
   a. By decreasing sweating and vasodilation
   b. By increasing shivering responses
   c. By promoting vasoconstriction
   d. By initiating sweating and vasodilation

Q17. A person working in a cold environment without proper protective clothing develops blisters and tissue damage on exposed skin areas. What cold-related injury is this indicative of?
   a. Frostbite
   b. Heat stroke
   c. Hypothermia
   d. Chilblains

Q18. What is the primary function of vasodilation during heat exposure?
   a. To reduce blood flow to the skin
   b. To decrease sweating
   c. To conserve heat
   d. To promote heat loss through radiation

Q19. A person participates in strenuous physical activity in hot weather and experiences cramps, headache, and dizziness. What condition is this indicative of?
   a. Hypothermia
   b. Heat stroke
   c. Frostbite
   d. Chilblains

Q20. What is the primary purpose of sweating during heat exposure?
   a. To increase metabolic rate
   b. To conserve heat
   c. To promote vasodilation
   d. To enhance heat loss through evaporation

## ANSWERS

1. c  2. c  3. c  4. b  5. c  6. d  7. b  8. c  9. c  10. c  11. c  12. a  13. d  14. c
15. b  16. d  17. a  18. d  19. b  20. d

# Physiology of Physical Activity
## (Sedentary Lifestyle and Exercise)

**CHAPTER 98**

> **COMPETENCY ADDRESSED**
>
> **PY11.4:** Describe and discuss cardiorespiratory and metabolic adjustments during exercise; physical training effects.
> **PY11.5:** Describe and discuss the physiological consequences of the sedentary lifestyle.
> **PY11.8:** Discuss and compare cardiorespiratory changes in exercise (isometric and isotonic) with that in the resting state and under different environmental conditions (heat and cold).

> **LEARNING OBJECTIVES**
>
> At the end of this chapter, the learner should be able to:
> - Understand the sedentary behavior and how it is distinct from lack of exercise or physical activity.
> - Recognize the sedentary behavior and its impact on physiological processes.
> - Explain the effect of reducing sedentary behavior.
> - Identify the differences between physical activity, exercise, and sports.
> - Describe the acute physiological responses of cardiovascular and respiratory adjustment during exercise.
> - Explain the changes in respiratory and cardiovascular systems due to regular indulgence in exercise and physical activity.
> - Understand the difference between isotonic/dynamic and isometric/static exercise.

The physical activity has a pronounced effect on our metabolism, cellular responses and the body physiology. Based on the levels of activity, the physical activity has been graded into a spectrum ranging from sedentary behavior to high intensity physical activity. Depending on the energy cost measured by the *indirect calorimetry or whole room calorimetry:*

- *Sedentary behavior* ranges between **1 to 1.5 MET** in healthy adults in postprandial states.
- *Low intensity duration exercise*, having **less than 3.0 MET**.
- *Moderate intensity exercise*, having **3.0 to 6.0 MET**.
- *High intensity exercise*, having **more than 6.0 MET**.

> - **MET stands for Metabolic Equivalent of Task,** which is a measure used to represent the energy cost of physical activities.
> - One MET is defined as the energy expended at rest, which is approximately equivalent to 1 kilocalorie per kilogram of body weight per hour for an average adult.

## RECOGNIZING SEDENTARY BEHAVIOR

Sedentary behavior and physical inactivity are often used interchangeably, but they represent different aspects of human movement. Sedentary behavior refers to prolonged periods of sitting or reclining with low energy expenditure. Physical inactivity denotes insufficient levels of moderate to vigorous intensity exercise or physical activity. The World Health Organization (WHO) has provided the following definitions as:

- **Sedentary behavior:** Sedentary behavior is defined as time spent sitting or lying with low energy expenditure (EE) (≤1.5 METs) while awake in the context of educational, home, and community settings and transportation.
- **Sedentary behavior pattern:** The manner in which sedentary behavior is accumulated, for example, timing of the day, duration, and frequency of bouts and breaks.
- **Passive standing:** Any waking activity characterized by an energy expenditure <2.0 METs while standing without ambulation.
- **Active standing:** Any waking activity characterized by an EE >2.0 METs while standing without ambulation.

Hence, individuals with sedentary behavior can be classified into four groups:
1. Physically active and highly sedentary
2. Physically active and slightly sedentary
3. Physically inactive and highly sedentary
4. Physically inactive and slightly sedentary

|  | Lying | Reclining | Sitting | Light PA 1.6 < 3.0 METs | Moderate PA 3.0 < 6.0 METs | Vigorous PA ≥6.0 METs |
|---|---|---|---|---|---|---|
| Sleep (<1 MET) | Sedentary behavior (1–1.5 METs) | | | Physical activity (>1.5 METS) | | |
| 24-hour movement and nonmovement behaviors | | | | | | |
| Continuum of human movement and nonmovement—refers to all behaviors, including sleep, sedentary behavior, standing, and physical activity at any intensity, that occur in the 24-hour interval. Behaviors comprised within the continuum differ in terms of type, posture, and physiological state—metabolic cost, oxygen consumption, heart rate, skeletal muscle activity, and blood flow—which may underpin health effects associated with each behavior. | | | | | | |

## Physiological Effects of Sedentary Lifestyle

A sedentary lifestyle can lead to various physiological effects, including increased risks of cardiovascular disease, obesity, and type 2 diabetes. Prolonged inactivity can also contribute to muscle atrophy, weakened bones, and poor circulation, significantly impacting overall health and well-being (Fig. 98.1 and Table 98.1).

After waking up in the morning, we first engage ourselves in some physical activity, moving muscles to

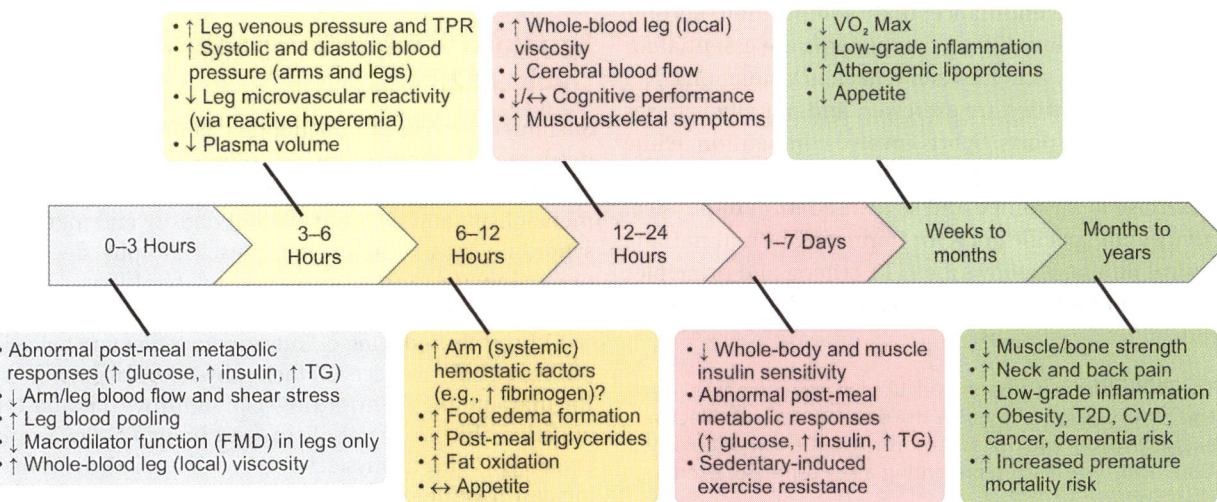

Fig. 98.1: Effects of sedentary lifestyle.

Table 98.1: Physiological responses to sedentary behavior.

| Physiological system | Changes |
|---|---|
| Metabolic changes | • Sedentary lifestyle shifts metabolism towards carbohydrate use over fat<br>• Low physical activity leads to low energy higher fasting triglycerides and lower fasting HDL (good cholesterol) levels<br>• Lack of activity can lower basal metabolic rate, worsening the energy surplus due to low energy utilization<br>• This imbalance can lead to weight gain and higher body fat percentage<br>• Prolonged sedentary behavior (SB) can lead to insulin resistance and glucose metabolism issues<br>• Poor glucose control increases cardiovascular disease risk, even in those without diabetes<br>• Chronic inactivity increases the risk of weight gain and other metabolic issues |
| Changes in cardiovascular system | • Impaired endothelial function due to reduction in blood flow and shear stress, potentially leading to atherosclerosis and cardiovascular diseases<br>• Extended periods of sitting have been associated with notable elevations in systolic blood pressure and mean arterial pressure in adults and older individuals |
| Respiratory system | Decline in $VO_2$ max |
| Musculoskeletal system | • Inactivity leads to muscle atrophy and changes in muscle fiber composition<br>• Shift in muscle fiber composition from oxidative to glycolytic types, decreasing muscle strength and function<br>• Loss of muscle strength and mass due to prolonged inactivity<br>• Decreased bone mineral density |
| CNS | • Reduced cerebral blood flow and impaired cognitive functions such as memory and executive function<br>• May lead to changes in brain structure and function, affecting neurogenesis and neurotransmitter levels<br>• Acute exposure to prolonged sedentary behavior can decrease cerebral blood flow velocity and cerebrovascular reactivity<br>• Prolonged sitting leads to impairment in dynamic cerebral autoregulation |

*Contd...*

Contd...

| Physiological system | Changes |
|---|---|
| Hematological changes | • Increased concentration of plasma C-reactive protein, IL-6, and TNF-α, contributing to systemic inflammation and chronic disease risk<br>• Influences the functioning of adaptive immunity, potentially impacting the body's ability to fight infections and diseases |

planned and unplanned activities utilizing the integrated circuitry of our organ systems. *This integration has made the human body extraordinary and unique. Do you know that, though physical activity and exercise are often used interchangeably, yet they are not the same? When we talk about sports, it also comes under physical activities, so what is physical activity?*

Physical fitness encompasses flexibility, muscle strength, muscle endurance, body composition, aerobic fitness, and balance. These components are essential for performing daily activities and emergency situations. Not all physical activities are exercises, and not all exercises are considered sports. Sports involve competition, while exercises are structured for improving fitness.

Exercise is a planned and structured form of physical activity with specific goals for improving or maintaining physical fitness. It follows the FITT criteria and principles like individuality, specificity, reversibility, progressive overload, and variations.

> The **FITT criteria** is a framework used in exercise physiology and fitness training to guide the development of effective exercise programs. It stands for Frequency, Intensity, Time, and Type, each representing a key aspect of exercise prescription.
> 1. **Frequency:** Refers to how often you exercise within a given timeframe, such as days per week.
> 2. **Intensity:** Relates to the level of exertion or difficulty of the exercise, often measured as a percentage of your maximum heart rate, perceived exertion, or weight lifted.
> 3. **Time:** Indicates the duration of each exercise session or the total duration of exercise per session.

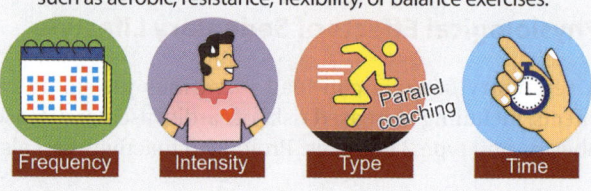

4. **Type:** Specifies the specific mode or kind of exercise performed, such as aerobic, resistance, flexibility, or balance exercises.

## Sustained vs Interrupting Sedentary Behavior (Table 98.2)

Sustained increases in sedentary behavior can lead to detrimental effects on various physiological parameters, such as reduced cardiovascular fitness, impaired glucose metabolism, and elevated risks of obesity and metabolic syndrome. It can also result in muscle atrophy, decreased bone density, and poorer mental health outcomes, including higher levels of anxiety and depression.

Conversely, reducing or interrupting sedentary behavior can have positive effects on these physiological parameters. Regular breaks from sitting can improve circulation, enhance glucose metabolism, and boost cardiovascular health. Engaging in physical activity can strengthen muscles, increase bone density, and contribute to better mental health by reducing stress and anxiety levels. These interruptions and reductions in sedentary behavior can significantly improve overall health and reduce the risk of chronic diseases.

## CLASSIFICATION OF EXERCISE

Exercise can be classified into several categories based on the type of activity and its primary benefits **(Table 98.3)**.

**Table 98.2:** Sustained effects of increasing sedentary behavior and reduction or interruption of sedentary behavior on various physiological parameters.

| Parameter | Sustained effects of increasing sedentary behavior | Sustained effects of reducing/interrupting sedentary behavior |
|---|---|---|
| Cerebrovascular blood flow | – | Increases |
| Mental well-being | – | Improves with activity |
| Cognitive performance | Lower | – |
| Waist circumference | Increases | Decreases |
| Body mass index | Increases | Decreases |
| Total body fat and adiposity | Increases | Decreases |
| Total fat-free mass | Decreases | Increases |
| Cardiorespiratory fitness | Increases | Decreases |
| Blood pressure | No significant change | Decreases |

Contd...

Contd...

| Parameter | Sustained effects of increasing sedentary behavior | Sustained effects of reducing/interrupting sedentary behavior |
|---|---|---|
| Fasting glucose and insulin concentration | Increases | Decreases |
| Postprandial glucose and insulin response | Increases | Decreases glucose variability |
| HbA1c | No significant change | Decreases |
| Insulin sensitivity | Decreases | Improves |
| Triglycerides | Increases | – |
| High-density lipoproteins | – | Decreases fasting levels |
| Carbohydrate oxidation | Increases | – |
| Lipid oxidation | Decreases | – |
| Vascular function | Increases vascular dysfunction (endothelin1 and nitric oxide secretion from endothelium getting affected) | Improves vascular functions |
| Muscle activity | Increases | Decreases |
| Muscle strength | Decreases | Increases |
| Bone mineral density | Decreases | Improves |
| Proinflammatory markers | Increases | – |
| Risk of depression | Increases (with mentally passive hours) | Improves |

**Table 98.3:** Classification of exercises.

| | | |
|---|---|---|
| By muscle contraction | Dynamic or isotonic | Muscle length changes during contraction involving joint movement, that can be either concentric or eccentric movement |
| | Static or isometric | Muscle contractions without a change in muscle length or joint movement |
| | Isokinetic | Performed with a constant speed of movement |
| By primary energy system | Aerobic | Exercise that relies on the use of oxygen to generate energy, i.e., oxidative phosphorylation in mitochondria—usually lower intensity and long duration |
| | Anaerobic | Exercise that does not use oxygen for ATP generation but glycogen lactate system—high intensity and short duration |
| By intensity and duration | Low-intensity PA | Exercises involving low oxygen consumption with less the 3.0 MET |
| | Moderate intensity PA | Exercises involving moderate oxygen consumption with 3.0 to 6.0 MET |
| | High-intensity PA | Exercises involving high oxygen consumption with more than 6.0 MET |
| By purpose | Strength training | Aimed at increasing muscular strength and size |
| | Endurance training | Designed to increase cardiovascular and muscular endurance |
| | Flexibility training | Focuses on improving the range of motion of joints |
| | Balance and coordination training | For enhancing balance and coordination |

## PHYSIOLOGICAL EFFECTS OF EXERCISE

Exercise exerts numerous positive physiological effects on the body, impacting various systems and promoting overall health **(Table 98.4)**.

**Table 98.4:** Effects of exercise on different physiological systems.

| | Isometric exercise | Isotonic exercise |
|---|---|---|
| Purpose | Muscle strengthening, and stabilization. It is used for rehabilitation due to the controlled nature of the exercise, which can minimize the risk of injury | Improves cardiovascular health, muscle strength, endurance, and coordination |
| | Strength training exercises | Endurance training/stamina building exercises |

Contd...

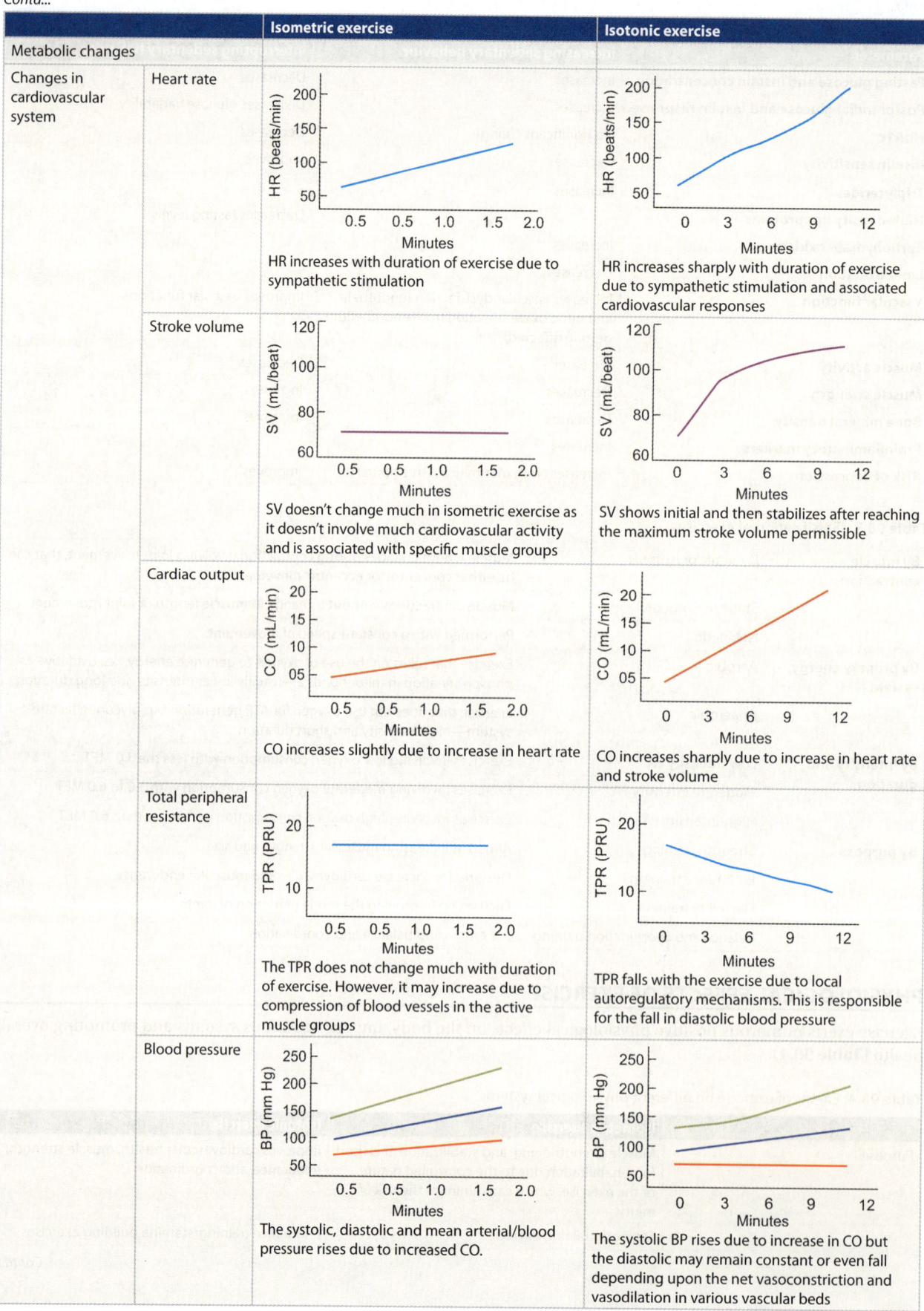

Contd...

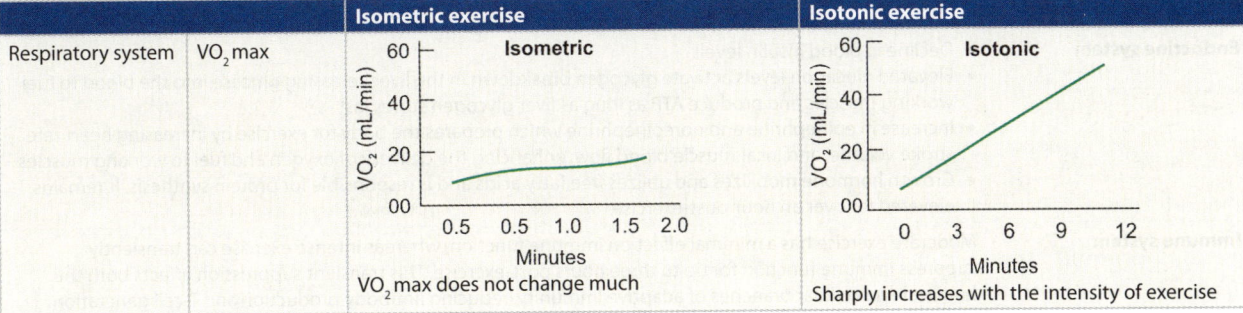

| | Isometric exercise | Isotonic exercise |
|---|---|---|
| Respiratory system | $VO_2$ max — $VO_2$ max does not change much | Sharply increases with the intensity of exercise |

## RESPONSE TO EXERCISE

During exercise, the body responds by increasing heart rate and blood flow to deliver more oxygen and nutrients to muscles, while the respiratory rate rises to enhance oxygen uptake and carbon dioxide removal. Additionally, energy production shifts to aerobic and anaerobic pathways to meet the heightened demand for ATP **(Table 98.5)**.

**Table 98.5:** Various responses to the exercise.

| | Acute response |
|---|---|
| **Respiratory response** | <ul><li>Increase in rate of respiration (from 12 breaths/min to 48 breaths/min)</li><li>Increase in depth of respiration (from 6 L/min to 192 L/min)</li><li>Increase in oxygen delivery to the tissues by more than 150 folds (from approximately 25 mL/min at rest to 4,000 mL/min)</li><li>$PO_2$ in working muscles is reduce to 20 mm Hg, leading to more pronounced unloading of oxygen from Hb</li><li>Increased blood oxygen carrying capacity</li><li>Removal of $CO_2$ increases by 40 folds</li><li>Diffusion capacity of increases significantly</li><li>Improved V/Q ratio</li></ul> |
| **Cardiovascular response** | <ul><li>The heart rate increases over time until it reaches the maximum heart rate</li><li>The stroke volume exhibits a linear increase at the beginning of exercise, but it may reach a plateau at submaximal workloads during graded exercise</li><li>The combination of increased heart rate and stroke volume leads to a consistent and proportional increase in cardiac output</li><li>Increased oxygen consumption</li><li>Redistribution of blood flow. Increased blood flow to active muscles (active hyperemia)</li><li>The systolic blood pressure increases steadily with an increase in exercise intensity in response to acute exercise, while diastolic blood pressure (DBP) remains relatively stable during aerobic exercise</li><li>During resistance exercise, both SBP and DBP can spike, especially during maneuvers like the Valsalva, sometimes reaching very high levels</li></ul> |
| **Blood volume** | <ul><li>RBC count increases in the initial duration of exercise, probably due to hemoconcentration</li><li>Increase in plasma volume, followed by a rise in red blood cell count</li><li>Increase in plasma volume is greater, leading to a decrease in hematocrit **(pseudo anemia of athletes)**</li><li>WBC count increases with strenuous exercise</li></ul> |
| **Nervous system** | Increase in sympathetic activity |
| **Thermoregulation** | Increased cutaneous blood flow to dissipate the heat and regulate the body temperature |
| **Musculoskeletal system** | <ul><li>Smaller motor units (with lower activation thresholds) are recruited first, followed by larger motor units (with higher activation thresholds) as force requirements increase to ensure a gradual increase in force output</li><li>Type I (slow twitch—oxidative and innervated by small diameter motor neuron with high conduction velocity)</li><li>Type II (fast twitch—glycolytic and innervated by large diameter motor neuron with low conduction velocity)<ul><li>Type IIa (fast-twitch—oxidative glycolytic) and</li><li>Type IIx (fast-twitch—glycolytic). Also called as power fibers are recruited during explosive movements like jumping, sprinting, and heavy lifting</li></ul></li></ul> |

Contd...

|  | Acute response |
|---|---|
| **Endocrine system** | • Decline in blood insulin levels<br>• Elevated glucagon levels activate glycogen breakdown in the liver, releasing glucose into the blood to fuel working muscles and produce ATP as long as liver glycogen stores last<br>• Increase in epinephrine and norepinephrine which prepares the body for exercise by increasing heart rate, stroke volume, and local muscle blood flow, enhancing the delivery of oxygen and fuel to working muscles<br>• Growth hormone mobilizes and utilizes free fatty acids and is responsible for protein synthesis. It remains elevated for over an hour post-exercise |
| **Immune system** | Moderate exercise has a minimal effect on immune function, whereas intense exercise can transiently suppress immune function for up to three hours post-exercise. This transient suppression affects both the humoral and cellular branches of adaptive immunity, reducing antibody production and T-cell generation. This phenomenon is described by the "Open Window Theory," which suggests that the immune system is temporarily weakened after intense exercise, increasing susceptibility to infections during the recovery period |

**Energy sources for exercise:**

The body utilizes three main energy systems to produce ATP, the primary source of energy for muscle contraction.

1. *The ATP-phosphocreatine-creatine system:* Provides immediate energy for high-intensity activities lasting up to 30 seconds. Phosphocreatine donates its phosphate group to convert ADP back into ATP in muscle tissue, replenishing depleted ATP levels. Most phosphocreatine stores can be restored within a 3-minute rest period.
2. *The glycogen-lactate system:* Also known as anaerobic metabolism or glycolysis, generates ATP in the absence of oxygen. Glucose is metabolized to pyruvate through glycolysis, producing two ATP molecules from glucose and three ATP molecules from glycogen. When oxygen levels are low, pyruvate is converted into lactate. This system serves as the primary energy source for activities lasting 1 to 3 minutes.
3. *The aerobic system:* Occurring within the mitochondria, utilizes oxidative phosphorylation to produce ATP. This process involves the Krebs cycle and the electron transport chain. In the presence of oxygen, pyruvate is converted into acetyl coenzyme A, which enters the Krebs cycle to produce ATP. Additionally, fats undergo lipolysis to produce glycerol and fatty acids, which are then converted into acetyl coenzyme A through beta-oxidation. Aerobic metabolism yields significantly more ATP compared to glycolysis and becomes the primary energy source for activities lasting longer than 3 minutes.

## LONG-TERM ADAPTATION OF EXERCISE (FIG. 98.2)

Long-term adaptation to exercise leads to improved cardiovascular efficiency, increased muscle strength and endurance, and enhanced metabolic function. These adaptations result in lower resting heart rate, increased stroke volume, greater mitochondrial density in muscles, and improved insulin sensitivity, contributing to overall enhanced physical fitness and health:

## EXERCISE IN EXTREME CLIMATE (HEAT AND COLD)

### In Hot Weather

In hot weather, exercise poses challenges to thermoregulation as the body copes with both metabolic heat from activity and environmental heat.
- Cardiovascular adjustments and increased sweating aid in dissipating heat through evaporative cooling.
- Exercising muscles and skin compete for blood flow, reducing stroke volume and increasing heart rate to maintain cardiac output.
- Reduced plasma volume from fluid loss can compromise aerobic capacity and lead to early fatigue.
- Vasoconstriction and vasodilation balance blood flow to active muscles and skin, potentially compromising visceral blood supply.
- Regulation of circulation prioritizes muscle blood flow over cooling, raising core temperature and risking heat-related illnesses.
- Factors like exercise intensity, duration, environmental conditions, and clothing affect dehydration risk.
- Dehydration impairs thermoregulation, reduces plasma volume, and increases cardiovascular strain.
- Even small fluid losses can impact performance, with severe dehydration severely limiting exercise capacity.
- Proper fluid replacement is crucial for maintaining performance and safety, especially in hot, humid environments.

### In Cold Weather

Exercising in cold environments presents challenges impacting performance and safety due to physiological responses:
- Muscle temperature decreases in the cold, affecting function and endurance, leading to degraded aerobic and strength performance.
- Maximal aerobic power can decrease significantly with dropping core temperatures, accompanied by lower heart rate and reduced muscle blood flow.
- Cold stress triggers vasoconstriction, shivering, and non-shivering thermogenesis to regulate core temperature.
- Peripheral vasoconstriction reduces blood flow to the skin and extremities, risking frostbite and impairing manual dexterity.

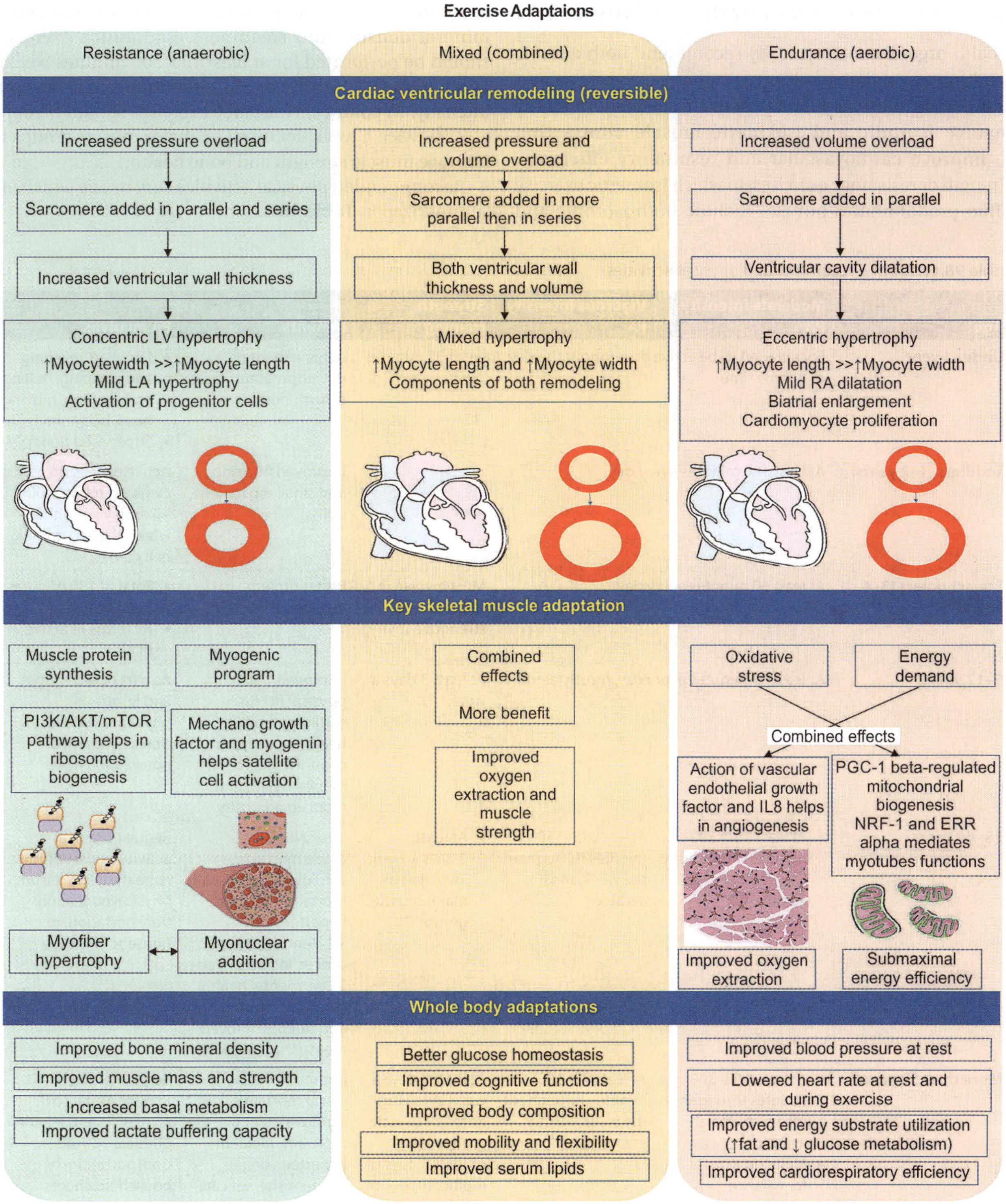

## Exercise Adaptations

### Resistance (anaerobic)

**Cardiac ventricular remodeling (reversible)**

Increased pressure overload → Sarcomere added in parallel and series → Increased ventricular wall thickness → Concentric LV hypertrophy
↑Myocyte width >> ↑Myocyte length
Mild LA hypertrophy
Activation of progenitor cells

**Key skeletal muscle adaptation**

- Muscle protein synthesis — PI3K/AKT/mTOR pathway helps in ribosomes biogenesis
- Myogenic program — Mechano growth factor and myogenin helps satellite cell activation
- Myofiber hypertrophy
- Myonuclear addition

**Whole body adaptations**

- Improved bone mineral density
- Improved muscle mass and strength
- Increased basal metabolism
- Improved lactate buffering capacity

### Mixed (combined)

**Cardiac ventricular remodeling (reversible)**

Increased pressure and volume overload → Sarcomere added in more parallel then in series → Both ventricular wall thickness and volume → Mixed hypertrophy
↑Myocyte length and ↑Myocyte width
Components of both remodeling

**Key skeletal muscle adaptation**

- Combined effects
- More benefit
- Improved oxygen extraction and muscle strength

**Whole body adaptations**

- Better glucose homeostasis
- Improved cognitive functions
- Improved body composition
- Improved mobility and flexibility
- Improved serum lipids

### Endurance (aerobic)

**Cardiac ventricular remodeling (reversible)**

Increased volume overload → Sarcomere added in parallel → Ventricular cavity dilatation → Eccentric hypertrophy
↑Myocyte length >> ↑Myocyte width
Mild RA dilatation
Biatrial enlargement
Cardiomyocyte proliferation

**Key skeletal muscle adaptation**

- Oxidative stress
- Energy demand

Combined effects:
- Action of vascular endothelial growth factor and IL8 helps in angiogenesis
- PGC-1 beta-regulated mitochondrial biogenesis; NRF-1 and ERR alpha mediates myotubes functions
- Improved oxygen extraction
- Submaximal energy efficiency

**Whole body adaptations**

- Improved blood pressure at rest
- Lowered heart rate at rest and during exercise
- Improved energy substrate utilization (↑fat and ↓glucose metabolism)
- Improved cardiorespiratory efficiency

**Fig. 98.2:** Adaptations to exercise.

- Chronic cold exposure can lead to "thermoregulatory fatigue," diminishing the body's heat maintenance abilities.
- Cold increases the metabolic cost of exercise, shifting metabolism towards anaerobic pathways quicker, leading to higher lactate levels and early fatigue.
- Cold-induced diuresis, respiratory fluid losses, and reduced fluid intake can lead to dehydration, impairing temperature regulation and performance.
- Proper hydration and carbohydrate intake are vital for maintaining performance and preventing hypothermia in cold conditions.

## Recommendations for Physical Activity

Health organizations typically recommend both aerobic (endurance) and anaerobic (resistance) exercises as part of a healthy lifestyle. Endurance exercises predominantly involve isotonic and isokinetic muscle contraction to improve cardiovascular and respiratory efficiency, strength or resistance exercises, in which isometric exercise often predominates but can include both isotonic and isometric exercises, help develop muscle strength, bone mineral density, and steadiness. Endurance exercises should be performed for at least 150–300 minutes weekly at a moderate intensity or 75–150 minutes at a vigorous intensity. In contrast, resistance exercises should be done at least twice a week, focusing on major muscle groups to improve muscle strength and bone health.

Recommended physical activities vary by age which are summarized in **Table 98.6**.

**Table 98.6:** Age and recommended physical activities.

| Age | Moderate intensity PA | Vigorous intensity PA | Strength training | Benefits | PA involves |
|---|---|---|---|---|---|
| **Under 1 year** | Encouraged to be active throughout the day. At least 30 minutes of tummy time | | | Achievement of developmental growth point | • Crawling, reaching and grasping, pulling and pushing, moving head, body and limbs<br>• Supervised floor play |
| **Toddlers (1–2 years)** | At least 180 minutes every day | | | Improved fine grip and small movement skills | Active play using a climbing frame, riding bike, playing in the water, chasing games, ball games, etc. |
| **Pre-schoolers (3–4 years)** | At least 60 minutes every day | | Must involve in some form of strength activity | Better growth milestone | • Total of 180 minutes per day<br>• All forms of active play |
| **5–17 years** | At least 60 minutes every day, mostly aerobic | | At least 3 days a week | Improved physical fitness, cardiometabolic health, bone health, cognitive outcome, mental health and reduced adiposity | As part of recreation and leisure, physical education, transportation, or household chores |
| **18–64 years** | • At least 150–300 minutes throughout the week, mostly aerobic | At least 75–150 minutes throughout the week, mostly aerobic | • At least 2 days a week involving all major muscle groups | Improved all-cause mortality, cardiovascular disease mortality, incident hypertension, incident site-specific cancer, incident type-2 DM, mental health, cognitive health, and sleep; improved measures of adiposity | Regular physical activity as part of recreation and leisure, physical education, transportation, or household chores |
| **More than 65 years** | • At least 150–300 minutes throughout the week, mostly aerobic<br>• Multicomponent PA for balance | At least 75–150 minutes throughout the week, mostly aerobic | At least 2 days a week involving all major muscle groups<br>At least 3 days of multicomponent activities to enhance functional capacity and prevent fall | Improved all-cause mortality, cardiovascular disease mortality, incident hypertension, incident site-specific cancer, incident type-2 DM, mental health, cognitive health, and sleep; improved measures of adiposity; help in falls and fall-related injuries and decline bone health and functional ability | Regular physical activity As part of recreation and leisure, physical education, transportation, or household chores |

*Contd...*

Contd...

| Age | Moderate intensity PA | Vigorous intensity PA | Strength training | Benefits | PA involves |
|---|---|---|---|---|---|
| Pregnant and postpartum women | • At least 150 minutes; incorporated aerobic and muscle strengthening activity; gentle stretch<br>• Women should continue their normal physical activity for which they are habitual | | | Decreased risk of pre-eclampsia, gestational diabetes, excessive gestational weight gain, delivery complications, and postpartum depression and fewer newborn complications, no adverse effect on birthweight; and no increase of stillbirth | Regular physical activity as part of recreation and leisure, physical education, transportation, or household chores |

A word of caution for exercise enthusiasts: Indulgence more than 2,000 min per week or 4 hours per day can have adverse effect on health.

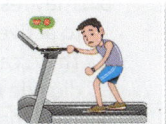

## SUMMARY

Sedentary behavior presents a significant public health concern, associated with a plethora of negative physiological outcomes such as cardiovascular diseases, metabolic dysfunction, and weight gain. During prolonged periods of sedentary behavior, the body's preference for carbohydrate over lipid oxidation can lead to energy imbalances and metabolic decline, exacerbating the risk of weight gain and insulin resistance. Furthermore, sedentary behavior adversely affects cardiovascular and cognitive functions, contributing to endothelial dysfunction and cognitive decline. Interventions aimed at reducing sedentary time, complemented by regular physical activity, offer synergistic health benefits. Interrupting prolonged sitting with light physical activity has been shown to improve metabolic responses and vascular function, emphasizing the importance of addressing sedentary behavior as a modifiable risk factor for improving health outcomes.

In contrast, physical activity, exercise, and sports are distinct entities with differing structures, purposes, and competitive natures. Exercise involves planned, structured movements with specific fitness goals aimed at improving physical fitness. These movements trigger acute adjustments in cardiovascular and respiratory systems, leading to adaptations improving efficiency and endurance over time. Metabolic responses to exercise involve the utilization of carbohydrates, fats, and proteins to meet energy demands. Additionally, environmental temperature influences physical activity responses, impacting performance and the risk of heat-related illnesses. Testing exercise capacity involves various methods, including maximal oxygen consumption ($VO_2$ max) testing and lactate threshold assessment, providing insights into an individual's fitness level and aerobic capacity.

## LET US SEE, HOW MUCH YOU HAVE LEARNT?

 *Review Questions*

### Long/Short Answer Questions

**Q1.** Describe the effect of sedentary lifestyle of metabolism.
**Q2.** Describe how the effects of sedentary lifestyle can be minimized?
**Q3.** Describe the cardiorespiratory changes occurring during exercise.
**Q4.** Describe the physiological adjustments occurring due to exercise.

 *Multiple Choice Questions*

**Q1.** Sedentary behavior refers to:
  a. Intense physical activity
  b. Prolonged periods of sitting or reclining with low energy expenditure
  c. Regular exercise routines
  d. Engaging in sports activities

**Q2.** Sedentary behavior is distinct from lack of exercise or physical activity because:
  a. Sedentary behavior involves intense physical activity
  b. Lack of exercise involves prolonged periods of sitting
  c. Sedentary behavior includes both sitting and standing activities

d. Lack of exercise refers to not engaging in structured physical activity

Q3. Which of the following health outcomes is NOT associated with sedentary behavior?
a. Obesity
b. Cardiovascular disease
c. Increased muscle strength
d. Type 2 diabetes

Q4. Interrupting prolonged sitting with short breaks or light physical activity can:
a. Increase the risk of chronic diseases
b. Improve blood flow and insulin sensitivity
c. Lead to muscle weakness
d. Have no impact on health outcomes

Q5. Sedentary behavior has been linked to an increased risk of:
a. Enhanced metabolic rate
b. Improved cardiovascular health
c. Type 1 diabetes
d. Metabolic syndrome

Q6. Which of the following is a strategy to reduce sedentary behavior?
a. Sitting for prolonged periods without breaks
b. Engaging in intense physical activity for long durations
c. Incorporating more movement throughout the day
d. Avoiding standing or walking activities

Q7. Public health interventions aimed at reducing sedentary behavior may include:
a. Encouraging prolonged sitting
b. Discouraging light physical activity breaks
c. Workplace interventions promoting sedentary behavior
d. Educational campaigns promoting movement breaks

Q8. Sedentary behavior is associated with negative changes in:
a. Muscle strength
b. Blood flow and insulin sensitivity
c. Increased metabolic rate
d. Improved cardiovascular health

Q9. Sedentary behavior and physical inactivity represent different aspects of human movement on the continuum of activity. (True/False)

Q10. Which of the following is NOT a potential consequence of sedentary behavior?
a. Increased risk of obesity
b. Improved cognitive function
c. Elevated risk of cardiovascular disease
d. Impaired blood flow

Q11. What characterizes an isotonic muscle contraction?
a. Static muscle length with no visible joint movement
b. Dynamic movement with changes in muscle length and joint movement
c. Muscle lengthening while generating force
d. No change in muscle length despite tension generation

Q12. During which type of muscle contraction does the muscle shorten as it contracts, generating force to move a load?
a. Isometric contraction
b. Eccentric contraction
c. Concentric contraction
d. Isotonic contraction

Q13. Which term describes a muscle contraction where the muscle lengthens while still generating force, often as it controls the movement of a load?
a. Isometric contraction
b. Eccentric contraction
c. Concentric contraction
d. Isotonic contraction

Q14. What is a characteristic systemic change during isotonic muscle contractions?
a. Sustained muscle contraction without visible joint movement
b. Static muscle length with dynamic joint movement
c. Increased blood pressure due to sustained muscle contraction
d. Decreased cardiovascular and respiratory responses

Q15. How do isotonic muscle contractions primarily affect cardiovascular responses during exercise?
a. They lead to decreased heart rate and blood pressure
b. They result in increased cardiac output and blood flow to active muscles
c. They cause decreased oxygen uptake and carbon dioxide removal
d. They have no significant impact on cardiovascular responses

Q16. What is a common physiological response to isometric muscle contractions?
a. Increased heart rate and blood flow to active muscles
b. Static muscle length with no visible joint movement
c. Decreased blood pressure due to decreased cardiac output
d. Rapid muscle fatigue and reduced endurance

Q17. How does blood pressure typically respond during isometric muscle contractions?
a. It decreases due to decreased cardiac output
b. It remains unchanged
c. It increases significantly due to sustained muscle contraction
d. It fluctuates randomly during muscle contraction

Q18. Which type of muscle contraction is often used in rehabilitation settings due to its controlled nature?
a. Isotonic contraction
b. Concentric contraction
c. Eccentric contraction
d. Isometric contraction

Q19. What is a primary benefit of isometric muscle contractions?
a. They improve cardiovascular fitness
b. They enhance muscle flexibility
c. They minimize the risk of injury
d. They strengthen muscles at specific joint angles

Q20. During isotonic muscle contractions, what happens to the muscle length?
a. It remains constant
b. It shortens as the muscle contracts
c. It lengthens while generating force
d. It fluctuates rapidly

Q21. What encompasses all bodily movements requiring energy expenditure?
a. Exercise
b. Sports
c. Physical activity
d. Rest

Q22. Which term refers to planned, structured, and repeated movements aimed at improving or maintaining physical fitness?
a. Physical activity
b. Sports
c. Exercise
d. Recreation

Q23. Which of the following may not meet the criteria for exercise?
a. Jogging for 30 minutes daily
b. Climbing stairs at work
c. Walking the dog
d. Playing basketball with friends

Q24. What are the acute adjustments in cardiovascular and respiratory systems during exercise primarily aimed at?
a. Reducing oxygen uptake
b. Decreasing heart rate
c. Meeting increased oxygen demand
d. Decreasing ventilation rate

Q25. Which physiological response increases during exercise to facilitate oxygen uptake and carbon dioxide removal?
a. Heart rate
b. Blood pressure
c. Respiratory rate and depth
d. Blood glucose levels

Q26. Regular exercise leads to adaptations in which systems, improving efficiency and endurance?
a. Cardiovascular and respiratory
b. Digestive and nervous
c. Skeletal and muscular
d. Endocrine and immune

Q27. Which cellular processes play crucial roles in providing energy during exercise?
a. Glycolysis, oxidative phosphorylation, and ATP production
b. DNA replication, transcription, and translation
c. Photosynthesis and respiration
d. Mitosis and meiosis

Q28. What are isotonic exercises characterized by?
a. Static contractions without visible joint movement
b. Dynamic movements with changes in muscle length and joint movement
c. Rapid muscle fatigue
d. Reduced heart rate

Q29. What is the primary difference between isotonic and isometric exercises?
a. Isotonic exercises involve dynamic movements, while isometric exercises involve static contractions
b. Isotonic exercises are performed in water, while isometric exercises are performed on land
c. Isotonic exercises are more intense than isometric exercises
d. Isotonic exercises primarily target flexibility, while isometric exercises primarily target strength

Q30. How does environmental temperature affect physical activity responses?
a. It has no impact on physical activity responses
b. It increases thermoregulation and sweat rate
c. It decreases heart rate and blood pressure
d. It enhances muscle strength and endurance

Q31. Which of the following is an acute physiological response to exercise?
a. Decreased heart rate
b. Decreased ventilation rate
c. Increased cardiac output
d. Decreased blood pressure

Q32. Isotonic exercises involve:
a. Static contractions without visible joint movement
b. Dynamic movements with changes in muscle length and joint movement
c. Rapid muscle fatigue
d. Reduced heart rate

## ANSWERS

1. b   2. d   3. c   4. b   5. d   6. c   7. d   8. b   9. T   10. b   11. b   12. c   13. b   14. b
15. b   16. b   17. c   18. d   19. d   20. c   21. c   22. c   23. c   24. c   25. c   26. a   27. a   28. b
29. a   30. b   31. c   32. b

# Physiology of Infancy

**CHAPTER 99**

### COMPETENCY ADDRESSED
**PY11.6:** Describe physiology of infancy.
**PY11.10:** Interpret anthropometric assessment of infants.

### LEARNING OBJECTIVES
**At the end of this chapter, the learner should be able to:**
- Describe the changes in anthropometric measurements of the infants.
- Describe the physiological changes in various systems after birth, during the period of infancy.

Infancy is the earliest stage of human life, typically spanning from birth to around one year of age. It represents a critical period characterized by rapid growth, development, and adaptation to the external environment. During infancy, infants undergo significant physiological changes as they transition from intrauterine life to independent existence outside the womb. This period is marked by unique milestones in physical, cognitive, motor, and social-emotional domains, laying the foundation for lifelong health and well-being.

## DEVELOPMENTAL MILESTONES

They refer to key achievements or abilities that infants typically reach at specific ages during the infancy period. These milestones encompass various aspects of development, including:
- Motor skills (such as rolling over, crawling, and walking)
- Cognitive skills (such as object permanence and language development)
- Social-emotional skills (such as bonding with caregivers and expressing emotions)
- Sensory-perceptual skills (such as responding to stimuli and exploring the environment).

Understanding developmental milestones is crucial for monitoring infant development, identifying potential delays or concerns, and providing appropriate support and intervention when needed.

## IMPORTANCE OF UNDERSTANDING INFANT PHYSIOLOGY

- **Growth and development:** Infancy is characterized by *rapid physical growth and development*, with infants doubling their birth weight by around six months and tripling it by one year. Understanding infant physiology helps healthcare providers and caregivers track growth parameters such as weight, length/height, and head circumference, ensuring that infants are progressing healthily **(Fig. 99.1)**.
- **Nutritional needs:** Infants have unique nutritional requirements to support their growth and development. Breastfeeding and the introduction of solid foods play crucial roles in meeting these needs. Knowledge of infant physiology helps caregivers make informed decisions about feeding practices, ensuring adequate nutrition, and promoting optimal health outcomes.
- **Health monitoring:** Infants are susceptible to various health issues, including infections, nutritional deficiencies, and developmental disorders. Understanding infant physiology enables healthcare providers to assess and monitor infants' health status, identify potential concerns, or risk factors early on, and intervene promptly to prevent or address health problems.
- **Parental guidance:** Parents and caregivers play a vital role in nurturing and supporting infant development. Understanding infant physiology empowers parents to

infant physiology. Research in areas such as neonatal medicine, developmental psychology, and nutritional science drives innovation in healthcare practices, interventions, and technologies aimed at improving infant health outcomes and promoting optimal development.

## Growth in Infancy

### Physical Growth

This can be assessed by monitoring the *anthropometric measurements* of the children.

### Weight Gain

Infancy is characterized by *rapid weight gain*, with infants typically doubling their birth weight by around six months and tripling it by one year of age. Weight gain serves as an essential indicator of infant health and nutritional status, reflecting the adequacy of feeding practices and growth trajectory.

Infant weight is one of the *most critical anthropometric measurements*. It is typically plotted on growth charts to track weight gain over time. Weight percentile curves are used to compare an infant's weight to that of other infants of the same age and sex. Adequate weight gain is essential for overall growth and development, while inadequate weight gain may indicate malnutrition or underlying health issues.

### Length/Height Gain

Along with the weight gain, infants experience significant growth in length or height during the infancy period. Length (for infants up to 2 years old) or height (for older infants) is another important anthropometric measurement. Length/height gain reflects skeletal growth and overall body development, contributing to the infant's physical stature and proportions. Monitoring length/height gain allows healthcare providers to *track linear growth patterns* and assess whether infants are growing proportionally and achieving appropriate developmental milestones.

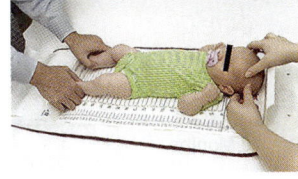

Length/height percentiles indicate whether an infant's growth is within the expected range for their age and sex.

### Head Circumference

Head circumference is measured around the infant's head at the widest part. It is also plotted on growth charts, with percentile curves indicating whether an infant's head size is typical for their age and sex. Deviations from the expected range may signal issues such as microcephaly or macrocephaly. Infants' head circumference

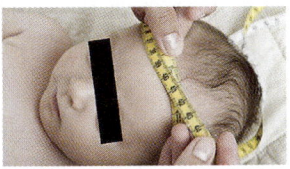

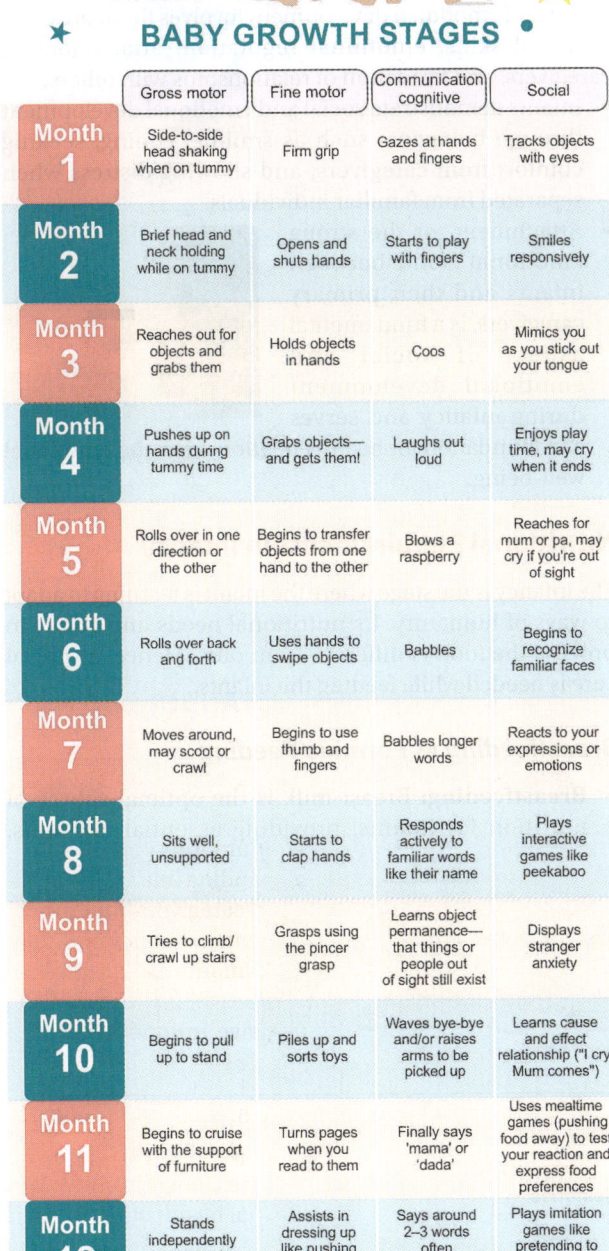

**Fig. 99.1:** Stages of growth and development.

recognize normal developmental milestones, provide appropriate care and stimulation, and seek assistance if developmental delays or health issues arise. It fosters positive parent-child interactions and promotes healthy attachment and bonding.

- **Research and innovation:** Advancements in neonatal and infant healthcare rely on a deep understanding of typically increases rapidly during the first few months of life, reflecting brain growth and expansion of the skull.

### Motor Development

Motor development refers to the progression of movement skills and abilities during infancy, including both gross motor skills (involving larger muscle groups) and fine motor skills (involving smaller muscle groups).

- Gross motor milestones include activities such as rolling over, sitting up, crawling, standing, and walking, which reflect the maturation of the central nervous system and musculoskeletal system (**Fig. 99.2**).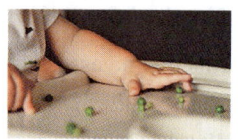
- Fine motor milestones encompass skills such as grasping objects, reaching for toys, and manipulating small objects, demonstrating the development of hand-eye coordination and manual dexterity.

### Cognitive Development

Cognitive development refers to the acquisition of mental processes and abilities, including perception, memory, problem-solving, language development, and understanding of the world.

- During infancy, cognitive development progresses rapidly, with infants demonstrating increasing awareness of their surroundings, recognition of familiar faces and objects, and engagement in simple problem-solving tasks.
- Key cognitive milestones include reaching for and manipulating objects, responding to stimuli, babbling and vocalizing, imitating sounds and gestures, and eventually understanding and producing words.

### Social and Emotional Development

Social and emotional development involves the acquisition of social skills, emotional regulation, attachment to caregivers, and formation of relationships with others.

- Infants demonstrate social and emotional development through behaviors such as smiling, cooing, seeking comfort from caregivers, and showing distress when separated from familiar individuals.
- Attachment, or the strong emotional bond between infants and their primary caregivers, is a fundamental aspect of social and emotional development during infancy and serves 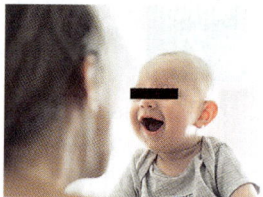 as a foundation for healthy relationships and emotional well-being.

## Nutritional Requirements in Infancy

The infancy is the stage where the infant is learning to adapt to ways of humanity. Its nutritional needs and ability to process the food is different from ours. Hence, a special care is needed while feeding the infants.

### Breastfeeding vs Formula Feeding

- **Breastfeeding:** Breast milk is the optimal source of nutrition for infants, providing essential nutrients,

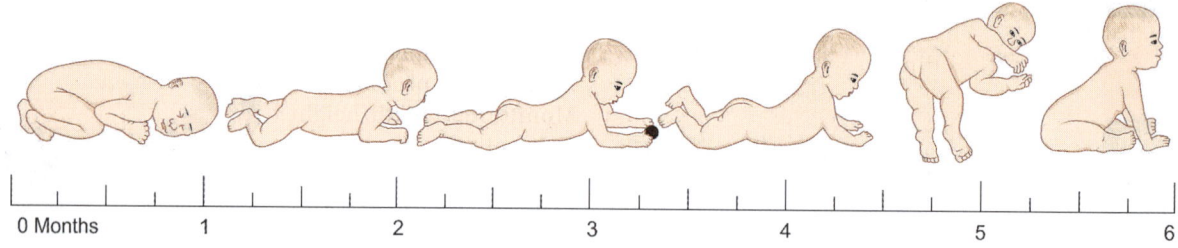
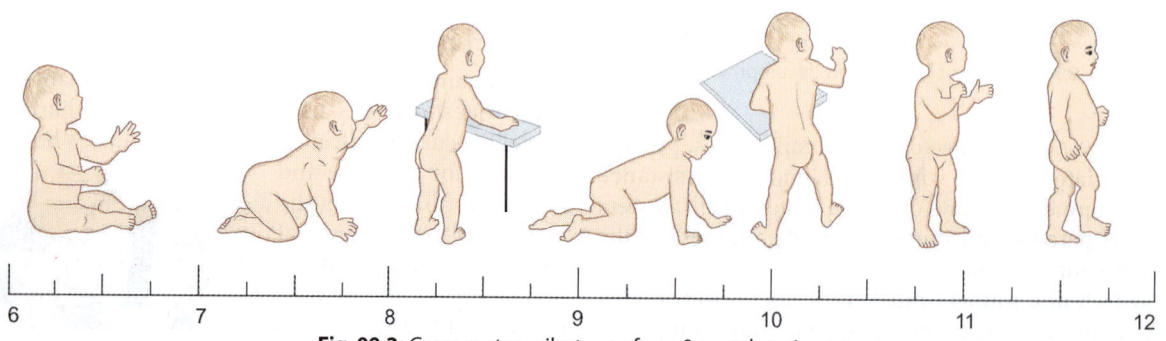

**Fig. 99.2:** Gross motor milestones from 0 month to 1 year.

antibodies, and hormones necessary for growth and development. Breastfeeding offers numerous health benefits for both infants and mothers, including reduced risk of infections, improved cognitive development, and bonding between mother and baby. The World Health Organization (WHO) recommends exclusive breastfeeding *for the first six months* of life, followed by continued breastfeeding alongside complementary foods for up to two years or beyond.
- **Formula feeding:** Formula feeding involves feeding infants with infant formula, which is formulated to mimic the nutritional composition of breast milk. While formula feeding can provide adequate nutrition for infants who are unable to breastfeed or when breastfeeding is not feasible, it lacks the immune-boosting properties and other benefits associated with breast milk. Commercially available infant formulas come in various types, including cow's milk-based, soy-based, hydrolyzed protein, and specialized formulas for specific medical conditions.

### Introduction of Solid Foods (Weaning)

The introduction of solid foods, also known as complementary feeding, typically begins around six months of age when infants show signs of readiness, such as sitting with support, showing interest in food, and loss of the tongue-thrust reflex. Complementary foods complement breast milk or formula and provide additional nutrients and energy to support the infant's growth and development. Common first foods include iron-fortified infant cereals, pureed fruits and vegetables, and mashed proteins such as meat, poultry, or legumes. Introducing a variety of nutrient-rich foods gradually helps infants develop taste preferences, motor skills, and chewing abilities while ensuring adequate nutrition.

### Micronutrient Needs

Infants have specific requirements for essential vitamins and minerals to support their rapid growth and development. Key micronutrients critical for infant health include iron, vitamin D, vitamin B12, zinc, and omega-3 fatty acids. Breast milk provides most of these nutrients in adequate amounts, although some infants may require supplementation based on individual needs or risk factors. Iron supplementation is often recommended for exclusively breastfed infants starting around four to six months of age, as breast milk alone may not provide sufficient iron to meet their needs. Vitamin D supplementation is recommended for all breastfed infants, as breast milk contains low levels of vitamin D.

### Factors Affecting Nutritional Status

Several factors influence infants' nutritional status and feeding practices, including maternal nutrition, breastfeeding support, socioeconomic status, cultural beliefs and practices, maternal employment, access to healthcare, and availability of nutritious foods.

Adequate maternal nutrition during pregnancy and lactation is essential for ensuring the production of high-quality breast milk and optimal infant growth and development.

Breastfeeding support from healthcare providers, lactation consultants, and community resources can help mothers overcome breastfeeding challenges and establish successful breastfeeding relationships.

Socioeconomic factors such as income level, education, and food insecurity may impact access to nutritious foods, infant feeding practices, and overall health outcomes for infants and their families.

Cultural beliefs and practices surrounding infant feeding, including traditional feeding rituals and taboos, influence caregivers' choices regarding breastfeeding, formula feeding, and introduction of solid foods.

Healthcare providers play a crucial role in addressing these factors and providing evidence-based guidance and support to promote optimal nutrition and health for infants and their families.

## PHYSIOLOGICAL CHANGES IN INFANTS

### Respiratory System

The respiratory system of infants undergoes rapid development and maturation during the prenatal and postnatal periods. At birth, infants transition from intrauterine to extrauterine life, necessitating significant adaptations in respiratory function.
- At birth, an infant's respiratory system is smaller and more delicate compared to that of adults. The airways, lungs, and chest cavity are all proportionally smaller. The trachea is shorter and narrower, and the airways have fewer branches. Over the first few years of life, the respiratory system continues to mature. Lung capacity increases, airway diameter enlarges, and the immune system strengthens, reducing the risk of respiratory illnesses.
- Newborns breathe through their noses, not their mouths. They have irregular breathing patterns, with periods of rapid breathing followed by brief pauses, known as periodic breathing. This is normal and usually resolves within a few weeks.
- Infants primarily use their diaphragm, the main muscle of respiration, to breathe. Their chest walls are more compliant, allowing them to rely more on diaphragmatic breathing rather than chest expansion.
- A normal respiratory rate for a newborn is typically between 30 to 60 breaths per minute. However, this can vary depending on factors such as activity level, crying, and temperature.

## Cardiovascular System

The cardiovascular system of infants undergoes significant changes during the transition from fetal to neonatal circulation.

- **Fetal circulation adaptation:** Before birth, the fetal cardiovascular system functions differently from the postnatal cardiovascular system. For instance, the fetal lungs are not used for oxygenation, and the placenta serves as the organ for gas exchange. The fetal circulation includes structures like the ductus arteriosus and the foramen ovale, which allow blood to bypass the non-functional lungs **(Fig. 99.3)**.

  After birth, as the infant starts breathing independently, the fetal shunts gradually close. The ductus arteriosus typically closes within the first few days to weeks of life, and the foramen ovale usually closes within the first year, allowing for normal separate pulmonary and systemic circulations **(Flowchart 99.1)**.

- A newborn's heart rate is higher than that of adults, typically ranging from *100 to 160 beats per minute.* The rhythm may be irregular initially but usually stabilizes within the first few days of life.

- Newborns and infants have a *higher blood volume* relative to their body weight compared to adults. The hemoglobin concentration of newborns is much higher than the adults due to the intrauterine hypoxia. However, during the infancy period, the hemoglobin level drops and can affect oxygen-carrying capacity.

- Vascular resistance in newborns is relatively high initially but decreases over the first weeks to months of life. Blood pressure in newborns is lower than in adults, with systolic and diastolic values typically around *60–80 mm Hg and 40–50 mm Hg*, respectively.

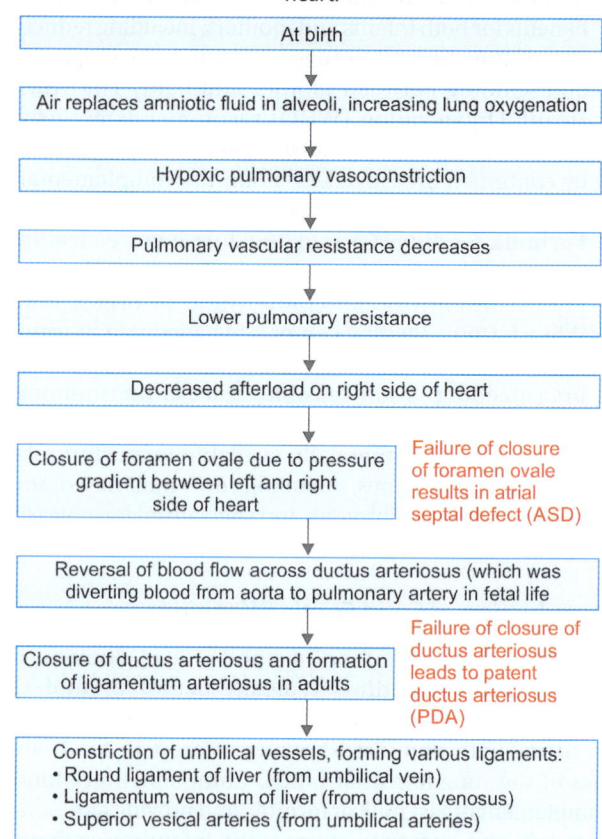

**Flowchart 99.1:** Changes in structures from newborn to infant heart.

- The blood vessels in newborns are *more compliant* and have less muscular tone compared to those in adults. Over time, the vessels mature, becoming more rigid and responsive to changes in blood pressure.

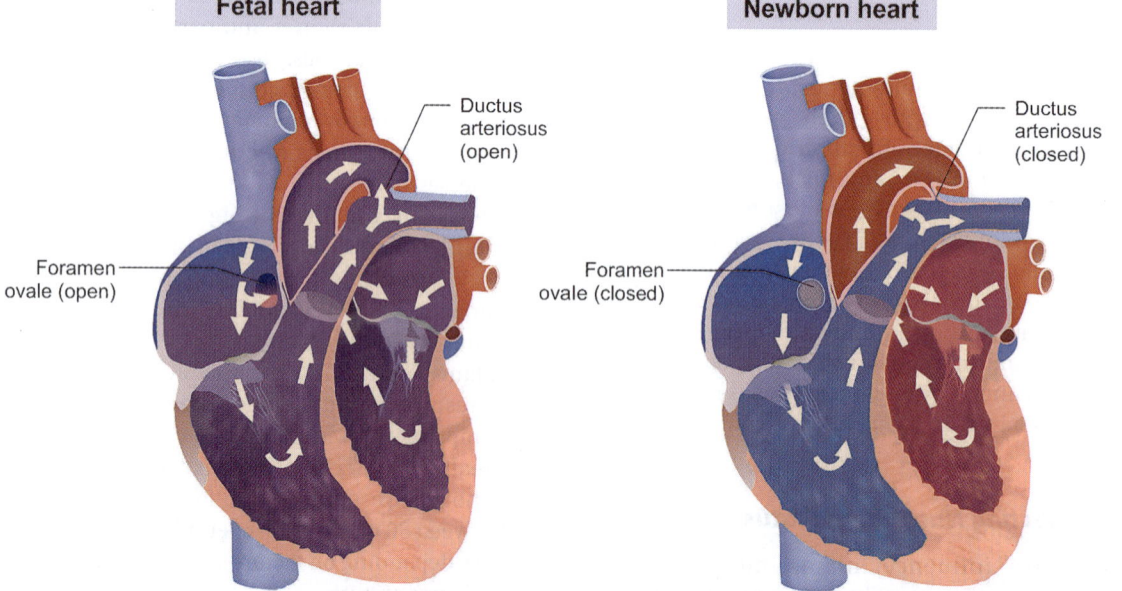

**Fig. 99.3:** Differences between fetal and newborn heart.

## Gastrointestinal System

The gastrointestinal tract (GIT) undergoes several significant physiological changes during the first year of life as infants transition from a liquid diet (breast milk or formula) to consuming solid foods.

- **Increased digestive enzyme production:** As infants grow, their digestive system matures, leading to increased production of digestive enzymes such as amylase, lipase, and protease. This enhances their ability to break down carbohydrates, fats, and proteins present in solid foods.
- **Development of intestinal motility:** Intestinal motility refers to the movement of food through the digestive tract. In newborns, intestinal motility is relatively slow, but it increases and becomes more coordinated during the first year of life. This improvement helps facilitate the digestion and absorption of nutrients from solid foods.
- **Expansion of intestinal surface area:** The surface area of the intestines increases through the development of intestinal villi and microvilli. This expansion allows for greater absorption of nutrients from the digestive tract into the bloodstream.
- **Transition to solid foods:** Around 4 to 6 months of age, infants begin transitioning from a diet consisting solely of breast milk or formula to consuming solid foods. This process, known as weaning or complementary feeding, introduces infants to a variety of tastes and textures, promoting the development of their taste preferences and oral motor skills.
- **Changes in stool characteristics:** As infants transition to solid foods, their stool characteristics change. Stools may become thicker, firmer, and more formed compared to the meconium and the loose, seedy stools of breastfed newborns. The frequency of bowel movements may also decrease.
- **Establishment of intestinal microbiota:** The gut microbiota, composed of trillions of bacteria, fungi, and other microorganisms, undergoes dynamic changes during infancy. Factors such as mode of delivery (vaginal birth versus cesarean section), feeding method (breastfeeding versus formula feeding), and introduction of solid foods influence the composition and diversity of the infant gut microbiota.
- **Immune system development:** The gut plays a crucial role in immune system development, as it is a primary site of interaction between the body and the external environment. During the first year of life, the infant's immune system matures and adapts to respond to various pathogens and antigens encountered through the GIT.
- **Teething:** Towards the end of the first year of life, many infants begin teething, which can lead to increased drooling, chewing on objects, and changes in appetite. While teething is not directly related to GIT physiology, it can affect feeding patterns and oral sensitivity. Introduction of solid foods typically begins around six months of age when infants show signs of readiness and can tolerate different textures and flavors. Early introduction of solid foods before six months of age may increase the risk of allergies and gastrointestinal problems.

## Renal System

The renal system undergoes several physiological changes during the first year of life as infants transition from intrauterine to extrauterine life and adapt to changes in fluid and electrolyte balance. Here are some key changes:

- **Kidney size and function:** At birth, the kidneys are proportionally larger relative to body size compared to adults. However, their functional capacity is still immature. Over the first year of life, the kidneys continue to grow and develop, increasing in both size and functional capacity.
- **Glomerular filtration rate (GFR):** Glomerular filtration rate, which measures the rate at which blood is filtered by the kidneys, undergoes significant changes during infancy. GFR is initially low in newborns but increases rapidly during the first weeks of life, reaching approximately half of adult levels by one year of age.
- **Tubular reabsorption and secretion:** The ability of the renal tubules to reabsorb and secrete substances also matures during the first year of life. Infants have higher renal thresholds for certain substances such as glucose and amino acids compared to adults, leading to increased excretion of these substances in the urine.
- **Renal blood flow:** Renal blood flow increases during the first year of life to meet the metabolic demands of growth and development. This increase in renal blood flow contributes to the maturation of renal function.
- **Fluid and electrolyte balance:** Infants have a higher percentage of total body water and a lower concentration of solutes compared to adults. As a result, they are more prone to dehydration and electrolyte imbalances, particularly in the early months of life. The kidneys play a crucial role in maintaining fluid and electrolyte balance during this time.
- **Urine concentration ability:** The ability of the kidneys to concentrate urine develops gradually during infancy. Newborns have limited ability to concentrate urine, leading to a relatively low urine osmolality. However, this ability improves over the first year of life, allowing infants to conserve water more effectively.
- **Renal response to hormones:** The renal system responds to hormonal signals such as antidiuretic hormone (ADH) and aldosterone, which regulate water and electrolyte balance. The responsiveness of the renal tubules to these hormones matures during infancy, contributing to the regulation of fluid and electrolyte homeostasis.
- **Development of renal structure:** The structural development of the kidneys continues during infancy, with ongoing maturation of nephrons and renal tubules.

This structural development supports the functional maturation of the kidneys and their ability to regulate body fluid and electrolyte balance.

## Immune System

The immune system undergoes significant physiological changes during the first year of life as infants transition from the protection provided by maternal antibodies to developing their own adaptive immune responses. Here are some key changes:

- **Maternal antibodies:** During pregnancy, maternal antibodies are transferred to the fetus through the placenta, providing passive immunity against certain infections. These antibodies offer protection to the newborn during the first few months of life until their own immune system matures.
- **Neonatal immune system:** At birth, the infant's immune system is relatively immature, with limited ability to mount an effective immune response to pathogens. However, innate immune cells such as macrophages, dendritic cells, and natural killer (NK) cells are present and functional, providing some degree of protection against infection.
- **Breastfeeding:** Breast milk contains antibodies, cytokines, and other immune factors that help protect the infant against infections. Breastfeeding provides passive immunity and supports the development of the infant's immune system.
- **Thymus development:** The thymus, an organ critical for the development of T lymphocytes (T cells), continues to grow and mature during the first year of life. T cells are essential for cell-mediated immunity and play a crucial role in fighting infections.
- **Adaptive immune responses:** Over the first year of life, the infant's immune system undergoes maturation, leading to the development of adaptive immune responses. B lymphocytes (B cells) begin to produce antibodies in response to specific pathogens, a process known as humoral immunity. T cells become more diverse and specialized, enabling the immune system to recognize and respond to a wide range of infectious agents.
- **Vaccination:** Vaccination plays a crucial role in stimulating the infant's immune system and providing protection against infectious diseases. The recommended vaccination schedule starts in the first few months of life and continues throughout infancy to build immunity against various pathogens.
- **Immune memory:** With each encounter with a pathogen or vaccination, the infant's immune system develops memory cells that provide long-lasting immunity against specific infections. This process, known as immunological memory, becomes more robust over the first year of life, contributing to the effectiveness of the immune response to subsequent exposures.
- **Decrease in maternal antibodies:** As maternal antibodies wane over time, usually by around 6 to 12 months of age, infants become increasingly reliant on their own immune responses for protection against infections. This period, known as the "window of vulnerability," may result in increased susceptibility to certain infections until the infant's immune system fully matures.

## Endocrine system

- **Hormonal transition at birth:** At birth, there is a rapid shift in hormone levels as the infant transitions from the intrauterine environment to independent life. Hormones such as cortisol, insulin, and thyroid hormones play critical roles in regulating metabolism, energy balance, and stress response during this transition period.
- **Thyroid development and function:** The thyroid gland continues to develop and mature during the first year of life. Thyroid hormones, such as thyroxine (T4) and triiodothyronine (T3), are essential for normal growth and development, including brain development. Newborn screening programs are in place to detect congenital hypothyroidism, a condition that can affect thyroid hormone production and lead to developmental delays if left untreated.
- **Growth hormone (GH) secretion:** Growth hormone plays a crucial role in stimulating growth and development, particularly during infancy and childhood. GH secretion is highest during the first year of life, contributing to rapid growth and weight gain in infants. Deficiencies or excesses of GH can lead to growth disorders such as growth hormone deficiency or gigantism.
- **Sex hormone production:** While the reproductive system is not fully developed at birth, the endocrine glands responsible for producing sex hormones begin to function during infancy. In boys, the testes produce testosterone, while in girls, the ovaries produce estrogen and progesterone. These hormones play important roles in sexual development and reproductive function, although their effects are not fully manifested until puberty.
- **Adrenal function:** The adrenal glands, located on top of the kidneys, produce hormones such as cortisol, aldosterone, and adrenaline. Cortisol, in particular, is important for regulating the stress response, metabolism, and immune function. Adrenal function matures during infancy, with cortisol levels responding to stressors and fluctuations in blood glucose levels.
- **Insulin sensitivity:** Insulin sensitivity, the body's response to insulin, changes during infancy. While infants are relatively insulin-sensitive compared to adults, insulin resistance may develop in some infants, particularly those born large for gestational age or with certain genetic predispositions. This can affect glucose metabolism and increase the risk of conditions such as type 2 diabetes later in life.
- **Maturation of endocrine organs:** Overall, the endocrine organs, including the pituitary gland, thyroid

gland, adrenal glands, pancreas, and gonads, continue to mature and develop throughout infancy. These organs gradually increase in size and functional capacity, supporting the growing demands of the infant's body.

## Nervous System

- **Brain growth and development:** The brain undergoes rapid growth and development during the first year of life. Neurogenesis, the formation of new neurons, occurs predominantly during fetal development but continues to some extent after birth, particularly in regions such as the hippocampus and olfactory bulb. Synaptogenesis, the formation of connections between neurons (synapses), also occurs at a rapid pace, allowing for the establishment of neural circuits and networks.
- **Myelination:** Myelination, the process by which nerve fibers are insulated with myelin sheaths, continues throughout infancy. Myelination enhances the speed and efficiency of nerve signal transmission and is particularly active in regions such as the cerebral cortex, which is involved in higher cognitive functions, and the spinal cord, which is involved in motor control.
- **Reflexes:** Newborn infants exhibit a variety of primitive reflexes, such as the Moro reflex (startle reflex) and the rooting reflex (turning the head in response to touch on the cheek). These reflexes are automatic responses to specific stimuli and help infants adapt to their environment. Many of these reflexes gradually disappear during the first year of life as higher brain centers mature.
- **Sensory development:** Sensory systems, including vision, hearing, touch, taste, and smell, continue to develop and refine during infancy. Visual acuity improves, allowing infants to discriminate between shapes, colors, and patterns. Auditory discrimination improves, enabling infants to differentiate between sounds and localize their sources. Tactile sensitivity increases, allowing infants to explore their environment through touch.
- **Motor development:** Motor development progresses rapidly during the first year of life. Infants initially exhibit involuntary movements, such as primitive reflexes, but gradually gain voluntary control over their movements. Motor milestones, such as lifting the head, rolling over, sitting up, crawling, and eventually walking, are achieved sequentially as motor skills develop.
- **Cognitive development:** Cognitive abilities, including attention, memory, learning, and problem-solving, develop rapidly during infancy. Infants demonstrate increasing awareness of their surroundings, recognition of familiar faces and objects, and responsiveness to social interactions. Cognitive development is influenced by both genetic factors and environmental experiences.
- **Language development:** Language development begins during infancy, with infants progressively acquiring receptive and expressive language skills. Infants initially communicate through crying, babbling, and cooing, and gradually develop the ability to understand and produce words. Language development is facilitated by exposure to spoken language and social interactions with caregivers.
- **Social and emotional development:** Social and emotional development is an integral aspect of nervous system development during infancy. Infants form attachments to caregivers, express emotions such as joy, sadness, and fear, and engage in social interactions with others. These early social experiences shape the development of neural circuits involved in emotional regulation and social cognition.

## SUMMARY

- The physiology of infancy encompasses a dynamic period of growth and development during the first year of life, characterized by significant changes in various physiological systems. This chapter provides an overview of the key physiological changes that occur during infancy, including those related to growth, nutrition, metabolism, cardiovascular function, respiratory function, immune function, endocrine regulation, nervous system development.
- Infants undergo rapid growth and development, with notable changes in weight, length/height, and head circumference monitored through anthropometric assessments. Nutrition plays a critical role in supporting growth and development during infancy, with breast milk or formula providing essential nutrients and immune factors. As infants transition to solid foods, their digestive system matures, and they develop the ability to digest and absorb nutrients from a wider variety of foods.
- Cardiovascular and respiratory function undergo adaptations to support the infant's increasing metabolic demands and oxygen requirements. The immune system matures during infancy, transitioning from passive immunity provided by maternal antibodies to active immune responses. Endocrine glands such as the thyroid, adrenal, and pancreas undergo maturation, regulating metabolism, stress response, and hormonal balance.
- The nervous system undergoes rapid development during infancy, with neurogenesis, myelination, and synaptic pruning contributing to the establishment of neural circuits and sensory processing pathways. Special senses, including vision, hearing, taste, smell, and touch, continue to develop and refine, shaping the infant's perception of the world.
- Understanding the physiology of infancy is essential for healthcare providers and caregivers to monitor growth and development, identify potential health issues or developmental delays, and provide appropriate support and interventions to optimize infant health and well-being. By promoting healthy nutrition, growth, and sensory experiences, caregivers can support infants' physiological development during this critical period of life.

# LET US SEE, HOW MUCH YOU HAVE LEARNT?

 **Review Questions**

Q1. Describe the anthropometric measurements required for the assessment of growth in an infant.
Q2. What physiological changes occur in the infants in first year of life?
Q3. What changes occur in the heart at the time of birth, when the lungs expand?

 **Multiple Choice Questions**

Q1. What is the primary source of nutrition for infants during the first year of life?
   a. Solid foods     b. Breast milk
   c. Cow's milk     d. Water

Q2. Which of the following is a physiological change in the cardiovascular system during infancy?
   a. Increase in pulmonary vascular resistance
   b. Decrease in heart rate
   c. Reduction in blood volume
   d. Development of collateral circulation

Q3. At what age do infants typically begin to transition to solid foods?
   a. 2–3 months     b. 6–8 months
   c. 12–14 months     d. 18–24 months

Q4. Which hormone is important for regulating metabolism and growth during infancy?
   a. Insulin     b. Growth hormone
   c. Thyroxine     d. Cortisol

Q5. What is the primary function of myelination in the nervous system during infancy?
   a. Enhancing nerve signal transmission
   b. Stimulating neurogenesis
   c. Suppressing synaptic activity
   d. Inhibiting axonal growth

Q6. What is the term for the automatic response to specific stimuli exhibited by newborn infants?
   a. Reflexes     b. Cognition
   c. Synaptogenesis     d. Myelination

Q7. Which of the following senses is typically the least developed at birth and continues to mature during infancy?
   a. Vision
   b. Hearing
   c. Taste
   d. Touch

Q8. What role does breast milk play in supporting infant immune function during the first year of life?
   a. It provides passive immunity through maternal antibodies
   b. It suppresses the infant's immune system
   c. It has no effect on immune function
   d. It stimulates the production of infant antibodies

Q9. What is the primary purpose of neonatal screening programs for congenital hypothyroidism?
   a. To assess visual acuity
   b. To monitor respiratory function
   c. To detect abnormalities in thyroid hormone production
   d. To evaluate cardiac function

Q10. Which of the following is a common reflex exhibited by newborn infants in response to a sudden loss of support or a loud noise?
   a. Rooting reflex     b. Moro reflex
   c. Babinski reflex     d. Grasping reflex

Q11. When do infants typically achieve the milestone of lifting their head while lying on their stomach?
   a. 1–2 months     b. 4–6 months
   c. 8–10 months     d. 12–14 months

Q12. What is the primary role of the thymus gland in infants?
   a. Regulation of blood glucose levels
   b. Production of insulin
   c. Maturation of T lymphocytes
   d. Synthesis of growth hormone

Q13. Which of the following is a characteristic of infants' taste preferences?
   a. Preference for bitter tastes
   b. Aversion to sweet tastes
   c. Preference for salty tastes
   d. Preference for sweet tastes

Q14. Which sensory system is involved in the perception of auditory stimuli?
   a. Visual system
   b. Auditory system
   c. Olfactory system
   d. Gustatory system

Q15. What is the primary mechanism by which infants regulate body temperature during the first year of life?
   a. Shivering
   b. Sweating
   c. Vasoconstriction
   d. Vasodilation

Q16. Which of the following hormones plays a crucial role in regulating stress response and metabolism in infants?
   a. Estrogen     b. Testosterone
   c. Cortisol     d. Insulin

Q17. What is the term for the process by which nerve fibers are insulated with myelin sheaths?
   a. Neurogenesis
   b. Myelination
   c. Synaptogenesis
   d. Neurotransmission

Q18. What is the primary function of the adrenal glands in infants?
   a. Regulation of blood pressure
   b. Production of sex hormones
   c. Production of cortisol and adrenaline
   d. Regulation of insulin secretion

Q19. Which of the following is a milestone of motor development typically achieved by infants around 6–8 months of age?
- a. Rolling over
- b. Sitting up without support
- c. Crawling
- d. Walking

Q20. Which sensory system is responsible for the perception of tactile sensations?
- a. Visual system
- b. Auditory system
- c. Olfactory system
- d. Somatosensory system

**ANSWERS**

1. b   2. d   3. b   4. b   5. a   6. a   7. d   8. a   9. c   10. b   11. a   12. c   13. d   14. b   15. b   16. c   17. b   18. c   19. b   20. d

# Physiology of Aging, Free Radicals and Antioxidants

**100 CHAPTER**

### COMPETENCY ADDRESSED
**PY11.7:** Describe and discuss physiology of aging; free radicals and antioxidants.

### LEARNING OBJECTIVES
**At the end of this chapter, the learner should be able to:**
- Define aging.
- Describe the theories of aging.
- Describe the physiological basis of aging.
- Describe the physiology of aging and oxidative stress.
- Describe the strategies to mitigate aging and oxidative stress.

Aging is a complex biological process characterized by the progressive deterioration of physiological functions and the increased vulnerability to age-related diseases and mortality. It is a natural and inevitable aspect of life that occurs across all living organisms, albeit at varying rates. Aging involves a multitude of interconnected cellular, molecular, and systemic changes that affect the structure and function of tissues and organs throughout the body.

At the cellular level, aging is marked by a decline in the regenerative capacity and efficiency of cells, as well as the accumulation of damage to cellular components such as DNA, proteins, and lipids. This accumulation of damage is often attributed to various intrinsic and extrinsic factors, including oxidative stress, inflammation, telomere shortening, and mitochondrial dysfunction.

## THEORIES OF AGING

They are frameworks that attempt to explain the underlying mechanisms driving the aging process.

### Oxidative Stress Theory

- Oxidative stress theory proposes that aging is primarily driven by the *accumulation of cellular damage caused by reactive oxygen species (ROS)* and other free radicals.
- ROS are highly reactive molecules produced during normal metabolic processes, such as mitochondrial respiration, as well as in response to external stressors such as UV radiation, pollution, and toxins.
- Over time, ROS can cause damage to cellular components including DNA, proteins, and lipids, leading to impaired cellular function and contributing to the aging process.
- Antioxidant defense mechanisms, including enzymes such as superoxide dismutase and catalase, as well as dietary antioxidants like vitamins C and E, help to neutralize ROS.

### Cellular Senescence Theory

- Cellular senescence theory proposes that aging is influenced by the *accumulation of senescent cells*, which are irreversibly arrested cells that have ceased to divide.
- Senescence can be triggered by various factors, including telomere shortening, DNA damage, oncogene activation, and oxidative stress.
- Senescent cells exhibit *alterations in gene expression*, secretion of inflammatory cytokines and growth factors (known as the senescence-associated secretory phenotype or SASP), and impaired function.
- While senescence initially serves as a protective mechanism to prevent the proliferation of damaged or potentially cancerous cells, the accumulation of senescent cells over time contributes to tissue dysfunction, inflammation, and age-related diseases.

# PHYSIOLOGICAL CHANGES ASSOCIATED WITH AGEING

Various physiological changes occur as a result of aging, affecting almost every organ system in the body. These changes contribute to the increased susceptibility to diseases, decline in functional capacity, and reduced resilience to stressors commonly observed in older adults.

## Cardiovascular System

- Structural changes in the heart, such as increased fibrosis and stiffening of the myocardium, leading to *reduced compliance and impaired diastolic function*.
- *Decreased elasticity* and *thickening of arterial walls*, resulting in arterial stiffness and elevated blood pressure (hypertension).
- Progressive *decline in cardiac output* and maximal heart rate, limiting the capacity to meet increased metabolic demands during physical activity.
- Increased prevalence of cardiovascular diseases such as atherosclerosis, coronary artery disease, heart failure, and arrhythmias.

## Respiratory System

- *Reduction in lung elasticity and compliance*, leading to decreased lung volumes and impaired gas exchange.
- Decline in respiratory muscle strength and endurance, resulting in *reduced respiratory reserve* and increased susceptibility to respiratory infections.
- Increased incidence of respiratory conditions such as chronic obstructive pulmonary disease (COPD), pneumonia, and respiratory failure.

## Musculoskeletal System

- *Loss of muscle mass and strength* (sarcopenia) due to decreased protein synthesis, increased protein breakdown, and altered muscle fiber composition.
- Reduction in bone density and mineral content *(osteopenia and osteoporosis)*, leading to increased risk of fractures and bone fragility.
- Degenerative changes in joints *(osteoarthritis)* characterized by cartilage loss, joint inflammation, and pain.

## Neurological System

- *Decline in cognitive function*, including memory, attention, processing speed, and executive function, due to changes in brain structure and function.
- *Reduction in neuronal density and synaptic connections*, accompanied by accumulation of abnormal protein aggregates (e.g., amyloid-beta, tau) implicated in neurodegenerative diseases such as Alzheimer's disease.
- Decreased sensory perception, including vision, hearing, taste, and smell, due to age-related changes in sensory organs and neural pathways.

## Endocrine System

- *Decline in hormonal production* and secretion by endocrine glands, including the pituitary, thyroid, adrenal, and gonadal glands.
- Alterations in hormonal regulation, including dysregulation of the hypothalamic-pituitary-adrenal (HPA) axis and the hypothalamic-pituitary-gonadal (HPG) axis, leading to hormonal imbalances.
- *Increased prevalence of endocrine disorders* such as diabetes mellitus, thyroid disorders, and adrenal insufficiency.

## Immune System

- Gradual decline in immune function (immune-senescence), characterized by decreased immune cell proliferation, reduced antibody production, and impaired immune response to pathogens.
- Chronic low-grade inflammation characterized by elevated levels of pro-inflammatory cytokines and mediators, contributing to age-related diseases and frailty.
- Increased susceptibility to infections, autoimmune diseases, and cancer due to compromised immune surveillance and response.

# ROLE OF FREE RADICALS

- Free radicals are highly reactive molecules that contain one or more unpaired electrons in their outer shell, making them unstable and prone to participate in chemical reactions.
- Common types of free radicals include oxygen-derived radicals such as *superoxide anion ($O_2^{\bullet-}$), hydroxyl radical ($\bullet OH$), and singlet oxygen ($^1O_2$), as well as nitrogen-derived radicals like nitric oxide ($\bullet NO$) and peroxynitrite ($ONOO^-$)*.

## Metabolic Processes

Free radicals are generated as byproducts of normal metabolic processes within the body, such as cellular respiration, mitochondrial electron transport chain reactions, and enzymatic reactions involved in metabolism. **Environmental factors:** External sources of free radicals include exposure to environmental pollutants, ultraviolet (UV) radiation from sunlight, ionizing radiation, tobacco smoke, air pollution, and certain chemicals in food and water. These factors can induce oxidative stress and increase free radical production in cells and tissues.

## Cellular Damage Caused by Free Radicals

- Free radicals can cause cellular damage through a process known as *oxidative stress*, which occurs when there is an imbalance between the production of free radicals and the antioxidant defense mechanisms that neutralize them.

- Oxidative damage to cellular components such as DNA, proteins, lipids, and carbohydrates can disrupt cellular function and integrity, leading to cellular dysfunction, inflammation, and cell death.
- DNA damage by free radicals can result in *mutations, chromosomal aberrations, and genomic instability*, which may contribute to the development of cancer and other age-related diseases.
- Protein oxidation can impair enzyme activity, disrupt cellular signaling pathways, and lead to the formation of protein aggregates implicated in neurodegenerative disorders such as Alzheimer's and Parkinson's disease.
- Lipid peroxidation of cell membranes can compromise membrane integrity and fluidity, disrupt cellular signaling, and generate toxic byproducts that contribute to tissue damage and inflammation.

### Role of Free Radicals in Aging Processes

- Free radicals have been implicated in the aging process through various mechanisms, including the accumulation of oxidative damage to cellular components over time.
- The oxidative stress theory of aging proposes that the progressive accumulation of oxidative damage by free radicals contributes to the functional decline and degenerative changes associated with aging.
- Free radicals can promote cellular senescence, apoptosis, and tissue degeneration by inducing DNA damage, protein oxidation, and lipid peroxidation, leading to impaired cellular function and tissue homeostasis.
- Age-related diseases such as cardiovascular disease, neurodegenerative disorders, cancer, diabetes, and inflammatory conditions are associated with increased oxidative stress and damage caused by free radicals.

## ANTIOXIDANTS: MECHANISMS AND IMPORTANCE

- Antioxidants are molecules that can neutralize or inhibit the harmful effects of free radicals by donating electrons or hydrogen atoms, thereby preventing oxidative damage to cellular components.
- There are various types of antioxidants, including:
  - *Enzymatic antioxidants:* These include enzymes such as superoxide dismutase (SOD), catalase, and glutathione peroxidase (GPx), which catalyze the breakdown of free radicals and reactive oxygen species (ROS) into less harmful substances.
  - *Nonenzymatic antioxidants:* These are small *molecules that scavenge free radicals directly or regenerate other antioxidants.* Examples include vitamins (e.g., vitamin C, vitamin E), minerals (e.g., selenium, zinc), phytochemicals (e.g., flavonoids, polyphenols), and endogenous molecules (e.g., glutathione, coenzyme Q10).

### Mechanisms of Antioxidant Action

- **Scavenging free radicals:** Antioxidants can directly neutralize free radicals by donating electrons or hydrogen atoms, thereby stabilizing the radicals and preventing them from causing oxidative damage to cellular components.
- **Enhancing enzyme activity:** Some antioxidants can enhance the activity of endogenous antioxidant enzymes such as *SOD, catalase, and GPx*, thereby augmenting the cellular defense against oxidative stress.
- **Regenerating other antioxidants:** Certain antioxidants have the ability to regenerate other antioxidants that have been oxidized during the process of neutralizing free radicals. For example, vitamin C can regenerate oxidized vitamin E, allowing it to continue its antioxidant function.

### Sources of Antioxidants

- **Dietary antioxidants:** Antioxidants can be obtained from a variety of plant-based foods, including fruits, vegetables, nuts, seeds, whole grains, and herbs. These foods are rich in vitamins, minerals, and phytochemicals with antioxidant properties.
- **Endogenous antioxidants:** The body also produces its own antioxidants, such as glutathione, coenzyme Q10, and uric acid, which play important roles in maintaining cellular redox balance and protecting against oxidative stress.

### Importance of Antioxidants in Mitigating Oxidative Stress and Aging-related Damage

- Antioxidants play a crucial role in mitigating oxidative stress by scavenging free radicals and preventing oxidative damage to cellular components such as DNA, proteins, lipids, and carbohydrates.
- By neutralizing free radicals and ROS, antioxidants help maintain cellular homeostasis, protect against oxidative damage, and preserve cellular function and integrity.
- Antioxidants have been implicated in various physiological processes, including immune function, inflammation, energy metabolism, and cell signaling, highlighting their importance in overall health and disease prevention.
- Deficiencies in antioxidants or impaired antioxidant defense mechanisms have been linked to increased susceptibility to oxidative stress-related diseases, aging-related degenerative disorders, and age-related decline in physiological function.
- Dietary intake of antioxidants from a balanced and varied diet rich in fruits, vegetables, and other antioxidant-rich foods is recommended as part of a healthy lifestyle to support optimal antioxidant status and protect against oxidative stress and aging-related damage.

## STRATEGIES TO MITIGATE AGING AND OXIDATIVE STRESS

### Lifestyle Interventions

- **Dietary modifications:** Consuming a balanced diet rich in antioxidant-rich foods such as fruits, vegetables, nuts, seeds, whole grains, and legumes can help combat oxidative stress and reduce the risk of age-related diseases. Emphasizing foods high in vitamins C and E, selenium, zinc, and phytochemicals can support optimal antioxidant status.
- **Regular exercise:** Engaging in regular physical activity and exercise has been shown to enhance antioxidant defense mechanisms, improve mitochondrial function, and reduce oxidative stress. Both aerobic exercise and resistance training can benefit overall health and promote healthy aging by reducing inflammation, enhancing cardiovascular fitness, and preserving muscle mass and function.

### Pharmacological Interventions

- **Antioxidant supplements:** While dietary antioxidants are preferred sources of antioxidants, supplementation with specific antioxidants such as vitamins C and E, coenzyme Q10, and polyphenols may be beneficial in individuals with inadequate dietary intake or increased oxidative stress. However, the efficacy of antioxidant supplements in preventing age-related diseases and promoting longevity remains controversial, and excessive supplementation may have adverse effects.
- **Mitochondrial-targeted therapies:** Strategies aimed at enhancing mitochondrial function and reducing mitochondrial oxidative stress are being explored as potential anti-aging interventions. Mitochondrial-targeted antioxidants, mitochondrial biogenesis inducers, and mitochondrial quality control enhancers are among the emerging pharmacological approaches to mitigate aging-related mitochondrial dysfunction and oxidative damage.

### Emerging Research on Anti-aging Therapies

- **Caloric restriction and intermittent fasting:** Caloric restriction and intermittent fasting have been shown to extend lifespan and improve healthspan in various organisms by enhancing cellular stress resistance, reducing oxidative stress, and activating longevity-promoting pathways such as *sirtuins and AMP-activated protein kinase (AMPK)*. Emerging research is investigating the underlying mechanisms and potential translational applications of these dietary interventions for promoting healthy aging in humans.
- **Senolytics and senomorphics:** Senolytics are compounds that selectively target and eliminate senescent cells, while senomorphics modulate the senescence-associated secretory phenotype (SASP) to reduce the pro-inflammatory effects of senescent cells. These emerging anti-aging therapies hold promise for delaying age-related functional decline, preventing age-related diseases, and promoting tissue regeneration and rejuvenation.
- **Epigenetic modulators:** Epigenetic modifications play a critical role in regulating gene expression patterns associated with aging and age-related diseases. Emerging research is investigating the potential of epigenetic modulators such as DNA methyltransferase inhibitors, histone deacetylase inhibitors, and microRNA modulators to reverse epigenetic changes associated with aging and restore youthful gene expression profiles.

---

### SUMMARY

- Aging is a complex biological process characterized by the progressive decline in physiological function and increased susceptibility to age-related diseases.
- Key physiological changes associated with aging include alterations in cellular function, tissue structure, organ function, and systemic homeostasis.
- Aging affects virtually all organ systems in the body, contributing to functional decline, impaired tissue repair, and decreased resilience to stressors.
- Free radicals are highly reactive molecules with unpaired electrons, generated as a by product of metabolic processes.
- Excessive production of free radicals can lead to oxidative stress, resulting in damage to cellular components such as DNA, proteins, lipids, and carbohydrates.
- Oxidative stress is implicated in the pathogenesis of various age-related diseases and contributes to the aging process by promoting cellular dysfunction, inflammation, and tissue degeneration.
- Antioxidants are molecules that neutralize free radicals and prevent oxidative damage by donating electrons or hydrogen atoms.
- Enzymatic antioxidants, such as superoxide dismutase and catalase, and nonenzymatic antioxidants, including vitamins C and E, play crucial roles in maintaining cellular redox balance and protecting against oxidative stress.
- Antioxidants are obtained from dietary sources such as fruits, vegetables, nuts, seeds, and whole grains, as well as through endogenous production within the body.
- Enhancing antioxidant defenses through dietary interventions, regular exercise, and supplementation may help mitigate oxidative stress and promote healthy aging.
- Understanding the physiology of aging, free radicals, and antioxidants is essential for developing strategies to promote healthy aging and prevent age-related diseases.
- Further research is needed to elucidate the mechanisms underlying the interplay between oxidative stress, antioxidant defenses, and the aging process.
- Integration of lifestyle modifications, pharmacological interventions, and emerging anti-aging therapies holds promise for enhancing overall well-being and extending health span in an aging population.

# LET US SEE, HOW MUCH YOU HAVE LEARNT?

## Review Questions

**Q1.** Describe the theories of ageing.
**Q2.** What are free radiclas? How are they responsible for the process of aging?
**Q3.** Describe the role of antioxidants in preventing the free radical injury/oxidative stress.
**Q4.** Describe the physiological changes occurring during the process of aging.

## Multiple Choice Questions

**Q1.** What is the primary role of antioxidants in mitigating oxidative stress?
 a. Enhancing ROS production
 b. Increasing cellular damage
 c. Neutralizing free radicals
 d. Stimulating inflammatory responses

**Q2.** Which of the following is NOT a lifestyle intervention to mitigate oxidative stress and aging?
 a. Regular exercise
 b. Caloric restriction
 c. Smoking cessation
 d. Increased alcohol consumption

**Q3.** What is the main source of free radicals in the body?
 a. Antioxidant supplements
 b. Environmental pollutants
 c. Cellular respiration
 d. Dietary antioxidants

**Q4.** Which enzyme is NOT considered an enzymatic antioxidant?
 a. Superoxide dismutase (SOD)
 b. Catalase
 c. Glutathione peroxidase (GPx)
 d. Glucose oxidase

**Q5.** What is the primary mechanism of action of antioxidant supplements?
 a. Stimulating ROS production
 b. Inhibiting antioxidant enzymes
 c. Enhancing mitochondrial function
 d. Scavenging free radicals

**Q6.** How does oxidative stress impact cellular function and aging?
 a. By promoting DNA repair mechanisms
 b. By reducing oxidative damage
 c. By inducing cellular senescence and dysfunction
 d. By increasing antioxidant defense mechanisms

**Q7.** Which dietary modification is recommended to combat oxidative stress?
 a. High intake of processed foods
 b. Low consumption of fruits and vegetables
 c. Increased intake of antioxidant-rich foods
 d. Excessive alcohol consumption

**Q8.** What is the primary goal of emerging antiaging therapies such as senolytics?
 a. To enhance cellular senescence
 b. To target and eliminate senescent cells
 c. To induce ROS production
 d. To promote inflammation

**Q9.** Which factor contributes to the decline in antioxidant defense mechanisms with aging?
 a. Increased synthesis of antioxidant enzymes
 b. Reduced activity of antioxidant enzymes
 c. Enhanced recycling of nonenzymatic antioxidants
 d. Upregulation of antioxidant-related genes

**Q10.** What is the primary implication of oxidative stress in age-related diseases?
 a. Protection against age-related diseases
 b. Promotion of cellular health
 c. Contribution to disease pathogenesis
 d. Preservation of tissue integrity

**ANSWERS**
 1. c  2. d  3. c  4. d  5. d  6. c  7. c  8. b  9. b  10. c

# Physiology of Yoga and Meditation

**101**
CHAPTER

**COMPETENCY ADDRESSED**

**PY11.12:** Discuss the physiological effects of meditation.

 **LEARNING OBJECTIVES**

**At the end of this chapter, you should be able to:**
- Describe the physiology of stress and implications of stress on health.
- Describe Yoga and its physiological effects.
- Describe the meditation and its physiological effects.

## YOGA AND MEDITATION

Yoga and meditation are ancient practices that have endured for millennia, rooted in the cultures of India and other Eastern civilizations. Yoga, derived from the Sanskrit word "Yuj," meaning to unite or yoke, encompasses a diverse range of physical, mental, and spiritual practices aimed at achieving harmony and balance in one's life. It is not merely a form of exercise but a holistic approach to well-being, integrating physical postures (asanas), breath control (pranayama), meditation, and ethical principles.

Meditation, on the other hand, is a practice of focusing the mind and cultivating awareness, often leading to a heightened state of mental clarity and inner peace. It involves various techniques such as mindfulness, concentration, and contemplation, each designed to quiet the mind and promote a sense of presence and tranquility.

Before we learn more about yoga, let us understand the physiology of stress.

## PHYSIOLOGY OF STRESS

### Definition and Types of Stress

Stress is a natural physiological response to perceived threats or challenges, triggering the body's "fight or flight" mechanism to mobilize resources for survival. While acute stress is a temporary and adaptive reaction to immediate stressors, chronic stress occurs when these stressors persist over an extended period, leading to sustained activation of the stress response system. There are various types of stress, including:

- **Acute stress:** This type of stress is short-term and typically triggered by specific events or situations, such as a deadline at work, a traffic jam, or a sudden illness. Acute stress activates the body's stress response temporarily, helping individuals cope with immediate challenges.
- **Episodic acute stress:** Some individuals experience frequent episodes of acute stress due to recurring life circumstances or personality traits characterized by high levels of worry and tension. Episodic acute stress can lead to a cycle of repeated stress responses and may contribute to health problems over time.
- **Chronic stress:** Chronic stress results from ongoing stressors, such as financial difficulties, relationship problems, work-related pressures, or traumatic experiences. Prolonged activation of the stress response system can have detrimental effects on physical, mental, and emotional well-being.

### Physiological Response to Stress

When confronted with a stressor, the body initiates a series of physiological responses orchestrated by the autonomic nervous system and the hypothalamic-pituitary-adrenal (HPA) axis. These responses are designed to mobilize energy and resources to cope with the perceived threat.

- **Activation of the sympathetic nervous system:** The sympathetic nervous system triggers the release of stress hormones, such as adrenaline and noradrenaline, leading to *increased heart rate, elevated blood pressure, and heightened alertness*. This prepares the body for action in response to perceived danger.
- **Release of cortisol:** The hypothalamo-pituitary axis stimulates the adrenal glands to release cortisol, often referred to as the *"stress hormone."* Cortisol helps regulate metabolism, immune function, and the body's response to inflammation. In the short term, *cortisol promotes adaptive responses to stress, but chronic elevation of cortisol levels can have deleterious effects on health*.
- **Suppression of nonessential functions:** During times of stress, the body prioritizes functions essential for survival, such as respiration and circulation, while suppressing nonessential activities, such as digestion, growth, and reproduction. This allocation of resources ensures that the body can respond effectively to immediate threats.

## Health Implications of Chronic Stress (Fig. 101.1)

Chronic stress has profound implications for physical and mental health, contributing to a wide range of disorders and conditions, including:

- **Cardiovascular disease:** Prolonged activation of the stress response system can lead to hypertension, atherosclerosis, and increased risk of heart attack or stroke.
- **Immune dysfunction:** Chronic stress suppresses immune function, making individuals more susceptible to infections, autoimmune disorders, and delayed wound healing.
- **Metabolic disorders:** Dysregulation of cortisol and other stress hormones can disrupt metabolism, leading to weight gain, insulin resistance, and an increased risk of type 2 diabetes.
- **Mental health disorders:** Chronic stress is strongly associated with anxiety disorders, depression, post-traumatic stress disorder (PTSD), and other psychiatric conditions.
- **Altered brain structure and function:** Prolonged exposure to stress hormones can impair neuroplasticity, reduce hippocampal volume, and disrupt neurotransmitter balance, contributing to cognitive decline and mood disturbances.

## YOGA

In the modern world the relevance of YOGA and MEDITATION in health and disease is so universal that it has become a necessity for one and all. A wide variety of common diseases such as coronary heart disease, hypertension, diabetes mellitus etc. Now being attributed to a faulty lifestyle. Yoga is probably the best lifestyle ever devised in the history of mankind. It is simply loving giving nonjudgmental way and view of life upon which people across cultures and countries have stumbled from time to time for centuries. Yoga is finding increasing acceptance as a non-pharmacological intervention for the prevention and treatment of several diseases. This piece of universal wisdom, which has been discovered and rediscovered several times in history as the ultimate prescription for health.

Yoga is a journey towards self-perfection. Improvement is the first step towards perfection and the journey towards perfection never ends. Different schools of yoga are shown in **Figure 101.2**.

**HATHA YOGA:** This aims primarily at perfection of the body. A perfect body means a strong and healthy body. Only a strong and healthy body can be an instrument to carry out the divine will. Advanced Hatha Yoga not only achieves this, but also gains mastery over the functions of the body which are normally considered uncontrollable. The result may be improvement in physical health without

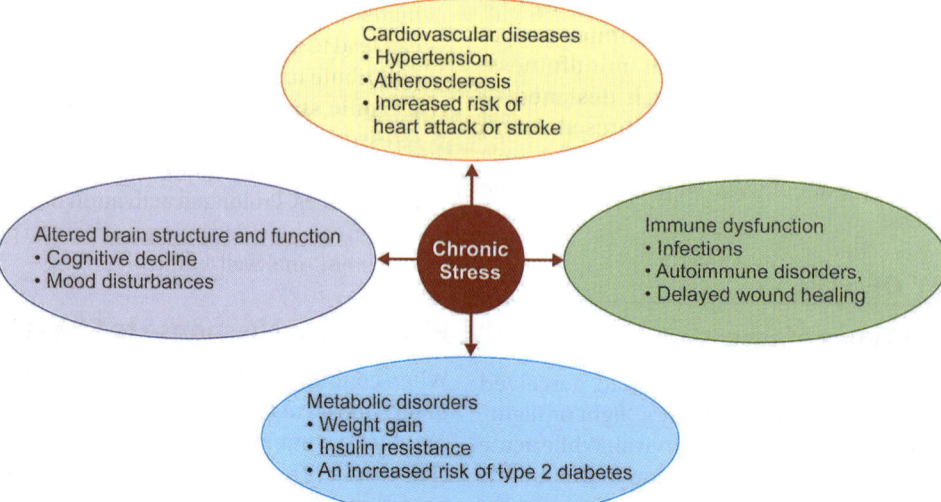

**Fig. 101.1:** Effects of chronic stress.

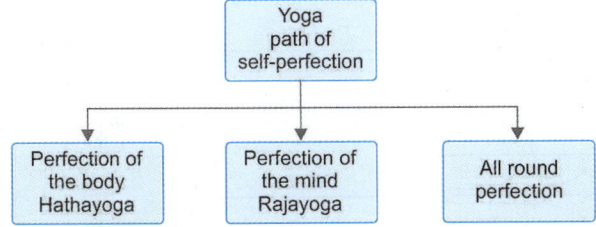

**Fig. 101.2:** Different schools of YOGA.

refinement of the mind. Top sided development of the body is a potential weakness of Hatha Yoga.

**RAJA YOGA:** Raja Yoga, literally the royal path, aims primarily at the perfection of the mind. A perfect mind is one that is not disturbed by ordinary thoughts and distractions.

The ordinary mind is very turbulent, but if these disturbances can be quietened the veil concealing the divine is lifted, a step towards union with the divine.

The basic technique of Raja Yoga is meditation. But Patanjali, the master of Raja Yoga, breaks the journey into light limbs also called Ashtanga Yoga.

**The eight limbs are:**
1. **Yama**
   Yama is essentially a set of five don'ts:
   a. Ahimsa (nonviolence)
   b. Satya (Truth)
   c. Asteya (non-stealing)
   d. Brahmacharya (celibacy)
   e. Aparigraha (non-receiving – no greed)
2. **Niyama**
   Niyama is essentially a set of five do's:
   a. Shaucha (cleanliness), i.e., internal and external purification
   b. Santosh (contentment), i.e., bringing satisfaction with what we are given.
   c. Tapas (austerities), i.e., disciplining or concentrating energies on our objective
   d. Swadhyaya (study), i.e., study of scriptures
   e. Ishvara pranidhan a (surrender to God), i.e., placing full trust in the will and wisdom of the divine
   Yama and Niyama are preparatory codes of conduct. They are followed by five specialized techniques. The last limb SAMADHI is an experiential state.
3. Asna, i.e., postures which are steady and comfortable
4. Pranayama, i.e., control of prana\breath
5. Pratyahara (gathering towards), i.e., restraint of the senses so as to free the mind
6. Dharana (concentration on a certain point): The point may be an object, sound or an idea
7. Dhyana (meditation), i.e., letting the mind flow towards the points of concentration
8. Samadhi, i.e., superconsciousness

**Raja Yoga** concentrates on perfection of the mind but doesn't neglect the body as only a healthy body can work on the oldest meditative practices and its goal is Chitta Vritti Nirodha, i.e., absence of the normal activities of the mind. The idea is not to have a blank mind but to have a more receptive mind.

## Physiological Effects of Yoga on Body

### Neurological Changes

- **Impact on brain structure:** Regular yoga practice can lead to structural changes in the brain, including increases in gray matter volume in regions associated with attention, memory, and emotional regulation. These changes suggest that yoga may *enhance cognitive function and promote brain health*.
- **Neurotransmitter regulation:** It has been found to modulate neurotransmitter activity in the brain, particularly *serotonin and gamma-aminobutyric acid (GABA)*. Increased levels of these neurotransmitters are associated with *improved mood, reduced anxiety, and enhanced stress resilience*, highlighting the potential therapeutic benefits of yoga for mental well-being.

### Endocrine System

- **Hormonal balance:** Yoga practice has been shown to influence the endocrine system, leading to more balanced hormone levels. For example, regular yoga practice has been associated with *lower levels of cortisol*, the primary stress hormone, as well as *increased production of oxytocin*, often referred to as the *"love hormone"* which promotes feelings of bonding and connection.
- **Stress response regulation:** Through its effects on the hypothalamic-pituitary-adrenal (HPA) axis, yoga helps regulate the body's stress response system. By reducing cortisol levels and promoting parasympathetic nervous system activity, yoga induces a relaxation response that counteracts the detrimental effects of chronic stress on health.

### Cardiovascular Health

- **Blood pressure regulation:** Numerous studies have demonstrated the beneficial effects of yoga on blood pressure regulation, with regular practice associated with *reductions in both systolic and diastolic blood pressure*. Yoga techniques such as asanas, pranayama, and meditation promote relaxation, improve circulation, and enhance endothelial function, contributing to cardiovascular health.
- **Heart rate variability:** Yoga practice has been shown to *increase heart rate variability* (HRV), which reflects the variability in the time interval between heartbeats. Higher HRV is indicative of *greater autonomic flexibility* and resilience to stress. By *enhancing parasympathetic tone and reducing sympathetic dominance*, yoga improves HRV and promotes cardiovascular resilience.

### Respiratory System

- **Breath awareness and control:** Through techniques such as pranayama (breath control exercises) and mindful breathing, individuals learn to regulate their breathing patterns, deepen their breath, and synchronize

breath with movement. This conscious breathing fosters ***relaxation, reduces anxiety***, and enhances overall respiratory function.
- **Lung function improvement:** Yoga postures and breathing exercises can improve lung function by *increasing lung capacity, enhancing respiratory muscle strength, and promoting efficient gas exchange*. Research suggests that yoga may be beneficial for individuals with respiratory conditions such as asthma, chronic obstructive pulmonary disease (COPD), and bronchitis, helping to alleviate symptoms and improve quality of life.

## PROCESS OF MEDITATION

Although meditation can be performed at any time and at any place, it is preferable to do it at nearly the same time and at a fixed place everyday. It can be done once or twice a day for about 20 minutes each time.

The best timings are dawn and dusk. The place should be quiet and a clean corner. If an altar is set up as a focal point in the chosen corner it helps to create the right mood and atmosphere. The altar could be a flower, a candle or a picture of God or guru.

- The first two limbs Yama and Niyama aim at moral purification which helps improve the receptivity to higher truths.
- The next limb is Asana. Meditation is usually performed sitting on the floor with the eyes closed. The recommended postures are PADMASANA, SUKHASANA, VAJRASANA. If sitting on a chair is more convenient than that is also acceptable. The basic principle of the posture for meditation is that it should be steady and comfortable. The body should be erect but not tense. It should be possible to stay relaxed and immobile in that posture for a considerable time without any discomfort. Lying down is not a suitable posture for meditation as it is too passive and may induce sleep.
- After assuming the right posture with the eyes closed the next step is to attend to the breathing. Take four or five slow and deep breaths. The rate of breathing should be about 6/min and its depth, slightly greater than usual, slow and deep breathing itself has a calming effect on the mind and facilitates meditation proper. A deep inspiration followed by a very slow exhalation is a simple form of pranayama. Observe the breath. Feel the cool air passing through the nostrils during inspiration, feel the warm air leaving the throat during expiration.
- The next step is pratyahara which means bringing together the mind, which is normally very restless. It is crowded with a multiplicity of thoughts running in various directions. But by a gentle effort and patience these thoughts can be suspended. When we do so we become aware of thoughts such as chirping of the birds. The whirring of the fan. These sounds were already there but were masked by our usual preoccupations. Perceiving these sounds is the first step. The next step is to ignore these sounds as well, sensory withdrawal is

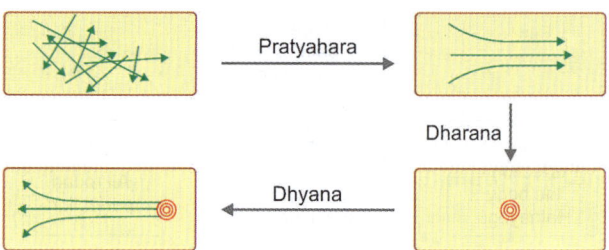

**Fig. 101.3:** Progressive steps in meditation.

an important part of pratyahara. We begin by cutting the unruly bunch of thoughts and then finally eliminating them and when total silence has been reached we are ready for the next step.
- The next step is Dharana. In addition to the concentration on breath which started during pranayama, we may choose an object to concentrate on. It could be a part of the body.
- A sound such as aum, amen, ameen or a mantra
- A picture of God, guru, a flower, a flame
- An idea or thought such as peace, love or beauty.
- The next step is Dhyana.

Dhyana or meditation proper means allowing the mind to divert from the object of concentration. Imagine concentrating on a problem. After some time, a solution to the problem may occur in the mind. Concentrating on the problem is dharana, the solution developing in the mind is dhyana.

Normally meditation should be for about 20 minutes. One should come out of the meditation gently and not use the alarm, timer, or bell to terminate meditation suddenly **(Fig. 101.3)**.

### Features of Meditation

- Sensory (afferent) attenuation, i.e., minimal sensory input
- Motor (efferent) attenuation, i.e., minimal motor output
- Nonanalytic attention, or nontargeted thinking, i.e., minimal cortical activity focusing the attention to a specific object or topic.

### Physiological Effects of Meditation

- Meditation results in a shift in autonomic balance in favor of the parasympathetic division as in.
  - Decrease in heart rate
  - Decrease in respiratory rate
  - Decrease in oxygen consumption
  - Decrease in blood pressure (if the basal blood pressure is high)
  - Increase in % time spent in alpha rhythm in EEG.
  - Decrease in muscle tension
  - Decrease in blood lactate level
- **Brain activity and neuroplasticity:** Meditation practices have been shown to induce changes in brain activity and promote neuroplasticity, the brain's ability to reorganize and adapt. Functional magnetic resonance

imaging (fMRI) studies have revealed alterations in brain regions associated with *attention, memory, emotional regulation, and self-awareness* among experienced meditators. These changes suggest that meditation may *enhance cognitive function, emotional resilience, and overall brain health*.

- **Immune system enhancement:** Regular meditation practice can have a positive impact on immune function, leading to enhanced immune response and reduced susceptibility to illness. Meditation has been associated with *increased activity of natural killer cells*, which play a critical role in immune surveillance and defense against pathogens. Moreover, meditation-induced *reductions in stress hormones* such as cortisol may contribute to immune system enhancement by mitigating the immunosuppressive effects of chronic stress.
- **Stress reduction:** One of the most well-established physiological effects of meditation is its ability to reduce stress levels and promote relaxation. Mindfulness-based meditation techniques, such as mindfulness meditation and loving-kindness meditation, have been shown to downregulate the sympathetic nervous system and activate the parasympathetic nervous system, inducing a state of deep relaxation known as the relaxation response. This results in *lowered heart rate, reduced blood pressure, decreased muscle tension, and alleviation of physiological markers of stress*.
- **Emotional regulation:** Meditation practices cultivate emotional regulation skills by promoting greater self-awareness, acceptance, and equanimity in the face of challenging emotions. Through mindfulness meditation, individuals learn to observe their thoughts and emotions without judgment, allowing them to *respond more skillfully to stressful situations and negative emotional experiences*. Functional imaging studies suggest that meditation strengthens connections between brain regions involved in emotional processing, leading to improved emotion regulation and emotional resilience over time.

Meditation is a wakeful hypometabolic state but differs from sleep and hibernation which are also physiological hypometabolic states. In sleep the fall in metabolic rate is much steeper and much greater and unlike hibernation there is no fall in rectal temperature during meditation.

Meditation to be truly effective, should facilitate bringing in the yogic attitude to everyday life. Meditation cannot help much if it is used merely as a relaxation technique leaving the rest of life completely unaffected. Twenty minutes of relaxation cannot compensate fully for day long tension and turmoil. It is only when the calming effect of meditation spills over into the rest of the day as a meditation spills over into the rest of the day as a meditative poise and brings true relaxation.

Yoga provides a new way of looking at life. The control that the person acquires does not consist predominantly of efforts to change circumstances and to change others. Instead the person tries to change his way of looking at circumstances and people, i.e., instead of learning to control circumstances, the person learns to gain liberation from circumstances. This approach works very well because our ability to change circumstances and people is very limited. On the other hand, the freedom to look at things the way we like is unlimited and nobody can take it away from us. This approach is recognized valid and is called cognitive reappraisal.

## INTEGRATING YOGA AND MEDITATION FOR HEALTH AND WELLNESS

### Synergistic Effects

Yoga and meditation are complementary practices that synergistically enhance each other's benefits when integrated into a holistic wellness regimen. Yoga provides a physical foundation through postures (asanas) and breath work (pranayama), promoting strength, flexibility, and body awareness. Meditation, on the other hand, cultivates mental clarity, emotional balance, and mindfulness, fostering inner peace and self-awareness.

Together, yoga and meditation offer a comprehensive approach to health and wellness, addressing the interconnectedness of mind, body, and spirit. By combining the physical and mental aspects of these practices, individuals can experience greater synergy and amplification of their therapeutic effects, leading to improved overall well-being.

### Practical Applications in Healthcare

The integration of yoga and meditation into healthcare settings has gained momentum in recent years, with growing recognition of their therapeutic potential for managing various health conditions and promoting preventive care. Healthcare providers are increasingly incorporating these practices into treatment plans for *chronic pain, anxiety, depression, cardiovascular disease, cancer, and other medical conditions*.

Yoga therapy programs, which tailor yoga practices to individual needs and health goals, have emerged as effective adjunctive therapies in rehabilitation, pain management, and mental health treatment. Similarly, mindfulness-based interventions, such as *mindfulness-based stress reduction (MBSR) and mindfulness-based cognitive therapy (MBCT)*, have been widely implemented in clinical settings to reduce stress, alleviate symptoms of mood disorders, and enhance overall well-being.

Furthermore, yoga and meditation programs are being integrated into corporate wellness initiatives, educational curricula, community health programs, and public health campaigns, extending their reach and impact across diverse populations.

## SUMMARY

- The chapter explores the profound physiological effects of yoga and meditation, highlighting their role in promoting health and well-being. Beginning with an overview of yoga and meditation, we have learned about the physiology of stress, emphasizing the importance of understanding the body's response to stressors.
- The physiological effects of yoga are then examined in detail, focusing on neurological changes, endocrine system modulation, cardiovascular health, and respiratory function. Yoga is shown to influence brain structure, neurotransmitter regulation, hormonal balance, blood pressure regulation, heart rate variability, breath awareness, and lung function, thereby enhancing overall physiological resilience and vitality.
- Similarly, the chapter explores the physiological effects of meditation, emphasizing its impact on brain activity, immune system function, stress reduction, and emotional regulation. Meditation is shown to promote neuroplasticity, immune system enhancement, stress resilience, and emotional balance, offering a holistic approach to fostering health and well-being from within.
- The chapter concludes by discussing the integration of yoga and meditation for health and wellness, highlighting their synergistic effects, practical applications in healthcare, and challenges to implementation. By combining the physical and mental aspects of these practices, healthcare providers can offer patients a comprehensive approach to healing and flourishing, addressing the interconnectedness of mind, body, and spirit in the pursuit of optimal health and well-being.

## LET US SEE, HOW MUCH YOU HAVE LEARNT?

### Review Questions

Q1. Describe the physiological effects of yoga and meditation.

Q2. Describe the role of yoga and meditation in relieving chronic stress.

### Multiple Choice Questions

Q1. Which of the following is NOT a component of yoga practice?
   a. Meditation
   b. Pranayama
   c. Cardiovascular exercise
   d. Asanas

Q2. Chronic stress is characterized by:
   a. Short-term activation of the stress response system
   b. Recurring episodes of acute stress
   c. Sustained activation of the stress response system over time
   d. Absence of any physiological response to stressors

Q3. What physiological response is triggered by the sympathetic nervous system during stress?
   a. Decreased heart rate
   b. Reduced blood pressure
   c. Release of cortisol
   d. Increased alertness

Q4. Which hormone is often referred to as the "stress hormone"?
   a. Serotonin
   b. Oxytocin
   c. Cortisol
   d. Adrenaline

Q5. How does yoga influence the endocrine system?
   a. By increasing cortisol levels
   b. By decreasing oxytocin production
   c. By promoting hormonal balance
   d. By suppressing the release of adrenaline

Q6. Which of the following is a physiological effect of meditation?
   a. Increased heart rate
   b. Enhanced immune system function
   c. Elevated blood pressure
   d. Decreased neuroplasticity

Q7. What is one of the main benefits of integrating yoga and meditation for health and wellness?
   a. Reduced physical activity
   b. Increased stress levels
   c. Enhanced overall well-being
   d. Worsened emotional regulation

Q8. What is the primary goal of yoga therapy programs?
   a. To standardize yoga practices
   b. To promote mindfulness meditation
   c. To tailor yoga practices to individual needs
   d. To exclude meditation from yoga practice

Q9. Which of the following is NOT a challenge associated with the integration of yoga and meditation into healthcare?
   a. Accessibility issues
   b. Standardization of instruction
   c. Cultural sensitivity and adaptation
   d. Lack of research evidence

Q10. What is the significance of neuroplasticity in the context of meditation?
   a. It refers to the brain's ability to adapt and reorganize in response to meditation practice
   b. It indicates a decrease in brain function due to meditation
   c. It highlights the importance of physical exercise over meditation for brain health
   d. It has no relevance to the effects of meditation on the brain

### ANSWERS
1. c   2. c   3. d   4. c   5. c   6. b   7. c   8. c   9. d   10. a

# Brain Death

**CHAPTER 102**

**COMPETENCY ADDRESSED**

**PY11.11:** Discuss the concept and criteria for diagnosis of brain death and its implications.

**LEARNING OBJECTIVES**

At the end of this chapter, you should be able to:
- Define brain death and discuss its concept.
- Discuss the diagnostic criteria for brain death.
- Describe the clinical implications of brain death.

## DEFINITION

Brain death is a state where there is a permanent and absolute halt in all brain functions, including the critical functions of the brainstem.

This status is irreversible, denoting a complete absence of neurological activity, which in turn results in the inability to sustain essential bodily functions autonomously.

It marks the end of all brain-related activities necessary for life, such as consciousness, cognition, and the regulation of vital processes like breathing and heart function.

## CONCEPT AND CRITERIA

There is a need to diagnose brain death with utmost accuracy and urgency. Major criterial to declare brain death are discussed below.

### Absent Brainstem Reflexes

These reflexes are mediated by the cranial nerves and are the main indicators of brainstem function. Absent light/pupillary reflex (both direct and consensual) is considered one of the most discriminant reflexes in BD diagnosis. Absence of other brain stem reflexes like corneal reflex, gag reflex etc. add to the diagnosis.

> **Pupils:** No response to bright light size: mid-position (4 mm) to dilated (9 mm) (absent light reflex, relation to dysfunctional cranial nerve II and III)

### Deep Unresponsive Coma

The diagnosis of deep unresponsive coma is a lack of spontaneous movements in addition to an absence of motor responses mediated by stimuli applied within the cranial nerve distribution.

### Atropine Test (AtT)

The atropine test assesses bulbar parasympathetic activity on heart activity in brain-dead patients. The method for this test consists in injecting 2 mg atropine under continuous monitoring of the ECG for 10 minutes. The atropine test is considered negative if heart rate is not increased by more than 3% compared with basal ECG records.

### Apnea Test

If absent respiratory effort is found by apnea test, it provides an essential sign of a complete loss of brainstem functions. But safely of the procedure is debatable in certain situation. If complete precautions are taken, the test can be done, and it can confirm brain death.

## IMPLICATIONS

- **Organ transplantation and procurement:** Early diagnosis of brain death can lead to better organ procurement and in turn organ transplantation benefits can be enhanced.

- **Judicious use of ventilators** and other advanced critical care facilities. Early and effective diagnosis of brain death will lead to the correct use of expensive critical care facilities including ventilators.
- **Medical research:** Brain death criteria are crucial for research on brain function and neurological disorders. Understanding brain death helps researchers develop treatments for conditions like traumatic brain injuries and strokes.
- **Ethical and legal decisions:** Brain death criteria guide ethical and legal decisions regarding life support, organ donation, and end-of-life care. Clear guidelines ensure respect for patient wishes and family decisions in challenging medical situations.

## SUMMARY

Brain death is a condition of permanent cessation of complete brain activity. In this condition, the person has absent brainstem reflexes which can be further confirmed by atropine test, apnea test etc. A brain-dead person with vegetative functions is an ideal donor for the procurement of organs for transplantation, following the appropriate ethical code and consent of the relatives of the patient.

## LET US SEE, HOW MUCH YOU HAVE LEARNT?

*Review Questions*

Q1. How would you confirm brain death in a patient?

Q2. What are the clinical implications of brain death?

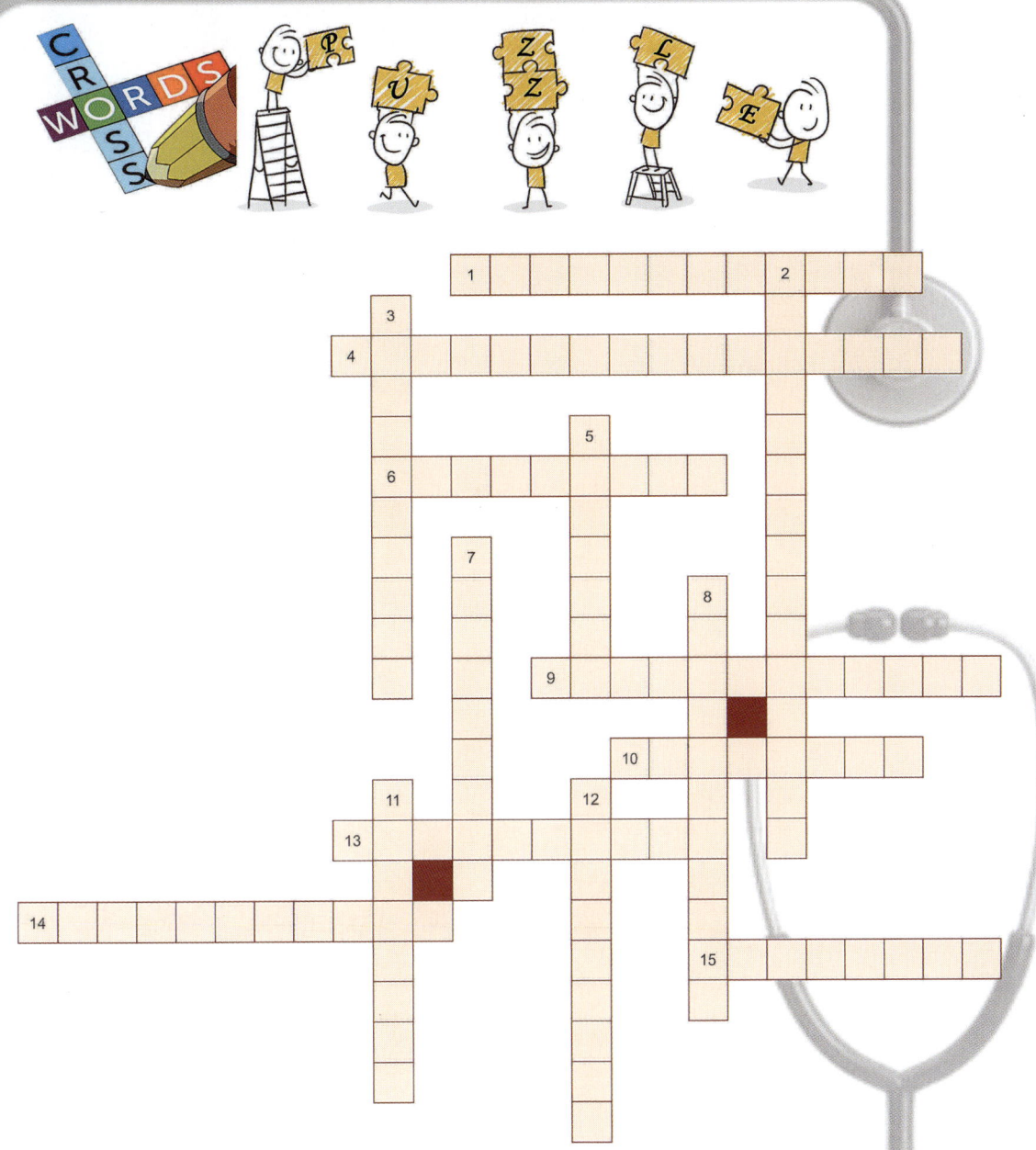

### Across

1. Compounds that inhibit oxidation and neutralize free radicals in the body
4. This physiological response helps to conserve heat in cold environments by reducing blood flow to the skin
6. This term describes exercises involving muscle contractions without movement
9. This gland plays a critical role in there gulation of body temperature
10. Regular meditation can reduce levels of this stress hormone
13. A severe and potentially fatal condition caused by prolonged exposure to high temperatures
14. The volume of air breathed in and out per minute during exercise
15. Exercise where muscle length changes while muscle tension remains constant

### Down

2. The body's process of adjusting to high temperatures over time
3. This molecule, produced during anaerobic metabolism, can cause muscle fatigue
5. The decrease in muscle mass and strength due to inactivity
7. The term for localized damage to the skin and other tissues due to extreme cold
8. This cytokine is known as anendogenous pyrogen, causing fever
11. The first stool of an infant, composed of materials ingested during the time the infant spends in the uterus
12. The absence of this reflex can be acriterion for brain death

# Appendix

## AETCOM 1: DOCTOR-PATIENT RELATIONSHIP

### COMPETENCY ADDRESSED
1. Enumerate and describe professional qualities and roles of a physician.
2. Demonstrate empathy in patient encounters.

### LEARNING OBJECTIVES
**At the end of this chapter, the learner should be able to:**
- Describe the duties of a physician to his patient, public, colleagues and himself.
- Describe the rights of the patients.
- Describe the doctor patient relationship and importance of building trust in it.
- Describe the boundaries of doctor patient relationship.

## MODULE-1: INTRODUCTION

Doctor patient relationship is established when a patient, suffering from a particular disease, at a given point of time, visits a doctor for his treatment. This relationship is based on four pillars viz. trust, knowledge, regard and loyalty.

As described by Chipidza and Wallwork,
*Knowledge refers to the doctor's knowledge of the patient as well as the patient's knowledge of the doctor. Trust involves the patient's faith in the doctor's competence and caring, as well as the doctor's trust in the patient and his or her beliefs and report of symptoms. Loyalty refers to the patient's willingness to forgive a doctor for any inconvenience or mistake and the doctor's commitment not to abandon a patient. Regard implies that the patients feel as though the doctor likes them as individuals and is "on their side."*

Though the doctor patient relationship is a mutual understanding of trust, it is vulnerable to turn stale due to some interferences mentioned below:
1. Any patient visiting the doctor for the first time, when the trust, knowledge and loyalty have not built up enough.
2. Any patient suffering from an untreatable disease with poor prognosis, the doctor instead of aiming at patient's quality of life, is over enthusiastically treating him. Communication with patient in such condition is very important in building trust and loyalty.
3. Over informed "Internet literate" patients typically try testing their doctor and question the knowledge of doctor. This obstructs building of trust between doctor and patient.
4. Family pressure, where the competence of the doctor is questioned and hampers the building of healthy doctor patient relationship.

| Models of doctor patient relationship | | | | |
|---|---|---|---|---|
| | *Paternalistic* | *Deliberative* | *Interpretive* | *Informative* |
| Patient's values | Objective: Shared by physician and patient | Open to development and revision through moral discussion | Inchoate and conflicting, requiring elucidation | Defined, fixed and known to the patient |
| Physician's obligation | Promoting patient's well-being irrespective of patient's preferences | Articulating and persuading the patient of the most admirable values as well as informing patient and implementing the patient's selected intervention | Elucidating and interpreting relevant patient values as well as informing the patient and implementing the patient's selected intervention | Providing relevant factual information and implementing patient's selected intervention |
| Conception of patient's autonomy | Asserting to objective values | Moral self-development relevant to medical care | Self-understanding relevant to medical care | Choice of and control over medical care |
| Conception of physician's role | Guardian | Friend or teacher | Councilor or advisor | Competent technical expert |

## MODULE-2: PANEL DISCUSSION/SYMPOSIUM

Visit the following links and answer the following questions:
a. https://www.mciindia.org/CMS/rules-regulations/code-of-medical-ethics-regulations-2002
b. http://www.cpso.on.ca/policies-publications/the-practice-guide-medicalprofessionalism-and-col/principles-of-practice-and-duties-of-physicians
   1. Keeping in view the principles of practice, what are the duties of a physician to an individual patient?
   2. What are the duties of a doctor to the public?
   3. What are the duties of a doctor to themselves and colleagues?

## MODULE-3: AETCOM MODULE REFERS TO THE PRESCRIBED SYLLABUS, GIVEN ON NMC WEBSITE

A 53-year-old man is seen by a cardiologist for chest pain lasting for a few minutes on accustomed exercise for the past 3 weeks. After a detailed history and physical examination, the doctor orders an ECG which was normal. He further orders an exercise stress test which showed reversible ischemia. The doctor orders an angiogram. At the time, the patient requests that he would like to have a second opinion. The cardiologist explains that he has done everything correctly and that the patient indeed requires an angiogram. The patient tells him that he cannot make a decision unless he talks to his family doctor of 20 years. The cardiologist is offended and tells the patient that he does not wish to see the patient any longer.

Answer the following questions from above scenario:
1. What are the rights of a patient?
2. What is the importance of trust in the doctor patient relationship?
3. Does the request for a second opinion provide sufficient grounds to terminate the doctor-patient relationship?

## MODULE-4: AETCOM MODULE REFERS TO THE PRESCRIBED SYLLABUS, GIVEN ON NMC WEBSITE

A young doctor has been taking care of an 86-year-old woman for the past 2 years. She had a fall 2 years ago and has been mostly bed ridden. She lives alone with just a caretaker and her children are abroad. She requires preventive care mostly and the doctor makes house visits once a week. The doctor spends time talking to her during each visit and makes her feel comfortable. One day during such a visit, the patient expresses the view that her children have been ungrateful to her and that she intends to call her lawyer today and divide her assets between the doctor and the caretaker after her death.

Answer the following questions from above scenario:
1. What should the doctor do?
2. What are the boundaries in the doctor-patient relationship?
3. What is value of trust and vulnerability in doctor-patient relationship?

## MODULE-5: REFLECTION

What Happened?
So what?
What next?

# AETCOM 2: THE FOUNDATIONS OF COMMUNICATION-I

## COMPETENCY ADDRESSED
Demonstrate ability to communicate to patients in a patient, respectful, nonthreatening, nonjudgmental and empathetic manner.

## LEARNING OBJECTIVES
**At the end of this chapter, the learner should be able to:**
- Describe the principles of communication.
- Describe the importance of effective communication for good doctor patient relationship.
- Communicate with a patient/subject to obtain the consent for examination of the patient/subject.

## MODULE-1: INTRODUCTION TO COMMUNICATION SKILLS

**Need to learn to communicate:** Formal training in developing communication skills is essential in the medical profession as it is essential for clinical practice where doctors have to deal with humans with sensitive needs and for avoiding medico-legal and ethical problems, arising out of communication failure.

**The process of communication:** It involves the transmission of message from the sender to receiver in the understandable manner.

### Components of Communication

- Verbal communication: (Speech and language). It is required in: Interpersonal communications.
- Sharing of knowledge (Lectures, presentations, seminars)
- Sharing of experiences, etc.

Nonverbal communication (Speech modulation, signs, gestures, expressions, body language, etc.).

**Effective communication "SKILL":** It involves the effective transmission of message from the sender to receiver in the understandable manner without changing the context and meaning of the message. It is combination of three skills:

1. **Conversational skill:** It involves *focusing, sharing information, clarifying, summarizing, paraphrasing, providing information, relevant questions, sharing humor.*
2. **Listening skill:** It involves active *listening, listening with purpose, feedback, using silence, acknowledgement of message.*
3. **Technical skill:** It involves *sharing empathy, feelings, observations and hopes, using nonverbal clues, appropriate use of touch and presenting reality.*

Key to good communication is:

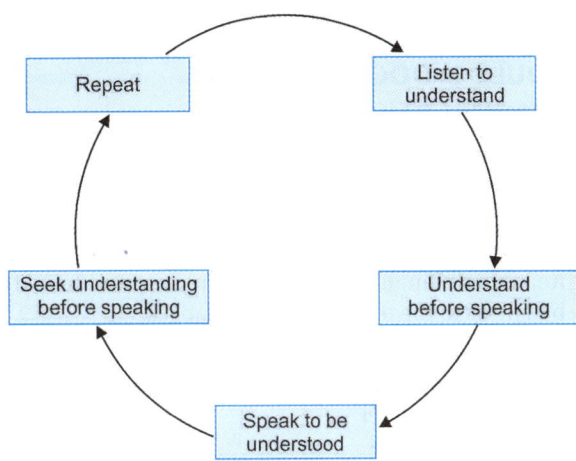

To sum up, effective communication should be:
*C*
- lear
- onsiderate
- omplete
- oncise
- ourteous
- orrect
- onsiderate

### Advantages of Effective Communication

- Understand person or situation in a better way
- Solves differences
- Builds the trust and respect
- Solves the misunderstandings
- Helps to connect well with everyone
- Helps in decision making.

### Barriers of Effective Communication

- Language
- Time constrain on physician
- Mental state of patient/relative of patient/psychological or emotional state
- Effect of medications on patient
- Personal attributes: Gender, race, etc.

### Overcoming the Barriers of Effective Communication

- Connecting with audience
- Use simple words
- Use nonverbal clues body language, gestures, etc.
- Show cultural and racial sensitivity
- Seek the participation of recipient
- Summarize whatever has been said and understood.

## MODULE-2: DOCTOR-PATIENT COMMUNICATION

a. ROLE-PLAY/Cinema-education (https://www.youtube.com/watch?v=UBpQ6YEAm6A).
b. A doctor will be required to communicate with the patient at the time of history taking, discussing the treatment plan, taking informed consent and breaking bad news to the patient or their relatives.

As per the literature, four models of doctor patient relationship have been described:
1. Paternalistic model
2. Informative model
3. Interpretive model
4. Deliberative model

Refer to the link given below and discuss each of these models:

https://www.researchgate.net/profile/Linda_Emanuel/publication/21598527_Four_Models_of_the_Physician-Patient_Relationship/links/0f3175398b5b75eb33000000/Four-Models-of-the-Physician-Patient-Relationship.pdf?origin=publication_detail

## MODULE-3: REFLECTION

What happened?
So what?
What next?

## COMMUNICATION SKILLS RATING SCALE ADAPTED FROM KALAMAZOO CONSENSUS STATEMENT

**Rating:** 1–3—Poor, 4–6—Satisfactory, 6–10—Superior

| Criteria | Score |
|---|---|
| Builds relationship | |
| Opens the discussion | |
| Gathers information | |
| Understands the patient's perspective | |
| Shares information | |
| Manages flow | |
| Overall rating | |

# Answers to Crossword Puzzles

##  Section 1: General Physiology

**Across**
- 4. Lysosome
- 7. Osmosis
- 9. Repolarization
- 11. Nitric
- 12. Cholesterol
- 14. Serotonin
- 15. Homeostasis
- 18. Phagocytosis
- 19. Glycerol
- 20. Desmosomes

**Down**
- 1. Acrosomes
- 2. Necrosis
- 3. Bicarbonate
- 5. Myosin
- 6. Centrioles
- 8. Microtubules
- 10. Endocytosis
- 13. Lactation
- 16. Crystalloids
- 17. Apoptosis

##  Section 4: Gastrointestinal Physiology

**Across**
- 1. Carboxypeptidase
- 6. Choleretics
- 10. Cholelithiasis
- 12. Duodenum
- 13. Defecation
- 14. Secretin
- 15. Deamination
- 18. Serosa
- 21. KupfferCells
- 22. Sialorrhea
- 24. Enterocytes
- 25. Hepatocytes

**Down**
- 2. Oxyntic
- 3. Cholesterol
- 4. Micelles
- 5. Glycogenesis
- 7. Chyme
- 8. Histamine
- 9. BirdBeak
- 11. Steatorrhea
- 16. Amylase
- 17. Haustrations
- 19. Cholecystokinin
- 20. Gastritis
- 23. Acini

##  Section 2: Hematology

**Across**
- 5. Platelets
- 6. Neutrophils
- 7. Interferons
- 8. Biliverdin
- 11. Monocytes
- 12. Hephaestin
- 13. Leukopoiesis
- 14. Phototherapy
- 19. Anticoagulants
- 20. Thrombopoietin
- 23. Stercobilinogen
- 24. Spectrin
- 27. Erythropoietin
- 28. Defensins
- 29. Hemoglobin
- 30. Hemophilia

**Down**
- 1. Immunoglobulin
- 2. Plasmapheresis
- 3. Agglutinins
- 4. Basophils
- 9. Hypoxia
- 10. Thalassemia
- 15. Hemosiderin
- 16. Reticulocyte
- 17. Pica
- 18. Albumin
- 21. Antibody
- 22. Carotenemia
- 25. Fibrinogen
- 26. Purpura

##  Section 5: Cardiovascular Physiology

**Across**
- 2. Pericardium
- 4. Vagus
- 6. CardiacOutput
- 7. PWave
- 11. Resistance
- 12. Ischemia
- 16. Baroreceptors
- 17. Angiotensin
- 21. Hypertension
- 22. Echocardiography

**Down**
- 1. Hemorrhage
- 3. Hypokalemia
- 4. Vasoconstriction
- 5. Atherosclerosis
- 7. Pulse
- 8. Arrhythmia
- 9. Endothelin
- 10. Atria
- 13. Angiography
- 14. Inverted
- 15. Technetium
- 16. Bradycardia
- 18. VenousPump
- 19. Diastole
- 20. Syncope

##  Section 3: Nerve Muscle Physiology

**Across**
- 3. Sarcolemma
- 5. Astrocytes
- 7. Caveolae
- 8. Sarcomere
- 10. Electromyography
- 12. Tetanus
- 15. Oligodendrocytes
- 17. Chromatolysis
- 18. Neurotemesis
- 19. Neuropraxia

**Down**
- 1. Tropomyosin
- 2. Dendrites
- 3. Synapsin
- 4. Physostigmine
- 6. Thymectomy
- 9. Neurotrophins
- 11. Tetrodotoxin
- 13. Hemicholinium
- 14. Crossbridges
- 16. Titin

##  Section 6: Respiratory Physiology

**Across**
- 3. Phosphatidylcholine
- 4. Emphysema
- 5. Alveoli
- 6. Oxidation
- 9. Compliance
- 13. BreathingReserve
- 15. PleuralEffusion
- 17. Hypoxia
- 18. Thoracentesis
- 19. Sympathetic
- 20. Apneustic

**Down**
- 1. Salbutamol
- 2. DeadSpaceAir
- 7. Acclimatization
- 8. Diaphragm
- 10. VitalCapacity
- 11. Bronchitis
- 12. Pneumocytes
- 14. Spirometer
- 16. Dyspnea

### Section 7: Renal Physiology

**Across**
2. Aldosterone
4. PlasmaClearance
8. Uremia
10. Vasopressin
11. GlomerularFiltration
13. Spironolactone
14. ObligatoryUrineVolume
17. Isosthenuria
18. Inulin
19. Frusemide

**Down**
1. FreeWaterClearance
2. AtonicBladder
3. Bradykinin
5. Nephron
6. GLUT
7. Fenestrae
9. VasaRecta
12. LoopOfHenle
15. Glomerulus
16. Dialysis

### Section 8: Endocrine Physiology

**Across**
3. Parathormone
4. Somatostatin
5. Acromegaly
7. Oxytocin
12. Thymosin
13. Hyperthermia
17. Osteoporosis
18. Panhypopituitarism
23. Kussamaul
27. Poikilothermia
28. Thyroglobulin
29. Insulin

**Down**
1. Osmoreceptors
2. AdrenalDiabetes
5. Aromatase
6. Brain
8. ChiefCells
9. Rickets
10. Chvostek
11. Neurohypophysis
14. Myxedema
15. Leptin
16. Korsakoff
19. Melatonin
20. Calcitonin
21. Potassium
22. Dyslipidemia
24. Dopamine
25. Somatotrophs
26. Transcortin

### Section 9: Reproductive Physiology

**Across**
3. Collagenase
6. Proliferative
8. Estrogen
10. Levonorgestrel
11. Implantation
13. Vasectomy
14. Menarche
16. Testes
19. Amenorrhea

**Down**
1. Spermiogenesis
2. Capacitation
4. Testosterone
5. Oxytocin
7. Trisomy
9. Spermatogenesis
12. Progesterone
14. Menstruation
15. Hyaluronidase
17. BarrBody
18. Puberty

### Section 10: Neurophysiology and Special Senses

**Across**
3. Agnosia
4. Basilar
7. Midbrain
10. Presbycusis
12. Otolith
13. CaudaEquina
16. Cataract
21. Spinothalamic
22. Muscarinic
23. Strychnine
25. Cochlea
27. Broadman
28. Wernicke
29. Delta
30. Corticospinal

**Down**
1. Mechanoreceptor
2. Dopamine
5. Synapse
6. Dyslexia
8. Macula
9. Arousal
11. Ishihara
14. Striatum
15. Rods
17. Tonometer
18. Nociceptor
19. BrocasArea
20. Vestibular
24. Fovea
26. Hippocampus

### Section 11: Integrated Physiology

**Across**
1. Antioxidants
4. Vasoconstriction
6. Isometric
9. Hypothalamus
10. Cortisol
13. Heatstroke
14. Ventilation
15. Isotonic

**Down**
2. Acclimatization
3. LacticAcid
5. Atrophy
7. Frostbite
8. Interleukin
11. Meconium
12. Brainstem

# Index

Page numbers followed by *f* refer to figure, *fc* refer to flowchart, and *t* refer to table

## A

A blood group 138
ABC test 885
Abdominal aorta, branches of 220*f*
Abdominal stria 614
ABO blood group system 138, 145
    agglutinins of 139*t*
    inheritance of 138
Absolute bone conduction test 884, 885*f*
Absorption 90, 240, 270, 274
    disorders of 279
Acclimatization 465, 862
Accommodation reflex 819, 865, 866
Acetazolamide 534
Acetone breath 622
Acetyl coenzyme A 718
Acetylcholine 213, 259, 339, 718, 787, 814
    receptor, serum 178
    release of 818*f*
Acetylcholinesterase inhibitors 176, 178
Acetylsalicylic acid 46
Achalasia 230
    cardia 230
    pathophysiology of 230
    potential complications of 230
Achlorhydria 240
Acid 837
Acid-base 34
    balance 40, 449
        clinical assessment of 44
        regulation of 402, 494
    disorders 445
    nomogram 46, 46*f*
Acidosis 45, 620, 622*fc*, 716
    effects of 45*t*
    hyperchloremic metabolic 46
    metabolic 40, 44, 45*f*, 386, 534, 537, 538
    respiratory 44, 449
Acidotic diets 573
Acini forms 245
Acquired immunity 110
    formation of 110
    maturation of 110
    types of 110*f*
Acquired immunodeficiency syndrome 117
Acromegalic facies 589
Acromegalic hand 590*f*
Acrosome 664
    reaction 681
Actin filament, molecular structure of 183*f*
Activated partial thromboplastin time 135
Actomyosin complex 192
Acute anaphylaxis reaction 116
Acute coronary artery occlusion 368
Acute kidney injury 534
    causes of 535
    clinical features of 536

Acute mountain sickness 466, 467
Acute renal failure 534
    causes of 535
    clinical features of 536
Acute respiratory distress syndrome 423, 438, 460
Adaptation, mechanism of 832
Addison's disease 611, 612
Addisonian crisis 613
Adenine nucleotides 367
Adenosine 220, 825
    diphosphate 147
    monophosphate 839
    triphosphate 202, 247
Adenylyl cyclase 20, 561, 570*f*
Adequate stimulus 725, 872
Adipokines 633
Adipose tissue 559, 826
    role of 633
Adiposity 900
Adjunctive therapy 533
Adolf's method 347
Adrenal cortex 559
    disorders of 612
Adrenal corticotropic hormone 586
Adrenal function 916
    tests 614
Adrenal gland 608*f*, 686
    anatomy of 608*f*
    biosynthesis of hormones of 607
    functional anatomy of 607
    hormone
        biosynthesis of 607
        hypersecretion of 607
        hyposecretion of 607
        physiological actions of 607
        secretion 607
    physiological anatomy of 607
    physiology of 607
Adrenal insufficiency 61, 612, 613, 615
    pathophysiology of 612*f*
    primary 37, 614
    secondary 613, 614
    tertiary 614
Adrenal medulla 607
Adrenaline 344, 497
Adrenarche 656
Adrenocortical hormones
    disorders of 612
    excretion of 608
    hypersecretion of 613
    hyposecretion of 612
    metabolism of 608
    secretion of 607
    transport of 607
Adrenocorticotropic hormone 611, 556
Adult respiratory distress syndrome 414
Aerobic system 904

Afferent arteriolar mechanism 500
Ageusia 841
Agglutinins 138, 139
Agglutinogen 138, 139
Aging, theories of 920
Agnosia 748
Agranular cells 500
Air
    filled lungs 410, 410*f*
    flow of 414
    liquid interface 413
    maximum amount of 427, 430
Airway
    epithelium 459
    management 479, 485
    obstruction 479, 484
    radius of 414
    resistance 411
        seat of 396, 414
    smooth muscle cells 459
Akinesia 765
Alanine
    aminotransferase 262
    transferase 99
Albumin 38, 69, 70, 76, 147, 262
    bilirubin complex 76
Albuminuria, physiological cause of 507
Alcohol 837
    intake, moderation of 634
Aldehydes 837
Aldosterone 513, 557, 608, 615
    antagonist 534
    deficiency 613
    effects of 609*f*
    escape 609, 609*f*
    hypersecretion of 609
    hyposecretion of 609
    mechanism 362
    physiological effects of 608
    secretion 609
        regulation of 609
    test 615
Alexia 746
Alkaline 237
    phosphatase 99, 262
    urine, excretion of 465
    yellow green 257
Alkaloids 838
Alkalosis 44, 45, 45*t*, 609
    metabolic 40, 44, 45*t*
    respiratory 44, 465
Allergic reactions 148
Allergic sensitization 482
Alpha actinin 185
Alpha cells 557
Alpha chain 74
Alpha gamma co-activation 728*f*
Alpha motor neuron, lesions of 778

Alpha neurons 706
Alpha waves 795, 800
   origin of 795
Alveolar air 421, 421*f*
   pressure, effects of 437*f*
Alveolar capillary membrane 402
Alveolar ducts 399
Alveolar epithelium 418
Alveolar macrophages, pulmonary 400, 401
Alveolar pressure 407, 407*f*, 408
Alveolar respiratory membrane 399*f*
Alveolar sac 399
Alveolar surfactant deficiency 413
Alveolar tissues, structure of 400*f*
Alveolar ventilation 422, 430
Alveoli 397-399, 402
   collapse of 411
   interdependence of 411
   level of 419*f*
Alveolus, microscopic structure of 400
Alzheimer's disease 25, 56, 222, 719, 795, 796*f*, 921
Amacrine cells 849, 850
Amenorrhea 685, 687*f*, 693
   temporary 689*f*
Amiloride 534, 838
Amine 718
   hormones 17, 559
   precursor uptake 400
Amino acids 69, 251, 274, 718
   conjugation of 259*fc*
   deamination of 256
   reabsorption of 510
Amino terminal 113
Aminopeptidase 247
Aminopyrine 34
Ammonia buffer 42, 44
Amnesia, anterograde 795
Amorphosynthesis 746
Amphetamines 719
Amygdala 790, 828, 830
   bilateral ablation of 790
Amylase, serum 252
Amyloid
   beta 921
   precursor protein 795
Anal canal 211
Analgesia
   pathway 783*f*
   system 781, 783
Anaphylactic reaction 148
Anaphylactic shock 116, 384, 535
   mechanism of 116*f*
Androgen 557, 607, 612, 645, 674
   binding protein 663
   pharmacological effects of 611
   resistance 651
Andropause 658
Androstenedione 674
Androsterone 646
Anemia 66, 77, 85, 141, 349, 367, 383, 458, 459, 477, 537, 538
   aplastic 122
   autoimmune 86
   chronic 82
   classification of 85, 86*t*
   clinical features of 86*f*
   hemolytic 79, 91, 93, 93*t*
   macrocytic 88, 91, 91*t*
   megaloblastic 88
   mild 85
   moderate 85
   morphological classification of 85*t*, 86*f*
   nonmegaloblastic 88
   pernicious 90, 236
   physiology of 85
   severe 85
   treatment of 147
Anemic hypoxia 476, 476*f*, 478
   effects of 476
Angina 368
   pectoris 368
Angiogenesis 330
Angiogram, coronary 366, 366*f*
Angiography 327
Angiotensin 330, 497, 501, 509
   concentration 609
   converting enzyme inhibitors 634
   receptor blockers 634
Angular gyrus 746, 792
   functions of 746
Anion
   channel 713
   exchanger 448
   gap 45, 46
   normal 46
Ankyrin 79
Anomia 748
Anomic aphasia 792
Anopia 854
Anorexia 579
Anosmia 832
   postinfluenza 833
Anoxia 478
Antagonist muscle 759
Anterior abdominal muscles 407
Anterior horn cells 778
Anterior pituitary gland 585, 588
   disorders of 588
Anterior semicircular canal 807
Anterior spinocerebellar tract 772
Anterior spinothalamic tract 771, 772, 773*f*
Anterior wall myocardial infarction 317
Anti-A antisera 141
Anti-acetylcholinesterase 176
Anti-aging therapies 923
Antianxiety drugs 720
Anti-B antisera 141
Antibiotics 271, 384
Antibody 112, 115, 138
   complement effects of 115
   elevated levels of 178
   maternal 916
Anticholinergics 270, 483
Anticlotting mechanism 132*f*
Anticoagulants 127*f*, 132, 133
   action of 133*f*
Anti-D antibody 139, 140
   injection of 141
Anti-D antisera 141
Anti-D prophylaxis, role of 140*f*
Antidepressant drugs 719
Antidiabetic medications 634
Antidiuretic hormone 37, 75, 513, 556, 590
   effects of 517*f*
   role of 516
   secretion, regulation of 590, 591*f*
Antifever effect 611
Antigen 112, 115, 138
   antibody reaction 113*f*
   binding site 113
   presenting cell 112, 112*f*
   viral 112
Antihypertensive agents 634
Anti-inflammatory medications 478
Antimotility agents 271
Antioxidants 922
   action, mechanism of 922
   endogenous 922
   nonenzymatic 922
   physiology of 920
   sources of 922
   supplements 923
   therapy 477
Antiplatelets drugs 124, 132
   mechanism of action of 124*f*
   role of 124*f*
Antiport 27*f*
Antithrombotic drugs, types of 133*f*
Antral follicle 673
   early 673
   formation of 673
Antrum 399
Anucleated cell 120
Anxiety 222, 536, 539, 635, 732, 927, 928
   disorders 926
Aorta 334, 375
   arch of 334
   coarctation of 299
Aortic bodies 457*f*, 458
Aortic valve 290
Apgar scores 413
Aphakia 846
Aphasia 792
   expressive 792
   global 792
   nonfluent 792
Apnea test 931
Apneusis 457, 481, 482*f*
Apneustic center 454, 456
Apoferritin 88
Apoptosis 23, 24, 24*t*, 25, 56
   absence of 24
   effects of dysregulated 25
   mechanism of 23
   pathological 24
   physiological 24
Appetite 601, 602, 801
   loss of 467
   regulation of 222
Aqueous flow 847
Aqueous humor 844, 846
   drainage of 846
   formation of 846*f*
Arachidonic acid, metabolites of 825
Arachnoid mater 769
Archicerebellum 757
Arcuate fasciculus 791, 792, 881
Arcuate nucleus 556, 578, 579
Argyll Robertson pupil 866
Arrhythmias 314, 370, 540
Arterial blood 40, 67, 825
Arterial circulation 375
Arterial gas embolism 472
Arterial pressure 299, 363, 501*f*, 609
   effects of 334*f*
   regulation of 494
Arterial pulse, characteristic of 375*f*
Arterial system 374*f*
Arterial tree, compliance of 375
Arteriole 324, 324*t*
Artery 324, 324*t*, 421
   distention of walls of 334
   hepatic 255
   left anterior descending 327, 365, 369
   occlusion 369*fc*

peripheral 375
    pulmonary 325, 434
    renal 372
    small 825
Artificial kidney 539
Ascending tracts, demyelination of 780
Ascites 379, 533
    treatment of 534
Asna 927
Aspartate aminotransferase 99, 262
Asphyxia 478, 479
    causes of 479$f$
Aspirin 46
Asthenozoospermia 666
Asthma 400, 411, 415, 423, 449
    bronchial 400, 482
    treatment of 400
Astigmatism 864
    physiological basis of 864, 864$f$
Astrocytes 157, 157$f$, 720
    fibrous 157
    protoplasmic 157
Atelectasis 409, 413
Atherosclerosis 368, 369, 622, 634, 641
Atherosclerotic plaques, development of 369
Athetosis 762
Atmospheric pressure 408, 464, 464$t$
Atonic bladder 546
    symptoms 547
Atria 287, 293
    depolarization of 304
Atrial contraction 297
Atrial natriuretic
    hormone 609
    peptide 37, 214, 234, 339, 513
Atrial repolarization 306
Atrial rhythm disorders 315$t$
Atrial septal defect 288, 299
Atrial stretch receptors 339
Atrial systole 295, 296
Atrial volume receptors 339
Atrial wall, stretching of 339
Atrioventricular block 317
Atrioventricular valves 288, 289, 289$t$, 299
Atrium 295
Atrophic rhinitis 833
Atropine test 931
Attachment proteins 185, 185$f$
Attenuation reflex 874
Auditory cortex 747, 747$f$
Auditory nerve fibers 880
Auditory pathway 870, 881
    ganglion of 881$t$
    nuclei of 881$t$
Auditory radiation 881
Auditory reflexes 881
Auditory tube 875
Auerbach's plexus 216
Augmented limb leads 309, 309$f$, 310
Auscultatory gap 360
Autacoids 509, 509$t$
Autoantibody 117, 157
Autoimmune diseases 537, 620, 628
Autoimmunity 116
Autologous transfusion 147
Automatic bladder
    features of 547
    function 547
Automatic involuntary system 454
Automatism 798
Autonomic functions, regulation of 578

Autonomic ganglia 814, 815, 818$f$
Autonomic nerves 367
Autonomic nervous system 217, 222, 333, 701, 814, 819, 925
    control of 818, 820$f$
    organization of 814, 814$f$
    role of 333
    working of 818
Autonomous bladder, features of 547
Autoregulation 496, 508$f$
    mechanism of 496
Axis deviation 319, 319$f$
Axon 170
    destruction of 163
    hillock 155
    length of 156
    structure of 161
Axonal loss 163
Axonal transport 162
Axonotemesis 167
Azoospermia 666
Azurophilic granules 101

# B

B blood group 138
Back pain 148
Bacteria 221
    role of 269
Bacterial infections, chronic 112
Bacteroides 222
Bainbridge reflex 333, 339
    mechanism 339$f$
Ballistic movements 758
    loss of 760
Ballistocardiography 348
Baram's loop 858
Barium swallow study 230
Barometric pressures 463
Baroreceptor 334
    discharge 334$f$
    location of 335$f$
    physiological significance of 335
    reflex 335, 344
        mechanism 333
Barr body 648
    significance of 648
Barrel chest 411
Barrier methods 693
Bartter syndrome 883
Basal acid output 242
Basal body temperature 675
Basal cell 828, 837
Basal ganglia 141, 719, 752, 755, 756, 761, 766
    anatomical location of 761$f$
    connections of 761, 762$f$
    direct pathway of 764$f$
    functioning of 763, 764, 764$f$
    indirect pathway of 764$f$
    lesions of 755
    location of 763$f$
    motor disorder of 719
    nuclei of 762$f$
    role of 755, 766
Basal metabolic rate 13, 601, 602, 799, 801, 892
Basement membrane 493, 493$f$, 506
Basilar membrane
    characteristics of 878
    frequency range of 880$f$
Basket cells 756, 758
Basophilic myeloblast 103

Basophils 102, 103
    lower number of 610
Bathmotropic effect 344
Becker muscular dystrophy 203
Behavior
    aggressive 581
    effects 578, 790
    functions 581
    reactions 790
Bell Magendie law 770
Beriberi 350
Beta agonists 483
Beta amyloid protein 795
Beta cell 557, 617, 619, 620$f$, 855
    development of 117$f$
    function declines 633
    pancreatic 619
Beta chain, position of 74
Beta waves 796
    origin of 796
Betamethasone 414
Beta-thalassemia 74, 76
    major 92
    minor 92
Bezold Jarish reflex 333, 339, 339$f$
Bicarbonate 278, 279
    buffer 42, 44
    excretion 44
    ion 34, 246, 449, 510
Biceps brachii, testing of 732
Bicuspid valve 288
Bile
    acidification of 258, 259$f$
    acids
        deficiency of 252
        secondary 259
    composition of 257
    concentration of 258
    deficiency of 259
    functions of 258
    role of 260, 277
    salt 259, 260$f$
        detergent-like action of 277
        functions of 259
        production 259$fc$
    secretion 258$f$, 260
        regulation of 258, 259$f$
    storage of 258
Biliary insufficiency 252
Biliary secretion 257
    mechanism of 258
Bilirubin 76, 96, 141
    conjugation of 98
    direct 99
    excretion of 258
    glucuronide 76
    indirect 99
    level, serum 93
    metabolism of 97$f$, 257
    unconjugated 76, 99
Biliverdin 76, 96
Bioactive compounds, synthesis of 221
Biochemical assays 56
Biological stimuli 781
Biomolecule, types of 18
Biots breathing 481
Biphasic recording, principle of 304$f$
Bipolar cells 849, 850
Bipolar limb leads 311
Bipolar neuron 156, 156$f$
Bird beak appearance 230

Bladder
  activity, unstable 545
  capacity 545
  contractions 545
  control 545
  decentralized 547
  distension 547
  fullness, loss of sensation of 546
  motor innervation of 543
  neck of 536
  posterior wall of 543
  regulation 544*fc*
  sensations 545
  sensory innervation of 543
Blast cells 66
Bleeding 540
  disorders 135, 135*t*
  gastrointestinal 525
  mucosal 123
  phase 675
  stoppage of 127
  tendencies 256
  time 123, 134
  types of 135
Blindness 746, 749
Blood 65, 66*f*, 399, 465, 475*f*
  banking 138, 145
    process of 145
  borne pathogen screening 146
  brain barrier
    formation of 157, 157*f*
    immature 141
  buffer system 42
  cells 610
  cleansing 257
  clots 438
  collection 145
  components 66, 67
    transfusion of 147
  composition of 65
  damming of 370
  delivery system 539
  deoxygenated 449*f*
  donation 145
  filtration of 257
  flow 6, 220, 255, 290, 290*f*, 326, 327*f*, 354, 366, 374, 423, 436, 495, 686, 824
    acute control of 329
    autoregulation of 329, 333, 339, 825
    control of 219*f*
    coronary 327, 365
    intermittent 377, 437
    long-term control of 330
    measurement of 326
    path of 496*f*
    pulmonary 436
    regulation of 329
    renal 494, 496*f*, 497, 497*fc*, 524, 528, 915
    types of 328
  functions of 65, 67
  glucose level 613, 826
  group 138, 138*t*, 139, 141, 142, 145
    antigens 80, 138, 139*f*
    physiological significance of 142
    prevalence of 142*t*
    testing 141, 141*t*
    types of 138
  investigations 538
  loss 86, 147
  osmolality of 67
  oxygen level dependent 824

  oxygenation of 449, 449*f*
  passing, amount of 326
  pH of 44, 44*f*, 65, 67
  physical characteristics of 67
  pressure 328, 334, 358, 358*f*, 360, 360*t*, 363, 459, 591, 799, 818, 900
    classification 362, 362*t*
    components of 358
    determinants of 358
    diastolic 297, 325, 358, 359*f*, 436, 927
    elevated 926
    high 500
    inhibits sympathetic outflow 334
    low 501
    measurement of 359, 359*f*
    regulation of 335, 335*fc*, 336, 336*fc*, 338*f*, 347, 358, 360, 819, 927
    short-term regulation of 360
    systolic 297, 325, 358, 375, 436, 927
  prevents damming of 339
  product management 148
  pumping of 290
  reservoir of 257
  sugar levels, regulation of 269
  supply 219, 398, 399
  testes barrier 661
  tests 145, 524
  transfusion 138, 139, 145, 147
    complications of 147
    incompatible 139
  urea 524
  urea nitrogen 525
  vessels 131, 182, 264, 333, 334, 459
    diameters 328*f*
    disorders of 133
    organization of 275*f*
    radius of 327
    small 435
    vasodilation of cutaneous 579
  viscosity of 327
  volume 34, 35, 220, 325, 356, 379, 383, 436, 591, 609, 903
Bloodstream 603
Blurred vision 863
Body 757*f*
  fat, total 900
  fluid 33, 40*t*
    compartments 33, 33*f*, 34, 34*t*, 35*f*, 36
  fluid
    loss of 384
    osmolality 35, 494
    pH of 40
    physical attributes of 34*t*
    volume 34, 37
  growth of acral parts of 590
  heat dissipating mechanisms of 892
  ipsilateral side of 760
  maintains equilibrium of 758
  mass index 900
  peripheral parts of 769
  plethysmography 426, 431
  righting reflex 737, 738
    types of 737*t*
  surface area 347
  systems 464, 600
  temperature 444, 445, 891, 891*f*, 894, 895*f*
    maintenance of 65
    normal 891
    regulation of 13*f*, 402, 579, 893*fc*, 894*fc*
  tissues 613
  water regulation 580
  weight 801

Bohr's effect 445
Bone 565*t*, 573, 611
  age 656
  composition of 565*f*
  endomysium of 379
  fluid 565
    calcium concentration falls 565
  formation of 566*f*
  marrow 80, 86
    yellow 80, 80*t*
  mineral density 901
  morphogenic protein 828
  regulation, physiology of 564
  resorption 538, 572
    mechanism of action of 565
  types of 565*f*
Botulinum toxin 176
  injection 230
Bötzinger complex 456
Bowel
  disease, inflammatory 221, 270
  wall, stretching of 251
Bowman's capsule 493, 507
  colloid osmotic pressure of 507
  structure of 493*f*
Bowman's glands 828
Boyle's law 470
Bradycardia 337*f*, 343, 344, 460, 602
Bradykinin 220, 330, 509
Brain 333, 454*f*, 618, 701, 782, 798
  activity 799, 928, 931
  attack 778
  death 931, 932
    diagnosis of 931
  derived neurotrophic factor 159, 222, 721
  development 917
  frontal regions of 796
  functional anatomy of 701
  growth 917
  gut
    axis dysfunction 271
    peptide 721
  health 927
  metabolism of 825
  parietal regions of 796
  parts of 702*f*
  regions, role of 832
  structure 927
  weight 795
Brainstem 333, 334*f*, 456, 456*f*, 482, 720, 735
  evoked potential 59
  median raphe of 719
  neuron of 719
  reflexes, absent 931
Breast
  cancers 57
  milk, role of 109
  parenchyma, regression of 24
Breastfeeding 912, 916
  support 913
Breath
  awareness 927
  control 925
  holding 460
  normal 454, 832*f*
  shortness of 86
  sounds 439
Breathing 405, 414, 443, 457
  apneustic 457
  capacity, maximum 430
  deep 622
  energy cost of 415, 415*f*

reserve 430, 431
techniques 478
Broad waxy casts 531
Broadman area 791
Broca's area 742, 744, 791, 791f, 792, 881
Bronchi 396, 397
histological section of 398f
Bronchial artery 435, 435f
system 399
Bronchial circulation 434
Bronchial secretion 399
Bronchial tone 400
Bronchioles
respiratory 396, 398, 399
terminal 396, 398
Bronchoprovocation test 426, 431
Bronchopulmonary anastomosis 435f
Bronze diabetes 88
Brown tumor 572, 572f
Brown-Sequard syndrome 780, 780f
Bruch lines, membrane of 845
Brunner's gland 249, 250
histology of 250f
Bucket handle movement 405, 406f
Buffalo hump 613
Buffer
nerves 334
systems 42
types of 40
Bulldog scalp 590f
Bumetanide 534

# C

C fibers 782
Caisson's disease 470
Cajal interstitial cells 213
Calcitonin 557, 569, 573, 575, 598
functions of 574
Calcitriol 574t
Calcium 131, 164, 192, 278, 279, 320, 564, 510
balance 569f
calmodulin complex 195
concentration 571fc
distribution of 564f
dysregulation 566
gluconate 569
homeostasis 573
hormonal regulation of 569f
induced calcium release 194, 195
influx 195, 213, 680
level
hormonal control of 569, 569t
serum 566, 573, 575
loss of 574
regulation, physiology of 564
release 195
sodium channels 213
spark 192
Calsequestrin 192
Cancer
cells 57, 438
pancreatic 253
Capillary
basement membrane 35, 418
circulation 376
endothelial membrane 418
endothelium 493, 506
exchange 437, 437f
filtration coefficient 377

fluid
dynamics 65, 71f, 377
exchange, Starling's equilibrium of 70f
shift mechanism 333, 338, 338f, 362
functions of 377
hydrostatic pressure 36, 70, 380, 507
membrane 36, 418
permeability of 380
Captopril 839
Carbachol 176
Carbamino hemoglobin 75, 448
Carbohydrate 6, 251, 274, 610f
absorption of 275, 275f, 276f
digestion of 240, 248, 248f, 275, 275f
metabolism 256, 257, 599, 609, 619, 620
oxidation 901
Carbon dioxide 75, 247, 442, 445, 447
accumulation of 459
concentration of 825
diffusion of 682
dissociation curves 448, 449f
narcosis 459
transport of 447, 447f, 448
Carbon monoxide 75, 420, 424, 426, 431, 446
poisoning 458, 472
Carbonic acid 449
Carbonic anhydrase 247
enzyme 80, 449
inhibitors 534
Carboxypeptidase 246, 247, 251
Cardiac activity 347
Cardiac arrhythmias 316
diagnosis of 309
Cardiac axis 314
diagnosis of 309
Cardiac catheterization 294
Cardiac complications 386
Cardiac cycle 293, 294, 295t, 297, 302
events of 298f
phases of 387, 437
time 293
Cardiac efficiency 299, 343
Cardiac failure 81, 386, 387, 535
classification of 387, 387t
pathophysiology of 387, 387f
treatment of 534
Cardiac function curves 351, 351f
Cardiac index 347
Cardiac metabolic derangements 349
Cardiac muscle 182, 183, 187, 188, 190f, 191t, 194f, 195, 196, 196f, 197, 198, 198f, 199, 343
action potential of 189
blood supply of 366f
contraction of 193, 200f
Cardiac output 336, 347-349, 351, 354, 355f, 367, 434, 818, 921
effects of 359fc
high 349
low 349
measurement of 347
regulation of 347, 350, 350fc
Cardiac receptors, role of 339
Cardiac sphincter 228
Cardiac tamponade 349
Cardiomyopathy 5
Cardiopulmonary exercise testing 426, 431
Cardiovascular abnormalities 653
Cardiovascular diseases 388, 634, 926
physiological basis of 383
reduced risk of 343

Cardiovascular efficiency 906
Cardiovascular function 46
Cardiovascular health 633, 927
Cardiovascular management 481
Cardiovascular mechanisms, regulation of 333t
Cardiovascular regulation 333, 339
Cardiovascular regulatory mechanisms 333
classification of 333
Cardiovascular system 45, 86, 285, 465, 600, 899, 902, 914, 921
functions of 290
Carotenemia 98, 602
Carotid
bodies 458, 459
sinus 334
Carpel tunnel syndrome 590
Carpopedal spasm 568, 568f
Carrier proteins 26
Cartilage 398
Castle's intrinsic factor, role of 236
Catalase 922
Cataract 846, 846f
Catecholamines 19, 351, 560
bronchodilator effect of 610
Catechol-o-methyltransferase 719
Cauda equina 705
Caudate circuit 763
lesions of 763
neural connections of 763
primary 763f
Caudate loop 766
Caveolae system 188f
Cavity, oral 211, 224, 228, 230, 275, 277
Celiac disease 270, 280
Celiac ganglions 217
Cell 3, 7, 56f, 112, 565, 608, 758
adhesion molecules 7
body 155, 167, 168f, 170, 840
cluster of 837
communications 16, 17f
complex 858
component isolation 56
constituents of 3t
counts 67
culture 56
cytoskeleton 5f
diameter 81
drinking 30
eating 30
fractionation 56
functions of 55
in vitro, growth of 56
malignant 112
mediated immune response 111f
mediated immunity 110, 111
functions of 112
membrane 3, 6, 7, 19, 27f, 35, 48, 418, 555, 838, 839, 939
functions of 6
proteins 7
selective permeability of 6
structure of 6f
morphology 81
nucleus 5f
organelles 7
functions of 7
structure of 7
removal of 66
types of 828, 849
Cellophane membranes 539

Cellular acclimatization 466
Cellular analysis, applications of 58
Cellular casts 531
Cellular communications 57
Cellular damage 921
   accumulation of 920
Cellular defense 109
Cellular dynamics, long-term observation of 57
Cellular epithelium 418
Cellular function 611
Cellular organelles 79
Cellular oxidoreductase enzymes 56
Cellular physiology, applications of 55
Cellular senescence theory 920
Central auditory pathway 881, 882$f$
Central canal, dilation of 780
Central nervous system 24, 45, 169, 217, 222, 240, 379, 600, 601, 701
   disorders 480
   embryonic development of 702$f$
   myelination of neurons of 157
   stimulation 614
Central venous pressure 378
Cephalic phase 214, 235, 235$f$, 249
Cerebellar function tests, abnormal 760
Cerebellar nuclei 756, 757$f$
Cerebellar nystagmus 760
Cerebellospinal tract 756
Cerebellum 704, 719, 755, 756, 757$f$, 789
   functional unit of 757, 757$f$, 759$f$
   functions of 758
   histology of 756$f$
   inferior surfaces of 756$f$
   lesions of 755, 760
   midsagittal section of 756$f$
   physiological division of 757
   role of 755, 766
   superior surfaces of 756$f$
Cerebral artery
   middle 825, 860
   posterior 825, 860
Cerebral association areas 744$f$
Cerebral blood flow 823, 824$fc$
   functional anatomy of 823
   measurement of 824
   physiology of 823
   regulation of 823, 825
Cerebral circulation, physiology of 824
Cerebral cortex 701, 719, 730, 738, 742, 743$t$, 763
   areas of 823$f$
   functional anatomy of 742
   functions of 752
   level of 738
   lobes of 743$f$
   motor connections of 755$f$
   parts of 755$f$
   structural organization of 743$f$
   superior view of 702$f$
Cerebral dominance 749
Cerebral edema 465, 467, 468, 533, 534
Cerebral hemispheres 749
Cerebral ischemia 465
Cerebral syndrome 467
Cerebration 602
Cerebrocerebellum 757
Cerebrospinal fluid 630
Cerebrovascular accidents 825
Cerebrovascular blood flow 900
Cerebrum 769
   basal view of 703$f$
   coronal section of 773$f$
   lobes of 742
   medial view of 703$f$
Ceruloplasmin 663
Cervical ganglia 343
Chamber enlargement 319
Charcot-Marie-Tooth disease 157
Chemical 531
   connections 17
   detoxification of 257
   messengers 18, 20
      classification of 18$t$
      mechanism of action of 17
   regulation 454, 457
   stimuli 781
   synapse 711
   thermogenesis 580
Chemoreceptor 337, 457$f$, 827, 838
   central 457, 457$f$
   location of 335$f$
   reflex 336, 344, 458
      mechanism 333
Chemoreflex
   coronary 333
   pulmonary 454, 460
Chemotaxis 106
Chemotherapy, cytotoxic 122
Chenodeoxycholic acid 259
Chest
   diameters of 404, 405$f$
   leads 309, 310, 310$f$
      place theory of 310$f$
   pain 299, 327
   tube insertion 440, 440$f$
   wall 410, 411
      deformities 411
      disorders 484
Chewing reflex 228
Cheyne-Stokes respiration 457, 480, 481, 482$f$
Chloride 278, 448, 526
   ion 34
   shift 448$f$
Chlorothiazide 534
Cholagogues 260
Cholangiopancreatography, endoscopic retrograde 253
Cholecystokinin 214, 218, 219, 236, 239, 249, 259, 558
Cholelithiasis 260, 261
Cholera 279
   infection 279$fc$
Choleretics 260
Cholesterol 259, 602, 680
   esterase 248
   esters, digestion of 278
   levels, management of 269
   stones 261
Cholesteryl ester hydrolase 251
Cholic acid 259
Choline 718
Chorea 762, 763
Choroid 845
Christmas disease 135
Chromium labelled red cells 80
Chromosomal aberrations 922
Chromosomal abnormality 649, 650, 650$t$
Chromosome 795
Chronaxie 164
Chronic hypoventilation syndrome 454
Chronic kidney disease 537
   causes of 537
   clinical features of 538
   management of 539
   pathophysiology of 538$f$
Chronic mountain sickness 466, 467
Chronic obstructive pulmonary disease 70, 399, 410, 411, 415, 420, 424, 445, 448, 449, 477, 483, 921
Chronic stress 925
   effects of 926$f$
   health implications of 926
Chronotropic effect 343
Chvostek's sign 568, 569$f$
Chylomicron formation 278
Chyme 238, 251
   pH of 249
Chymotrypsin 246, 247, 251
Cilia 398
Ciliary body 845
Ciliary escalator action 401
Ciliary muscles 845
Ciliary neurotrophic factor 160
Cineradiography 294
Circadian rhythm 719
   maintenance of 801
   regulation of 581, 629
Circular smooth muscles, layers of 211
Circulation 324, 325$f$
   phase 103
Circulatory system 324, 468
   components of 324$fc$
Circumoral numbness 568
Circumvallate papillae 836
Citric acid 665
Clara cells 400
Clarke's column 770
Clasp knife spasticity 739$f$
Clathrin 30
   mediated vesicular transport 163$f$
Climax 680
Close off nasopharynx 229
Closed circuit method 428
Clot
   formation, disorders of 133
   retraction 122, 123, 131
      time 131, 134
   stabilization of 131
Cloudy dialysate 540
Cocaine 719
Cochlea 875
   structure of 876, 876$f$
Cochlear nerve 879$f$
Cochlear nuclei 881
Coenzyme Q10 922, 923
Cognitive development 917
Cognitive function 801, 921
Cognitive performance 900
Cognitive skills 910
Cold
   clammy skin 386
   injury 895
      mechanism of 895
   intolerance 602
Collagen 182, 506
   meshwork of 493
Collecting duct 44, 494, 499
Colliculus, inferior 881
Colloidal suspension 67
Colloids 38
   droplets 599
   natural 38
   osmotic pressure 69, 70, 377, 380, 507
   synthetic 38

Colon 269
    distal portion of 271
Colonic motility 266
Colonoileal reflex 217
Color vision 844, 853
    defects 854t
        types of 853, 854
    photochemistry of 853
    tests for 854
    theories of 853
    Young-Helmholtz theory of 853
Coma 459
    hyperosmolar
        nonketonuric 622
        nonketotic 622
Comatose 716
Combined estrogen-progesterone pill 694
Common bile duct 97
Complement system 115
    pathway of 116f
Complete airway blockage 422
Complete androgen insensitivity syndrome 657
Complete cord transaction 779
Complete perfusion blockage 422
Complex biological process 920
Complex somatic sensation 723
Compliance loop 409f
Concave lens 863f
Concentration
    high 591, 603, 605
    ionic 50
Conception, physiology of 679
Conduction, disorders of 317
Cone
    cell 847
    spectral sensitivity of 853
Congenital disorders 454
Congenital immunodeficiency syndromes 117
Congestion
    degree of 411
    pulmonary 459
Conn syndrome 614
Consciousness, impaired 798
Consensual light reflex 865, 866f
Constipation 233, 269, 272
Constricted kidney response 362
Constrictor pupillae 845
Contraception 692
    methods of 692, 692fc, 694
Contraceptives pills, oral 694
Contraction 201
    propulsive 251
    summation of 196, 197f
    velocity of 200f
Cord transaction 778
Core temperature 891
Cornea 844, 845
Corneal calcification 573
Corona radiata 680
Coronary artery 367f
    disease 368
    phasic blood flow of 367f
    syndrome 622
Coronary blood flow 327, 365
    measurement of 366
    pecularities of 366
    regulation of 367, 368fc
Coronary circulation 365, 365f, 367
Corpus
    albicans 674
    callosum 702, 703f, 749
        functions of 749
    hemorrhagicum 674
    luteum 558, 674, 684
        functions of 674
        granulosa cells of 558
    striatum 761
        stimulation of 764
Cortex
    contralateral 798
    renal 494
    temporal 881
Corti organ 876
Corti rods 877
Cortical collecting duct 494
    role of 511
Cortical nephrons 494, 495, 495t
Cortical reaction 681, 681f
Corticonuclear fibers 756
Cortico-olivo-cerebellar fiber 756
Cortico-ponto-cerebellar fibers 756
Cortico-reticular-cerebellar fibers 756
Corticorubral fibers 756
Corticospinal pathway 707
Corticospinal tract 454, 763f, 775, 776
    anterior 776, 776f
    functions of 776
    lateral 776
    lesion 779
Corticosteroid 178, 607
    pharmacological actions of 607
Corticosterone 607, 609
Corticostriate pathway 763
Corticotrophs 556, 585
Corticotropin-releasing hormone 556
    secretion of 611
Cortico-vestibulo-cerebellar fibers 756
Cortisol 609
    antiallergic effect of 611
    anti-inflammatory effect of 611
    antistress effect of 611
    effects of 610f
    levels 615
    lower levels of 927
    permissive action of 610
    physiological effects of 609
    release of 926
    secretion, regulation of 611
Cough 148, 460
    reflex 402
Counter current exchanger system 514, 515, 516f
Counter current multiplier system 514, 515f
    complement effects of 515f
Cramps 536, 568
Cranial nerve nuclei 818
Cranium 379
Creatine phosphate 202
Creatinine 526
    clearance method 527
    production 528
Cretinism 602
Critical anthropometric measurements 911
Critical care support 485
Critical closing pressure 327
Crossbridge 184
Crossed extensor reflex 734f
Crude touch
    expressions of 774f
    physiological significance of 773
Cryoprecipitate 147

Cryopreservation 146
Cryptorchidism 666
Crystalline lens 845, 845f, 846f
Crystalloids 37
    hypertonic 38
    isotonic 38
Cupula, movement of 808f
Cushing's disease 613
Cushing's reflex 333, 337, 337f
Cushing's syndrome 574, 613-615
    clinical features of 614f
    pathophysiology of 613f
Cyanide 458
    ions oxidize 75
    poisoning 329, 477
Cyanosis 386, 413, 439, 479
    central 480
    peripheral 480
Cyclic adenosine monophosphate 831, 839
Cyclic guanosine monophosphate 839
Cylindrical lens 864
Cystic fibrosis 252
Cystometry, static 546
Cytokines 159
Cytolysis 112
Cytoplasm 3, 101
Cytoplasmic characteristics 81
Cytoskeleton 3, 4, 4t
Cytotoxic reaction 116
Cytotoxicity 111

## D

D antigen 139
Dampness, degree of 375
Dark urine 148
Darrow-Yannet diagram 35
Dead space
    air 423
    measurement of 423
Deafness
    conductive 883, 885
    physiology of 883
Decarboxylation cells store 400
Decompression sickness 470, 472
Deep brain stimulation 766
Deep sleep 797, 801
Deep tendon reflexes 177
Deep unresponsive coma 931
    diagnosis of 931
Deep-sea diving 470
Defecation 265, 267
    reflex 218, 267, 267t, 268f
        process of 268fc
Defensins 106
Defibrillator, mechanism of action of 315f
Degenerative brain disease 796
Deglutition
    apnea 229
    buccal phase of 228f
    esophageal phase of 229, 229f
    involuntary phase of 229f
    pharyngeal phase of 229f
    reflex 217, 819
Dehydration 33-35, 279fc, 525
    acute 70
    signs of 622
Dehydroepiandrosterone 646
    sulfate test 615
Delta cells 557
Delta chain 74

Delta waves 797, 801
　origin of 797
Demyelinating disorders 164
Dendrites 155
Dendritic spines 793
Denervation disuse atrophy 778
Dentate
　gyrus 790
　nucleus 756
Dentato-rubro-olivo-cerebello-dentate loop 766
Dento-thalamo-cortical fibers 756
Deoxyribonucleic acid 3
　synthesis 89f
　transcription of 587
Depolarization 213
　phases of 195
　receptor potential 831
Depolarizing blockers 176
Depressed mood 658
Depression 222, 635, 719, 926
　risk of 901
Descending tracts 775, 780
Desmin 185
Desmosomes 16
Desynchronized sleep 799, 801
Detrusor muscle function 546
Deuteranopia 854
Deuterium oxide 34
Development 272, 599
Dexamethasone suppression test 614
Dextran 38
Dhyana 927
Di George syndrome 572
Diabetes insipidus 517, 534, 591
　nephrogenic 518, 591
　neurogenic 591
　types of 591
Diabetes mellitus 75, 257, 369, 507, 534, 537, 619, 622
　complications of 622
　pathogenesis of 620, 621fc
　pituitary 589
　stage of 620
　treatment of 622
　type 1 621t
　type 2 621t, 634
Diabetic control, long-term 75
Diabetic ketoacidosis 622
　treatment of 623
Diabetic retinopathy 622
Diadochokinesia 761f
Dialysate 539
Dialysis, principle of 539f
Dialyzer 539
Diapedesis 106
Diaphragm 405
　central tendinous portion of 405
　peripheral part of 405
Diaphragmatic descent leads 405
Diarrhea 35, 233, 166, 270, 295
　chronic 280
　psychogenic 271
　treatment of 271
Diencephalon 702
Dietary antioxidants 922
Dietary deficiency 89
Dietary fiber 269
　role of 233, 245
Diffusion 26
　capacity 420, 426

Digestion 221, 222, 228, 231f, 233, 245, 264, 274, 277
　disorders of 279
　physiology of 274
Digestive disorders, prevention of 269
Digestive enzyme 5, 247, 252
　pancreatic 249
　production 915
Digestive functions 247
Digestive health 269
Digestive system 274, 465
　functions of 211
　structure of 211
Dihydropyridine 192
　receptors 192
Dihydrotestosterone 646
Dilator pupillae 845
Dipalmitoylphosphatidylcholine 411
Diplegia 781
Diploid chromosomes 648
Dipole, principle of 302f
Direct light reflex 865
Direct nerve stimulation 59
Disequilibrium syndrome 540
Dissolved oxygen, calculate concentration of 443
Distal colon 264
Distal convoluted tubule 493, 499
　role of 511
Distant vision 862
Disulfide bonds 113
Diuretics 478, 533
　mechanism of action of 533, 534fc
　osmotic 534
　physiological basis of 533
　use of 533
Diurnal variation 360, 891
Divalent metal transporter 88
Diver's paralysis 470
Divergence 707, 714
Dominant cerebral hemisphere, angular gyrus of 792
Donan effect 28
Donor
　registration of 145
　screening 148
Dopamine 556, 559, 719
　receptors 719
　secreting fetal cells, transplantation of 765
Dopaminergic neurons 719
　selective loss of 719
Doppler's principle 326
Dorsal column 90
　medial lemniscal system 774
　tract 772, 774f
Dorsal nucleus, lateral 753
Dorsal respiratory group 454-456
Dorsal spinocerebellar tracts 775f
Dorsiflexion 736f
Double vision, intermittent 176
Down's syndrome 651
　clinical features of 652
Dromotropic effect 343
Drowning 479
Drowsiness 459
Drug
　absorption of 402, 438
　blocking ACh-gated sodium receptors 176
　detoxification of 257
　effects of 716
　overdose 484

Dry vaginal lining 658
d-tubocurarine 176
Duchenne muscular dystrophy 203
Duct 661
Ductal cells 247f
Ductal dilatation 253
Ductal obstruction, pancreatic 253
Dumping syndrome 240, 241
Duodenal distension 267
Duodenal mucosa 249
　irritation of 250
Duodenum 213, 245, 249, 251, 275, 276
Dwarfism, pituitary 603
Dye relation, concentration of 348f
Dynamic lung volumes 427, 429, 429f
Dynamin 30
Dynein 7f
Dysarthria 760
Dysautonomia, familial 841
Dysbarism 470
Dysdiadochokinesia 760
Dysgeusia 841
Dyslexia 746
Dyslipidemia 261, 632, 633
　impact of 633
Dysmetria 760
Dysosmia 833
Dysphagia 765
Dyspnea 148, 438, 439, 465, 477
Dyspneic index 431
Dystrophin 185

# E

Ear
　functional anatomy of 872
　muscles, sudden contraction of 874
　ossicles 873
　　functions of 874
Early dumping syndrome 241
Echocardiography 293, 294
Ectoderm 845
Ectopic calcification 573
Edema 459, 533, 537, 538, 590
　pulmonary 438, 460, 465, 468
Edinger-Westphal nucleus 845
Edridge green lantern 855f
Edrophonium test 177, 178
Effector 731
Efferent arteriolar mechanism 500
Einthoven's law 308
Einthoven's triangle 308, 308f
Ejaculation 680, 819
Elastase 106
Elastic recoil, loss of 409
Elastin 182
Electrical activity, genesis of 850
Electrical synapse 711
　structure of 711f
Electrocardiogram 307, 311, 319, 319t, 320t
　physiology of 302
Electrocardiography 59, 293, 302, 307
　basics of 302
　jelly 308
　leads 308
　　types of 308fc
　paper 307, 307f
Electrodes 308, 308f
　placement 303, 797f
Electrodiagnostic test 178

Electroencephalography
  physiology of 795
  waves, types of 795
Electrolyte 246, 320
  absorption of 258, 265
  balance 46, 915
    regulation of 494
  disturbances 314, 319, 320t
  imbalance 538, 540
    detection 311
  obligatory reabsorption of 510
Electromagnetic flowmeter 326, 349
Electromyography 170
Electron
  loss of 75
  microscopy 55
Electrophysiological techniques 59
Electrophysiology 59
Embolus formation, pathogenesis of 368f
Embryo, sex differentiation of 648
Embryonic development 702f, 702t
Emission 679
Emmetropia 862, 862f
Emotional stimulus 237
Emotions 360
  physiology of 789
  regulation of 222
Emphysema 411, 415, 445, 448
Emulsification, functions of 277
End-diastolic volume 296, 297
Endocardium 288
Endocrine disorder 574t
  prevalence of 921
  primary 561, 562, 574
  principle of 561
  secondary 561, 562, 574
  tertiary 562
Endocrine dysfunction 5
Endocrine functions 235, 257, 494, 578, 790
Endocrine gland 555, 556, 556t
Endocrine hormones
  disorders of
    hypersecretion of 561t
    hyposecretion of 561t
Endocrine organs, maturation of 916
Endocrine pancreas 617
  role of 617
Endocrine physiology 553
Endocrine system 555, 555f, 904, 916, 921, 927
Endocrinology, reproductive 641
Endocytosis 30
  receptor-mediated 30, 30f
Endolymph 876
Endomysium 182
Endopeptidases 247
Endothelial cells 132
Endothelial derived relaxation factor 368
Endothelial dysfunction 633
Endothelial surface, smoothness of 132
Endothelin 330, 509
Endothelium 124, 130
  derived factor 329, 329f
End-systolic volume 296, 297
Endurance exercises 906
Energy
  fat utilization for 587
  production, glycolytic pathway for 79
  release, hormone of 623
  system, primary 901
Enkephalins 720
Enteric nervous system 215, 217, 222, 235
Enteritis 266

Enterochromaffin cells 234
Enterocytes 250
Enteroendocrine cells 234
Enterogastric reflex 217, 239, 240f
Enterohepatic circulation 260, 260f
Enterokinase 248
Entorhinal cortex 830, 832
Envelope synapses 157
Enzymatic antioxidants 922
Enzyme 19, 19f, 106, 138
  activity 46
    assays 56
  clotting 665
  linked
    cytokine receptors 561
    immunosorbent assay 57
  pancreatic 246, 248f
  premature activation of 252
  proteolytic 664, 666
Eosinophils 102
Ependymal cells 157, 157f
Epicritic sensations 746
Epigenetic modulators 923
Epiglottis 840
Epilepsy 716
  psychomotor 798, 798f
  treatment of 799
Epileptic seizures, types of 797
Epimysium 182
Epinephrine 330, 509, 557, 559, 719
Epithelial basement membrane 418
Epithelial cells 55f, 250
  layers of 493, 506
Epithelial sodium channels 513
Epithelium 398
Epsilon chain 74
Erectile dysfunction 658
Erection 819
  female 680
Erlanger Gasser's classification 162, 162f, 162t, 165
Erythroblast
  immature 140
  stage 81
Erythroblastosis fetalis 140
Erythrocytes 67, 79, 81
  formation 79
  functions of 79, 80
  sedimentation rate 87
Erythroid series, formation of 101
Erythropoiesis 80
  prime regulator of 80
  regulation of 80
  site of 80
Erythropoietin 80, 81, 465, 558, 561
  decreased production of 538
  formation of 82f
  gene 81, 466
  level peak 465
  mechanism of action of 82
  stimulates 82
  synthesis of 81
Esophageal manometry 230
Esophageal sphincter 240
Esophagogastroduodenoscopy 230
Esophagus 211, 224
  functional anatomy of 228
Estradiol 646
Estriol 643, 646
Estrogen 557, 558, 643, 663, 664, 674, 683
  formation of 645f
Estrone 643

Ethacrynic acid 534
Ethmoid bone, cribriform plate of 828
Ethylene glycol poisoning 46
Eustachian tube 873
Exacerbations, management of 483
Exchange transfusion 141, 141f
Excitation contraction coupling theory 192, 192f, 193fc
Excitotoxicity, glutamate-induced 720
Excretory function 235, 257, 494
Excretory products, diffusion of 683
Excretory system 491f
Exercise 349, 360, 892
  classification of 900, 901t
  effects of 360t, 901t
  energy sources for 904
  induced bronchoconstriction 482
  intolerance 5
  isotonic 901
  lack of 898
  long-term adaptation of 904
  mild 336, 360
  moderate 336, 360
  physiological effects of 901
  physiology 445
  severe 360
  stress testing 311
Exocytosis 30, 31
  constitutive 30
Exopeptidases 247
Exophthalmos 601
Expiration
  maximum speed of 430
  mechanism of 407
  muscles of 407
  process of 408f
Expiratory capacity 426, 427
Expiratory flow rates 430
Expiratory reserve volume 426, 427
Extensive mucosal foldings 274f
Extensor muscles 780
External auditory canal 872
External ear 872, 873f
  functions of 872
External intercostal muscles 405
Extracellular fluid 26, 33, 34, 40, 838, 839
  composition of 34
  ionic
    changes, effects of 164f
    composition of 164
  volume 609
    measurement of 34, 35
Extracellular potassium ion 609
Extracorpuscular defect 86, 93
Extraglomerular mesangial cells 500
Extrapyramidal tract 775, 776, 777t, 778
  lesion 779
  functions of 777
Extremities, gangrene of 622
Extrinsic innervation 215, 216f
Extrinsic mechanism 509
Extrinsic pathway 130
Extrinsic protein 6
Eye 844
  anatomy of 844
  closure of 800
  external anatomy of 844f
  functional anatomy of 844
  fundus of 848f
  movements 865
Eyeball 844, 845
  internal structure of 845f

## F

Faces, recognition of 748
Facial nerve 840
   lesions of 841
Facultative reabsorption 511
Fåhræus-Lindqvist effect 327, 327$f$
Fallopian tubes 670
Farsightedness 863
Fast pain 782, 782$t$
   sensation of 782
Fastigial nucleus 757
Fat 240, 251, 274, 610
   absorption of 277, 278
   cells 438
   digestion of 248, 260, 277
   emulsification of 277
   globule, emulsification of 260$f$
   malabsorption 252
   metabolism 69, 70, 257, 599, 610, 619, 620
   mobilization of 587, 610
   redistribution of 610
Fate 76$f$
Fatigability 178
Fatigue 5, 201
Fatty acids, beta-oxidation of 257
Fatty liver disease, nonalcoholic 634
Fatty stools 259, 280
Fecal elastase 253
Fecal incontinence 267
Fecal material, storage of 265
Fecal stercobilinogen 99
Feces
   composition of 269
   formation of 265
Feed forward
   control systems 14
   mechanism 11$f$, 12, 12$f$, 13$f$
Feedback
   control systems 14
   mechanism 11$f$
Feeding, regulation of 579
Female genotype 649
   development of 649$t$
Female reproductive system 670$f$
   functional anatomy of 670
   organs of 670
Female sexual cycle 671
Fenestrae 493
Ferguson reflex 592$f$, 593
Fern test 675
Ferric reductase 88
Ferritin levels, serum 87
Ferroportin 88
Fertile period, onset of 693
Fertilization 664, 665, 680
Fetal circulation adaptation 914
Fetoplacental circulation 682
   anatomy of 682$f$
   process of 682$fc$
Fetoplacental unit 684
Fetus, conception of 679
Fever 148, 540
   mechanism of 895, 895$fc$
   termination of 895, 895$fc$
Fibers 162, 758
   parasympathetic 816
   postganglionic 343
      parasympathetic 818$f$
   preganglionic 815
   types of 724, 742

Fibrillation potential 170
Fibrin
   clot, stabilization of 131
   formation of 131
   stabilizing factor 122, 131
Fibrinogen 67, 69, 70, 131, 665
Fibrinolytic mechanism 402
Fibrinolytic system 131, 132$f$
Fibroblast growth factor 160, 561
Fibrosa 844
Fibrosis 410
   pulmonary 410
Fick's principle 326, 347, 347$f$, 348, 351, 824
Fight response 818$f$, 819$f$
Filaments 4
   intermediate 4, 186
Filiform papillae 837
Filtration
   forces, sum of 378
   fraction 505
   membrane 506
Fingers, precise movements of 776
Finger-to-nose test 760
Firmicutes 222
Fishberg test 524, 529
Fissure, lateral 701
Flaccid paralysis 778
   lower motor neuron type of 780
Flagellum 664
   functions of 664
Flexion 568
Flexor muscles 780
Flexor reflex 733, 733$f$
   develops 780
Flight response 818$f$, 819$f$
Flow, velocity of 325, 414
Flowmeter 349
Fluent aphasia 792
Fluid 680
   absorption of 258
   accumulation 536
   across capillary membrane 378
      reabsorption of 378
   balance 915
   connective tissue 65
   drainage of 440$f$
   dynamics 378$t$, 437, 437$f$
      Starling's equilibrium of 377
   exchange 438
   lining alveolus, layers of 418
   movement 412$f$
      across compartments 35
      regulation of 36$f$
   osmolality of 510
   overload 438
   removal of 402
   replacement therapy 37
   retention 36, 537, 538
   surface tension of 411
   types of 37
   volume
      distribution of 33$f$
      regulation of 33
Fluorescence microscopy 55, 58$f$
Focal seizures 797, 798
   propagation of 798$f$
Foliate papillae 836
Folic acid 82, 89$f$
   deficiency 89
      causes of 89$f$
   role of 89$f$

Follicle
   primary 671
   stimulating hormone 556, 586, 642, 663
      role of 673, 673$f$
Follicular cells 645$f$
Follicular development 671
   stage of 674$f$
Food
   allergies 116
   digestion of 230
   intake 894
   poisoning 270
   storage of 238$fc$
Foodborne illnesses 270
Forced expiratory
   time 429
   volume 429
      significance of 429
Forced oscillation technique 432
Forced vital capacity 430
Forebrain structures 818
Formula feeding 912, 913
Foul-smelling 272
Fovea 848$f$
   centralis 847, 848$f$, 850$f$
   diameter of 862
Fragility, osmotic 67
Frank Starling's law 199
   mechanism of 199$f$
Free radicals
   injuries 5
   physiology of 920
   role of 921, 922
Frequency discrimination, volley principle of 880
Fresh frozen
   plasma 147
   tissue samples 58
Frontal lobe
   functions of 744
   orbital surface of 829
   parts of 743$f$
Frostbite 895
Frusemide 534
Functional magnetic resonance imaging 824
Functional residual capacity 427, 428
   measurement of 428
   significance of 429
Fundus oculi 847
Fungi 221
Fungiform papillae 836

## G

G forces, effects of 468$f$
G protein coupled receptors 19, 560
Gain, interpretation of 14, 15
Gait 765
   drunken 761
   festinating 765
   reeling 761
   spastic 778$f$
Galactose 138
Galactosyl transferase 138
Gallbladder 258, 258$f$, 258$t$, 259$f$
   bile 258
   cause contraction of 260
   disorders of 260
Gallstone 261
   formation, causes of 261
   pathophysiology of 261$f$

Gametes, fate of 680
Gamma chain 74
Gamma efferent discharge 728*f*
    control of 732
Gamma neurons 706
Gamma-aminobutyric acid 222, 720, 927
Gammaglobulin 113
Gamma-glutamyl transferase 99, 262
Ganglia
    collateral 816
    prevertebral 216
    terminal 816
Ganglion
    cell 272, 847, 850, 850*f*, 855
        absence of 271
        large 855
        layer 850
        types of 855
    geniculate 840
    mesenteric 217
Gap junctions 16, 183, 186, 212
Gas
    bubbles 438
    diffusion 418, 466
        coefficient of 419
    gangrene 472
    transport of 395
Gaseous exchange 418
    limitations of 420
Gastric acid
    neutralization of 258
    secretion 241, 242, 611
        evaluation of 242
        tests 241
Gastric bypass surgery 280
Gastric emptying 238
    normal 238
    process of 239*f*
    regulation of 239
    study 241
    time 238
Gastric function tests 241
Gastric glands 233
Gastric inhibitory peptide 214, 218, 236, 251, 558
Gastric juice 235, 236
    composition of 235
    mechanism of secretion of 236
Gastric manometry 242
Gastric motility studies 237, 242
Gastric mucosa 275
    superficial inflammation of 240
Gastric mucosal biopsy 242
Gastric pH capsule monitoring 242
Gastric phase 214, 236, 236*f*, 249
Gastric secretion 235, 235*f*, 236, 236*f*, 237, 237*t*
    composition of 235
    phases of 235
    regulation of 237
Gastric surgery 241
Gastric volume 239
Gastrin 218, 239, 558
    overproduction 241
Gastrinomas 241
Gastritis 240
    autoimmune 90
Gastrocnemius, testing of 732
Gastrocolic reflex 217, 235, 267
Gastroesophageal reflex disease 233, 240
    physiology of 240
Gastroesophageal sphincter 228

Gastroileal reflex 235
Gastrointestinal blood supply, anatomy of 218
Gastrointestinal dysfunction 5
Gastrointestinal motility, general principles of 215
Gastrointestinal secretions
    general principles of 213
    inhibition of 818
    phases of 214
Gastrointestinal system 45, 209, 219*f*, 915
    anatomy of 211
    nervous control of 216*f*
    organization of 211
    physiological anatomy of 211
Gastrointestinal tract 217, 264, 265*f*, 279*f*
    effects of 601
    functions
        hormonal control of 217
        regulation of 215
    smooth muscles 212*f*
        electrical activity of 212
Gastrointestinal wall 211
    histology of 211
Gastrosalivary reflex 235
Gene expression 920
    analysis 57
    regulation 466
Generalized tonic clonic seizure 798, 799*f*
    propagation of 798*f*
Genetic predisposition 369, 482
Geniculate body, lateral 752, 857, 858, 862, 866
Genital differentiation 649
Genital ridge 650*f*
Genitalia
    external 649
    internal 649
Genomic instability 922
Germinal cells, division of 663
Gibbs-Donnan effect 28, 28*f*, 48
Gigantism 589, 589*f*
Glands 561, 661
    complex 214
    mucous 398
    secreting hormone, parts of 556
    serous 398
    types of 214
Glaucoma 533, 847
Glia 720
Glial cell 458, 458*f*, 590
    line-derived neurotrophic factors 160
    types of 157
Glial tissues 850
Globin chains 75
Globulin 69, 70
Globus pallidus 761, 764
Glomerular capillary 496, 496*t*, 507, 507*f*
    colloid osmotic pressure of 507
    filtration coefficient 507
    membrane 493, 506
        basic structure of 506*f*
Glomerular filtration rate 500, 505, 507, 509, 526, 915
    autoregulation of 507
    calculation of 527*f*
    myogenic autoregulation of 509*f*
Glomerulonephritis 537
Glomerulotubular balance 496, 500, 509
Glomerulotubular feedback mechanism 512
Glomerulus 493, 493*f*, 505
Glomus, mechanism of 458*f*
Glossopharyngeal nerve 334, 816

Glucagon 351, 557, 617, 623
    like peptide-1 receptor agonists 634
Glucocorticoids 384, 557, 566, 607, 609-612, 628
    deficiency 612
        symptoms of 612
    excess, symptoms of 612
    mechanism of action of 610*f*
Gluconeogenesis 494, 609, 619
    inhibition of 619
    stimulation of 620
Glucose 34, 526, 534
    6-phosphate dehydrogenase deficiency, pathophysiology of 92*f*
    effects of 497*fc*
    fasting 901
    homeostasis 617
    intolerance 632, 633
    postprandial 901
    reabsorption of 510
    tolerance test 253
    transport maximum of 512
    transporter 275
    tubular reabsorption of 524, 528
Glucosuria 512
Glucuronic acid 76
Glutamate 720, 783
    receptor, metabotropic 838
Glutamine 720
    replaces glutamic acid 74
Glutaminergic pathways 763
Glutathione 922
    peroxidase 922
Gluten
    free diet 280
    sensitivity 280
Glycerol 534
Glycine 720
Glycogen
    lactate system 904
    phosphorylase 203
Glycogenesis 619, 620
Glycogenolysis 609, 623
Glycols 837
Glycolysis 619, 620
Glycolytic enzyme genes 466
Glycoprotein 6, 81, 559
    hormone 642
    receptors 121
Glycosaminoglycans, accumulation of 602
Goblet cells 214, 214*f*, 234, 250
Goiter, endemic 603, 604
Goldman-Hodgkin Katz equation 49, 50
Golgi cell 756, 758
Golgi neurons 156
Golgi tendon organ 732, 733*f*
Gonadal dysgenesis 653
    partial 657
Gonadectomy 657
Gonadotrophs 556, 585
Gonadotropin releasing hormone 556, 642
Gonads, removal of 657
G-protein 20*f*, 21, 838
Graafian follicle 673
    growth of 673
    late 673
Graft-versus-host disease 148
Grand mal epilepsy 798
Granular casts 531
Granular cell layer 756
Granular pneumocytes 400

Granule 101, 104
    cell 756, 758, 828
    primary 101
Granulocytes, mature 103
Granulosa cells 558, 645$f$, 670, 673, 674
    interaction of 645$f$
Graves' disease 600, 601
Gravity 360
Gray rami communicantes 816$f$
Great arteries 295
Growth 80, 159, 272, 599, 911
    hormone 20, 556, 561, 586, 589, 664
        hypersecretion of 589
        inhibiting hormone 556
        metabolic effects of 589$fc$
        physiological actions of 586, 587$t$
        releasing hormone 556
        secretion 916
    linear 587
    metabolic effects of 587
    neuronal 160
    spurt 655
    stage of 911$f$
Guanosine monophosphate 839
Guanylyl cyclase cyclic guanosine
    monophosphate pathway 679
Guillain-Barré syndrome 157, 164
Gunshot blast 872
Gustation 836
Gustatory sensation 836
Gustatory stimuli, transduction of 838
Gustatory transduction 840$f$
    mechanism of 839, 840$fc$
Gustducin 838
Gut
    brain axis 211, 221, 221$f$
        functions of 222
    immune apparatus of 211, 220
    immunity, dysregulation of 221
    law of 215
    microbiota 221
        dysbiosis 222, 271
        regulation of 269
Gymnemic acid 839
Gynecomastia 257
Gyri, narrowing of 795

## H

Hageman factor 131
Hagen Poiseuille's equation 326, 326$f$
Hair
    cell 877
        hyperpolarization of 878
        inner 877
        innervations 877$f$
        orientation detection of 808$f$
        outer 877, 881
        resting potential of 877, 878$f$
        structure of 806$f$
    loss 602
    thinning of 602
Haldane effect 449
Hands
    athetotic movements of 762$f$
    phalanges of 572
    precise movements of 776
Hard palate 840
Hatha yoga 926
Haustral contractions, mechanism of 266$f$
Haustrations 265, 266

Head
    circumference 911
    injury 548
    righting reflex 737
Headaches 459
Health monitoring 910
Hearing 875
    defects 883
        physiology of 883
    importance of 872
    physiology of 870
    place theory of 878
    system 883
    test 870, 883, 885
Heart 290, 290$f$, 290$t$, 296, 297, 302, 333, 334,
    344, 914$f$
    anatomy 287
        surface features of 288$f$
    attack 634
    base of 287
    block 317
        complete 317, 318$f$
        first degree 317
        second degree 317
    blood supply of 365$f$
    disease
        ischemic 25, 368
        valvular 299
    failure 379, 383, 388, 437, 438, 460, 480,
        525, 533
        congestive 387, 439
        types of 388
    fetal 914$f$
    functional
        abnormality of 309
        anatomy of 287
    horizontal plane 311
    hypereffective 351
    hypoeffective 351
    layers of 289$f$
    nerve supply of 342$f$
    obscured emptying of 384
    obscured filling of 384
    rate 314, 336, 342, 344, 244$t$, 344$t$, 349, 350,
        355, 360, 367, 436, 459, 799, 818, 926,
        914, 927, 929
        generation of 344
        normal 344
        regulation of 344
        variability 927
    sounds 294, 294$t$, 295, 296$f$
        abnormal 299
    valve of 288, 289$f$, 290
    walls of 288
Heat
    dissipation 201, 893$f$
        mechanisms 893
    gain 893
    intolerance 601
    loss mechanisms 892
    production 892$f$, 892$t$, 893
        mechanisms 892
    stroke 895
        mechanism of 895
Height gain 911
*Helicobacter pylori* 240
Helium dilution method 428, 428$f$
Helper T cells 111
Hematocrit 67
Hematology 63
Hematuria, evaluation of 530

Heme
    carrier protein 88
    oxygenase 76, 88, 96
Hemianopia
    bitemporal 589, 589$f$
    homonymous 860
Hemiballismus 762, 763
Hemicholinium 176
Hemidesmosomes 16
Hemineglect syndrome 746, 746$f$
Hemiplegia, contralateral 778$f$
Hemiretina, temporal 860
Hemochromatosis 88
Hemocytoblast 81
Hemodialysis 539, 540
Hemodynamics 324, 326
Hemoglobin 73, 74$t$, 80, 81, 86, 92, 447
    abnormal 74
    breakdown of 76
    content 87, 91
    deoxygenated 449
    excretion of 76$f$
    fate of 97$f$
    fetal 445
    formation of 74$f$
    forms of 75
    functions of 75
    glycated 75
    molecule, structure of 73, 74$f$
    normal types of 74
    oxygen saturation of 447$f$
    oxygenation of 443
    saturation of 443
    synthesis of 73
    types of 74
Hemoglobinopathies 74
Hemolysis 86, 146
Hemolytic disease 140
    grades of 140, 140$t$
    pathophysiology of 140, 140$f$
    treatment of 141
Hemolytic reaction 147, 148
    delayed 148
Hemophilia 134
    A 135
    B 135
Hemorrhage 349, 736, 738
    postpartum 688
    pulmonary 414
Hemosiderin 88
Hemostasis 121, 127, 129$f$, 130
    disorders 133, 134$f$, 147
    mechanism of 121$f$, 127
    primary 127, 128$f$
    secondary 130
    temporary 127, 128, 128$f$, 129$f$
Hemostatic regulatory mechanism 10$f$
Henle loop 493, 493$f$, 499, 511, 514
Henry's law 442
Heparin 132
    overdose of 540
Hepatic architecture 255$f$
Hepatitis
    A 98
    B 98
    C 98
    E 98
    viral 98
Hepatobiliary system, physiology of 255
Hepatocyte growth factor 561
Hepatosplenomegaly 141

Hephaestin 88
Hering's opponent color theory 854
Hering-Breuer inflation reflex 456, 456f
Hermaphroditism, true 651
Hexagonal pattern 185
High altitude 349, 475, 480, 484
    cerebral edema 466, 467
    illness 466
    periodic breathing 481
    physiology 464
    pulmonary edema 438, 466, 467, 476
    sickness, symptoms of 467
High gain systems 14
High pressure
    nervous syndrome 472
    system 325
High protein
    concentration 256
    diet 516, 525
        effects of 509
High total plasma cortisol levels 612
Higher intellectual functions 747
Higher vagal tone 343
    physiological significance of 343
Hippocampus
    functions of 790
    lesions of 795
Hirschsprung's disease 217, 233, 271, 272
    management of 272
Histamine 330, 339, 719
    massive amounts of 116
Histidine 719
Histotoxic hypoxia 477, 478
Hodgkin's cycle 52, 52f
Holmgren's wool test kit 854, 855f
Homeostasis 10, 13
Homeostatic control
    gain in 13
    mechanism 10, 11, 13, 13f
Homometric regulation 350
Hopping reaction 738, 738f
Horizontal cells 849, 850
Hormone 17f, 65, 218, 237, 367, 509, 509t, 555, 556, 560, 561, 569, 586, 619, 642, 665, 683, 915
    abnormalities 649
    action, mechanism of 555
    balance 927
    biosynthesis of 607, 608f
    catabolic 623
    classification of 17t, 555
    concentrations 604
    control 251, 330, 569, 569t
    dependent tissues, involution of 24
    distribution of 324
    effects of 351
    feedback regulation 645f
    gonadal 559, 642
    imbalance 652, 801
    mechanism of action of 18
    pituitary 586t
    production 921
    receptor complex 19
    regulation 239, 248, 259, 333, 339, 496, 569f
        of secretion of 588, 646
    regulatory elements 19
    release of 579f, 591f, 598
    reproductive 641, 642t
    response elements 19
    role of 37
    secretion of 617
    sensitive lipase 619, 620
    synthesis of 402, 591f, 645
    thrombopoietin 120
    types of 556, 559t, 586
    vasoconstriction 497
    vasodilatation 497
Horner's syndrome 817
Hot
    fluids, ingestion of 893
    flushes 658
Human chorionic gonadotropin 674, 683
    level of 685f
Human chorionic somatomammotropin 683
Human placental lactogen 683
Humoral immunity 110, 112
    mechanism of 112, 113f
Hung up ankle reflex 602
Hunger pangs 238
Huntington's chorea 762, 763
Hyaline casts 531
Hyaluronidase 664, 681f
    enzyme 666, 681
Hydrochloric acid secretion, mechanism of 237, 237f
Hydrochlorothiazide 534
Hydrops fetalis 140
Hydrostatic pressure 377, 437f, 507
    gradients, role of 436
Hydroxyethyl starch 38
Hyperactive deep tendon reflexes 778
Hyperadrenalism 613
Hyperaldosteronism 614
Hyperbaric oxygen therapy 472, 477
    side effects of 472
Hypercalcemia 320f, 533, 572
    effects of 567f
Hypercapnic respiratory failure 484
Hyperchloremia 46
Hyperchromia 85
Hypercomplex cells 859
Hyperdynamic state 86
Hypereffective heart 351
    causes of 351t
Hyperemia
    active 329
    reactive 329
Hyperestrinism 646
Hyperexcitability, neuromuscular 566, 567f, 568f
Hyperglycemia 609, 620, 622, 633
    persistent 620
Hyperinsulinemia 632, 633
Hyperkalemia 317, 320f, 533, 537, 612, 620
Hyperlipoproteinemia 369
Hypermetropia 863
    physiological basis of 863
Hypernatremia 36, 609
Hyperopia 863f
    correction of 864f
Hyperorality 748
Hyperosmotic renal medulla 514
Hyperparathyroidism 538, 572-574
Hyperphagia 748
Hyperpigmentation 611
Hyperplasia, adrenal 615
Hyperpolarization 213, 878, 880f
    phases of 190
Hyperreflexia 91, 601
Hyper-responsiveness 561
Hypersecretion 561
    disorders of 561t
Hypersensitivity 116
    delayed 111, 116
    denervation 169
    visceral 271
Hypersexuality 748
Hypersomnia 602
Hypersplenism 122
Hypertension 362, 369, 502f, 507, 533, 534, 537, 538, 613, 614, 632, 633, 685
    blood pressure classification of 362t
    medications 502
    physiological cause of 501
    pregnancy induced 685
    pulmonary 354, 421
Hyperthermia 579
Hyperthyroidism 349, 600
    physiological basis of 601
    primary 600, 601, 601t
    secondary 601, 601t
Hypertonia 730, 778
Hypertonic fluid 67
Hypertonic saline 38
Hypertrophy, ventricular 200f, 319
Hypnogram 800, 800f
Hypoadrenalism 611, 612
Hypocalcemia 320, 320f, 536, 566, 567f, 572, 573, 573f, 574
    effects of 567f, 571fc
    management of 569
Hypocalcemic tetany 465
Hypochlorhydria 240
Hypochromic 85
Hypocretin 802
Hypoeffective heart 351
    causes of 351t
Hypogeusia 841
Hypoglycemia, postprandial 241
Hypoglycemics, oral 619
Hypogonadism 652
    hypergonadotropic 657
    hypogonadotropic 657
    late-onset 658
Hypokalemia 320, 320f, 609, 614
Hyponatremia 36, 320, 536
Hypoparathyroidism 566, 568f, 571, 574
Hypophosphatemia 572, 574
Hypoproteinemia 69, 71, 71f, 82
    deficiency of 70
Hyporesponsiveness 561
Hyposecretion 561
    disorders of 561t
Hyposmia 832
Hypotension 148, 363, 386, 460, 540, 591
    causes of 363
    severe 328, 337
Hypothalamic nuclei 577, 577f, 580f
Hypothalamic-pituitary
    adrenal axis 925
    gonadal axis 694f
    thyroid axis 600f
Hypothalamic-releasing hormones 720
Hypothalamo-hypophyseal
    gland axis 579f
    neural tract 578, 579f, 587f
    portal system 578, 578f, 587f
Hypothalamo-pituitary-gonadal axis 641, 642f
Hypothalamus 577, 611, 611f, 752, 790, 802, 828, 832
    anterior 578
    arcuate nuclei of 642, 719
    functions of 578

lateral 579
location of 577f
neuron of 719
paraventricular nucleus of 557, 585, 720
physiology of 577
posterior 578, 579, 818
role of 894f
supraoptic nucleus of 557, 585
vegetative functions of 579
Hypothermia 386, 472
Hypothyroidism 270, 601, 602
  primary 601, 603, 603t
  secondary 601, 603, 603t
  tertiary 601
Hypotonia 730, 760
Hypotonic crystalloids 38
Hypotonic fluid 37, 67
  loss of 36f
Hypovolemia 349, 356, 535, 591
Hypoxemia 439
Hypoxia 80, 162, 383, 466, 475, 478t, 709fc
  classification of 475
  cytotoxic 477f
  effects of 436, 464, 715
  etiopathogenesis of 475
  inducible factor 81, 82, 465
  mechanism of effect of 436fc
  moderate 465
  response element 81, 466
  sensitive glomus cells 337
  severity of 464
  stimulates chemoreceptors 465
Hypoxic damage 495
Hypoxic effects, severe 465
Hypoxic hypoxia 475, 478
  effects of 476
Hysteresis 409
  loop 410

## I

I band shortens 191
I-cells 494
Icterus gravis neonatorum 140, 141
Idiopathic thrombocytopenic purpura 133
Idioventricular rhythm 317
Ileum 213, 245
Immune
  complex disease 116
  dysfunction 926
  memory 916
  regulation 221
  response
    primary 114, 115, 115f
    secondary 115, 115f
  system 904, 916, 921
    development 915
    enhancement 929
    neonatal 916
    parts of 157
    support 630
  thrombocytopenia 122
  tolerance 117, 627
Immunity 65, 611
  acquired 110
  adaptive 110
  applications of 116
  basics of 109
  cell mediated 110, 111
  classification of 109, 110f
  functions of 109

humoral 110, 112
innate 109
Immunocytochemistry 58
Immunodeficiency 117
Immunoglobulin 111, 113
  structure of 113, 113f
Immunohistochemistry 58
Immunomodulatory effects 147, 611
Immunosuppressive therapy 179, 541
Immunotherapy 483
Implantation 682
Impulse 155
  across neuromuscular junction,
    transmission of 174
  conduction of 164f
  generation, inherent rate of 344
  transmission of 163, 831
*In vitro* growth conditions 56
Inclusion bodies 3
Incus 873
Indicator dye dilution method 348, 348f
Infant respiratory distress syndrome 413
Infections 133, 270, 438, 539, 546
  fungal 112
  parasitic 112
  respiratory 401, 482, 483
  viral 112, 122, 780, 781f
Infectious diseases 664
Inferior retina fibers 858
Infertility 652, 666
Inflammation 24, 242, 633
Inflammatory cells, death of 24
Inflammatory disorders 574
Inhibin 663, 664
Inhibition, loss of 548
Inhibitory cells 756
Inhibitory postsynaptic potentials 707, 713, 713f
Injury
  current of 307
  level of 779
  location of 170
  management of 147
  severity of 169
Innate immunity 109
  limitations of 110
Inner circular layer 264
Inner ear, structure of 875f
Inner granular layer 743
Inner nuclear layer 847, 849
Inner plexiform layer 847, 850
Inner synaptic layer 850
Inner white matter 756
Inorganic ions 65
Inositol trisphosphate 839
  production 838
Inotropic effect 344
Insomnia 802
Inspiration 404
  mechanism of 405
  process of 408f
Inspiratory capacity 426, 427
Inspiratory muscles 405
Inspiratory ramp
  controls switch off point of 456
  signal 454
Inspiratory reserve volume 427
Inspired air 421
Insulin 557, 561, 617, 628, 826
  actions of 618
  concentration 901

deficiency 620
  effects of 620t
effects of 619, 619t, 620
  action of 618f
like growth factor 160, 587
metabolism of 617
release of 617, 619, 620f
resistance 632, 633
secretion 619fc
  regulation of 619
sensitivity 901, 916
storage of 617
synthesis of 617, 618f
tolerance test 614
Intensity 871, 900, 901
Intention tremor 760
Intercellular cement 681
Intercellular connections 16, 16f
Interferons 111, 112
Interleukin 80, 111, 633
  stimulate thrombopoietin 120
Internal intercostal muscles 405, 407
Internal limiting membrane 850
Internal organs, genital development 649t
Interneurons 156, 828, 829
Interoreceptors 723
Interphalangeal joints, extension of 568
Interstitial fluid 34, 40, 195, 377, 447
  colloid osmotic pressure of 70
  hydrostatic pressure 70
  pressure 380
  volume, measurement of 34, 35
Interstitial space 418
Interventricular septum 288
Intestinal cells 279f
Intestinal damage 280
Intestinal disorders 270, 279
Intestinal flora 221
Intestinal juice, mechanism of secretion of 250
Intestinal lumen 276f
Intestinal microbiota 915
  disruption of 270
Intestinal microvilli 219, 220f
Intestinal motility, regulation of 251
Intestinal phase 214, 236, 236f, 249
Intestinal secretion 270
  composition of 250
Intestinal villi 274
Intestine, parts of 235
Intoxication 35
Intra-abdominal pressure 407
Intracardiac electrophysiology studies 59
Intracellular calcium 330
Intracellular fluid 26, 33, 34, 40, 838, 839
  composition of 34
  volume 33
    measurement of 34, 35
Intracellular neurofibrillary tangles 795
Intracellular receptors 18, 555
Intracorpuscular defect 86, 91
Intracranial lesions 832
Intragastric pressure 242
Intralaminar nuclei 753
Intraluminal pressure 213f, 237
Intranuclear receptors 555
Intraocular fluid 846
Intraocular pressure 847
Intraocular tension, lower 534
Intrapleural pressure 406, 407, 407f, 408
Intrapulmonary pressure 407
Intrathoracic pressure 355, 406-408, 414f

Intrathoracic volume 405
Intrauterine device 693, 694*f*
Intravenous pyelogram 530*f*
   procedure of 530*f*
Intraventricular pressure 296
Intravesical pressure 546
Intrinsic defecation reflex 267
Intrinsic neuronal excitability 709
Intrinsic protein 6
Intrinsic pump failure 386
Inulin 526
   properties of 527
Inverse stretch reflex 732, 732*f*
Iodide
   high concentration of 603
   trapping 598
Iodine uptake, radioactive 604
Ionic balance around neurons 157
Ionic channel activity 713*f*
Ionic distribution 34*t*
Ionizable salts, anion of 837
Ions
   diffusion of 27
   distribution of 48*f*
   effects of 367
   exchange of 279*f*
   role of 330
Iris 845
Iron
   absorption of 88, 88*f*
   atom, coordination bonds of 75
   deficiency anemia 86, 87*t*
   dietary sources of 87
Irritable bowel syndrome 222, 270, 271
Irritation
   gastrointestinal 228
   small bowel of 251
Ischemic heart disease 25, 368
   pathogenesis of 369
Ishihara's color plates 854, 855*f*
Isometric contraction 201, 201*f*, 201*t*
Isometric exercise 901
Iso-osmotic fluid 67
Isosthenuria 538
Isotonic alkaline fluid 246
Isotonic contraction 201, 201*f*, 201*t*
Isotonic fluid 67
   loss of 36*f*
Isovolumetric contraction 295, 297
Isovolumetric relaxation 295
Ito cells 255

## J

J receptors 459
   location of 459*f*
J reflex 459
Jacksonian march 798
Jaeger's chart 862
Janus kinase 21, 21*f*
   enzyme 561
Jargon aphasia 792
Jaundice 77, 96, 98, 99*t*, 141, 260, 261
   classification of 97
   diagnosis of 98
   hepatic 97, 98
   neonatal 140, 141
   obstructive 97, 98
   physiological 98
   physiology of 96
   posthepatic 97, 98

   prehepatic 97
   types of 97*f*
Jejunum 213, 245, 276
Jet lag 630
Jod-Basedow phenomenon 602, 603
Joint pains 590
Juxtacapillary receptors 459
Juxtaglomerular apparatus 499-502
   structure of 499*f*
Juxtaglomerular cells 499

## K

Kainite receptors 720
Kallmann's syndrome 833
Kartagener syndrome 401
K-complexes 800
Keratocyte 55*f*
Keratotomy, astigmatic 864
Kerckring folds 274, 274*f*
Kernicterus 98, 141
Ketogenic effect 587
Ketone 531
   bodies 257
Ketonemia 257
Ketosis 620, 622*fc*
Kety's method 366, 824
Kidney 465, 491
   disease 533
      chronic 537
      end stage 573
   function 494, 915
      impaired 525
      loss of 537
      maternal 686
   functional anatomy of 491
   infections, recurrent 537
   injury, acute 534
   role of 37, 41
   size 915
   stone formation, prevention of 533
   structure of 492*f*
   tissue 58*f*, 494
Kinesin 7*f*
Klinefelter syndrome 650-652
   clinical features of 652, 652*f*
Klüver-Bucy syndrome 748, 790
Knee
   heel test 760
   jerk 732
Koilonychia 87, 87*f*
Korotkoff's sound 359, 359*f*
Korsakoff psychosis 795
Krauze's end bulb 724
Kupffer cells 255
Kwashiorkor, effect of 588
Kyphosis 590*f*

## L

Labyrinthine 739
   righting reflex 737
Lacis cells 500
Lactation 11, 688, 689*f*
   physiology of 679
Lactational amenorrhea method 689, 693
Lactic acid 41
Lactic acidosis 46
Lactoferrin 106
Lactotrophs 556, 585

Lag phase 115
Lambert-Eaton myasthenic syndrome 179
   pathogenesis of 179*f*
Lamina X 771
Laminar blood flow 328, 328*f*
Laminin 7
   stains 58*f*
Landsteiner's law, second part of 139
Langerhans islet 245, 617
Language development 917
Large intestine 264, 266*f*
   absorption of 269
   anatomical parts of 265*f*
   digestion of 269
   disorders 269
   functional anatomy of 264
   functions of 265
   histology of 264
   inflammation of 266
   mucosa of 265
   secretion of 265
Largest kinocilium 806, 807
Laryngeal stridor 568
Laryngopharynx 396
Latch bridge mechanism 199, 200*f*
Late dumping syndrome 241
Lateral geniculate body 752, 857, 858, 862, 866
   layers of 858*f*
Lateral hypothalamus 579
   stimulation of 581
Lateral spinothalamic tract 771, 772, 773*f*
   composition of 780
Leads 308, 308*f*
   pipe 765
Lean body mass 587
Learning, physiology of 792
Lecithin 277
Left atrial pressure 299, 436
Left circumflex artery 365
Left coronary artery 365
Left ventricular
   failure 387
   volume pressure loop 297*f*
Leg cramps 86
Length gain 911
Lens
   opacity of 846*f*
   transparency 846
Leptin 561, 633
Lesions
   effects of 456
   features of 457*t*
Lethargy 459
Leukemia 106
   classification of 106, 107*f*
   inhibitory factor 160
Leukocytes 65, 66, 67, 101, 104*t*, 147
   accumulation 147
   classification of 102*f*
   formation of 101
   general structure of 101
   life cycle of 103*t*
Leukocytic blast cells 106
Leukocytosis 101, 106
Leukopoiesis
   regulation of 102, 103*f*
   stage of 102, 103*f*
Levi-Laron dwarfs 588
Leydig cells 558, 662*f*, 663
Lie detector polygraph test 337
Lieberkühn crypts 214*f*, 250, 250*f*

Ligand gated ion channels 19f
Light 860
　　adaptation 852f
　　chains 184
　　effects of 852
　　microscopic structure 183
　　microscopy 55
　　reflex 844
Limb
　　leads, directions of 309f
　　proximal portions of 776
Limbic system 789, 789f, 790, 818
　　function of 791
　　parts of 790
　　physiology of 789
Linear acceleration, detection of 807
Linear movements 806f
Linear velocity detection 808
Lingual nerve 840
Linker protein ankyrin, deficiency of 91
Lipase 252
Lipid 6
　　absorption of 277f
　　digestion of 248f, 277f
　　lowering medications 634
　　metabolism 257
　　molecule
　　　　nonpolar ends of 6f
　　　　polar ends of 6f
　　oxidation 901
　　solubility 18, 377
　　soluble 830
　　　　hormones 555
Lipolytic 610
Lipophilic molecules, small 831
Lipoproteins 6
　　high-density 256, 633, 901
　　intermediate density 256
　　lipase 258, 619, 620
　　low density 256
　　very low-density 133, 256
Liquefaction 666
Liraglutide 634
Liver 214, 256, 258f, 258t, 623
　　adipose 826
　　bile 258
　　cell injury 261
　　disease 256, 439
　　disorders of 260
　　endocrine functions of 257
　　enzymes, lack of 98
　　failure 257
　　　　leads 257
　　function 256, 257
　　　　tests 262
　　functional anatomy of 255
　　lymph flows out of 255
　　macrophage system 257
　　metabolic function of 256
　　regeneration of 256
　　special features of 255
Locus coeruleus 719
Long loop reflexes 217
Long QT syndrome 883
Loop diuretics 534
Love hormone 927
Low gain systems 14
Low molecular weight substances 506
Low voltage high frequency waves 799
Lower esophageal sphincter 228, 230
Lower motor neuron 705, 779

　　damage 781f
　　lesion 778, 779t
Lubrication 680
Lumen diameter 325
Luminal border 247
Luminal pH 251
Lumirubin, water soluble 141
Lundh test 253
Lung 406, 410
　　capacities 426
　　compliance 408, 413
　　defense systems 401
　　diffusion capacity of 426, 431
　　disease 81
　　　　interstitial 421
　　elastic fibers of 410
　　elasticity 921
　　endocrine functions of 402
　　function improvement 928
　　immaturity 413
　　infections 439
　　injury, acute 148
　　metabolic function of 402
　　parenchymal disease 484
　　parts of 436f
　　role of 41
　　thorax system 409
　　tissue
　　　　elasticity of 410
　　　　resistance 409
　　volume 414, 426
　　　　abnormal 429f
　　　　change of 410, 427
　　　　effects of 409
Lutein cells 674
Luteinizing hormone 11, 556, 586, 642, 663
　　levels of 11
　　role of 673, 673f
　　surge 11
Lymph
　　collection of 380f
　　flow 380
　　formation of 380
　　protein content of 380
Lymphatic
　　capillaries 380f
　　circulation 374, 379, 379f, 380, 435, 823
　　　　functions of 380
　　flow 380
　　pump 380
　　system 435
Lymphedema 653
Lymphoblasts 103
Lymphocytes 111
　　self-reactive 24
Lymphoid
　　organs
　　　　primary 110
　　　　secondary 110
　　stem cells 101
　　tissue, gut-associated 220, 222
Lymphotoxin 112
Lysosomal storage diseases 5
Lysosomes 5
Lysozyme 106

# M

Macrophages 255
Macrosomatics 827

Macula
　　densa cells 500
　　detect 806
　　lutea 847
　　nutrition of 847
Magnesium 510
Magnocellular neurons 585
Magnocellular pathway 859
Major circulatory systems 434
Major metabolic pathways 619t, 620t
Major somatic receptors 724t
Malabsorption syndrome 90, 270, 279, 280
　　causes of 279
　　pathogenesis of 280
Male genotype 649
　　development of 649t
Male reproductive system 661, 662f
　　anatomy of 661
Malignancy 439, 798
Malignant lesions 601
Malnutrition, severe 574
Mamillary bodies 578
Mammalian cell 3
　　functional organization of 4f
Mammillary body 579
Mannitol 534
Marey's law 333, 339
Mass movements 266
　　mechanism of 267f
Mass reflex appears 780
Massa intermedia 752
Mast cells 402
　　degranulation of 116
Mastication, physiology of 228, 228f
Mastoid antrum 873
Maximal acid output 242
Maximal expiratory flow rate 430
Maximal mid-expiatory flow rate 430
Maximum hemoglobin saturation 447
Maximum potential difference, magnitude
　　of 303
Maximum ventilatory capacity 431
Maximum voluntary ventilation 430
McArdle syndrome 203
Mean aortic pressure 367
Mean arterial pressure 358, 379, 825
Mean capillary fluid pressures 378
Mean cardiac axis 308
Mean corpuscular volume 85
Mean platelet volume 134
Mean pressure 325f, 436
Mean pulmonary capillary pressure 325
Mean systemic filling pressure 354, 354f, 356
Meaningless jargons 792
Mechanical papillae 837
Mechanical ventilation 459, 484
Mechanoreceptors 723
Meconium aspiration syndrome 413
Medial geniculate body 752, 753
Medial occipital lobe 748f
Medial rectus 865
Medial superior olivary nucleus 881
Medial vestibular nucleus 810
Mediodorsal nucleus 753
Meditation 925, 929
　　physiological effects of 925, 928
　　process of 928
Medulla
　　oblongata 456, 731, 735f
　　　　level of 735
　　reticular nuclei of 783

Medullary collecting duct 494
    role of 511
Medullary reticular formation 787*f*
Meissner's corpuscle 724
Meissner's plexus 216, 217, 250
Melatonin 558, 629, 802
    functions of 629
    mechanism of secretion of 629, 629*f*
Membrane, presynaptic 172
Membranous labyrinth 805*f*
Memory 748, 789, 790, 801, 929
    cells, formation of 113, 141
    classification of 792, 793*f*
    consolidation of 793, 794*f*, 801
    intermediate long-term 793, 794*f*
    long-term 793, 801
    physiological basis of 789
    physiology of 792
    short-term 793
    T cells 111
    trace 792
Menarche 655, 671
Mendelian inheritance 138
Ménière's disease 811
    cause of 811
Menopause 658, 671
Menstrual cycle 671, 672*f*, 675*f*, 693*f*
    phases of 672*t*
Menstruation, causes of 24
Mental
    confusion 459
    functions 704, 705, 826
    health disorders 926
Merkel's disc 724
Mesencephalon 702, 783
Mesenchymal cells 55*f*
Meta arterioles, terminal 376
Metabolic disorders 449, 926
Metabolic disturbances 590
Metabolic function 221, 257
Metabolic rate 599
Metabolic regulation 367
Metabolic syndrome 261, 632-635
    clinical features of 632
    management of 634
    pathogenesis of 632
Metabolic theory 329
Metabolic waste products 801
Metabolism 45, 599
    active 375
    heat of 892
Metacarpophalangeal joints 568
Metaencephalon 702
Metalloproteinases 106
Metamyelocytes 103
Methacholine 176
    challenge test 426
Methanol poisoning 46
Methemoglobinemia 480
Meyer's loop 858
Micelles 278
    formation of 278
Microcirculation, characteristics of 376
Microcytic hypochromic cells 76*f*
Microfilaments 4
Microglia 157
Micro-organism, killing of 106
Microsomatics 827
Microtubules based molecular motor 7
Micturition
    frequent 548

reflex 545, 545*f*, 819
    excitation of 548
    inhibition of 818
Midbrain
    arteries of 825
    preparation 738
Middle ear 873
    functions of 874
        muscles of 874
    mechanics 873
    muscles 873
Midget cells 855
Migrating motor complex 213
Milk
    let down reflex 592*f*, 593, 688, 689*f*
    process of formation of 688*fc*
Mind, resting state of 795
Mineral 82
    absorption of 278, 279*f*
    digestion of 279*f*
    metabolism 610
Mineralocorticoid 557, 607, 608, 612
    deficiency 612
Mini pill 694
Minute to minute respiration 458
Minute ventilation 430
Miosis 845
Mitochondria 3
    enzymes, blockage of 477
    targeted therapies 923
Mitochondrion 5*f*
Mitral cells 828, 829
Mitral regurgitation 299, 436
Mitral stenosis 299, 436
Mitral valve 288
Mixed cell population 55*f*
Mobilize labile proteins 611
Molecular biology techniques 57
Molecular motors 7, 7*f*, 8
    actin based 7
Molecular oxygen, conversion of 471
Molecule
    neurotransmitters 718
        large 720
    transport of 69
Monge's disease 466, 467
Monoamine oxidase 719
    inhibitors 765
Monocyte 102
    macrophage system 106
        components of 106
        functions of 106
Monosaccharides 274
Monosomy 650
Monosynaptic reflex 731
Mood
    regulation of 222
    swings 658
Moon shaped face 613
Morning after pill 694
Mossy fibers 758
Motilin 218, 238, 251, 558
Motility 270
    causes of 238
    patterns 242
Motion sickness 812
Motor activity
    execution of 766*f*
    planning of 764
    programming of 764
Motor aphasia 792

Motor cortex 742, 744, 744*f*
    role of 766, 766*f*
Motor development 912, 917
Motor dysfunction 765
Motor fiber 731
Motor homunculus 704
Motor horn 771
Motor neurons 156, 706
    monitor muscle length 728
Motor paralytic bladder 546
Motor root 706
Motor skills 910
Motor speech area 744, 791
Motor tracts 775
Motor unit
    properties of 188
    recruitment of 188
    size of 188
Mouse eye cells 55*f*
Mouth 224
Movement, execution of learned patterns of 762
Mucosa 211, 233, 245, 264
    irritation of 251
Mucosal lining, integrity of 401
Mucus
    bicarbonate layer 236
    cells 234
Muller's cells 850
Mullerian duct 24
    inhibitory substance 649, 663
Multiple ions, effects of 49
Multiple motor subprograms, coordinates simultaneous performance of 766
Multiple system atrophy 815
Multipolar neurons 156, 156*f*
Murmur 299
    systolic 86
    types of 299, 299*t*
Muscarinic receptors 818*f*
Muscle 187*t*, 196, 197*t*, 199, 200*f*, 201, 405, 611, 818, 873
    activity 894, 901
    circular 234
    contractile proteins 611
    contraction 182, 194*f*, 199, 564, 901
        efficient 200
        energy sources of 182, 202
        isokinetic 906
        isometric 200, 201
        isotonic 200, 906
        mode of 182
        molecular mechanism of 192
        physiology of 182, 190
        types of 200
    disorders of 203, 203*t*
    electrical
        properties of 188
        stimulation of 192
    endomysium of 379
    expiratory 405
    fibers 186, 199, 201
        types of 182, 186
    functional unit of 185
    length of 199, 199*f*, 201
    longitudinal 234
    lose 801
    mass, loss of 921
    papillary 306
    physiology 153
    postural 730
    preloaded 200

proteins 182
pump 379
sarcotubular system of 187
spindle 160, 726, 726f, 727
  activation of 727f, 828f
  active stretching of 728
  functions of 728
  innervation of 727
  passive stretching of 727
  structure of 726f
  tonic discharge of 727f
  working of 727, 727f
strength 177, 901
stretching of 217
structural unit of 185
structure of 182
tone 758, 800
twitching 459
types of 182, 183t, 187t
weakness 91, 178, 609, 611
  physiological basis of 609
  proximal 179
Muscular activity 892
  gradation of 182
Muscular coat, intermittent 376
Muscular dystrophy 182, 203
  disorders of 203
Muscular exercise 344
Muscular tissue 48
Muscularis externa 234, 246, 264
Muscularis mucosa 212, 234
Muscularis propria, layers of 211
Musculoskeletal system 45, 899, 903, 921
Mushroom poisoning 817
Mutation 157, 922
Myasthenia gravis 178
  parts of 628
  pathophysiology of 172
Mydriasis 818
Myelencephalon 702
Myelin sheath 157
Myelinated nerve fiber 161, 161f, 163
Myelination 917
Myelocytes 103
Myeloid stem cells 101
Myeloperoxidase enzyme 106
Myenteric plexus 216
Myocardial action potentials 303f
Myocardial cells 369, 369fc
Myocardial contraction 302
Myocardial infarction 319, 319f, 368, 369, 472, 634
Myocardial ischemic syndrome 368
Myocardial oxygen demand 350, 367
Myocarditis 317
Myocardium 288, 302
  hypertrophy of 351
Myofilaments 186
  structure of 186f
  types of 186
Myogenic mechanism 496
Myogenic theory 329, 329fc
Myoglobin 445
  oxygen dissociation curve of 446f
Myomesin 185
Myopathy 182
Myopia 863
  correction of 863f
  physiological basis of 863
  physiology of 863f
Myosin 7f, 184
  ATPase activity 195

chain, dephosphorylation of 195
filament
  molecular structure of 184f
  organization of 184, 184f
head 184
light chain
  kinase 195
  phosphatase 195
linked contraction 195
Myotatic reflex 731
Myotomy, surgical 230
Myxedema 601, 602
  gelatinous nonpitting pretibial 602

# N

N-acetylgalactosamine 138
Narrow-band noise 883
Nasal breathing 396
Nasal cavity
  upper one-third of 827
  warm 396
Nasal flaring 413
Nasal hemiretina 860
Nasal obstruction 832
Nasopharynx 396
Natural family planning techniques 696
Natural killer cells 112
  increased activity of 929
Nausea 386
Nebulin 185
Neck
  proprioceptors 739
  righting reflex 737
Necrosis 24, 24t
Negative pressure filling 406f
Neocerebellum 757
Neocortex 832
Neologisms 792
Neospinothalamic pathway 782
  course of 783f
  origin of 783f
  termination of 783f
Neostigmine 176
Nephritis, interstitial 536, 537
Nephrons 492, 508f
  juxtamedullary 494, 495, 495t
  progressive loss of 539
  structure of 492, 492f
  types of 494
Nephrosis 612
Nerve
  action potential of 50, 189f
  cells 165
  conduction
    studies 163, 170
    velocity of 164
  deafness 885
  factors influencing regeneration of 169
  fiber 161, 880
    classification of 162
    diameter of 163
    Erlanger Gasser's classification of 162f, 162t
    functions of 161
    numerical classification of 162, 162t
    physioclinical classification of 162t
    properties of 161, 163
    types of 161, 162, 165
growth factor 159, 721

injury
  diagnosis of 170
  grades of 167, 168f
physiology 153
supply 399
Nervous regulation 215, 226, 454
Nervous system 465, 611, 719, 903, 917
  function 46
  organization of 701
Nervous tissue 48
Net filtration pressure 507, 507f
Neural analysis 881
Neural maturation 801
Neural regulation 239, 248, 259, 368
Neural transmission 872
Neurogenic bladder 546, 547
  dysfunction 548
Neuroglia 155, 156, 158
Neurohypophysis 590
Neurological damage 546, 547
Neurological disorders 547
Neurological symptoms 5, 90
Neurological system 921
Neuroma 170
  formation of 169f
Neuromuscular blocking agents 172
Neuromuscular disorders 484
Neuromuscular junction 172, 176, 177f
  anatomy of 172
  disorders of 176
  physiological anatomy of 172
  site of 172f
  structure of 172, 173f
Neuron 155, 158, 704, 720, 802, 826
  cell body of 167
  cholinergic 719
  circuits 708
  classification of 156
  depolarization of 713
  discharge 455
  distal stump of 168f, 169
  dorsal respiratory group of 454
  facilitatory 735
  first order 772, 840
  functions of 156
  postganglionic 814
    sympathetic 719
  preganglionic 814
  proprioceptor 160
  proximal stump of 168f
  pseudounipolar 156, 156f
  responses of 857
  second order 772, 840
  structure of 155, 155f
  system of 771
  third order 772, 841
  types of 742
  ventral respiratory group of 454
Neuronal density 921
Neuronal function 826
Neuronal pool 707f, 708
  organization of 707f
  processing of 707
Neuropeptide
  pituitary 720
  Y 556
Neuroplasticity 928
Neuropraxia 167
  compound muscle action potential 170
Neurotemesis 167
Neurotensin 721

Neurotransmitter 175, 718, 764f, 801, 814, 855
    classification of 18t
    drug blocking release of 176
    excitatory 713, 719, 720
    presynaptic release of 712fc
    regulation 927
Neurotrophins 159, 170
Neutral lipids 412
Neutral molecules, diffusion of 27
Neutrophil 102, 106
    extracellular trap formation 106
    hypersegmented nucleus of 89
    increases number of 610
    mechanism of action of 105f
Newton's third law 411
Nicotinamide adenine dinucleotide phosphate oxidase 56, 106
Nicotine 458
Nicotinic receptors 818f
Nicotinic type 815
Nigrostriatal pathway 719
Nitric oxide 132, 720, 825
    endothelial derived 509
    fractional exhalation of 431
    genes 466
    release of 230
Nitrogen
    narcosis 470
    washout method 428, 428f
Nitroglycerin 439
Nitrous oxide 366, 420
Niyama 927
Nocturnal enuresis 802
Noise 883
Noncellular casts 531
Nonchemical regulation 454, 459
Non-excretory functions 494
Noninvasive pulmonary function test 432
Nonrapid eye movement sleep 799, 801
Nonspirometric lung volume 426, 427
Nonsteroidal anti-inflammatory drugs 538
Nonthrombocytopenic purpura 123
Nonvolatile acids 41
Norepinephrine 330, 509, 719
Normal lung volumes 429f
Normoblast
    early 81
    late 81
Normochloremia 46
Nose, olfactory mucosa of 827
Nuclear
    bag fibers 726
    characteristics 81
Nuclei
    functional classification of 752
    lateral group of 577
    medial group of 577
Nucleus 3, 101, 183, 849, 881
    anterior 753
    emboliform 756
    globose 756
    interpositus 756
    paraventricular 556, 557, 581
    tractus solitarius 840
Nutrient
    absorption of 274
    deficiency of 86, 839
    diffusion of 682
    lack theory 329
    metabolism 221
    transportation of 682fc
Nystagmus 811
    central 811
    peripheral 811

# O

Obesity 478, 482, 632, 635
    hypothalamic 579
    truncal 613
Obstruction, intestinal 383
Obstructive sleep apnea 802
Occipital lobe 748
Ocular muscles 865f
Oculomotor nerve 816, 845
Odorant binding protein 831
Odorant molecule
    binding of 831
    features of 830
Odorant stimuli, types of 830
Odoriferous stimulus 830
Ohm's law 327
Olfaction 402
    mechanism of 828, 829fc
    physiology of 827
    site of 827, 827f
Olfactometer 833, 833f
Olfactory bulb 828, 829f
    contralateral 829
Olfactory cells 831
Olfactory cortex 829, 831
Olfactory fibers 830
Olfactory mucosa 827, 828f
    histology of 828
    nerve supply of 828
Olfactory nerves 828
Olfactory nucleus, anterior 829
Olfactory pathway 828
    components, functions of 830
Olfactory receptors 402, 831
    adaptation of 832
    neurons 831
Olfactory rods 828
Olfactory sensation
    conversion of 830
    processing of 831
Olfactory stria 829
Olfactory sulcus 829
Olfactory tract 829, 830f
Olfactory transduction 830, 831f
Oligoasthenoteratozoospermia 666
Oligodendrocyte 157, 157f
Oligozoospermia 666
Oliguric phase 536
Olivary nucleus, superior 881
Olivocochlear bundle 881
Ondine's curse 454
Oocyte
    maturation inhibiting factor 671
    meiotic division of 681
    primary 670
Oogenesis 670
Oogonia 670
Ophthalmologic abnormalities 5
Ophthalmoscope 847
Opioid 270
    peptides 720
Opisthotonus 736, 737f
Optic
    chiasma 860
    cup 848f
    disc 847
    nerve 850, 857
        stretching of 601
    principle of 860
    tract 858
Optical righting reflex 737
Oral cavity 211, 224, 228, 230, 275, 277
    digestion of 224
    parts of 225, 225f
Orbitofrontal cortex 830, 832
Orchitis, bilateral 666
Orexins 556
Organ
    allocation 540
    perfusion of 65
    procurement 540
    transplantation 931
Organelle disorders, physiological basis of 8
Organic bone matrix 574
Organophosphorus compound 176
    poisoning 719, 817
Organum vasculosum 591
Orgasm
    female 680
    male 680
Oropharynx 396
Orthograde transport 162
Oscillometry, forced 426
Osmolality 34, 514
Osmoreceptors 591
Osmosis 29
Osmotic lysis 112
Ossicular lever action 874, 874f
Osteitis fibrosa cystica 572, 572f
Osteoarthritis 921
Osteoblast 565
Osteoclast 565
Osteocyte 565
Osteocytic membrane
    pump 565
    system 565
Osteodystrophy, renal 538
Osteolysis 565
    mechanism of 567f
Osteomalacia 574
Osteomyelitis 472
Osteopenia 921
Osteoporosis 565, 566, 574, 614, 641, 658, 921
Otolith reflexes 811
Outer limiting membrane 849, 850
Outer molecular layer 743, 756
Outer nuclear layer 847, 849
Outer plexiform layer 847
Ovalocytosis 79
Ovarian follicle 558
    granulosa cells of 558
Ovary 670, 671, 674f
    atresia of follicles of 24
Overflow incontinence 546
Ovulation
    indicators of 675
    mechanism of 674f
Ovum 680
    fertilization of 680
    formation of 670, 671f
    zona pellucida of 664
Oxidation 75
Oxidative stress 5, 920, 922, 923
    physiology of 920
    theory 920
Oxygen 442, 442t
    affinity of 443f

concentration 220, 337, 825
consumption 447, 494, 496f
diffusion of 682, 683f
exchange of 683f
hemoglobin dissociation curve 443, 444f, 446f
saturation, measurement of 447
therapy 384, 439, 477-481, 483, 484
   long-term 483
toxicity 471
transport of 75, 442
vehicles for transport of 447
Oxyhemoglobin 75
Oxyntic glands 233
   anatomy 234f
Oxytocin 556, 586, 590, 593, 720
   increased production of 927

# P

P ganglion cells 749
P wave 304
Pacemaker cells 213
Pacinian corpuscle 724
Packed cell volume 65, 66, 87
Paget's disease 574
Pain 781, 782, 782t
   abdominal 272, 540, 622
   acute 782
   causes of 781
   chronic 782
   colicky 568
   fibers, types of 783
   labor 688
   pathways 782
   receptors, localization of 782
   referred 784
   slow 782
   types of 782
   visceral 784
Paleocerebellum 757
Paleospinothalamic pathway 783
   course of 783f
   origin of 783f
   termination of 783f
Pancreas 214, 245, 248
   anatomy of 245
   autodigestion of 252
   disorders of 252
   endocrine 617
   exocrine 247, 617
   functional anatomy of 245, 246f
   secretions of 246
Pancreatic amylase 248, 251
   action of 251
Pancreatic enzyme 246, 248f
   activation of 248f
   stimulation tests 252
Pancreatic function tests 252
Pancreatic juice 246, 278
   composition of 246
   formation of 247f
   functions of 247
   mechanism of formation of 247
   pH of 246
Pancreatic lipase 248, 251, 278
Pancreatic secretion 246, 249
   phases of 249
   regulation of 248, 249f
Pancreatitis 252
   acute 252, 536
   chronic 252, 253

Pancreozymin 249
Panhypopituitarism 588
Papillae
   distribution of 836f
   types of 836
Para-aminohippuric acid 326
Paracellular transport 510f
Paradoxical sleep 799, 801
Paraffin 58
Parafollicular cells 557, 573
Paragigantocellular nuclei 784
Parahippocampal gyrus 795
Parallel vascular circuits 327
Paralysis
   agitans 765
   types of 781
Paraolfactory area 790
Paraplegia 780, 781
Parasomia 833
Parasthesias 568
Parasympathetic defecation reflex 267
Parasympathetic inhibition 351
Parasympathetic innervation 343
Parasympathetic nervous system 333, 815, 815t
   organization of 815f
Parasympathetic stimulation 217, 220
   effects of 343
Parasympathetic tone 927
Parathormone 557, 569, 570, 574t
   actions of 570
   mechanism of action of 570, 570f
   role of 573
   synthesis of 570f
Parathyroid gland 570, 570f, 686
   abnormality of 571
Parathyroid hormone
   role of 573f
   secretion, regulation of 571, 572f
Paravertebral sympathetic chain 816
Paresthesia, circumoral 568
Parietal cells 234
Parkinson's disease 25, 222, 270, 719, 763, 765, 765f
Parosmia 833
Pars
   flaccida 873
   tensa 873
Parturition reflex 11, 592f, 593, 687, 687f
Parvocellular layer 858
Parvocellular pathway 859
Pascal's law 470
Patent ductus arteriosus 299
P-cells 494, 855
Pea sized gland 585
Pelvic floor dysfunction 270
Pelvic parasympathetic nerves 679
Pendred syndrome 883
Penicillamine 839
Penile erection 679
Pentagastrin 242
   stimulation test 241
Pepper pot skull 572, 572f
Pepsinogen 240
Peptic ulcer 233, 240, 572
   formation 241
Peptide 721
   bonds 599
   hormone 17, 19, 559, 560, 573
Periaqueductal gray matter 783, 784
Pericardium 288
   layers of 289f

Periglomerular cells 828
Perilymph 876
Perimenopause 658
Perimysium 182
Periodic breathing
   drug-induced 481
   patterns, types of 481f
Periodic limb movement disorders 802
Peripheral blood film 87, 92f, 93, 93f
Peripheral chemoreceptors 337, 453, 458
   stimulation of 458
Peripheral circulatory system changes 466
Peripheral nerves
   degeneration of 167
   regeneration of 167
Peripheral nervous system 169, 701
Peristalsis 238, 238f, 267f
   primary 229
   secondary 229
Peristaltic rush 251
Peritoneal dialysis 540
   complications of 540
Peritoneointestinal reflex 269
Peritubular capillaries 496, 496t
Periventricular nuclei 720, 784
Peroxisomes 5
Peroxynitrite 921
Petit mal epilepsy 799
pH 40, 44, 445, 531
   effects of 716
   regulation 494
Phagocytosis 30, 106
Phalanges 572f
Phantom limb syndrome 704
Pharynx 396, 840
Phasic blood flow 366
Phenotype 139
   sex differentiation 649
Pheochromocytoma 817
Pheromones 828
Phonocardiogram 293, 294
Phosphate 510, 526
   buffer 42, 44
Phosphatidylcholine 412
Phosphatidylethanolamine 412
Phosphatidylglycerol 411, 412
Phosphatidylinositol 412
Phosphodiesterase 839
Phospholipase 248, 251, 839
Phospholipid 6f, 278, 412
Phosphoric acid 41
Phosphorylates myosin head 195
Phosphorylation, oxidative 202
Photoreceptors
   membrane 851f
   segment of 849
Phototherapy 99, 141
Physical cell connections, types of 16t
Physical stress, lack of 574
Physiological shunt 423, 423f
Physostigmine 176
Pigment
   epithelium, cell of 849
   stones 261
Piloerection 580
Pineal gland 629
   functions of 629
   physiologic anatomy of 629
   physiology of 627, 629
   secretion, disturbance of 630
Pinna 872
Pinocytosis 30

Piriform cortex 832
Pitch discrimination 878
   duplex theory of 881
Pits 214
Pituicytes 590
Pituitary gland 585, 585f, 686
   histology of 586f
   hormone of 585, 590
   physiology of 585
Placenta 114, 558
   role of 685
Placental diffusion, process of 682fc
Placental hormone 683, 683t, 685f
   formation of 684
Placental membrane 682, 683, 683f
Placidity 748, 791
Plasma 34, 65, 66, 66f, 146, 337, 447, 447f
   calcium levels 570
   cells 112
   clearance 524, 526t
      principle of 526f
   concentration of 70
   glucose 512
      level 619, 620
   level 512, 598
   membrane 6, 18
      receptors of 560
   osmolarity 590
   phosphate levels 570
   proteins 66, 69, 70t, 564
      deficiency of 70
      functions of 69
      levels of 69-70
      origin of 69
      pools of 69f
      types of 69, 70
   skimming effect 327
   thromboplastin antecedent 131
   ultrafiltrate of 505, 506
   volume
      loss of 384
      measurement of 34, 35
Plasmapheresis 71
Plasmolytic system 132f
Plasticity
   peculiar property of 199
   physiological basis of 199
Plateau phase 191, 444
Platelets 65-67, 120, 146, 147, 610
   activation 128
   adhesion 121, 121f, 128
   aggregation 121f, 128, 825
      test 123, 134
   constituents of 122
   count 123, 124, 134
      low 123t
   defects 135
   derived growth factor 122
   disorder 122f
      diagnosis of 123
   dysfunction 537, 538
   facilitates aggregation of 121
   formation of 120
   function 121, 134
      analyzer 123
      tests 123
   functional structure of 120
   granules, types of 121f
   growth factor 160
   life span of 120
   plug formation 128, 129f, 133
      disorders of 133

   rich plasma 66
   structure of 121f
Plethysmography 326
Pleura 400
Pleural effusion 439, 439f
Pleural fluid 401
Pleuritic chest pain 439
Pleurodesis 440
Pneumatic dilation 230
Pneumocyte cells 411
Pneumonia 410, 439, 921
Pneumotaxic center 454, 455, 455f, 457
Pneumothorax 414
Podocytes 493, 506
   arrangement of 493f
Poikilothermia 579
Poliomyelitis 780
Polycystic kidney disease 537
Polypeptide 251
   hormone 623
Polyphenols 923
Polysaccharides 230, 274, 275
Polyspermy block 681
Polyuria 518, 622
Porphyrin ring 75
Positive airway pressure therapy 481
Positive feedback mechanism, characteristics of 12
Positive pressure filling 406, 406f
Positive supporting reaction 733, 735
Post-central gyrus 841
Posterior column tract 772, 774
Posterior hypothalamus 578, 579, 818
   lesions of 579
Posterior pituitary
   extract 344
   gland 586, 591f
Posterior semicircular canal 807
Postexercise oxygen consumption 202
Postprandial alkaline tide 237
Post-seizure depression 798
Postsynaptic membrane 172, 175, 175f
Post-traumatic stress disorder 926
Postural movements 758
Postural reflexes 730, 731, 735, 737, 738
Posture, effects of 349
Potassium 164, 320, 510, 526, 622
   channels 608
   ion 34, 825
      secretion of 608
   role of 623
Power stroke 192
Pranayama 925, 927
Pratyahara 927
Pre-Bötzinger complex 454, 455
Preconception and Prenatal Diagnostic Techniques Act 649
Precursor cell 101
Pre-excitation syndrome 318
Prefrontal cortex 742, 744
Preganglionic sympathetic fibers 343
Pregnancy 90, 344, 349, 379, 681, 685, 687fc
   corpus luteum of 674, 684
   physiology of 679
   test 684
Pregnanediol 646
Presbycusis 883
Presbyopia 864
   physiological basis of 865
Pressure 435
   pulse 375
   system, low 325

   transduction of 725f
   volume curve 374f
Prestin, role of 880f
Presupplementary motor area 766
Presynaptic dendritic spines 793
Presynaptic inhibition 793
Primary follicles 671
   formation of 671
Primary visual cortex 748, 748f, 858
   histology of 749
   layers of 749f
Primordial follicle 670, 671
Primordial ova 670
Proaccelerin 131
Proconvertin 131
Proerythroblast 82
   pronormoblast 81
Progesterone 558, 644, 646, 674, 683, 684
Progesterone-only pill 694
Prolactin 556, 561, 586
   inhibiting hormone 556
Promonocytes 103
Promyelocytes 103
Pronucleus
   female 681
   male 681
Properdin 115
Proptosis 601
Propulsive peristaltic movements 215, 215f
Prosencephalon 702
Prosopagnosia 748
Prostacyclin 132
Prostaglandins 339, 509, 665
Prostate
   gland 665
   specific antigen, increased levels of 57
Prostatic fluid 665
Protanopia 854
Proteases 106, 681f
Protective reflex 456, 874
Protein 6, 6f, 26, 240, 248f, 251, 274, 610f, 795
   absorption of 276, 276f, 277
   arrangement of 6
   breakdown, increases rate of 610
   buffer 42
   C 132
   catabolism 587
   channels 17
   chemical digestion of 276
   complement 115
   deposition of 587
   digestion of 247, 276, 276f
   energy malnutrition, severe 588
   hormone 560f, 642, 644, 645
   hydrophobic 412
   integral 6
   metabolism 256, 257, 600, 610, 619, 620
   misfolded 24
   peripheral 6
   quantification 56
   regulatory 184, 185f
   S 132
   sparing effect 587
   structural 201
   surfactant 412
   synthesis 402
Proteoglycan fibrillae 493, 506
Prothrombin 130
   activator, formation of 130
   time 134, 262
Proximal colon 264
Proximal convoluted tubule 27, 493, 499, 510

Pseudohermaphroditism 651
    female 651
    male 651
Pseudo-isochromatic chart test 854
Psychiatry component 635
Psychic blindness 748
Psychosocial health 540
Ptosis 176
    bilateral 176
    temporary improvement of 177
Puberty
    central precocious 657
    delayed 657
    precocious 657
    stage of 655, 656, 656$t$
Pulmonary artery 325, 434
    pressure 436
    system 399
Pulmonary blood flow 436
Pulmonary capillary 399, 411
    pressure 435, 436
Pulmonary circulation 290$f$, 291, 291$t$, 325, 434, 434$f$, 435, 436$t$, 437
    facilitates fluid exchange 438
    functions of 402, 438
    physiological anatomy of 434
Pulmonary diffusion 395
Pulmonary edema 438, 460, 465, 468
    treatment of 534
Pulmonary embolism 423, 439
Pulmonary function
    evaluation of 421
    tests 426
        assessment of 431
Pulmonary valve 288
Pulmonary ventilation 395, 418, 430, 465
    mechanics of 404
Pulse
    abnormal 376, 376$t$
    contours, abnormality of 375
    jugular venous 293, 294
    mechanism of transmission of 375$fc$
    pressure 358
Pump
    failure 383, 384
    handle movement 405, 406$f$
Pupil 845
    dilatation of 845$f$
    physiology of 844
Pupillary dilator muscle 845
Pupillary light reflex 819, 858, 865
Pupillary response, abnormal 866
Purkinje cell 758
    layer 756
Purpura 133
    kinds of 123
Putamen circuit 762
    lesions of 762
Pyloric gland anatomy 234, 234$f$
Pyramidal cell, layers of 743
Pyramidal tract 775, 776
    functions of 776
    lesions of 778
Pyridostigmine 178

## Q

Q waves, appearance of 319
QRS complex
    direction of 310
    pattern of 310$f$

Quadriceps femoris 732
Quadriplegia 781

## R

R wave 306
Radiation 122, 893
Radiographic technique 529
Raised intra-abdominal pressure 379
Raised intracranial tension 337
Raja yoga 927
Ranvier node 163, 167
Raphe
    magnus nuclei of 784
    nucleus 784
Rapid breathing 386, 622
Rapid eye movement 799
    sleep 718, 799, 801
Real-time visualization techniques 57
Receptive relaxation 200, 237, 238$f$
Receptor
    cell 828, 837
        depolarization of 831$f$
    classification of 723$t$
    sensitivity 561, 562
Rectangular hyperbola 445
Red blood cell 65, 67, 79, 80, 146, 610
    count 82$f$, 87, 91
    membrane 139$f$
    structure of 79$f$
Red bone marrow 80, 80$t$
Red cell 81$t$
    decreased synthesis of 86
    differentiation of 80
    enzymes 86
    increased breakdown of 86
    indices 87, 91
    membrane 86, 138
        proteins 92$f$
    volume 79
Red-green color blindness 854
Reflex 237, 737, 739, 917
    action 235
    bladder 547
    duodenocolic 267
    features of 547
    gastrointestinal 217
    inference of 732$t$
    observation of 732$t$
    properties of 730
    respiratory 453
    superficial 776
Refraction
    errors of 863
    principle of 861$f$
Refractive indexes 861$f$
Regional blood flow 494
Regulatory mechanisms
    classification of 360
    long-term 361
Regurgitation 299
    aortic 299
Rehabilitation, pulmonary 478, 483
Relaxation 928
Renal arterial pressure, normalization of 363
Renal artery 372
    stenosis 535
Renal blood flow 494, 496$f$, 497, 497$fc$, 524, 528, 915
    autoregulation of 500
    estimation of 528

    hormonal regulation of 497$t$
    measurement of 497
    regulation of 495
Renal buffer system 42
Renal disease
    chronic 81
    end-stage 540
Renal disorders, physiological basis of 533
Renal failure
    acute 534
    chronic 46, 494, 537, 573
    treatment of 534
Renal function 492
    evaluation of 529
    tests 524
Renal medulla 494, 495, 515
Renal nerves, stimulation of 496
Renal osteodystrophy 538
    development of 538
Renal structure, development of 915
Renal system 45, 915
Renal transplantation 540
Renal tubular
    acidosis 44
    function tests 524, 528
Renin 558
    test 615
Renin-angiotensin aldosterone system 362, 499, 501, 633
    blockers 502
    excessive activation of 614
Renin-angiotensin mechanism 333, 338, 362
Renointestinal reflex 269
Repetitive nerve stimulation 178$f$
Repolarization, phases of 190, 191
Reproductive hormones 641, 642$t$
    regulation of 630
Reproductive physiology 639, 641, 661, 670
    life cycle of 655
Reproductive system 611, 661, 662$f$
Respiration 395, 453, 453$fc$, 456$f$, 463
    chemical regulation of 458
    control of 455$f$
    depth of 458, 465
    effects of 355
    external 395
    internal 395
    involuntary autonomic control of 454
    maternal 686
    mechanics of 404
    modes of 404
    muscles of 405, 405$t$
    rate of 456
    regulatory controls of 453
    voluntary inhibition of 460
Respiratory airways zones 397$f$
Respiratory buffer system 42
Respiratory burst 106
Respiratory centers 453, 454, 456
Respiratory depression, drug-induced 480
Respiratory diseases 445
Respiratory disorder 46, 448, 449, 475
    physiological basis of 475
Respiratory distress
    signs of 413
    syndrome 410, 413
        pathophysiology of 414$f$
Respiratory failure 479, 484, 921
    classification of 484$f$
    hypoxemic 484
Respiratory function 46, 460

Respiratory gases 65, 80
　exchange of 418
　transport of 442
Respiratory membrane 399, 418
　thickness of 419
Respiratory minute volume 430
Respiratory muscles activity 892
Respiratory physiology 393
Respiratory pump 356, 408
Respiratory rate 202, 799, 818
Respiratory supportive measures 485
Respiratory symptoms 148
Respiratory system 395, 396f, 454, 465, 476, 899, 913, 921, 927
　effects of 601
　epithelial lining of 401f
　functional anatomy of 395
　nonrespiratory functions of 401
Respiratory tract, functional anatomy of 395
Respiratory unit 399, 399f
Respiratory zone 395, 397
Resting membrane potential 48, 50, 51, 212, 303, 568
Resuscitation
　cardiopulmonary 479
　neonatal 479
Reticular activating system 735, 787
　anatomy of 787
　functions of 787
　structure of 787
Reticular ascending system 787f
Reticular excitatory area, gigantocellular neurons of 787
Reticular formation 787
　ascending 787
Reticular nucleus 753
Reticulocyte 81
Reticuloendothelial system 106
Reticulospinal tract 777
Retina 847, 849, 850, 855, 858f, 861, 863
　anatomy of layers of 844
　contralateral 858
　fibers, superior 858
　front of 863
　layers of 848f
Retinal cells 844
Retinal M ganglion cells 749
Retinal sensitivity, recovery of 853f
Retinitis pigmentosa 849
Retrograde amnesia, amount of 795
Retro-orbital connective tissues, swelling of 601
Retropulsion, phenomenon of 765
Reverberatory circuits 708, 709, 793
Reverse enterogastric reflex 237, 239
Rh
　blood grouping system 139
　factor 146
　incompatibility 139, 140
　system 138
Rheobase 164
Rhesus monkey 139
Rhodopsin 852, 854
Rhombencephalon 702
Rhomberg's test 761
Rhythm
　abnormality of 314
　disorders of 316
　method 692, 693f
Rib
　outward movement of 405
　upward movement of 405

Rickets 574
Right atrial pressure 354, 378, 379
　direct reflection of 293
Right ventricular failure 354
Rigor mortis 192
Ringer's solution, lactated 38
Rinne's test 884, 885
Road traffic accident 328f
Rocket launching pad 872
Rods 849
Rotational thromboelastometry 123
Rubrospinal tract 756, 777, 777f
Ruffini's endings 724
Ryanodine receptors 192

# S

Saccades 865
Saccule 805
Sacral micturition pathway 545f
Saline
　filled lungs 410, 410f
　normal 38
Saliva 231
　functions of 245
　mechanism of secretion of 245
　regulation of 245
　secretion of 226, 226f
Salivary glands 214
　anatomy of 226f
Salivary secretion 225, 227f
　nervous regulation of 227f
　physiology of 225
　regulation of 226
Salty sensation 837
　mechanism of 839f
Salty tastants 838
Sarcolemma 172
Sarcomere, structure of 186f
Sarcoplasmic endoplasmic reticulum calcium ATPase 192, 193
Sarcoplasmic reticulum, longitudinal 187
Sarcotubular system 187, 187t
Saturation kinetics 29f
Scar tissue 798
Schizophrenia 719
Schlemm canal 847
Schwabach's test 884, 885, 885f
Schwann cells 157
Sclera 844
Sclerosis, multiple 164, 780
Scuba equipment 471f
Secretin 218, 249, 251, 259, 558, 559
Secretin-cerulein test 252
Secretions, disorders of 561
Secretory cells 48
Secretory function 234, 257
Seddon's classification 167
Sedentary behavior 898, 899t, 900, 900t
Sedentary lifestyle 898
　effects of 899f
　physiological effects of 899
Segmentation peristaltic movements 215, 215f
Seizures 716
　absence 799f
　complex partial 798
　focal 797, 798
　generalized 797
　　epileptic 798
　　tonic clonic 799f
　partial 797
　simple partial 798

Selective taste blindness 841
Self-regenerative reflex 545f
Sella turcica 585
Semen 665, 680
　analysis 666t
　composition of 665
　fate of 666
　increases bulk of 665
Semicircular canal 807, 875
　lateral 807
Semilunar valve 288, 289, 289t, 299
Seminal fluid 665
Seminal vesicle 665
Semipermeable membrane 28, 49f, 539
Senescent cells, accumulation of 920
Senomorphics 923
Sensation, loss of 546
Sense organ 731
Sensorineural deafness 883
Sensory aphasia 748
Sensory development 917
Sensory feedback, role of 766
Sensory fiber 731
Sensory homunculus 704
Sensory horn 770
Sensory inputs 790
Sensory loss 90, 546
Sensory motor coordination 776
Sensory nerve 216, 217
Sensory neurons 156, 704
　maintenance of 159
Sensory perceptual skills 910
Sensory receptors, physiology of 723
Sensory root 706
Sensory speech 747
　area 791
Sensory stimuli, transduction of 724
Sensory tracts 769, 771
Sepsis 535, 539
Septicemia 350
Septum 790, 827
　left endocardial surface of 304
Series elastic
　component 201, 202f
　elements, stretching of 201
Serosa 211, 234, 246, 265
Serotonin 122, 222, 559, 719, 927
Sertoli cells 661, 662f
　functions of 661
Serum creatinine 525
　levels 538
Sex 838
　chromosomes 648f, 649
　determination 648
　differentiation 649, 650f
　　stage of 649
　genotype, identification of 648
　hormone
　　effects of male 661
　　physiological effects of 661
　　production 916
　steroids 557, 607
Sexual development
　disorders of 649, 657
　fetus 24
Sexual maturity, Tanner's classification of 655, 656f
Sheehan's syndrome 588
Shivering thermogenesis 892
Shock 220, 383, 384t, 388
　absorbers 201
　anaphylactic 116, 384, 535

cardiac 370
cardiogenic 383, 384
clinical manifestations of 384, 386t
complications of 386
distributive 383, 384, 386
hypovolemic 383, 384
management of 384
neurogenic 384
obstructive 383, 384
pathogenesis of 384, 386f
physiology, stage of 385f
septic 384
severe 611
spinal 547, 548
stage of 384
Short loop reflexes 217
Short stature 652
Short-chain fatty acids
direct absorption of 278
fermentation of 265
production of 265
Short-term memory 793
physiological basis of 793
Shy-Drager syndrome 815
Sialorrhea 227, 231
Sick sinus syndrome 318
Sickle cell anemia 93, 93f
Signal through synapse, convergence of 714f
Signal transduction pathways 832
Simple cells 858
Single cell mucous glands 214
Singlet oxygen 921
Sinus
arrhythmia 314
bradycardia 314
paranasal 396
rhythm 314f
tachycardia 314
Six-minute walk test 431
Sjögren syndrome 227
Skeletal motor nervous axis 702, 704, 705f
Skeletal muscle 182, 183, 186-188, 189f, 190, 190t, 194f, 195, 196, 196f, 197, 197f, 198f, 199, 727, 826
action potential of 189
fiber 187t
fiber, surface membrane of 187f
pump 356
Skin 379
flushing of 459
Skull, base of 585
Sleep 360, 892
apnea 635
disorders 802
disturbances 658
functions of 801
induction 630
neurohormonal control of 801, 801f
physiology of 799
spindles 800, 801f
stage of 800f, 801
types of 799
wake cycle 629
Sliding filament theory 191, 191f
Slow wave sleep 799
Small bowel 251
secretions, regulation of 250
Small fibrin 438
Small ganglion cells 855
Small intestine 211, 213f, 245, 277
absorption of 251

anatomy of 245
digestion of 251
disorders of 252
first part of 251
functional anatomy of 245
layers of 246f
motility of 251
secretions of 246, 249
Small molecule neurotransmitters 718
types of 718t
Small parathyroid glands embedded 570
Smell, sense of 833
Smoker voice 602
Smoking cessation 483, 634
Smooth muscle 182, 183, 186-188, 188f, 191f, 191t, 196, 197, 199, 780
contraction 194
molecular mechanism of 195
electrical properties of 190
longitudinal 211
mechanism of contraction of 195fc
true action potential of 213
Snellen's chart 862
Social-emotional skills 910
Sodium 164, 278, 320, 510, 513, 526
absorption 278, 513
balance 278
bicarbonate
solution 247
role of 248
channel 52f
glucose
cotransporter inhibitors 275, 634
linked transport 26, 510
ion 34
linked cotransport 277
low 622
potassium ATPase pump 608
reabsorption of 608
retention 633
Soft palate 840
Soleus, testing of 732
Solid foods 913
Solitary tract, nucleus of 335
Soma, condition of 170
Somatic receptors, classification of 723
Somatic sensation 723, 747f, 769
simple 723
Somatic senses 723
Somatomedins 587
Somatosensory cortex 704
Somatosensory evoked potential 59
Somatosensory nervous axis 702, 704, 704f
Somatostatin 556, 557, 617, 623
Somnambulism 802
Sound 870, 872, 878
causes of 294
character of 294
conduction 873
intensity of 872t
location of 881
loudness of 881
pressure level 872
properties of 871t
speed of 871
stimuli, relative intensity of 881
transduction of 878, 879f
transmission of 873f
vibrations
mechanism of transmission of 875
pathway of 875f

waves 870, 870f, 874
amplitude of 871f
frequency of 871f
transmission 874f
Sour sensation 837
mechanism of 839f
Sour tastants 838
Spastic paralysis 778
Spatial summation 715
Special senses 723
Special sensory nerve fibers 837
Specific nerve energies, Muller's doctrine of 704
Speech 402, 789
disorders of 765, 792
physiology of 791
Sperm 665, 680
banks 666
binding ZP receptors, internalization of 681
capacitation of 666
count 667
formation of 663
maturation of 664, 665f
morphological abnormalities 667, 667f
structure of 664, 664f
Spermatogenesis 663, 663f, 666
hormonal regulation of 663
regulation of 663
stage of 664t
Spermatozoa 680, 681
capacitation of 666
Spherocytosis 79, 92f
hereditary 92f
Sphincter, external 543
Sphygmomanometer 359f
Spike potential 190, 212, 213
Spinal cord 328, 705, 706f, 719, 720, 769, 770f, 772f, 773, 773f
anterior gray
column of 780
horns of 781f
ascending tracts of 771, 772f
descending tracts of 775
disorders 547
dorsal horn of 720
functional anatomy of 701, 769
hemisection of 780
lesions of 547, 778
level of 731
organization of 769, 769f
reflexes 545
structure of 706f
transaction, effects of 733
tumors, intramedullary 773
Spinal reflex 731, 733, 736
pathways 547
Spinal roots 770
Spinal segments
T12-L1 680
T12-L2 679
Spinal shock 547, 548
stage of 735, 779
Spinal tracts 771f
Spinnbarkeit test 675
Spinocerebellar tracts 90, 775
Spinocerebellum 757
Spino-olivary tract 775
Spinoreticular tracts 772
Spinotectal tract 775
Spinothalamic tract 780

anterolateral 772
lateral 771, 772, 773f
Spinovisual reflex 737
Spiral ganglion 881
nerve 879f
Spirometer, simple 426, 426f
Spirometric lung volumes 426
Spirometry 426
Spironolactone 534
Splanchnic circulation 211
functions of 218
physiology of 218
Spotty pigmentation 612
Squamous flat cells 400
ST segment depression 319
Stagnant hypoxia 476, 477f, 478
Starling's equilibrium 377
Static equilibrium, maintenance of 807
Static lung volumes 427, 428f
Statins 634
Statoconia 806
Steatohepatitis, nonalcoholic 260, 634
Steatorrhea 252, 259, 280
Stellate cells 255, 756, 758
Stenosis, aortic 299
Stercobilin 76
Stercobilinogen 76, 96
Stereognosis 746
Stereopsis, mechanism of 749
Steroid 614
hormone 17, 18, 559, 642-644, 646f
formation 645f
hyposecretion of essential 612
mechanism of action of 18f
Steroidogenesis 645f
Stimulate bone resorption 611
Stimuli, types of 837
Stimulus 267, 334, 458, 460, 707f, 731, 737-739
intensity 725
movement of 859
velocity of 859
Stokes-Adams syndrome 317
Stomach 211, 233, 235f, 238fc, 240, 276, 611
absorption of 239
digestion of 239
digestive functions of 234
disorders of 240
functional anatomy of 233
functions of 234
histological layers of 234f
histology of 233
motor functions of 234
oxyntic glands of 214f
regions of 233f
Stones, renal 572
Streamline flow 328
Stress 664, 925
acute 925
chronic 925
emotional 796
episodic acute 925
harmful effects of 612
hormone 926, 929
implications of 925
physiology of 925
reduction 929
response 222
regulation 927
types of 925
Stretch receptor 456
Stretch reflex 731, 731f

Stria vascularis 876
Stroke 634, 778, 825
hemorrhagic 825
ischemic 634, 825
volume 343, 347, 349, 350, 359, 436, 602
index 347
output 375
Subcellular respiratory organelles 5
Subcutaneous tissue 602
Subiculum 790
Subliminal fringe 715, 715f
Submucosa 211, 234, 246
Submucosal plexus 217
Subneural cleft 173
Substance, molecular size of 377
Substantia
gelatinosa 770
nigra 761
pars compacta 764
pars reticularis 764
propria 770
Subthalamic nuclei 761, 764
Succinylcholine 176
Sucrose 534
Suffocation 479
Suicide 23
Sulfonylureas 634
Sulphuric acid 41
Sunderland's classification 167
Superior colliculus 738, 858
Superoxide
anion 921
dismutase 922
Supplemental oxygen therapy 459
Supplementary motor area 766
Support cellular metabolism 477
Supporting cells 837, 877, 877f
Suprachiasmatic nucleus 581, 629, 858
Supraoptic nucleus 556, 557, 581, 585
Surface tension 411, 411f
Surfactant
deficiency 412f
consequences of 413
formation of 402
functions of 412
mechanism of action of 412, 412f
molecules 409
replacement therapy 413
Sustentacular cells 828
Swallowing deglutition, physiology of 228
Sweating 36, 580, 658
Sweet sensation 837
mechanism of 838f
Sweet tastants 838
Swelling 148, 601
Sympathetic discharge, effects of 328
Sympathetic fiber 629, 816
Sympathetic nervous system 333, 633, 815, 815t, 825, 926
mass activation of 818
organization of 815f
Sympathetic neuron 160
maintenance of 159
Sympathetic stimulation 217, 220, 350, 351, 680
effects of 325, 343, 355
stimulates 355
Sympathetic vasoconstrictor tone 328f
Sympathomimetic drugs 384
Symport 27f
Symptomatic therapy 179

Synapse 24, 711, 715f
electrical 711
functioning of 712
location of 711, 712f
properties of 713, 730
structure of 712, 712f
types of 711, 712f
Synaptic body 849
Synaptic cleft 172, 174, 175f, 712
Synaptic delay 714
Synaptic fatigue 714
Synaptic gutter 172
Synaptic insulation 157f
Synaptic knob 155, 172
Synaptic plasticity 159
Synaptic transmission 716
Synaptic vesicles 155, 172, 793
inhibits docking of 176
recycling of 163, 163f
synthesis of 173f
Synaptobrevin 174, 176
Syntaxin 173, 174
Synthetic functions 257
Syringomyelia 780, 781f
Systemic circulation 290f, 291, 291t
components of 374
Systolic stretch 370, 370f

# T

T cell
activation of 112
cytotoxic 111
development of 117f
differentiation 627
functions of 111
proliferation of 112
T tubules 193
T wave 306
inversion 319
significance of 306
Tachybrady syndrome 318
Tachycardia 86, 148, 344
Tachypnea 413
Tactile fremitus 439
Taenia coli 265
Tanner's classification 655, 656f
Target cell responsiveness, disorders of 561
Tastant, temperature of 838
Taste
buds 837
innervation of 837
structure of 837, 837f
cells 837
cortex 841
molecules 838
pathway 440, 840f, 840fc
three-order neurons of 840
producing substances 839
receptor cell 841
salivary reflex 841
sensation 838
clinical assessment of 836
disorders of 836
distribution of 837f
mechanism 836
physiology of 836
site of 836
sense of 836
Tectorial membrane 876, 877f

Tectospinal tract 777, 881
Telencephalon 702
Telereceptors 827
Temperature 164, 360, 367, 445, 664
    adaptation 891, 893*t*
    control mechanisms 893
    regulation 891
        mechanism of 891
Temporal lobe 746, 747*f*, 798
    epilepsy 795
        limbic seizures 798
    parts of 747*f*
Temporary hemostasis 127, 128, 128*f*, 129*f*
    disorders of 133
    mechanism of 129*f*
Tendons 201
Tensilon test 177, 178
Tension 201
Tensor tympani 873
Teratozoospermia 666
Testis 665*f*
    functions of 663
    microscopic anatomy of 661
    structure of 662*f*
Testosterone 82, 558, 642, 646, 663, 674
    abnormal secretion of 667
    level 643
Tetanus
    genesis of 196
    physiological significance of 198
    types of 198*f*
Tetany 568
Tetrodotoxin 176
Thalamic nuclei 752, 753*f*
Thalamic pain syndrome 753
Thalamic projections 798
Thalamocortical system 796
Thalamostriatal projection 763
Thalamus 704, 752, 762, 797
    generalized nuclei of 753
        medial geniculate nucleus of 881
    nuclei of 752
    structure of 752
Thalassemia 76, 92
Thallium 366
    radionucleotide scan 366*f*
Theca cells 673, 674
    interaction of 645*f*
Theca externa 673
Thelarche 655
Thermal stimuli 781
Thermodilution method 348, 348*f*
Thermoreceptors 723, 893
Thermoregulation 324, 893, 894*f*, 903
Theta waves 796
Thiazides 534
Thiazolidinediones 634
Thick ascending limb 514
Thick filaments 186
    arrangement of 185, 186*f*
Thin ascending limb 514
Thin descending limb 514
Thin filaments 186
    arrangement of 185, 186*f*
Thirst 386
    mechanism 37
Thoracentesis 440
Thoracic aorta 435*f*
Thoracic duct 380
Thoracolumbar division 343
Threshold stimulus 707, 715

Thrombin
    formation of 130
    thrombomodulin complex 132
Thrombocytes 66
Thrombocytopenia 122, 133
    causes of 120, 122
    idiopathic 122, 123
Thrombocytopenic purpura 123
Thrombocytosis 122
    essential 122
    primary 122
    reactive 122
    secondary 122
Thromboelastography 123
Thrombopoiesis, formation of 120
Thrombotic thrombocytopenic purpura 122
Thrombus 825
    formation, pathogenesis of 368*f*
Thumb, adduction of 568
Thymectomy 178, 179, 628
Thymus 627, 628
    anatomy of 627*f*
    development 916
    gland, physiology of 627
    involvement 178
Thyroglobulin
    secretion of 598
    synthesis of 598
Thyroid
    adenoma 600
    carcinoma 600
    damage, tests for 604
    development 916
    dwarfism 603
    function 916
        tests 604
    gland 573, 597, 597*f*, 598, 686
        disorders of 600
        enlargement of 603, 604
        functional anatomy of 597
        hormone of 597
        microanatomy of 597*f*
        posterior surface of 570*f*
    hormone 19, 598, 599
        actions of 599
        biosynthesis of 598, 598*f*
        level lowering drugs 601
        mechanism of action of 18*f*, 599, 599*f*, 628*f*
        metabolism of 600
        overproduction of 603
        regulation of secretion of 11*f*
        release of 598, 599
        secretion, regulation of 600
        synthesis, transient inhibition of 603
    secretes 598
    stimulating
        antibody, long acting 600
        hormone 11, 556, 586
        immunoglobulin 600
    suppression tests 604
Thyroidectomy 601
Thyrotoxic myopathy 601
Thyrotoxicosis 600
Thyrotrophs 556, 585
Thyrotropin-releasing hormone 11, 556
    stimulating tests 604
Thyroxine 19, 82, 344, 351, 557, 599
    binding globulin 599
    decreased production of 601
    half-life of 599

Tidal inspiration, emulsification of normal 427
Tidal volume 427, 456
Tingling 90
Tiredness 602
Tissue 475*f*
    damage 252
    decreased oxygenation of 383
    fluid 34
    growth 828
    level of 419*f*
    necrosis factor 111
    oxygen demand 351
    phase 103
    pool 103
    respiration 395
    thromboplastin 131
T-lymphocytes 111
Tongue 836*f*, 837*f*
    functional anatomy of 836
Tonic contraction 213
Tonic labyrinthine reflexes 736, 736*f*
Tonic neck reflex 735, 735*f*, 736*f*
Tonometer 847
Tonotopic maps 747
Total body water 33
    measurement of 34, 35
Total fat free mass 900
Total leukocyte count 103, 106
Total lung
    capacity 427
    collapse 409
Total pancreatic secretion 249
Total plasma cortisol, low 612
Total protein 262
Total renal blood flow 494
Toxic nodular goiter 600
Toxicity 471
Toxicology management 479
Toxin, detoxification of 257
Trace elements, absorption of 278
Trachea 396-398
    histological section of 398*f*
Tracheobronchial tree 396, 396*f*, 397, 397*f*, 398, 398*t*
Track linear growth patterns 911
Tractus solitaries 840
Transcellular fluid 34
Transcytosis 31
Transferrin 88, 663
Transforming growth factor 160
Transfusion
    associated circulatory overload 148
    massive 147
    role of 147
    transmitted infections 148
Transient ischemic attacks 634
Transmembrane protein 6
    band 91
Transmission electron microscope 56*f*
Transport across cell membrane 26
    mechanism of 26
    mode of 27*t*
Transport maximum 512, 513
Transpulmonary pressure 406, 407
    change of 410
Transverse diameter 404
Trauma 147, 547, 548
Traveler's diarrhea 270
Tremor 765
Triamterene 534
Triceps, testing of 732

Trichromatic color theory 853
Tricuspid valve 288, 378
Triglycerides 240, 274, 901
    digestion of 278
    elevated 633
Triiodothyronine 19, 557
Trilineage stem cells 101
Triploidy 651
Trisomy 650
Tritanopia 854
Tritium oxide 34
Tropomyosin 183$f$, 184
    binding site 183
Troponin 183$f$, 184, 186
    binding site 183
    tropomyosin interaction, role of 194$f$
Trousseau's sign 568, 569$f$
Truncal ataxia 760
Trunk, control of muscles of 776
Trypsin 247, 251
    inhibitor 248
Tryptophan 719
T-tubules 187
Tubal ligation 694
Tubectomy 694
Tubular glands 214
Tubular necrosis, acute 536
Tubular reabsorption 505, 509, 915
    hormonal control of 513$f$
    secretion, regulation of 512$f$
Tubular secretion 505, 509, 915
    hormonal control of 513
    physiological control of 512
Tubule 4
    transverse 187
Tubuloglomerular feedback mechanism 496, 500, 500$f$, 508, 508$fc$, 509$f$
Tufted cells 828, 829
Tumor 736, 738
    abdominal 379
    acidophilic 585
    adrenal 615
    cells 112
    extramedullary lesions 773
    intracranial 833
    necrosis factor-alpha 633
Tunica
    externa 844
    fibrosa 844
    intima 847
Tuning fork test 883
Turbulence 414
Turbulent blood flow 328, 328$f$
Turner's syndrome 650, 652
    clinical features of 652, 652$f$
    diagnosis of 649
Tympanic membrane 872, 873, 873$f$
    functions of 874
Tympanic reflex 874
Tyrosine
    kinase 561
        A receptors 159
        B receptors 159
    iodination of 598

## U

Ultrasonographic flowmeter 326, 326$f$
Ultrasound, endoscopic 253
Umami sensation 838
Umami taste 838

Unipolar leads 309
Unipolar neuron 156, 156$f$
Uniport 27$f$
Unmyelinated nerve fiber 163
Unstable angina 368
Upper esophageal sphincter 228
Upper motor neuron 705, 778, 779
    lesion 778, 779$t$
    inhibitory influence of 778
Upper thoracic ganglia 343
Urea 526
    recycling 516
    recycling, process of 516$f$
Uremia 525, 538
Ureters 491
Urethra 491
    narrowing of 536
Uric acid 41
    serum 525
Uridine diphosphate glucuronic acid 96
Urinary bilirubin 96, 99
Urinary bladder 491, 543
    functional anatomy of 543, 544$f$
    innervation of 543, 544$f$
Urinary excretion rate 505
Urinary free cortisol test 614
Urinary hesitancy 547
Urinary retention 546
Urinary sphincters 543, 544$fc$
Urinary tract
    infections 547
    obstruction of 525
Urinary urobilinogen 99
Urine 40
    accumulation 536
    analysis 530
    collection 528
    color, abnormal 530
    concentration 505, 514
        test 524, 529
    dilution test 524, 529
    formation 505, 511
        process of 506$f$
    minimum amount of 516
    output 386, 536
    volume, obligatory 516
Urobilin 76
Urobilinogen 76, 96
Urodynamic studies 545
Uropathy, obstructive 537
Uterine changes 675, 675$f$
Uterus 670
Utricle 805, 875
    role of 806$f$

## V

Vaccination 916
Vagal stimulation 250
Vagal tone 343, 351
    higher 343
Vagina 666
Vaginal discharge 675
Vagotomy 457
Vagus 343
    intact 457
    nerve 399, 456
        endings 249
Valine 75
Valve status 295
Valvulae conniventes 274

Valvular incompetence 299
Valvular stenosis 299
Van den Bergh reaction 99
Vascular capacitance 374
Vascular disease 135
    pulmonary 421
Vascular endothelial growth factor 561
    genes 466
Vascular function 901
Vascular resistance 327, 914
Vascular wall tension 327
Vasculature
    pulmonary 423
    stress relaxation of 200, 333, 338, 362
Vasectomy 694
Vasoactive intestinal peptide 218, 219, 230, 400, 679
Vasoconstrictor 330
    hormones 340
    system, control of 334$f$
Vasodilator 330, 439, 478
    hormones 339
    substances, accumulation of 329
    theory 329
Vasomotion 377
Vasomotor center 333, 334$f$
Vasopressin 330, 556, 590, 610, 720
Vater ampulla 250
Veins 324, 324$t$, 374, 421
    collapse of 356
    obstruction of large 349
    pulmonary 325
    systemic 374
Velocity, effects of 328
Vena cava 325, 339
Venous blood 40
    pH of 67
Venous circulation 378
    functions of 379
Venous pressure 378, 378$f$
Venous pump 379
    functions of 378
Venous return 349, 350, 354, 356, 383, 436
Venous system 374$f$
Venous tone 356
Venous valves, role of 379
Ventilation management 449
Ventilation perfusion
    disturbances 422$f$
    mismatch 413, 422
    ratio 422
        values of 422$f$
Ventilation
    normal 422
    pulmonary 395, 418, 430, 465
    support 479
Ventilator, judicious use of 932
Ventral anterior nucleus 753
Ventral posterior medial nucleus 841
Ventral respiratory group 454, 455
Ventral spinocerebellar tracts 775$f$
Ventricle 287, 288, 293, 295
    enlargement of 795
    pressure 436
    repolarization of 306
Ventricular depolarization 306
Ventricular failure 387
Ventricular muscles 288
Ventricular pressure 299, 366
Ventricular repolarization 306
Ventricular rhythm disorders 315$t$

Ventricular septal defect 299
Ventroanterior nucleus 752
Ventrobasal complex 753
Ventroflexion 736f
Ventrolateral nucleus 752, 753, 578, 579
Vero cells 57
Vertebrae, fracture of 468
Vertical diameter 405
Vertigo, benign paroxysmal positional 811
Vesicointestinal reflex 269
Vesicular membrane 174
Vesicular transport 30
    types of 30, 30f
Vessels, pulmonary 434, 435f
Vestibular apparatus 805, 811
    functions of 807
Vestibular nucleus 735, 735f, 809, 810
    connections of 810, 810f
    lateral 810
    parts of 810f
    superior 810
Vestibular pathways 809
Vestibular reflexes 810
Vestibular system 805, 812
    central connections of 809f
Vestibulo-autonomic reflexes 811
Vestibulocerebellum 757
Vestibulocollic reflex 811
Vestibulo-ocular reflex 810
Vestibulospinal reflex 811
Vestibulospinal tract 777
Villi 274, 275f
Viruses 221
Visceral afferent nucleus 771
Visceral pleura 401
Visceral sensation 723
Viscosity 67
Vision
    field of 860
    loss of 749
    photochemistry of 852
    physiology of 844
Visual acuity 850f, 861, 862, 862f
Visual agnosia 748
Visual cortex 857, 858, 860
    primary 748, 748f, 858
    secondary 749
Visual cycle 852f
Visual evoked potential 59, 844
Visual field 860
    defect 869, 590, 860f
Visual information, parallel processing of 850
Visual pathway 844, 857, 858, 859f, 865
Visual righting reflexes 737
Visual signal processing 856f, 859
Vital capacity 426, 427
Vital signs 413

Vitamin 82, 257, 922
    B12 82, 89f, 90
        absorption of 90, 90f
        deficiency 89, 89f, 122, 123
    C 477, 922
        lack of 574
    D 279, 575
        resistant rickets 574
        supplementation 913
    D3 569, 574t
        action of 574f
        deficiency 566, 574
        formation of 574f
        levels 573
        role of 573
    E 477
    K 256, 265
        production of 265
Vitreous body 846
Vitreous humor 846
Volatile acids 41
Voltage-gated calcium channels 52, 173, 174, 192
    disruption of 176
Vomeronasal organ 827, 828
Vomiting 233, 386, 467
    reflex 218, 219f, 819
von Willebrand disease 135
von Willebrand factor 121, 134
    function of 135

## W

Waist circumference 900
Wakefulness 800
Walking movements 733, 735, 736f
Wall thickness 325
Wallerian degeneration 169
Warfarin 133
Waste products 65
    accumulation of 351
Water
    absorption of 265, 278
    balance, maintenance of 402
    distribution of 33f
    homeostasis, regulation of 494
    metabolism 610
    obligatory reabsorption of 510
    permeability 513
    reabsorption 513, 608
    retention 36, 37f
        treatment of 534
Waves 303
    patterns, normal 309, 310t
    physiological basis of 304f, 305f
Weak platelet plug, formation of 128
Weak urinary stream 547

Weakness 5, 602, 614
    severe 613
Weber's test 884, 884f, 885
Weight
    gain 602, 686, 911
    loss 601
        medications 634
    management 269
Wenckebach phenomenon 317
Wernicke's area 747, 747f, 791, 792, 881
    lesions of 748
White blood cells 65, 67, 101
White rami communicantes 816f
Whole blood 146, 447
    composition of 66f
Wigger's diagram 296
Willis circle 824f
Windkessel effect 324, 325, 326f, 358
Withdrawal reflex 733
Wolff-Chaikoff effect 602
Wolff-Parkinson-white syndrome 317, 318
Wolfian duct 24
Wound healing
    delayed 614
    long term 122
Wrist 568

## X

X-chromosomes 854
Xerostomia 227

## Y

Yama 927
Yoga 925, 926, 929
    different schools of 927f
    physiological effects of 927
    physiology of 925
Young-Helmholtz theory 853

## Z

Zellweger syndrome 5
Zero surface tension compliance 410
Zeta chain 74
Zollinger-Ellison syndrome 240, 241
Zona
    adherens 16
    fasciculata 557, 607
    glomerulosa 557, 607
    occludens 16
    pellucida 664, 673, 681
    reticularis 557, 607
Zwischen line 185
Zygote, formation of 682f